P9-CKV-984

Brief Contents

ELSEVIER evolve

YOU'VE JUST PURCHASED MORE THAN A TEXTBOOK!*

Evolve Student Resources for *Mosby's Essentials for Nursing Assistants, Fifth Edition,* include the following:

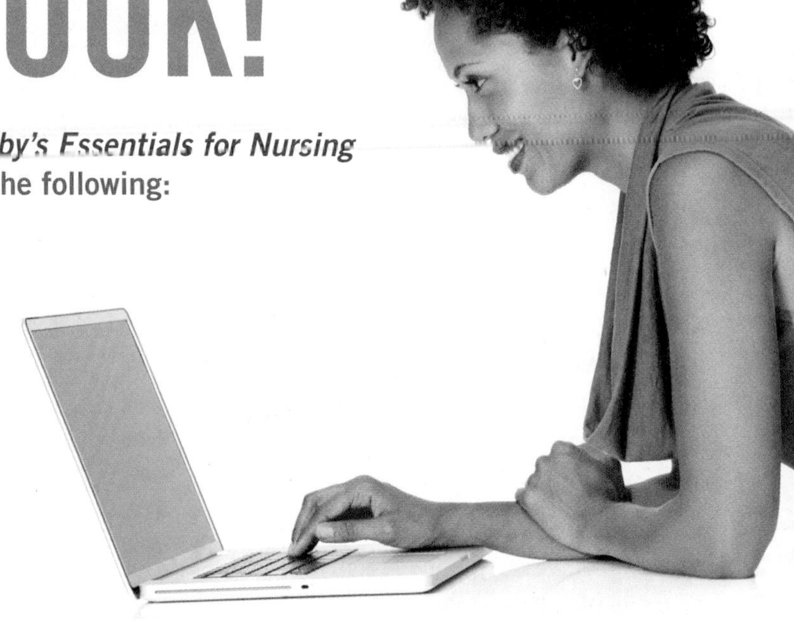

- Video Clips
- Audio Glossary
- Spanish Vocabulary and Phrases Audio Glossary
- Skills Evaluation Review
- Procedure Checklists
- Body Spectrum

Activate the complete learning experience that comes with each *NEW* textbook purchase by registering with your scratch-off access code at

http://evolve.elsevier.com/Sorrentino/essentials/

If you purchased a used book and the scratch-off code at the right has already been revealed, the code may have been used and cannot be re-used for registration. To purchase a new code to access these valuable study resources, simply follow the link above.

Sorrentino
Scratch Gently to Reveal Code

REGISTER TODAY!

You can now purchase Elsevier products on Evolve!
Go to evolve.elsevier.com/html/shop-promo.html to search and browse for products.

* Evolve Student Resources are provided free with each *NEW* book purchase only.

5 EDITION

MOSBY'S ESSENTIALS FOR NURSING ASSISTANTS

SHEILA A. SORRENTINO, PhD, RN
Delegation Consultant
Anthem, Arizona

LEIGHANN N. REMMERT, MS, RN
Health Occupations Instructor
Lincolnland Technical Education Center
Lincoln, Illinois

ELSEVIER

ELSEVIER
MOSBY

3251 Riverport Lane
St. Louis, Missouri 63043

MOSBY'S ESSENTIALS FOR NURSING ASSISTANTS ISBN: 978-0-323-11317-5

Copyright © 2014 by Mosby, an imprint of Elsevier Inc.
Previous editions copyright © 2010, 2006, 2001, 1997 by Mosby, Inc., an affiliate of Elsevier Inc.

All rights reserved. No part of this publication may be reproduced or transmitted in any form or by any means, electronic or mechanical, including photocopying, recording, or any information storage and retrieval system, without permission in writing from the publisher. Details on how to seek permission, further information about the Publisher's permissions policies and our arrangements with organizations such as the Copyright Clearance Center and the Copyright Licensing Agency, can be found at our website: www.elsevier.com/permissions.

This book and the individual contributions contained in it are protected under copyright by the Publisher (other than as may be noted herein).

Notices

The content and procedures in this book are based on information currently available. They were reviewed by instructors and practicing professionals in various regions of the United States. However, agency policies and procedures may vary from the information and procedures in this book. In addition, research and new information may require changes in standards and practices.

Standards and guidelines from the Centers for Disease Control and Prevention (CDC) and the Occupational Safety and Health Administration (OSHA) may change as new information becomes available. Other federal and state agencies also may issue new standards and guidelines. So may accrediting agencies and national organizations.

You are responsible for following the policies and procedures of your employer and the most current standards, practices, and guidelines as they relate to the safety of your work.

To the fullest extent of the law, neither the Publisher nor the authors or editors assume any liability for any injury and/or damage to persons or property as a matter of products liability, negligence or otherwise, or from any use or operation of any methods, products, instructions, or ideas contained in the material herein.

Library of Congress Cataloging-in-Publication Data

Sorrentino, Sheila A., author.
Mosby's essentials for nursing assistants / Sheila A. Sorrentino, Leighann N. Remmert.—5th edition.
p. ; cm.
Essentials for nursing assistants
Includes index.
ISBN 978-0-323-11317-5 (pbk. : alk. paper)
I. Remmert, Leighann N., author. II. Title. III. Title: Essentials for nursing assistants.
[DNLM: 1. Nurses' Aides. 2. Nursing Care–methods. WY 193]
RT84
610.7306'98–dc23

2013030270

Content Strategist: Nancy O'Brien
Senior Content Development Specialist: Maria Broeker
Publishing Services Manager: Jeff Patterson
Project Manager: Bill Drone
Designer: Brian Salisbury

Printed in Canada

Last digit is the print number: 9 8 7 6 5 4 3 2 1

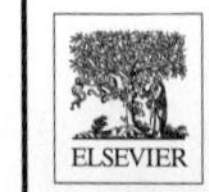

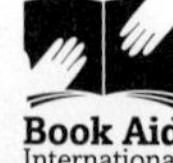

Working together to grow libraries in developing countries
www.elsevier.com • www.bookaid.org

Dedication

To my brother Tony's children:

Carly Marie Sorrentino, BS (Accounting), MA (Accounting), CPA (Certified Public Accountant),
Anthony Louis Sorrentino, Certificate in Automotive Technology, and
Michael Matthew Sorrentino, BS (Kinesiology and Sports Studies)

From babies to now successful, young adults, they bring much joy and laughter.
Wishing them a lifetime of health, happiness, and love.

With much love,
Aunt Sheila

Heartfelt congratulations to my sister, Jenn, and brother, Ryan, on the birth of their sons:

Sawyer Thomas Phillips
and
Connor Reilly Dennison

May these boys grow to be wise and discerning men.
Wishing their expanding families abundant blessings.

With love,
Leighann

About The Authors

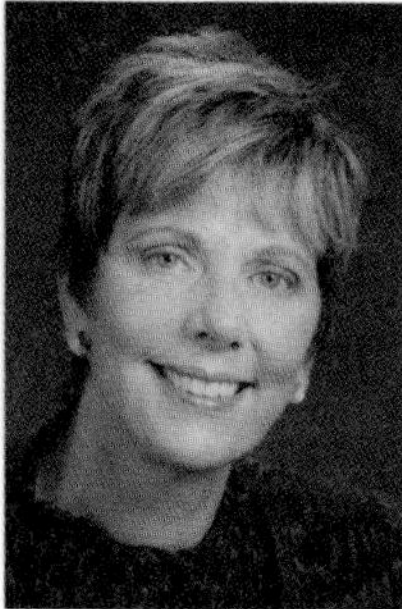

Sheila A. Sorrentino is currently a consultant focusing on effective delegation and partnering with nursing assistive personnel in health care settings. Her conference presentations focus on delegation and other issues relating to nursing assistive personnel.

Dr. Sorrentino was instrumental in the development and approval of CNA-PN-ADN career-ladder programs in the Illinois community college system and has taught at various levels of nursing education—nursing assistant, practical nursing, associate degree nursing, and baccalaureate and higher-degree programs. Her career includes experiences in nursing practice and higher education—nursing assistant, staff nurse, charge and head nurse, nursing faculty, program director, assistant dean, and dean.

A Mosby author and co-author of several nursing assistant titles since 1982, Dr. Sorrentino has a Bachelor of Science degree in nursing, a Master of Arts degree in education, a Master of Science degree in nursing, and a PhD in higher education administration. She is a member of Sigma Theta Tau International, the Honor Society of Nursing and the Rotary Club of Anthem (Anthem, Arizona). Her past community activities include serving as a board member on the Provena Senior Services Board of Directors (Mokena, Illinois), the Central Illinois Higher Education Health Care Task Force, the Iowa-Illinois Safety Council Board of Directors, and the Board of Directors of Our Lady of Victory Nursing Center (Bourbonnais, Illinois).

She received an alumni achievement award from Lewis University for outstanding leadership and dedication in nursing education. She is also a member of the Illinois State University College of Education Hall of Fame.

Dr. Sorrentino sponsors two nursing scholarships. One is awarded to a senior student from her high school alma mater who intends to major in nursing. The other is awarded to a nursing assistant who intends to major or is majoring in nursing and employed at one of the three agencies in which she worked during and after college—Heritage Health (Peru, Illinois), Illinois Valley Community Hospital (Peru, Illinois), and St. Margaret's Hospital (Spring Valley, Illinois).

Mike Spinelli Photography, Phoenix, Arizona

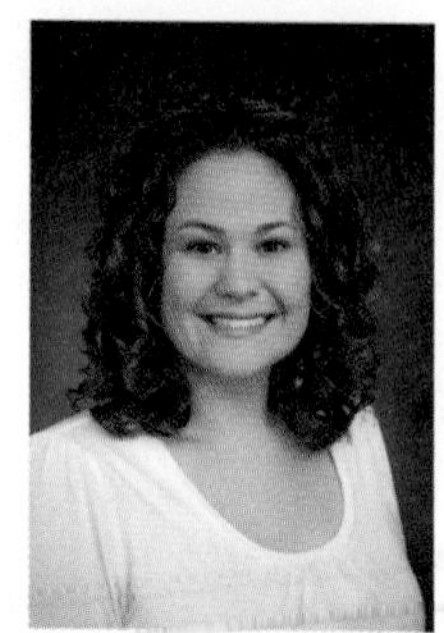

Leighann N. Remmert is a Health Occupations Instructor at Lincolnland Technical Education Center in Lincoln, Illinois. She teaches high school nursing assistant students in the clinical setting and instructs nursing assistant courses for adult learners.

Leighann has a Bachelor of Science degree in nursing from Bradley University (Peoria, Illinois) and a Master of Science degree in nursing education from Southern Illinois University Edwardsville (Edwardsville, Illinois). Leighann's clinical background includes the roles of nursing assistant/tech, nurse extern, staff nurse, charge nurse, nurse preceptor, and trauma nurse specialist. As an RN, Leighann concentrated in the area of emergency nursing at Memorial Medical Center (Springfield, Illinois). She is a member of Sigma Theta Tau International, the Honor Society of Nursing and the Certified Nursing Assistant Educator's Association (Illinois, Central Region).

Leighann has supervised, instructed, and evaluated student learning in long-term care and acute care settings as a clinical nursing instructor at the Capital Area School of Practical Nursing (Springfield, Illinois). In her current position at Lincolnland Technical Education Center, Leighann guides students in acquiring the skills and knowledge they need to succeed as nursing assistants. Through her teaching, she emphasizes the importance of professionalism and work ethics, safety, teamwork, communication, and accountability. Valuing the role of the nursing assistant and treating the person with dignity, care, and respect are integral to her instruction in the classroom and clinical settings.

Leighann is co-author of *Mosby's Textbook for Medication Assistants*, *Mosby's Essentials for Nursing Assistants* (4e), and *Mosby's Textbook for Nursing Assistants* (8e). She was a consultant on *Mosby's Textbook for Long-Term Care Nursing Assistants* (6e).

Leighann and her husband, Shane, have one daughter, Olivia. Leighann and Shane are active in various ministry areas at Elkhart Christian Church (Elkhart, Illinois). Leighann is certified as a Basic Life Support instructor and teaches CPR courses for the church and community.

Terry Farmer Photography, Springfield, Illinois

Reviewers

Carrie Adams, RN, MSN
Adjunct Instructor – Nursing/Nursing Assistant
Mesa Community College
Mesa, Arizona

Clare DeVries, RN, BSN
CNA Instructor
Joliet Junior College
Joliet, Illinois

JoAnne M. Franz, RN, MS
CNA Instructor
Joliet Junior College
Joliet, Illinois
Mohave Community College
Bullhead City, Arizona

Mary Therese Galka, RN, BSN
BNAT Instructor and Program Coordinator
Moraine Valley Community College
Palos Hills, Illinois

Karrie Pater, RN, BSN
Instructor, Certified Nurse Aide Course
Director of Nursing
North Central Michigan College, Bortz Health Care of Petoskey
Petoskey, Michigan

Linda Skroch, RN, BSN
School Nurse/CNA Instructor
NASN
Yerington, Nevada

Acknowledgments

As authors, we rely on others to provide assistance and to fulfill their respective roles and responsibilities to ensure an accurate, up-to-date, and timely publication. Therefore we extend a "thank you" and appreciation to the following individuals.

- The reviewers who spent time reading, commenting on, and making suggestions to improve our textbook. We found their thoughts and ideas insightful and useful.
  - Carrie Adams, RN, MSN
  - Clare DeVries, RN, BSN
  - JoAnne M. Franz, RN, MS
  - Mary Therese Galka, RN, BSN
  - Karrie Pater, RN, BSN
  - Linda Skroch, RN, BSN
- Susan Broadhurst (Rochester, New York) for her role as copy editor. She accommodates our style well.
- Jody McBride for her proofreading efforts. The task requires attention to detail and special talents.
- The artists at Graphic World (St. Louis, Missouri). They made sense out of "roughs."
- And finally to the Elsevier/Mosby staff involved:
  - Nancy O'Brien, Content Strategist
  - Maria Broeker, Senior Content Development Specialist
  - Kelly Albright, Content Coordinator
  - Jeff Patterson, Publishing Services Manager
  - Bill Drone, Project Manager, Book Production
  - Brian Salisbury, Designer
  - Emily Ogle, Producer

To all individuals who contributed to this effort in any way, we are sincerely grateful.

Sheila A. Sorrentino and Leighann N. Remmert

Instructor Preface

The fifth edition of *Mosby's Essentials for Nursing Assistants* serves several purposes. As authors, we believe the book:

- Prepares students to function as nursing assistants in nursing centers and hospitals.
- Serves the needs of students and instructors in educational settings offering nursing assistant courses.
- Is a valuable resource for individuals preparing for the competency evaluation.
- Is a useful reference as the certified (licensed or registered) nursing assistant seeks to review or learn new information for safe care.

Foundational principles and concepts are presented in specific chapters while values, objectives, and organizational strategies are intertwined and integrated in content and key features throughout the book. (See "Student Preface" p. xii for key features.)

- Patients and residents are presented as *persons* with dignity who have a past, a present, and a future. Such persons are physical, social, psychological, and spiritual beings with basic needs and protected rights. Their culture and religion influence health and illness practices.
- Nursing assistant roles, range of functions, and limitations are defined and described by federal and state laws and are dependent on effective delegation and good work ethics.
- Promoting safety and comfort is central to the nursing assistant role. Body structure and function, body mechanics, preventing infection, safety practices, and comfort measures form the essential knowledge base.
- Communication skills are needed to communicate effectively with the nursing and health teams, patients and residents, and families and visitors.
- The nursing process is the basis for planning and delivering nursing care. Nursing assistants play a key role in assisting with the nursing process.

Content Issues

Every edition requires revision and content decisions. Changes in laws or in guidelines and standards issued by government or accrediting agencies are accommodated. So are changes to state curricula and competency evaluations. Every attempt is made to publish an up-to-date book. Often changes are made right before publication.

Student learning needs and abilities, instructor desires, work-related issues, course/program and book length, and student cost are among the many factors considered. With such issues in mind, new and expanded content and figures are listed in this section.

Chapter 2: The Person's Rights *(NEW!)*

- FOCUS ON SURVEYS: Residents' Rights
- FOCUS ON COMMUNICATION: Information
- FOCUS ON COMMUNICATION: Quality of Life
- FOCUS ON COMMUNICATION: Activities
- FOCUS ON SURVEYS: Activities

Chapter 3: The Nursing Assistant

- Nurse Practice Acts
- Nursing Assistants
- FOCUS ON COMMUNICATION: The Training Program
- Certification
- FOCUS ON SURVEYS: Maintaining Competence
- FOCUS ON COMMUNICATION: Job Description
- FOCUS ON COMMUNICATION: Refusing a Task
- FOCUS ON COMMUNICATION: Professional Boundaries
- FOCUS ON COMMUNICATION: Intentional Torts (Invasion of Privacy)
- FOCUS ON COMMUNICATION: Reporting Abuse
- FOCUS ON SURVEYS: Reporting Abuse
- Child Abuse and Neglect
- Domestic Abuse

Chapter 4: Work Ethics

- FOCUS ON COMMUNICATION: Attendance

Chapter 5: Communicating With the Health Team

- FOCUS ON SURVEYS: The Comprehensive Care Plan
- Box 5-4 The 24-Hour Clock

Chapter 6: Understanding the Person

- FOCUS ON COMMUNICATION: Culture and Religion
- Paraphrasing
- Persons With Bariatric Needs

Chapter 7: Body Structure and Function

- The Lymphatic System

Chapter 8: Care of the Older Person

- FOCUS ON COMMUNICATION: Social Relationships

Chapter 9: Assisting With Safety

- PROMOTING SAFETY AND COMFORT: Assisting With Safety
- FOCUS ON SURVEYS: Assisting With Safety
- FOCUS ON COMMUNICATION: Identifying the Person
- Box 9-2 Choking—Chest Thrusts for Obese or Pregnant Persons
- FOCUS ON OLDER PERSONS: Choking
- PROMOTING SAFETY AND COMFORT: Preventing Equipment Accidents
- FOCUS ON SURVEYS: Disasters

Chapter 10: Assisting With Fall Prevention
- FOCUS ON SURVEYS: Assisting With Fall Prevention
- FOCUS ON COMMUNICATION: Transfer/Gait Belts

Chapter 11: Restraint Alternatives and Safe Restraint Use
- Enablers

Chapter 12: Preventing Infection
- FOCUS ON SURVEYS: Infection
- PROCEDURE: Using an Alcohol-Based Hand Rub
- FOCUS ON SURVEYS: Transmission-Based Precautions
- Collecting Specimens
- Transporting Persons
- FOCUS ON COMMUNICATION: Meeting Basic Needs
- FOCUS ON SURVEYS: Laundry

Chapter 14: Assisting With Moving and Transfers
- FOCUS ON SURVEYS: Protecting the Skin
- FOCUS ON SURVEYS: Bed to Chair or Wheelchair Transfers
- Slings

Chapter 15: Assisting With Comfort
- FOCUS ON COMMUNICATION: Comfort
- FOCUS ON COMMUNICATION: Noise
- FOCUS ON SURVEYS: Noise
- PROMOTING SAFETY AND COMFORT: The Call System
- PROMOTING SAFETY AND COMFORT: Closet and Drawer Space
- FOCUS ON SURVEYS: Linens
- FOCUS ON SURVEYS: Pain

Chapter 16: Assisting With Hygiene
- FOCUS ON COMMUNICATION: Assisting With Hygiene
- PROMOTING SAFETY AND COMFORT: Assisting With Hygiene
- FOCUS ON COMMUNICATION: Mouth Care for the Unconscious Person

Chapter 17: Assisting With Grooming
- FOCUS ON SURVEYS: Assisting with Grooming
- FOCUS ON OLDER PERSONS: Shampooing
- PROMOTING SAFETY AND COMFORT: Dressing and Undressing

Chapter 18: Assisting With Urinary Elimination
- PROMOTING SAFETY AND COMFORT: Assisting With Urinary Elimination
- Managing Incontinence
- FOCUS ON SURVEYS: Managing Incontinence
- Applying Incontinence Products
- FOCUS ON COMMUNICATION: Applying Incontinence Products
- DELEGATION GUIDELINES: Applying Incontinence Products

Chapter 18: Assisting With Urinary Elimination—cont'd
- PROMOTING SAFETY AND COMFORT: Applying Incontinence Products
- PROCEDURE: Applying an Incontinence Brief
- FOCUS ON SURVEYS: Catheters

Chapter 19: Assisting With Bowel Elimination
- DELEGATION GUIDELINES: Assisting With Bowel Elimination
- PROMOTING SAFETY AND COMFORT: Assisting With Bowel Elimination
- FOCUS ON COMMUNICATION: Safety and Comfort
- FOCUS ON OLDER PERSONS: Diarrhea

Chapter 20: Assisting With Nutrition and Fluids
- FOCUS ON SURVEYS: Assisting With Nutrition and Fluids
- FOCUS ON OLDER PERSONS: Factors Affecting Eating and Nutrition
- FOCUS ON SURVEYS: Feeding the Person
- FOCUS ON COMMUNICATION: Providing Drinking Water
- FOCUS ON COMMUNICATION: Assisting With IV Therapy

Chapter 21: Assisting With Assessment
- FOCUS ON COMMUNICATION: Temperature Sites
- FOCUS ON OLDER PERSONS: Temperature Sites
- FOCUS ON COMMUNICATION: Normal and Abnormal Blood Pressures
- FOCUS ON OLDER PERSONS: Signs and Symptoms of Pain
- FOCUS ON COMMUNICATION: Weight and Height

Chapter 22: Assisting With Specimens
- The 24-Hour Urine Specimen

Chapter 23: Assisting With Exercise and Activity
- FOCUS ON SURVEYS: Range-of-Motion Exercises
- PROMOTING SAFETY AND COMFORT: Walkers

Chapter 24: Assisting With Wound Care
- DELEGATION GUIDELINES: Assisting With Wound Care
- FOCUS ON OLDER PERSONS: Applying Dressings
- FOCUS ON OLDER PERSONS: Heat and Cold Applications

Chapter 25: Assisting With Pressure Ulcers *(NEW!)*

Chapter 26: Assisting With Oxygen Needs
- Pulse Oximetry
- DELEGATION GUIDELINES: Pulse Oximetry
- PROCEDURE: Using a Pulse Oximeter

Chapter 28: Caring for Persons With Common Health Problems

- FOCUS ON COMMUNICATION: The Person's Needs
- Influenza
- FOCUS ON OLDER PERSONS: Influenza
- FOCUS ON OLDER PERSONS: Sexually Transmitted Diseases
- Autoimmune Disorders
- FOCUS ON OLDER PERSONS: Acquired Immunodeficiency Syndrome
- Skin Disorders
- Shingles

Chapter 29: Caring for Persons With Mental Health Disorders

- FOCUS ON OLDER PERSONS: Alcoholism and Alcohol Abuse
- Eating Disorders
- FOCUS ON OLDER PERSONS: Suicide

Chapter 30: Caring for Persons With Confusion and Dementia

- Box 30-4 Signs and Symptoms of Delirium
- Box 30-6 Alzheimer's Disease and Normal Aging
- Box 30-7 Three Stages of Alzheimer's Disease—National Institute on Aging
- Box 30-8 Seven Stages of Alzheimer's Disease—Alzheimer's Association
- PROMOTING SAFETY AND COMFORT: Behaviors and Problems
- PROMOTING SAFETY AND COMFORT: Wandering and Getting Lost
- Paranoia
- PROMOTING SAFETY AND COMFORT: Paranoia
- Communication Problems
- CARING ABOUT CULTURE: Communication Problems
- FOCUS ON COMMUNICATION: Communication Problems
- Rummaging and Hiding Things
- FOCUS ON OLDER PERSONS: Care of Persons With AD and Other Dementias
- FOCUS ON SURVEYS: Care of Persons with AD and Other Dementias
- Box 30-11 Family Caregivers—Taking Care of Yourself

Chapter 32: Assisting With End-of-Life Care

- Types of Care
- FOCUS ON OLDER PERSONS: Comfort Needs
- Pain
- Breathing Problems
- Nutrition
- Mental and Emotional Needs
- FOCUS ON SURVEYS: Advance Directives

New Figures

Figure 5-3	The nursing process is continuous.
Figure 5-4	Sample assignment sheet. Note: This assignment sheet is a computer printout.
Figure 7-18	The lymphatic system.
Figure 11-9	The restraint is secured to the moveable part of the bed frame.
Figure 12-3	Sneezing into the upper arm.
Figure 12-6	The fingers are interlaced to clean between the fingers.
Figure 12-10	Using an alcohol-based hand rub.
Figure 14-21	Parts of a mechanical lift.
Figure 15-21	**A,** Waterproof pad. **B,** Disposable bed protector.
Figure 17-1	Head lice.
Figure 17-2	Scabies.
Figure 17-7	Electric shaver and safety razor.
Figure 18-10	Applying an incontinence brief.
Figure 18-15	The clamp is closed and positioned in the holder on the drainage bag
Figure 20-6	Water mug with straw. The mug is marked in milliliters (mL) and ounces (oz).
Figure 21-19	Reading the manometer. Long lines mark 10 mm Hg values. Short lines mark 2 mm Hg values.
Figure 24-1	Skin tear.
Figure 24-3	Arterial ulcer.
Figure 24-4	Foot problems common with diabetes.
Figure 24-13	Compression garment.
Figure 25-4	Pressure ulcer stages.
Figure 26-13	Cannula prongs are inserted. The prong openings face downward.
Figure 28-30	Enlarged prostate. The prostate presses against the urethra. Urine flow is obstructed.
Figure 28-31	Shingles rash.
Figure 30-2	**A,** Normal brain. **B,** Dark patches show damage to brain tissue.
Figure 30-3	**A,** Very early AD. **B,** Mild to moderate AD. **C,** Severe AD.
Figure 30-7	Safety covers are on stove knobs.

Features and Design

Besides content issues, attention is given to improving the book's features and designs. To make the book readable and user friendly, new features and design elements are added while others are retained or modified. See "Student Preface," p. xii.

May this book serve you and your students well. Our intent is to provide the current information needed to teach and learn safe and effective care during this time of dynamic change in health care.

Sheila A. Sorrentino, BSN, MA, MSN, PhD, RN
Leighann N. Remmert, BSN, MS, RN

Student Preface

This book was designed for you. It was designed to help you learn. The book is a useful resource as you gain experience and expand your knowledge.

This preface gives study guidelines and helps you use the book. For a reading assignment, do you read from the first page to the last page without stopping? What do you remember? To learn more, use a study system with these steps.

- Survey or preview
- Question
- Read and record
- Recite and review

Survey or Preview

First, preview or survey the reading assignment for a few minutes. This gives an idea of what the assignment covers. It also helps in recalling what you know about the subject. Carefully look over the assignment. Preview the chapter title, objectives, key terms and abbreviations, headings, subheadings, and key ideas in italics. Also survey the boxes and review questions at the end of the chapter.

Question

Next, form questions to answer while reading. Questions should relate to how the information applies to giving care or what might be asked on a test. Use the headings and subheadings to form questions. Questions starting with what, how, or why are helpful. Avoid questions with one-word answers. If a question does not help you study, just change the question. Questioning sets a purpose for reading. Changing a question makes this step more useful.

Read and Record

Reading is the next step. You need to:

- Gain new information.
- Connect new information to what you already know.
- Find answers to your questions.

Break the assignment into small parts. Then answer your questions as you read each part. Also underline or highlight important information. This reminds you of what you need to learn. Review the marked parts later. Also make notes for more immediate learning. To make notes, write down important information in the margins or in a notebook. Use words and statements to jog your memory about the material.

To remember what you read, work with the information. Organize information into a study guide. Study guides have many forms. Diagrams or charts show relationships or steps in a process. Note taking in outline format is also very useful. A sample outline follows.

1 Main heading
  A Second level
  B Second level
    (1) Third level
    (2) Third level

Recite and Review

Finally, recite and review. Use your notes and study guides. Answer questions and others that came up when reading and answering the "Review Questions" at the end of a chapter. Answer all questions out loud (recite).

Reviewing is more about when to study rather than what to study. You decided what to study during your preview, question, and reading steps. It is best to review right after the first study session, 1 week later, and before a quiz or test.

This book was designed to help you study. Special features are described on the next pages.

We hope you enjoy learning and your work. You and your work are important. You and the care you give make a difference in the person's life!

Sheila A. Sorrentino
Leighann N. Remmert

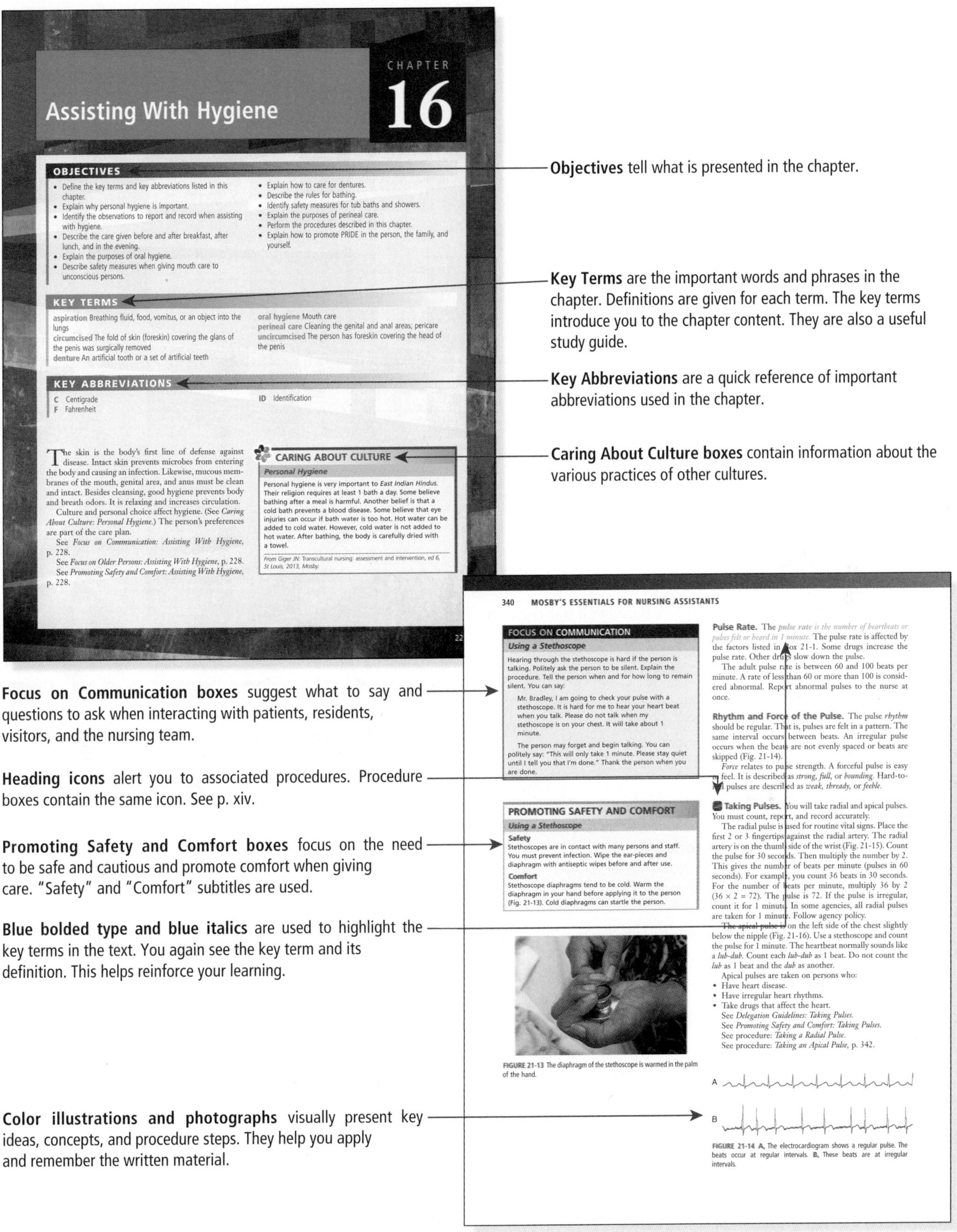

CHAPTER 16

Assisting With Hygiene

OBJECTIVES

- Define the key terms and key abbreviations listed in this chapter.
- Explain why personal hygiene is important.
- Identify the observations to report and record when assisting with hygiene.
- Describe the care given before and after breakfast, after lunch, and in the evening.
- Explain the purposes of oral hygiene.
- Describe safety measures when giving mouth care to unconscious persons.
- Explain how to care for dentures.
- Describe the rules for bathing.
- Identify safety measures for tub baths and showers.
- Explain the purposes of perineal care.
- Perform the procedures described in this chapter.
- Explain how to promote PRIDE in the person, the family, and yourself.

KEY TERMS

aspiration Breathing fluid, food, vomitus, or an object into the lungs
circumcised The fold of skin (foreskin) covering the glans of the penis was surgically removed
denture An artificial tooth or a set of artificial teeth
oral hygiene Mouth care
perineal care Cleaning the genital and anal areas; pericare
uncircumcised The person has foreskin covering the head of the penis

KEY ABBREVIATIONS

C Centigrade
F Fahrenheit
ID Identification

The skin is the body's first line of defense against disease. Intact skin prevents microbes from entering the body and causing an infection. Likewise, mucous membranes of the mouth, genital area, and anus must be clean and intact. Besides cleansing, good hygiene prevents body and breath odors. It is relaxing and increases circulation.

Culture and personal choice affect hygiene. (See *Caring About Culture: Personal Hygiene.*) The person's preferences are part of the care plan.

See *Focus on Communication: Assisting With Hygiene,* p. 228.

See *Focus on Older Persons: Assisting With Hygiene,* p. 228.

See *Promoting Safety and Comfort: Assisting With Hygiene,* p. 228.

CARING ABOUT CULTURE

Personal Hygiene

Personal hygiene is very important to *East Indian Hindus.* Their religion requires at least 1 bath a day. Some believe bathing after a meal is harmful. Another belief is that a cold bath prevents a blood disease. Some believe that eye injuries can occur if bath water is too hot. Hot water can be added to cold water. However, cold water is not added to hot water. After bathing, the body is carefully dried with a towel.

From Giger JN: *Transcultural nursing: assessment and intervention,* ed 6, St Louis, 2013, Mosby.

340 MOSBY'S ESSENTIALS FOR NURSING ASSISTANTS

FOCUS ON COMMUNICATION

Using a Stethoscope

Hearing through the stethoscope is hard if the person is talking. Politely ask the person to be silent. Explain the procedure. Tell the person when and for how long to remain silent. You can say:

Mr. Bradley, I am going to check your pulse with a stethoscope. It is hard for me to hear your heart beat when you talk. Please do not talk when my stethoscope is on your chest. It will take about 1 minute.

The person may forget and begin talking. You can politely say: "This will only take 1 minute. Please stay quiet until I tell you that I'm done." Thank the person when you are done.

PROMOTING SAFETY AND COMFORT

Using a Stethoscope

Safety

Stethoscopes are in contact with many persons and staff. You must prevent infection. Wipe the ear-pieces and diaphragm with antiseptic wipes before and after use.

Comfort

Stethoscope diaphragms tend to be cold. Warm the diaphragm in your hand before applying it to the person (Fig. 21-13). Cold diaphragms can startle the person.

FIGURE 21-13 The diaphragm of the stethoscope is warmed in the palm of the hand.

Pulse Rate. The *pulse rate is the number of heartbeats or pulses felt or heard in 1 minute.* The pulse rate is affected by the factors listed in Box 21-1. Some drugs increase the pulse rate. Other drugs slow down the pulse.

The adult pulse rate is between 60 and 100 beats per minute. A rate of less than 60 or more than 100 is considered abnormal. Report abnormal pulses to the nurse at once.

Rhythm and Force of the Pulse. The pulse *rhythm* should be regular. That is, pulses are felt in a pattern. The same interval occurs between beats. An irregular pulse occurs when the beats are not evenly spaced or beats are skipped (Fig. 21-14).

Force relates to pulse strength. A forceful pulse is easy to feel. It is described as *strong, full,* or *bounding.* Hard-to-feel pulses are described as *weak, thready,* or *feeble.*

Taking Pulses. You will take radial and apical pulses. You must count, report, and record accurately.

The radial pulse is used for routine vital signs. Place the first 2 or 3 fingertips against the radial artery. The radial artery is on the thumb side of the wrist (Fig. 21-15). Count the pulse for 30 seconds. Then multiply the number by 2. This gives the number of beats per minute (pulses in 60 seconds). For example, you count 36 beats in 30 seconds. For the number of beats per minute, multiply 36 by 2 (36 × 2 = 72). The pulse is 72. If the pulse is irregular, count it for 1 minute. In some agencies, all radial pulses are taken for 1 minute. Follow agency policy.

The apical pulse is on the left side of the chest slightly below the nipple (Fig. 21-16). Use a stethoscope and count the pulse for 1 minute. The heartbeat normally sounds like a *lub-dub.* Count each *lub-dub* as 1 beat. Do not count the *lub* as 1 beat and the *dub* as another.

Apical pulses are taken on persons who:

- Have heart disease.
- Have irregular heart rhythms.
- Take drugs that affect the heart.

See *Delegation Guidelines: Taking Pulses.*
See *Promoting Safety and Comfort: Taking Pulses.*
See procedure: *Taking a Radial Pulse.*
See procedure: *Taking an Apical Pulse,* p. 342.

FIGURE 21-14 **A,** The electrocardiogram shows a regular pulse. The beats occur at regular intervals. **B,** These beats are at irregular intervals.

Objectives tell what is presented in the chapter.

Key Terms are the important words and phrases in the chapter. Definitions are given for each term. The key terms introduce you to the chapter content. They are also a useful study guide.

Key Abbreviations are a quick reference of important abbreviations used in the chapter.

Caring About Culture boxes contain information about the various practices of other cultures.

Focus on Communication boxes suggest what to say and questions to ask when interacting with patients, residents, visitors, and the nursing team.

Heading icons alert you to associated procedures. Procedure boxes contain the same icon. See p. xiv.

Promoting Safety and Comfort boxes focus on the need to be safe and cautious and promote comfort when giving care. "Safety" and "Comfort" subtitles are used.

Blue bolded type and blue italics are used to highlight the key terms in the text. You again see the key term and its definition. This helps reinforce your learning.

Color illustrations and photographs visually present key ideas, concepts, and procedure steps. They help you apply and remember the written material.

Boxes and tables list important rules, principles, guidelines, signs and symptoms, nursing measures, and other information. They identify important information and are useful study guides.

Focus on Older Persons boxes provide information about the needs, considerations, and special circumstances of older persons. These sections also provide useful information about persons with Alzheimer's disease and other dementias.

Delegation Guidelines describe the information you need from the nurse and the care plan before performing a procedure. They also tell you the observations to report and record.

Title Bar Icons:

- **NNAAP®** in the procedure title bar alerts you to the skills that are part of the *National Nurse Aide Assessment Program* (NNAAP®). Note: Not all states participate in NNAAP®. Ask your instructor for a list of the skills tested in your state.
- **CD icons** appear in the procedure box title bar for the skills included on the CD-ROM in the book.
- **Video clip icons** in the procedure title bar alert you to related video clips available on-line on *Evolve Student Learning Resources*.
- **Video icons** in the procedure title bar alert you to procedures included in *Mosby's Nursing Assistant Video Skills 3.0.*

Procedure icons in the procedure title bar alert you to associated content areas. Heading icons (see p. xiii) and procedure icons are the same.

Procedure boxes are written in a step-by-step format. They are divided into *Quality of Life, Pre-Procedure, Procedure*, and *Post-Procedure* sections for easy studying. The *Quality of Life* sections list 6 simple courtesies that show respect for the patient or resident as a person.

---

140 MOSBY'S ESSENTIALS FOR NURSING ASSISTANTS

An *infection is a disease state resulting from the invasion and growth of microbes in the body.* Infection is a major safety and health hazard. Minor infections cause short illnesses. A serious infection can cause death. Older and disabled persons are at risk. The health team follows certain *practices and procedures to prevent the spread of infection (infection control).* The goal is to protect patients, residents, visitors, and staff from infection.

MICROORGANISMS

A *microorganism (microbe) is a small (micro) living thing (organism). It is seen only with a microscope.* Microbes are everywhere—mouth, nose, respiratory tract, stomach, and intestines. They are on the skin and in the air, soil, water, and food. They are on animals, clothing, and furniture.

Microbes that are harmful and can cause infections are called pathogens. Non-pathogens are microbes that do not usually cause an infection.

Requirements of Microbes

Microbes need a *reservoir (host)*. The reservoir is the place where the microbe lives and grows. People, plants, animals, the soil, food, and water are examples. Microbes need *water* and *nourishment* from the reservoir. Most need *oxygen* to live. A *warm* and *dark* environment is needed. Most grow best at body temperature. They are destroyed by heat and light.

Multidrug-Resistant Organisms

Multidrug-resistant organisms (MDROs) are microbes that can resist the effects of antibiotics. *Antibiotics are drugs that kill certain pathogens.* Some pathogens can change their structures. This makes them harder to kill. They can live in the presence of antibiotics. Therefore the infections they cause are hard to treat.

MDROs are caused by prescribing antibiotics when not needed (over-prescribing). Not taking antibiotics for the length of time prescribed is another cause. Common MDROs are:

- *Methicillin-resistant* Staphylococcus aureus *(MRSA). Staphylococcus aureus* ("staph") is a bacterium normally found in the nose and on the skin. MRSA is resistant to antibiotics often used for "staph" infections. MRSA can cause pneumonia and serious wound and bloodstream infections.
- *Vancomycin-resistant* Enterococci *(VRE). Enterococcus* is a bacterium normally found in the intestines and in feces. It can be transmitted to others by contaminated hands, toilet seats, care equipment, and other items that the hands touch. When not in their natural site (the intestines), enterococci can cause urinary tract, wound, pelvic, and other infections. Enterococci resistant to the antibiotic vancomycin are called vancomycin-resistant *Enterococci* (VRE).

INFECTION

A *local infection* is in a body part. A *systemic infection* involves the whole body. (*Systemic* means *entire.*) The person has some or all of the signs and symptoms listed in Box 12-1.

See *Focus on Older Persons: Infection.*

See *Focus on Surveys: Infection.*

BOX 12-1 Signs and Symptoms of Infection

- Fever (elevated body temperature)
- Chills
- Pulse rate: increased
- Respiratory rate: increased
- Pain or tenderness
- Fatigue and loss of energy
- Appetite: loss of *(anorexia)*
- Nausea
- Vomiting
- Diarrhea
- Rash
- Sores on mucous membranes
- Redness and swelling of a body part
- Discharge or drainage from the infected area
- Heat or warmth in a body part
- Limited use of a body part
- Headache
- Muscle aches
- Joint pain
- Confusion

FOCUS ON OLDER PERSONS

Infection

The immune system protects the body from disease and infection (Chapter 7). Changes occur in this system with aging. Therefore older persons are at risk for infection.

An older person may not show the signs and symptoms of infection listed in Box 12-1. The person may have only a slight fever or no fever at all. Redness and swelling may be slight. The person may not complain of pain. Confusion and delirium may occur (Chapter 30).

An infection can become life-threatening before the older person has obvious signs and symptoms. Report minor changes in the person's behavior or condition at once.

Healing takes longer in older persons. Therefore an infection can prolong the rehabilitation process. Independence and quality of life are affected.

FOCUS ON SURVEYS

Infection

Infection control practices are a major focus of surveys. You may be asked:

- What do you do when you observe signs and symptoms of an infection?
- Who do you tell when you observe signs and symptoms of an infection?

CHAPTER 21 Assisting With Assessment 341

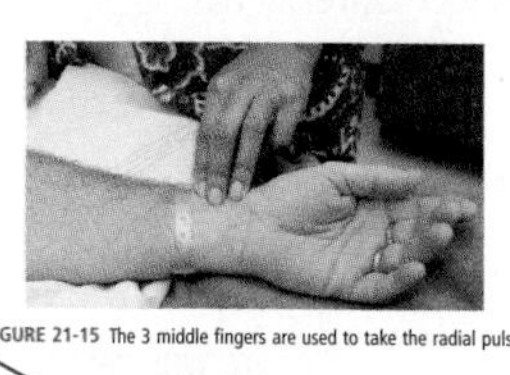

FIGURE 21-15 The 3 middle fingers are used to take the radial pulse.

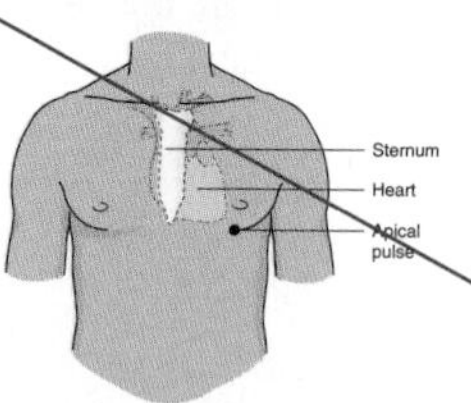

FIGURE 21-16 The apical pulse is located 2 to 3 inches to the left of the sternum (breastbone) and below the left nipple.

DELEGATION GUIDELINES

Taking Pulses

Before taking a pulse, you need this information from the nurse and the care plan.

- What pulse to take for each person—radial or apical
- When to take the pulse
- What other vital signs to measure
- How long to count the pulse—30 seconds or 1 minute
- If the nurse has concerns about certain patients or residents
- What observations to report and record:
  - The pulse site
  - The pulse rate—report a pulse rate less than 60 (bradycardia) or more than 100 (tachycardia) beats per minute at once
  - If the pulse is regular or irregular
  - Pulse force—strong, full, bounding, weak, thready, or feeble
- When to report the pulse rate
- What patient or resident concerns to report at once

PROMOTING SAFETY AND COMFORT

Taking Pulses

Safety

Use your first 2 or 3 fingertips to take a pulse. Do not use your thumb. The thumb has a pulse. You could mistake the pulse in your thumb for the person's pulse. Reporting and recording the wrong pulse rate can harm the person.

Taking a Radial Pulse NNAAP CD VIDEO CLIP VIDEO

QUALITY OF LIFE

- Knock before entering the person's room.
- Address the person by name.
- Introduce yourself by name and title.
- Explain the procedure before starting and during the procedure.
- Protect the person's rights during the procedure.
- Handle the person gently during the procedure.

PRE-PROCEDURE

1 Follow *Delegation Guidelines: Taking Pulses.* See *Promoting Safety and Comfort: Taking Pulses.*
2 Practice hand hygiene.
3 Identify the person. Check the ID bracelet against the assignment sheet. Also call the person by name.
4 Provide for privacy.

PROCEDURE

5 Have the person sit or lie down.
6 Locate the radial pulse on the thumb side of the person's wrist. Use your first 2 or 3 middle fingertips (see Fig. 21-15).
7 Note if the pulse is strong or weak, and regular or irregular.
8 Count the pulse for 30 seconds. Multiply the number of beats by 2 for the number of pulses in 60 seconds (1 minute). (For example, you count 45 beats in 30 seconds. Multiply 45 by 2. 45 × 2 = 90. The pulse is 90 beats per minute.)
9 Count the pulse for 1 minute if:
  a Directed by the nurse and the care plan.
  b Required by agency policy.
  c The pulse was irregular.
  d Required for your state competency test.
10 Note the following on your note pad or assignment sheet.
  a The person's name
  b Pulse rate
  c Pulse strength
  d If the pulse was regular or irregular

POST-PROCEDURE

11 Provide for comfort. (See the inside of the front cover.)
12 Place the call light within reach.
13 Unscreen the person.
14 Complete a safety check of the room. (See the inside of the front cover.)
15 Practice hand hygiene.
16 Report and record the pulse rate and your observations. Report an abnormal pulse at once.

CHAPTER 1 Hospitals and Nursing Centers 7

The Survey Process

Surveys are done to see if the agency meets set standards. A survey team will:

- Review policies, procedures, and medical records.
- Interview staff, patients and residents, and families.
- Observe how care is given.
- Observe if dignity and privacy are promoted.
- Check for cleanliness and safety.
- Make sure staff meet state requirements. (Are doctors and nurses licensed? Are nursing assistants on the state registry?)

The survey team decides if the agency meets the standards. Sometimes problems are found. A problem is called a *deficiency.* The agency usually has 60 days to correct the problem. Sometimes less time is given. The agency can be fined for uncorrected or serious deficiencies. Or it can lose its license, certification, or accreditation.

Your Role

You have an important role in meeting standards and in the survey process. You must:

- Provide quality care.
- Protect the person's rights.
- Provide for the person's and your own safety.
- Help keep the agency clean and safe.
- Conduct yourself in a professional manner.
- Have good work ethics.
- Follow agency policies and procedures.
- Answer questions honestly and completely.

See *Focus on Surveys: Your Role.*

FOCUS ON SURVEYS

Your Role

Survey teams are made up of surveyors. A *surveyor* is a person who collects information by observing and asking questions.

A surveyor may ask you questions. If so, be polite. Avoid seeming annoyed or upset. Answer the questions honestly and thoroughly. If you do not understand the question, ask the surveyor to re-phrase it. Do not guess at an answer. Tell the surveyor where you can find the answer. You can say: "I am unsure, but I would ask the nurse."

For example, a surveyor approaches you:

Surveyor: "Do you have a moment? May I ask you a few questions?"

You: "Yes. I am happy to answer your questions."

Surveyor: "Thank you. First, when should you practice hand hygiene?"

You: "I wash my hands before and after contact with a patient. I also wash my hands when they are dirty and after I take off my gloves."

Surveyor: "Thank you. Next, what are 2 appropriate patient identifiers?"

You: "I'm not sure I understand the question. Can you re-phrase it?"

Surveyor: "Yes. Name 2 things you can use to identify a patient."

You: "Okay. Thank you. I can use the patient's full name and date of birth. I cannot use the room number."

Surveyor: "Thank you. I have 1 last question. In a disaster, where would you find the Emergency Preparedness Plan?"

You: "Well, I'm not sure where the plan is located. I will ask my supervising nurse or the charge nurse where to find it."

FOCUS ON PRIDE

The Person, Family, and Yourself

Personal and Professional Responsibility

Health care is a rewarding profession. The health team works hard to provide quality care. You are an important part of that team. You will spend most of your time giving care. Remember to show patience, compassion, dignity, and respect. You have a great impact on the quality of care each person receives.

Rights and Respect

Many hospitals and nursing centers conduct employee satisfaction surveys. The surveys ask what employees think about their jobs.

All staff are expected to complete and return the form. You may need to note the area you work in or your role in the agency. Identifying information, such as your name, is usually not given. This helps protect your identity. You have the right to voice your true thoughts on a survey. When filling out a survey:

- Be honest. Positive and negative comments are important.
- Take the survey seriously. Do not rush. Answer the questions completely.
- Complete and return the form in a timely manner.

Surveys are one way hospitals and nursing centers show respect for employees. Comments are used to make changes. Take pride in your ideas. Your thoughts matter.

Independence and Social Interaction

People who rely on others for care often feel frustrated, useless, sad, and a burden to others. A common goal is to return persons to their highest level of functioning. Physical, occupational, and speech therapists work together with doctors, the nursing team, and others to promote independence (see Table 1-1). Independence promotes feelings of improvement and success. Help the person take pride in working to restore independence.

Delegation and Teamwork

Each health team member has a certain role. Everyone must work together to provide quality care. Offer to help team members when you can. Helping others shows you are dependable and value teamwork.

Ethics and Laws

Nursing team members have different levels of training and responsibilities. RN, LPN/LVN, and nursing assistant roles vary. Federal and state laws determine the legal limits of these roles. See Chapter 3 for your role limits. Functions may also vary among agencies. A job description (Chapter 3) describes the agency's expectations. To protect yourself and others, know the limits of your role in your state and agency.

Focus on Surveys boxes (*NEW!*) alert you to questions that surveyors may ask you. The boxes also include what surveyors may observe you doing.

Focus on PRIDE: The Person, Family, and Yourself boxes build on the concepts and principles presented in the chapter to help you promote *pride* in the person, the family, and yourself. *PRIDE* is spelled out in the first letter of each section.

- ***Personal and Professional Responsibility***—how you can have pride in yourself through personal and professional behaviors and development.
- ***Rights and Respect***—how to promote the person's rights and respect him or her as a person with dignity and value.
- ***Independence and Social Interaction***—ways to help the person remain or attain independence and interact socially with others.
- ***Delegation and Teamwork***—how to work efficiently with and help other nursing team members.
- ***Ethics and Laws***—laws affecting nursing care and doing the right thing when dealing with patients, residents, and co-workers.

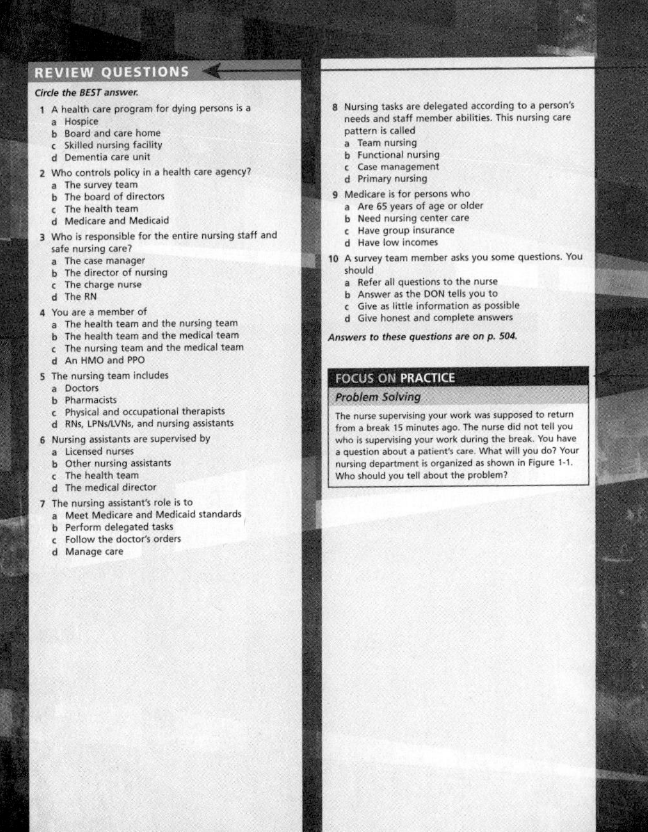

REVIEW QUESTIONS

Circle the BEST answer.

1 A health care program for dying persons is a
 a Hospice
 b Board and care home
 c Skilled nursing facility
 d Dementia care unit

2 Who controls policy in a health care agency?
 a The survey team
 b The board of directors
 c The health team
 d Medicare and Medicaid

3 Who is responsible for the entire nursing staff and safe nursing care?
 a The case manager
 b The director of nursing
 c The charge nurse
 d The RN

4 You are a member of
 a The health team and the nursing team
 b The health team and the medical team
 c The nursing team and the medical team
 d An HMO and PPO

5 The nursing team includes
 a Doctors
 b Pharmacists
 c Physical and occupational therapists
 d RNs, LPNs/LVNs, and nursing assistants

6 Nursing assistants are supervised by
 a Licensed nurses
 b Other nursing assistants
 c The health team
 d The medical director

7 The nursing assistant's role is to
 a Meet Medicare and Medicaid standards
 b Perform delegated tasks
 c Follow the doctor's orders
 d Manage care

8 Nursing tasks are delegated according to a person's needs and staff member abilities. This nursing care pattern is called
 a Team nursing
 b Functional nursing
 c Case management
 d Primary nursing

9 Medicare is for persons who
 a Are 65 years of age or older
 b Need nursing center care
 c Have group insurance
 d Have low incomes

10 A survey team member asks you some questions. You should
 a Refer all questions to the nurse
 b Answer as the DON tells you to
 c Give as little information as possible
 d Give honest and complete answers

Answers to these questions are on p. 504.

FOCUS ON PRACTICE

Problem Solving

The nurse supervising your work was supposed to return from a break 15 minutes ago. The nurse did not tell you who is supervising your work during the break. You have a question about a patient's care. What will you do? Your nursing department is organized as shown in Figure 1-1. Who should you tell about the problem?

8

Review Questions are useful study guides. They help in reviewing what you have learned. You can also use them to study for a test or for the competency evaluation. Answers are given at the back of the book. See p. 504.

Focus on Practice: Problem Solving boxes (*NEW!*) at the end of each chapter present a situation with a patient or resident that you may encounter as a student or in the work setting. Intended for classroom discussion or self-study, questions that follow ask about what you should do, how you should act, or how you can improve the situation.

Contents

CHAPTER

1

Hospitals and Nursing Centers

OBJECTIVES

- Define the key terms and key abbreviations listed in this chapter.
- Describe hospitals and long-term care centers.
- Describe the persons cared for in long-term care centers.
- Describe the members of the health team and nursing team.
- Describe 5 nursing care patterns.
- Describe the programs that pay for health care.
- Explain your role in meeting standards.
- Explain how to promote PRIDE in the person, the family, and yourself.

KEY TERMS

acute illness A sudden illness from which a person is expected to recover

assisted living residence (ALR) Provides housing, personal care, support services, health care, and social activities in a home-like setting for persons needing help with daily activities

chronic illness An on-going illness, slow or gradual in onset; it has no known cure; it can be controlled and complications prevented with proper treatment

health team The many health care workers whose skills and knowledge focus on the person's total care; interdisciplinary health care team

hospice A health care agency or program for persons who are dying

licensed practical nurse (LPN) A nurse who has completed a 1-year nursing program and has passed a licensing test; called *licensed vocational nurse (LVN)* in some states

licensed vocational nurse (LVN) See "licensed practical nurse (LPN)"

nursing assistant A person who has passed a nursing assistant training and competency evaluation program; performs delegated nursing tasks under the supervision of a licensed nurse

nursing team Those who provide nursing care—RNs, LPNs/LVNs, and nursing assistants

registered nurse (RN) A nurse who has completed a 2-, 3-, or 4-year nursing program and has passed a licensing test

terminal illness An illness or injury from which the person will not likely recover

KEY ABBREVIATIONS

ALR Assisted living residence
DON Director of nursing
HMO Health maintenance organization
LPN Licensed practical nurse
LVN Licensed vocational nurse
PPO Preferred provider organization
RN Registered nurse
SNF Skilled nursing facility

Hospitals and long-term care centers provide health care. Staff members use their knowledge and skills to meet the person's needs. The *person* is always the focus of care.

HOSPITALS

Hospitals provide emergency care, surgery, nursing care, x-ray procedures and treatments, and laboratory testing. They also provide respiratory, physical, occupational, speech, and other therapies.

People of all ages need hospital care. They have babies, surgery, physical and mental health disorders, and broken bones. Some people need hospital care when dying.

Persons cared for in hospitals are called *patients.* Hospital patients have acute, chronic, or terminal illnesses.

- ***Acute illness*** *is a sudden illness from which the person is expected to recover.* A heart attack is an example.
- ***Chronic illness*** *is an on-going illness that is slow or gradual in onset. There is no known cure. The illness can be controlled and complications prevented with proper treatment.* Diabetes is an example.
- ***Terminal illness*** *is an illness or injury from which the person will not likely recover.* The person will die (Chapter 32). Cancers that do not respond to treatment are examples.

LONG-TERM CARE CENTERS

Some persons cannot care for themselves at home but do not need hospital care. Long-term care centers are designed to meet their needs. Care needs range from simple to complex. Medical, nursing, dietary, recreation, rehabilitation, and social services are provided.

Persons in long-term care centers are called *residents.* They are not *patients.* This is because the center is their temporary or permanent home.

Most residents are older. They may have chronic diseases, poor nutrition, memory problems, or poor health. Not all residents are old. Some are disabled from birth defects, accidents, or disease. Hospital patients are often discharged while still recovering from illness or surgery. Some residents recover and return home. Others need nursing care until death.

Long-term care centers meet the needs of:

- *Alert, oriented persons.* They know who they are, where they are, the year, and the time of day. They have physical problems. Disability level affects the care required. Some require complete care. Others need help with daily activities.
- *Confused and disoriented persons.* They are mildly to severely confused and disoriented. Some cannot remember names or dates. Others do not know who or where they are. They cannot dress or feed themselves. Sometimes the problem is short-term. Some persons have Alzheimer's disease and other dementias. Confusion and disorientation are permanent and become worse (Chapter 30).
- *Persons needing complete care.* They are very disabled, confused, or disoriented. They cannot meet any of their own needs. Some cannot say what they need or want.
- *Short-term residents.* These people need to recover from illness, surgery, fractures, and other injuries. Often they are younger than most residents. They usually recover and return home.
- *Persons needing respite care.* Some people cared for at home go to nursing centers for short stays. This is *respite care. Respite* means *rest* or *relief.* The caregiver can take a trip, tend to business, or simply rest. Respite care may be from a few days to several weeks.
- *Life-long residents.* Birth defects and childhood injuries and diseases can cause disabilities. A disability occurring before 22 years of age is called a *developmental disability*. It may be a physical impairment, intellectual impairment, or both. The person has limited function in at least 3 of these areas: self-care, understanding or expressing language, learning, mobility, or self-direction. The person needs life-long assistance, support, and special devices. Some nursing centers admit developmentally disabled children and adults.
- *Residents who are mentally ill.* Behavior and function are affected. In severe cases, self-care and independent living are impaired. Some persons also have physical illnesses.
- *Terminally ill persons.* Some are alert and oriented. If in a coma (Chapter 6), they cannot respond to what people say to them. But they may still feel pain. Terminally ill persons may need hospice care. The goal is quality end-of-life care for persons who are dying.

Board and Care Homes

Board and care homes (group homes) provide a room, meals, laundry, and supervision. Some homes are for older persons. Others are for people with certain problems. Dementia, mental health disorders, and developmental disabilities are examples.

Homes vary in size—from housing 4 to 10 people or more. Residents share common living areas and eat together. A safe setting is provided but not 24-hour nursing care. Residents can usually dress themselves and meet grooming and elimination needs with little help.

Assisted Living Residences

An ***assisted living residence (ALR)*** *provides housing, personal care, support services, health care, and social activities in a home-like setting for persons needing help with daily activities.* ALR residents may need help with taking drugs and with bathing, dressing, elimination, and eating. Many have problems with thinking, reasoning, and judgment.

Mobility is often required. The person walks or uses a wheelchair or motor scooter. The person is able to leave the building in an emergency. Stable health also is required. The person needs limited health care or treatment.

A home-like, secure setting is provided. Residents have 24-hour supervision and 3 meals a day. They have laundry, housekeeping, transportation, social, recreational, and some health services. Services are added or reduced as the person's needs change.

Some ALRs are part of nursing centers or retirement communities. Others are separate facilities. ALRs must follow state laws and rules.

Nursing Centers

A *nursing center (nursing facility, nursing home)* provides health care services to persons who need regular or continuous care. Licensed nurses are required. Medical, nursing, dietary, recreation, rehabilitation, and social services are provided.

Skilled nursing facilities (SNFs) provide complex care for severe health problems. They are part of hospitals or nursing centers. SNF residents need time to recover or rehabilitation. Others never go home.

Some nursing centers and hospitals provide subacute care. *Subacute care* is complex medical care or rehabilitation when hospital care is no longer needed. Often called *patients*, they may have nervous system injuries, bone or joint surgeries or injuries, or wounds that are not healing. Short stays are common.

The Omnibus Budget Reconciliation Act of 1987 and "Residents' Rights" are discussed in Chapter 2.

Hospices

A ***hospice*** *is a health care agency or program for persons who are dying.* Such persons no longer respond to treatments aimed at cures. Usually they have less than 6 months to live.

The physical, emotional, social, and spiritual needs of the person and family are met. The focus is on comfort, not cure. Hospice care is provided by hospitals, nursing centers, and home care agencies.

Alzheimer's Units (Dementia Care Units)

An Alzheimer's unit is designed for persons with Alzheimer's disease and other dementias (Chapter 30). Such persons suffer increasing memory loss and confusion. Over time, they cannot tend to simple personal needs. Often they wander and may become agitated and combative. The unit is usually closed off from other parts of the center. The closed unit provides a safe setting where residents can wander freely.

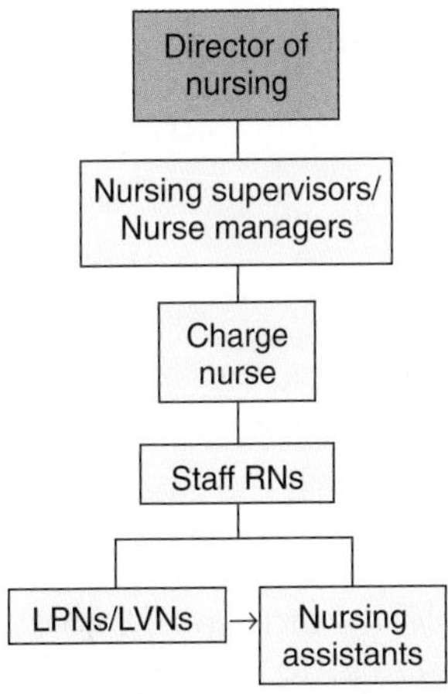

FIGURE 1-1 Sample organizational chart of the nursing department. (*LPN*—licensed practical nurse; *LVN*—licensed vocational nurse; *RN*—registered nurse.)

ORGANIZATION

A hospital has a governing body called the *board of trustees* or *board of directors.* The board makes policies. It makes sure that safe care is given at the lowest possible cost. Local, state, and federal laws are followed.

An administrator manages the agency. He or she reports directly to the board. Directors or department heads manage certain areas (Fig. 1-1).

Nursing centers are usually owned by an individual or a corporation. Some are owned by county or state health departments. The U.S. Department of Veterans Affairs (Veterans Administration; VA) also has nursing centers.

Each center has an administrator. Department directors report to the administrator. Nursing centers have nursing, therapy, and food service departments. They also have social service, activity, and other departments.

Hospitals, nursing centers, and other health care agencies must follow local, state, and federal laws and rules. This is to ensure safe care.

The Health Team

The ***health team*** *(interdisciplinary health care team) involves the many health care workers whose skills and knowledge focus on the person's total care.* Some members of the health team are described in Table 1-1, p. 4. The goal is to provide quality care. The person is the focus of care.

Many team members are involved in the care of each person. Coordinated care is needed. An RN leads this team.

See *Focus on Communication: The Health Team*, p. 4.

TABLE 1-1 Health Team Members

Title	Description
Activities director	Assesses, plans, and implements recreational needs.
Audiologist	Tests hearing; prescribes hearing aids; works with persons who are hard-of-hearing.
Cleric (clergyman; clergywoman)	Assists with spiritual needs.
Clinical nurse specialist	Provides nursing care and consults in a nursing specialty. Geriatrics, critical care, diabetes, rehabilitation, and wound care are examples.
Dietitian and nutritionist	Assesses and plans for nutritional needs; teaches good nutrition, food selection, and preparation.
Licensed practical/vocational nurse (LPN/LVN)	Provides direct nursing care, including giving drugs, under the direction of an RN.
Medical or clinical laboratory technician	Collects specimens and performs laboratory tests on blood, urine, and other body fluids, secretions, and excretions.
Medication assistant-certified (MA-C)	Gives drugs as allowed by state law under the supervision of a licensed nurse.
Nurse practitioner	Plans and provides care with the health team; does physical exams, health assessments, and health education.
Nursing assistant	Assists nurses and gives care; supervised by a licensed nurse.
Occupational therapist registered (OTR)	Assists persons to learn or retain skills needed to perform daily activities; designs adaptive equipment for daily living.
Physical therapist (PT)	Assists persons with musculo-skeletal problems to restore function and prevent disability.
Physician (doctor)	Diagnoses and treats diseases and injuries.
Podiatrist	Prevents, diagnoses, and treats foot disorders.
Radiographer/radiologic technologist	Takes x-rays; processes film for viewing.
Registered nurse (RN)	Assesses, makes nursing diagnoses, plans, implements, and evaluates nursing care; supervises LPNs/LVNs and nursing assistants.
Respiratory therapist (RT)	Assists in treating lung and heart disorders; gives respiratory treatments and therapies.
Social worker	Deals with social, emotional, and environmental issues affecting illness and recovery; coordinates community agencies to assist patients, residents, and families.
Speech-language pathologist	Evaluates speech and language and treats persons with speech, voice, hearing, communication, and swallowing disorders.

Modified from Bureau of Labor Statistics, U.S. Department of Labor: Occupational outlook handbook, 2012-2013 edition.

FOCUS ON COMMUNICATION

The Health Team

Many staff members work together to provide a person's care. Each member has different roles. Health team members must communicate often. You may have questions or concerns about a person and his or her care. Tell the team leader. The leader will communicate with other health team members.

Nursing Service

Nursing service is a large department (see Fig. 1-1). The director of nursing (DON) is an RN. (*Director of nursing services*, *chief nurse executive*, *vice president of nursing*, and *vice president of patient services* are some other titles.) The DON is responsible for the entire nursing staff and the care given.

Nursing supervisors and nurse managers oversee a work shift, a nursing area, or a certain function. Functions include staff development, restorative nursing, infection control, and continuous quality care. Nurse supervisors or managers are responsible for all nursing care and the actions of nursing staff in their areas.

Nursing areas usually have charge nurses for each shift. Usually RNs, some states allow LPNs/LVNs to be charge nurses. The charge nurse is responsible for all nursing care and for the actions of nursing staff during that shift. Staff RNs report to the charge nurse. LPNs/LVNs report to staff RNs or to the charge nurse. You report to the nurse supervising your work.

Nursing education (staff development) is part of nursing service. Nursing education staff:

- Plan and present educational programs (in-service programs). This includes programs that meet federal and state educational requirements.
- Provide new and changing information.
- Show how to use new equipment and supplies.
- Review policies and procedures on a regular basis.
- Educate and train nursing assistants.
- Conduct new employee orientation programs.

THE NURSING TEAM

The ***nursing team*** *involves those who provide nursing care—RNs, LPNs/LVNs, and nursing assistants.* All focus on the physical, social, emotional, and spiritual needs of the person and family.

Registered Nurses

A ***registered nurse (RN)*** *has completed a 2-, 3-, or 4-year nursing program and has passed a licensing test.*

- Community college programs—2 years
- Hospital-based diploma programs—2 or 3 years
- College or university programs—4 years

Graduate nurses take a licensing test offered by their state board of nursing. They receive a license and become *registered* when the test is passed. RNs must have a license recognized by the state in which they work.

RNs assess, make nursing diagnoses, plan, implement, and evaluate nursing care (Chapter 5). They develop care plans, provide care, and delegate (Chapter 3) nursing care and tasks to the nursing team. They evaluate how care plans and nursing care affect each person. RNs teach the person and family how to improve health and independence.

RNs follow the doctor's orders. They may delegate them to other nursing team members. RNs do not prescribe treatments or drugs. However, RNs can become *clinical nurse specialists* or *nurse practitioners.* These RNs have limited diagnosing and prescribing functions.

Licensed Practical Nurses and Licensed Vocational Nurses

A ***licensed practical nurse (LPN)*** *has completed a 1-year nursing program and has passed a licensing test.* Hospitals, community colleges, vocational schools, and technical schools offer programs. Some programs are 10 months long; others take 18 months. Some high schools offer 2-year programs.

Graduates take a licensing test for practical nursing. After passing the test, they receive a license to practice and the title of *licensed practical nurse.* ***Licensed vocational nurse (LVN)*** *is used in some states.* LPNs/LVNs must have a license recognized by the state in which they work.

LPNs/LVNs are supervised by RNs, licensed doctors, and licensed dentists. They have fewer responsibilities and functions than RNs do. They need little supervision when the person's condition is stable and care is simple. They assist RNs in caring for acutely ill persons and with complex procedures.

Nursing Assistants

A ***nursing assistant*** *has passed a nursing assistant training and competency evaluation program (NATCEP).* Nursing assistants *perform delegated tasks under the supervision of a licensed nurse.* Nursing assistants are discussed in Chapter 3.

NURSING CARE PATTERNS

Nursing care is given in many ways. The pattern used depends on how many persons need care, the staff, and the cost.

- *Functional nursing* focuses on tasks and jobs. Each nursing team member has certain tasks and jobs to do. For example, one nurse gives all drugs. Another gives all treatments. Nursing assistants give baths, make beds, and serve meals.
- *Team nursing* involves a team of nursing staff led by an RN. Called the "team leader," he or she delegates the care of certain persons to other nurses and nursing assistants. Delegation (Chapter 3) is based on the person's needs and team member abilities. Team members report observations and the care given to the team leader.
- *Primary nursing* involves total care. An RN is responsible for the person's total care. The nursing team assists as needed. The RN ("primary nurse") gives nursing care and makes discharge plans. The RN teaches and counsels the person and family.
- *Case management* is like primary nursing. A case manager (an RN) coordinates a person's care from admission through discharge and into the home or long-term care setting. He or she communicates with the person's doctor and the health team. There also is communication with insurance companies and community agencies as needed. Some case managers work with certain doctors. Others deal with certain health problems. Heart diseases, diabetes, and cancer are examples.
- *Patient-focused care* is when services are moved from departments to the bedside. The nursing team performs basic skills usually done by other health team members. For example, an RN may draw a blood sample. The number of people caring for each person is reduced. This reduces care costs.

PAYING FOR HEALTH CARE

Health care is costly. Most people cannot afford these costs. Some avoid health care because they cannot pay. Others pay doctor bills but go without food or drugs. If the person has insurance, some costs are covered. Rarely are all costs covered.

These programs help pay for health care.

- *Private insurance* is bought by individuals and families. The insurance company pays for some or all health care costs.
- *Group insurance* is bought by groups or organizations for individuals. This is often an employee benefit.
- *Medicare* is a federal health insurance program for persons 65 years of age or older. Some younger people with certain disabilities are covered. Part A pays for some hospital, SNF, hospice, and home care costs. Part B helps pay for doctor's services, out-patient hospital care, physical and occupational therapists, some home care, and many other services. Part B is voluntary. The person pays a monthly premium.
- *Medicaid* is a health care payment program. Sponsored by the federal government, it is run by the states. People with low incomes usually qualify. So do some children and some older, blind, and disabled persons. There is no insurance premium. The amount paid for covered services is limited.

See *Promoting Safety and Comfort: Paying for Health Care.*

Prospective Payment Systems

Prospective payment systems limit the amount paid by insurers, Medicare, and Medicaid. *Prospective* means *before*. The amount paid for services is determined before giving care.

- Medicare severity-adjusted diagnosis-related groups (MS-DRGs) are used for hospital costs.
- Resource utilization groups (RUGs) are used for SNF payments.
- Case mix groups (CMGs) are used for rehabilitation centers.

Length of stay and treatment costs are determined for each group. If costs are less than the amount paid, the agency keeps the extra money. If costs are greater, the agency takes the loss.

Managed Care

Managed care deals with health care delivery and payment (Box 1-1). Insurers contract with doctors and hospitals for reduced rates or discounts. The insured person uses doctors and agencies providing the lower rates. The person pays for costs not covered by insurance.

Managed care limits the choice of where to go for health care. It also limits the care that doctors provide. Many states require managed care for Medicare and Medicaid coverage.

MEETING STANDARDS

Health care agencies must meet certain standards. Standards are set by the federal and state governments and accrediting agencies. Standards relate to policies and procedures, budget and finances, and quality of care.

PROMOTING SAFETY AND COMFORT

Paying for Health Care

Safety

Some conditions can be prevented with proper care. Medicare pays a lower rate for such conditions if they are acquired during a hospital stay. Pressure ulcers (Chapter 25) and certain types of falls, trauma, and infections are examples. You must help the nursing and health teams prevent such conditions.

BOX 1-1 Types of Managed Care

Health maintenance organization (HMO). For a pre-paid fee, the person receives needed services offered by the HMO. Some have a yearly exam. Others need hospital care. HMOs stress preventing disease and maintaining health. Keeping someone healthy costs far less than treating illness.

Preferred provider organization (PPO). A group of doctors and hospitals provides health care at reduced rates. Usually the agreement is between the PPO and an employer or an insurance company. Employees or those insured have reduced rates for the services used. The person can choose any doctor or hospital in the PPO.

The Survey Process

Surveys are done to see if the agency meets set standards. A survey team will:

- Review policies, procedures, and medical records.
- Interview staff, patients and residents, and families.
- Observe how care is given.
- Observe if dignity and privacy are promoted.
- Check for cleanliness and safety.
- Make sure staff meet state requirements. (Are doctors and nurses licensed? Are nursing assistants on the state registry?)

The survey team decides if the agency meets the standards. Sometimes problems are found. A problem is called a *deficiency*. The agency usually has 60 days to correct the problem. Sometimes less time is given. The agency can be fined for uncorrected or serious deficiencies. Or it can lose its license, certification, or accreditation.

Your Role

You have an important role in meeting standards and in the survey process. You must:

- Provide quality care.
- Protect the person's rights.
- Provide for the person's and your own safety.
- Help keep the agency clean and safe.
- Conduct yourself in a professional manner.
- Have good work ethics.
- Follow agency policies and procedures.
- Answer questions honestly and completely.

See *Focus on Surveys: Your Role.*

FOCUS ON SURVEYS

Your Role

Survey teams are made up of surveyors. A *surveyor* is a person who collects information by observing and asking questions.

A surveyor may ask you questions. If so, be polite. Avoid seeming annoyed or upset. Answer the questions honestly and thoroughly. If you do not understand the question, ask the surveyor to re-phrase it. Do not guess at an answer. Tell the surveyor where you can find the answer. You can say: "I am unsure, but I would ask the nurse."

For example, a surveyor approaches you:

Surveyor: "Do you have a moment? May I ask you a few questions?"

You: "Yes. I am happy to answer your questions."

Surveyor: "Thank you. First, when should you practice hand hygiene?"

You: "I wash my hands before and after contact with a patient. I also wash my hands when they are dirty and after I take off my gloves."

Surveyor: "Thank you. Next, what are 2 appropriate patient identifiers?"

You: "I'm not sure I understand the question. Can you re-phrase it?"

Surveyor: "Yes. Name 2 things you can use to identify a patient."

You: "Okay. Thank you. I can use the patient's full name and date of birth. I cannot use the room number."

Surveyor: "Thank you. I have 1 last question. In a disaster, where would you find the Emergency Preparedness Plan?"

You: "Well, I'm not sure where the plan is located. I will ask my supervising nurse or the charge nurse where to find it."

FOCUS ON PRIDE

The Person, Family, and Yourself

Personal and Professional Responsibility

Health care is a rewarding profession. The health team works hard to provide quality care. You are an important part of that team. You will spend most of your time giving care. Remember to show patience, compassion, dignity, and respect. You have a great impact on the quality of care each person receives.

Rights and Respect

Many hospitals and nursing centers conduct employee satisfaction surveys. The surveys ask what employees think about their jobs.

All staff are expected to complete and return the form. You may need to note the area you work in or your role in the agency. Identifying information, such as your name, is usually not given. This helps protect your identity. You have the right to voice your true thoughts on a survey. When filling out a survey:

- Be honest. Positive and negative comments are important.
- Take the survey seriously. Do not rush. Answer the questions completely.
- Complete and return the form in a timely manner.

Surveys are one way hospitals and nursing centers show respect for employees. Comments are used to make changes. Take pride in your ideas. Your thoughts matter.

Independence and Social Interaction

People who rely on others for care often feel frustrated, useless, sad, and a burden to others. A common goal is to return persons to their highest level of functioning. Physical, occupational, and speech therapists work together with doctors, the nursing team, and others to promote independence (see Table 1-1). Independence promotes feelings of improvement and success. Help the person take pride in working to restore independence.

Delegation and Teamwork

Each health team member has a certain role. Everyone must work together to provide quality care. Offer to help team members when you can. Helping others shows you are dependable and value teamwork.

Ethics and Laws

Nursing team members have different levels of training and responsibilities. RN, LPN/LVN, and nursing assistant roles vary. Federal and state laws determine the legal limits of these roles. See Chapter 3 for your role limits. Functions may also vary among agencies. A job description (Chapter 3) describes the agency's expectations. To protect yourself and others, know the limits of your role in your state and agency.

REVIEW QUESTIONS

Circle the BEST answer.

1 A health care program for dying persons is a
  a Hospice
  b Board and care home
  c Skilled nursing facility
  d Dementia care unit

2 Who controls policy in a health care agency?
  a The survey team
  b The board of directors
  c The health team
  d Medicare and Medicaid

3 Who is responsible for the entire nursing staff and safe nursing care?
  a The case manager
  b The director of nursing
  c The charge nurse
  d The RN

4 You are a member of
  a The health team and the nursing team
  b The health team and the medical team
  c The nursing team and the medical team
  d An HMO and PPO

5 The nursing team includes
  a Doctors
  b Pharmacists
  c Physical and occupational therapists
  d RNs, LPNs/LVNs, and nursing assistants

6 Nursing assistants are supervised by
  a Licensed nurses
  b Other nursing assistants
  c The health team
  d The medical director

7 The nursing assistant's role is to
  a Meet Medicare and Medicaid standards
  b Perform delegated tasks
  c Follow the doctor's orders
  d Manage care

8 Nursing tasks are delegated according to a person's needs and staff member abilities. This nursing care pattern is called
  a Team nursing
  b Functional nursing
  c Case management
  d Primary nursing

9 Medicare is for persons who
  a Are 65 years of age or older
  b Need nursing center care
  c Have group insurance
  d Have low incomes

10 A survey team member asks you some questions. You should
  a Refer all questions to the nurse
  b Answer as the DON tells you to
  c Give as little information as possible
  d Give honest and complete answers

Answers to these questions are on p. 504.

FOCUS ON PRACTICE

Problem Solving

The nurse supervising your work was supposed to return from a break 15 minutes ago. The nurse did not tell you who is supervising your work during the break. You have a question about a patient's care. What will you do? Your nursing department is organized as shown in Figure 1-1. Who should you tell about the problem?

CHAPTER 2

The Person's Rights

OBJECTIVES

- Define the key terms and key abbreviation listed in this chapter.
- Explain the purpose of *The Patient Care Partnership: Understanding Expectations, Rights, and Responsibilities.*
- Describe the purposes and requirements of the Omnibus Budget Reconciliation Act of 1987 (OBRA).
- Identify the person's rights under OBRA.
- Explain how to protect the person's rights.
- Explain the ombudsman role.
- Explain how to promote PRIDE in the person, the family, and yourself.

KEY TERMS

involuntary seclusion Separating a person from others against his or her will, keeping the person to a certain area, or keeping the person away from his or her room without consent

ombudsman Someone who supports or promotes the needs and interests of another person

representative A person who has the legal right to act on the patient's or resident's behalf when he or she cannot do so for himself or herself

treatment The care provided to maintain or restore health, improve function, or relieve symptoms

KEY ABBREVIATION

OBRA Omnibus Budget Reconciliation Act of 1987

People want information about their health problems and treatment. They want to understand and be involved in treatment decisions. As patients and residents, they have certain rights.

PATIENTS' RIGHTS

In April 2003 the American Hospital Association adopted *The Patient Care Partnership: Understanding Expectations, Rights, and Responsibilities* (Appendix A). The document explains the person's rights and expectations during hospital stays. The relationship between the doctor, health team, and patient is stressed.

RESIDENTS' RIGHTS

The Omnibus Budget Reconciliation Act of 1987 (OBRA) is a federal law. It applies to all 50 states. Nursing centers must provide care in a manner and in a setting that maintains or improves each person's quality of life, health, and safety. Nursing assistant training and competency evaluation are part of OBRA (Chapter 3). Resident rights are a major part of OBRA.

Residents have rights as United States citizens. They also have rights relating to their everyday lives and care in a nursing center. Some residents cannot exercise their rights. A representative (partner, adult child, court-appointed guardian) does so for them. A ***representative*** *is a person who has the legal right to act on the patient's or resident's behalf when he or she cannot do so for himself or herself.*

Nursing centers must inform residents of their rights. This is done orally and in writing before or during admission to the center. It is given in the language the person uses and understands. An interpreter is used if the person speaks and understands a foreign language or communicates by sign language. Resident rights also are posted throughout the center.

See *Focus on Surveys: Residents' Rights*, p. 10.

FOCUS ON SURVEYS

Residents' Rights

Resident rights are a major focus of surveys. Surveyors observe staff behaviors and actions. They listen to staff comments and remarks. You may not know they are doing so. What you say and do must promote the person's quality of life, health, and safety. For example, a surveyor may observe:

- How you prevent unnecessary exposure of the person's body
- How you help a person dress for the season and time of day
- How you label clothing
- If you knock on a person's door before entering the room
- If you change a person's radio or TV without permission
- If you move a person's personal items without permission
- How you address and speak to a person

You will learn how to protect the person's rights as you study this and other chapters. You must always act and speak in a professional manner.

Information

The *right to information* means access to all records about the person. They include the medical record, contracts, incident reports, and financial records. The request can be oral or written.

The person has the right to be fully informed of his or her health condition. The person must also have information about his or her doctor. This includes the doctor's name and specialty and how to contact the doctor.

Report any request for information to the nurse. *You do not give the information described above to the person or family* (Chapter 3).

See *Focus on Communication: Information.*

FOCUS ON COMMUNICATION

Information

You may be asked for information about a person's care. You must not give out information. This is the nurse's responsibility. You can say: "I am sorry. I am not allowed to give any information. I will report your request to the nurse." Communicate the person's request promptly. You can tell the person: "I told the nurse about your question. The nurse will come and speak with you soon."

Refusing Treatment

The person has the *right to refuse treatment. Treatment means the care provided to maintain or restore health, improve function, or relieve symptoms.* A person who does not give consent (Chapter 3) or refuses treatment cannot be treated against his or her wishes. The center must find out what the person is refusing and why. The center must:

- Find out the reason for the refusal.
- Explain the problems that can result from the refusal.
- Offer other treatment options.
- Continue to provide all other services.

Advance directives are part of the right to refuse treatment (Chapter 32). They include living wills and instructions about life support. *Advance directives* are written instructions about health care when the person is not able to make such decisions.

Report any treatment refusal to the nurse. The nurse may change the person's care plan (Chapter 5).

Privacy and Confidentiality

Residents have the *right to personal privacy.* Expose the person's body only as necessary. Only staff directly involved in care and treatment are present. Consent is needed for others to be present.

A person has the right to use the bathroom in private. Privacy is maintained for all personal care measures. Bathing, dressing, and elimination are examples. Residents have the right to visit with others in private—in areas where others cannot see or hear them. This includes phone calls (Fig. 2-1). If requested, the center must provide private space. Offices, chapels, dining rooms, and meeting rooms are used as needed.

The right to privacy also involves mail. No one can open mail the person sends or receives without his or her consent.

Information about the person's care, treatment, and condition is kept confidential. So are medical and financial records.

Privacy and confidentiality are discussed in Chapters 4 and 5.

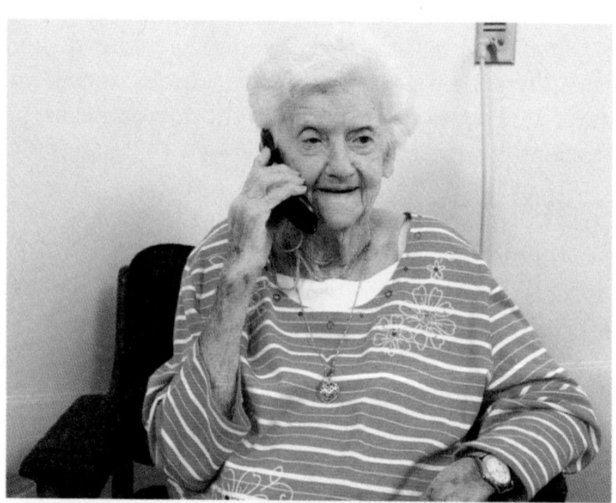

FIGURE 2-1 A resident is talking privately on the phone.

Personal Choice

Residents have the *right to make their own choices.* They can choose their own doctors. They also help plan and decide about their care and treatment. They can choose activities, schedules, and care. They can choose when to get up and go to bed, what to wear, how to spend time, and what to eat (Fig. 2-2). They can choose friends and visitors inside and outside the center. Allow personal choice whenever possible.

Grievances

Residents have the *right to voice concerns, questions, and complaints about treatment and care.* The problem may involve another person. It may be about care that was given or not given. The center must promptly try to correct the matter. No one can punish the person in any way for voicing the grievance.

Work

The person does not work for care, care items, or other things or privileges. The person is not required to perform services for the center.

However, the person has the *right to work or perform services if he or she wants to do so.* Some people like to garden, repair or build things, clean, sew, mend, or cook. Other persons need work for rehabilitation or activity reasons. The desire or need for work is part of the person's care plan.

Taking Part in Resident Groups

The person has *the right to form and take part in resident groups.* Families have the right to meet with other families. These groups can discuss concerns and suggest center improvements. They can provide support and comfort to group members.

Residents have the *right to take part in social, cultural, religious, and community events.* They have the *right to help in getting to and from events of their choice.*

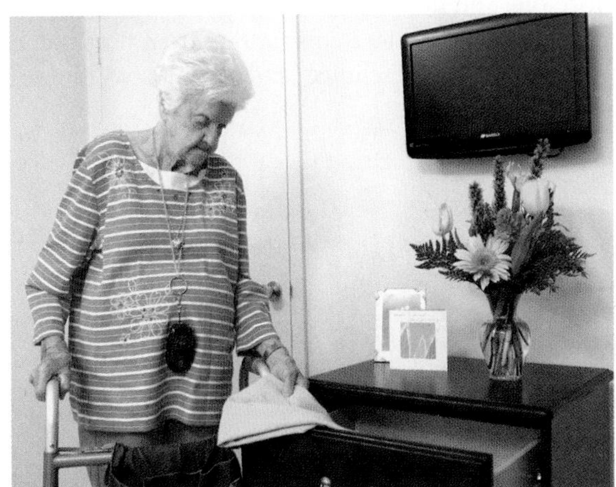

FIGURE 2-2 A resident is choosing what clothing to wear.

Personal Items

Residents have the *right to keep and use personal items.* Treat the person's property with care and respect. The items may not have value to you but have meaning to the person. They also relate to personal choice, dignity, a home-like setting, and quality of life.

The person's property is protected. Items are labeled with the person's name. The center must investigate reports of lost, stolen, or damaged items. Police help is sometimes needed.

Protect yourself and the center from being accused of stealing a person's property. Do not go through a person's closet, drawers, purse, or other space without the person's knowledge and consent. A nurse may ask you to inspect closets and drawers. Center policy should require that a co-worker and the person or legal representative be present. They witness your actions.

Freedom From Abuse, Mistreatment, and Neglect

Residents have the *right to be free from verbal, sexual, physical, and mental abuse* (Chapter 3). They also have the right to be free from ***involuntary seclusion.***

- *Separating the person from others against his or her will*
- *Keeping the person to a certain area*
- *Keeping the person away from his or her room without consent*

No one can abuse, neglect, or mistreat a resident. This includes center staff, volunteers, other residents, family members, visitors, and legal representatives. Centers must investigate suspected or reported cases of abuse. They cannot employ persons who:

- Were found guilty of abusing, neglecting, or mistreating others by a court of law.
- Have a finding entered into the state's nursing assistant registry (Chapter 3) about abuse, neglect, mistreatment, or wrongful acts involving the person's money or property. A *finding* means that a state has determined that the employee abused, neglected, mistreated, or wrongfully used the person's money or property.

Freedom From Restraint

Residents have the *right not to have body movements restricted.* Restraints and certain drugs can restrict body movements (Chapter 11). Some drugs are restraints because they affect mood, behavior, and mental function. Sometimes residents are restrained to protect them from harming themselves or others. A doctor's order is needed for restraint use. Restraints are not used for staff convenience or to discipline a person.

BOX 2-1 OBRA-Required Actions to Promote Dignity and Privacy

Courteous and Dignified Interactions
- Use the right tone of voice.
- Use good eye contact.
- Stand or sit close enough as needed.
- Use the person's proper name and title. For example: "Mrs. Crane."
- Gain the person's attention before interacting with him or her.
- Use touch if the person approves.
- Respect the person's social status.
- Listen with interest to what the person is saying.
- Do not yell at, scold, or embarrass the person.

Courteous and Dignified Care
- Groom hair, beards, and nails as the person wishes.
- Assist with dressing in the right clothing for time of day and personal choice.
- Promote independence and dignity in dining.
- Respect private space and property. For example, change radio or TV stations only with the person's consent.
- Assist with walking and transfers. Do not interfere with independence.
- Assist with bathing and hygiene preferences. Do not interfere with independence.
  - Appearance is neat and clean.
  - The person is clean shaven or has a groomed beard and mustache.
  - Nails are trimmed and clean.
  - Dentures, hearing aids, eyeglasses, and other devices are used correctly.
  - Clothing is clean.
  - Clothing is properly fitted and fastened.
  - Shoes, hose, and socks are properly applied and fastened.
  - Extra clothing is worn for warmth as needed. Sweaters and lap blankets are examples.

Privacy and Self-Determination
- Drape properly during care and procedures to avoid exposure and embarrassment.
- Drape properly in a chair.
- Use privacy curtains or screens during care and procedures.
- Close the room door during care and procedures as the person desires. Also close window coverings.
- Knock on the door before entering. Wait to be asked in.
- Close the bathroom door when the person uses the bathroom.

Personal Choice and Independence
- Person smokes in allowed areas.
- Person takes part in activities according to his or her interests.
- Person takes part in scheduling activities and care.
- Person gives input into the care plan about preferences and independence.
- Person is involved in room or roommate change.
- The person's items are moved or inspected only with the person's consent.

Quality of Life

Residents have the *right to quality of life.* They must be cared for in a manner and in a setting that promotes dignity and respect for self. Care must promote physical, mental, and social well-being. Protecting resident rights promotes quality of life. It shows respect for the person.

Speak to the person in a polite and courteous manner. Good, honest, and thoughtful care enhances the person's quality of life. Box 2-1 lists OBRA-required actions that promote dignity and privacy.

See *Focus on Communication: Quality of Life.*

FOCUS ON COMMUNICATION

Quality of Life

Every person deserves to be addressed in a manner that conveys dignity and respect. When speaking with a patient or resident, address the person by his or her title and last name. For example: Mr. Baker, Mrs. Harty, or Dr. Collins. Do not address a person by his or her first name or another name unless the person requests it. Avoid the use of terms like *Sweetheart, Honey, Grandpa,* and *Dear.*

Activities. Residents have the *right to activities that enhance each person's physical, mental, and psycho-social well-being.* Centers must provide religious services for spiritual health.

You assist residents to and from activity programs. You may need to help them with activities.

See *Focus on Communication: Activities.*

See *Focus on Surveys: Activities.*

Environment. Residents have the right to a safe, clean, comfortable, and home-like setting. The person is allowed to have and use personal items to the extent possible. Such items allow personal choice and promote a home-like setting.

FOCUS ON COMMUNICATION

Activities

You may need help assisting residents to and from activity programs. Politely ask a co-worker to help you. Share the following with your co-worker.

- What time you need the help.
- How much of the co-worker's time you need.
- The residents you need help with.
- If the person walks or uses a wheelchair.
- What assistive devices are used. Eyeglasses, hearing aids, canes, and walkers are examples.

Always say "please" when asking for help. And thank the person for helping you. For example:

Jane, can you please help me assist 2 residents to the concert? It starts at 1:00, so I'll need your help at 12:45. Mr. Harris needs his glasses and hearing aid. He'll use a walker. Mrs. Janz uses a wheelchair. She needs her glasses and a blanket for her lap. The blanket is in her wheelchair. The concert is over at 2:00. Can you help me then, too? Thanks so much for helping me.

FOCUS ON SURVEYS

Activities

The Centers for Medicare & Medicaid Services' (CMS) *State Operations Manual* has guidelines for surveyors. This includes the nursing assistant interview about helping residents with activities. You may be asked about:

- Your role in helping residents get ready for a group activity.
  - How do you make sure the person is out of bed, dressed, and ready to take part in the activity?
  - How do you provide needed transportation?
- Your role in providing help with activities of daily living during an activity. For example, does the person need to use the bathroom? Does the person need help with eating?
- Your role in helping a person with an individual activity. For example, you play cards with a person. Do you have needed supplies? Is the person properly positioned? Do you provide good lighting?
- How are activities provided when the activities staff is not available?

FOCUS ON PRIDE

The Person, Family, and Yourself

Personal and Professional Responsibility

OBRA is concerned with quality of life, health, and safety. All care must maintain or improve each person's quality of life. You are responsible for the care you give. To provide quality care:

- Protect the person's rights.
- Provide for safety (Chapter 9) and prevent falls (Chapter 10).
- Help keep the agency clean and safe.
- Act in a professional manner.
- Have good work ethics (Chapter 4).
- Follow agency policies and procedures.

Take pride in the work you do. The care you give helps improve each person's quality of life, health, and safety.

Rights and Respect

Every person has the right to refuse treatment. This does not mean that all treatment stops. The health team offers other treatment options. For example, the doctor suggests short-term placement in a nursing center. The person refuses. The family agrees to help the person at home. A social worker helps the person and family arrange for home health care and respite care. Respite care relieves caregivers of daily care for a short time.

Independence and Social Interaction

Many patients and residents feel a loss of independence and social interaction. Promote independence by having the person choose food, clothing, visitors, activities, and schedules.

Encourage social interaction by telling the person about activities and offering help to and from activities. Also respect the person's right to privacy when visiting with others and making phone calls. These actions help improve independence, self-worth, and quality of life.

Delegation and Teamwork

Health care agencies must meet the person's needs and preferences. Schedules, care assignments, and room arrangements may need changing to meet the person's needs. Flexibility, good teamwork, and communication are required to provide quality care.

For example, Mrs. Gordon needs help with bathing. She likes to bathe at night. She says bathing at night helps her rest better. However, the day shift gives baths. You share her preference with the nurse. The daytime and evening staffs work together so Mrs. Gordon can bathe when she chooses.

Ethics and Laws

The Older Americans Act is a federal law. It requires a long-term care ombudsman program in every state. An ***ombudsman*** *is someone who supports or promotes the needs and interests of another person.* Ombudsmen act on behalf of persons receiving health care at home and in hospitals, nursing centers, assisted living residences, adult day care, and other settings.

Ombudsmen protect a person's health, safety, welfare, and rights. They:

- Investigate and resolve complaints.
- Provide services to assist the person.
- Provide information about long-term care services.
- Monitor nursing care and nursing center conditions.
- Provide support to resident and family groups.
- Help resolve family conflicts.
- Help the center manage difficult problems.

Nursing centers must post contact information for local and state ombudsmen. A resident or family may share a concern with you. You must know state and center policies and procedures for contacting an ombudsman. Ombudsman services are useful when:

- There is concern about a person's care or treatment.
- Someone interferes with a person's rights, health, safety, or welfare.

REVIEW QUESTIONS

Circle* T *if the statement is TRUE or* F *if it is FALSE.

1 **T F** OBRA applies to all 50 states.

2 **T F** Nursing center residents have rights as U.S. citizens.

3 **T F** Residents are informed of their rights only in writing.

4 **T F** Residents must provide some type of work for the center.

5 **T F** Resident groups can discuss ideas for activity programs.

6 **T F** An employee was found guilty of abusing a resident. The center can continue to employ the person.

7 **T F** You can restrain a resident to provide care.

Circle the BEST answer.

8 The *Patient Care Partnership: Understanding Expectations, Rights, and Responsibilities* is concerned with
  - a Hospital care
  - b Home care
  - c Long-term care
  - d All health care agencies and settings

9 OBRA is a
  - a State law
  - b Federal law
  - c State agency
  - d Federal agency

10 A son has the legal right to act on his mother's behalf. The son is his mother's legal
  - a Ombudsman
  - b Representative
  - c Caregiver
  - d Health care provider

11 A daughter wants to read her father's medical record. What should you do?
  - a Give her the medical record.
  - b Ask the resident if you can give the daughter the record.
  - c Tell the nurse.
  - d Tell her that she cannot do so.

12 A resident refuses to have a shower. What should you do?
  - a Tell her that she cannot refuse a shower.
  - b Tell her daughter.
  - c Comply, but tell her she must have a shower tomorrow.
  - d Tell the nurse.

13 Which violates the person's right to privacy?
  - a Closing the bathroom door when the person uses the bathroom
  - b Opening the window blinds when assisting with bathing
  - c Covering the person when giving personal care
  - d Asking the person's permission to observe a treatment

14 A resident has a phone and wants to make a call. What should you do?
  - a Leave the room.
  - b Tell the nurse.
  - c Ask the person to use the phone at the nurses' station.
  - d Close the privacy curtain so you can stay in the room to finish your tasks.

15 Who decides how to style a person's hair?
  - a The person
  - b The nurse
  - c You
  - d The ombudsman

16 Residents do not have the right to
  - a Bring weapons into the center
  - b Choose when to bathe
  - c Voice a complaint about care
  - d Choose a doctor

17 Residents have the right to be free from the following *except*
  - a Disease
  - b Abuse
  - c Involuntary seclusion
  - d Neglect

18 Who selects activities for a resident?
  - a The nurse
  - b You
  - c The person's representative
  - d The person

19 A nursing center must provide
  - a A safe, clean, and comfortable setting
  - b A private bathroom
  - c A bed near a window
  - d A noise-free setting

20 Which is the correct way to address a person?
  - a "Hello, sweetie."
  - b "Hello, Mrs. Smith."
  - c "Hello, Jim."
  - d "Hello, Grandpa."

21 Which does *not* promote dignity or privacy?
  - a Knocking before entering the person's room
  - b Closing the privacy curtain for a procedure
  - c Assisting with bathing and hygiene preferences
  - d Moving the person's items as you prefer

Answers to these questions are on p. 504.

FOCUS ON **PRACTICE**

Problem Solving

You are assisting a resident with feeding. The resident refuses to eat. What will you do? Does the resident have the right to refuse to eat? What is the nursing center's responsibility?

CHAPTER 3

The Nursing Assistant

OBJECTIVES

- Define the key terms and key abbreviations listed in this chapter.
- List the reasons for denying, suspending, or revoking a nursing assistant's certification, license, or registration.
- Describe the training and competency evaluation requirements for nursing assistants.
- Identify the information in the nursing assistant registry.
- Describe what nursing assistants can do and their role limits.
- Describe the standards for nursing assistants developed by the National Council of State Boards of Nursing.
- Explain why a job description is important.
- Describe the delegation process and your role.
- Explain how to accept or refuse a delegated task.
- Give examples of intentional and unintentional torts.
- Explain how to protect the right to privacy.
- Explain the importance of informed consent.
- Describe elder abuse.
- Explain how to promote PRIDE in the person, the family, and yourself.

KEY TERMS

abuse The willful infliction of injury, unreasonable confinement, intimidation, or punishment that results in physical harm, pain, or mental anguish; depriving the person (or the person's caregiver) of the goods or services needed to attain or maintain well-being

assault Intentionally attempting or threatening to touch a person's body without the person's consent

battery Touching a person's body without his or her consent

boundary crossing A brief act or behavior outside of the helpful zone

boundary sign An act, behavior, or thought that warns of a boundary crossing or boundary violation

boundary violation An act or behavior that meets your needs, not the person's

civil law Laws concerned with relationships between people

crime An act that violates a criminal law

criminal law Laws concerned with offenses against the public and society in general

defamation Injuring a person's name or reputation by making false statements to a third person

delegate To authorize another person to perform a nursing task in a certain situation

elder abuse Any knowing, intentional, or negligent act by a caregiver or any other person to an older adult; the act causes harm or serious risk of harm

ethics Knowledge of what is right conduct and wrong conduct

false imprisonment Unlawful restraint or restriction of a person's freedom of movement

fraud Saying or doing something to trick, fool, or deceive a person

invasion of privacy Violating a person's right not to have his or her name, photo, or private affairs exposed or made public without giving consent

job description A document that describes what the agency expects you to do

law A rule of conduct made by a government body

libel Making false statements in print, in writing, or through pictures or drawings

malpractice Negligence by a professional person

neglect Failure to provide the person with the goods or services needed to avoid physical harm, mental anguish, or mental illness

negligence An unintentional wrong in which a person did not act in a reasonable and careful manner and a person or the person's property was harmed

nursing task Nursing care or a nursing function, procedure, activity, or work that can be delegated to nursing assistants when it does not require an RN's professional knowledge or judgment

professional boundary That which separates helpful behaviors from behaviors that are not helpful

professional sexual misconduct An act, behavior, or comment that is sexual in nature

protected health information Identifying information and information about the person's health care that is maintained or sent in any form (paper, electronic, oral)

self-neglect A person's behaviors and way of living that threaten his or her health, safety, and well-being

slander Making false statements orally

vulnerable adult A person 18 years old or older who has a disability or condition that makes him or her at risk to be wounded, attacked, or damaged

KEY ABBREVIATIONS

HIPAA	Health Insurance Portability and Accountability Act of 1996
LPN	Licensed practical nurse
LVN	Licensed vocational nurse
NATCEP	Nursing assistant training and competency evaluation program
NCSBN	National Council of State Boards of Nursing
OBRA	Omnibus Budget Reconciliation Act of 1987
RN	Registered nurse

Federal and state laws and agency policies combine to define your roles and functions. To protect patients and residents from harm, you need to know:

- What you can and cannot do
- What is right conduct and wrong conduct
- Rules and standards of conduct affecting your work
- Your legal limits

Laws, job descriptions, and the person's condition shape your work. So does the amount of supervision you need.

NURSE PRACTICE ACTS

Each state has a nurse practice act. A nurse practice act:

- Defines RN and LPN/LVN and their scope of practice.
- Describes education and licensing requirements for RNs and LPNs/LVNs.
- Protects the public from persons practicing nursing without a license. Persons who do not meet the state's requirements cannot perform nursing functions.

The law allows for denying, revoking, or suspending a nursing license. The intent is to protect the public from unsafe nurses.

Nursing Assistants

A state's nurse practice act is used to decide what nursing assistants can do. Some nurse practice acts also regulate nursing assistant roles, functions, education, and certification requirements. Other states have separate laws for nursing assistants.

If you do something beyond the legal limits of your role, you could be practicing nursing without a license. This creates serious legal problems for you, your supervisor, and your employer.

Nursing assistants must be able to function with skill and safety. Like nurses, nursing assistants can have their certification (license, registration) denied, revoked, or suspended. (See "Certification.")

THE OMNIBUS BUDGET RECONCILIATION ACT OF 1987

The Omnibus Budget Reconciliation Act of 1987 (OBRA) is a federal law. It applies to all 50 states. Each state must have a nursing assistant training and competency evaluation program (NATCEP). A nursing assistant must successfully complete a NATCEP to work in a nursing center, hospital long-term care unit, or home care agency receiving Medicare funds.

The Training Program

OBRA requires at least 75 hours of instruction. Some states require more hours. Classroom and at least 16 hours of supervised practical training are required. Practical training (clinical practicum or clinical experience) occurs in a laboratory or clinical setting. Students perform nursing tasks on another person. A nurse supervises this training.

See *Focus on Communication: The Training Program.*

> **FOCUS ON COMMUNICATION**
>
> ***The Training Program***
>
> In many training programs, clinical experiences take place in a real clinical setting. Care is practiced on real patients or residents. The patient or resident has the right to know who is providing care. When you meet the person, introduce yourself. Tell the person you are a student. For example: "Hello. My name is Jennifer Smith. I am a nursing assistant student. I will be working with your nurse, Mr. Kline, today."

Competency Evaluation

The competency evaluation has a written test and a skills test (Appendix B). The written test has multiple-choice questions. The skills test involves performing certain skills learned in your training program.

You take the competency evaluation after your training program. Your instructor tells you the testing service used in your state and when and where the tests are given. He or she helps you complete the application. Or you can go to the testing service website to complete the application on-line. The evaluation has a fee. If working in a nursing center, the employer pays the fee. Otherwise you pay the fee.

If you listen, study hard, and practice safe care, you should do well. If the first attempt was not successful, you can retest. OBRA allows 3 attempts to successfully complete the evaluation.

Nursing Assistant Registry

OBRA requires a nursing assistant registry in each state. It is an official record or listing of persons who have successfully completed a NATCEP. The registry has information about each nursing assistant.

- Full name, including maiden name and any married names.
- Last known home address.
- Registry number and the date it expires.
- Date of birth.
- Last known employer, date hired, and date employment ended.
- Date the competency evaluation was passed.
- Information about findings of abuse, neglect, or dishonest use of property. It includes the nature of the offense and supporting evidence. If a hearing was held, the date and its outcome are included. The person has the right to include a statement disputing the finding. All information stays in the registry for at least 5 years.

Any health care agency can access registry information. You also receive a copy of your registry information. The copy is sent when the first entry is made and when information is changed or added. You can correct wrong information.

Certification. After successfully completing your state's NATCEP, you have the title used in your state.

- Certified nursing assistant (CNA) or certified nurse aide (CNA). CNA is used in most states.
- Licensed nursing assistant (LNA).
- Registered nurse aide (RNA).
- State tested nurse aide (STNA).

Nursing assistants can have their certifications (licenses, registrations) denied, revoked, or suspended. See Box 3-1 for the reasons listed by the National Council of State Boards of Nursing (NCSBN).

To work in another state, you must meet that state's NATCEP requirements.

Maintaining Competence

Re-training and a new competency evaluation program are required for nursing assistants who have not worked for 24 months. It does not matter how long you worked as a nursing assistant before. What matters is how long you did *not* work. States can require:

- A new competency evaluation
- Both re-training and a new competency evaluation

Agencies must provide 12 hours of educational programs to nursing assistants every year. Performance reviews also are required. That is, your work is evaluated. These requirements help ensure that you have the current knowledge and skills to give safe, effective care.

See *Focus on Surveys: Maintaining Competence.*

BOX 3-1 Losing Certification, a License, or Registration

The National Council of State Boards of Nursing (NCSBN) lists these reasons for doing so.

- Substance abuse or dependency.
- Abandoning, abusing, or neglecting a person.
- Fraud or deceit. Examples are:
  - Filing false personal information
  - Providing false information when applying for initial certification, re-instatement, or renewal
- Violating professional boundaries (p. 25).
- Giving unsafe care.
- Performing acts beyond the nursing assistant role.
- Misappropriation (stealing, theft) or mis-using property.
- Obtaining money or property from a patient or resident. This can be done through fraud, falsely representing oneself, or by force.
- Being convicted of a crime. Examples include murder, assault, kidnapping, rape or sexual assault, robbery, sexual crimes involving children, criminal mistreatment of children or a vulnerable adult (p. 28), drug trafficking, embezzlement (to take a person's property for one's own use), theft, and arson (starting fires).
- Failing to conform to the standards of nursing assistants (p. 18).
- Putting patients and residents at risk for harm.
- Violating a person's privacy.
- Failing to maintain the confidentiality of patient or resident information.

FOCUS ON SURVEYS

Maintaining Competence

Surveyors must make sure that nursing assistants are competent to safely care for residents. They will:

- Check if all nursing assistants have completed a NATCEP.
- Ask nursing assistants:
  - Where they received their training
  - The length of their training
  - How long they have worked in the agency
- Observe if nursing assistants are able to:
  - Maintain or improve the person's independent functioning.
  - Perform range-of-motion exercises (Chapter 23).
  - Transfer the person from bed to a wheelchair (Chapter 14).
  - Observe, describe, and report the person's behavior and condition to the nurse (Chapter 5).
  - Follow instructions.
  - Practice infection control (Chapter 12) and safety measures (Chapters 9 and 10).

ROLES AND RESPONSIBILITIES

Nurse practice acts, OBRA, state laws, and legal and advisory opinions direct what you can do. To protect persons from harm, you must understand what you can do, what you cannot do, and the legal limits of your role. In some states, this is called *scope of practice.* The NCSBN calls it *range of functions.*

Licensed nurses supervise your work. You perform nursing tasks related to the person's care. A ***nursing task*** *is the nursing care or a nursing function, procedure, activity, or work that can be delegated to nursing assistants when it does not require an RN's professional knowledge or judgment.* Often you function without a nurse in the room. At other times you help nurses give care. The rules in Box 3-2 will help you understand your role.

The range of functions for nursing assistants varies among states and agencies. Before you perform a nursing task make sure that:

- Your state allows nursing assistants to do so.
- It is in your job description.
- You have the necessary education and training.
- A nurse is available to answer questions and to supervise you.

You perform nursing tasks to meet the person's hygiene, safety, comfort, nutrition, exercise, and elimination needs. You also move and transfer persons and make observations. You also measure temperatures, pulses, respirations, and blood pressures. And you help promote the person's mental comfort.

Box 3-3 describes the limits of your role—the tasks that you should never do. State laws differ. Know what you can do in the state in which you are working.

State laws and rules limit nursing assistant functions. Your job description reflects those laws and rules. An agency can further limit what you can do. So can a nurse based on the person's needs. However, no agency or nurse can expand your range of functions beyond what your state's laws and rules allow.

Nursing Assistant Standards

OBRA defines the basic range of functions for nursing assistants. All NATCEPs include those functions. Some states allow other functions. NATCEPs also prepare nursing assistants to meet the standards listed in Box 3-4.

BOX 3-2 Rules for Nursing Assistants

- You are an assistant to the nurse.
- A nurse assigns and supervises your work.
- You report observations about the person's physical and mental status to the nurse (Chapter 5). Report changes in the person's condition or behavior at once.
- The nurse decides what is done for a person. The nurse decides what should not be done for a person. You do not make these decisions.
- Review directions and the care plan with the nurse before going to the person.
- Perform only those nursing tasks that you are trained to do.
- Ask a nurse to supervise you if you are not comfortable performing a nursing task.
- Perform only the nursing tasks that your state and job description allow.

BOX 3-3 Role Limits

- *Never give drugs.* Nurses give drugs. Many states allow nursing assistants to give drugs after completing a state-approved medication assistant training program.
- *Never insert tubes or objects into body openings. Do not remove them from the body.* Exceptions to this rule are the procedures you will study during your training. Giving enemas is an example.
- *Never take oral or phone orders from doctors.* Politely give your name and title, and ask the doctor to wait for a nurse. Promptly find a nurse to speak with the doctor.
- *Never perform procedures that require sterile technique.* With sterile technique, all objects in contact with the person are free of microorganisms (Chapter 12). You can assist a nurse with a sterile procedure. However, you will not perform the procedure yourself.
- *Never tell the person or family the person's diagnosis or medical or surgical treatment plans.* This is the doctor's responsibility. Nurses may clarify what the doctor has said.
- *Never diagnose or prescribe treatments or drugs for anyone.* Doctors diagnose and prescribe.
- *Never supervise others including other nursing assistants.* This is a nurse's responsibility. You will not be trained to supervise others. Supervising others can have serious legal problems.
- *Never ignore an order or request to do something.* This includes nursing tasks that you can do, those you cannot do, and those beyond your legal limits. Promptly and politely explain to the nurse why you cannot carry out the order or request. The nurse assumes you are doing what you were told to do unless you explain otherwise. You cannot neglect the person's care.

Job Description

The ***job description*** *is a document that describes what the agency expects you to do* (Fig. 3-1, pp. 20–21). It also states educational requirements.

Always obtain a written job description when you apply for a job. Ask questions about it during your job interview. Before accepting a job, tell the employer about:

- Functions you did not learn
- Functions you cannot do for moral or religious reasons

Clearly understand what is expected before taking a job. Do not take a job that requires you to:

- Act beyond the legal limits of your role.
- Function beyond your training limits.
- Perform acts that are against your morals or religion.

No one can force you to do something beyond the legal limits of your role. Sometimes jobs are threatened for refusing to follow a nurse's orders. Often staff obey out of fear. That is why you must understand:

- Your roles and responsibilities
- What you can safely do
- The things you should never do
- Your job description
- The ethical and legal aspects of your role

See *Focus on Communication: Job Description.*

DELEGATION

Delegate *means to authorize another person to perform a nursing task in a certain situation.* The person must be competent to perform the task in a given situation. For example, you know how to give a bed bath. However, Mr. Jones is a new resident. The RN wants to spend time with him and assess his nursing needs. You do not assess. Therefore the RN gives the bath.

Who Can Delegate

RNs can delegate tasks to LPNs/LVNs and nursing assistants. In some states, LPNs/LVNs can delegate tasks to nursing assistants. Delegation decisions must protect the person's health and safety.

The delegating nurse must make sure that the task was completed safely and correctly. If the RN delegates, the RN is responsible for the delegated task. If the LPN/LVN delegates, he or she is responsible for the delegated task. The RN also supervises LPNs/LVNs. Therefore the RN is legally responsible for the tasks that LPNs/LVNs delegate to nursing assistants. The RN is responsible for all nursing care.

Nursing assistants cannot delegate. You cannot delegate any task to other nursing assistants or to any other worker. You can ask someone to help you. But you cannot ask or tell someone to do your work.

Text continued on p. 22

BOX 3-4 Nursing Assistant Standards

The nursing assistant:

- Performs nursing tasks within the range of functions allowed by the state's nurse practice act and its rules.
- Is honest and shows integrity in performing nursing tasks. (*Integrity* involves following a code of ethics. See p. 24.)
- Bases nursing tasks on his or her education and training. Also bases them on the nurse's directions.
- Is accountable for his or her behavior and actions while assisting the nurse and helping patients and residents.
- Performs delegated aspects of the person's nursing care.
- Assists the nurse in observing patients and residents. Also assists in identifying their needs.
- Communicates:
  - Progress toward completing delegated nursing tasks
  - Problems in completing delegated nursing tasks
  - Changes in the person's status
- Asks the nurse to clarify what is expected when unsure.
- Uses educational and training opportunities as available.
- Practices safety measures to protect the person, others, and self.
- Respects the person's rights, concerns, decisions, and dignity.
- Functions as a member of the health team. Helps implement the care plan (Chapter 5).
- Respects the person's property and the property of others.
- Protects confidential information unless required by law to share the information.

Modified from National Council of State Boards of Nursing, Inc.: Model nursing practice act and model administrative rules, *Chicago, 2006, Author.*

FOCUS ON COMMUNICATION

Job Description

Your training prepares you to perform certain nursing tasks. The agency may not let you do everything you learned. Other agencies may want you to do things that you did not learn. Use your job description to discuss these issues with the nurse.

For example, Mr. Wey is in the bathroom when the nurse brings a drug to him. The nurse tells you to give him the drug when he comes out of the bathroom. If you give the drug, you are performing a task and responsibility outside the legal limits of your role. With respect, firmly refuse to follow the nurse's direction. You can say: "I'm sorry, but I cannot give Mr. Wey that drug. I was not trained to give drugs, and that task is not in my job description. I'll let you know when Mr. Wey comes out of the bathroom."

POSITION DESCRIPTION/PERFORMANCE EVALUATION

Job Title: LTC Certified Nursing Assistant (CNA)
Prepared by: ____________________
Date: ____________________

Supervised by: CNA Coordinator, Charge Nurse
Approved by: ____________________
Date: ____________________

Job Summary: Provides direct and indirect resident care activities under the direction of an RN or LPN/LVN. Assists residents with activities of daily living, provides for personal care and comfort, and assists in the maintenance of a safe and clean environment for an assigned group of residents.

DUTIES AND RESPONSIBILITIES:

3 = Exceeds Performance 2 = Expected Performance 1 = Needs Improvement

Demonstrates Competency in the Following Areas:

Assists in the preparation for admission of residents.	3	2	1
Assists in and accompanies residents in the admission, transfer and discharge procedures.	3	2	1
Provides morning care, which may include bed bath, shower or whirlpool, oral hygiene, combing hair, back care, dressing residents, changing bed linen, cleaning overbed table and bedside stand, straightening room and other general care as necessary throughout the day.	3	2	1
Provides evening care which includes hands/face washing as needed, oral hygiene, back rubs, peri-care, freshening linen, cleaning overbed tables, straightening room and other general care as needed.	3	2	1
Notifies appropriate licensed staff when resident complains of pain.	3	2	1
Provides postmortem care and assists in transporting bodies to the morgue.	3	2	1
Assists LPN/LVN in treatment procedures.	3	2	1
Provides general nursing care such as positioning residents, lifting and turning residents, applying/utilizing special equipment, assisting in use of bedpan or commode and ambulating the residents.	3	2	1
Performs all aspects of resident care in an environment that optimizes resident safety and reduces the likelihood of medical/health care errors.	3	2	1
Supports and maintains a culture of safety and quality.	3	2	1
Takes and records temperature, pulse, respiration, weight, blood pressure and intake-output.	3	2	1
Makes rounds with outgoing shift; knows whereabouts of assigned residents.	3	2	1
Makes rounds with oncoming shift to ensure the unit is left in good condition.	3	2	1
Adheres to policies and procedures of the facility and the Nursing Department.	3	2	1
Participates in socialization activities on the unit.	3	2	1
Turns and positions residents as ordered and/or as needed, making sure no rough surfaces are in direct contact with the body. Lifts and turns with proper and safe body mechanics and with available resources.	3	2	1
Checks for reddened areas or skin breakdown and reports to RN or LPN/LVN.	3	2	1
Ensures residents are dressed properly and assists, as necessary. Ensures that used clothing is properly stored in bedside stand or on hangers in closet. Ensures that all residents are clean and dry at all times.	3	2	1
Checks unit for adequate linen. Folds neatly and arranges linen in linen closet. Cleans linen cart. Provides clean linen and clothing. Makes beds.	3	2	1
Treats residents and their families with respect and dignity.	3	2	1
Restrains residents properly, when ordered.	3	2	1
Accompanies residents to appointments, as directed.	3	2	1
Provides reality orientation in daily care.	3	2	1
Prepares residents for meals; serves and removes food trays and assists with meals or feeds residents, if necessary.	3	2	1
Distributes drinking water and other nourishments to residents.	3	2	1
Performs general care activities for residents in isolation.	3	2	1
Answers residents' call lights, anticipates residents' needs and makes rounds to assigned residents.	3	2	1
Assists residents with handling and care of clothing and other personal property (including dentures, glasses, contact lenses, hearing aids and prosthetic devices).	3	2	1
Transports residents to and from various departments, as requested.	3	2	1
Reports and, when appropriate, records any changes observed in condition or behavior of residents and unusual incidents.	3	2	1
Participates in and contributes to interdisciplinary care conferences.	3	2	1
Must be able to follow directions, both oral and written, and work cooperatively with other staff members.	3	2	1

FIGURE 3-1 A sample nursing assistant job description. Note that the job description is also a performance evaluation.

POSITION DESCRIPTION/PERFORMANCE EVALUATION—cont'd

Must have the ability to acquire knowledge of and develop skills in basic nursing procedures and simple charting.	3	2	1
Establishes and maintains interpersonal relationship with residents, family members and other facility staff while assuring confidentiality of resident information.	3	2	1
Attends inservice education programs, as assigned, to learn new treatments, procedures, developmental skills, etc.	3	2	1
Practices careful, efficient and nonwasteful use of supplies and linen and follows established charge procedure for resident charge items.	3	2	1
Maintains personal health in order to prevent absence from work due to health problems.	3	2	1
Possesses a genuine interest and concern for geriatric and disabled persons.	3	2	1
Professional Requirements:			
Adheres to dress code, appearance is neat and clean.	3	2	1
Completes annual education requirements.	3	2	1
Maintains regulatory requirements.	3	2	1
Maintains resident confidentiality at all times.	3	2	1
Reports to work on time and as scheduled, completes work within designated time.	3	2	1
Wears identification while on duty, uses computerized punch time system correctly.	3	2	1
Completes inservices and returns in a timely fashion.	3	2	1
Attends annual review and department inservices, as scheduled.	3	2	1
Attends at least ____ staff meetings annually, reads and returns all monthly staff meeting minutes.	3	2	1
Represents the organization in a positive and professional manner.	3	2	1
Actively participates in performance improvement and continuous quality improvement (CQI) activities.	3	2	1
Complies with all organizational policies regarding ethical business practices.	3	2	1
Communicates the mission, ethics and goals of the facility.	3	2	1
TOTAL POINTS	______	______	______

Regulatory Requirements:

- High School graduate or equivalent.
- Current Certified Nursing Assistant (CNA) certification in State of ______________ for Long Term Care Facilities.
- Current Basic Cardiac Life Support certification within three (3) months of hire date.

Language Skills:

- Able to communicate effectively in English, both verbally and in writing.
- Additional languages preferred.

Skills:

- Basic computer knowledge.

Physical Demands:

- For physical demands of position, including vision, hearing, repetitive motion and environment, see following description.

Reasonable accommodations may be made to enable individuals with disabilities to perform the essential functions of the position without compromising patient care.

I have received, read and understand the Position Description/Performance Evaluation above.

______________________________ ______________________

Name/Signature Date Signed

FIGURE 3-1, cont'd

Delegation Process

To make delegation decisions, the nurse follows a process. The person's needs, the nursing task, and the staff member doing the task must fit. The nurse decides if the task will be delegated to you. The person's needs and the task may require a nurse's knowledge, judgment, and skill. You may be asked to assist.

Delegation decisions must result in the best care for the person. Otherwise the person's health and safety are at risk. The NCSBN describes the delegation process in 4 steps.

Step 1—Assess and Plan. The nurse needs to understand the person's needs. And the nurse needs to know your knowledge, skills, and job description.

When assessing the person's needs, the nurse answers these questions.

- What is the nature of the person's needs? How complex are they? How can they vary? How urgent are the care needs?
- What are the most important long-term needs? What are the most important short-term needs?
- How much judgment is needed to meet the person's needs and give care?
- How predictable is the person's health status? How does the person respond to health care?
- What problems might arise from the nursing task? How severe might they be?
- What actions are needed if a problem arises? How complex are those actions?
- What emergencies or incidents might arise? How likely might they occur?
- How involved is the person in health care decisions? How involved is the family?
- How will delegating the nursing task help the person? What are the risks to the person?

To assess your knowledge and skills, the nurse answers these questions.

- What knowledge and skills are needed to safely perform the nursing task?
- What is your role in the agency? What is in your job description?
- What are the conditions under which the nursing task will be performed?
- What is expected after the nursing task is performed?
- What problems can arise from the nursing task? What problems might the person develop during the nursing task?

The nurse then decides if it is safe to delegate the nursing task. It must be safe for the person and safe for you. If unsafe, the nurse stops the delegation process. If it is safe for the person and you, the nurse moves to step 2.

Step 2—Communication. This step involves the nurse and you. The nurse must provide clear and complete directions about:

- How to perform and complete the task
- What observations to report and record
- When to report observations
- What specific patient and resident concerns to report at once
- Priorities for nursing tasks
- What to do if the person's condition changes or needs change

The nurse must make sure that you understand the directions to give safe care. The nurse asks you questions to make sure you understand. He or she may ask you to explain what you are going to do. Do not be insulted by such questions. The intent is to protect the person and you.

Before performing a delegated task, it is important that you discuss the task with the nurse. Make sure that you:

- Ask questions about the delegated task.
- Ask questions about what you are expected to do.
- Tell the nurse if you have not done the task before or not often.
- Ask for needed training or supervision.
- Re-state what is expected of you.
- Re-state what specific patient or resident concerns to report to the nurse.
- Explain how and when you will report your progress in completing the task.
- Know how to contact the nurse for an emergency.
- Know what the nurse wants you to do during an emergency.

After completing a delegated task, you report and record the care given. You also report and record your observations. See "Reporting and Recording" in Chapter 5.

Step 3—Surveillance and Supervision. *Surveillance* means *to keep a close watch over someone or something. Supervise* means *to oversee, direct, or manage.* In this step, the nurse:

- Observes the care you give.
- Makes sure that you complete the task correctly.
- Observes the person's condition and response to care.

How often the nurse makes observations depends on:

- The person's health status and needs
- If the person's condition is stable or unstable
- If the nurse can predict the person's responses and risks to care
- The setting where the task occurs
- The resources and support available
- If the task is simple or complex

The nurse must follow up on any problems or concerns. For example, the nurse takes action if:

- You did not complete the task in a timely manner.
- The task did not meet expectations.
- There is an unexpected change in the person's condition.

The nurse is alert for signs and symptoms that signal a possible change in the person's condition. This way the nurse, with your help, can take action before the person's condition changes in a major way.

Sometimes problems arise during a nursing task. By supervising you, the nurse can detect and solve problems early. This helps you complete the task safely and on time.

After you complete the task, the nurse may review and discuss what happened with you. This helps you learn. If a similar situation happens again, you have ideas about how to adjust.

Step 4—Evaluation and Feedback. This step is done by the nurse. *Evaluate* means *to judge.* The nurse decides if the delegation was successful. The nurse answers these questions.

- Was the task done correctly?
- Did the person respond to the task as expected?
- Was the outcome (the result) as desired? Was it a good or bad result?
- Was communication between you and the nurse timely and effective?
- What went well? What were the problems?
- Does the care plan need to change (Chapter 5)? Or can the plan stay the same?
- Did the task present ways for the nurse or you to learn?
- Did the nurse give you the right feedback? *Feedback* means *to respond.* The nurse tells you what you did correctly. If you did something wrong, the nurse tells you that too. Feedback is another way for you to learn and improve the care you give.
- Did the nurse thank you for completing the task?

The Five Rights of Delegation

The NCSBN's *Five Rights of Delegation* is another way to view the delegation process. The nurse answers questions listed in the 4 steps described under "Delegation Process." The *Five Rights of Delegation* are:

- *The right task.* Can the task be delegated? Is the nurse allowed to delegate the task? Is the task in your job description?
- *The right circumstances.* What are the person's physical, mental, emotional, and spiritual needs at this time?
- *The right person.* Do you have the training and experience to safely perform the task for this person?
- *The right directions and communication.* The nurse must give clear directions. The nurse tells you what to do and when to do it. The nurse tells you what observations to make and when to report back. The nurse allows questions and helps you set priorities.
- *The right supervision.* In this step, the nurse:
  - Guides, directs, and evaluates the care you give.
  - Demonstrates tasks as necessary and is available to answer questions. The less experience you have with a task, the more supervision you need. Complex tasks require more supervision than do basic tasks. Also, the person's circumstances affect how much supervision you need.
  - Assesses how the task affected the person and how well you performed the task.
  - Tells you what you did well and how to improve your work. This helps you learn and give better care.

Your Role in Delegation

You perform delegated tasks for or on *a person.* You must protect the person from harm. You have 2 choices when a task is delegated to you. You either *agree* or *refuse* to do a task. Use the *Five Rights of Delegation* in Box 3-5.

BOX 3-5 The *Five Rights of Delegation* for Nursing Assistants

The Right Task

- Does your state allow you to perform the task?
- Were you trained to do the task?
- Do you have experience performing the task?
- Is the task in your job description?

The Right Circumstances

- Do you have experience with the task given the person's condition and needs?
- Do you understand the purposes of the task for the person?
- Can you perform the task safely under the current circumstances?
- Do you have the equipment and supplies to safely complete the task?
- Do you know how to use the equipment and supplies?

The Right Person

- Are you comfortable performing the task?
- Do you have concerns about performing the task?

The Right Directions and Communication

- Did the nurse give clear directions and instructions?
- Did you review the task with the nurse?
- Do you understand what the nurse expects?

The Right Supervision

- Is a nurse available to answer questions?
- Is a nurse available if the person's condition changes or if problems occur?

Modified from the National Council of State Boards of Nursing, Inc.: The five rights of delegation, *Chicago, 1997, Author.*

Accepting a Task. When you agree to perform a task, you are responsible for your own actions. What you do or fail to do can harm the person. *You must complete the task safely.* Ask for help when you are unsure or have questions about a task. Report to the nurse what you did and the observations you made.

Refusing a Task. You have the right to say "no." Sometimes refusing to follow the nurse's directions is your right and duty. You should refuse to perform a task when:

- The task is beyond the legal limits of your role.
- The task is not in your job description.
- You were not trained to perform the task.
- The task could harm the person.
- The person's condition has changed.
- You do not know how to use the supplies or equipment.
- Directions are not ethical or legal.
- Directions are against agency policies.
- Directions are not clear or complete.
- A nurse is not available for supervision.

Use common sense. This protects you and the person. Ask yourself if what you are doing is safe for the person.

Never ignore an order or a request to do something. Tell the nurse about your concerns. If the task is within the legal limits of your role and in your job description, the nurse can help increase your comfort with the task. The nurse can:

- Answer your questions.
- Demonstrate the task.
- Show you how to use supplies and equipment.
- Help you as needed.
- Observe you performing the task.
- Check on you often.
- Arrange for needed training.

Do not refuse a task because you do not like it or do not want to do it. You must have sound reasons. Otherwise, you place the person at risk for harm. You could lose your job.

See *Focus on Communication: Refusing a Task.*

FOCUS ON COMMUNICATION

Refusing a Task

A nurse may delegate a task that you did not learn in your training program. The task is in your job description. You can say: "I know this task is in my job description, but I did not learn it in school. Can you show me what to do and then observe me doing it? That would really help me."

A nurse may ask you to do something that is *not* in your job description. With respect, you must firmly refuse the nurse's request. You can say: "I'm sorry. That task is not in my job description. Can I help you with something else?"

ETHICAL ASPECTS

Ethics is knowledge of what is right conduct and wrong conduct. Morals are involved. It also deals with choices or judgments about what should or should not be done. An ethical person behaves and acts in the right way. He or she does not cause a person harm.

Ethical behavior also involves not being prejudiced or biased. To be *prejudiced* or *biased* means *making judgments and having views before knowing the facts.* Judgments and views usually are based on one's values and standards. They are based on the person's culture, religion, education, and experiences. The person's situation may be very different from your own. For example:

- Children think their mother needs nursing home care. In your culture, children care for older parents at home.
- A person has many tattoos. You do not like tattoos.

Do not judge the person by your values and standards. Do not avoid persons whose standards and values differ from your own.

Ethical problems involve making choices. You must decide what is the right thing to do.

Professional groups have codes of ethics. The code has rules, or standards of conduct, for group members to follow. The rules of conduct in Box 3-6 can guide your thinking and behavior. See Chapter 4 for ethics in the workplace.

Boundaries

A *boundary* limits or separates something. A fence forms a boundary. You stay inside or outside of the fenced area. As a nursing assistant, you help patients, residents, and families. Therefore you enter into a helping relationship with them. The helping relationship has professional boundaries.

BOX 3-6 Code of Conduct for Nursing Assistants

- Respect each person as an individual.
- Know the limits of your role and knowledge.
- Perform only those tasks within the legal limits of your role.
- Perform only those tasks that you were trained to do.
- Perform no act that will harm the person.
- Take drugs only if prescribed and supervised by your doctor.
- Follow the directions and instructions of the nurse to your best possible ability.
- Follow the agency's policies and procedures.
- Complete each task safely.
- Be loyal to your employer and co-workers.
- Act as a responsible citizen at all times.
- Keep the person's information confidential.
- Protect the person's privacy.
- Protect the person's property.
- Consider the person's needs to be more important than your own.
- Report errors and incidents at once.
- Be accountable for your actions.

Professional boundaries *separate helpful behaviors from behaviors that are not helpful* (Fig. 3-2). The boundaries create a helpful zone. If your behaviors are outside of the helpful zone, you are over-involved with the person or under-involved. The following can occur.

- ***Boundary crossing*** *is a brief act or behavior outside of the helpful zone.* The act or behavior may be thoughtless or something you did not mean to do. Or it could have purpose if it meets the person's needs. For example, you give a crying patient a hug. The hug meets the person's needs at the time. If giving a hug meets your needs, the act is wrong. Also, it is wrong to hug the person every time you see him or her.
- ***Boundary violation*** *is an act or behavior that meets your needs, not the person's.* The act or behavior is not ethical. It violates the code of conduct in Box 3-6. The person can be harmed. Boundary violations include:
  - Abuse (p. 27).
  - Giving a lot of information about yourself. You tell the person about your personal relationships or problems.
  - Keeping secrets with the person.
- ***Professional sexual misconduct*** *is an act, behavior, or comment that is sexual in nature.* It is sexual misconduct even if the person consents or makes the first move.

Some boundary violations and some types of professional sexual misconduct also are crimes (p. 26). To maintain professional boundaries, follow the rules in Box 3-7. Be alert to boundary signs. ***Boundary signs*** *are acts, behaviors, or thoughts that warn of a boundary crossing or boundary violation.* Examples include:

- You spend free time with the person.
- You give more attention to the person at the expense of other patients and residents.
- The person gives you gifts or money. Or you give the person gifts or money.
- You flirt with the person.
- You make comments that have a sexual message.
- You notice more touch between you and the person.

See *Focus on Communication: Professional Boundaries.*

FOCUS ON COMMUNICATION

Professional Boundaries

Some patients, residents, and families want to thank the staff for the care given. Some send thank-you cards and letters. Some offer gifts—candy, cookies, money, gift certificates, flowers, and so on. Accepting gifts is a boundary violation. When offered a gift, you can say:

- "Thank you so much for thinking of me. It's very kind of you. However, it is against center policy to accept gifts of any kind. I do appreciate your offer."
- "Thank you for wanting me to have the flowers from your friend. They are lovely. However, it is against hospital policy to receive gifts. Let me help you find a way to take them home."

PROFESSIONAL BOUNDARIES

Under-involved	Helpful zone	Over-involved

FIGURE 3-2 Professional boundaries.

BOX 3-7 Maintaining Professional Boundaries

- Follow the code of conduct listed in Box 3-6.
- Talk to the nurse if you sense a boundary sign, crossing, or violation.
- Avoid caring for family, friends, and people with whom you do business. This may be hard to do in a small community. Always tell the nurse if you know the person. The nurse may change your assignment.
- Do not make sexual comments or jokes.
- Do not use offensive language.
- Use touch correctly (Chapter 6). Touch or handle sexual and genital areas only when necessary to give care. Such areas include the breasts, nipples, perineum, buttocks, and anus.
- Do not visit or spend extra time with a patient or resident who is not part of your assignment.
- The following apply to patients, residents, and family members.
  - Do not date, flirt with, kiss, or have a sexual relationship with them.
  - Do not discuss your sexual relationships with them.
  - Do not say or write things that could suggest a romantic or sexual relationship with them.
  - Do not accept gifts, loans, money, credit cards, or other valuables from them.
  - Do not give gifts, loans, money, credit cards, or other valuables to them.
  - Do not borrow from them. This includes money, personal items, and transportation.
  - Maintain a professional relationship at all times. Do not develop any personal relationship or friendship with them.
  - Do not share personal or financial information with them.
  - Do not help them with their finances.
  - Do not take a person home with you. This includes for holidays or other events.
- Ask these questions before you date or marry a person whom you cared for. Be aware of the risk for professional sexual misconduct.
  - How long ago did you assist with the person's care?
  - Was the person's care short-term or long-term?
  - What kind and how much information do you have about the person? How will that information affect your relationship with the person?
  - Will the person need more care in the future?
  - Does dating or marrying the person place the person at risk for harm?

LEGAL ASPECTS

A *law is a rule of conduct made by a government body.* The U.S. Congress and state legislatures make laws. Enforced by the government, laws protect the public welfare.

Criminal laws *are concerned with offenses against the public and society in general. An act that violates a criminal law is called a* ***crime.*** A person found guilty of a crime is fined or sent to prison. Murder, robbery, rape, kidnapping, and abuse are crimes.

Civil laws *are concerned with relationships between people.* Examples are those that involve contracts and nursing practice. A person found guilty of breaking a civil law usually has to pay a sum of money to the injured person.

Tort comes from the French word meaning *wrong.* Torts are part of civil law. A *tort* is a wrong committed against a person or the person's property. Some torts are unintentional. Harm was not intended. Some torts are intentional. Harm was intended.

Unintentional Torts

Negligence *is an unintentional wrong. The negligent person did not act in a reasonable and careful manner. As a result, a person or the person's property was harmed.* The person causing the harm did not intend or mean to cause harm. The person failed to do what a reasonable and careful person would have done. Or he or she did what a reasonable and careful person would not have done.

Malpractice *is negligence by a professional person.* A person has professional status because of training and the service provided. Nurses, doctors, dentists, and pharmacists are examples.

What you do or do not do can lead to a lawsuit if a person or property is harmed.

You are legally responsible *(liable)* for your own actions. The nurse is liable as your supervisor. However, you have personal liability. Sometimes refusing to follow the nurse's directions is your right and duty.

Intentional Torts

Intentional torts are acts meant to be harmful.

- ***Defamation*** *is injuring a person's name or reputation by making false statements to a third person.* ***Libel*** *is making false statements in print, in writing, or through pictures or drawings.* ***Slander*** *is making false statements orally.*
- ***False imprisonment*** *is the unlawful restraint or restriction of a person's freedom of movement.* It involves:
  - Threatening to restrain a person
  - Restraining a person
  - Preventing a person from leaving the agency
- ***Invasion of privacy*** *is violating a person's right not to have his or her name, photo, or private affairs exposed or made public without giving consent.* You must treat the person with respect and ensure privacy. Only staff involved in the person's care should see, handle, or examine his or her body. See Box 3-8 for measures to protect privacy.
- ***Fraud*** *is saying or doing something to trick, fool, or deceive a person.* The act is fraud if it does or could harm a person or the person's property. Telling a person or family that you are a nurse is fraud. So is giving wrong or incomplete information on a job application.
- ***Assault*** *is intentionally attempting or threatening to touch a person's body without the person's consent.* The person fears bodily harm.
- ***Battery*** *is touching a person's body without his or her consent.* The person must consent to any procedure, treatment, or other act that involves touching the body. The person has the right to withdraw consent at any time.

See *Focus on Communication: Intentional Torts (Invasion of Privacy).*

BOX 3-8 The Right to Privacy

- Keep all information about the person confidential.
- Cover the person when he or she is being moved in hallways.
- Screen the person. Close the privacy curtain as in Figure 3-3. Close the door when giving care. Also close window coverings.
- Expose only the body part involved in a task.
- Do not discuss the person or the person's treatment with anyone except the nurse supervising your work. "Shop talk" is a common cause of invasion of privacy.
- Ask visitors to leave the room when care is given.
- Do not open the person's mail.
- Allow the person to visit with others in private.
- Allow the person to use the phone in private.
- Follow agency policies and procedures required to protect privacy.

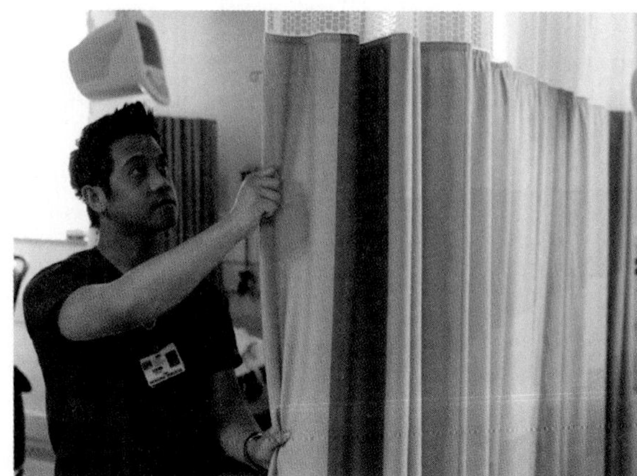

FIGURE 3-3 Pulling the privacy curtain around the bed helps protect the person's privacy.

FOCUS ON COMMUNICATION

Intentional Torts (Invasion of Privacy)

The Health Insurance Portability and Accountability Act of 1996 (HIPAA) protects the privacy and security of a person's health information. ***Protected health information*** *refers to identifying information and information about the person's health care that is maintained or sent in any form (paper, electronic, oral).* Failure to comply with HIPAA rules can result in fines, penalties, and criminal action including jail time. You must follow agency policies and procedures. For example, you must never take photos of patients or residents. Sharing photos or posting them on social media websites is a very serious violation of HIPAA. So is sharing or posting patient or resident information.

You may be asked questions about the person or the person's care. Direct questions to the nurse. Also follow the rules for using computers and other electronic devices (Chapter 5).

Informed Consent

A person has the right to decide what will be done to his or her body and who can touch his or her body. The doctor is responsible for informing the person about all aspects of treatment. Consent is informed when the person clearly understands all aspects of treatment.

Persons under legal age (usually 18 years) cannot give consent. Nor can persons who are mentally incompetent. Such persons are unconscious, sedated, or confused. Or they have certain mental health disorders. Informed consent is given by a responsible party—a wife, husband, parent, daughter, son, or legal representative.

Nurses often obtain written consent. *You are never responsible for obtaining written consent.* In some agencies, you can witness the signing of a consent. When a witness, you are present when the person signs the consent.

See *Focus on Communication: Informed Consent.*

FOCUS ON COMMUNICATION

Informed Consent

There are different ways to give consent.

- *Written consent.* The person signs a form agreeing to a treatment or procedure. You are not responsible for obtaining written consent.
- *Verbal consent.* The person says aloud that he or she consents. "Yes" and "okay" are examples.
- *Implied consent.* For example, you ask Mr. Jones if you can check his blood pressure. He extends his arm. His movement implies consent.

Before any procedure, explain the steps to the person. That is how you obtain verbal or implied consent. Also explain each step during a procedure. That allows the person the chance to refuse at any time.

REPORTING ABUSE

Abuse *is:*

- *The willful infliction of injury, unreasonable confinement, intimidation, or punishment that results in physical harm, pain, or mental anguish.* ***Intimidation*** *means to make afraid with threats of force or violence.*
- *Depriving the person (or the person's caregiver) of the goods or services needed to attain or maintain well-being.*

Abuse includes involuntary seclusion (Chapter 2). Abuse is a crime. It can occur at home or in a health care agency. All persons must be protected from abuse. This includes persons in a coma.

The abuser is usually a family member or caregiver—spouse, partner, adult child, and others. The abuser can be a friend, neighbor, landlord, or other person. Both men and women are abusers. Both men and women are abused.

See *Focus on Communication: Reporting Abuse.*

See *Focus on Surveys: Reporting Abuse.*

FOCUS ON COMMUNICATION

Reporting Abuse

Persons being abused may confide in you. They may ask you to keep it a secret. For example, a person says: "If I tell you something, will you promise not to tell anyone?" Never promise to keep abuse a secret. You must also be honest. Do not tell the person you will keep a secret and then report it to the nurse. You can say: "For your safety, some things I must tell the nurse. What did you want to tell me?" If the person refuses to tell you, notify the nurse.

If you suspect abuse, tell the nurse what you observed. Give as much detail as you can. For example: "I am concerned about Ms. Sloan. She has been very quiet today. When I asked about her afternoon out with her niece, she didn't respond. She refused her bath. And when I helped her to the bathroom, I noticed bruises on her back."

FOCUS ON SURVEYS

Reporting Abuse

Abuse is a major focus of surveys. Surveyors will look for any signs of abuse through interviews, observations, and medical record reviews.

The Centers for Medicare & Medicaid Services (CMS) requires that agencies have procedures to:

- Screen staff applicants for a history of abuse, neglect, or mistreatment of residents. This includes:
  - Information from previous or current employers
  - Checking nursing assistant registries or licensing boards
- Train staff on how to prevent abuse.
- Identify and correct situations in which abuse is more likely to occur.
- Identify events, patterns, and trends that may signal abuse. Bruises, falls, and staff yelling are examples.
- Investigate abuse.
- Protect residents from harm during an investigation.
- Report and respond to claims of abuse or actual abuse.

Vulnerable Adults

Vulnerable comes from the Latin word *vulnerare*, which means *to wound*. ***Vulnerable adults*** *are persons 18 years old or older who have disabilities or conditions that make them at risk to be wounded, attacked, or damaged.* They have problems caring for or protecting themselves due to:

- A mental, emotional, physical, or developmental disability
- Brain damage
- Changes from aging

All patients and residents, regardless of age, are vulnerable. Older persons and children are at risk for abuse.

See *Focus on Older Persons: Vulnerable Adults*.

FOCUS ON OLDER PERSONS

Vulnerable Adults

Some persons have behaviors and ways of living that threaten their health, safety, and well-being. This is called ***self-neglect.*** Causes include declining health and chronic disease. Other causes are disorders that impair judgment or memory—Alzheimer's disease, dementia, depression, and drug or alcohol abuse.

Report warning signs of self-neglect to the nurse.

- Hoarding—saving, hiding, or storing things. For example, the person saves newspapers, magazines, food containers, shopping bags, and so on.
- Not eating enough food. Weight loss.
- Absence of food, water, heat, and other necessities.
- Failing to take needed drugs.
- Refusing to seek medical treatment for serious illnesses.
- Dehydration—poor urinary output, dry skin, dry mouth, confusion.
- Poor hygiene—dirty hair, nails, or skin. He or she smells of urine or feces.
- Skin rashes.
- Pressure ulcers (Chapter 25).
- Not wearing the correct clothing for the weather. Or wearing dirty or torn clothing.
- Not having dentures, eyeglasses, hearing aids, walkers, wheelchairs, commodes, or other needed devices.
- Confusion, disorientation, hallucinations, or delusions (Chapter 30).
- Not attending to or not being able to attend to housekeeping.
- Safety hazards in the home (Chapter 9).
- Mis-using drugs or alcohol.

Elder Abuse

Elder abuse *is any knowing, intentional, or negligent act by a caregiver or any other person to an older adult. The act causes harm or serious risk of harm.* Elder abuse can take these forms.

- *Physical abuse.* This involves inflicting, or threatening to inflict, physical pain or injury. Grabbing, hitting, slapping, kicking, pinching, hair-pulling, or beating are examples. It also includes *corporal punishment*—punishment inflicted directly on the body. Beatings, lashings, and whippings are examples. Depriving the person of a basic need also is physical abuse.
- *Neglect. Failure to provide the person with the goods or services needed to avoid physical harm, mental anguish, or mental illness is called* ***neglect.*** This includes failure to provide health care or treatment, food, clothing, hygiene, shelter, or other needs. In health care, neglect includes but is not limited to:
  - Leaving the person lying or sitting in urine or feces
  - Keeping persons alone in their rooms or other areas
  - Failing to answer call lights
- *Verbal abuse.* Verbal abuse is using oral or written words or statements that speak badly of, sneer at, criticize, or condemn the person. It includes unkind gestures, threats of harm, or saying things to frighten the person. For example, a person is told that he or she will never see family members again.
- *Involuntary seclusion.* This involves confining the person to a certain area. People have been locked in closets, basements, attics, bathrooms, and other spaces.
- *Financial exploitation or misappropriation.* To *exploit* means *to use unjustly. Misappropriate* means *to dishonestly, unfairly, or wrongly take for one's own use.* The older person's resources (money, property, assets) are mis-used by another person. Or the resources are used for the other person's profit or benefit. The person's money is stolen or used by another person. It is also mis-using a person's property. For example, children sell their mother's house without her consent.
- *Emotional or mental abuse.* This involves inflicting mental pain, anguish, or distress through verbal or nonverbal acts. Humiliation, harassment, ridicule, and threats of punishment are examples. It includes being deprived of needs such as food, clothing, care, a home, or a place to sleep.
- *Sexual abuse.* The person is harassed about sex or is attacked sexually. The person may be forced to perform sexual acts out of fear of punishment or physical harm.

- *Abandonment. Abandon* means *to leave or desert someone.* The person is deserted by someone who is supposed to give his or her care. Abandonment involves the following 4 points:
  - You accept an assignment to care for a person or group of persons.
  - You accept that assignment for a certain time period.
  - You remove yourself from the care setting—hospital, nursing center, or other agency.
  - You do not report off to a staff member who will assume responsibility for your assignment.

There are many signs of elder abuse. The abused person may show only some of the signs in Box 3-9.

Federal and state laws require the reporting of elder abuse. You may suspect abuse. If so, discuss the matter and your observations with the nurse. Give as many details as possible. The nurse contacts health team members as needed. The nurse also contacts community agencies that investigate elder abuse. They act at once if the problem is life-threatening. Sometimes the police or courts are involved.

OBRA Requirements. State laws, accrediting agencies, and the Omnibus Budget Reconciliation Act of 1987 (OBRA) do not allow agencies to employ persons who were convicted of abuse, neglect, or mistreatment. Before hiring, the agency must thoroughly check the applicant's work history. All references are checked. Efforts must be made to find out about any criminal records.

The agency also checks the nursing assistant registry for findings of abuse, neglect, or mistreatment. It also is checked for mis-using or stealing a person's property.

OBRA requires these actions if abuse is suspected within the center.

- The matter is reported at once to:
  - The administrator
  - Other officials as required by federal and state laws
- All claims of abuse are thoroughly investigated.
- The center must prevent further potential for abuse while the investigation is in progress.
- Investigation results are reported to the center administrator within 5 days of the incident. They also are reported to other officials as required by federal and state laws.
- Corrective actions are taken if the claim is found to be true.

Child Abuse and Neglect

All states require the reporting of suspected child abuse and neglect. Abuse can be in the form of physical, sexual, or emotional abuse; substance abuse; or abandonment. You must be alert for signs and symptoms of child abuse. Report any changes in the child's body or behavior. Share your concerns with the nurse. Give as much detail as you can. The nurse contacts health team members and child protection agencies as needed.

BOX 3-9 Signs of Elder Abuse

- Living conditions are unsafe, unclean, or inadequate.
- Personal hygiene is lacking. The person is not clean. Clothes are dirty.
- Weight loss—there are signs of poor nutrition and poor fluid intake.
- Assistive devices are missing or broken—eyeglasses, hearing aids, dentures, cane, walker, and so on.
- Medical needs are not met.
- Frequent injuries—conditions behind the injuries are strange or seem impossible.
- Old and new injuries—bruises, pressure marks, welts, scars, fractures, punctures, and so on.
- Complaints of pain or itching in the genital area.
- Bleeding and bruising around the breasts or in the genital area.
- Burns on the feet, hands, buttocks, or other parts of the body. Cigarettes and cigars cause small circle-like burns.
- Pressure ulcers (Chapter 25) or contractures (Chapter 23).
- The person seems very quiet or withdrawn.
- Unexplained withdrawal from normal activities.
- The person seems fearful, anxious, or agitated.
- Sudden changes in alertness.
- Depression.
- Sudden changes in finances.
- The person does not seem to want to talk or answer questions.
- The person is restrained. Or the person is locked in a certain area for long periods.
- The person cannot reach toilet facilities, food, water, and other needed items.
- Private conversations are not allowed. The caregiver is present during all conversations.
- Strained or tense relationships with a caregiver.
- Frequent arguments with a caregiver.
- The person seems anxious to please the caregiver.
- Drugs are not taken properly. Drugs are not bought. Or too much or too little of the drug is taken.
- Emergency visits may be frequent.
- The person may change doctors often. Some people do not have a doctor.

Domestic Abuse

Domestic abuse occurs in relationships. One partner has power and control over the other through abuse—physical, sexual, verbal, economic, or social abuse. The victim often hides the abuse. He or she may protect the abuser. State laws vary about reporting domestic abuse. However, the health team has an ethical duty to give information about safety and community resources. If you suspect domestic abuse, share your concerns with the nurse. The nurse gathers information to help the person.

OTHER LAWS

See "Ethics and Laws" in the *Focus on PRIDE: The Person, Family, and Yourself* boxes at the end of each chapter. They describe other laws affecting your work as a nursing assistant.

FOCUS ON PRIDE

The Person, Family, and Yourself

Personal and Professional Responsibility
Health care is constantly changing. New career opportunities are common. For example, some states have advanced levels of nursing assistants. Medication Assistant-Certified (MA-C) is an example. MA-Cs are nursing assistants with extra training. Supervised by a licensed nurse, they give drugs as allowed by state law.

Continuing education increases your skills and knowledge and helps you provide safe, quality care. Agency in-services, staff meetings, and conferences offer learning opportunities. Continuing to learn is a personal and professional responsibility.

Your current training is the start of a life-time of learning and possibilities. Take advantage of options in your state and agency. Be proud of your training. And never stop learning!

Rights and Respect
Most training programs involve practice in a real clinical setting. Sometimes a patient or resident refuses to have a student. Or the person refuses to allow a student to watch a procedure. The person's right to refuse must be respected.

If this happens to you, you may feel disappointed and rejected. Or you may feel that you did something wrong. Kindly accept the person's request. Try not to be ashamed or upset. Tell your instructor. Do not speak badly about the patient or resident. The person may have had a bad experience. This had nothing to do with you. Respect the person's right to choose who is involved in his or her care.

Independence and Social Interaction
You will interact closely with patients, residents, and families. You may begin to know them well. Social and professional relationships differ. To maintain professional boundaries:

- Follow the "Code of Conduct" in Box 3-6.
- Maintain professional boundaries (see Box 3-7).
- Monitor for boundary signs.
- Ask the nurse if you have a question about an interaction.

Use good judgment when interacting with patients, residents, and families. Take pride in being professional.

Delegation and Teamwork
You may be delegated several tasks at a time. This can be overwhelming. For example, you are asked to:

- Take Mr. Austin's temperature.
- Get Ms. Sams a glass of water.
- Turn and re-position Mr. Mason.
- Assist Mrs. Philips to the bathroom.

When delegated several tasks, stay calm. Keep a positive attitude. Communicate with the nurse. Ask the nurse to help you set priorities. Also, good teamwork is needed. When others have many delegated tasks, offer to help. Thank others when they help you.

Ethics and Laws
Some nursing assistants are also emergency medical technicians (EMTs). EMTs give emergency care outside of health care settings. State laws and rules for EMTs and nursing assistants differ. For example, your state laws allow EMTs to start intravenous (IV) lines. Nursing assistants do not start IVs.

The ability to do something does not give the right to do so in all settings. There are legal limits to your role. Be proud of your other skills and training. But when working as a nursing assistant, follow your state's laws and rules for nursing assistants.

REVIEW QUESTIONS

Circle the BEST answer.

1 What state law affects what nursing assistants can do?
  a HIPAA
  b OBRA
  c Nurse practice act
  d Medicaid

2 Your nursing assistant certification can be revoked for
  a Refusing a nursing task
  b Asking the nurse questions
  c Performing acts beyond your role
  d Keeping the person's information confidential

3 Which requires a training and competency evaluation program for nursing assistants?
  a Medicare
  b Medicaid
  c NCSBN
  d OBRA

4 As a nursing assistant, you
  a Must accept all tasks delegated by the nurse
  b Make decisions about a person's care
  c Need a written job description before employment
  d Give a drug when a nurse tells you to

5 As a nursing assistant, you
  a Can take verbal or phone orders from doctors
  b Are responsible for your own actions
  c Can remove tubes from the person's body
  d Can ignore a nursing task if it is not in your job description

6 Who assigns and supervises your work?
  a Other nursing assistants
  b The health team
  c Nurses
  d Doctors

7 You are responsible for
  a Supervising other nursing assistants
  b Delegation decisions
  c Completing delegated tasks safely
  d Deciding what treatments are needed

8 You perform a task not allowed by your state. Which is *true?*
  a If a nurse delegated the task, there is no legal problem.
  b You could be practicing nursing without a license.
  c You can perform the task if it is in your job description.
  d If you complete the task safely, there is no legal problem.

9 These statements are about delegation. Which is *false?*
  a Nurses can delegate their responsibilities to you.
  b A delegated task must be safe for the person.
  c The delegated task must be in your job description.
  d The delegating nurse is responsible for the safe completion of the task.

10 A task is in your job description. Which is *false?*
  a The nurse must delegate the task to you.
  b The nurse can delegate the task if the person's circumstances are right.
  c You must have the necessary education and training to complete the task.
  d You must have clear directions before you perform the task.

11 A nurse delegates a task to you. You must
  a Complete the task
  b Decide to accept or refuse the task
  c Delegate the task if you are busy
  d Ignore the request if you do not know what to do

12 You can refuse to perform a task if
  a The task is within the legal limits of your role
  b The task is in your job description
  c You do not like the task
  d A nurse is not available to supervise you

13 You decide to refuse a task. What should you do?
  a Delegate the task to a nursing assistant.
  b Communicate your concerns to the nurse.
  c Ignore the request.
  d Talk to the director of nursing.

14 Ethics is
  a Making judgments before you have the facts
  b Knowledge of right and wrong conduct
  c A behavior that meets your needs, not the person's
  d A health team member's skill, care, and judgment

15 Which is ethical behavior?
  a Sharing information about a person with a friend
  b Accepting gifts from a resident's family
  c Reporting errors
  d Calling your family before answering a call light

16 To maintain professional boundaries, your behaviors must
  a Help the person
  b Meet your needs
  c Be biased
  d Show that you care

17 You help with a friend's hospital care. This is a
  a Professional boundary
  b Boundary crossing
  c Tort
  d Crime

18 These statements are about negligence. Which is *true?*
  a It is an intentional tort.
  b The negligent person acted in a reasonable manner.
  c The person or the person's property was harmed.
  d A prison term is likely.

19 Threatening to touch the person's body without the person's consent is
  a Assault
  b Battery
  c Defamation
  d False imprisonment

20 Restraining a person's freedom of movement is
  a Assault
  b Battery
  c Defamation
  d False imprisonment

21 You tell others that you are nurse. This is
  a Negligence
  b Fraud
  c Libel
  d Slander

22 Informed consent is when the person
  a Fully understands all aspects of his or her treatment
  b Signs a consent form
  c Is admitted to the agency
  d Decides what to do with property after his or her death

23 Self-neglect is when
  a A caregiver harms a person
  b The person's behaviors put him or her at risk for harm
  c A person is deprived of food, clothing, hygiene, and shelter
  d The person does not receive attention or affection

24 You scold an older person for not eating lunch. This is
  a Physical abuse
  b Neglect
  c Battery
  d Verbal abuse

25 Which is a sign of elder abuse?
  a Stiff joints and joint pain
  b Weight gain
  c Poor personal hygiene
  d Forgetfulness

26 You suspect a person was abused. What should you do?
  a Tell the family.
  b Call the police.
  c Tell the nurse.
  d Ask the person about the abuse.

Answers to these questions are on p. 504.

FOCUS ON **PRACTICE**

Problem Solving

A resident in your nursing center asks you to visit on your day off. The resident wants you to bring your children to visit. How do you respond? How do professional boundaries protect the person? How do these actions affect professional boundaries?

CHAPTER

4 Work Ethics

OBJECTIVES

- Define the key terms and key abbreviation listed in this chapter.
- Describe the practices for good health, hygiene, and a professional appearance.
- Describe the qualities and traits of a successful nursing assistant.
- Explain how to get a job.
- Explain how to plan for childcare and transportation.
- Describe ethical behavior on the job.
- Explain how to manage stress.
- Explain the aspects of harassment.
- Explain how to resign from a job.
- Identify the common reasons for losing a job.
- Explain the reasons for drug testing.
- Explain how to promote PRIDE in the person, the family, and yourself.

KEY TERMS

confidentiality Trusting others with personal and private information
gossip To spread rumors or talk about the private matters of others
harassment To trouble, torment, offend, or worry a person by one's behavior or comments
preceptor A staff member who guides another staff member; mentor
priority The most important thing at the time
professionalism Following laws, being ethical, having good work ethics, and having the skills to do your work
stress The response or change in the body caused by any emotional, physical, social, or economic factor
teamwork Staff members work together as a group; each person does his or her part to provide safe and effective care
work ethics Behavior in the workplace

KEY ABBREVIATION

NATCEP Nursing assistant training and competency evaluation program

As a student and a nursing assistant, you must act and function in a professional manner. *Professionalism involves following laws, being ethical, having good work ethics, and having the skills to do your work.* Certain behaviors (conduct), choices, and judgments are expected in health care agencies. *Work ethics deals with behavior in the workplace.* Your conduct reflects your choices and judgments. Work ethics involves:

- How you look
- What you say
- How you behave
- How you treat others
- How you work with others

Much of the content in this chapter applies while you are a student. Always practice good work ethics.

HEALTH, HYGIENE, AND APPEARANCE

Patients, residents, families, and visitors expect you to look and act healthy. For example, a person is told to stop smoking. Yet you are seen smoking. If you are not clean, people wonder if you give good care. Your health, appearance, and hygiene need careful attention.

Your Health

To give safe and effective care, you must be physically and mentally healthy.

- *Diet.* You need a balanced diet (Chapter 20) for good nutrition.
- *Sleep and rest.* Most adults need 7 to 8 hours of sleep daily.
- *Body mechanics.* You will bend, carry heavy objects, and move and turn persons. Use your muscles correctly (Chapter 13).
- *Exercise.* Exercise is needed for muscle tone, circulation, and weight loss.
- *Your eyes.* You will read instructions and take measurements. Wrong readings can cause the person harm. Have your eyes checked. Wear needed eyeglasses or contact lenses. Provide enough light for reading and fine work.
- *Smoking.* Smoking causes lung, heart, and circulatory disorders. Smoke odors stay on your breath, hands, clothing, and hair. Hand washing and good hygiene are needed.
- *Drugs.* Some drugs affect thinking, feeling, behavior, and function. Working under the influence of drugs affects the person's safety. Take only those drugs ordered by your doctor.
- *Alcohol.* Alcohol is a drug that affects thinking, balance, coordination, and alertness. Never report to work under the influence of alcohol. Do not drink alcohol while working.

Your Hygiene

Your hygiene needs careful attention. Bathe daily. Use a deodorant or antiperspirant to prevent body odors. Brush your teeth upon awakening, before and after meals, and at bedtime. Use a mouthwash to prevent breath odors. Shampoo often. Style hair in a simple, attractive way. Keep fingernails clean, short, and neatly shaped.

Menstrual hygiene is important. Change tampons or sanitary pads often, especially for heavy flow. Wash your genital area with soap and water at least twice a day. Also practice good hand washing.

Foot care prevents odors and infection. Wash your feet daily. Dry thoroughly between the toes. Cut toenails straight across after bathing or soaking them.

Your Appearance

Good health and hygiene practices help you look and feel well. Follow the practices in Box 4-1. They help you look clean, neat, and professional (Fig. 4-1, p. 34).

BOX 4-1 Practices for a Professional Appearance

- Practice good hygiene.
- Wear uniforms that fit well. They are modest in length and style. Follow the agency's dress code.
- Keep uniforms clean, pressed, and mended. Sew on buttons. Repair zippers, tears, and hems.
- Wear a clean uniform daily.
- Wear your name badge or photo ID (identification) at all times when on duty. Make sure it can be seen. Wear it according to agency policy. It is best to wear it above your waist. Agencies may use first names only or first and last names. The agency may let you decide what to have on your name badge. For security reasons, some staff choose the first name only option.
- Wear undergarments that are clean and fit properly. Change them daily.
- Wear undergarments in the correct color for your skin tone. Do not wear colored (red, pink, blue, and so on) ones. They can be seen through white and light-colored uniforms.
- Cover tattoos (body art). They may offend others.
- Follow the agency's dress code for jewelry. Wedding and engagement rings may be allowed. Rings and bracelets can scratch a person. Confused or combative persons can easily pull on jewelry (necklaces, dangling earrings). So can young children.
- Do not wear jewelry in pierced eyebrows, nose, lips, or tongue while on duty.
- Follow the agency's dress code for earrings. Usually small, simple earrings are allowed. For multiple ear piercings, usually only 1 set of earrings is allowed.
- Wear a wristwatch with a second (sweep) hand.
- Wear clean stockings and socks that fit well. Change them daily.
- Wear shoes that fit properly, are comfortable, give needed support, and have non-skid soles. Do not wear sandals or open-toed shoes.
- Clean and polish shoes often. Wash and replace laces as needed.
- Keep fingernails clean, short, and neatly shaped. Long nails can scratch a person. Nails must be natural.
- Do not wear nail polish. Chipped nail polish may provide a place for microbes to grow.
- Have a simple, attractive hairstyle. Hair is off your collar and away from your face. Use simple pins, combs, barrettes, and bands to keep long hair up and in place.
- Keep beards and mustaches clean and trimmed.
- Use make-up that is modest in amount and moderate in color. Avoid a painted and severe look.
- Do not wear perfume, cologne, or after-shave lotion. The scents may offend, nauseate, or cause breathing problems in patients and residents.

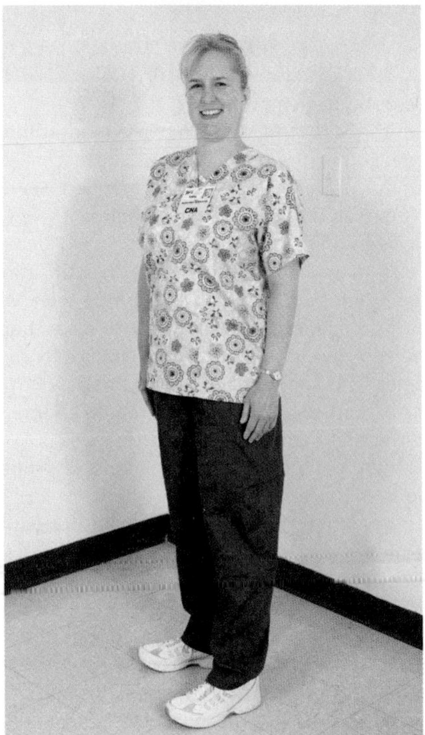

FIGURE 4-1 The nursing assistant is well-groomed. Her uniform and shoes are clean. Her hair has a simple style. It is away from her face and off of her collar. She does not wear jewelry.

BOX 4-2 Qualities and Traits for Good Work Ethics

- *Caring.* Have concern for the person. Help make the person's life happier, easier, or less painful.
- *Dependable.* Report to work on time and when scheduled. Perform delegated tasks. Keep obligations and promises.
- *Considerate.* Respect the person's physical and emotional feelings. Be gentle and kind toward patients, residents, families, and co-workers.
- *Cheerful.* Greet and talk to people in a pleasant manner. Do not be moody, bad-tempered, or unhappy while at work.
- *Empathetic.* Empathy is seeing things from the person's point of view—putting yourself in the person's place. How would you feel if you had the person's problems?
- *Trustworthy.* Patients, residents, families, and staff have confidence in you. They believe you will keep information confidential. They trust you not to gossip about patients, residents, families, or the health team.
- *Respectful.* Patients and residents have rights, values, beliefs, and feelings. They may differ from yours. Do not judge or condemn the person. Treat the person with respect and dignity at all times. Also show respect for the health team.
- *Courteous.* Be polite and courteous to patients, residents, families, visitors, and co-workers. See p. 39 for common courtesies in the workplace.
- *Conscientious.* Be careful, alert, and exact in following instructions. Give thorough care. Do not lose or damage the person's property.
- *Honest.* Accurately report the care given, your observations, and any errors.
- *Cooperative.* Willingly help and work with others. Also take that "extra step" during busy and stressful times.
- *Enthusiastic.* Be eager, interested, and excited about your work. Your work is important.
- *Self-aware.* Know your feelings, strengths, and weaknesses. You need to understand yourself before you can understand patients and residents.

GETTING A JOB

There are easy ways to find out about jobs and places to work.

- Newspaper ads
- Local and state employment services
- Agencies you would like to work at
- Phone book yellow pages
- People you know—your instructor, family, and friends
- The Internet
- Your school's or college's job placement counselors
- Your clinical experience site

What Employers Look For

If you owned a business, who would you hire? Your answer helps you understand the employer's point of view. Employers want people who:

- Are dependable.
- Are well-groomed.
- Have needed job skills and training.
- Have values and attitudes that fit with the agency.
- Have the qualities and traits described in Box 4-2.

You must be at work on time and when scheduled. Undependable people cause everyone problems. Other staff take on extra work. Fewer people give care. Quality of care suffers. You want co-workers to work when scheduled. Otherwise, you have extra work. You have less time to spend with patients and residents. Likewise, co-workers also expect you to work when scheduled.

Job Skills and Training. The employer checks the nursing assistant registry and requests proof that you completed a nursing assistant training and competency evaluation program (NATCEP).

- A certificate of program completion
- A high school, college, or technical school transcript
- An official grade report (report card)

Give the employer a *copy* of the document. Never give the original to anyone. Keep it in a safe place for future use. The employer may want a transcript sent directly from the school or college. A criminal background check and drug testing are common requirements.

Job Applications

You get a job application (Appendix C) from the *personnel office* or *human resources office*. You can complete the application there. Or take it home for return by mail or in person. Be well-groomed and behave pleasantly when seeking or returning a job application. It may be your first chance to make a good impression.

To complete a job application, see Box 4-3. A neat, readable, and complete application gives a good image. A sloppy or incomplete one does not.

Some agencies have job applications on-line. Follow the instructions for completing an on-line application.

BOX 4-3 Completing a Job Application

- Read and follow the directions. They may ask you to print using black ink. You must follow directions on the job. Employers look at job applications to see if you can follow directions.
- Write neatly. Writing must be readable. A messy application gives a bad image. Readable writing gives the correct information. The agency cannot contact you if unable to read your phone number. You may miss getting the job.
- Complete the entire form. Something may not apply to you. If so, write "N/A" for non-applicable. Or draw a line through the space. This shows that you read the section. It also shows that you did not skip the item on purpose.
- Report any felony arrests or convictions as directed. Write "no" or "none" as appropriate. Criminal background and fingerprint checks are common requirements.
- Give information about employment gaps. If you did not work for a time, the employer wonders why. Providing this information shows you are honest. Some reasons are an illness, going to school, raising your children, or caring for an ill or older family member.
- Tell why you left a job, if asked. Be brief, but honest. People leave jobs for one that pays better. Some leave for career advancement. Others leave for reasons given for employment gaps. If you were fired from a job, give an honest but positive response. Do not talk badly about a former employer.
- Provide references. Be prepared to give names, titles, addresses, and phone numbers of at least 4 non-family references. Have this information written down before completing an application. (Always ask references if an employer can contact them.) If references are missing or not complete, the employer waits for all the information. This wastes your time and the employer's time. Also, the employer wonders if you are hiding something with incomplete reference information.
- Be prepared to provide the following.
  - Social Security number
  - Proof of citizenship or legal residency
  - Proof of successful NATCEP completion
  - Identification—driver's license or government-issued ID card
- Give honest responses. Lying on an application is fraud. It is grounds for being fired.
- Keep a file of your education and work history.

The Job Interview

A job interview is when the employer gets to know and evaluate you. You also learn about the agency.

The interview may be when you complete the job application. Some agencies schedule interviews after reviewing applications. Write down the interviewer's name and the interview date and time. If you need directions to the agency, ask for them at this time.

Preparing for the Interview. Box 4-4, p. 36 lists common interview questions. Prepare your answers ahead of time. Also prepare a list of your skills.

You must be neat, clean, and well-groomed (Fig. 4-2). Follow the guidelines in Box 4-5, p. 36.

Be on time. It shows you are dependable. Go to the agency some day before your interview. Note how long it takes and where to park. Also find the personnel office. A *dry run* (practice run) gives an idea of how long it takes to get from your home to the personnel office.

When you arrive for an interview, turn off your wireless phone and other electronic devices. Tell the receptionist your name and the interviewer's name. Then sit quietly in the waiting area. Do not smoke, chew gum, or use your phone. Review your answers to the interview questions. Waiting may be part of the interview. The interviewer may ask the receptionist about how you acted while waiting. Smile, and be polite and friendly.

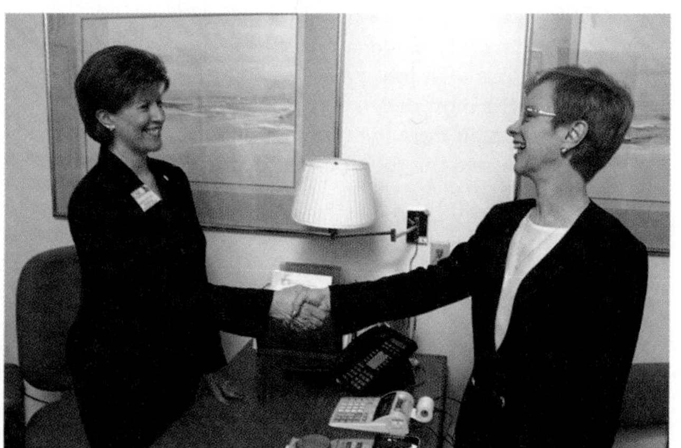
A

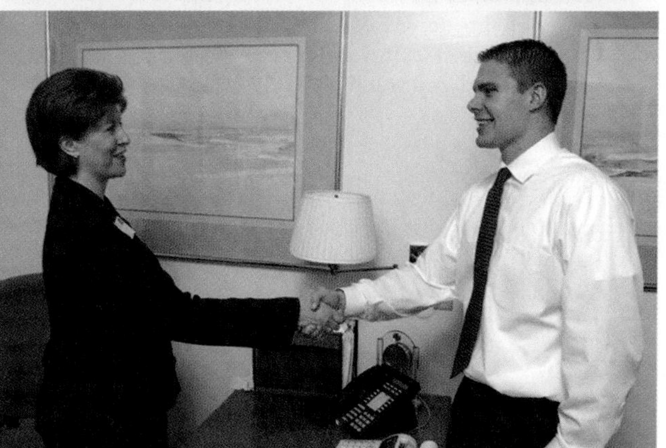
B

FIGURE 4-2 **A,** A simple suit is worn for a job interview. **B,** This man wears slacks and a shirt and tie for his interview.

BOX 4-4 Common Interview Questions

Questions for You
- Tell me about yourself.
- Tell me about your career goals.
- What are you doing to reach these goals?
- Describe what *professional* behavior means to you.
- Tell me about your last job. Why did you leave?
- What did you like the most about your last job? What did you like the least?
- What would your supervisor and co-workers tell me about you? Your dependability? Your skills? Your flexibility?
- Which functions are the hardest for you? How do you handle this difficulty?
- How do you set your priorities?
- How have your experiences prepared you for this job?
- What would you like to change about your last job?
- How do you handle problems with patients, residents, families, and co-workers?
- Why do you want to work here?
- Why should this agency hire you?

Questions for the Interviewer
- Which job functions do you think are the most important?
- What employee qualities and traits are the most important to you?
- What nursing care pattern is used here (Chapter 1)?
- Who will I work with?
- When are performance evaluations done? Who does them? How are they done?
- What performance factors are evaluated?
- How does the supervisor handle problems?
- What are the most common reasons that nursing assistants lose their jobs here?
- What are the most common reasons that nursing assistants resign from their jobs here?
- How do you see this job in the next year? In the next 5 years?
- What is the greatest reward from this job?
- What is the greatest challenge from this job?
- What do you like the most about nursing assistants who work here? What do you like the least?
- Why should I work here rather than in another agency?
- Why are you interested in hiring me?
- How much will I make an hour?
- What hours will I work?
- What uniforms are required?
- What benefits do you offer?
  - Health and disability insurance?
  - Continuing education?
  - Vacation time?
- Does the agency have a new employee orientation program? How long is it?
- May I have a tour of the agency and the unit I will work on? Will you introduce me to the nurse manager and unit staff?
- Can I have a few minutes to talk to the nurse manager?

BOX 4-5 Grooming and Dressing for an Interview

- Bathe and brush your teeth. Wash your hair.
- Use deodorant or antiperspirant.
- Make sure your hands and fingernails are clean.
- Apply make-up in a simple, attractive manner.
- Style your hair in a neat and attractive way. Wear it as you would for work.
- Do not wear jeans, shorts, tank tops, halter tops, or other casual clothing.
- Iron clothing. Sew on loose buttons and mend garments as needed.
- Wear clothing that covers tattoos (body art).
- Wear a simple dress, skirt and blouse, or suit (women). Wear a suit or dark slacks and a shirt and tie (men). A jacket is optional. A long-sleeved white or light blue shirt is best.
- Wear socks (men and women) or hose (women). Hose should be free of runs and snags.
- Make sure shoes are clean and in good repair.
- Avoid heavy perfumes, colognes, and after-shave lotions. A light fragrance is okay.
- Wear only simple jewelry that complements your clothes. Avoid adornments in body piercings. If you have multiple ear piercings, wear only 1 set of earrings.
- Stop in the restroom when you arrive for the interview. Check your hair, make-up, and clothes.

During the Interview. Politely greet the interviewer. A firm hand-shake is correct for men and women. Address the interviewer as Miss, Mrs., Ms., Mr., or Doctor. Stand until asked to sit. Sit with good posture and in a professional way. If offered a beverage, you may accept. Be sure to thank the person.

Look directly at the interviewer when you answer or ask questions. Poor eye contact sends negative information—being shy, insecure, dishonest, or lacking interest.

Watch your body language (Chapter 6). Body language involves facial expressions, gestures, posture, and body movements. What you say is important. However, how you use and move your body also tells a great deal. Avoid distracting habits—biting nails; playing with jewelry, clothing, or your hair; crossing your arms; and swinging your legs back and forth.

Give complete and honest answers. Speak clearly and with confidence. Avoid short and long answers. "Yes" and "no" answers give little information. Briefly explain "yes" and "no" responses.

The interviewer will ask about your skills. Share your skills list. You may be asked about a skill not on your list. Explain that you are willing to learn the skill if your state allows nursing assistants to perform the task.

Box 4-4 lists some questions for you to ask at the end of the interview. Review the job description with the interviewer. Ask any questions at this time. Advise the interviewer of functions you cannot perform because of training, legal, ethical, or religious reasons.

You may be offered a job at this time. Or you are told when to expect a call or letter. Follow-up is acceptable. Ask when you can check on your application. Before leaving, thank the interviewer and shake hands. Say that you look forward to hearing from him or her.

After the Interview. Write a thank-you letter or note within 24 hours after the interview. Use a computer if your writing is hard to read. The thank-you note should include:

- The date
- The interviewer's formal name using Miss, Ms., Mrs., Mr., or Dr.
- A statement thanking the person for the interview
- Comments about the interview, the agency, and your eagerness to hear about the job
- Your signature using your first and last names

Accepting a Job

When you accept a job, agree on a starting date, pay rate, and work hours. Ask where to report on your first day. Ask for such information in writing. Use the written offer later if questions arise. Also ask for the employee handbook and other agency information. Read everything before you start working.

New Employee Orientation

Agencies have orientation programs for new employees. The policy and procedure manual is reviewed. Your skills are checked for safety and correctness. Also, you are shown how to use the agency's supplies and equipment.

Preceptor programs are common. A ***preceptor*** *(mentor) is a staff member who guides another staff member.* A nurse or nursing assistant:

- Helps you learn the agency's layout and where to find things.
- Introduces you to patients, residents, and staff.
- Helps you organize your work.
- Helps you feel like part of the nursing team.
- Answers questions about the policy and procedure manual.

A nursing assistant preceptor is not your supervisor. Only nurses can supervise.

A preceptor program usually lasts 2 to 4 weeks. When the program ends, you should feel comfortable with the setting and your role. If not, ask for more orientation time.

PREPARING FOR WORK

To keep your job, you must function well and work well with others. You must:

- Work when scheduled.
- Get to work on time.
- Stay the entire shift.

Absences and tardiness (being late) are common reasons for losing a job. Childcare and transportation issues often interfere with getting to work. They need careful planning.

Childcare

Someone needs to care for your children when you leave for work, while you are at work, and before you get home. Also plan for emergencies.

- Your childcare provider is ill or cannot care for your children that day.
- A child becomes ill or injured while you are at work.
- You will be late getting home from work.

Transportation

Plan for getting to and from work. If you drive, keep your car in good working order. Keep enough gas in the car. Or leave early to get gas.

Carpooling is an option. Carpool members depend on each other. If the driver is late leaving, everyone is late for work. If one person is not ready when the driver arrives, everyone is late for work. Carpool with members you trust to be ready on time. Be on time as a driver or a passenger.

Know your bus or train schedule. Know what other bus or train to take if delays occur. Always carry enough money for fares to and from work.

Always have a back-up plan for getting to work. Your car may not start, the carpool driver may not go to work, or public transportation may not run.

TEAMWORK

Teamwork *means that staff members work together as a group. Each person does his or her part to provide safe and effective care.* Teamwork involves:

- Working when scheduled.
- Being cheerful and friendly.
- Performing delegated tasks.
- Being available to help others. Help willingly.
- Being kind to others.

You are an important member of the nursing and health teams. Quality of care is affected by how you work with others and how you feel about your job.

Attendance

Report to work when scheduled and on time. The entire unit is affected when just one person is late. Call the agency if you will be late or cannot go to work. Follow the attendance policy in your employee handbook. Poor attendance can cause you to lose your job.

Be *ready to work* when your shift starts.

- Store your belongings before your shift starts.
- Use the restroom when you arrive at the agency.
- Arrive on your nursing unit a few minutes early. This gives you time to greet others and settle yourself.

You must stay the entire shift. You may need to work over-time. When it is time to leave, report off duty to the nurse.

See *Focus on Communication: Attendance.*

Your Attitude

You need a good attitude. Show that you enjoy your work. Listen to others. Be willing to learn. Stay busy, and use your time well.

Always think before you speak. These statements signal a bad attitude.

- "That's not my resident (patient)."
- "I can't. I'm too busy."
- "I didn't do it."
- "I don't feel like it."
- "It's not my fault."
- "Don't blame me."
- "It's not my turn. I did it yesterday."
- "Nobody told me."
- "That's not my job."
- "You didn't say that you needed it right away."
- "I work harder than anyone else."
- "No one appreciates what I do."
- "I'm tired of this place."
- "Is it time to leave yet?"
- "Good luck. I had a horrible day."

Gossip

To ***gossip*** *means to spread rumors or talk about the private matters of others.* Gossiping is unprofessional and hurtful. To avoid being part of gossip:

- Remove yourself from a group or setting where people are gossiping.
- Do not make or repeat any comment that can hurt a person, family member, visitor, co-worker, or the agency.
- Do not make or repeat any comment that you do not know is true. Making or writing false statements about another person is defamation (Chapter 3).
- Do not talk about patients, residents, family members, visitors, co-workers, or the agency at home or in social settings, by e-mail, instant messaging, text messages, or social networking sites (Twitter, Facebook, MySpace, and others).

Confidentiality

The person's information is private and personal. ***Confidentiality*** *means trusting others with personal and private information.* The person's information is shared only among staff involved in his or her care. The person has the right to privacy and confidentiality. Agency, family, and co-worker information also is confidential.

Share information only with the nurse. Avoid talking about patients, residents, families, the agency, or co-workers when others are present. Do not talk about them in hallways, elevators, dining areas, or outside the agency. Others may over-hear you. Do not eavesdrop. To *eavesdrop* means *to listen in or over-hear what others are saying.* It invades a person's privacy.

Many agencies have intercom systems. They allow for communication between the bedside and the nurses' station (Chapter 15). Be careful what you say over the intercom. It is like a loud speaker. Others nearby can hear what you are saying.

See *Focus on Communication: Confidentiality.*

FOCUS ON COMMUNICATION

Attendance

You may have days that you cannot work. Illness, a family death, and other emergencies are reasons. You must communicate with the agency about your absence. Otherwise you could lose your job. To report an absence:

- *Call well before your shift begins.* See the attendance policy in your employee handbook for how far in advance you should call. Calling 2 hours before your shift starts is common.
- *Know who to call.* A charge nurse, nurse manager, or supervisor often handles absences. You may need your call transferred. For example: "Hello. This is Erin Jones. Please transfer me to the charge nurse." You must give information to the right person.
- *Give the reason for your absence.* Be honest. You can say: "I am sorry. I will be absent from work today. I have a fever and a cough."
- *Communicate how long you expect to be absent.* People often miss 1 or 2 days for illness or a family emergency. Longer absences or uncertain time frames require more communication.

FOCUS ON COMMUNICATION

Confidentiality

Your family and friends may ask you about patients, residents, families, or employees. For example, your mother says: "Mrs. Drew goes to our church. I heard she's in your nursing home. What's wrong with her?"

Do not share any information with your family and friends. Doing so violates the person's right to privacy and confidentiality (Chapters 2 and 3). You can say: "I'm sorry, but I can't tell you about anyone in the center. It is unprofessional and against center policies. And it violates the person's right to privacy and confidentiality. Please don't ask me about anyone in the center."

Hygiene and Appearance

Home and social attire is not proper at work. You cannot wear jeans, halter tops, tank tops, or short skirts. Clothing must not be tight, revealing, or sexual. Women cannot show cleavage, the tops of breasts, or upper thighs. Men must avoid tight pants and exposing their chests. Only the top shirt button is open. Follow the practices in Box 4-1.

Speech and Language

Your speech and language must be professional. Words used in home and social settings may not be proper at work. Words used with family and friends may offend patients, residents, families, visitors, and co-workers. Remember:

- Do not swear or use foul, vulgar, slang, or abusive language.
- Speak softly and gently.
- Speak clearly. Hearing problems are common.
- Do not shout or yell.
- Do not fight or argue with a person, family member, visitor, or co-worker.

Courtesies

A *courtesy* is a polite, considerate, or helpful comment or act. Courtesies take little time or energy. And they mean so much to people.

- Address others by Miss, Mrs., Ms., Mr., or Doctor. Use a first name only if the person asks you to do so.
- Begin or end each request with "please."
- Say "thank you" whenever someone does something for you.
- Apologize. Say "I'm sorry" when you make a mistake or hurt someone. Even little things—like bumping someone in the hallway—need an apology.
- Hold doors open for others. If you are at the door first, open the door and let others pass through.
- Hold elevator doors open for others coming down the hallway.
- Let patients, residents, families, and visitors enter elevators first.
- Help others willingly when asked.
- Give praise. If you see a co-worker do or say something that impresses you, tell that person. Also tell your co-workers.

Personal Matters

Personal matters cannot interfere with your job. Otherwise care is neglected. You could lose your job. To keep personal matters out of the workplace:

- Make phone calls during meals and breaks. Use a pay phone or your wireless phone.
- Do not let family and friends visit you on the unit. If they must see you, have them meet you during a meal or break.
- Make appointments (doctor, dentist, lawyer, and others) for your days off.
- Do not use agency computers, printers, fax machines, copiers, or other equipment for your personal use.
- Do not take the agency's supplies (pens, paper, and others) for your personal use.
- Do not discuss personal problems.
- Control your emotions. If you need to cry or express anger, do so in private. Get yourself together quickly and return to your work.
- Do not borrow money from or lend it to co-workers.
- Do not sell things or engage in fund-raising.
- Turn off wireless phones and other electronic devices.
- Do not send or check text messages.

Meals and Breaks

Meal breaks are usually 30 minutes. Other breaks are usually 15 minutes. Meals and breaks are scheduled so some staff are always on the unit. Staff remaining on the unit cover for the staff on break.

Staff members depend on each other. Leave for and return from breaks on time. That way other staff can have their turn. Do not take longer than allowed. Tell the nurse when you leave and return to the unit.

Job Safety

You must protect patients, residents, families, visitors, co-workers, and yourself from harm. Negligent acts affect the safety of others (Chapter 3). Safety practices are presented throughout this book. These guidelines apply to everything you do.

- Understand the roles, functions, and responsibilities in your job description.
- Follow agency rules, policies, and procedures.
- Know what is right and wrong conduct.
- Know what you can and cannot do.
- Develop the desired qualities and traits in Box 4-2.
- Follow the nurse's directions and instructions.
- Question unclear directions and things you do not understand.
- Help others willingly when asked.
- Ask for any training you might need.
- Report measurements, observations, the care given, the person's complaints, and any errors accurately (Chapters 5 and 9).
- Accept responsibility for your actions. Admit when you are wrong or make mistakes. Do not blame others. Do not make excuses for your actions. Learn what you did wrong and why. Always try to learn from your mistakes.
- Handle the person's property carefully and prevent damage.
- Follow the safety measures in Chapter 9 and throughout this book.

Planning Your Work

You will give care and perform routine tasks on the nursing unit. Some tasks are done at certain times. Others are done at the end of the shift.

The nurse, the Kardex, the care plan, and your assignment sheet help you decide what to do and when (Chapter 5). This is called *priority setting.* A ***priority*** *is the most important thing at the time.* Setting priorities involves deciding:

- Which person has the greatest or most life-threatening needs
- What task the nurse or person needs done first
- What tasks need to be done at a certain time
- What tasks need to be done when your shift starts
- What tasks need to be done at the end of your shift
- How much time it takes to complete a task
- How much help you need to complete a task
- Who can help you and when

Priorities change as the person's needs change. A person's condition can improve or worsen. New patients and residents are admitted. Others are transferred to other nursing units or discharged. These and many other factors can change priorities.

Setting priorities is hard at first. It becomes easier with experience. You can ask the nurse to help you set priorities. Plan your work to give safe, thorough care and to make good use of your time (Box 4-6).

BOX 4-6 Planning Your Work

- Discuss priorities with the nurse.
- Know the routine of your shift and nursing unit.
- Follow unit policies for shift reports.
- List tasks that are on a schedule. For example, some persons are turned or offered the bedpan every 2 hours.
- Judge how much time you need for each person and task.
- Identify the tasks to do while patients and residents are eating, visiting, or involved with activities or therapies.
- Plan care around meal times, visiting hours, and therapies. Also consider recreation and social activities.
- Identify when you will need help from a co-worker. Ask a co-worker to help you. Give the time when you will need help and for how long.
- Schedule equipment or rooms for the person's use. The shower room is an example.
- Review delegated tasks. Gather needed supplies ahead of time.
- Do not waste time. Stay focused on your work.
- Leave a clean work area. Make sure rooms are neat and orderly. Also clean utility areas.
- Be a self-starter. Have initiative. Ask others if they need help. Follow unit routines, stock supply areas, and clean utility rooms. Stay busy.

MANAGING STRESS

Stress *is the response or change in the body caused by any emotional, physical, social, or economic factor.* Stress is normal. It occurs every minute of every day. It occurs in everything you do. No matter the cause—pleasant or unpleasant—stress affects the whole person.

- *Physically*—sweating, increased heart rate, faster and deeper breathing, increased blood pressure, dry mouth, and so on
- *Mentally*—anxiety, fear, anger, dread, apprehension, and using defense mechanisms (Chapter 29)
- *Socially*—changes in relationships, avoiding others, needing others, blaming others, and so on
- *Spiritually*—changes in beliefs and values and strengthening or questioning one's beliefs in God or a higher power

Prolonged or frequent stress threatens physical and mental health. Some problems are minor—headaches, stomach upset, sleep problems, muscle tension, and so on. Others are life-threatening—high blood pressure, heart attack, stroke, ulcers, and so on.

Job stresses affect your family and friends. Stress in your personal life affects your work. Stress affects you, the care you give, the person's quality of life, and how you relate to co-workers. To reduce or cope with stress:

- Exercise regularly.
- Get enough rest and sleep.
- Eat healthy.
- Plan personal and quiet time for you.
- Use common sense about what you can and cannot do. Do not try to do everything that family and friends ask you to do.
- Do 1 thing at a time. Set priorities.
- Do not judge yourself harshly. Do not try to be perfect or expect too much from yourself.
- Give yourself praise. You do good and wonderful things every day.
- Have a sense of humor. Laugh at yourself. Laugh with others. Spend time with those who make you laugh.
- Talk to the nurse if your work or a person is causing too much stress. The nurse can help you deal with the matter.

HARASSMENT

Harassment means to trouble, torment, offend, or worry a person by one's behavior or comments. Harassment can be sexual. Or it can involve age, race, ethnic background, religion, or disability. Respect others. Do not offend others by your gestures, remarks, or use of touch. Do not offend others with jokes, photos, or other pictures (drawings, cartoons, and so on). Harassment is not legal in the workplace.

See *Focus on Communication: Harassment.*

FOCUS ON COMMUNICATION

Harassment

You have the right to feel safe and not threatened. If someone's comments make you uncomfortable, you can say: "Please don't say things like that. It's unprofessional." If someone's actions make you uneasy, you can say: "Please don't do that. It's unprofessional." Leave the area. Report the person's statements or actions to the nurse.

Sexual Harassment

Sexual harassment involves unwanted sexual behaviors by another. The behavior may be a sexual advance. Or it may be a request for a sexual favor. Some remarks, comments, and touching are sexual. The behavior affects the person's work and comfort. In extreme cases, the person's job is threatened if sexual favors are not granted.

Victims of sexual harassment may be men or women. Men harass women or men. Women harass men or women. You might feel that you are being harassed. If so, report the matter to the nurse and the human resources officer.

Even innocent remarks and behaviors can be viewed as harassment. Employee orientation programs address harassment. You might not be sure about your own or another person's remarks or behaviors. If so, talk to the nurse. You cannot be too careful.

RESIGNING FROM A JOB

Whatever your reason for resigning, tell your employer. Do 1 of the following.

- Give a written notice.
- Write a resignation letter.
- Complete a form in the human resources office.

A 2-week notice is a good practice. Do not leave a job without notice. Include the following in your notice.

- Reason for leaving
- The last date you will work
- Comments thanking the employer for the opportunity to work in the agency

LOSING A JOB

You must perform your job well and protect patients and residents from harm. No pay raise or losing your job results from poor performance. Failing to follow agency policy is often grounds for termination. So is failure to get along with others. Box 4-7 lists the many reasons why you can lose your job. To protect your job, function at your best. Always practice good work ethics.

DRUG TESTING

Drug and alcohol use affect patient, resident, and staff safety. Quality of care suffers. Those who use drugs or alcohol are late to work or absent more often than staff who do not use such substances. Therefore drug testing policies are common. Review your agency's policy for when and how you might be tested.

BOX 4-7 Common Reasons for Losing a Job

- Poor attendance—not going to work or excessive tardiness (being late).
- Abandonment—leaving the job during your shift.
- Falsifying a record—job application or a person's record.
- Violent behavior in the workplace.
- Having weapons in the workplace—guns, knives, explosives, or other dangerous items.
- Having, using, or distributing alcohol in the work setting.
- Having or using drugs in the work setting. This excludes drugs ordered by your doctor.
- Distributing drugs in the workplace.
- Taking a person's drugs for your own use or giving them to others.
- Harassment.
- Using offensive speech and language.
- Stealing or destroying the agency's or a person's property.
- Showing disrespect to patients, residents, families, visitors, co-workers, or supervisors.
- Abusing or neglecting a person.
- Invading a person's privacy.
- Failing to maintain patient, resident, family, agency, or co-worker confidentiality. This includes access to computer and other electronic information.
- Using the agency's supplies and equipment for your own use.
- Defamation—see Chapter 3 and "Gossip" (p. 38).
- Abusing meal breaks and break periods.
- Sleeping on the job.
- Violating the agency's dress code.
- Violating any agency policy or care procedure.
- Tending to personal matters while on duty.

FOCUS ON PRIDE

The Person, Family, and Yourself

Personal and Professional Responsibility

As a nursing assistant, you are responsible for following the ethical guidelines in this chapter. Patients, residents, families, visitors, and co-workers depend on you to give safe and effective care. They trust that you will:

- Work when scheduled.
- Arrive at work on time.
- Stay the entire shift.
- Complete your assignments.
- Work safely.
- Be pleasant and courteous.

Your job as a nursing assistant is important. You can help persons feel safe, secure, loved, and cared for. By practicing good work ethics, you can make others' lives happier, easier, and less painful. Take pride in your work ethics. Your work affects quality of life.

Rights and Respect

Your attitude affects how you feel about your job. So do the attitudes of others. You will work with many different personalities. You may be more comfortable with some than with others. Your attitude and ability to work with others affect quality care.

Sometimes you may work without enough staff. Or you may work with a challenging person. Do not complain about or put down another staff member. For example, do not say: "She calls in sick all the time. You know she's not sick."

Every team member has value. Treat everyone with respect. Try to work well with everyone. Take pride in keeping a positive attitude.

Independence and Social Interaction

Social interaction is a vital part of your job. Employers look for good social skills. During an interview, smile, give a firm hand-shake, make eye contact, and answer questions confidently.

At work, smile and greet patients and residents by name. Politely introduce yourself. Do not appear hurried. Display a caring and friendly manner all the time. Remain calm and helpful in stressful situations. These actions promote good relationships and reflect well on you and the agency.

Delegation and Teamwork

Your work ethics affects the team. Greet co-workers pleasantly. Help others willingly when asked. Offer to help others if you can. After completing tasks, ask the nurse if you can help with anything else. Be available. Stay where you can easily be found. If you will be in one area for a while, tell the nurse.

When you would like a break, ask the nurse. Return from breaks on time. Help others so they may take a break. Set a positive example with your behavior. Your actions help build a strong team.

Ethics and Laws

To be professional, you must be safe. You must follow federal, state, and agency laws and rules. Many agencies require a background check and drug testing before hiring.

Show good judgment with your actions inside and outside the workplace. Be honest and give accurate information to employers. Giving wrong or incomplete information is fraud (Chapter 3).

REVIEW QUESTIONS

Circle T if the statement is TRUE and F if it is FALSE.

1 **T F** You wear needed eyeglasses. This helps protect the person's safety.

2 **T F** Childcare requires planning before you go to work.

3 **T F** Being on time for work means arriving at the agency when your shift begins.

4 **T F** You share information about a patient with a friend. You could lose your job.

5 **T F** You wear jeans to work. You could lose your job.

6 **T F** You can use the agency's computer for your homework.

7 **T F** You must know the agency's attendance policy.

8 **T F** Harassment is legal in the workplace.

Circle the BEST answer.

9 Which will help you do your job well?
- **a** Sleeping 3 to 4 hours daily
- **b** Avoiding exercise
- **c** Using drugs and alcohol
- **d** Having good nutrition

10 Which is a good hygiene practice?
- **a** Bathing weekly
- **b** Wearing strongly scented perfume or cologne
- **c** Brushing teeth after meals
- **d** Having long and polished fingernails

11 When should you ask questions about your job description?
- **a** After completing the job application
- **b** Before completing the job application
- **c** When your interview is scheduled
- **d** During the interview

12 Lying on a job application is
- **a** Negligence
- **b** Fraud
- **c** Libel
- **d** Defamation

13 When completing a job application
- **a** Do not report felony arrests and convictions
- **b** Provide references
- **c** Leave out information about employment gaps
- **d** Leave spaces blank that do not apply to you

14 Which of the following do employers look for the *most?*
- **a** Cooperation
- **b** Courtesy
- **c** Dependability
- **d** Empathy

15 What should you wear to a job interview?
- **a** A uniform
- **b** Party clothes
- **c** A simple dress or suit
- **d** Whatever is most comfortable

16 Which is poor behavior during a job interview?
- **a** Good eye contact with the interviewer
- **b** Shaking hands with the interviewer
- **c** Asking the interviewer questions
- **d** Crossing your arms and legs

17 Which is the *best* response to an interview question?
- **a** "Yes" or "no"
- **b** Long answers
- **c** Brief explanations
- **d** A written response

18 Which statement reflects a good work attitude?
- **a** "It's not my fault."
- **b** "I'm sorry. I didn't know."
- **c** "That's not my job."
- **d** "I did it yesterday. It's your turn."

19 A co-worker says that a doctor and nurse are dating. This is
- **a** Gossip
- **b** Eavesdropping
- **c** Confidential information
- **d** Sexual harassment

20 Which is professional speech and language
- **a** Speaking clearly
- **b** Using vulgar words
- **c** Shouting
- **d** Arguing

21 Which is *not* a courteous act?
- **a** Saying "please" and "thank you"
- **b** Wanting others to open doors for you
- **c** Saying "I'm sorry"
- **d** Complimenting others

22 You are on a meal break. Which is *true?*
- **a** You cannot make personal phone calls.
- **b** Family members cannot meet you.
- **c** You can take a few extra minutes if needed.
- **d** The nurse needs to know that you are off the unit.

23 When planning your work
- **a** Discuss priorities with the nurse
- **b** Skip the shift report to allow more time for work
- **c** Do not ask co-workers for help
- **d** Plan care so that you can watch the person's TV

24 Which helps to reduce stress?
- **a** Exercise, rest, and sleep
- **b** Blaming others for things you did not do
- **c** Putting off quiet time to get work done
- **d** Agreeing to do everything others ask

25 Which is *not* harassment?
- **a** Asking for a sexual favor
- **b** Joking about a person's religion
- **c** Using touch to comfort a person
- **d** Acting like a disabled person

26 Which is *not* a reason for losing your job?
- **a** Leaving the job during your shift
- **b** Using alcohol in the work setting
- **c** Sleeping on the job
- **d** Taking a meal break

Answers to these questions are on p. 504.

FOCUS ON **PRACTICE**

Problem Solving

A co-worker did not show up for work. You and the other staff members have extra work. How do you respond? Do you complain or keep a positive attitude? How will you plan, prioritize, and manage the extra work?

CHAPTER 5

Communicating With the Health Team

OBJECTIVES

- Define the key terms and key abbreviations listed in this chapter.
- Describe the rules for good communication.
- Describe the legal and ethical aspects of medical records.
- Identify common parts of the medical record.
- Explain your role in the nursing process.
- List the information you need to report to the nurse.
- List the rules for recording.
- Use the 24-hour clock, medical terminology, and medical abbreviations.
- Explain how computers and other electronic devices are used in health care.
- Explain how to protect the right to privacy when using computers and other electronic devices.
- Describe how to answer phones.
- Explain how to problem solve and deal with conflict.
- Explain how to promote PRIDE in the person, the family, and yourself.

KEY TERMS

chart See "medical record"
communication The exchange of information—a message sent is received and correctly interpreted by the intended person
end-of-shift report A report that the nurse gives at the end of the shift to the on-coming shift; change-of-shift report
medical record The legal account of a person's condition and response to treatment and care; chart
nursing care plan A written guide about the person's nursing care; care plan
nursing diagnosis A health problem that can be treated by nursing measures
nursing process The method nurses use to plan and deliver nursing care; its 5 steps are assessment, nursing diagnosis, planning, implementation, and evaluation
objective data Information that is seen, heard, felt, or smelled by an observer; signs
observation Using the senses of sight, hearing, touch, and smell to collect information
planning Setting priorities and goals
recording The written account of care and observations; charting
reporting The oral account of care and observations
signs See "objective data"
subjective data Things a person tells you about that you cannot observe through your senses; symptoms
symptoms See "subjective data"

KEY ABBREVIATIONS

ADL	Activities of daily living
EPHI; ePHI	Electronic protected health information
OBRA	Omnibus Budget Reconciliation Act of 1987
PHI	Protected health information

Health team members communicate with each other to give coordinated and effective care. They share information about:

- What was done for the person
- What needs to be done for the person
- The person's response to treatment

COMMUNICATION

Communication is the exchange of information—a message sent is received and correctly interpreted by the intended person. For good communication:

- Use words that mean the same thing to you and the message receiver. Avoid words with more than 1 meaning. What does "far" mean—50 feet or 100 feet?

- Use familiar words. Avoid terms that the person and family do not understand.
- Be brief and concise. Do not add unrelated or unnecessary information. Stay on the subject. Do not wander in thought or get wordy.
- Give information in a logical and orderly way. Organize your thoughts. Present them step-by-step.
- Give facts and be specific. You report a pulse rate of 110. It is more specific and factual than saying the "pulse is fast."

THE MEDICAL RECORD

The ***medical record (chart)*** *is the legal account of a person's condition and response to treatment and care.* The health team uses it to share information about the person. The record is a permanent legal document. It can be used in court as legal evidence of the person's problems, treatment, and care.

Agencies have policies about medical records and who can access them. Policies address:

- Who records. In some agencies, nursing assistants record observations and care.
- When to record.
- Abbreviations.
- How to make entries.
- How to correct errors.

Professional staff involved in the person's care can review charts. If you have access to charts, you have an ethical and legal duty to keep information confidential. If not involved in the person's care, you have no right to review the person's chart. Doing so is an invasion of privacy.

Common parts of the record include:

- *Admission information*—is gathered when the person is admitted to the agency. It includes the person's identifying information.
- *Health history*—is completed by the nurse. The nurse asks about current and past illnesses, signs and symptoms, allergies, and drugs.
- *Flow sheets and graphic sheets*—are used to record care measures, observations, and measurements made daily, every shift, or 3 to 4 times a day (Fig. 5-1). Information includes vital signs (blood pressure, temperature, pulse, respirations), weight, intake and output (Chapter 20), bowel movements, doctor visits, and everyday activities.
- *Progress notes and nurses' notes*—are used to describe observations, the care given, and the person's response and progress. They are used to record information about treatments, some drugs, and procedures. In long-term care, summaries of care describe the person's progress toward meeting goals and response to care.

Activities of Daily Living Flow Sheet

		JAN		FEB		MAR		APR		
ORDER/INSTRUCTION	**TIME**	**1**	**2**	**3**	**4**	**5**	**6**	**7**	**8**	**9**
Bowel Movements L = Large M = Medium S = Small IC = Incontinent	11-7	M								
	7-3			L						
	3-11									
Urinary Elimination I = Independent IC = Incontinent FC = Foley catheter	11-7	I	I	I	I					
	7-3	I	I	I	I					
	3-11	I	IC	I	I					
Weight Bearing Status TT = Toe touch AT = As tol. P = Partial F = Full NWB = No weight bearing	11-7	AT	AT	AT	AT					
	7-3	AT	AT	AT	AT					
	3-11	AT	AT	AT	AT					
Transfer Status ML = Mech lift SBA = Stand by assist; Assist of 1 or 2 (A-1, A-2)	11-7	SBA	SBA	SBA	SBA					
	7-3	SBA	SBA	SBA	SBA					
	3-11	SBA	SBA	SBA	A-1					
Activity A = Ambulate GC = Gerichair T = Turn every 2 hrs. W/C = Wheelchair	11-7	T	T	T	T					
	7-3	A	A	A	A					
	3-11	A	A	A	A					
Safety LT = Lap tray BR – Bed rails BA = Bed alarm SB = Seat belt	11-7									
	7-3									
	3-11									
Feeding Status I = Independent S = Set up F = Staff feed SP = Swallow precautions TL = Thickened liquids	Breakfast	S	S	S	S					
	Lunch	S	S	S	S					
	Supper	S	S	S	S					
Amount of food taken in %	Breakfast	75	100	100	75					
	Lunch	75	75	100	75					
	Supper	50	50	50	75					
Bath and Shampoo every Monday & Thursday on 7-3 shift T = Tub S = Shower B = Bed bath	11-7									
	7-3		T							
	3-11									
Oral Care Own/(Dentures)/No teeth I = Independent S = Set up A = Assist	11-7	S	S	S	S					
	7-3	S	S	S	S					
	3-11	S	S	S	S					
Dressing I = Independent S = Set up A = Assist T = Total care	11-7	A	A	S	S					
	7-3									
	3-11	A	A	A	A					
Grooming: Washing Face and Hands Combing Hair I = Independent S = Set up A = Assist T = Total care	11-7	A	A	A	A					
	7-3	A	A	A	A					
	3-11	A	A	A	A					
Trim Fingernails weekly Thursday	11-7									
	7-3		✓							
	3-11									
Lotion Arms and Legs twice daily	11-7									
	7-3	✓	✓	✓	✓					
	3-11	✓	✓	✓	✓					
Shave Men daily Shave (Women) every Monday & Thursday on 7-3 shift	11-7									
	7-3		✓							
	3-11									
Amount Between-Meal Nourishment taken in %	AM	100	75	100	50					
	PM	100	100	75	75					
	HS	50	75	75	75					
Intake and Output	11-7									
	7-3									
	3-11									
Vital Signs Every Thursday	11-7									
	7-3		✓							
	3-11									
Weight Every Thursday	11-7		✓							
	7-3									
	3-11									

FIGURE 5-1 A sample flow sheet. This form shows some items on an activities of daily living flow sheet.

THE KARDEX OR CARE SUMMARY

The *Kardex* or *care summary* provides a quick, easy reference to the person's drugs, treatments, diagnoses, care measures, equipment, and special needs. The Kardex is a type of card file (Fig. 5-2). With computer systems, the person's information is organized in a care summary. The summary can be printed for reference when providing care.

THE NURSING PROCESS

The ***nursing process*** *is the method nurses use to plan and deliver nursing care. It has 5 steps.*

- *Assessment*
- *Nursing diagnosis*
- *Planning*
- *Implementation*
- *Evaluation*

The nursing process focuses on the person's nursing needs. All nursing team members do the same things for the person. They have the same goals.

DIET
Regular
Hold:

NOURISHMENT/SPECIAL FEEDING
Health shake at Bedtime

INTAKE/OUTPUT
Encourage/(Restrict) Fluids 2000 mL/24 Hr.
7-3 1000 3-11 800 11-7 200

FUNCTIONAL STATUS

	SELF	ASSIST	TOTAL	OTHER	SPECIFY
Feeding	☐	☒	☐	☐	
Bathing	☐	☒	☐	☐	
Toileting	☐	☒	☐	☐	
Oral Care	☐	☒	☐	☐	
Positioning	☒	☐	☐	☐	
Transferring	☒	☐	☐	☐	
Wheeling	☐	☐	☐	☐	
Walking	☒	☐	☐	☐	
	☐	☐	☐	☐	

ACTIVITIES
Bedrest & BRP
Bedside Commode
Up ad Lib X
Chair
Ambulatory X
Ambulate & Assist
Turn
Dangle
Mode of Travel

ELIMINATION
Urinary - Cont. / (Incont.)
Catheter
Date Changed
Irrigations
Bowel - (Cont.) / Incont.
Ostomy
Irrigations

VITALS
Temp. daily
Pulse daily
Resp. daily
BP daily
Weight daily
Other: Pulse OX daily

COMMUNICATION DEFICITS ☐ None
Hearing Hard-of-hearing
Vision Impaired
Speech
Language Impaired

SPECIAL CONDITIONS (Paralysis, Pressure Ulcers, Etc.)

SAFETY/SUPPORTIVE MEASURES
Bed rails: ☒ Nights Only ☐ Constant ☐ No Need
Restraints:
Support Devices: ☐ PRN ☐ Constant

RESPIRATORY THERAPY
Aerosol
IPPB
Ultrasonic
Rx Med

OXYGEN
2 Liter/Minute
☒ PRN ☐ Constant
___ Tent ___ Catheter
___ Mask X Cannula

PROSTHESIS ☐ None
Glasses X Dentures X
Contacts Limb
Hearing Aid L ear

SPECIAL EQUIPMENT/PROCEDURES/ANCILLARY SERVICES/ETC.
Speech therapy 3 times/wk.

ORDERED	SCHEDULED	COMPLETED	X-RAY AND SPECIAL DIAGNOSTIC EXAMS
10-20	10-20	10-20	Chest x-ray

DATE	TREATMENTS

DATE	TIME	SCHEDULED MEDICATIONS
10-19		Lasix 40 mg PO daily
10-19		Lanoxin 0.25 mg PO daily

DATE	TIME	PRN MEDICATIONS

MISCELLANEOUS

ALLERGIES:
☒ None Known

NURSING ALERTS:
fall prevention

EMERGENCY CONTACT:
Name: Parker, Marie
Relationship: Wife
Telephone No. Home: 555-1212 Bus:

ROOM	NAME	PHYSICIAN	ADMITTING DIAGNOSIS/PROBLEM	HOSP. NO.
310	Parker, Edwin	Dr. S Epstein	1. CHF 2. Dementia	1035B

FIGURE 5-2 A sample Kardex.

The nursing process is on-going. New information is gathered and the person's needs may change. However, the steps are the same. You will see how the nursing process is continuous as each step is explained (Fig. 5-3).

You have a key role in the nursing process. Your observations are used for the assessment step. You may help develop the care plan. In the implementation step, you perform tasks in the care plan. Your assignment sheet (p. 51) tells you what to do. Your observations are used for the evaluation step.

Assessment

Assessment involves collecting information about the person. A health history is taken about current and past health problems. The family's health history is important. Information from the doctor is reviewed. So are test results from past medical records.

An RN (registered nurse) assesses the person's body systems and mental status. You assist with assessment. You make many observations as you give care and talk to the person.

Observation *is using the senses of sight, hearing, touch, and smell to collect information.*

- You *see* how the person lies, sits, or walks. You see flushed or pale skin. You see red and swollen body areas.
- You *listen* to the person breathe, talk, and cough. You use a stethoscope to measure blood pressure.
- Through *touch*, you feel if the skin is hot or cold, or moist or dry. You use touch to take the person's pulse.
- *Smell* is used to detect body, wound, and breath odors. You also smell odors from urine and bowel movements.

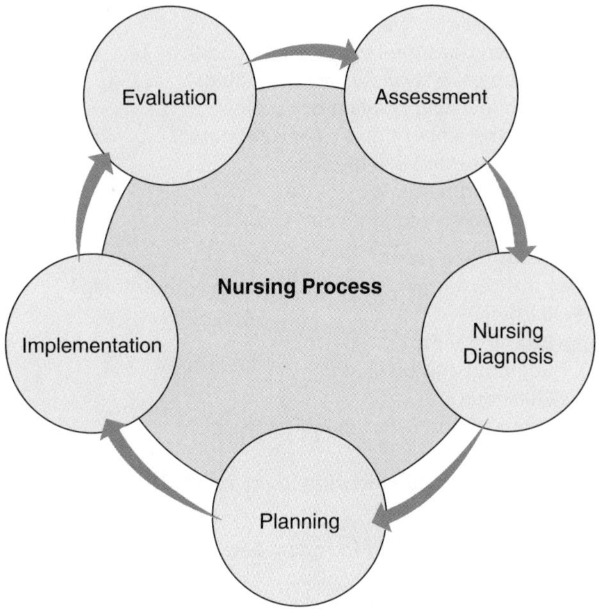

Evaluation → Assessment → Nursing Diagnosis → Planning → Implementation → Evaluation (Nursing Process)

FIGURE 5-3 The nursing process is continuous.

Objective data (signs) *are seen, heard, felt, or smelled by an observer.* You can feel a pulse. You can see urine color. ***Subjective data (symptoms)*** *are things a person tells you about that you cannot observe through your senses.* You cannot feel or see the person's pain, fear, or nausea.

Box 5-1 lists the observations to report at once. Box 5-2, p. 48 lists the observations you need to make and report to the nurse. Make notes of your observations. Use them to report and record observations. Carry a note pad and pen in your pocket. Note your observations as you make them.

The Minimum Data Set. The Omnibus Budget Reconciliation Act of 1987 (OBRA) requires the Minimum Data Set (MDS) for nursing center residents (Appendix D). It provides extensive information about the person. Examples include memory, communication, hearing and vision, physical function, and activities.

The nurse uses your observations to complete the MDS. The MDS is started when the person is admitted to the center. It is updated before each care conference. A new MDS is completed once a year and whenever a significant change occurs in the person's health status.

Nursing Diagnosis

The RN uses assessment information to make a nursing diagnosis. A ***nursing diagnosis*** *describes a health problem that can be treated by nursing measures* (Box 5-3, p. 49). It is different from a *medical diagnosis*—the identification of a disease or condition by a doctor. Cancer, stroke, heart attack, and diabetes are examples of medical diagnoses.

A person can have many nursing diagnoses. They may change as assessment information changes. For example, "Acute pain" is added after surgery.

BOX 5-1 Observations to Report at Once

- A change in the person's ability to respond
  - A responsive person no longer responds.
  - A non-responsive person now responds.
- A change in the person's mobility
  - The person cannot move a body part.
  - The person can now move a body part.
- Complaints of sudden, severe pain
- A sore or reddened area on the person's skin
- Complaints of a sudden change in vision
- Complaints of pain or difficulty breathing
- Abnormal respirations
- Complaints of or signs of difficulty swallowing
- Vomiting
- Bleeding
- Dizziness
- Vital signs outside their normal ranges (temperature, pulse, respirations, and blood pressure)

BOX 5-2 Basic Observations

Ability to Respond
- Is the person easy or hard to wake up?
- Can the person give his or her name, the time, and location when asked?
- Does the person identify others correctly?
- Does the person answer questions correctly?
- Does the person speak clearly?
- Are instructions followed correctly?
- Is the person calm, restless, or excited?
- Is the person conversing, quiet, or talking a lot?

Movement
- Can the person squeeze your fingers with each hand?
- Can the person move arms and legs?
- Are the person's movements shaky or jerky?
- Does the person complain of stiff or painful joints?

Pain or Discomfort
- Where is the pain located? (Ask the person to point to the pain.)
- Does the pain go anywhere else?
- How does the person rate the severity of the pain—mild, moderate, severe?
- How does the person rate the pain on a scale of 0 to 10 (Chapter 15)?
- When did the pain begin?
- What was the person doing when the pain began?
- How long does the pain last?
- How does the person describe the pain?
  - Sharp
  - Severe
  - Knife-like
  - Dull
  - Burning
  - Aching
  - Comes and goes
  - Depends on position
- Was a pain-relief drug given?
- Did the pain-relief drug relieve pain? Is the pain still present?
- Is the person able to sleep and rest?
- What is the position of comfort?

Skin
- Is the skin pale or flushed?
- Is the skin cool, warm, or hot?
- Is the skin moist or dry?
- Does the skin appear mottled (blotchy, spotted with color)?
- What color are the lips and nail beds?
- Is the skin intact? Are there broken areas? If yes, where?
- Are sores or reddened areas present? If yes, where?
- Are bruises present? Where are they located?
- Does the person complain of itching? If yes, where?

Eyes, Ears, Nose, and Mouth
- Is there drainage from the eyes? What color is the drainage?
- Are the eyelids closed? Do they stay open?
- Are the eyes reddened?
- Does the person complain of spots, flashes, or blurring?
- Is the person sensitive to bright lights?
- Is there drainage from the ears? What color is the drainage?

Eyes, Ears, Nose, and Mouth—cont'd
- Can the person hear? Is repeating necessary? Are questions answered appropriately?
- Is there drainage from the nose? What color is the drainage?
- Can the person breathe through the nose?
- Is there breath odor?
- Does the person complain of a bad taste in the mouth?
- Does the person complain of painful gums or teeth?

Respirations
- Do both sides of the person's chest rise and fall with respirations?
- Is breathing noisy?
- Does the person complain of pain or difficulty breathing?
- What is the amount and color of sputum?
- What is the frequency of the person's cough? Is it dry or productive?

Bowels and Bladder
- Is the abdomen firm or soft?
- Does the person complain of gas?
- Which does the person use: toilet, commode, bedpan, or urinal?
- What are the amount, color, and consistency of bowel movements?
- What is the frequency of bowel movements?
- Can the person control bowel movements?
- Does the person have pain or difficulty urinating?
- What is the amount of urine?
- What is the color of urine?
- Is the urine clear? Are there particles in the urine?
- Does urine have a foul smell?
- Can the person control the passage of urine?
- What is the frequency of urination?

Appetite
- Does the person like the food served?
- How much of the meal is eaten?
- What foods does the person like?
- Can the person chew food?
- What is the amount of fluid taken?
- What fluids does the person like?
- How often does the person drink fluids?
- Can the person swallow food and fluids?
- Does the person complain of nausea?
- What is the amount and color of vomitus?
- Does the person have hiccups?
- Is the person belching?
- Does the person cough when swallowing?

Activities of Daily Living
- Can the person perform personal care without help?
  - Bathing?
  - Brushing teeth?
  - Combing and brushing hair?
  - Shaving?
- Does the person feed himself or herself?
- Can the person walk?
- What amount and kind of help are needed?

Bleeding
- Is the person bleeding from any body part? If yes, where and how much?

Planning

Planning *involves setting priorities and goals.* Priorities are what is most important for the person. Goals are aimed at the person's highest level of well-being and function—physical, emotional, social, and spiritual. Goals promote health and prevent health problems.

A *nursing intervention* is an action or measure taken by the nursing team to help the person reach a goal. *Nursing intervention, nursing action,* and *nursing measure* mean the same thing. A nursing intervention does not need a doctor's order.

The ***nursing care plan*** *(care plan) is a written guide about the person's nursing care.* It has the person's nursing diagnoses and goals. It also has measures or actions for each goal. The care plan is a communication tool. Nursing staff use it to see what care to give. The care plan helps ensure that nursing team members give the same care.

Each agency has a care plan form. It is found in the medical record. The plan is carried out. It may change as the person's nursing diagnoses change.

BOX 5-3 Some Nursing Diagnoses Approved by the North American Nursing Diagnosis Association International (NANDA-I)

- Activity Intolerance; Activity Intolerance, Risk for
- Airway Clearance, Ineffective
- Allergy Response, Risk for
- Anxiety
- Aspiration, Risk for
- Bathing Self-Care Deficit
- Bleeding, Risk for
- Blood Glucose Level, Risk for Unstable
- Body Image, Disturbed
- Body Temperature, Risk for Imbalanced
- Breathing Pattern, Ineffective
- Comfort: Impaired, Readiness for Enhanced
- Communication: Impaired Verbal, Readiness for Enhanced
- Confusion: Acute, Chronic, Risk for Acute
- Constipation; Constipation: Perceived, Risk for
- Contamination; Contamination, Risk for
- Coping: Defensive, Ineffective, Readiness for Enhanced
- Death Anxiety
- Decisional Conflict
- Denial, Ineffective
- Dentition, Impaired
- Diarrhea
- Disuse Syndrome, Risk for
- Diversional Activity, Deficient
- Dressing Self-Care Deficit
- Failure to Thrive, Adult
- Falls, Risk for
- Family Coping: Compromised, Disabled, Readiness for Enhanced
- Fatigue
- Fear
- Feeding Self-Care Deficit
- Fluid Balance, Readiness for Enhanced
- Fluid Volume: Deficient, Excess, Risk for Deficient, Risk for Imbalanced
- Grieving; Grieving: Complicated, Risk for Complicated
- Health Behavior, Risk-Prone
- Health Maintenance, Ineffective
- Hopelessness
- Human Dignity, Risk for Compromised
- Incontinence, Bowel
- Incontinence, Urinary: Functional; Overflow; Reflex; Stress; Urge; Urge, Risk for
- Infection, Risk for
- Injury, Risk for
- Insomnia
- Knowledge: Deficient, Readiness for Enhanced
- Latex Allergy Response; Latex Allergy Response, Risk for
- Loneliness, Risk for
- Memory, Impaired
- Mobility: Impaired Bed, Impaired Physical, Impaired Wheelchair
- Nausea
- Nutrition, Imbalanced: Less Than Body Requirements; More Than Body Requirements; More Than Body Requirements, Risk for
- Nutrition, Readiness for Enhanced
- Oral Mucous Membrane, Impaired
- Pain: Acute, Chronic
- Post-Trauma Syndrome; Post-Trauma Syndrome, Risk for
- Powerlessness; Powerlessness, Risk for
- Protection, Ineffective
- Relocation Stress Syndrome; Relocation Stress Syndrome, Risk for
- Self-Care, Readiness for Enhanced
- Self-Esteem: Chronic Low; Chronic Low, Risk for; Situational Low; Situational Low, Risk for
- Self-Neglect
- Sexuality Pattern, Ineffective
- Skin Integrity: Impaired, Risk for Impaired
- Sleep Deprivation
- Sleep Pattern, Disturbed
- Sleep, Readiness for Enhanced
- Social Interaction, Impaired
- Social Isolation
- Sorrow, Chronic
- Spiritual Distress; Spiritual Distress, Risk for
- Stress, Overload
- Suffocation, Risk for
- Suicide, Risk for
- Surgical Recovery, Delayed
- Swallowing, Impaired
- Thermal Injury, Risk for
- Tissue Integrity, Impaired
- Toileting Self-Care Deficit
- Transfer Ability, Impaired
- Trauma, Risk for: Trauma, Risk for Vascular
- Urinary Elimination: Impaired, Readiness for Enhanced
- Urinary Retention
- Violence: Risk for Other-Directed, Risk for Self-Directed
- Walking, Impaired
- Wandering

NANDA International Nursing Diagnoses: Definitions and Classifications 2012–2014; *Herdman T.H. (ED); copyright © 2012, 1994-2012 NANDA International; used by arrangement with John Wiley & Sons, Limited. In order to make safe and effective judgments using NANDA-I nursing diagnoses it is essential that nurses refer to the definitions and defining characteristics of the diagnoses listed in this work.*

Care Conferences. The RN may conduct a care conference to share information and ideas about the person's care. The purpose is to develop or revise the person's nursing care plan. Effective care is the goal. Nursing assistants may take part in the conference.

See *Focus on Communication: Care Conferences.*

The Comprehensive Care Plan. OBRA requires a *comprehensive care plan.* It is a written guide about the person's care. The plan has the person's problems, goals for care, and actions to take.

For example, Mr. Woo is weak from illness and no exercise. The MDS shows that he cannot do activities of daily living (ADL). A care plan is developed to solve the problem. The goal is for Mr. Woo to do his own ADL. Actions to help Mr. Woo reach the goal are:

- Occupational therapy to work with Mr. Woo on ADL daily
- Physical therapy to work with Mr. Woo on exercises daily
- Nursing staff to walk Mr. Woo 20 yards twice daily

The comprehensive care plan also states the person's strengths. For example, Mr. Woo can feed himself. This strength increases his independence. The health team helps Mr. Woo continue to feed himself.

See *Focus on Surveys: The Comprehensive Care Plan.*

FOCUS ON COMMUNICATION

Care Conferences

You see what patients and residents like and do not like. You see what they can and cannot do. Patients and residents talk to you. They tell you about their families and interests. You make observations every time you are with them. Share this information during care conferences. Also share ideas about the person's care. For example, you can say:

- "Mr. Antonio misses the fresh green beans and broccoli from his garden. Can he have those more often?"
- "Mrs. Clark can use her feet to propel her wheelchair. Why do we have to push her wheelchair?"
- "Miss Walsh never talks when her family visits. Yet she talks to her roommate all the time."

FOCUS ON SURVEYS

The Comprehensive Care Plan

During a survey, you may be asked questions about the person's comprehensive care plan. Give honest and complete answers. You may be asked about:

- The person's goals
- Care measures
- How the care measures are carried out
- How you give input about the person's care needs and your observations

Assignment Sheet

Date: 9–10
Shift: Day
Nursing assistant: John Reed
Supervisor: Mary Adams, RN

Breaks: *1000* *1400*
Lunch: *1230*
Unit Tasks: *Pass drinking water at 0900*
Clean utility room at 1430

***Check the care plan for other care measures and information**

	Functional status/other care measures and procedures
Room # 501A Name: Mrs. Ann Lopez ID Number: S1514491530 Date of birth: 11/04/1925 VS: Daily at 0700 T ______ P ______ R ______ BP ______ Wt: Weekly (Monday at 0700) Intake ______ Output ______ BM ______ Bath: Portable tub Shampoo Bed rails	Total assist with ADL Stand-pivot transfers Uses w/c Incontinent of bowel and bladder – uses briefs Bilateral passive ROM exercises to extremities twice daily Turn and re-position q2h when in bed Wears eyeglasses and dentures Diet: High fiber (Total Assist)
Room # 510B Name: Mr. Mark Lee ID Number: D4468947762 Date of birth: 12/29/1926 VS: 2 times daily, at 0700 and 1500 0700: T ______ P ______ R ______ BP ______ 1500: T ______ P ______ R ______ BP ______ Wt: Daily at 0700 Intake ______ Output ______ BM ______ Bath: Shower	**Functional status/other care measures and procedures** Independent with ADL Independent with ambulation Attends exercise group every morning Continent of bowel and bladder – q4h bathroom schedule to maintain continence Wears eyeglasses Coughing and deep breathing exercises q4h Diet: Sodium-controlled (Independent)

FIGURE 5-4 A sample assignment sheet. NOTE: This assignment sheet is a computer printout.

Implementation

To *implement* means *to perform* or *carry out*. The *implementation* step is performing or carrying out nursing measures (interventions) in the care plan. Care is given. The nurse delegates tasks within your legal limits and job description.

Assignment Sheets. The nurse uses an assignment sheet to communicate delegated measures and tasks to you (Fig. 5-4). The assignment sheet tells you about:

- Each person's care.
- What measures and tasks need to be done.
- Which nursing unit tasks to do. Cleaning utility rooms and stocking shower rooms are examples.

Talk to the nurse about an unclear assignment. Also check the care plan and Kardex or care summary if you need more information.

See *Focus on Communication: Assignment Sheets.*

Evaluation

Evaluate means *to measure*. The *evaluation* step involves measuring if the goals in the planning step were met. Progress is evaluated. Changes in nursing diagnoses, goals, and the care plan may result.

FOCUS ON COMMUNICATION

Assignment Sheets

Assignment sheets provide a summary of the information you need to give care. The sheets communicate information clearly and in an organized way. Use your assignment sheet when receiving a report from the nurse. Add any new information. Ask the nurse if you have questions. For example:

I have a question about Mr. Lee. My assignment sheet does not mention any assistive devices. Last week physical therapy was helping him use a walker instead of his cane. Which is he using now?

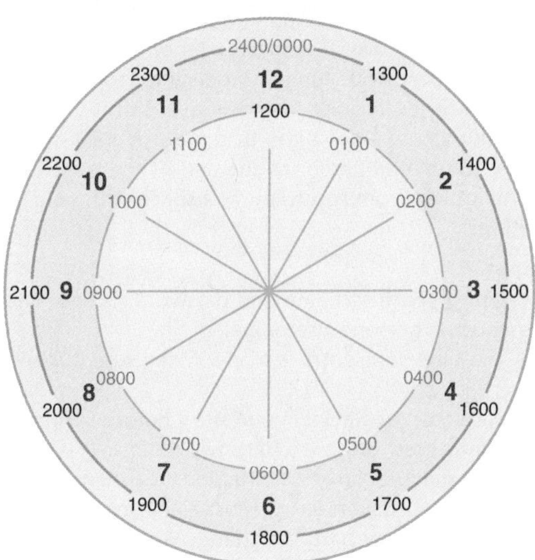

FIGURE 5-5 The 24-hour clock. The AM times are in orange. The PM times are in purple. NOTE: 12 noon is 1200; 12 midnight is 2400 or 0000.

REPORTING AND RECORDING

The health team communicates by reporting and recording. ***Reporting*** *is the oral account of care and observations.* ***Recording*** *(charting) is the written account of care and observations.*

Reporting and Recording Time

The 24-hour clock (military time or international time) has four digits (Fig. 5-5). The first two digits are for the hours: 0100 = 1:00 AM; 1300 = 1:00 PM. The last two digits are for minutes: 0110 = 1:10 AM. Colons and AM and PM are not used.

Box 5-4 shows how "conventional time" is written in "24-hour time." To change conventional time to 24-hour time with 4 digits, do the following:

- When an AM time has 3 digits (from 1:00 AM to 9:59 AM), remove the colon and add 0 as the first digit. For example:
  - Add 0 to 1:00 AM for 0100.
  - Add 0 to 7:30 AM for 0730.
  - Add 0 to 9:59 AM for 0959.
- When an AM or 12:00 PM time has 4 digits (10:00 AM to 12:59 PM), simply remove the colon. For example:
  - 10:00 AM becomes 1000.
  - 11:15 AM becomes 1115.
  - 12:59 PM becomes 1259.
- For PM times, remove the colon and add 1200 to the time. For example:
  - 1:00 PM becomes 1300 by adding 100 and 1200 (100 + 1200 = 1300).
  - 4:30 PM becomes 1630 by adding 430 and 1200 (430 + 1200 = 1630).
  - 10:40 PM becomes 2240 by adding 1040 and 1200 (1040 + 1200 = 2240).

Some agencies use 0000 for midnight. Others use 2400. Follow agency policy.

See *Promoting Safety and Comfort: Reporting and Recording Time*, p. 52.

BOX 5-4 24-Hour Clock

AM		PM	
Conventional Time	24-Hour Time	Conventional Time	24-Hour Time
12:00 MIDNIGHT	0000 or 2400	12:00 NOON	1200
1:00 AM	0100	1:00 PM	1300
2:00 AM	0200	2:00 PM	1400
3:00 AM	0300	3:00 PM	1500
4:00 AM	0400	4:00 PM	1600
5:00 AM	0500	5:00 PM	1700
6:00 AM	0600	6:00 PM	1800
7:00 AM	0700	7:00 PM	1900
8:00 AM	0800	8:00 PM	2000
9:00 AM	0900	9:00 PM	2100
10:00 AM	1000	10:00 PM	2200
11:00 AM	1100	11:00 PM	2300

PROMOTING SAFETY AND COMFORT

Reporting and Recording Time

Safety

Communication is better with the 24-hour clock. You must use AM and PM with conventional time. Someone may forget to use AM or PM. Writing may be unclear. This means that the correct time is not communicated. Harm to the person could result.

Reporting

You report care and observations to the nurse. Report:

- Whenever there is a change from normal or a change in the person's condition. Report these changes at once (see Box 5-1).
- When the nurse asks you to do so.
- When you leave the unit for meals, breaks, or other reasons.
- Before the end-of-shift report.

When reporting, follow the rules in Box 5-5.

End-of-Shift Report. *The nurse gives a report at the end of the shift to the on-coming shift. This is called the* ***end-of-shift report*** *or change-of-shift report.* The nurse reports about:

- The care given
- The care to give during other shifts
- The person's current condition
- Likely changes in the person's condition

In some agencies, the entire nursing team hears the end-of-shift report as they come on duty. In other agencies, only nurses hear the report. After the report, information is shared with nursing assistants.

See *Promoting Safety and Comfort: End-of-Shift Report.*

BOX 5-5 Reporting and Recording

Reporting

- Be prompt, thorough, and accurate.
- Give the person's name and room and bed number.
- Give the time your observations were made or the care was given. Use conventional time (AM or PM) or 24-hour clock time according to agency policy.
- Report only what you observed and did yourself.
- Report care measures that you expect the person to need. For example, the person may need the bedpan during your meal break.
- Report expected changes in the person's condition. For example, the person may be tired after lunch.
- Give reports as often as the person's condition requires. Or give them when the nurse asks you to.
- Report any changes from normal or changes in the person's condition. Report these changes at once.
- Use your written notes to give a specific, concise, and clear report.

Recording

General Rules

- Follow agency policies and procedures for recording. Ask for needed training.
- Include the date and time for every recording. Use conventional time (AM or PM) or 24-hour clock time according to agency policy.
- Use only agency-approved abbreviations (p. 55).
- Use correct spelling, grammar, and punctuation.
- Do not use ditto (//) marks.
- Sign or save all entries as required by agency policy.
- Make sure each form has the person's name and other identifying information.
- Check the name and identifying information on the chart. You must record on the correct chart.
- Record only what you observed and did yourself. Do not record for another person.
- Never chart a procedure, treatment, or care measure until after it is completed.
- Be accurate, concise, and factual. Do not record judgments or interpretations.
- Record in a logical manner and in sequence.

Recording—cont'd

General Rules—cont'd

- Be descriptive. Avoid terms with more than 1 meaning.
- Use the person's exact words whenever possible. Use quotation marks ("...") to show that the statement is a direct quote.
- Chart any changes from normal or changes in the person's condition. Also chart that you told the nurse (include the nurse's name), what you said, and the time you made the report.
- Do not omit information.
- Record safety measures. Examples include placing the call light within reach, assisting the person when up, or reminding a person not to get out of bed.

On Paper

- Always use ink. Use the ink color required by the agency.
- Make sure writing is readable and neat.
- Never erase or use correction fluid. Draw a line through the incorrect part. Date and initial the line. Write "mistaken entry" over it if this is agency policy. Then re-write the part. Follow agency policy for correcting errors.
- Sign your entries. Include your name and title.
- Do not skip lines. Draw a line through the blank space of a partially completed line or to the end of the page. This prevents others from recording in a space with your signature.

On Computer

- Log in using your username and password. Do not chart using another person's username.
- Check the time your entry is made. Make sure it is the right time.
- Check for accuracy. Review your entry before saving.
- Save your entries. Un-saved data will be lost.
- Follow the manufacturer's instructions for changing or un-charting a mistaken entry. Most electronic systems keep a record of an entry before a change was made. The first entry is still visible.
- Log off when done charting. This prevents others from charting under your username.

PROMOTING SAFETY AND COMFORT

End-of-Shift Report

Safety

You may not hear the end-of-shift report as you come on duty. Yet you answer call lights and give care before the nurse shares information with you. For safe care:

- Check the care plan and Kardex or care summary before granting a request. The person's condition or care plan may have changed. There may be new doctor's orders.
- Ask a nurse about the care needs of new patients or residents. If necessary, politely interrupt the end-of-shift report to ask your questions.
- Do not take directions or orders from other nursing assistants. Remember, nursing assistants cannot supervise or delegate to other nursing assistants.

FOCUS ON COMMUNICATION

Recording

"Small," "moderate," "large," "long," and "short" mean different things to different people. Is small the size of a dime or the size of a quarter? Different meanings can cause serious problems. Give accurate descriptions and measurements. If you have a question, ask the nurse to look at what you are trying to describe.

Recording

When making notes on flow sheets or recording on the person's chart, communicate clearly and thoroughly. Follow the rules in Box 5-5. Anyone who reads your notes or charting should know:

- What you observed
- What you did
- The person's response

See *Focus on Communication: Recording.*

MEDICAL TERMS AND ABBREVIATIONS

Medical terms and abbreviations are used in health care. Like all words, medical terms are made up of parts of words or *word elements*—prefixes, roots, and suffixes (Box 5-6, pp. 54-55). Most are from Greek or Latin. They are combined to form medical terms. To translate a term, the word is separated into its elements.

Prefixes, Roots, and Suffixes

A *prefix* is a word element placed before a root. It changes the meaning of the word. The prefix *olig* (scant, small amount) is placed before the root *uria* (urine) to make *oliguria.* It means a scant amount of urine. Prefixes are used with other word elements. Prefixes are never used alone.

The *root* is the word element that contains the basic meaning of the word. It is combined with another root, prefixes, and suffixes. A vowel (an *o* or an *i*) is added when 2 roots are combined or when a suffix is added to a root. The vowel makes the word easier to pronounce.

A *suffix* is a word element placed after a root. It changes the meaning of the word. Suffixes are not used alone. When translating medical terms, begin with the suffix. For example, *nephritis* means inflammation of the kidney. It was formed by combining *nephro* (kidney) and *itis* (inflammation).

Medical terms are formed by combining word elements. Remember, prefixes always come before roots. Suffixes always come after roots. A root can be combined with prefixes, roots, and suffixes. For example:

- The prefix *dys* (difficult) is combined with the root *pnea* (breathing). This forms *dyspnea.* It means difficulty breathing.
- The root *mast* (breast) combined with the suffix *ectomy* (excision or removal) forms *mastectomy.* It means removal of a breast.
- Endocarditis has the prefix *endo* (inner), the root *card* (heart), and the suffix *itis* (inflammation). *Endocarditis* means inflammation of the inner part of the heart.

Directional Terms

Certain terms describe the position of 1 body part in relation to another. These terms give the direction of the body part when a person is standing and facing forward (Fig. 5-6).

- *Anterior (ventral)*—at or toward the front of the body or body part
- *Posterior (dorsal)*—at or toward the back of the body or body part
- *Proximal*—the part nearest to the center or to the point of attachment
- *Distal*—the part farthest from the center or from the point of attachment
- *Lateral*—away from the mid-line; at the side of the body or body part
- *Medial*—at or near the middle or mid-line of the body or body part

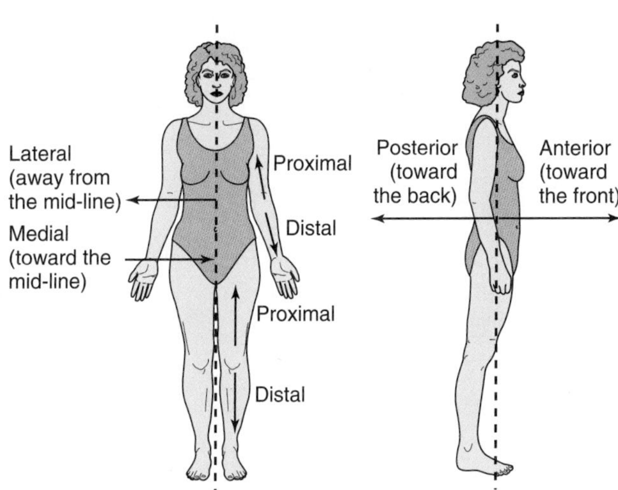

FIGURE 5-6 Directional terms describe the position of 1 part of the body in relation to another.

BOX 5-6 Medical Terminology

Prefix	Meaning
a-, an-	without, not, lack of
ab-	away from
ad-	to, toward, near
ante-	before, forward, in front of
anti-	against
auto-	self
bi-	double, two, twice
brady-	slow
circum-	around
contra-	against, opposite
de-	down, from
dia-	across, through, apart
dis-	apart, free from
dys-	bad, difficult, abnormal
ecto-	outer, outside
en-	in, into, within
endo-	inner, inside
epi-	over, on, upon
eryth-	red
eu-	normal, good, well, healthy
ex-	out, out of, from, away from
hemi-	half
hyper-	excessive, too much, high
hypo-	under, decreased, less than normal
in-	in, into, within, not
inter-	between
intra-	within
intro-	into, within
leuk-	white
macro-	large
mal-	bad, illness, disease
meg-	large
micro-	small
mono-	one, single
neo-	new
non-	not
olig-	small, scant
para-	beside, beyond, after
per-	by, through
peri-	around
poly-	many, much
post-	after, behind
pre-	before, in front of, prior to
pro-	before, in front of
re-	again, backward
retro-	backward, behind
semi-	half
sub-	under, beneath
super-	above, over, excess
supra-	above, over
tachy-	fast, rapid
trans-	across
uni-	one

Root (Combining Vowel)	Meaning
abdomin (o)	abdomen
aden (o)	gland
adren (o)	adrenal gland
angi (o)	vessel
arteri (o)	artery
arthr (o)	joint
bronch (o)	bronchus, bronchi
card, cardi (o)	heart
cephal (o)	head
chole, chol (o)	bile
chondr (o)	cartilage
colo	colon, large intestine
cost (o)	rib
crani (o)	skull
cyan (o)	blue
cyst (o)	bladder, cyst
cyt (o)	cell
dent (o)	tooth
derma	skin
duoden (o)	duodenum
encephal (o)	brain
enter (o)	intestines
fibr (o)	fiber, fibrous
gastr (o)	stomach
gloss (o)	tongue
gluc (o)	sweetness, glucose
glyc (o)	sugar
gyn, gyne, gyneco	woman
hem, hema, hemo, hemat (o)	blood
hepat (o)	liver
hydr (o)	water
hyster (o)	uterus
ile (o), ili (o)	ileum
laparo	abdomen, loin, flank
laryng (o)	larynx
lith (o)	stone
mamm (o)	breast, mammary gland
mast (o)	mammary gland, breast
meno	menstruation
my (o)	muscle
myel (o)	spinal cord, bone marrow
necro	death
nephr (o)	kidney
neur (o)	nerve
ocul (o)	eye
oophor (o)	ovary
ophthalm (o)	eye
orth (o)	straight, normal, correct
oste (o)	bone
ot (o)	ear
ped (o)	child, foot
pharyng (o)	pharynx
phleb (o)	vein
pnea	breathing, respiration
pneum (o)	lung, air, gas
proct (o)	rectum
psych (o)	mind
pulmo	lung
py (o)	pus
rect (o)	rectum
rhin (o)	nose
salping (o)	eustachian tube, fallopian tube
splen (o)	spleen
sten (o)	narrow, constriction
stern (o)	sternum
stomat (o)	mouth
therm (o)	heat

BOX 5-6 Medical Terminology—cont'd

Root (Combining Vowel)	Meaning
thoraco	chest
thromb (o)	clot, thrombus
thyr (o)	thyroid
toxic (o)	poison, poisonous
toxo	poison
trache (o)	trachea
urethr (o)	urethra
urin (o)	urine
uro	urine, urinary tract, urination
uter (o)	uterus
vas (o)	blood vessel, vas deferens
ven (o)	vein
vertebr (o)	spine, vertebrae

Suffix	Meaning
-algia	pain
-asis	condition, usually abnormal
-cele	hernia, herniation, pouching
-centesis	puncture and aspiration of
-cyte	cell
-ectasis	dilation, stretching
-ectomy	excision, removal of
-emia	blood condition
-genesis	development, production, creation
-genic	producing, causing
-gram	record
-graph	a diagram, a recording instrument
-graphy	making a recording
-iasis	condition of
-ism	a condition
-itis	inflammation
-logy	the study of
-lysis	destruction of, decomposition
-megaly	enlargement
-meter	measuring instrument
-oma	tumor
-osis	condition
-pathy	disease
-penia	lack, deficiency
-phagia	to eat or consume, swallowing
-phasia	speaking
-phobia	an exaggerated fear
-plasty	surgical repair or re-shaping
-plegia	paralysis
-ptosis	falling, sagging, dropping down
-rrhage, rrhagia	excessive flow
-rrhaphy	stitching, suturing
-rrhea	flow, discharge
-scope	examination instrument
-scopy	examination using a scope
-stasis	maintenance, maintaining a constant level
-stomy, -ostomy	creation of an opening
-tomy, -otomy	incision, cutting into
-uria	condition of the urine

Abbreviations

Abbreviations are shortened forms of words or phrases. They save time and space when recording. Each agency has a list of accepted abbreviations. Obtain the list when you are hired. Use only those on the list. If not sure about using an abbreviation, write the term out in full. This promotes accurate communication.

Common abbreviations are listed on the inside of the back cover for easy use.

COMPUTERS AND OTHER ELECTRONIC DEVICES

Computer systems collect, send, record, and store information (data). Many agencies store charts and care plans on computers. Entering data on a computer is often easier and faster than paper charting.

Computers and faxes are used to send messages and reports to the nursing unit. This reduces clerical work and phone calls. And data are sent with greater speed and accuracy.

Computers and other electronic devices save time. Quality care and safety are increased. Fewer errors are made in recording. Records are more complete. Staff is more efficient.

Each staff member using computers and other electronic devices is issued a username and password. They are used to access, send, receive, or store protected health information (PHI).

You must follow the agency's policies when using computers and other electronic devices. You must keep PHI and electronic protected health information (EPHI, ePHI) confidential. Follow the rules in Box 5-7, p. 56 and the ethical and legal rules about privacy, confidentiality, and defamation (Chapters 3 and 4).

PHONE COMMUNICATIONS

You will answer phones at the nurses' station or in the person's room. You need good communication skills. The caller cannot see you. But you give much information by your tone of voice, how clearly you speak, and your attitude. Act as if speaking to someone face-to-face. Be professional and courteous. Also practice good work ethics. Follow the agency's policy and the guidelines in Box 5-8, p. 56.

DEALING WITH CONFLICT

People bring their values, attitudes, opinions, experiences, and expectations to the work setting. Differences often lead to *conflict—a clash between opposing interests or ideas.* People disagree and argue. There are misunderstandings and unrest.

Conflicts arise over issues or events. Work schedules, absences, and the amount and quality of work performed are examples. The problems must be worked out. Otherwise, unkind words or actions may occur. The work setting becomes unpleasant. Care is affected.

BOX 5-7 Computers and Other Electronic Devices

Computers

- Do not tell anyone your username or password. If someone has your information, he or she can access, record, send, receive, or store EPHI (ePHI) under your name. It will be hard to prove that someone else did so and not you.
- Do not write down, post, or expose your username or password. This is for your security. For example, do not write them on a note pad or post them at your work station.
- Change your password often. Follow agency policy.
- Do not use another person's username or password.
- Follow the rules for recording (see Box 5-5).
- Enter data carefully. Double-check your entries.
- Prevent others from seeing what is on the screen:
  - Position the monitor so the screen cannot be seen in the hallway or by others.
  - Be aware of anyone standing behind you.
  - Stand or sit with your back to the wall if using a mobile computer unit.
  - Do not leave the computer unattended.
- Log off after making an entry.
- Do not leave printouts where others can read them or pick them up.
- Shred or destroy computer-printed documents or worksheets. Follow agency policy.
- Send e-mail and messages only to those needing the information.
- Do not use e-mail for information or messages that require immediate reporting. Give the report in person. The person may not read the e-mail in a timely manner.
- Do not use e-mail or messages to report confidential information. This includes addresses, phone numbers, Social Security numbers, and insurance numbers. The computer system may not be secure.
- Remember that any communication can be read or heard by someone other than the intended person.
- Remember that deleted communications can be retrieved by authorized staff.

Computers—cont'd

- Do not use the agency's computer for your personal use. Do not:
  - Send personal e-mail messages.
  - Send or receive e-mail or messages that are offensive, not legal, or sexual.
  - Send or receive e-mail for illegal activities, jokes, politics, gambling (including football and other pools), chain letters, or other non-work activities.
  - Post information, opinions, or comments on Internet message boards or social networking sites (Twitter, Facebook, MySpace, and others).
  - Take part in Internet discussion groups.
  - Upload, download, or send materials containing a copyright, trademark, or patent.
- Remember that the agency has the right to monitor your use of computers or other electronic devices. This includes Internet use.
- Do not open another person's e-mail or messages.
- Follow agency policy for mis-directed e-mails.

Faxes

- Use the agency's approved "cover sheet." The sheet has instructions about:
  - The confidentiality of PHI (EPHI; ePHI)
  - The receiver's responsibilities concerning PHI (EPHI; ePHI)
  - The receiver's responsibilities if the fax is received in error (mis-directed fax)
- Complete the "cover sheet" according to agency policy. The following is common.
  - Name of the person to receive the fax
  - Receiver's fax number
  - Date
  - Number of pages being faxed
  - Department name
  - Name and phone number of the employee sending the fax
- Follow agency policy for a mis-directed fax.
- Do not leave sent or received faxes unattended in the fax machine or lying around.

BOX 5-8 Answering Phones

- Answer the call after the first ring if possible. Be sure to answer by the fourth ring.
- Do not answer the phone in a rushed or hasty manner.
- Give a courteous greeting. Identify the nursing unit, and give your name and title. For example, "Good morning, Three center. Mark Wills, nursing assistant."
- Write this information when taking a message.
  - The caller's name and phone number (include the area code and extension number)
  - The date and time
  - The message
- Repeat the message and phone number back to the caller.
- Ask the caller to "Please hold" if necessary. First find out who is calling and the caller's number. Then ask if the caller can hold. Do not put callers with an emergency on hold.
- Do not lay the phone down or cover the receiver with your hand when not speaking to the caller. The caller may over-hear confidential conversations.
- Return to a caller on hold within 30 seconds. Ask if the caller can wait longer or if the call can be returned.
- Do not give confidential information to any caller. Patient, resident, and employee information is confidential. Refer such calls to the nurse.
- Transfer the call if appropriate.
  - Tell the caller that you are going to transfer the call.
  - Give the name of the department or the person's name who should answer if appropriate.
  - Get the caller's name and number in case the call gets disconnected.
  - Give the caller the phone number in case the call gets disconnected or the line is busy.
- End the conversation politely. Thank the person for calling, and say good-bye.
- Give the message to the appropriate person.

Resolving Conflict

To resolve conflict, identify the real problem. This is part of *problem solving*. The problem solving process involves these steps.

- Step 1: Define the problem. *A nurse ignores me.*
- Step 2: Collect information about the problem. Do not include unrelated information. *The nurse does not look at me. The nurse does not talk to me. The nurse does not respond when I ask for help. The nurse does not ask me to help with tasks that require 2 people. The nurse talks to other staff members.*
- Step 3: Identify possible solutions. *Ignore the nurse. Talk to my supervisor. Talk to co-workers about the problem. Change jobs.*
- Step 4: Select the best solution. *Talk to my supervisor.*
- Step 5: Carry out the solution. *See below.*
- Step 6: Evaluate the results. *See below.*

Communication and good work ethics help prevent and resolve conflicts. Identify and solve problems before they become major issues. To deal with conflict:

- Ask your supervisor for some time to talk privately. Explain the problem. Give facts and specific examples. Ask for advice in solving the problem.
- Approach the person with whom you have the conflict. Ask to talk privately. Be polite and professional.
- Agree on a time and place to talk.
- Talk in a private setting. No one should hear you or the other person.
- Explain the problem and what is bothering you. Give facts and specific behaviors. Focus on the problem. Do not focus on the person.
- Listen to the person. Do not interrupt.
- Identify ways to solve the problem. Offer your thoughts. Ask for the co-worker's ideas.
- Set a date and time to review the matter.
- Thank the person for meeting with you.
- Carry out the solution.
- Review the matter as scheduled.

See *Focus on Communication: Resolving Conflict.*

FOCUS ON COMMUNICATION

Resolving Conflict

You may find it hard to talk to someone with whom you have a conflict. This is hard for many people. However, letting the problem or issue continue only makes the matter worse. The following may help you start talking to the person.

- "You say 'no' when I ask you to help me. I help you when you ask me to. This really bothers me. Can we talk privately for a few minutes?"
- "I heard you tell John that you saw me sitting in Mrs. Gordon's room. You seemed angry when you said it. Can we talk privately? I want to explain why I was sitting and find out why that bothers you."
- "The new schedule shows me working every weekend this month. Please tell me why. The employee handbook says that we work every other weekend."

FOCUS ON PRIDE

The Person, Family, and Yourself

Personal and Professional Responsibility

You are responsible for the information you report and record. It must be accurate. False or incomplete information can harm the person. If your agency allows you to chart:

- Chart what you do. If not charted, there is no proof that you completed a task.
- Never falsify charting. Never chart that something was done when it really was not.
- Only chart after completing a delegated task. If events change, your charting is wrong.
- Ask the nurse if you have questions about what or how to chart.

Rights and Respect

Conflict among co-workers will arise. Dealing with conflict can be hard. But, it must be addressed. Deal with conflict in a respectful and mature way. Do not gossip, put others down, or talk about people behind their backs. These are not professional behaviors.

Everyone, including you, deserves to be treated with respect. If you feel someone has wronged you, address the issue. Politely ask to talk to the person in private. Speak calmly and respectfully. Focus on the problem and the solution. Do not attack the person's character. For example, do not say: "You are so mean. I can't believe you were talking about me behind my back." Instead, you can say: "It bothers me that you didn't come to me about this. Next time could you talk to me first?" For good working relationships, identify and resolve the conflict in a respectful and professional manner.

Independence and Social Interaction

Communication with the health team is not limited to reporting and recording. You also interact in the nurses' station, hallways, break room, cafeteria, parking lot, and so on. Your informal interactions carry over into working relationships. Treat co-workers with kindness and respect. Have a good attitude. Be someone others enjoy working with!

Delegation and Teamwork

You are responsible for your speech, actions, and charting. This is called being accountable. For example, you are delegated a task. You must complete the task and report or record its completion. If the task was not done, you must tell the nurse why.

Do not be offended when asked if you completed a task or charted. This is part of accountability. The delegating nurse must know what was done and what was not done. Show you are accountable by:

- Completing tasks in a timely manner
- Recording accurately
- Reporting when you complete a task
- Telling the nurse if a task was not done and why

Ethics and Laws

Assignment sheets contain confidential information. Keep your sheets with you at all times. Do not leave them lying around for others to find. This violates the Health Insurance Portability and Accountability Act of 1996 (Chapter 3). Before leaving work, place your assignment sheets in a wastebasket marked CONFIDENTIAL INFORMATION for shredding. Take pride in protecting the privacy and security of protected health information.

REVIEW QUESTIONS

Circle T if the statement is TRUE and F if it is FALSE.

1 **T F** You help with Mrs. Gordon's care. Reading her medical record violates her right to privacy.

2 **T F** You can access all records in the agency.

3 **T F** When using a computer, the person's privacy must be protected.

4 **T F** All employees have the same password for computer use.

5 **T F** You can give information about the person over the phone.

6 **T F** You should leave faxes in the fax machine for the nurse to read.

Circle the BEST answer.

7 To communicate well, you should
- a Use terms with many meanings
- b Give long descriptions
- c Use unfamiliar terms
- d Give facts and be specific

8 What happens during assessment?
- a Goals are set.
- b Information is collected.
- c Nursing measures are carried out.
- d Progress is evaluated.

9 Which is a symptom?
- a Redness
- b Vomiting
- c Pain
- d Pulse rate of 78

10 Which should you report at once?
- a The person had a bowel movement.
- b The person complains of sudden, severe pain.
- c The person does not like the food served.
- d The person complains of stiff, painful joints.

11 The nursing care plan is
- a Written by the doctor
- b The nursing measures to help the person
- c The same for all persons
- d Also called the Kardex

12 To communicate delegated tasks to you, the nurse uses
- a The care plan
- b The Kardex
- c An assignment sheet
- d Care conferences

13 These statements are about recording. Which is *false?*
- a Use the person's exact words when possible.
- b Record only what you did and observed.
- c Sign your initials to a mistaken entry.
- d Chart a procedure before completing it.

14 In the evening the clock shows 9:26. In 24-hour time this is
- a 9:26 PM
- b 1926
- c 0926
- d 2126

15 A suffix is
- a Placed at the beginning of a word
- b Placed after a root
- c A shortened form of a word or phrase
- d The main meaning of the word

16 Which word means a blood condition involving too much sugar?
- a Hepat-itis
- b Tachy-cardia
- c Hyper-glyc-emia
- d A-phasia

17 You are asked to complete a task *stat.* Stat means
- a At once, immediately
- b As desired
- c Without moving the person
- d When necessary, as needed

18 Which term relates to the side of the body?
- a Anterior
- b Lateral
- c Posterior
- d Proximal

19 You have access to the agency's computer. Which is *true?*
- a E-mail and messages are sent only to those needing the information.
- b E-mail is used for reports the nurse needs at once.
- c You can open another person's e-mail.
- d You can use the computer for your personal needs.

20 You answer a person's phone in a nursing center. How should you answer?
- a "Good morning. Mrs. Park's room."
- b "Good morning. Third floor."
- c "Hello."
- d "Good morning. Tammy Brown, nursing assistant, speaking."

21 You have extra work because a co-worker is often late for work. To resolve the conflict
- a Explain the problem to your supervisor
- b Discuss the matter during the end-of-shift report
- c Ignore the problem
- d Complain about the person to co-workers

Answers to these questions are on p. 504.

FOCUS ON PRACTICE

Problem Solving

A resident complains of nausea. You measure the resident's vital signs and report to the nurse. What do you record in the person's chart? What rules must you follow when reporting and recording? You made a mistake while recording. How do you correct the error?

CHAPTER 6

Understanding the Person

OBJECTIVES

- Define the key terms listed in this chapter.
- Identify the parts that make up the whole person.
- Explain how to properly address the person.
- Explain Abraham Maslow's theory of basic needs.
- Explain how culture and religion influence health and illness.
- Explain how to deal with behavior issues.
- Identify the elements needed for good communication.
- Describe how to use verbal and nonverbal communication.
- Explain the methods and barriers to good communication.
- Explain how to communicate with persons who have behavioral problems.
- Explain why family and visitors are important to the person.
- Identify courtesies given to the person, family, and friends.
- Explain how to promote PRIDE in the person, the family, and yourself.

KEY TERMS

body language Messages sent through facial expressions, gestures, posture, hand and body movements, gait, eye contact, and appearance

comatose Being unable to respond to stimuli

culture The characteristics of a group of people—language, values, beliefs, habits, likes, dislikes, customs—passed from one generation to the next

disability Any lost, absent, or impaired physical or mental function

holism A concept that considers the whole person; the whole person has physical, social, psychological, and spiritual parts that are woven together and cannot be separated

need Something necessary or desired for maintaining life and mental well-being

nonverbal communication Communication that does not use words

religion Spiritual beliefs, needs, and practices

verbal communication Communication that uses written or spoken words

The patient or resident is the most important person in the agency. Each person has value. Each has needs, fears, and rights. Each has suffered losses—loss of home, family, friends, and body functions.

CARING FOR THE PERSON

Holism means *whole*. ***Holism*** *is a concept that considers the whole person. The whole person has physical, social, psychological, and spiritual parts. These parts are woven together and cannot be separated* (Fig. 6-1).

Each part relates to and depends on the others. As a social being, a person speaks and communicates with others. Physically, the brain, mouth, tongue, lips, and throat structures must function for speech. Communication is also psychological. It involves thinking and reasoning.

To consider only the physical part is to ignore the person's ability to think, make decisions, and interact with others. It also ignores the person's experiences, life-style, culture, religion, joys, sorrows, and needs.

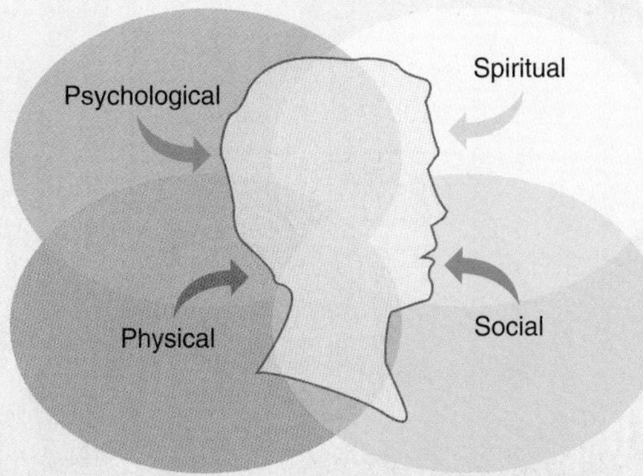

FIGURE 6-1 A person is a physical, psychological, social, and spiritual being. The parts overlap and cannot be separated.

Addressing the Person

You must know and respect the whole person for effective, quality care. Too often a person is referred to as a room number. For example: "12A needs the bedpan" rather than "Mrs. Brown in 12A needs the bedpan."

To address patients and residents with dignity and respect:

- Use their titles—Mrs. Jones, Mr. Smith, Miss Turner, Ms. Beal, or Dr. Gonzalez.
- Do not call them by their first names unless they ask you to.
- Do not call them by any other name unless they ask you to.
- Do not call them Grandma, Papa, Sweetheart, Honey, or other names.

BASIC NEEDS

A ***need*** *is something necessary or desired for maintaining life and mental well-being.* According to psychologist Abraham Maslow, basic needs must be met for a person to survive and function. These needs are arranged in order of importance (Fig. 6-2). Lower-level needs must be met before the higher-level needs. Basic needs, from the lowest level to the highest level, are:

- *Physical needs.* Oxygen, food, water, elimination, rest, and shelter are needed for life and to survive. A person dies within minutes without oxygen. Without food or water, a person feels weak and ill within a few hours. The kidneys and intestines must function. Otherwise, poisonous wastes build up in the blood and can cause death. Without enough rest and sleep, a person becomes very tired. Without shelter, the person is exposed to extremes of heat and cold.

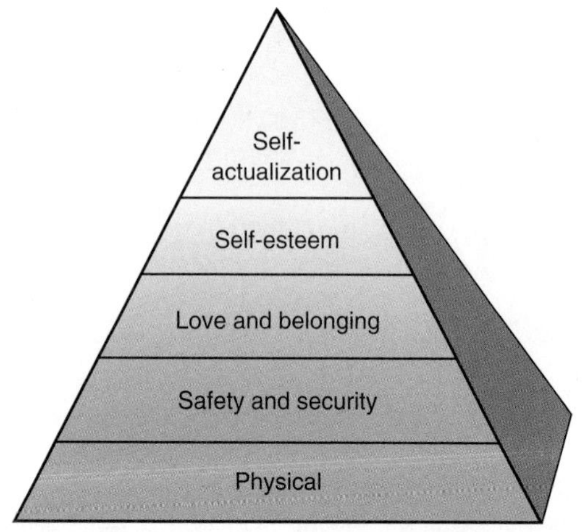

FIGURE 6-2 Basic needs for life as described by Maslow.

- *Safety and security needs.* The person needs to feel safe from harm, danger, and fear. Health care agencies are strange places with strange routines and equipment. Some care causes pain or discomfort. People feel safe and more secure if they know what will happen. For every task, the person should know:
  - Why it is needed
  - Who will do it
  - How it will be done
  - What sensations or feelings to expect
- *Love and belonging needs.* These needs relate to love, closeness, affection, and meaningful relationships with others. Some people become weaker or die from the lack of love and belonging. This is seen in older persons who have out-lived family and friends.
- *Self-esteem needs. Self-esteem* means *to think well of oneself and to see oneself as useful and having value.* People often lack self-esteem when ill, injured, older, or disabled.
- *The need for self-actualization. Self-actualization* means *experiencing one's potential.* It involves learning, understanding, and creating to the limit of a person's capacity. This is the highest need. Rarely, if ever, is it totally met. Most people constantly try to learn and understand more. This need can be postponed and life will continue.

CULTURE AND RELIGION

Culture *is the characteristics of a group of people—language, values, beliefs, habits, likes, dislikes, and customs. They are passed from one generation to the next.* The person's culture influences health beliefs and practices. Culture also affects thinking and behavior during illness.

People come from many cultures, races, and nationalities. Their family practices and food choices may differ from yours. So might their hygiene habits and clothing styles. Some speak a foreign language. Some cultures have beliefs about what causes and cures illness. (See *Caring About Culture: Health Care Beliefs.*) They may perform rituals to rid the body of disease. (See *Caring About Culture: Sick Care Practices.*) Many cultures have health beliefs and rituals about dying and death (Chapter 32). Culture also is a factor in communication.

Religion *relates to spiritual beliefs, needs, and practices.* Religions may have beliefs about daily living, behaviors, relationships with others, diet, healing, days of worship, birth and birth control, drugs, and death.

Many people find comfort and strength from religion during illness. They may want to pray and observe religious practices. Assist the person to attend services as needed.

A person may not follow all the beliefs and practices of his or her culture or religion. Some people do not practice a religion. Each person is unique. Do not judge the person by your standards. And do not force your ideas on the person.

See *Focus on Communication: Culture and Religion.*

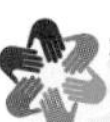

CARING ABOUT CULTURE

Health Care Beliefs

Some *Mexican Americans* believe that illness is caused by prolonged exposure to hot or cold. If hot causes illness, cold is used for cure. Likewise, hot is used for illnesses caused by cold. Hot and cold are found in body organs, medicines (drugs), the air, and food. Hot conditions include fever, infection, rashes, sore throat, diarrhea, and constipation. Cold conditions include cancer, joint pain, earache, and stomach cramps.

The hot-cold balance is also a belief of some *Vietnamese Americans.* Illnesses, food, drugs, and herbs are hot or cold. Hot is given to balance cold illnesses. Cold is given for hot illnesses.

Modified from Giger JN: Transcultural nursing: assessment and intervention, *ed 6, St Louis, 2013, Mosby.*

CARING ABOUT CULTURE

Sick Care Practices

Folk practices are common among some *Vietnamese Americans.* They include *cao gio* ("rub wind")—rubbing the skin with a coin to treat the common cold. Skin pinching (*bat gio*—"catch wind") is for headaches and sore throats. Herbs, oils, and soups are used for many signs and symptoms.

Some *Russian Americans* practice folk medicine. Herbs are taken through drinks or enemas. For headaches, an ointment is placed behind the ears and temples and at the back of the neck. Treatment for back pain involves placing a dough of dark rye flour and honey on the spine.

Some *Mexican Americans* use folk healers. They may or may not be family members. A *yerbero* uses herbs and spices to prevent or cure disease. A *curandero* (*curandera* if female) deals with serious physical and mental illnesses. Witches use magic. A *brujos* is a male witch. A *brujas* is a female witch.

Modified from Giger JN: Transcultural nursing: assessment and intervention, *ed 6, St Louis, 2013, Mosby.*

FOCUS ON COMMUNICATION

Culture and Religion

Hospitals and nursing centers ask about culture and religion on admission. The care plan communicates practices to include in the person's care. Check the care plan for the person's preferences. You can also ask: "Do you have any cultural or religious practices that should be included in your care?"

BEHAVIOR ISSUES

People do not choose illness, injury, or disability. A ***disability*** *is any lost, absent, or impaired physical or mental function.* It may be temporary or permanent.

Many people accept illness, injury, and disability. Others do not adjust well. They have some of the following behaviors. These behaviors are new for some people. For others, they are life-long. They are part of one's personality.

- *Anger.* Anger is a common emotion. Causes include fear, pain, and dying and death. Loss of function and loss of control over health and life are causes. Anger is a symptom of some diseases that affect thinking and behavior. Some people are generally angry. Anger is communicated verbally and nonverbally. Verbal outbursts, shouting, raised voices, and rapid speech are common. Some people are silent. Others are not cooperative. They may refuse to answer questions. Nonverbal signs include rapid movements, pacing, clenched fists, and a red face. Glaring and getting close to you when speaking are other signs. Violent behaviors can occur.
- *Demanding behavior.* Nothing seems to please the person. The person is critical of others. He or she wants care given at a certain time and in a certain way. Loss of independence, loss of health, and loss of control of life are causes. So are unmet needs.
- *Self-centered behavior.* The person cares only about his or her own needs. The needs of others are ignored. The person demands the time and attention of others. The person becomes impatient if needs are not met.
- *Aggressive behavior.* The person may swear, bite, hit, pinch, scratch, or kick. Fear, anger, pain, and dementia (Chapter 30) are causes. Protect the person, others, and yourself from harm (Chapter 9).
- *Withdrawal.* The person has little or no contact with family, friends, and staff. He or she spends time alone and does not take part in social or group activities. This may signal physical illness or depression. Some people are not social. They prefer to be alone.
- *Inappropriate sexual behavior.* Some people make inappropriate sexual remarks. Or they touch others in the wrong way. Some disrobe or masturbate in public. These behaviors may be on purpose. Or they are caused by disease, confusion, dementia, or drug side effects.

Some behaviors are not pleasant. You cannot avoid the person or lose control. Good communication is needed. Behaviors are addressed in the care plan. The care plan may include some of the guidelines in Box 6-1, p. 62.

See *Focus on Communication: Behavior Issues*, p. 62.

BOX 6-1 Dealing With Behavior Issues

- Recognize frustrating and frightening situations. How would you feel in the person's situation? How would you want to be treated?
- Treat the person with dignity and respect.
- Answer questions clearly and thoroughly. Ask the nurse to answer questions you cannot answer.
- Keep the person informed. Tell the person what you are going to do and when.
- Do not keep the person waiting. Answer call lights promptly. If you tell the person that you will do something for him or her, do it promptly.
- Explain the reason for long waits. Ask how you can increase the person's comfort.
- Stay calm and professional, especially if the person is angry or hostile. Often the person is not angry with you. He or she is angry with another person or situation.
- Do not argue with the person.
- Listen and use silence (p. 66). The person may feel better if able to express feelings.
- Protect yourself from violent behaviors (Chapter 9).
- Report the person's behavior to the nurse. Discuss how to deal with the person.

FOCUS ON COMMUNICATION

Behavior Issues

Anger is a common response to illness and disability. Patients and residents may be angry with their situation. A person may direct anger at you. You might have problems dealing with the person's anger. You must continue to act in a professional manner. Remain calm. Do not yell at or insult the person. Listen to his or her concerns. Provide needed care. Try not to take his or her statements personally. If a person says hurtful things, you can kindly say: "Please don't say those things. I'm trying to help you." Tell the nurse about the person's behavior.

Caring for demanding or angry persons can be hard. Ask the nurse or co-workers to help if needed.

COMMUNICATING WITH THE PERSON

You communicate with the person. You give information to the person. The person gives information to you. For effective communication between you and the person, you must:

- Follow the rules of communication (Chapter 5).
  - Use words that have the same meaning for you and the person.
  - Avoid medical terms and words not familiar to the person.
  - Communicate in a logical and orderly manner. Do not wander in thought.
  - Give facts and be specific.
  - Be brief and concise.
- Understand and respect the patient or resident as a person.
- View the person as a physical, psychological, social, and spiritual human being.
- Appreciate the person's problems and frustrations.
- Respect the person's rights, religion, and culture.
- Give the person time to understand the information that you give.
- Repeat information as often as needed. Repeat what you said. Use the exact same words. Do not give the person a new message to process. If the person does not seem to understand after repeating, try re-phrasing the message. This is very important for persons with hearing problems.
- Ask questions to see if the person understood you.
- Be patient. People with memory problems may ask the same question many times. Do not say that you are repeating information.
- Include the person in conversations when others are present. This includes when a co-worker is assisting with care.

See *Focus on Older Persons: Communicating With the Person.*

FOCUS ON OLDER PERSONS

Communicating With the Person

Communicating with persons who have dementia is often hard. The Alzheimer's Disease Education and Referral Center (ADEAR) recommends the following.

- Gain the person's attention before speaking. Call the person by name.
- Choose simple words and short sentences.
- Use a gentle, calm voice.
- Do not talk to the person as you would a baby.
- Do not talk about the person as if he or she is not there.
- Keep distractions and noise to a minimum.
- Help the person focus on what you are saying.
- Allow the person time to respond. Do not interrupt him or her.
- Try to provide the word the person is struggling to find.
- State questions and instructions in a positive way.

Verbal Communication

***Verbal communication** uses written or spoken words.* You talk to the person. You share information and find out how the person feels. Most verbal communication involves the spoken word. Follow these rules.

- Face the person. Look directly at the person.
- Position yourself at the person's eye level. Sit or squat by the person as needed.
- Control the loudness and tone of your voice.
- Speak clearly, slowly, and distinctly.
- Do not use slang or vulgar words.
- Repeat information as needed.
- Ask 1 question at a time. Wait for an answer.
- Do not shout, whisper, or mumble.
- Be kind, courteous, and friendly.

You use the written word when the person cannot speak or hear but can read. The nurse and care plan tell you how to communicate with the person. The devices in Figure 6-3 are often used. The person may have poor vision. When writing messages:

- Keep them simple and brief.
- Use a black felt pen on white paper.
- Print in large letters.

Some persons cannot speak or read. Ask questions that have "yes" or "no" answers. The person can nod, blink, or use other gestures for "yes" and "no." Follow the care plan. Persons who are deaf may use sign language. See Chapter 28.

Nonverbal Communication

***Nonverbal communication** does not use words.* Messages are sent with gestures, facial expressions, posture, body movements, touch, and smell. Nonverbal messages more accurately reflect a person's feelings than words do. They are usually involuntary and hard to control. A person may say one thing but act another way. Watch the person's eyes, hand movements, gestures, posture, and other actions. Sometimes they tell you more than words.

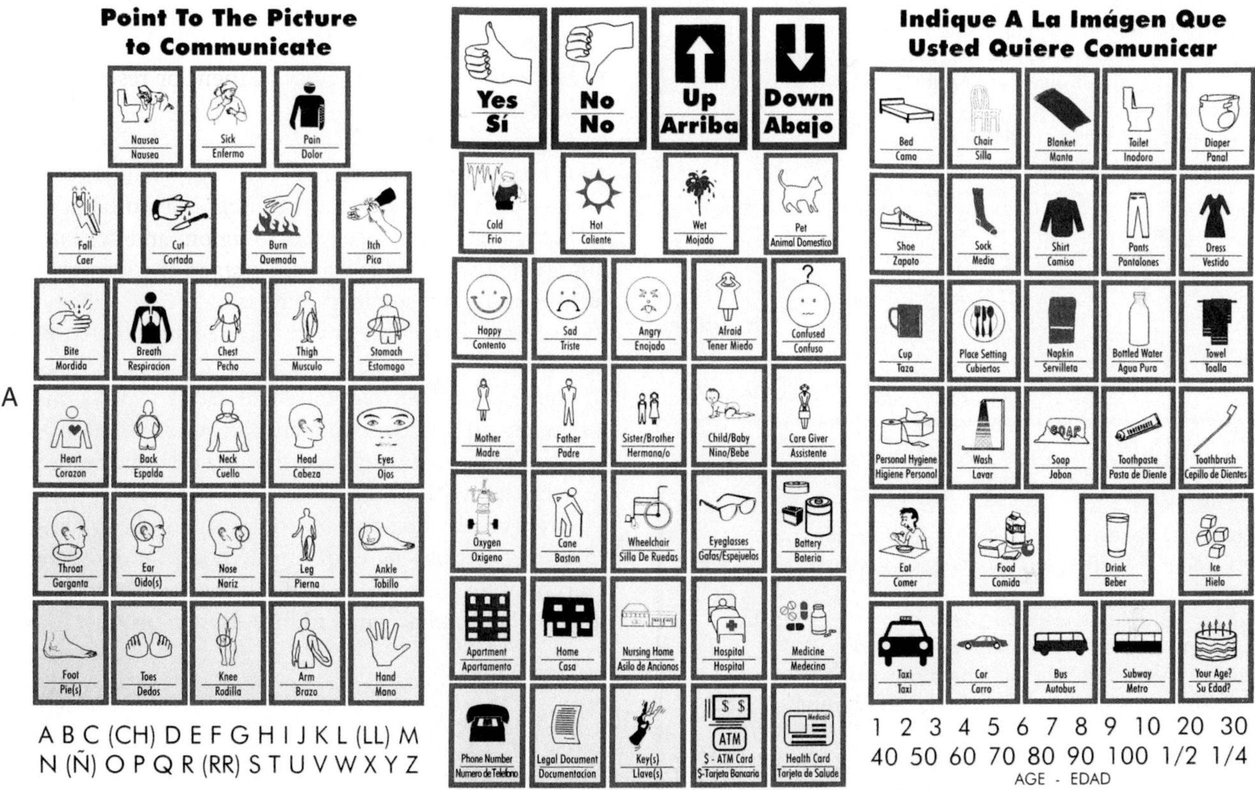

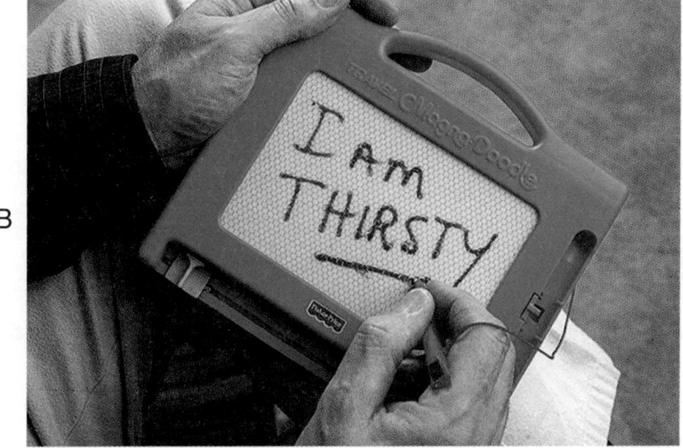

FIGURE 6-3 Communication aids. **A,** Picture board in English and Spanish. **B,** Magic Slate.

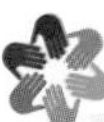

CARING ABOUT CULTURE

Touch Practices

Touch practices vary among cultural groups. Touch is a friendly gesture in the *Philippine* culture. Touch is often used in *Mexico.* Some people believe that using touch while complimenting a person is important. It is thought to neutralize the power of the evil eye *(mal de ojo).*

Persons from the *United Kingdom* tend to reserve touch for persons they know well. Within limits, touch is acceptable in *Poland.* Its use depends on age, gender, and relationship.

In *India,* men shake hands with other men but not with women. For women, they place their palms together and bow slightly. As a sign of respect or to seek a blessing, people touch the feet of older adults.

In *Vietnam,* a person's head is touched by others. It is considered the center of the soul. Men do not touch women they do not know. Men commonly shake hands with men.

People from *China* do not like touching by strangers. A nod or slight bow is given during introductions. Health care workers of the same gender are preferred.

In *Ireland,* a firm handshake is preferred. Only family and close friends are embraced.

Modified from D'Avanzo CE, Geisler EM: Pocket guide to cultural health assessment, *ed 4, St Louis, 2008, Mosby.*

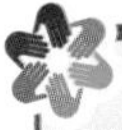

CARING ABOUT CULTURE

Facial Expressions

Through facial expressions, Americans communicate:

- *Coldness*—there is a constant stare. Face muscles do not move.
- *Fear*—eyes are wide open. Eyebrows are raised. The mouth is tense with the lips drawn back.
- *Anger*—eyes are fixed in a hard stare. Upper lids are lowered. Eyebrows are drawn down. Lips are slightly compressed.
- *Tiredness*—eyes are rolled upward.
- *Disapproval*—eyes are rolled upward.
- *Disgust*—narrowed eyes. The upper lip is curled. There are nose movements.
- *Embarrassment*—eyes are turned away or down. The face is flushed. The person pretends to smile. He or she rubs the eyes, nose, or face. He or she twitches the hair, beard, or mustache.
- *Surprise*—direct gaze with raised eyebrows.

Italian, Jewish, African-American, and *Hispanic* persons smile readily. They use many facial expressions and gestures for happiness, pain, or displeasure. *Irish, English,* and *Northern European* persons tend to have less facial expression.

In some cultures, facial expressions mean the opposite of what the person is feeling. For example, *Asians* may conceal negative emotions with a smile.

Modified from Giger JN: Transcultural nursing: assessment and intervention, *ed 6, St Louis, 2013, Mosby.*

Touch. Touch is a very important form of nonverbal communication. It shows comfort, caring, love, affection, interest, trust, concern, and reassurance. Touch means different things to different people. The meaning depends on age, gender (male or female), experiences, and culture. (See *Caring About Culture: Touch Practices.*)

Some people do not like being touched. However, stroking or holding a hand can comfort a person. Touch should be gentle—not hurried, rough, or sexual. To use touch, follow the person's care plan. Remember to maintain professional boundaries.

Body Language

People send messages through their ***body language.***

- *Facial expressions* (see *Caring About Culture: Facial Expressions*)
- *Gestures*
- *Posture*
- *Hand and body movements*
- *Gait*
- *Eye contact*
- *Appearance* (dress, hygiene, jewelry, perfume, cosmetics, body art and piercings, and so on)

Many messages are sent through body language. Slumped posture may mean the person is not happy or not feeling well. A person may deny pain. Yet he or she protects the affected body part by standing, lying, or sitting in a certain way.

Your actions, movements, and facial expressions send messages. So do how you stand, sit, walk, and look at the person. Your body language should show interest, caring, respect, and enthusiasm.

Often you will need to control your body language. Control reactions to odors from body fluids, secretions, excretions, or the person's body. The person cannot control some odors. Embarrassment increases if you react to odors.

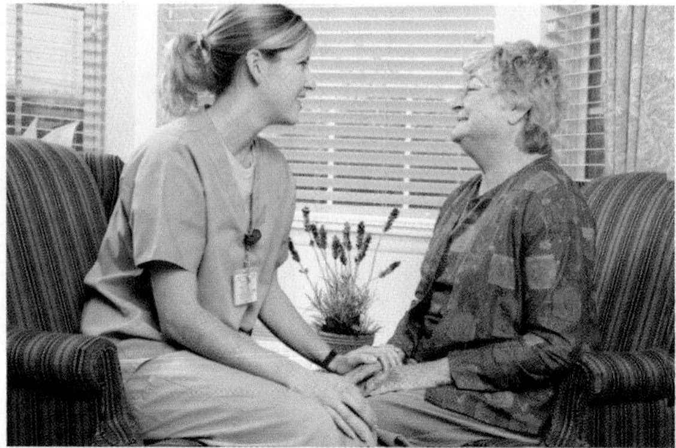

FIGURE 6-4 Listen by facing the person. Have good eye contact. Lean toward the person.

Communication Methods

Certain methods help you communicate with others. They result in better relationships. More information is gained for the nursing process.

Listening. Listening means to focus on verbal and nonverbal communication. You use sight, hearing, touch, and smell. You focus on what the person is saying. You observe nonverbal clues. They can support what the person says. Or they can show other feelings. For example, Mrs. Hayes says, "I want to stay here. That way my son won't have to care for me." You see tears, and she looks away from you. Her verbal says *happy*. Her nonverbal shows *sadness*.

Listening requires that you care and have interest. Follow these guidelines.

- Face the person.
- Have good eye contact with the person. See *Caring About Culture: Eye Contact Practices*.
- Lean toward the person (Fig. 6-4). Do not sit back with your arms crossed.
- Respond to the person. Nod your head. Say "uh huh," "mmm," and "I see." Repeat what the person says. Ask questions.
- Avoid communication barriers.

CARING ABOUT CULTURE

Eye Contact Practices

In the *American* culture, eye contact signals a good self-concept. It also shows openness, interest in others, attention, honesty, and warmth. Lack of eye contact can mean:

- Shyness
- Lack of interest
- Humility
- Guilt
- Embarrassment
- Low self-esteem
- Rudeness
- Dishonesty

For some *Asian* and *American Indian* cultures, eye contact is impolite. It is an invasion of privacy. In certain *Indian* cultures, eye contact is avoided with persons of higher or lower socio-economic class. It is also given a special sexual meaning.

In *Iraq*, men and women avoid direct eye contact. Long, direct eye contact is rude in *Mexico*. In rural parts of *Vietnam*, it is not respectful to look at another person while talking. Blinking means that a message is received. In the *United Kingdom*, looking directly at a speaker means the listener is paying attention.

Modified from Giger JN: Transcultural nursing: assessment and intervention, *ed 6, St Louis, 2013, Mosby; and D'Avanzo CE, Geissler EM:* Pocket guide to cultural health assessment, *ed 4, St Louis, 2008, Mosby.*

Paraphrasing. Paraphrasing is re-stating the person's message in your own words. You use fewer words than the person did. The person usually responds to your statement. For example:

Mrs. Hayes: My son was crying after he spoke with the doctor. I don't know what they talked about.
You: You don't know why your son was crying.
Mrs. Hayes: The doctor must have said that I have a tumor.

Direct Questions. Direct questions focus on certain information. You ask the person something you need to know. Some direct questions have "yes" or "no" answers. Others require more information. For example:

You: Mrs. Hayes, do you want to shower this morning?
Mrs. Hayes: Yes.
You: Mrs. Hayes, when would you like to do that?
Mrs. Hayes: Could we start in 15 minutes? I'd like to call my son first.
You: Yes, we can start in 15 minutes. Did you have a bowel movement today?
Mrs. Hayes: No.
You: You said you didn't eat well this morning. Can you tell me what you ate?
Mrs. Hayes: I only had toast and coffee. I just don't feel like eating this morning.

Open-Ended Questions. Open-ended questions lead or invite the person to share thoughts, feelings, or ideas. The person chooses what to talk about. He or she controls the topic and the information given. Answers require more than a "yes" or "no." For example:

- "What do you like about living with your son?"
- "What was your husband like?"
- "What do you like about being retired?"

Clarifying. Clarifying lets you make sure that you understand the message. You can ask the person to repeat the message, say you do not understand, or re-state the message. For example:

- "Could you say that again?"
- "I'm sorry, Mrs. Hayes. I don't understand what you mean."
- "Are you saying that you want to go home?"

Focusing. Focusing is dealing with a certain topic. It is useful when a person rambles or wanders in thought. For example, Mrs. Hayes talks at length about food and places to eat. You need to know why she did not eat much breakfast. To focus on breakfast you say: "Let's talk about breakfast. You said you don't feel like eating."

Silence. Silence is a very powerful way to communicate. Sometimes you do not need to say anything. This is true during sad times. Just being there shows you care. At other times, silence gives time to think, organize thoughts, or choose words. It also helps when the person is upset and needs to gain control. Silence on your part shows caring and respect for the person's situation and feelings.

Sometimes pauses or long silences are uncomfortable. You do not need to talk when the person is silent. The person may need silence. See *Caring About Culture: The Meaning of Silence.*

CARING ABOUT CULTURE

The Meaning of Silence

In the *English* and *Arabic* cultures, silence is used for privacy. Among *Russian, French,* and *Spanish* cultures, silence means agreement between parties. In some *Asian* cultures, silence is a sign of respect, particularly to an older person.

Modified from Giger JN: Transcultural nursing: assessment and intervention, *ed 6, St Louis, 2013, Mosby.*

Communication Barriers

Communication barriers prevent the sending and receiving of messages. Communication fails.

- *Unfamiliar language.* You and the person must use and understand the same language. If not, messages are not accurately interpreted. See Evolve Student Learning Resources or *Mosby's Nursing Assistant Companion CD*, included with this textbook, for a Spanish Vocabulary and Phrases Glossary.
- *Cultural differences.* The person may attach different meanings to verbal and nonverbal communication. See *Caring About Culture: Communicating With Persons From Other Cultures.*
- *Changing the subject.* Someone changes the subject when the topic is uncomfortable. Avoid changing the subject whenever possible.
- *Giving your opinion.* Opinions involve judging values, behaviors, or feelings. Let others express feelings and concerns without adding your opinion. Do not make judgments or jump to conclusions.
- *Talking a lot when others are silent.* Talking too much is usually because of nervousness and discomfort with silence.
- *Failure to listen.* Do not pretend to listen. It shows lack of interest and caring. This causes poor responses. You miss important complaints or symptoms that you must report to the nurse.
- *Pat answers.* "Don't worry." "Everything will be okay." "Your doctor knows best." These make the person feel that you do not care about his or her concerns, feelings, and fears.
- *Illness and disability.* Speech, hearing, vision, cognitive function, and body movements are often affected. Verbal and nonverbal communication is affected.
- *Age.* Values and communication styles vary among age-groups.

See *Focus on Communication: Communication Barriers.*

CARING ABOUT CULTURE

Communicating With Persons From Other Cultures

To communicate with persons from other cultures:

- Ask the nurse about the beliefs and values of the person's culture. You can also ask the person and family. Learn as much as you can about the person's culture.
- Do not judge the person by your attitudes, values, beliefs, and ideas.
- Follow the person's care plan. It includes the person's cultural beliefs and customs.
- Do the following when communicating with foreign-speaking persons.
  - Convey comfort by your tone of voice and body language.
  - Do not speak loudly or shout. It will not help the person understand English.
  - Speak slowly and distinctly.
  - Keep messages short and simple.
  - Be alert for words the person seems to understand.
  - Use gestures and pictures.
  - Repeat the message in other ways.
  - Avoid using medical terms and abbreviations.
  - Be alert for signs the persons is pretending to understand. Nodding and answering "yes" to all questions are signs that the person does not understand what you are saying.

Modified from Giger JN: Transcultural nursing: assessment and intervention, *ed 6, St Louis, 2013, Mosby.*

FOCUS ON COMMUNICATION

Communication Barriers

Persons from different cultures may speak a language you do not understand. This is a barrier to communication. Such persons may normally have family or friends translate. In the health care setting, the nurse may prefer to use a translator from the agency.

Trained translators know medical terms. Family or friends may not know a term. They may state something other than what was meant. There is a risk of giving wrong information. Also, having family or friends translate violates the right to privacy. The Health Insurance Portability and Accountability Act of 1996 (HIPAA) protects the right to privacy and security of a person's health information (Chapter 3). Privacy is protected when using a translator from the agency.

PERSONS WITH SPECIAL NEEDS

Each person is unique. Special knowledge and skills may be required to meet the person's needs.

Persons With Disabilities

A person may acquire a disability any time from birth through old age. Disease and injury are common causes. Common courtesies and manners *(etiquette)* apply to any person with a disability. See Box 6-2 for disability etiquette.

The Person Who Is Comatose

Comatose means being unable to respond to stimuli. The person who is comatose is unconscious. He or she cannot respond to others. Often the person can hear and can feel touch and pain. Pain may be shown by grimacing or groaning. Assume that the person hears and understands you. Use touch and give care gently. Practice these measures.

- Knock before entering the person's room.
- Tell the person your name, the time, and the place each time you enter the room.
- Give care on the same schedule every day.
- Explain what you are going to do. Explain care measures step-by-step as you do them.
- Tell the person when you are finishing care.
- Use touch to communicate care, concern, and comfort.
- Tell the person what time you will be back to check on him or her.
- Tell the person when you are leaving the room.

BOX 6-2 Disability Etiquette

- Extend the same courtesies to the person as you would to anyone else.
- Provide for privacy.
- Do not hang on or lean on a person's wheelchair.
- Treat adults as adults. Use the person's first name only if he or she asks you to do so.
- Do not pat a person who is in a wheelchair on the head.
- Speak directly to the person. Do not address questions for the person to his or her companion.
- Do not be embarrassed if you use words relating to the disability. For example, you say: "Did you see that?" to a person with a vision problem.
- Sit or squat to talk to a person in a wheelchair or in a chair. This puts you and the person at eye level.
- Ask the person if he or she needs help before acting. If the person says "no," respect the person's wishes. If the person wants help, ask what to do and how to do it.
- Think before giving directions to a person in a wheelchair. Think about distances, weather conditions, stairs, curbs, steep hills, and other obstacles.
- Allow the person extra time to say or do things. Let the person set the pace in walking, talking, or other activities.

Modified from Easter Seals: Disability etiquette. *2012.*

Persons With Bariatric Needs

Bariatrics focuses on *the treatment and control of obesity. Obesity* means *having an excess amount of total body fat.* Bariatric persons are at risk for many serious health problems. Heart disease, high blood pressure, stroke, cancer, and diabetes are examples. Physical and emotional needs are common. Special equipment and furniture are needed to meet the person's needs.

FAMILY AND FRIENDS

Family and friends help meet basic needs. They lessen loneliness. Some also help with care. The presence or absence of family or friends affects the person's quality of life.

The person has the right to visit with family and friends in private and without unnecessary interruptions. You may need to give care when visitors are there. Protect the right to privacy. Do not expose the person's body in front of them. Politely ask them to leave the room. Show them where to wait. Promptly tell them when they can return. A partner or family member may want to help you. If the patient or resident consents, you may allow the person to stay.

Treat family and friends with courtesy and respect. They have concerns about the person's condition and care. They need support and understanding. However, do not discuss the person's condition with them. Refer their questions to the nurse.

Visiting rules depend on agency policy and the person's condition. Know your agency's visiting policies and what is allowed for the person.

Visitors may have questions about the chapel, gift shop, lounge, dining room, or business office. Know the locations, special rules, and hours of these areas.

A visitor may upset or tire a person. Report your observations to the nurse. The nurse will speak with the visitor about the person's needs.

See *Caring About Culture: Family Roles in Sick Care.*

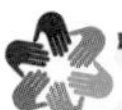

CARING ABOUT CULTURE

Family Roles in Sick Care

In *Vietnam,* family members are involved in the person's hospital care. They stay at the bedside and sleep in the person's bed or on straw mats. In *Vietnam* and *China,* family members provide food, hygiene, and comfort.

In *Pakistan,* hospitals have different sections for females and males. Adult family members of the opposite sex are not allowed to stay overnight.

Modified from D'Avanzo CE, Geissler EM: Pocket guide to cultural health assessment, *ed 4, St Louis, 2008, Mosby.*

FOCUS ON PRIDE

The Person, Family, and Yourself

Personal and Professional Responsibility

Improving communication is an on-going process. You may be uncomfortable with patient or resident interactions at first. You will have many chances to develop communication skills. You are responsible for taking advantage of these opportunities. To improve your communication:

- Use methods such as listening and clarifying.
- Pay attention to the nonverbal messages you may be sending.
- Avoid communication barriers.
- Know where your agency keeps resources to aid with communication. These may include devices like those shown in Figure 6-3 or translation lists with useful words or phrases (see Evolve Student Learning Resources or *Mosby's Nursing Assistant Companion CD* provided in this textbook).
- Learn from your mistakes.

With practice, you will communicate more effectively. This is a valuable skill.

Rights and Respect

You may care for young and old persons, ill and disabled persons, persons who are obese, and those from other cultures. Each person is different. Each has his or her own needs and concerns.

Avoid labeling the person or making assumptions. For example, a person is obese. That does not mean the person is lazy or lacks control. Or a person is elderly. Myths about older persons are common.

Each person is unique and has value. Try to understand the person. Listen and use good communication. Treat the person with dignity and respect.

Independence and Social Interaction

Fear and anxiety are common emotions for patients and residents. Nursing center residents may feel lonely or abandoned by family and friends. Patients may fear loss of function that will have social effects. For example, a stroke can cause loss of function on 1 side of the body. The person may lose the ability to work, live at home, perform daily activities, walk, drive a car, and so on. Feeling abandoned or worthless affects self-esteem and over-all health.

To provide a sense of identity, worth, and belonging:

- Greet each person by name.
- Talk to the person while providing care.
- Take an extra minute to visit or just listen.
- Treat each person with dignity and respect.
- Encourage as much independence as possible.
- Focus on the person's abilities, not his or her disabilities.
- Allow private time with visitors.

Delegation and Teamwork

Caring for persons with behavior issues requires great teamwork. Staff members may become frustrated. But the person's quality of care must not be lowered. The health team must work together to manage such persons. Care assignments may rotate to allow breaks.

When not assigned to such a person, assist your co-worker with the person or other tasks. When you interact with the person, be respectful. Treat the person as nicely as you treat others. Often when treated kindly, the person's behavior will improve. A supportive and encouraging team makes caring for difficult persons easier.

Ethics and Laws

You will care for persons with different ideas, values, and lifestyles. These shape the person's character and identity. It is not ethical to:

- Force your views and beliefs on another person.
- Make negative comments or insult the person's customs.
- Argue with a person about health care or religious beliefs.

Respect the person as a whole. This includes his or her cultural and religious practices.

REVIEW QUESTIONS

Circle the BEST answer.

1 You work in a health care agency. You focus on
  a The person's care plan
  b The person's physical, safety and security, and self-esteem needs
  c The person as a physical, psychological, social, and spiritual being
  d The person's cultural and spiritual needs

2 Which basic need is the *most* essential?
  a Self-actualization
  b Self-esteem
  c Love and belonging
  d Safety and security

3 A person says, "What are they doing to me?" Which basic needs are *not* being met?
  a Physical needs
  b Safety and security needs
  c Love and belonging needs
  d Self-esteem needs

4 A person wants care given at a certain time and in a certain way. Nothing seems to please the person. The person is most likely demonstrating
  a Angry behavior
  b Demanding behavior
  c Withdrawn behavior
  d Aggressive behavior

5 A person is demonstrating problem behavior. You should do the following *except*
  a Put yourself in the person's situation
  b Tell the person what you are going to do and when
  c Ask the person to be nicer
  d Listen and use silence

6 Which is *false?*
  a Verbal communication uses the written or spoken word.
  b Verbal communication is the truest reflection of a person's feelings.
  c Messages are sent by facial expressions, gestures, posture, and body movements.
  d Touch means different things to different people.

7 To communicate with the person you should
  a Use medical words and phrases
  b Change the subject often
  c Give your opinions
  d Be quiet when the person is silent

8 Which might mean that you are *not* listening?
  a You sit facing the person.
  b You have good eye contact with the person.
  c You sit with your arms crossed.
  d You ask questions.

9 Which is an open-ended question?
  a "What hobbies do you enjoy?"
  b "Do you want to wear your red sweater?"
  c "Would you like eggs and toast for breakfast?"
  d "Do you want to sit in your chair?"

10 Which promotes communication?
  a "Don't worry."
  b "Everything will be just fine."
  c "This is a good nursing center."
  d "Why are you crying?"

11 Which is a barrier to communication?
  a Pretending to listen
  b Asking questions
  c Focusing
  d Using familiar language

12 A person uses a wheelchair. For effective communication, you should
  a Lean on the wheelchair
  b Pat the person on the head
  c Direct questions to the companion
  d Sit or squat next to the person

13 A person is comatose. Which action is *not* correct?
  a Assume that the person can hear and can feel touch.
  b Explain what you are going to do.
  c Use listening and silence to communicate.
  d Tell the person when you are leaving the room.

14 A visitor seems to tire a person. What should you do?
  a Ask the person to leave.
  b Tell the nurse.
  c Stay in the room to observe the person and visitor.
  d Find out the visitor's relationship to the person.

Answers to these questions are on p. 504.

FOCUS ON PRACTICE

Problem Solving

Mr. Hawn is a new resident. He was admitted to the center last month after his wife died. He could not care for himself at home. Mr. Hawn is withdrawn and angry toward the staff. He is impatient and agitated when his needs are not met right away. Explain possible reasons for these behaviors. How will you manage his behaviors and provide quality care?

CHAPTER

7 Body Structure and Function

OBJECTIVES

- Define the key terms and key abbreviations listed in this chapter.
- Identify the basic structures of the cell.
- Explain how cells divide.
- Describe 4 types of tissues.
- Identify the structures of each body system.
- Identify the functions of each body system.
- Explain how to promote PRIDE in the person, the family, and yourself.

KEY TERMS

artery A blood vessel that carries blood away from the heart
capillary A tiny blood vessel; food, oxygen, and other substances pass from the capillaries into the cells
cell The basic unit of body structure
digestion The process that breaks down food physically and chemically so it can be absorbed for use by the cells
hemoglobin The substance in red blood cells that carries oxygen and gives blood its red color
hormone A chemical substance secreted by the endocrine glands into the bloodstream
immunity Protection against a disease or condition; the person will not get or be affected by the disease
joint The point at which 2 or more bones meet to allow movement
menstruation The process in which the lining of the uterus *(endometrium)* breaks up and is discharged from the body through the vagina
metabolism The burning of food for heat and energy by the cells
organ Groups of tissue with the same function
peristalsis Involuntary muscle contractions in the digestive system that move food down the esophagus through the alimentary canal
respiration The process of supplying the cells with oxygen and removing carbon dioxide from them
system Organs that work together to perform special functions
tissue A group of cells with similar functions
vein A blood vessel that returns blood to the heart

KEY ABBREVIATIONS

CNS Central nervous system
GI Gastro-intestinal
mL Milliliter
RBC Red blood cell
WBC White blood cell

Ideally, the human body is in a steady state called *homeostasis.* (*Homeo* means *sameness. Stasis* means *standing still*). Various body functions and processes work to promote health and survival. Homeostasis is affected by illness, disease, and injury.

You help residents meet their basic needs. Your care promotes comfort, healing, and recovery. Therefore you need to know the body's normal structure *(anatomy)* and function *(physiology)*. They will help you understand signs, symptoms, and the reasons for care and procedures. You will give safe and more effective care.

See Chapter 8 for the changes in body structure and function that occur with aging.

CELLS, TISSUES, AND ORGANS

The basic unit of body structure is the ***cell.*** Cells have the same basic structure. Function, size, and shape may differ. Cells are very small. You need a microscope to see them. Cells need food, water, and oxygen to live and function.

Figure 7-1 shows the cell and its structures. The *cell membrane* is the outer covering. It encloses the cell and helps to hold its shape. The *nucleus* is the control center of the cell. It directs the cell's activities. The nucleus is in the center of the cell. The *cytoplasm* surrounds the nucleus. Cytoplasm contains smaller structures that perform cell functions. *Protoplasm* means "living substance." It refers to all structures, substances, and water within the cell. Protoplasm is a semi-liquid substance much like an egg white.

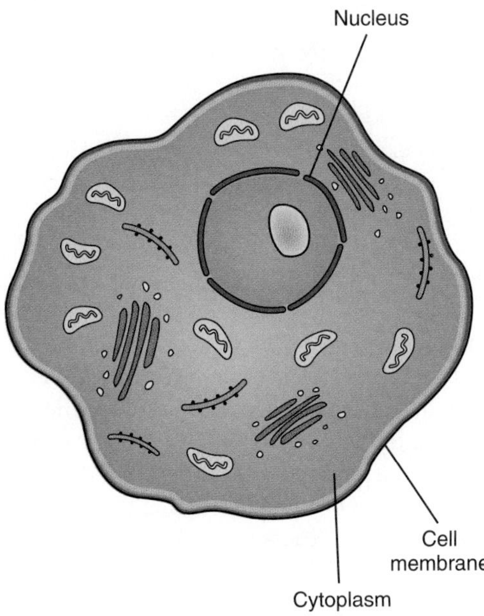

FIGURE 7-1 Parts of a cell.

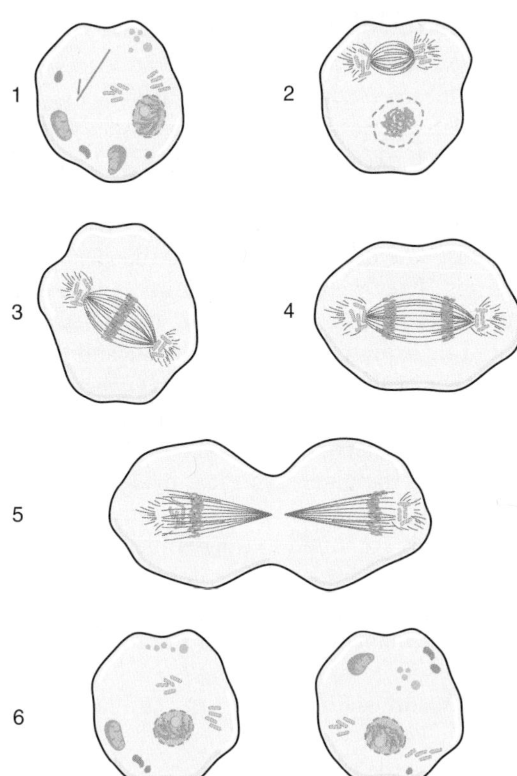

FIGURE 7-2 Cell division.

Chromosomes are thread-like structures in the nucleus. Each cell has 46 chromosomes. Chromosomes contain *genes.* Genes control the traits children inherit from their parents. Height, eye color, and skin color are examples.

The nucleus controls cell reproduction. Cells reproduce by dividing in half. The process of cell division is called *mitosis.* It is needed for tissue growth and repair. During mitosis, the 46 chromosomes arrange themselves in 23 pairs. As the cell divides, the 23 pairs are pulled in half. The 2 new cells are identical. Each has 46 chromosomes (Fig. 7-2).

Cells are the body's building blocks. *Groups of cells with similar functions combine to form* ***tissues.***

- *Epithelial tissue* covers internal and external body surfaces. Tissue lining the nose, mouth, respiratory tract, stomach, and intestines is epithelial tissue. So are the skin, hair, nails, and glands.
- *Connective tissue* anchors, connects, and supports other tissues. It is in every part of the body. Bones, tendons, ligaments, and cartilage are connective tissue. Blood is a form of connective tissue.
- *Muscle tissue* stretches and contracts to let the body move.
- *Nerve tissue* receives and carries impulses to the brain and back to body parts.

Groups of tissue with the same function form ***organs.*** An organ has 1 or more functions. Examples of organs are the heart, brain, liver, lungs, and kidneys. ***Systems*** *are formed by organs that work together to perform special functions* (Fig. 7-3).

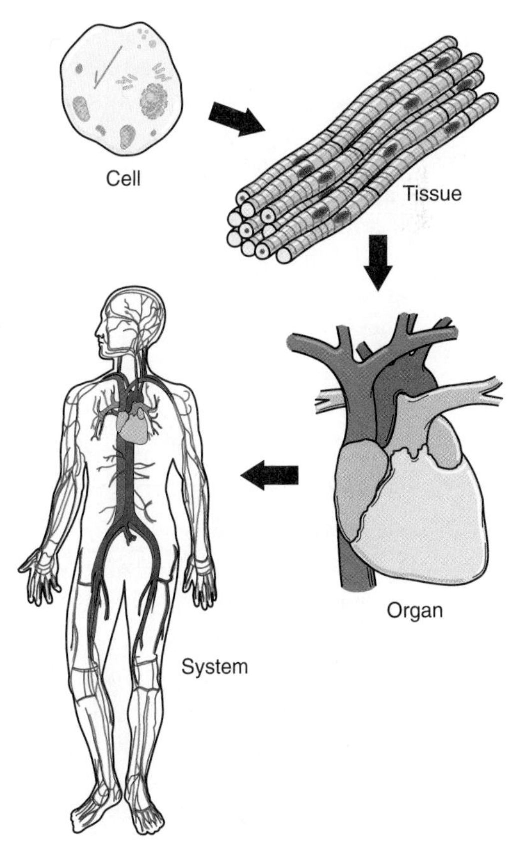

FIGURE 7-3 Organization of the body.

THE INTEGUMENTARY SYSTEM

The *integumentary system*, or *skin*, is the largest system. *Integument* means *covering*. The skin covers the body. It has epithelial, connective, and nerve tissue. It also has oil glands and sweat glands. There are 2 skin layers (Fig. 7-4).

- The *epidermis* is the outer layer. It has living cells and dead cells. The dead cells were once deeper in the epidermis. They were pushed upward as the cells divided. Dead cells constantly flake off. They are replaced by living cells. Living cells die and flake off. Living cells of the epidermis contain *pigment*. Pigment gives skin its color. The epidermis has no blood vessels and few nerve endings.
- The *dermis* is the inner layer. It is made up of connective tissue. Blood vessels, nerves, sweat glands, and oil glands are found in the dermis. So are hair roots.

The epidermis and dermis are supported by *subcutaneous tissue*. The subcutaneous tissue is a thick layer of fat and connective tissue.

Oil glands and *sweat glands*, *hair*, and *nails* are skin appendages.

- Hair—covers the entire body, except the palms of the hands and the soles of the feet. Hair in the nose and ears and around the eyes protects these organs from dust, insects, and other foreign objects.
- Nails—protect the tips of the fingers and toes. Nails help fingers pick up and handle small objects.
- Sweat glands (sudoriferous glands)—help the body regulate temperature. Sweat consists of water, salt, and a small amount of wastes. Sweat is secreted through pores in the skin. The body is cooled as sweat evaporates.
- Oil glands (sebaceous glands)—lie near the hair shafts. They secrete an oily substance into the space near the hair shaft. Oil travels to the skin surface. This helps keep the hair and skin soft and shiny.

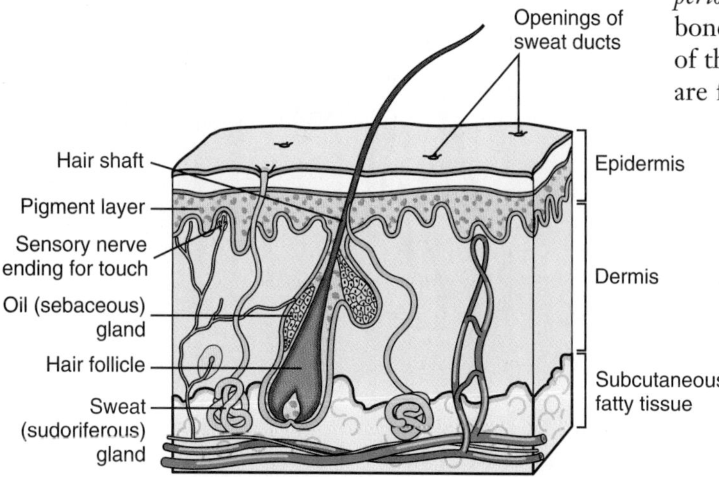

FIGURE 7-4 Layers of the skin.

The skin has many functions.

- It is the body's protective covering.
- It prevents microorganisms and other substances from entering the body.
- It prevents excess amounts of water from leaving the body.
- It protects organs from injury.
- Nerve endings in the skin sense both pleasant and unpleasant stimulation. Nerve endings are over the entire body. They sense cold, pain, touch, and pressure to protect the body from injury.
- It helps regulate body temperature. Blood vessels dilate (widen) when temperature outside the body is high. More blood is brought to the body surface for cooling during evaporation. When blood vessels constrict (narrow), the body retains heat. This is because less blood reaches the skin.
- It stores fat and water.

THE MUSCULO-SKELETAL SYSTEM

The *musculo-skeletal system* provides the framework for the body. It lets the body move. This system also protects internal organs and gives the body shape.

Bones

The human body has 206 *bones* (Fig. 7-5). There are 4 types of bones.

- *Long bones* bear the body's weight. Leg bones are long bones.
- *Short bones* allow skill and ease in movement. Bones in the wrists, fingers, ankles, and toes are short bones.
- *Flat bones* protect the organs. They include the ribs, skull, pelvic bones, and shoulder blades.
- *Irregular bones* are the vertebrae in the spinal column. They allow various degrees of movement and flexibility.

Bones are hard, rigid structures. They are made up of living cells. Calcium and phosphorus are needed for bone formation and strength. Bones store these minerals for use by the body. Bones are covered by a membrane called *periosteum*. Periosteum contains blood vessels that supply bone cells with oxygen and food. Inside the hollow centers of the bones is a substance called *bone marrow*. Blood cells are formed in the bone marrow.

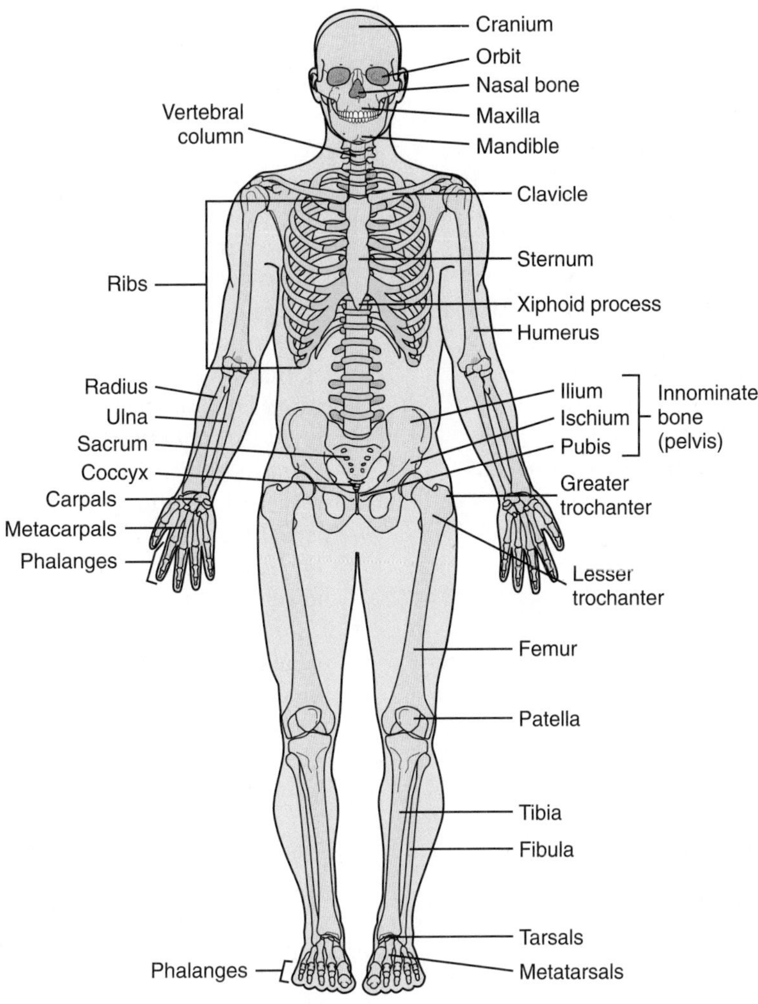

FIGURE 7-5 Bones of the body.

Joints

A ***joint*** *is the point at which 2 or more bones meet. Joints allow movement* (Chapter 23). *Cartilage* is connective tissue at the end of the long bones. It cushions the joint so that the bone ends do not rub together. The *synovial membrane* lines the joints. It secretes *synovial fluid.* Synovial fluid acts as a lubricant so the joint can move smoothly. Bones are held together at the joint by strong bands of connective tissue called *ligaments.*

There are 3 major types of joints (Fig. 7-6).

- A *ball-and-socket joint* allows movement in all directions. It is made of the rounded end of 1 bone and the hollow end of another bone. The rounded end of 1 fits into the hollow end of the other. The joints of the hips and shoulders are ball-and-socket joints.
- A *hinge joint* allows movement in 1 direction. The elbow is a hinge joint.
- A *pivot joint* allows turning from side to side. A pivot joint connects the skull to the spine.

Some joints are immovable. They connect the bones of the skull.

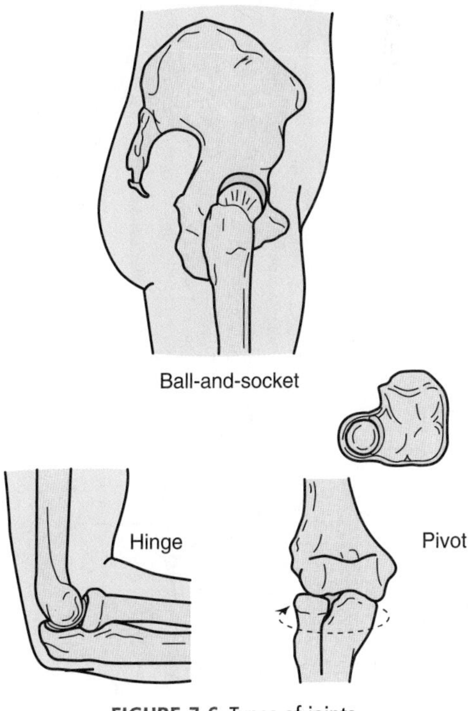

FIGURE 7-6 Types of joints.

Muscles

The human body has more than 500 *muscles* (Figs. 7-7 and 7-8). Some are voluntary. Others are involuntary.

- *Voluntary muscles* can be consciously controlled. Muscles attached to bones *(skeletal muscles)* are voluntary. Arm muscles do not work unless you move your arm; likewise for leg muscles. Skeletal muscles are *striated.* That is, they look striped or streaked.
- *Involuntary muscles* work automatically. You cannot control them. They control the action of the stomach, intestines, blood vessels, and other body organs. Involuntary muscles also are called *smooth muscles.* They look smooth, not streaked or striped.
- *Cardiac muscle* is in the heart. It is an involuntary muscle. However, it appears striated like skeletal muscle.

Muscles have 3 functions:

- Movement of body parts
- Maintenance of posture or muscle tone
- Production of body heat

Strong, tough connective tissues called *tendons* connect muscles to bones. When muscles contract (shorten), tendons at each end of the muscle cause the bone to move. The body has many tendons. See the Achilles tendon in Figure 7-8. Some muscles constantly contract to maintain the body's posture. When muscles contract, they burn food for energy. Heat is produced. The more muscle activity, the greater the amount of heat produced. Shivering is how the body produces heat when exposed to cold. Shivering is from rapid, general muscle contractions.

Sphincters are circular bands of muscle fibers. They constrict (narrow) a passage. Or they close a natural body opening. For example:

- The *pyloric sphincter* (Fig. 7-9) is an opening from the stomach into the small intestine. Closed, it holds food in the stomach for partial digestion. It opens to allow partially digested food to enter the small intestine.
- The *anal sphincter* keeps the anus closed. It opens for a bowel movement.
- *Urethral sphincters* seal off the bladder. This allows urine to collect in the bladder. The sphincters open for urination.

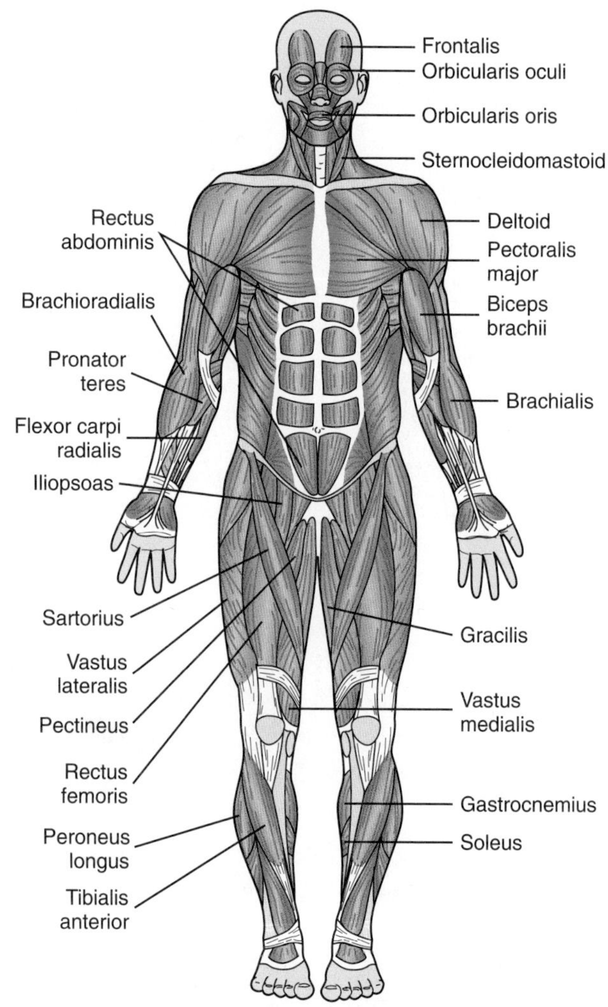

FIGURE 7-7 Anterior view of the muscles of the body.

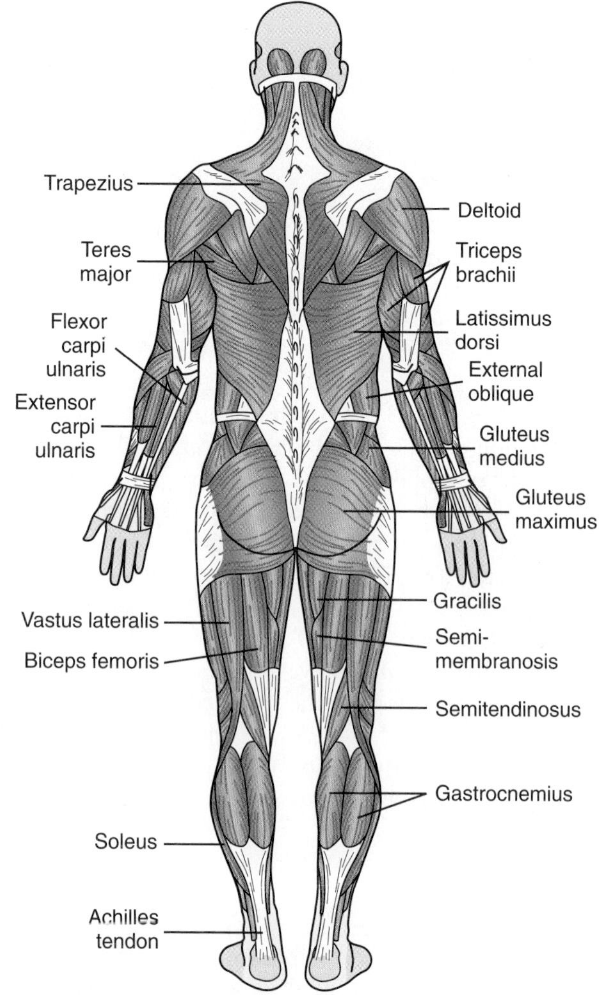

FIGURE 7-8 Posterior view of the muscles of the body.

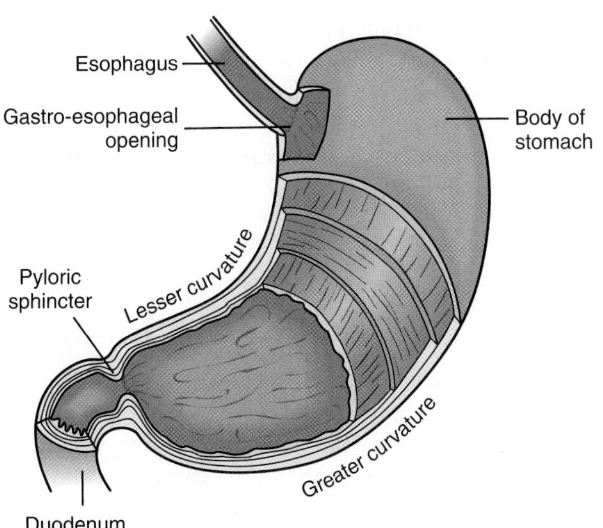

FIGURE 7-9 Pyloric sphincter.

THE NERVOUS SYSTEM

The *nervous system* controls, directs, and coordinates body functions. Its 2 main divisions are:

- The *central nervous system* (CNS). It consists of the brain and spinal cord (Fig. 7-10).
- The *peripheral nervous system.* It involves the nerves throughout the body (Fig. 7-11).

Nerves connect to the spinal cord. Nerves carry messages or impulses to and from the brain. A *stimulus* causes a nerve impulse. A stimulus is anything that excites or causes a body part to function, become active, or respond. A *reflex* is the body's response (functioning or movement) to a stimulus. Reflexes are involuntary, unconscious, and immediate. The person cannot control reflexes.

Nerves are easily damaged and take a long time to heal. Some nerve fibers have a protective covering called a *myelin sheath.* The myelin sheath also insulates the nerve fiber. Nerve fibers covered with myelin conduct impulses faster than those fibers without it.

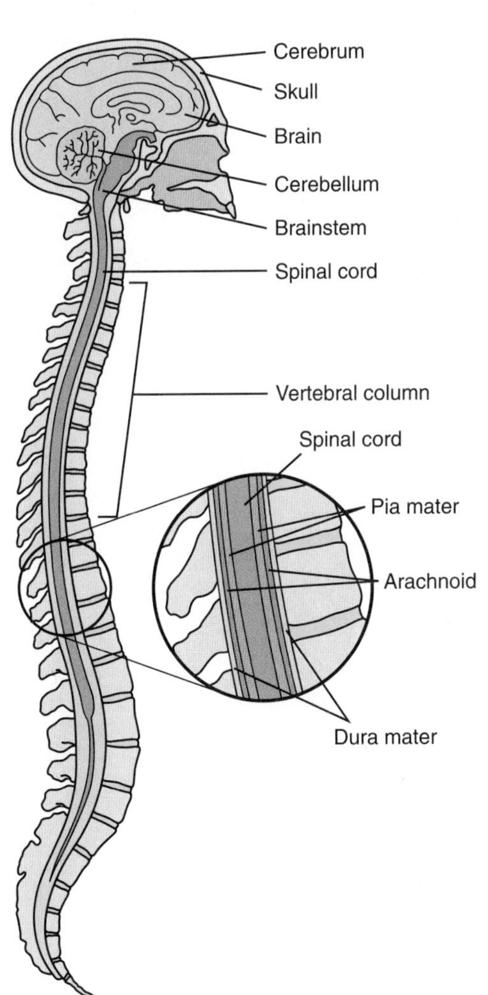

FIGURE 7-10 Central nervous system.

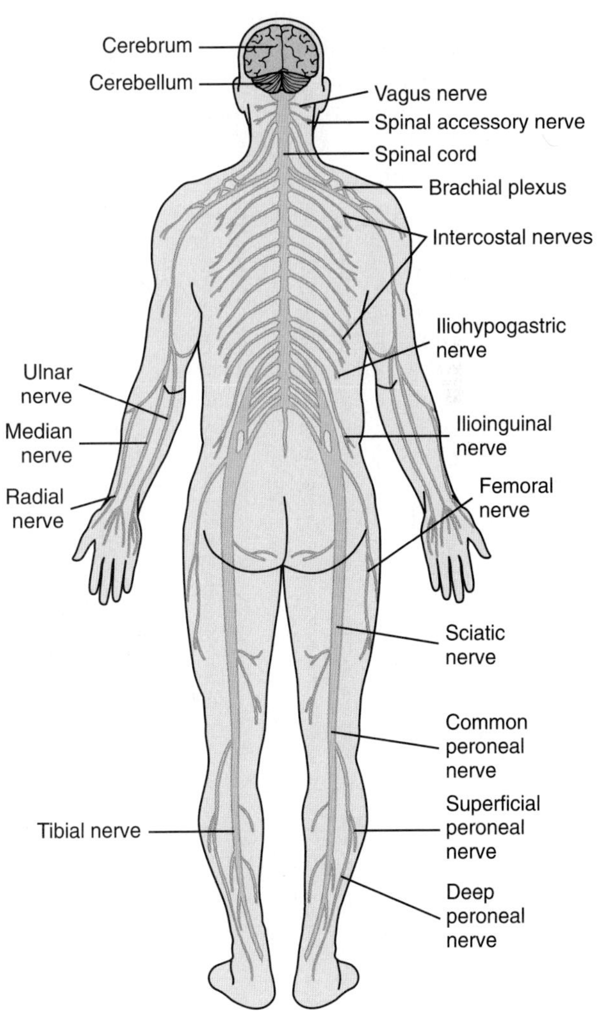

FIGURE 7-11 Peripheral nervous system.

The Central Nervous System

The *brain* and *spinal cord* make up the central nervous system. The brain is covered by the skull. The 3 main parts of the brain are the *cerebrum*, the *cerebellum*, and the *brainstem* (Fig. 7-12).

The cerebrum is the largest part of the brain. It is the center of thought and intelligence. The cerebrum is divided into 2 halves called *right* and *left hemispheres*. The right hemisphere controls movement and activities on the body's left side. The left hemisphere controls the right side.

The outside of the cerebrum is called the *cerebral cortex*. It controls the highest functions of the brain. These include reasoning, memory, consciousness, speech, voluntary muscle movement, vision, hearing, sensation, and other activities.

The cerebellum regulates and coordinates body movements. It controls balance and the smooth movements of voluntary muscles. Injury to the cerebellum results in jerky movements, loss of coordination, and muscle weakness.

The brainstem connects the cerebrum to the spinal cord. The brainstem contains the *midbrain*, *pons*, and *medulla*. The midbrain and pons relay messages between the medulla and the cerebrum. The medulla is below the pons. The medulla controls heart rate, breathing, blood vessel size, swallowing, coughing, and vomiting. The brain connects to the spinal cord at the lower end of the medulla.

The spinal cord lies within the spinal column. The cord is 17 to 18 inches long. It contains pathways that conduct messages to and from the brain.

The brain and spinal cord are covered and protected by 3 layers of connective tissue called meninges.

- The outer layer lies next to the skull. It is a tough covering called the *dura mater*.
- The middle layer is the *arachnoid*.
- The inner layer is the *pia mater*.

The space between the middle layer (arachnoid) and inner layer (pia mater) is the *arachnoid space*. The space is filled with *cerebrospinal fluid*. It circulates around the brain and spinal cord. Cerebrospinal fluid protects the central nervous system. It cushions shocks that could easily injure brain and spinal cord structures.

The Peripheral Nervous System

The peripheral nervous system has 12 pairs of *cranial nerves* and 31 pairs of *spinal nerves*. Cranial nerves conduct impulses between the brain and the head, neck, chest, and abdomen. They conduct impulses for smell, vision, hearing, pain, touch, temperature, and pressure. They also conduct impulses for voluntary and involuntary muscles. Spinal nerves carry impulses from the skin, extremities, and internal structures not supplied by the cranial nerves.

Some peripheral nerves form the *autonomic nervous system*. This system controls involuntary muscles and certain body functions. The functions include the heartbeat, blood pressure, intestinal contractions, and glandular secretions. These functions occur automatically.

The autonomic nervous system is divided into the *sympathetic nervous system* and the *parasympathetic nervous system*. They balance each other. The sympathetic nervous system speeds up functions. The parasympathetic nervous system slows functions. When you are angry, scared, excited, or exercising, the sympathetic nervous system is stimulated. The parasympathetic system is activated when you relax or when the sympathetic system is stimulated for too long.

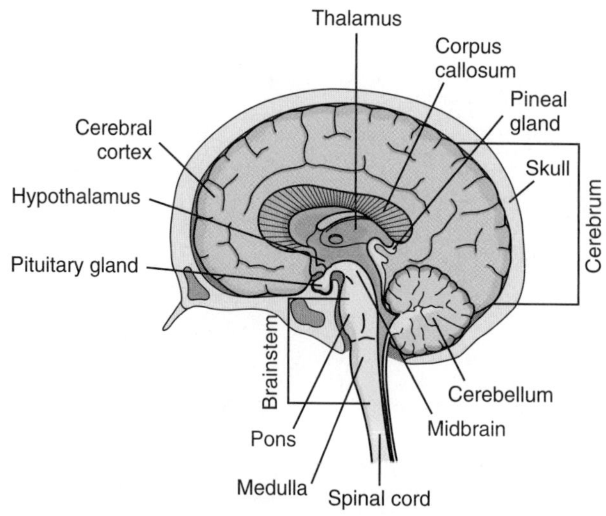

FIGURE 7-12 The brain.

The Sense Organs

The 5 senses are *sight*, *hearing*, *taste*, *smell*, and *touch*. Receptors for taste are in the tongue. They are called taste buds. Receptors for smell are in the nose. Touch receptors are in the dermis, especially in the toes and fingertips.

The Eye. Receptors for vision are in the eyes (Fig. 7-13). The eye is easily injured. Bones of the skull, eyelids and eyelashes, and tears protect the eyes from injury. The eye has 3 layers.

- The *sclera*, the white of the eye, is the outer layer. It is made of tough connective tissue.
- The *choroid* is the second layer. Blood vessels, the *ciliary muscle*, and the *iris* make up the choroid. The iris gives the eye its color. The opening in the middle of the iris is the *pupil*. Pupil size varies with the amount of light entering the eye. The pupil constricts (narrows) in bright light. It dilates (widens) in dim or dark places.
- The *retina* is the inner layer. It has receptors for vision and the nerve fibers of the *optic nerve*.

Light enters the eye through the *cornea*. It is the transparent part of the outer layer that lies over the eye. Light rays pass to the *lens*, which lies behind the pupil. The light is then reflected to the retina. Light is carried to the brain by the optic nerve.

The *aqueous chamber* separates the cornea from the lens. The chamber is filled with a fluid called *aqueous humor*. The fluid helps the cornea keep its shape and position. The *vitreous humor* is behind the lens. It is a gelatin-like substance that supports the retina and maintains the eye's shape.

The Ear

The *ear* is a sense organ (Fig. 7-14). It functions in hearing and balance. It has 3 parts: the *external ear*, *middle ear*, and *inner ear*.

The external ear (outer part) is called the *pinna* or *auricle*. Sound waves are guided through the external ear into the *auditory canal*. Glands in the auditory canal secrete a waxy substance called *cerumen*. The auditory canal extends about 1 inch into the *eardrum*. The eardrum *(tympanic membrane)* separates the external and middle ear.

The middle ear is a small space. It contains the *eustachian tube* and 3 small bones called *ossicles*. The eustachian tube connects the middle ear and the throat. Air enters the eustachian tube so there is equal pressure on both sides of the eardrum. The ossicles amplify sound received from the eardrum and transmit the sound to the inner ear. The 3 ossicles are:

- The *malleus*. It looks like a hammer.
- The *incus*. It looks like an anvil.
- The *stapes*. It is shaped like a stirrup.

The inner ear consists of *semicircular canals* and the *cochlea*. The cochlea looks like a snail shell. It contains fluid. The fluid carries sound waves from the middle ear to the *acoustic nerve*. The acoustic nerve then carries messages to the brain.

The 3 semicircular canals are involved with balance. They sense the head's position and changes in position. They send messages to the brain.

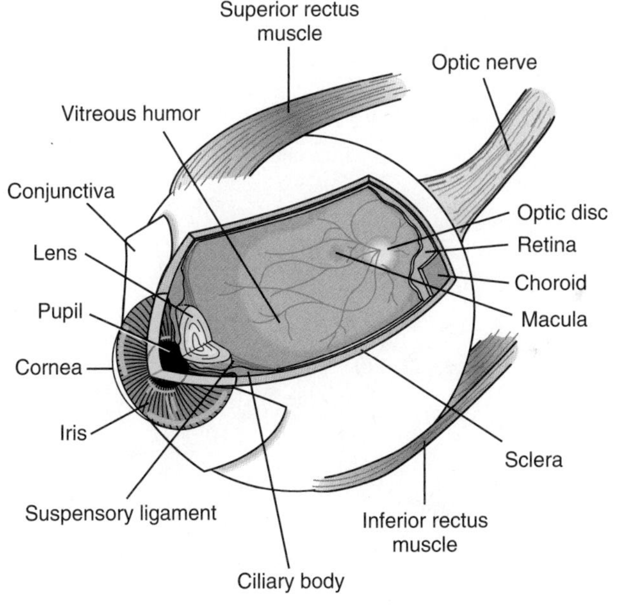

FIGURE 7-13 The eye.

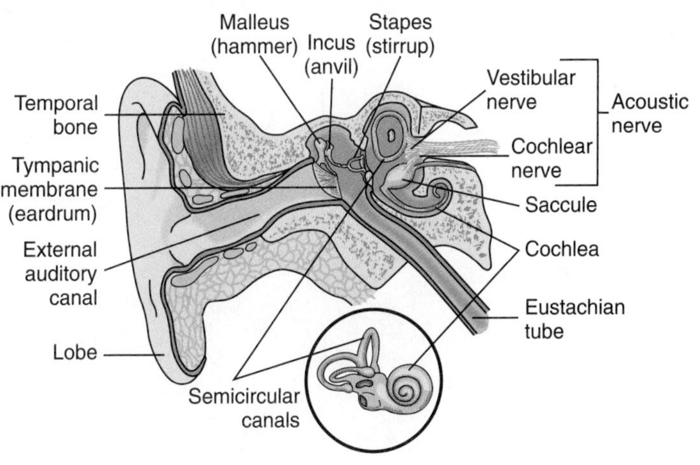

FIGURE 7-14 The ear.

THE CIRCULATORY SYSTEM

The *circulatory system* is made up of the *blood, heart,* and *blood vessels.* The heart pumps blood through the blood vessels. The circulatory system has many functions.

- Blood carries food, hormones, and other substances to the cells.
- Blood transports (carries) the gases of respiration (p. 81). It brings oxygen to the cells.
- Blood removes waste products from cells.
- Blood plays a role in maintaining the body's fluid balance.
- Blood and blood vessels help regulate body temperature. The blood carries heat from muscle activity to other body parts. Blood vessels in the skin dilate to cool the body. They constrict to retain heat.
- The system produces and carries cells that defend the body from microbes that cause disease.

The Blood

The *blood* consists of blood cells and *plasma.* Plasma is mostly water. It carries blood cells to other body cells. Plasma also carries substances that cells need to function. This includes food (proteins, fats, and carbohydrates), hormones (p. 85), and chemicals.

Red blood cells (RBCs) are called *erythrocytes.* *Hemoglobin is the substance in RBCs that carries oxygen and gives blood its red color.* As RBCs circulate through the lungs, hemoglobin picks up oxygen. Hemoglobin carries oxygen to the cells. When blood is bright red, hemoglobin in the RBCs is saturated (filled) with oxygen. As blood circulates through the body, oxygen is given to the cells. Cells release carbon dioxide (a waste product). It is picked up by the hemoglobin. RBCs saturated with carbon dioxide make the blood look dark red.

The body has about 25 trillion (25,000,000,000,000) RBCs. About 4½ to 5 million cells are in a cubic millimeter of blood (the size of a tiny drop). RBCs live for 3 to 4 months. They are destroyed by the liver and spleen as they wear out. New RBCs are formed in the bone marrow. About 1 million RBCs are produced every second.

White blood cells (WBCs) are called *leukocytes.* They have no color. They protect the body against infection. There are about 5,000 to 10,000 WBCs in a cubic millimeter of blood. At the first sign of infection, WBCs rush to the infection site. There they multiply rapidly. The number of WBCs increases when there is an infection. WBCs are formed by the bone marrow. They live about 9 days.

Platelets (thrombocytes) are needed for blood clotting. They are formed by the bone marrow. There are about 200,000 to 400,000 platelets in a cubic millimeter of blood. A platelet lives about 4 days.

The Heart

The *heart* is a muscle. It pumps blood through the blood vessels to the tissues and cells. The heart lies in the middle to lower part of the chest cavity toward the left side (Fig. 7-15). The heart is hollow and has 3 layers (Fig. 7-16).

- The *pericardium* is the outer layer. It is a thin sac covering the heart.
- The *myocardium* is the second layer. It is the thick, muscular part of the heart.
- The *endocardium* is the inner layer. A membrane, it lines the inner surface of the heart.

The heart has 4 chambers (see Fig. 7-16). Upper chambers receive blood and are called *atria.* The *right atrium* receives blood from body tissues. The *left atrium* receives blood from the lungs. Lower chambers are called *ventricles.* Ventricles pump blood. The *right ventricle* pumps blood to the lungs for oxygen. The *left ventricle* pumps blood to all parts of the body.

Valves are between the atria and ventricles. The valves allow blood flow in 1 direction. They prevent blood from flowing back into the atria from the ventricles. The *tricuspid valve* is between the right atrium and the right ventricle. The *mitral valve (bicuspid valve)* is between the left atrium and left ventricle.

Heart action has 2 phases.

- *Diastole.* It is the resting phase. Heart chambers fill with blood.
- *Systole.* It is the working phase. The heart contracts. Blood is pumped through the blood vessels when the heart contracts.

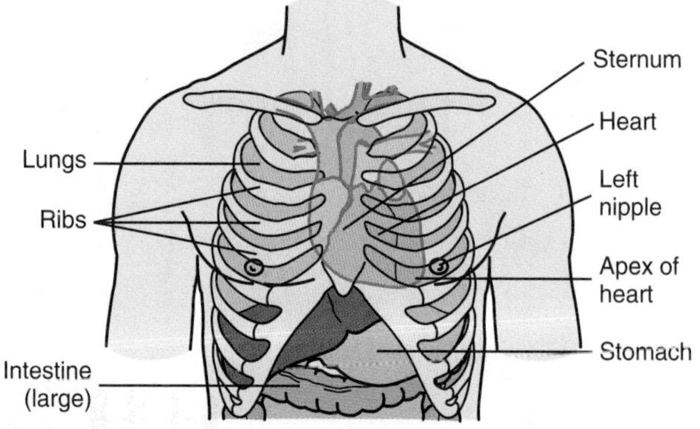

FIGURE 7-15 Location of the heart in the chest cavity.

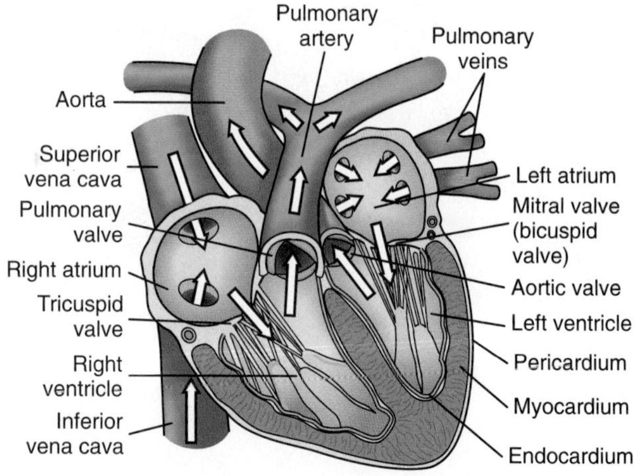

FIGURE 7-16 Structures of the heart.

The Blood Vessels

Blood flows to body tissues and cells through the blood vessels. There are 3 groups of blood vessels: arteries, capillaries, and veins.

***Arteries** carry blood away from the heart.* Arterial blood is rich in oxygen. The *aorta* is the largest artery. It receives blood directly from the left ventricle. The aorta branches into other arteries that carry blood to all parts of the body (Fig. 7-17). These arteries branch into smaller parts within the tissues. The smallest branch of an artery is an *arteriole.*

Arterioles connect to capillaries. ***Capillaries** are very tiny blood vessels. Food, oxygen, and other substances pass from capillaries into the cells.* The capillaries pick up waste products (including carbon dioxide) from the cells. Veins carry waste products back to the heart.

***Veins** return blood to the heart.* They connect to the capillaries by *venules.* Venules are small veins. Venules branch together to form veins. The many veins also branch together as they near the heart to form 2 main veins (see Fig. 7-17). The 2 main veins are the *inferior vena cava* and the *superior vena cava.* Both empty into the right atrium. The inferior vena cava carries blood from the legs and trunk. The superior vena cava carries blood from the head and arms. Venous blood is dark red. It has little oxygen and a lot of carbon dioxide.

Blood flow through the circulatory system is shown in Fig. 7-16. The path of blood flow is as follows.

- Venous blood, poor in oxygen, empties into the right atrium.
- Blood flows through the tricuspid valve into the right ventricle.
- The right ventricle pumps blood into the lungs to pick up oxygen.
- Oxygen-rich blood from the lungs enters the left atrium.
- Blood from the left atrium passes through the mitral valve into the left ventricle.
- The left ventricle pumps the blood into the aorta. It branches off to form other arteries.
- Arterial blood is carried to the tissues by arterioles and to the cells by capillaries.
- Cells and capillaries exchange oxygen and nutrients for carbon dioxide and waste products.
- Capillaries connect with venules. Venules carry blood that has carbon dioxide and waste products.
- Venules form veins.
- Veins return blood to the heart.

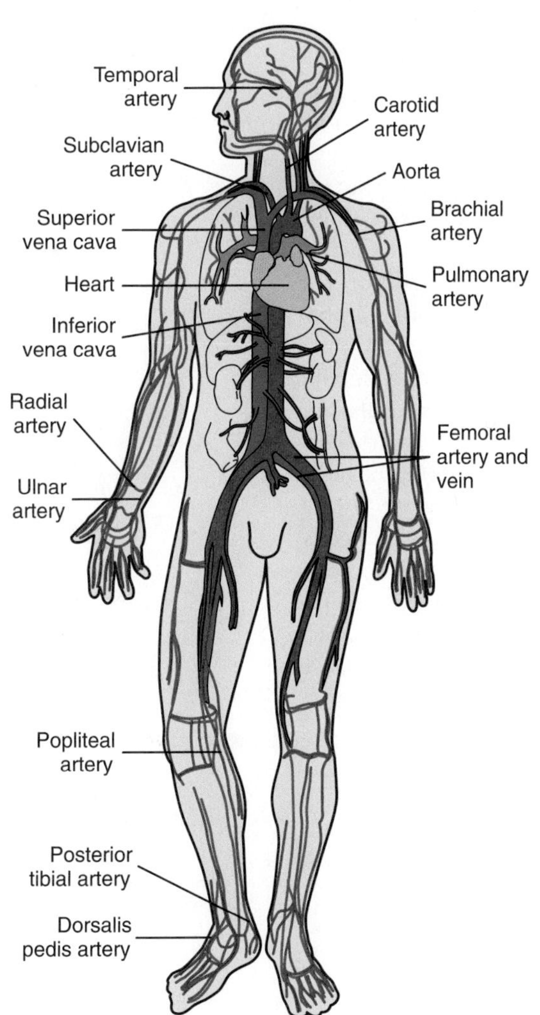

FIGURE 7-17 Arterial (red) and venous (blue) systems.

THE LYMPHATIC SYSTEM

The lymphatic (lymph) system is a complex network that transports lymph throughout the body (Fig. 7-18). *Lymph* is a clear, thin, watery fluid. Lymph contains proteins and fats from the intestines. Lymph also contains white blood cells (WBCs).

The lymphatic system:

- Collects extra lymph from the tissues and returns it to the blood. This helps maintain fluid balance. Water, proteins, and other substances normally leak out of the capillaries into surrounding tissues. The lymphatic system drains the extra fluid from the tissues. Otherwise, the tissues swell.
- Defends the body against infection by producing lymphocytes. *Lymphocytes* are a type of WBC that defends the body against microorganisms that cause infection (Chapter 12).
- Absorbs fats from the intestines and transports them to the blood.

Lymph is formed in the tissues. Lymph is transported by *lymphatic vessels*—lymphatic capillaries to lymphatic venules to the right lymphatic duct and the thoracic duct. Lymph then enters the blood in veins near the neck.

- The *right lymphatic duct* collects lymph from the right arm and from the right side of the head, neck, and chest. It empties into a vein on the right side of the neck.
- The *thoracic duct* collects lymph from the pelvis, abdomen, lower chest, and rest of the body. It empties into a vein on the left side of the neck.

Lymph nodes are shaped like beans. They range from the size of a pinhead to as large as a lima bean. They are found in the neck, underarms, groin area, chest, abdomen, pelvis, and behind the knees. Usually, you cannot see or feel lymph nodes. They swell when producing more lymphocytes to fight infection.

Lymph enters lymph nodes through the lymphatic vessels. The lymph nodes filter bacteria, cancer cells, and damaged cells from the lymph. This prevents such substances from entering and circulating throughout the body.

See Figure 7-18 for the location of the *thymus (thymus gland)*. Certain lymphocytes—T lymphocytes (T cells) develop in the thymus. Such lymphocytes are important for immune system function (p. 86). The thymus reaches full growth at puberty. Then thymus tissue is slowly replaced by fat and connective tissue. By age 80, it is usually gone.

The *tonsils* are in the back of the throat. *Adenoids* are behind the nose. These structures trap microorganisms in the mouth and nose to help prevent infection.

The *spleen* is the largest structure in the lymphatic system. It is about the size of a fist. The spleen has a rich blood supply—about 500 milliliters (mL) (1 pint) of blood. The spleen:

- Filters and removes bacteria and other substances.
- Destroys old red blood cells (RBCs).
- Saves the iron found in hemoglobin when RBCs are destroyed.
- Stores blood. When needed, the blood is returned to the circulatory system.

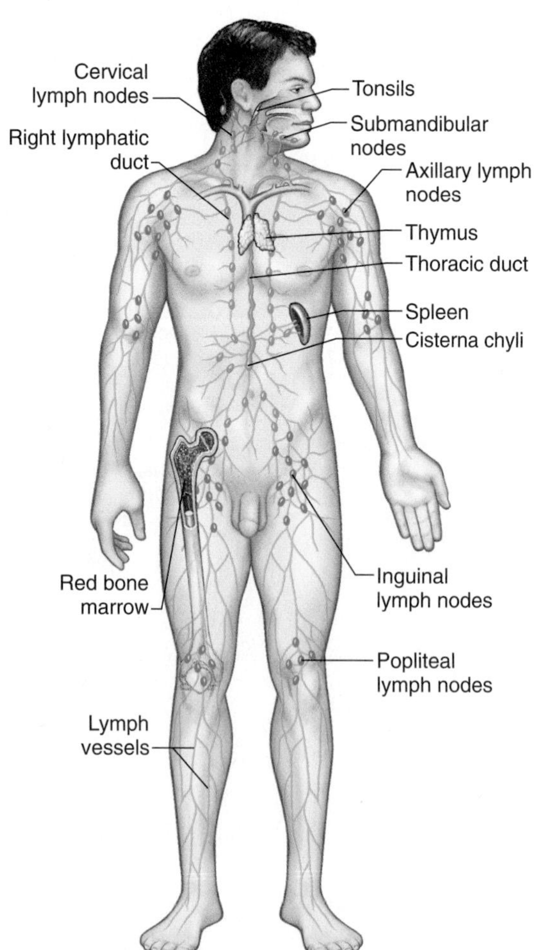

FIGURE 7-18 Lymphatic system.

THE RESPIRATORY SYSTEM

Oxygen is needed to live. Every cell needs oxygen. Air contains about 21% oxygen. This meets the body's needs under normal conditions. The respiratory system (Fig. 7-19) brings oxygen into the lungs and removes carbon dioxide. ***Respiration** is the process of supplying the cells with oxygen and removing carbon dioxide from them.* Respiration involves *inhalation* (breathing in) and *exhalation* (breathing out). The terms *inspiration* (breathing in) and *expiration* (breathing out) also are used.

Air enters the body through the *nose*. The air then passes into the *pharynx* (throat). It is a tube-shaped passageway for air and food. Air passes from the pharynx into the *larynx* (voice box). A piece of cartilage, the *epiglottis*, acts like a lid over the larynx. The epiglottis prevents food from entering the airway during swallowing. During inhalation the epiglottis lifts up to let air pass over the larynx. Air passes from the larynx into the *trachea* (windpipe).

The trachea divides at its lower end into the *right bronchus* and the *left bronchus*. Each bronchus enters a lung. Upon entering the lungs, the bronchi divide many times into smaller branches called *bronchioles*. Eventually the bronchioles subdivide. They end up in tiny one-celled air sacs called *alveoli*.

Alveoli look like small clusters of grapes. They are supplied by capillaries. Oxygen and carbon dioxide are exchanged between the alveoli and capillaries. Blood in the capillaries picks up oxygen from the alveoli. Then the blood is returned to the left side of the heart and pumped to the rest of the body. Alveoli pick up carbon dioxide from the capillaries for exhalation.

The lungs are spongy tissues. They are filled with alveoli, blood vessels, and nerves. Each lung is divided into lobes. The right lung has 3 lobes; the left lung has 2. The lungs are separated from the abdominal cavity by a muscle called the *diaphragm*.

Each lung is covered by a 2-layered sac called the *pleura*. One layer is attached to the lung and the other to the chest wall. The pleura secretes a very thin fluid that fills the space between the layers. The fluid prevents the layers from rubbing together during inhalation and exhalation. A bony framework made up of the ribs, sternum, and vertebrae protects the lungs.

THE DIGESTIVE SYSTEM

***Digestion** is the process that breaks down food physically and chemically so it can be absorbed for use by the cells.* The digestive system is also called the gastro-intestinal (GI) system. The system also removes solid wastes from the body.

The digestive system involves the *alimentary canal (GI tract)* and the accessory organs of digestion (Fig. 7-20). The alimentary canal is a long tube. It extends from the mouth to the anus. Its major parts are the mouth, pharynx, esophagus, stomach, small intestine, and large intestine. Accessory organs are the teeth, tongue, salivary glands, liver, gallbladder, and pancreas.

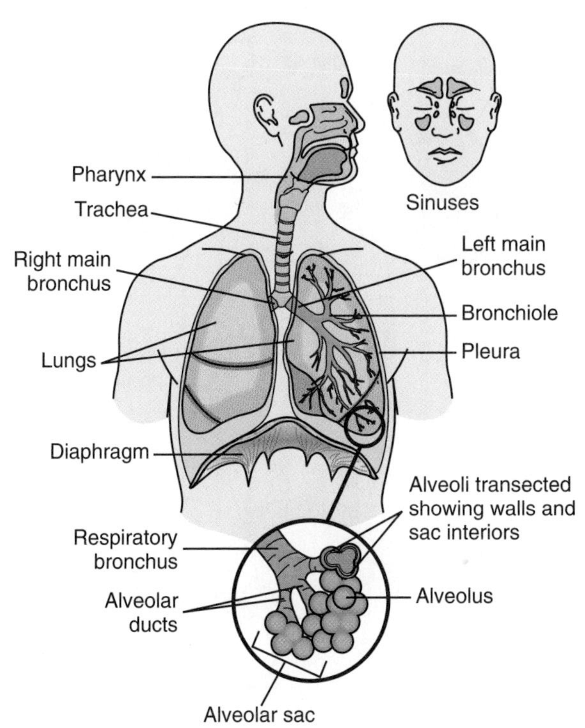

FIGURE 7-19 Respiratory system.

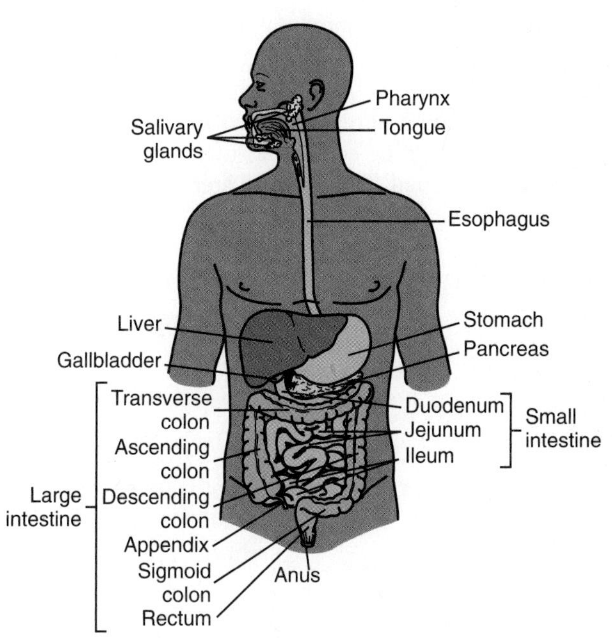

FIGURE 7-20 Digestive system.

Digestion begins in the *mouth (oral cavity)*. It receives food and prepares it for digestion. Using chewing motions, the *teeth* cut, chop, and grind food into small particles for digestion and swallowing. The *tongue* aids in chewing and swallowing. *Taste buds* on the tongue's surface contain nerve endings. Taste buds allow sweet, sour, bitter, and salty tastes to be sensed. *Salivary glands* in the mouth secrete *saliva*. Saliva moistens food particles to ease swallowing and begin digestion. During swallowing, the tongue pushes food into the *pharynx*.

The pharynx (throat) is a muscular tube. Swallowing continues as the pharynx contracts. Contraction of the pharynx pushes food into the *esophagus*. The esophagus is a muscular tube about 10 inches long. It extends from the pharynx to the *stomach*. *Involuntary muscle contractions move food down the esophagus through the alimentary canal* ***(peristalsis)***.

The stomach is a muscular, pouch-like sac. It is in the upper left part of the abdominal cavity. Strong stomach muscles stir and churn food to break it up into even smaller particles. A mucous membrane lines the stomach. It contains glands that secrete *gastric juices*. Food is mixed and churned with the gastric juices to form a semi-liquid substance called *chyme*. Through peristalsis, the chyme is pushed from the stomach into the small intestine.

The *small intestine* is about 20 feet long. It has 3 parts. The first part is the *duodenum*. There more digestive juices are added to the chyme. One is called *bile*. Bile is a greenish liquid made in the *liver*. Bile is stored in the *gallbladder*. Juices from the *pancreas* and small intestine are added to the chyme. Digestive juices chemically break down food so it can be absorbed.

Peristalsis moves the chyme through the 2 other parts of the small intestine: the *jejunum* and the *ileum*. Tiny projections called *villi* line the small intestine. Villi absorb the digested food into the capillaries. Most food absorption takes place in the jejunum and the ileum.

Some chyme is not digested. Undigested chyme passes from the small intestine into the large *intestine* (*large bowel* or *colon*). The colon absorbs most of the water from the chyme. The remaining semi-solid material is called *feces*. Feces contain a small amount of water, solid wastes, and some mucus and germs. These are the waste products of digestion. Feces pass through the colon into the *rectum* by peristalsis. Feces pass out of the body through the *anus*.

THE URINARY SYSTEM

The digestive system rids the body of solid wastes. The lungs rid the body of carbon dioxide. Water and other substances leave the body through sweat. There are other waste products in the blood from cells burning food for energy. The urinary system (Fig. 7-21):

- Removes waste products from the blood.
- Maintains water balance within the body.
- Maintains electrolyte balance. *Electrolytes* are substances that dissolve in water—sodium, potassium, and calcium.
  - Sodium is needed for fluid balance. The body retains water if sodium levels are high. Loss of sodium (through vomiting, diarrhea, some drugs, and so on) can result in dehydration.
  - Potassium and calcium are needed for the proper function of skeletal and cardiac muscles.
- Maintains acid-base balance. A pH scale measures if a substance is acidic, neutral, or basic. A pH of 7 is neutral. Anything below 7 is acidic. Anything above 7 is basic. The blood must remain within a certain pH range (7.35-7.45) for the body to function normally.

The *kidneys* are two bean-shaped organs in the upper abdomen. They lie against the back muscles on each side of the spine. They are protected by the lower edge of the rib cage.

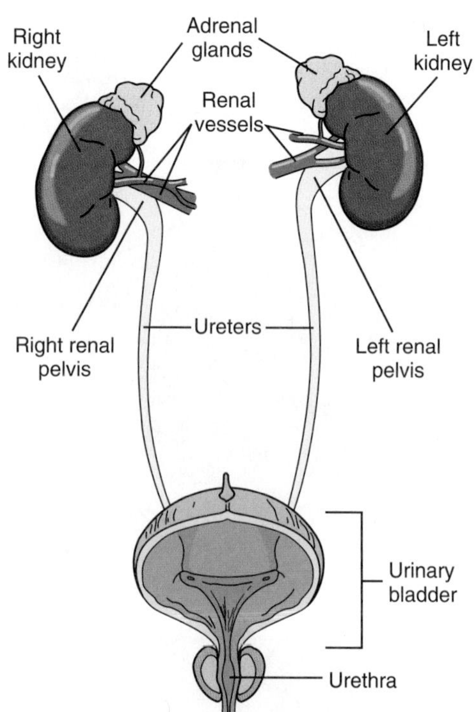

FIGURE 7-21 Urinary system.

Each kidney has over a million tiny *nephrons* (Fig. 7-22). Each nephron is the basic working unit of the kidney. Each nephron has a *convoluted tubule*, which is a tiny coiled tubule. Each convoluted tubule has a *Bowman's capsule* at one end. The capsule partly surrounds a cluster of capillaries called a *glomerulus*. Blood passes through the glomerulus and is filtered by the capillaries. The fluid part of the blood is squeezed into the Bowman's capsule. The fluid then passes into the tubule. Most of the water and other needed substances are re-absorbed by the blood. The rest of the fluid and the waste products form *urine* in the tubule. Urine flows through the tubule to a *collecting tubule*. All collecting tubules drain into the *renal pelvis* in the kidney.

A tube called the *ureter* is attached to the renal pelvis of the kidney. Each ureter is about 10 to 12 inches long. The ureters carry urine from the kidneys to the *bladder*. The bladder is a hollow, muscular sac. It lies toward the front in the lower part of the abdominal cavity.

Urine is stored in the bladder until the need to urinate is felt. This usually occurs when there is about a half pint (250 mL) of urine in the bladder. Urine passes from the bladder through the *urethra*. The opening at the end of the urethra is called the *meatus*. Urine passes from the body through the meatus. Urine is a clear, yellowish fluid.

THE REPRODUCTIVE SYSTEM

Human reproduction results from the union of a male sex cell and a female sex cell. The male and female reproductive systems are different. This allows for the process of reproduction.

The Male Reproductive System

The male reproductive system is shown in Figure 7-23. The *testes (testicles)* are the male sex glands. Sex glands also are called *gonads*. The 2 testes are oval or almond-shaped glands. Male sex cells are produced in the testes. Male sex cells are called *sperm* cells.

Testosterone, the male hormone, is produced in the testes. This hormone is needed for reproductive organ function. It also is needed for the development of the male secondary sex characteristics. There is facial hair; pubic and axillary (underarm) hair; and hair on the arms, chest, and legs. Neck and shoulder sizes increase.

The testes are suspended between the thighs in a sac called the *scrotum*. The scrotum is made of skin and muscle.

Sperm travel from the testis to the *epididymis*. The epididymis is a coiled tube on top and to the side of the testis. From the epididymis, sperm travel through a tube called the *vas deferens*. Each vas deferens joins a *seminal vesicle*. The 2 seminal vesicles store sperm and produce *semen*. Semen is a fluid that carries sperm from the male reproductive tract. The ducts of the seminal vesicles unite to form the *ejaculatory duct*. It passes through the *prostate gland*.

The prostate gland lies just below the bladder. It is shaped like a donut. The gland secretes fluid into the semen. As the ejaculatory ducts leave the prostate, they join the *urethra*. The urethra runs through the prostate gland. The urethra is the outlet for urine and semen. The urethra is contained within the *penis*.

The penis is outside of the body. The *glans* is at the end of the penis. The urethra opens at the end of the glans. A fold of skin (*prepuce* or *foreskin*) is at the end of the penis (Chapters 16 and 18).

The penis has *erectile* tissue. When a man is sexually excited, blood fills the erectile tissue. The penis enlarges and becomes hard and erect. The erect penis can enter a female's vagina. *Cowper's glands* are 2 pea-sized glands under the prostate. They produce a clear, colorless fluid before ejaculation (release of semen). The fluid cleanses the urethra, protects sperm from damage, and provides some lubrication for intercourse. With ejaculation, semen—containing sperm—is released into the vagina.

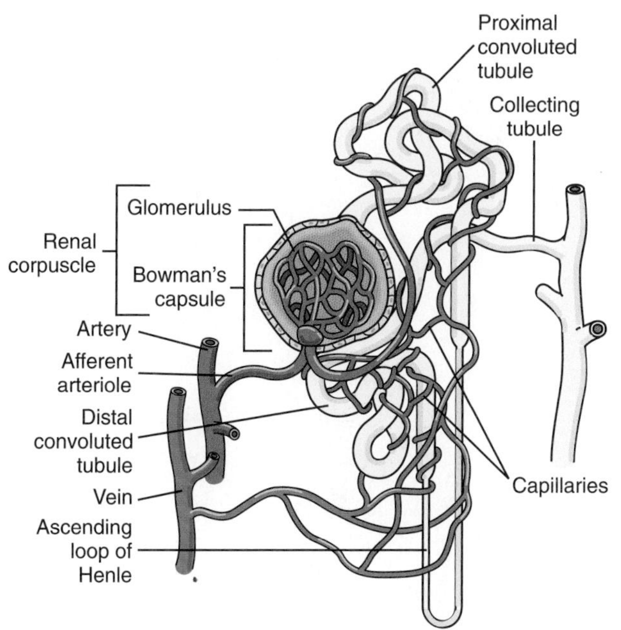

FIGURE 7-22 A nephron.

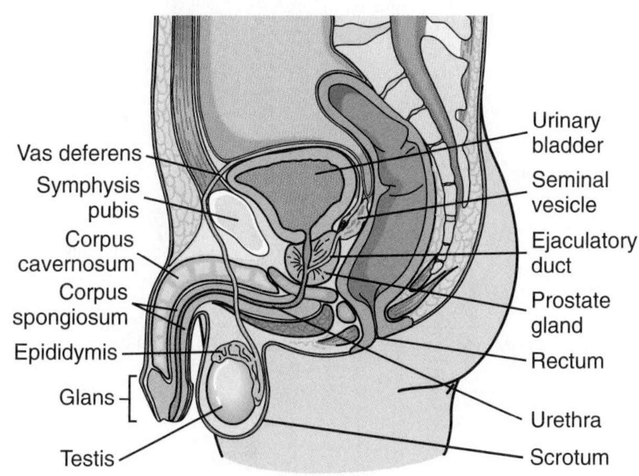

FIGURE 7-23 Male reproductive system.

The Female Reproductive System

Figure 7-24 shows the female reproductive system. The female gonads are 2 almond-shaped glands called *ovaries.* An ovary is on each side of the uterus in the abdominal cavity.

The ovaries contain *ova* or eggs. Ova are the female sex cells. One ovum (egg) is released monthly during the woman's reproductive years. Release of an ovum is called *ovulation.*

The ovaries secrete the female hormones *estrogen* and *progesterone.* These hormones are needed for reproductive system function. They also are needed for the development of secondary sex characteristics in the female. These include increased breast size, pubic and axillary (underarm) hair, slight deepening of the voice, and widening and rounding of the hips.

When an ovum is released from an ovary, it travels through a *fallopian tube.* There are 2 fallopian tubes, 1 on each side. The tubes are attached at one end to the *uterus.* The ovum travels through the fallopian tube to the uterus.

The uterus is a hollow, muscular organ shaped like a pear. It is in the center of the pelvic cavity behind the bladder and in front of the rectum. The main part of the uterus is the *fundus.* The neck or narrow section of the uterus is the *cervix.* Tissue lining the uterus is the *endometrium.* The endometrium has many blood vessels. If sex cells from the male and female unite into 1 cell, that cell implants into the endometrium. There the cell grows into a *fetus* (unborn baby) and receives nourishment.

The cervix of the uterus projects into a muscular canal called the *vagina.* The vagina opens to the outside of the body. It is just behind the urethra. The vagina receives the penis during intercourse. It also is part of the birth canal. Glands in the vaginal wall keep it moistened with secretions. The Bartholin's glands are examples. In young girls, the external vaginal opening is partially closed by a membrane called the *hymen.* The hymen ruptures when the female has intercourse for the first time.

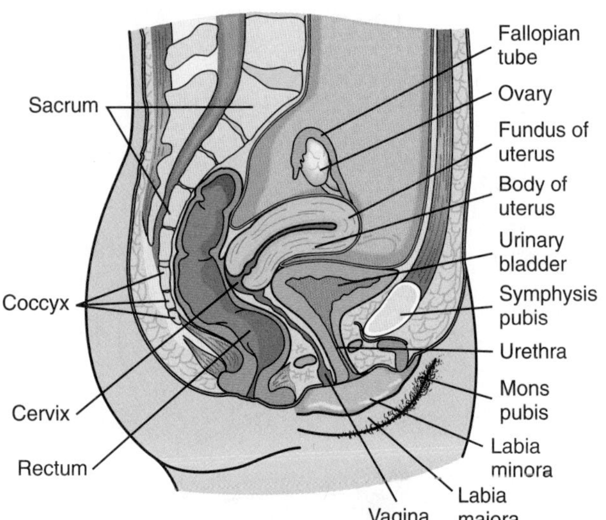

FIGURE 7-24 Female reproductive system.

The external female genitalia are called the vulva (Fig. 7-25).

- The *mons pubis* is a rounded, fatty pad over a bone called the *symphysis pubis.* The mons pubis is covered with hair in the adult female.
- The *labia majora* and *labia minora* are 2 folds of tissue on each side of the vaginal opening.
- The *clitoris* is a small organ composed of erectile tissue. It becomes hard when sexually stimulated.

The *mammary glands (breasts)* secrete milk after childbirth. The glands are on the outside of the chest. They are made up of glandular tissue and fat (Fig. 7-26). The milk drains into ducts that open onto the *nipple.*

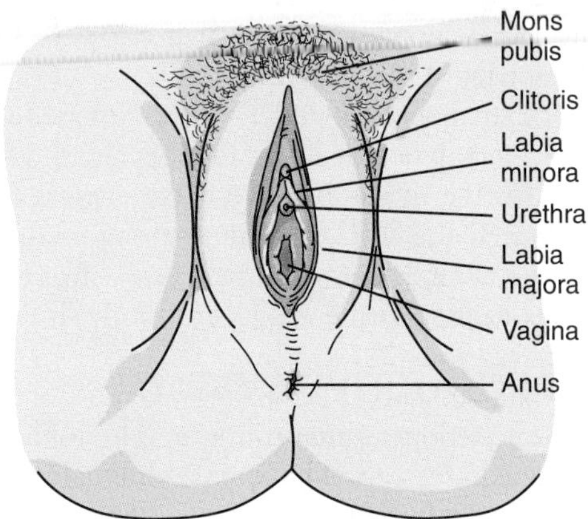

FIGURE 7-25 External female genitalia.

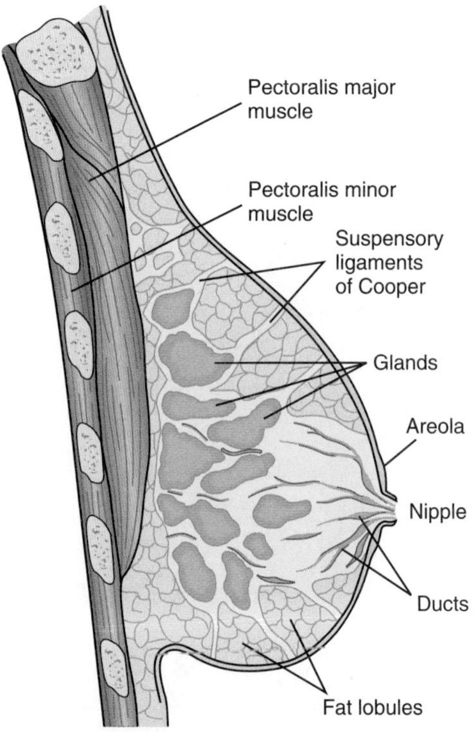

FIGURE 7-26 The female breast.

Menstruation. The endometrium is rich in blood to nourish the cell that grows into a fetus. If pregnancy does not occur, menstruation begins. ***Menstruation** is the process in which the lining of the uterus* (endometrium) *breaks up and is discharged from the body through the vagina.* It occurs about every 28 days. Therefore it is called the *menstrual cycle.*

The first day of the menstrual cycle begins with menstruation. Blood flows from the uterus through the vaginal opening. Menstrual flow usually lasts 3 to 7 days. Ovulation occurs during the next phase. An ovum matures in an ovary and is released. Ovulation usually occurs on or about day 14 of the cycle.

Meanwhile, estrogen and progesterone (the female hormones) are secreted by the ovaries. These hormones cause the endometrium to thicken for pregnancy. If pregnancy does not occur, the hormones decrease in amount. This causes the blood supply to the endometrium to decrease. The endometrium breaks up. It is discharged through the vagina. Another menstrual cycle begins.

Fertilization

To reproduce, a male sex cell (sperm) must unite with a female sex cell (ovum). The uniting of the sperm and ovum into 1 cell is called *fertilization.* A sperm has 23 chromosomes. An ovum has 23 chromosomes. When the 2 cells unite, the fertilized cell has 46 chromosomes.

During intercourse, millions of sperm are deposited into the vagina. Sperm travel up the cervix, through the uterus, and into the fallopian tubes. If a sperm and an ovum unite in a fallopian tube, fertilization results. Pregnancy occurs. The fertilized cell travels down the fallopian tube to the uterus. After a short time, the fertilized cell implants into the thick endometrium and grows during pregnancy.

THE ENDOCRINE SYSTEM

The endocrine system is made up of glands called the *endocrine glands* (Fig. 7-27). *The endocrine glands secrete chemical substances called **hormones** into the bloodstream.* Hormones regulate the activities of other organs and glands in the body.

The *pituitary gland* is called the *master gland.* About the size of a cherry, it is at the base of the brain behind the eyes. The pituitary gland is divided into the *anterior pituitary lobe* and the *posterior pituitary lobe.* The anterior pituitary lobe secretes:

- *Growth hormone (GH)*—needed for growth of muscles, bones, and other organs. It is needed throughout life to maintain normal-sized bones and muscles. Growth is stunted if a baby is born with deficient amounts of growth hormones. Too much of the hormone causes excessive growth.
- *Thyroid-stimulating hormone (TSH)*—needed for thyroid gland function.
- *Adrenocorticotropic hormone (ACTH)*—stimulates the adrenal glands.

The anterior lobe also secretes hormones that regulate growth, development, and function of the male and female reproductive systems.

The posterior pituitary lobe secretes *antidiuretic hormone (ADH)* and *oxytocin.* ADH prevents the kidneys from excreting excessive amounts of water. Oxytocin causes uterine muscles to contract during childbirth.

The *thyroid gland,* shaped like a butterfly, is in the neck in front of the larynx. *Thyroid hormone (TH, thyroxine)* is secreted by the thyroid gland. It regulates metabolism. ***Metabolism** is the burning of food for heat and energy by the cells.* Too little TH results in slowed body processes, slowed movements, and weight gain. Too much TH causes increased metabolism, excess energy, and weight loss. Some babies are born with deficient amounts of TH. Their physical growth and mental growth are stunted.

The 4 *parathyroid glands* secrete *parathormone.* Two lie on each side of the thyroid gland. Parathormone regulates calcium use. Calcium is needed for nerve and muscle function. Insufficient amounts of calcium cause *tetany.* Tetany is a state of severe muscle contraction and spasm. If untreated, tetany can cause death.

The *thymus* secretes the hormone *thymosin.* This hormone is important for the development and function of the immune system.

The *pancreas* secretes *insulin.* Insulin regulates the amount of sugar in the blood available for use by the cells. Insulin is needed for sugar to enter the cells. If there is too little insulin, sugar cannot enter the cells. If sugar cannot enter the cells, excess amounts build up in the blood. This condition is called *diabetes.*

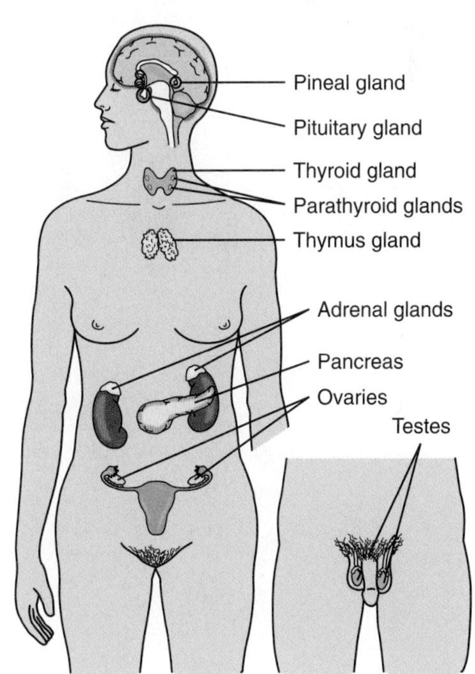

FIGURE 7-27 Endocrine system.

There are 2 *adrenal glands*. An adrenal gland is on the top of each kidney. The adrenal gland has 2 parts: the *adrenal medulla* and the *adrenal cortex*. The adrenal medulla secretes *epinephrine* and *norepinephrine*. These hormones stimulate the body to quickly produce energy during emergencies. Heart rate, blood pressure, muscle power, and energy all increase.

The adrenal cortex secretes 3 groups of hormones needed for life.

- *Glucocorticoids*—regulate metabolism of carbohydrates. They also control the body's response to stress and inflammation.
- *Mineralocorticoids*—regulate the amount of salt and water that is absorbed and lost by the kidneys.
- Small amounts of male and female sex hormones are secreted.

The *gonads* are the glands of human reproduction. Male sex glands (testes) secrete *testosterone*. Female sex glands (ovaries) secrete *estrogen* and *progesterone*.

THE IMMUNE SYSTEM

The immune system protects the body from disease and infection. Abnormal body cells can grow into tumors. Sometimes the body produces substances that cause the body to attack itself. Microorganisms (bacteria, viruses, and other germs) can cause an infection. The immune system defends against threats inside and outside the body.

The immune system gives the body immunity. ***Immunity*** *means that a person has protection against a disease or condition. The person will not get or be affected by the disease.*

- *Specific immunity* is the body's reaction to a certain threat.
- *Non-specific immunity* is the body's reaction to anything it does not recognize as a normal body substance.

Special cells and substances function to produce immunity:

- *Antibodies*—normal body substances that recognize other substances. They are involved in destroying abnormal or unwanted substances.
- *Antigens*—substances that cause an immune response. Antibodies recognize and bind with unwanted antigens. This leads to the destruction of unwanted substances and the production of more antibodies.
- *Phagocytes*—white blood cells (WBCs) that digest and destroy microorganisms and other unwanted substances (Fig. 7-28).
- *Lymphocytes*—WBCs that produce antibodies. Lymphocyte production increases as the body responds to an infection.
  - *B lymphocytes (B cells)*—cause the production of antibodies that circulate in the plasma. The antibodies react to specific antigens.
  - *T lymphocytes (T cells)*—destroy invading cells. *Killer T cells* produce poisons near the invading cells. Some T cells attract other cells. The other cells destroy the invaders.

When the body senses an antigen from an unwanted substance, the immune system acts. Phagocyte and lymphocyte production increases. Phagocytes destroy the invaders through digestion. The lymphocytes produce antibodies that identify and destroy the unwanted substances.

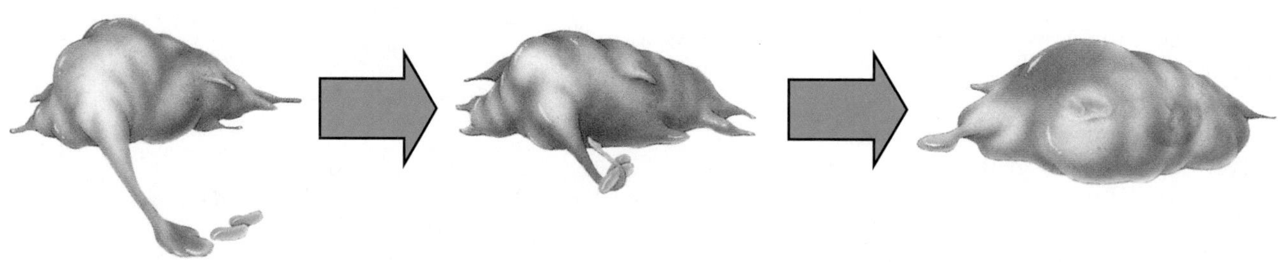

FIGURE 7-28 A phagocyte digests and destroys a microorganism.

FOCUS ON PRIDE

The Person, Family, and Yourself

Personal and Professional Responsibility

Taking care of yourself is a personal and professional responsibility. To care for others you need a strong and healthy body.

- Eat a healthy diet (Chapter 20), exercise, and get enough rest.
- See your doctor for a check-up at least once a year. Or do so sooner if you have a concern.
- Take prescription or over-the-counter drugs only as instructed.
- Keep your immunizations up to date. For example, get a tetanus booster every 10 years.
- Protect your bones and muscles from injury by using good body mechanics (Chapter 13).
- Protect yourself from infection. Follow Standard Precautions and practice good hand hygiene (Chapter 12).

Rights and Respect

Patients and residents have the right to make decisions about their bodies. You may not agree with those decisions. But you must respect the person's choices. If the decision will cause no harm, comply with the request. For example, Mr. Ferris does not want to wear his hearing aid today. He says: "I don't need that thing." His request will not harm him. Respect his choice. Tell the nurse.

If the person's decision may cause harm, tell the nurse at once. For example, Ms. Lane's kidneys do not function. She goes to dialysis 3 times a week. (*Dialysis* is the process of artificially removing wastes from the blood when the kidneys do not function.) Ms. Lane does not want to go today. She says: "I just can't sit there for that long." You know the importance of the urinary system. Without dialysis, she will become very sick. You tell the nurse. Ms. Lane cannot be forced to go to dialysis. But the nurse can talk with Ms. Lane about her decision, the consequences, and possible solutions.

Independence and Social Interaction

The body does not always work right. People become ill or injured. Some illnesses cannot be cured. Sometimes the health team cannot prevent loss of function. However, patients and residents are helped to maintain their optimal level of function. This is the person's highest potential for mental and physical performance.

To help maintain the person's optimal level of function:

- Do not treat the person as a sick, dependent person. This reduces quality of life.
- Encourage the person to be as independent as possible.
- Always focus on the person's abilities, not disabilities.
- Tell the person when you notice progress.
- Promote social interaction. This improves mental performance.

Take pride in helping each person regain or maintain the highest level of functioning possible.

Delegation and Teamwork

The body works like a team. Each system has independent functions. But all systems interact and depend on each other. They work together to keep the body functioning. When a person has a problem with 1 body system, other systems are affected. Understanding each system and how the systems interact helps you provide better care.

Ethics and Laws

Sometimes a person is not able to make decisions about his or her own body. For example, the person has dementia. Or the person is unconscious or affected by drugs or alcohol. Maybe the person thinks about harming himself or herself. Or the person is a child. Ethical issues may arise over who makes decisions for such persons.

Spouses, parents, family members, or legal guardians may make decisions. Some persons have an advance directive (Chapter 32). This document states a person's wishes about health care when that person is unable to make such decisions. In cases such as drug and alcohol abuse or attempts of harm, the person's safety is the priority. Sometimes the court appoints a guardian for a short time. Finally, the agency's ethics committee may address complex issues. The person's safety and best interests must guide the care given.

REVIEW QUESTIONS

Circle the BEST answer.

1 The basic unit of body structure is the
   a Cell
   b Neuron
   c Nephron
   d Ovum

2 The outer layer of the skin is called the
   a Dermis
   b Epidermis
   c Integument
   d Myelin

3 Which is a function of the skin?
   a Provides the protective covering for the body
   b Transports lymph
   c Forms blood cells
   d Provides the shape and framework for the body

4 Which allows movement?
   a Bone marrow
   b Synovial membrane
   c Joints
   d Ligaments

5 Skeletal muscles
   a Are under involuntary control
   b Appear smooth
   c Are under voluntary control
   d Appear striped and smooth

6 The highest functions in the brain take place in the
   a Cerebral cortex
   b Medulla
   c Brainstem
   d Spinal nerves

7 The ear is involved with
   a Regulating body movements
   b Balance
   c Smoothness of body movements
   d Controlling involuntary muscles

8 The liquid part of blood is the
   a Hemoglobin
   b Red blood cell
   c Plasma
   d White blood cell

9 Which part of the heart pumps blood to the body?
   a Right atrium
   b Left atrium
   c Right ventricle
   d Left ventricle

10 Which carry blood away from the heart?
   a Capillaries
   b Veins
   c Venules
   d Arteries

11 Oxygen and carbon dioxide are exchanged
   a In the bronchi
   b Between the alveoli and capillaries
   c Between the lungs and pleura
   d In the trachea

12 Digestion begins in the
   a Mouth
   b Stomach
   c Small intestine
   d Colon

13 Most food absorption takes place in the
   a Stomach
   b Small intestine
   c Colon
   d Large intestine

14 Urine is formed by the
   a Jejunum
   b Kidneys
   c Bladder
   d Liver

15 Urine passes from the body through the
   a Ureters
   b Urethra
   c Anus
   d Nephrons

16 The male sex gland is called the
   a Penis
   b Semen
   c Testis
   d Scrotum

17 The male sex cell is the
   a Semen
   b Ovum
   c Gonad
   d Sperm

18 The female sex gland is the
   a Ovary
   b Cervix
   c Uterus
   d Vagina

19 The discharge of the lining of the uterus is called
   a The endometrium
   b Ovulation
   c Fertilization
   d Menstruation

20 The endocrine glands secrete
   a Hormones
   b Mucus
   c Semen
   d Insulin

21 The immune system protects the body from
   a Low blood sugar
   b Disease and infection
   c Loss of fluid
   d Stunted growth

Answers to these questions are on p. 504.

FOCUS ON PRACTICE

Problem Solving

A patient has a disorder that affects the immune system. How does this affect body function? How will you provide care in a way that protects the person?

CHAPTER 8

Care of the Older Person

OBJECTIVES

- Define the key terms and key abbreviation listed in this chapter.
- Identify the developmental tasks of each age-group.
- Identify the social changes common in older adulthood.
- Describe the physical changes from aging and the care required.
- Describe the gains and losses related to long-term care.
- Describe the sexual changes and needs of older persons.
- Explain how to deal with sexually aggressive persons.
- Explain how to promote PRIDE in the person, the family, and yourself.

KEY TERMS

development Changes in mental, emotional, and social function

developmental task A skill that must be completed during a stage of development

geriatrics The care of aging people

gerontology The study of the aging process

growth The physical changes that are measured and that occur in a steady and orderly manner

menopause The time when menstruation stops and menstrual cycles end; there has been at least 1 year without a menstrual period

sexuality The physical, emotional, social, cultural, and spiritual factors that affect a person's feelings and attitudes about his or her sex

KEY ABBREVIATION

OBRA Omnibus Budget Reconciliation Act of 1987

People live longer than ever before. They are healthier and more active. Late adulthood ranges from 65 years of age and older. Most older people live with a partner, children, or other family. Some live alone or with friends. Still others live in assisted living residences or nursing centers.

Gerontology *is the study of the aging process.* ***Geriatrics*** *is the care of aging people.* Aging is normal. It is not a disease. Normal changes occur in body structure and function. They increase the risk for illness, injury, and disability. Psychological and social changes also occur. Often changes are slow. Most people adjust well to these changes. They lead happy, meaningful lives.

GROWTH AND DEVELOPMENT

People grow and develop throughout life. ***Growth*** *is the physical changes that are measured and that occur in a steady and orderly manner.* Growth is measured in weight, height, and changes in appearance and body functions.

Development *relates to changes in mental, emotional, and social function.* A person behaves and thinks in certain ways in each stage of development. A 2-year-old thinks in simple terms. A primary caregiver is needed for basic needs. A 40-year-old thinks in complex ways. Basic needs are met without help.

Growth and development occur in a sequence, order, and pattern. Certain skills must be completed during each stage. A ***developmental task*** *is a skill that must be completed during a stage of development.* A stage cannot be skipped. Each stage has its own characteristics and developmental tasks (Box 8-1, p. 90).

BOX 8-1 Growth and Development: Developmental Tasks

Infancy (Birth to 1 Year)
- Learning to walk
- Learning to eat solid foods
- Beginning to talk and communicate with others
- Learning to trust
- Beginning to have emotional relationships with parents, brothers, and sisters
- Developing stable sleep and feeding patterns

Toddlerhood (1 to 3 Years)
- Tolerating separation from the primary caregiver
- Gaining control of bowel and bladder function
- Using words to communicate
- Becoming less dependent on the primary caregiver

Preschool (3 to 6 Years)
- Increasing the ability to communicate and understand others
- Performing self-care
- Learning gender differences and developing sexual modesty
- Learning right from wrong and good from bad
- Learning to play with others
- Developing family relationships

School Age (6 to 9 or 10 Years)
- Developing the social and physical skills needed for playing games
- Learning to get along with persons of the same age and background (peers)
- Learning gender-appropriate behaviors and attitudes
- Learning basic reading, writing, and math skills
- Developing a conscience and morals
- Developing a good feeling and attitude about oneself

Late Childhood (9 or 10 to 12 Years)
- Becoming independent of adults and learning to depend on oneself
- Developing and keeping friendships with peers
- Understanding the physical, psychological, and social roles of one's sex
- Developing moral and ethical behavior
- Developing greater muscular strength, coordination, and balance
- Learning how to study

Adolescence (12 to 18 Years)
- Accepting changes in the body and appearance
- Developing appropriate relationships with males and females of the same age
- Accepting the male or female role appropriate for one's age
- Becoming independent from parents and adults
- Preparing for marriage and family life
- Preparing for a career
- Developing the morals, attitudes, and values needed to function in society

Young Adulthood (18 to 40 Years)
- Choosing education and a career
- Selecting a partner
- Learning to live with a partner
- Becoming a parent and raising children
- Developing a satisfactory sex life

Middle Adulthood (40 to 65 Years)
- Adjusting to physical changes
- Having grown children
- Developing leisure-time activities
- Adjusting to aging parents

Late Adulthood (65 Years and Older)
- Adjusting to decreased strength and loss of health
- Adjusting to retirement and reduced income
- Coping with a partner's death
- Developing new friends and relationships
- Preparing for one's own death

SOCIAL CHANGES

People cope with aging in their own way. The following social changes occur with aging.

- *Retirement.* Retirement is a reward for a life-time of work. The person can relax and enjoy life. Some people retire because of poor health or disability. Retired people may have part-time jobs or do volunteer work (Fig. 8-1). Work helps meet love, belonging, and self-esteem needs. The person feels fulfilled and useful. Friendships form with co-workers.
- *Reduced income.* Retirement often means reduced income. Social Security may provide the only income. Rent or house payments continue. Food, clothing, utility bills, and taxes are other expenses. Car expenses, home repairs, drugs, and health care are other costs. Severe money problems can result. Some people have income from savings, investments, retirement plans, and insurance.
- *Social relationships.* Social relationships change throughout life. Children grow up, leave home, and have their own families. Some live far away. Older family members and friends die, move away, or are disabled. Yet most older people have regular contact with children, grandchildren, family, and friends (Fig. 8-2). Others are lonely. Separation from children is a common cause. So is lack of companionship with people their own age (Fig. 8-3). Hobbies, religious and community events, and new friends help prevent loneliness. So do family times.
- *Children as caregivers.* Parents and children change roles. The child cares for the parent. Some older persons feel more secure. Others feel unwanted, in the way, and useless. Some lose dignity and self-respect. Tensions may occur among the child, parent, and other household members. Lack of privacy is a cause. So are disagreements and criticisms about housekeeping, raising children, cooking, and friends.

- *Death of a partner.* A person may try to prepare for a partner's death. When death occurs, the loss is crushing. No amount of preparation is ever enough for the emptiness and changes that result. The person loses a lover, friend, companion, and confidant. Grief may be very great. The person's life will likely change. Serious physical and mental health disorders result. Some lose the will to live. Some attempt suicide. See *Focus on Communication: Social Relationships.*

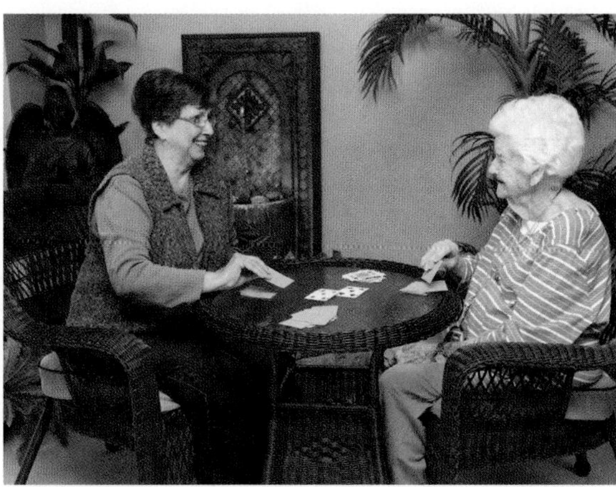

FIGURE 8-1 This retired woman is a nursing center volunteer.

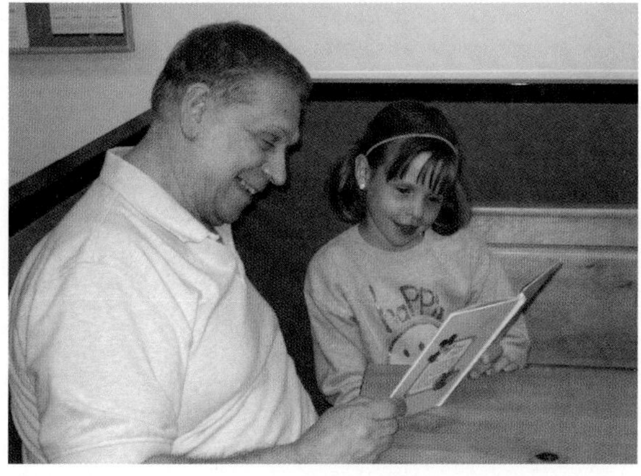

FIGURE 8-2 An older man reads to his grandchild.

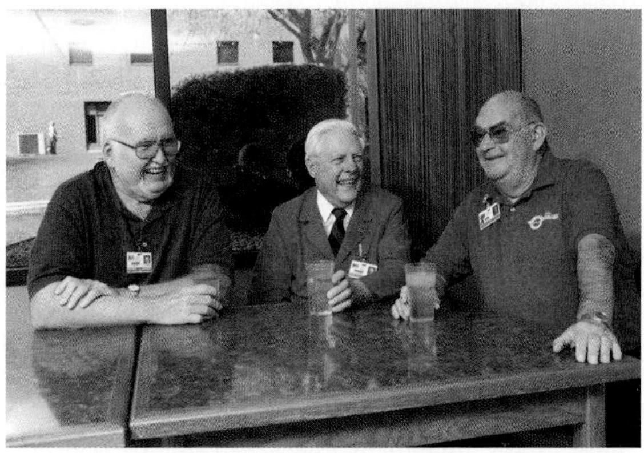

FIGURE 8-3 Older people enjoy being with others of their own age.

FOCUS ON COMMUNICATION

Social Relationships

The social changes of aging can cause loneliness. With nursing center care, the loneliness can seem even greater. To help the person feel less lonely, you can:

- Suggest that the person call a family member or friend. Offer to help with phone numbers and dialing.
- Keep the phone within the person's reach. He or she can place or answer calls with greater ease.
- Suggest that the person read cards and letters. Offer to assist.
- Visit with the person during your shift.
- Introduce new residents to other residents and staff.

PHYSICAL CHANGES

Physical changes occur with aging. Body processes slow down. Energy level and body efficiency decline. Changes are slow over many years. Often they are not seen for a long time.

The Integumentary System

The skin loses its elasticity, strength, and fatty tissue layer. The skin thins and sags. Wrinkles appear. Secretions from oil and sweat glands decrease. Dry skin and itching occur. The skin is fragile and easily injured. The skin's blood vessels are fragile, increasing the risk for:

- Skin breakdown
- Skin tears (Chapter 24)
- Pressure ulcers (Chapter 25)
- Bruising
- Delayed healing

Brown spots ("age spots" or "liver spots") appear on sun-exposed areas. They are common on the wrists and hands.

Loss of the skin's fatty tissue layer affects body temperature. More sensitive to cold, protect the person from drafts and cold. Sweaters, lap blankets, socks, extra blankets, and higher thermostat settings are helpful.

Dry skin causes itching. It is easily damaged. A shower or bath twice a week is enough for hygiene. Partial baths are taken at other times. Mild soaps or soap substitutes clean the underarms, genitals, and under the breasts. Often soap is not used on the face, arms, legs, back, chest, and abdomen. Lotions and creams prevent drying and itching. Deodorants may not be needed because sweat gland secretion is decreased.

Nails become thick and tough. Feet usually have poor circulation. A nick or cut can lead to a serious infection.

The skin has fewer nerve endings. This affects sensing heat, cold, pressure, and pain. Burns are great risks because of fragile skin, poor circulation, and decreased sensing of heat and cold. Complaints of cold feet are common. Socks provide warmth. Do not use hot water bottles and heating pads because of the risk for burns.

White or gray hair is common. Hair loss occurs in men. Hair thins on men and women—on the head, in the pubic area, and under the arms. Women and men may wear wigs. Some color hair to cover graying. Facial hair (lip and chin) may occur in women.

Hair is drier from decreases in scalp oils. Brushing promotes circulation and oil production. Shampoo frequency usually decreases with age. It is done as needed for hygiene and comfort.

The Musculo-Skeletal System

Muscle cells decrease in number. Muscles *atrophy* (shrink). They decrease in strength.

Bones lose minerals, especially calcium. Bones lose strength. They become brittle and break easily. Sometimes just turning in bed can cause fractures (broken bones).

Vertebrae shorten. Joints become stiff and painful. Hip and knee joints flex (bend) slightly. These changes cause gradual loss of height and strength. Mobility also decreases.

Activity, exercise, and diet help prevent bone loss and loss of muscle strength. Walking is good exercise. Exercise groups and range-of-motion exercises are helpful (Chapter 23). A diet high in protein, calcium, and vitamins is needed.

Protect the person from injury and falls (Chapters 9 and 10). Turn and move the person gently and carefully (Chapter 14). Some persons need help and support getting out of bed. Some need help walking.

The Nervous System

Nerve cells are lost. Nerve conduction and reflexes slow. Responses are slower.

Blood flow to the brain is reduced. Dizziness may occur. It increases the risk for falls. Practice measures to prevent falls (Chapter 10).

Changes occur in brain cells. This affects personality and mental function. So does the reduced blood flow to the brain. Memory is shorter. Forgetfulness increases. Responses slow. Confusion, dizziness, and fatigue may occur. Long ago events are easier to recall than recent ones. Older people who are mentally active and involved in current events show fewer personality and mental changes.

Sleep patterns change. Falling asleep is harder. Sleep periods are shorter. They wake often at night. Less sleep is needed. Loss of energy and decreased blood flow may cause fatigue. They may rest or nap during the day. They may go to bed early and get up early.

The Senses. Hearing and vision losses occur (Chapter 28). Taste and smell dull, decreasing appetite. Touch and sensitivity to pain and pressure are reduced. So is sensing heat and cold. These changes increase the risk for injury. The person may not notice painful injuries or diseases. Or the person feels minor pain. You need to:

- Protect older persons from injury (Chapters 9 and 10).
- Check for signs of skin breakdown (Chapters 16, 24, and 25).
- Give good skin care (Chapter 16).
- Prevent skin tears (Chapter 24) and pressure ulcers (Chapter 25).
- Follow safety measures for heat and cold (Chapter 24).

The Circulatory System

The heart muscle weakens. It pumps blood with less force. Activity, exercise, excitement, and illness increase the body's need for oxygen and nutrients. A damaged or weak heart cannot meet these needs.

Arteries narrow and are less elastic. Less blood flows through them. Poor circulation occurs in many body parts. A weak heart works harder to pump blood through narrowed vessels.

The number of red blood cells decreases. This can cause fatigue.

The Respiratory System

Respiratory muscles weaken. Lung tissue becomes less elastic. Difficult, labored, or painful breathing *(dyspnea)* may occur with activity. (*Dys* means *difficult. Pnea* means *breathing*.) The person may lack strength to cough and clear the airway of secretions. Respiratory infections and diseases may develop. These can threaten life.

Normal breathing is promoted. Avoid heavy bed linens over the chest. They prevent normal chest expansion. Turning, re-positioning, and deep breathing are important. Breathing usually is easier in semi-Fowler's position (Chapter 15). The person should be as active as possible.

The Digestive System

Salivary glands produce less saliva. This can cause difficulty swallowing *(dysphagia)*. (*Dys* means *difficult. Phagia* means *swallowing*.) Dry foods may be hard to swallow.

Secretion of digestive juices decreases. Fried and fatty foods are hard to digest. They may cause indigestion.

Loss of teeth and ill-fitting dentures cause chewing problems. Hard-to-chew foods are avoided. Ground, chopped, or pureed meat is easier to chew and swallow.

Peristalsis decreases. The stomach and colon empty slower. Flatulence and constipation can occur (Chapter 19).

Dry, fried, and fatty foods are avoided. This aids swallowing and digestion. Oral hygiene improves taste (Chapter 16). Some people do not have teeth or dentures.

High-fiber foods are hard to chew and can irritate the intestines. They include apricots, celery, and fruits and vegetables with skins and seeds. Persons with chewing problems or constipation often need foods that provide soft bulk. They include whole-grain cereals and cooked fruits and vegetables.

The Urinary System

Kidney function decreases. The kidneys shrink *(atrophy)*. Blood flow to the kidneys is reduced. Waste removal is less efficient.

The ureters, bladder, and urethra lose tone and elasticity. Bladder muscles weaken. Bladder size decreases, storing less urine. Urinary frequency or urgency may occur. Many older persons have to urinate (void) during the night. Urinary incontinence (the loss of bladder control) may occur (Chapter 18).

In men, the prostate gland enlarges. This puts pressure on the urethra. Difficulty voiding or frequent urination occurs.

Urinary tract infections are risks. Adequate fluids are needed—water, juices, milk, and gelatin. Follow the care plan. Most fluids should be taken before 1700 (5:00 PM). This reduces the need to void during the night.

Persons with incontinence may need bladder training programs. Sometimes catheters are needed (Chapter 18).

The Reproductive System

Reproductive organs change with aging.

- *Men.* The hormone *testosterone* decreases slightly. It affects strength, sperm production, and reproductive tissues. These changes affect sexual activity. An erection takes longer. The phase between erection and orgasm also is longer. Orgasm is less forceful than when younger. Erections are lost quickly. The time between erections also is longer.
- *Women.* ***Menopause*** *is when menstruation stops and menstrual cycles end. There has been at least 1 year without a menstrual period.* The woman can no longer have children. This occurs between 45 and 55 years of age. Female hormones (*estrogen* and *progesterone*) decrease. The uterus, vagina, and genitalia shrink *(atrophy)*. Vaginal walls thin. There is vaginal dryness. These make intercourse uncomfortable or painful. Arousal takes longer. Orgasm is less intense.

NEEDING NURSING CENTER CARE

Some older persons cannot care for themselves. Nursing centers are options for them (Chapter 1). Some people stay in nursing centers until death. Others return home. While there, the nursing center is the person's home. The setting is as home-like as possible.

The person needing nursing center care may suffer some or all of these losses.

- Loss of identity as a productive member of a family and community
- Loss of possessions—home, household items, car, and so on
- Loss of independence
- Loss of real-world experiences—shopping, traveling, cooking, driving, hobbies, and so on
- Loss of health and mobility

The person may feel useless, powerless, and hopeless. The health team helps the person cope with loss and improve quality of life. Treat the person with dignity and respect. Also practice good communication skills. Follow the care plan.

SEXUALITY

Sexuality *is the physical, emotional, social, cultural, and spiritual factors that affect a person's feelings and attitudes about his or her sex.* Sexuality involves the personality and the body. It affects how a person behaves, thinks, dresses, and responds to others.

Love, affection, and intimacy are needed throughout life (Fig. 8-4). Attitudes and sex needs change with aging and life events. These include injury, illness, surgery, divorce, death of a partner, and relationship break-ups. Yet older persons love and fall in love.

Frequency of sex decreases for many older persons. Besides life events, reasons relate to weakness, fatigue, and pain. Reduced mobility, aging, and chronic illness are factors.

Some older people do not have intercourse. This does not mean loss of sexual needs or desires. Often needs are expressed in other ways. They hold hands, touch, caress, and embrace. These bring closeness and intimacy.

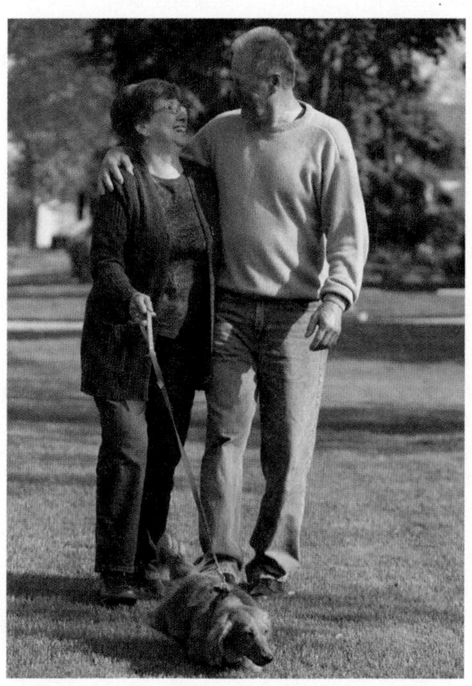

FIGURE 8-4 Love and affection are important to people of all ages.

Meeting Sexual Needs

The nursing team promotes the meeting of sexual needs. The measures in Box 8-2 may be part of the person's care plan.

Married couples in nursing centers can share the same room. This is a requirement of the Omnibus Budget Reconciliation Act of 1987 (OBRA). They can share the same bed if their conditions permit.

Single nursing center residents may develop relationships. They are allowed time together, not kept apart.

The Sexually Aggressive Person

Some patients and residents flirt or make sexual advances or comments. Some expose themselves, masturbate, or touch other staff. Often there are reasons for the person's behavior. Understanding this helps you deal with the matter.

Sexually aggressive behaviors have many causes. They include:

- Nervous system disorders
- Confusion, disorientation, and dementia
- Drug side effects
- Fever
- Poor vision

The person may confuse someone with his or her partner. Or the person cannot control the behavior. The healthy person controls sexual urges. Changes in the brain and mental function make control difficult. Sexual behavior in these cases is usually innocent.

Sometimes touch is used to gain attention. For example, Mr. Green cannot speak or move his right side. Your buttocks are near him. To get your attention, he touches your buttocks. His behavior is not sexual.

Sometimes masturbation is a sexually aggressive behavior. Some persons touch and fondle the genitals for sexual pleasure. However, urinary or reproductive system disorders can cause genital soreness and itching. So can poor hygiene and being wet or soiled from urine or feces. Touching genitals could signal a health problem.

Sometimes touch is sexual. For example, a person wants to prove that he or she is sexually attractive. You must be professional about the matter.

- Ask the person not to touch you. State the places where you were touched.
- Tell the person that you will not do what he or she wants.
- Tell the person what behaviors make you uncomfortable. Politely ask the person not to act that way.
- Allow privacy if the person is becoming aroused. Provide for safety. Complete a safety check of the room (see the inside of the front cover). Tell the person when you will return.
- Discuss the matter with the nurse. The nurse can help you understand the behavior.
- Follow the care plan. It has measures to deal with sexually aggressive behaviors. They are based on the cause of the behavior.

See *Focus on Communication: The Sexually Aggressive Person.*

BOX 8-2 Promoting Sexuality

- Allow grooming routines. Assist as needed. For women, this includes applying make-up, nail polish, and cologne. Many women shave their legs and underarms and pluck eyebrows. Men may use after-shave lotion and cologne. Hair care is important to men and women.
- Allow clothing choices. Street clothes are worn if the person's condition permits.
- Protect the right to privacy. Do not expose the person. Drape and screen the person.
- Show respect. The person may not share your sexual attitudes, values, or practices. The person may have a homosexual, premarital, or extramarital relationship. Do not judge or gossip about relationships.
- Allow privacy. If the person has a private room, close the door for privacy. Some agencies have DO NOT DISTURB signs for doors. Let the person and partner know how much time they have alone. Remind them about meal times, drugs, and treatments. Tell other staff that the person wants time alone.
- Knock before you enter any room. This simple courtesy shows respect for privacy.
- Consider the person's roommate. Privacy curtains do not block sound. Arrange for privacy when the roommate is out of the room. A roommate may offer to leave for a while. Or the nurse finds a private area.
- Allow privacy for masturbation. It is a normal form of sexual expression. Close the privacy curtain and the door. Knock before you enter any room. This saves you and the person embarrassment. Sometimes confused persons masturbate in public areas. Lead the person to a private area. Or distract him or her with an activity.

FOCUS ON COMMUNICATION

The Sexually Aggressive Person

Dealing with the sexually aggressive person is hard. This is true for young and older staff and for new and experienced staff. Ask yourself these questions.

- Does the person have a health problem that affects impulse control? If yes, the behavior may not have a sexual purpose.
- Is the person's behavior on purpose? Is the intent sexual? If yes, you must deal with the behavior. Be direct and matter-of-fact. For example, you can say:
  - "You brushed your hand across my breast (or other body part) 2 times this morning. Please don't do that again."
  - "No, I cannot kiss you. It would be unprofessional."
  - "You exposed yourself to me again today. Please do not do that again."

The sexually aggressive person needs the nurse's attention. Report what happened and when. Also report what you said and did. The nurse must deal with the problem. If other staff are reporting such behaviors, the nurse views the problem in a broader way.

Protecting the Person

The person must be protected from unwanted sexual comments and advances. This is sexual abuse (Chapter 3). Tell the nurse right away. No one should be allowed to sexually abuse another person. This includes staff members, patients, residents, family members or other visitors, and volunteers.

FOCUS ON PRIDE

The Person, Family, and Yourself

Personal and Professional Responsibility

Some people believe that all older persons have decreased mental and physical function. For example, they are hard-of-hearing, confused, or move slowly. Others think the elderly cannot care for themselves. Or they lose interest in activities.

Your beliefs affect the care you give. Each person is unique. Treat each person as an individual. This is a personal and professional responsibility.

Rights and Respect

The person's sexual attitudes, values, or practices may differ from yours. For example, you may not agree with a person's sexual relationship. Your feelings must not affect the person's care. Do not avoid the person. Do not judge or gossip about the person. Treat the person with dignity and respect.

Independence and Social Interaction

Older persons may feel lonely and isolated. Loss of friends and loved ones, a new home setting, reduced income, and physical changes are causes. To promote social interaction:

- Encourage the person to talk about friends and family.
- Ask about the person's hobbies and interests.
- Use touch to show caring. For example, gently place your hand on the person's shoulder or arm. Remember to maintain professional boundaries (Chapter 3).
- Take time to listen. Avoid seeming rushed.

Some persons prefer quiet and privacy. They may avoid social contacts. Respect their wishes for privacy. Take pride in considering their social needs.

Delegation and Teamwork

A person may have sexually aggressive behaviors. The health team must try to determine the cause. If the cause can be treated, the behavior may stop. When the cause cannot be treated, the health team follows the care plan to manage the behavior. A professional response is always needed.

Tell the nurse if you notice sexually aggressive behaviors. The problem cannot be ignored. Rely on the nursing team for advice, guidance, and support.

Ethics and Laws

A nursing center provides a temporary or permanent residence for some persons. The setting must promote quality of life. It must be clean, safe, comfortable, and as home-like as possible. Give care that reflects these principles. To do so:

- Make sure the person and his or her clothes and linens are clean and dry.
- Keep the person's room clean and orderly.
- Place soiled linens in the correct containers. Empty the containers often. Do not let them over-flow.
- Clean up your work area and the bathroom after giving care.
- Help the person display personal items if asked. Do not touch the person's items without permission.
- Treat the person as if you were in his or her home.

Respect the person and his or her setting. Take pride in providing quality care.

REVIEW QUESTIONS

Circle the BEST answer.

1 Which is a developmental task of late adulthood?
  a Accepting changes in appearance
  b Adjusting to decreased strength
  c Developing a satisfactory sex life
  d Performing self-care

2 Retirement usually means
  a Lowered income
  b Changes from aging
  c Less free time
  d Financial security

3 Which causes loneliness in older persons?
  a Children moving away
  b Having hobbies
  c Attending community events
  d Contact with other older persons

4 These statements are about a partner's death. Which is *false?*
  a The person loses a lover, friend, and companion.
  b Preparing for the event lessens grief.
  c The survivor may develop health problems.
  d The survivor's life will likely change.

5 Skin changes occur with aging. Care should include
  a Keeping the room cool
  b A daily bath with soap
  c Applying lotion
  d Bathing in hot water

6 Aging causes changes in the musculo-skeletal system. Which is *false?*
  a Bones become brittle. They can break easily.
  b Exercise slows musculo-skeletal changes.
  c Joints become stiff and painful.
  d Bedrest is needed for loss of strength.

7 Nervous system changes occur with aging. Which is *true?*
  a Less sleep is needed than when younger.
  b The person forgets events from long ago.
  c Sensitivity to pain increases.
  d Confusion occurs in all older persons.

8 An older person has circulatory changes. Care includes the following *except*
  a Placing needed items nearby
  b A moderate amount of daily exercise
  c Avoiding exertion
  d Long walks

9 Respiratory changes occur with aging. Which is *true?*
  a Heavy bed linens are used.
  b The person is turned often if on bedrest.
  c The side-lying position is best for breathing.
  d The person should be as inactive as possible.

10 Older persons should avoid dry foods because of
  a Decreases in saliva
  b Loss of teeth or ill-fitting dentures
  c Decreased amounts of digestive juices
  d Decreased peristalsis

11 The doctor orders increased fluid intake for an older person. You should
  a Give most of the fluid before 1700 (5:00 PM)
  b Provide mostly water
  c Start a bladder training program
  d Insert a catheter

12 Changes occur in the reproductive system. Which is *true?*
  a Men experience menopause.
  b Orgasms do not occur.
  c Hormones decrease.
  d The prostate gland decreases in size.

13 A person is masturbating in the dining room. You should do the following *except*
  a Cover the person and quietly take the person to his or her room
  b Scold the person
  c Provide for privacy
  d Tell the nurse

14 A person touches you sexually and asks for a kiss. You should
  a Avoid the person for the rest of your shift
  b Do what the person asks
  c Ignore the behavior
  d Ask the person not to touch you and tell the nurse

Answers to these questions are on p. 504.

FOCUS ON PRACTICE

Problem Solving

Ms. Hild has urinary incontinence and chewing and swallowing problems due to changes from aging. A co-worker uses the term "diaper" to describe her incontinence product and "bib" for her clothing protector. The co-worker swipes spilled food from Ms. Hild's face with a spoon and threatens to withhold privileges if she does not finish meals. Explain why it is important to treat the person as an adult and not a child. Describe ways to provide age-appropriate care. How will you respond to your co-worker's statements and actions?

CHAPTER 9

Assisting With Safety

OBJECTIVES

- Define the key terms and key abbreviations listed in this chapter.
- Describe accident risk factors.
- Explain why you identify a person before giving care.
- Explain how to correctly identify a person.
- Describe the safety measures to prevent burns, poisoning, and suffocation.
- Identify the signs and causes of choking.
- Explain how to prevent equipment accidents.
- Explain wheelchair and stretcher safety.
- Explain how to handle hazardous substances.
- Identify natural and human-made disasters.
- Describe fire prevention measures and oxygen safety.
- Explain what to do during a fire.
- Explain how to protect yourself from workplace violence.
- Describe your role in risk management.
- Perform the procedures described in this chapter.
- Explain how to promote PRIDE in the person, the family, and yourself.

KEY TERMS

coma A state of being unaware of one's setting and being unable to react or respond to people, places, or things

dementia The loss of cognitive function and social function caused by changes in the brain

disaster A sudden catastrophic event in which people are injured and killed and property is destroyed

hazardous substance Any chemical in the workplace that can cause harm

paralysis Loss of muscle function, sensation, or both

poison Any substance harmful to the body when ingested, inhaled, injected, or absorbed through the skin

suffocation When breathing stops from the lack of oxygen

workplace violence Violent acts (including assault or threat of assault) directed toward persons at work or while on duty

KEY ABBREVIATIONS

AED	Automated external defibrillator
CPR	Cardiopulmonary resuscitation
EMS	Emergency Medical Services
ID	Identification
MSDS	Material safety data sheet
OSHA	Occupational Safety and Health Administration
PASS	*Pull* the safety pin, *aim* low, *squeeze* the lever, *sweep* back and forth
RACE	Rescue, alarm, confine, extinguish
RRT	Rapid Response Team

Safety is a basic need. Patients and residents are at great risk for accidents and falls. (See Chapter 10 for falls.) Some accidents and injuries cause death.

You must protect patients, residents, visitors, co-workers, and yourself. The safety measures in this chapter apply to all health care settings and everyday life.

The goal is to decrease the person's risk of accidents and injuries without limiting mobility and independence. The care plan lists other safety measures for the person.

See *Promoting Safety and Comfort: Assisting With Safety*, p. 98

See *Focus on Surveys: Assisting With Safety*, p. 98.

PROMOTING SAFETY AND COMFORT

Assisting With Safety

Safety

You may see something unsafe. Correct the matter right away if it is something you can do. For example:

- Wipe up spills right away. Do so even if you did not cause the spill.
- A person is sliding out of a wheelchair. Position the person correctly in the chair. Do so even if a co-worker is responsible for the person's care.
- A person is having problems holding a cup of coffee. Offer to help the person.

You cannot correct some safety issues. Follow agency policy to report such problems. They include:

- Electrical outlets or switches coming out of the wall
- Electrical outlets that do not work
- Water leaks from windows, doors, ceilings, pipes, faucets, tubs, showers, toilets, water heaters, and other sources
- Toilets that do not work properly
- Water from faucets that does not warm up or that is very hot
- Broken or damaged windows or furniture
- Windows and doors that do not work properly
- Hand rails and grab bars that are loose or need repair
- Odd smells, odors, and sounds
- Signs of rodents, flies, ants, or other pests
- Lights and lamps that do not work or have burnt-out bulbs
- Flooring (carpeting, tiles) needing repair

FOCUS ON SURVEYS

Assisting With Safety

A survey team will observe the agency setting and patient or resident rooms. They observe:

- For potential or actual hazards. *A hazard* is something that could cause injury or illness. Examples include spills, loose hand rails, unanswered call lights, burnt-out bulbs, unsafe equipment, and other safety issues described in this chapter.
- For how staff respond to potential or actual hazards.
- If the care plan was followed on each shift for persons at risk.
- How staff supervise persons at risk.
- If the staff has removed or changed an identified hazard.

The survey team will interview staff. A surveyor may ask you:

- About measures in the person's care plan to reduce the person's risk for an accident.
- When and how you report risks and hazards.
- When and how you act to correct an immediate hazard. A spill is an example.
- The agency's procedures for removing or reducing a hazard.

You must provide for safety at all times. And you must know what to do if you find a hazard. Remember to give surveyors complete and honest answers. The goal of a survey is to protect patients and residents.

ACCIDENT RISK FACTORS

Some people cannot protect themselves. They rely on others for safety. Certain factors increase the risk of accidents and injuries. Follow the person's care plan.

- *Age.* Body changes occur with aging. Many older persons have decreased strength, move slowly, and are unsteady. Often balance is affected. Older persons also are less sensitive to heat and cold. They have poor vision, hearing problems, and a dulled sense of smell. Confusion, poor judgment, memory problems, and disorientation may occur (Chapter 30). Children are also at risk for injuries.
- *Awareness of surroundings.* ***Coma*** *is a state of being unaware of one's setting and being unable to react or respond to people, places, or things.* The person relies on others for protection. Confused and disoriented persons may not understand what is happening to and around them.
- *Agitated and aggressive behaviors.* Pain can cause these behaviors. So can confusion, decreased awareness of surroundings, and fear of what may happen.
- *Vision loss.* Persons with poor vision may not see toys, rugs, equipment, furniture, and cords. Some cannot read labels on containers. Poisoning can result.
- *Hearing loss.* Persons with hearing loss have problems hearing explanations and instructions. They may not hear warning signals or fire alarms. Some cannot hear approaching meal carts, drug carts, stretchers, or people in wheelchairs. They do not know to move to safety.
- *Impaired smell and touch.* Illness and aging affect smell and touch. The person may not detect smoke or gas odors. Burns are a risk from impaired touch. The person has problems sensing heat and cold. Some people have a decreased sense of pain. They may be unaware of injury.
- *Impaired mobility.* Some diseases and injuries affect mobility. A person may know there is danger but cannot move to safety. Some persons cannot walk or propel wheelchairs. Some persons are paralyzed. ***Paralysis*** *means loss of muscle function, sensation, or both.*
- *Drugs.* Drug side effects may include loss of balance, drowsiness, and lack of coordination. Reduced awareness, confusion, and disorientation occur.

See *Focus on Older Persons: Accident Risk Factors (Age).*

FOCUS ON OLDER PERSONS

Accident Risk Factors (Age)

Dementia *is the loss of cognitive function and social function caused by changes in the brain* (Chapter 30). (*Cognitive* relates to *knowledge*.) Memory and the ability to think and reason are lost. Persons with dementia are confused and disoriented. Their awareness of surroundings is reduced. They may not understand what is happening to and around them. Judgment is poor. They no longer know what is safe and what are dangers. They may access closets, cupboards, or other unsafe and unlocked areas. They may eat or drink cleaning products, drugs, or poisons. Accidents and injuries are great risks.

IDENTIFYING THE PERSON

Each person has different treatments, therapies, and activity limits. Life and health are threatened if the wrong care is given.

The person may receive an identification (ID) bracelet when admitted to the agency (Fig. 9-1). The bracelet has the person's name, room and bed number, birth date, age, doctor, and other identifying information.

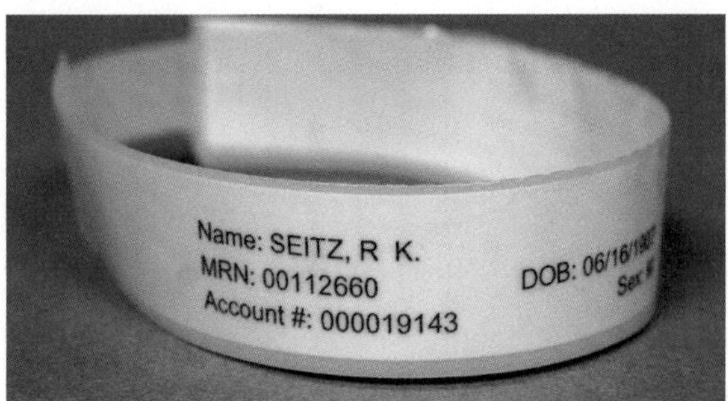

FIGURE 9-1 ID bracelet.

You use the bracelet to identify the person before giving care. The assignment sheet states what care to give. To identify the person:

- Compare identifying information on the assignment sheet with that on the ID bracelet (Fig. 9-2). Carefully check the information. Some people have the same first and last names. For example, John Smith is a very common name.
- Use at least 2 identifiers. An identifier cannot be the person's room or bed number. Some agencies require that the person state and spell his or her name and give his or her birth date. Others require using the person's ID number. Always follow agency policy.
- Call the person by name when checking the ID bracelet. This is a courtesy given as you touch the person and before giving care. Just calling the person by name is not enough to identify him or her. Confused, disoriented, drowsy, hard-of-hearing, or distracted persons may answer to any name.

See *Focus on Communication: Identifying the Person.*
See *Promoting Safety and Comfort: Identifying the Person.*

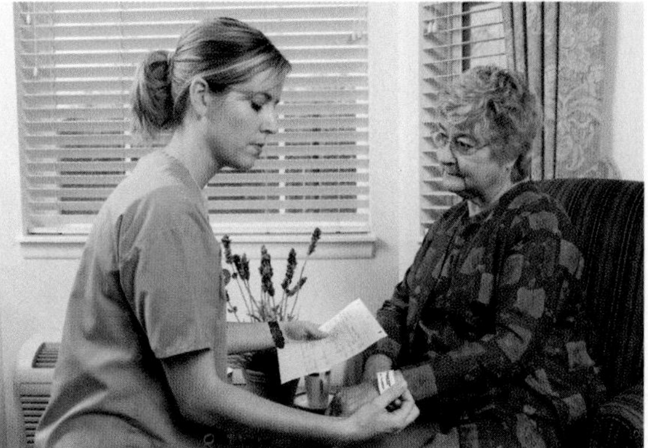

FIGURE 9-2 The ID bracelet is checked against the assignment sheet to accurately identify the person.

FOCUS ON COMMUNICATION

Identifying the Person

To identify the person, call the person by name. Ask to see his or her ID bracelet. For example: "Hello, Mr. Hall. May I see your ID bracelet?" Then ask for 2 identifiers. You can say: "Please tell me your full name and birth date." Compare the identifiers with the information on the ID bracelet and your assignment sheet.

For some persons, identifying themselves is annoying. The person may say: "Do I have to say it again? You know who I am." Be polite. Explain why you check the person's identity. You can say: "It is important to check so I give care to the right person. It is for your safety." Thank the person. Use his or her title and name. For example: "Thank you, Mr. Green."

PROMOTING SAFETY AND COMFORT

Identifying the Person

Safety

Always identify the person before starting a task or procedure. Do not identify the person and then leave the room for supplies and equipment. You could go to the wrong room and give care to the wrong person. And the person for whom the care was intended would not receive it. This too could cause harm.

Sometimes ID bracelets are damaged from water, spilled food and fluids, and everyday wear and tear. If you cannot read the information on the ID bracelet, tell the nurse. The nurse can have a new bracelet made for the person.

Comfort

Make sure ID bracelets are not too loose or too tight. You should be able to slide 1 or 2 fingers under a bracelet. If it is too loose or too tight, tell the nurse.

Identifying Nursing Center Residents

Alert and oriented residents may choose not to wear ID bracelets. This is noted on the person's care plan. Follow center policy and the care plan to identify the person.

Some nursing centers have photo ID systems (Fig. 9-3). The person's photo is taken on admission. Then it is placed in the person's medical record. If your center uses such a system, learn to use it safely.

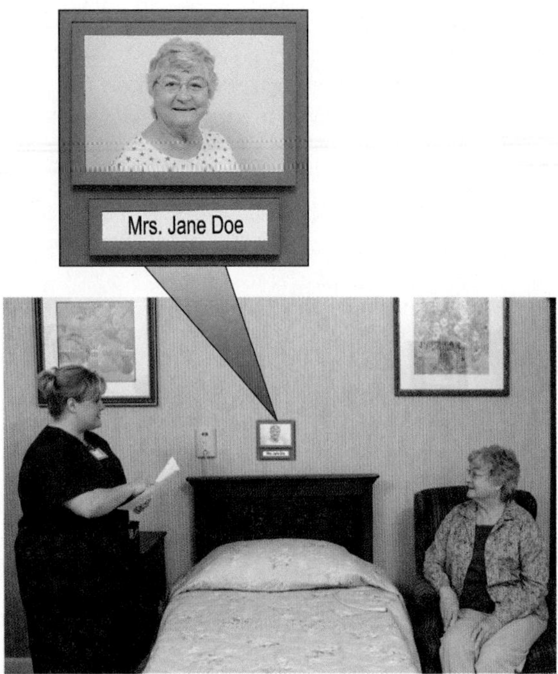

FIGURE 9-3 The person's photo is at the head-board. Her name is under the photo. The nursing assistant uses the photo to identify the person.

PREVENTING BURNS

Smoking, spilled hot liquids, electrical items, and very hot water (sinks, tubs, showers) are common causes of burns. To prevent burns:

- Assist with eating and drinking as needed. Spilled hot food or fluids can cause burns.
- Be careful when carrying hot food and fluids, especially when near patients or residents.
- Keep hot food and fluids away from counter and table edges.
- Do not pour hot liquids near a person.
- Turn on cold water first, then hot water. Turn off hot water first, then cold water.
- Measure bath or shower water temperature (Chapter 16). Check it before a person gets into the tub or shower.
- Check for "hot spots" in bath water. Move your hand back and forth.
- Do not let the person sleep with a heating pad or an electric blanket.
- Follow safety guidelines when applying heat and cold (Chapter 24).
- Provide safety measures for persons who smoke.
  - Be sure people smoke only in smoking areas.
  - Do not leave smoking materials at the bedside.
  - Supervise the smoking of persons who cannot protect themselves.
  - Do not allow smoking in bed.
  - Do not allow smoking where oxygen is used or stored (Chapter 26).
  - Be alert to ashes that may fall onto a person.

PREVENTING POISONING

A ***poison*** *is any substance harmful to the body when ingested, inhaled, injected, or absorbed through the skin.* Drugs and household products are common poisons. Poisoning in adults may be from carelessness, confusion, or poor vision when reading labels. To prevent poisoning:

- Make sure patients and residents cannot reach hazardous materials (p. 106).
- Follow agency policy for storing personal care items. Shampoo, mouthwash, lotion, perfume, and deodorant are examples. These products are harmful when swallowed.
- Keep harmful products in their original containers.
- Leave the original label on harmful products.
- Read all labels carefully before using a product.

PREVENTING SUFFOCATION

Suffocation *is when breathing stops from the lack of oxygen.* Death occurs if the person does not start breathing. Common causes include choking, drowning, inhaling gas or smoke, strangulation, and electrical shock (p. 105).

Measures to prevent suffocation are listed in Box 9-1. Clear the airway if the person is choking.

Choking

Foreign bodies can obstruct the airway. This is called *choking* or *foreign-body airway obstruction (FBAO).* Air cannot pass through the airways into the lungs. The body does not get enough oxygen. Death can result.

Choking often occurs during eating. A large, poorly chewed piece of meat is the most common cause. Laughing and talking while eating also are common causes. So is excessive alcohol intake.

Unconscious persons can choke. Common causes are aspiration of vomitus and the tongue falling back into the airway.

Foreign bodies can cause mild or severe airway obstruction. With *mild airway obstruction,* some air moves in and out of the lungs. The person is conscious and usually can speak. Often forceful coughing can remove the object. Breathing may sound like wheezing between coughs. For mild airway obstruction:

- Stay with the person.
- Encourage the person to keep coughing to expel the object.
- Do not interrupt the person's efforts to clear the airway. If the person is breathing and coughing, abdominal thrusts are not needed.
- If the obstruction persists, call for help.

A person with *severe airway obstruction* has difficulty breathing. Air does not move in and out of the lungs. The person may not be able to breathe, speak, or cough. If able to cough, the cough is of poor quality. When the person tries to inhale, there is no noise or a high-pitched noise. The person may appear pale and cyanotic (bluish color).

The conscious person clutches at the throat (Fig. 9-4). Clutching at the throat is often called the "universal sign of choking." The conscious person is very frightened. If the obstruction is not removed, the person will die. Severe airway obstruction is an emergency.

BOX 9-1 Preventing Suffocation

- Cut food into small, bite-sized pieces for persons who cannot do so themselves.
- Make sure dentures fit properly and are in place.
- Make sure the person can chew and swallow the food served.
- Report loose teeth or dentures.
- Check the care plan for swallowing problems before serving food (including snacks) or fluids. The person may ask for something that he or she cannot swallow.
- Tell the nurse at once if the person has swallowing problems.
- Do not give oral foods or fluids to persons with feeding tubes (Chapter 20).
- Follow aspiration precautions (Chapter 20).
- Do not leave a person unattended in a bathtub or shower.
- Move all persons from the area if you smell smoke.
- Position the person in bed properly (Chapter 15).
- Use bed rails correctly (Chapter 10).
- Use restraints correctly (Chapter 11).
- Prevent entrapment in the bed system (Chapter 15).
- Do not use power strips for care equipment.
- See "Preventing Equipment Accidents" (p. 104).

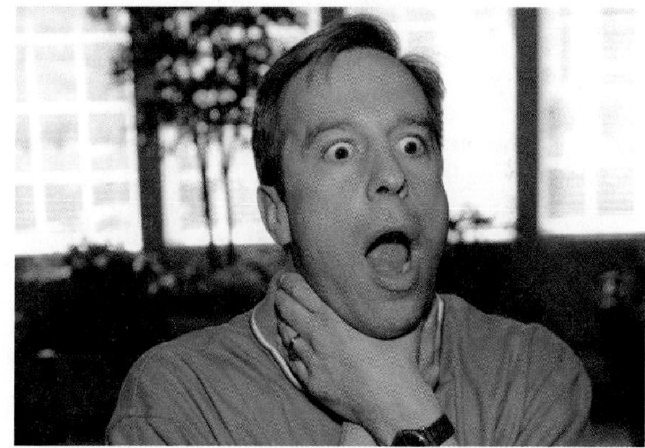

FIGURE 9-4 A choking person clutches at the throat.

Relieving Choking. Abdominal thrusts are used to relieve severe airway obstruction. Abdominal thrusts are quick, upward thrusts to the abdomen. They force air out of the lungs and create an artificial cough. They are done to try to expel the foreign body from the airway.

Abdominal thrusts are not used for very obese persons or pregnant women. Chest thrusts are used (Box 9-2 and Fig. 9-5).

You may observe a person choking. And you may perform emergency measures to relieve choking. Relief of choking occurs when the foreign body is removed. Or it occurs when you feel air move and see the chest rise and fall when giving rescue breaths. The person may still be unresponsive.

If you assist a choking person, report and record what happened. Include what you did and the person's response.

See *Focus on Older Persons: Choking.*

See procedure: *Relieving Choking—Adult or Child (Over 1 Year of Age).*

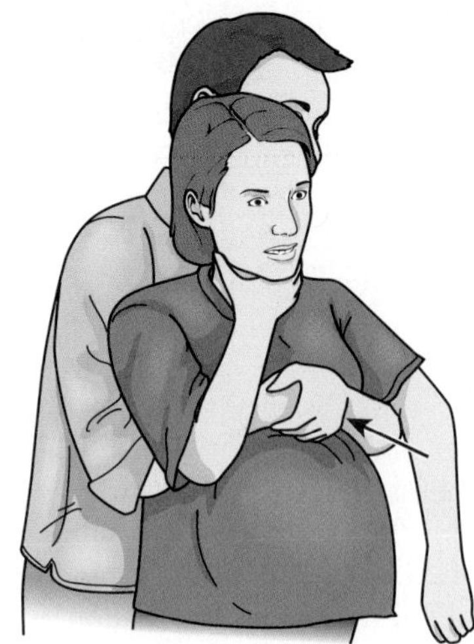

FIGURE 9-5 Chest thrusts to relieve choking in a pregnant woman.

BOX 9-2 Choking—Chest Thrusts for Obese or Pregnant Persons

1 Stand behind the person.
2 Place your arms under the person's underarms. Wrap your arms around the person's chest.
3 Make a fist. Place the thumb side of the fist on the middle of the sternum (breastbone).
4 Grasp the fist with your other hand.
5 Give chest thrusts until the object is expelled or the person becomes unresponsive.
6 If the person becomes unresponsive, activate the Emergency Medical Services (EMS) system or the agency's Rapid Response Team (RRT). This team quickly responds to give care in life-threatening situations. Start cardiopulmonary resuscitation (CPR). See Chapter 31.

FOCUS ON OLDER PERSONS

Choking

Older persons are at risk for choking. Weakness, dentures that fit poorly, dysphagia (difficulty swallowing), and chronic illness are common causes.

A

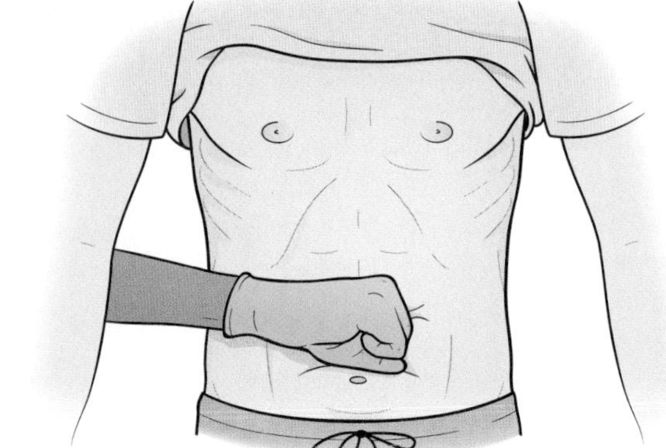

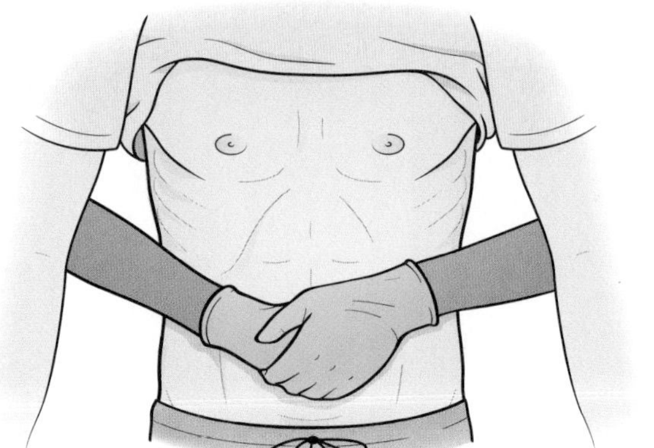

B

FIGURE 9-6 Hand positioning for abdominal thrusts. **A,** The fist is slightly above the navel in the mid-line of the abdomen. **B,** The other hand clasps the fist.

Relieving Choking—Adult or Child (Over 1 Year of Age)

PROCEDURE

1 Ask the person if he or she is choking. Help the person if he or she nods "yes" and cannot talk.
2 Have someone call for help.
  a *In a public area,* have someone activate the EMS system by calling 911. Send someone to get an automated external defibrillator (AED) (Chapter 31).
  b *In an agency,* have someone call the agency's RRT and get an AED.
3 Give abdominal thrusts.
  a Stand or kneel behind the person.
  b Wrap your arms around the person's waist.
  c Make a fist with 1 hand.
  d Place the thumb side of the fist against the abdomen. The fist is slightly above the navel in the middle of the abdomen and well below the end of the sternum (breastbone). See Figure 9-6, *A*.
  e Grasp the fist with your other hand (Fig. 9-6, *B*).
  f Press your fist into the person's abdomen with a quick, upward thrust (Fig. 9-7).
  g Repeat thrusts until the object is expelled or the person becomes unresponsive.
4 *If the object is dislodged,* encourage the person to go to the hospital. Injuries can occur from abdominal thrusts.
5 *If the person becomes unresponsive,* lower the person to the floor or ground. Position the person supine (lying flat on the back). Make sure the EMS or RRT was called. If alone, provide 5 cycles (2 minutes) of CPR first. Then call the EMS or RRT.
6 Start CPR. See Chapter 31.
  a Do not check for a pulse. Begin with compressions. Give 30 compressions. Chest compressions can help dislodge an obstruction.
  b Use the head tilt–chin lift method to open the airway (Fig. 9-8). Open the person's mouth. The mouth should be wide open. Look for an object. Remove the object if you can see it and can remove it easily. Use your fingers.
  c Give 2 breaths.
  d Continue cycles of 30 compressions and 2 breaths. Look for an object every time you open the airway for rescue breaths.
7 *If you relieve choking in an unresponsive person:*
  a Check for a response, breathing, and a pulse.
    1 *If no response, no normal breathing, and no pulse*—continue CPR. Attach an AED (Chapter 31).
    2 *If no response and no normal breathing but there is a pulse*—give rescue breaths. For an adult, give 1 breath every 5 to 6 seconds (10 to 12 breaths per minute). For a child, give 1 breath every 3 to 5 seconds (12 to 20 breaths per minute). Check for a pulse every 2 minutes. If no pulse, begin CPR.
    3 *If the person has normal breathing and a pulse*—place the person in the recovery position if there is no response (Chapter 31). Continue to check the person until help arrives. Encourage the person to go to the hospital if the person responds.

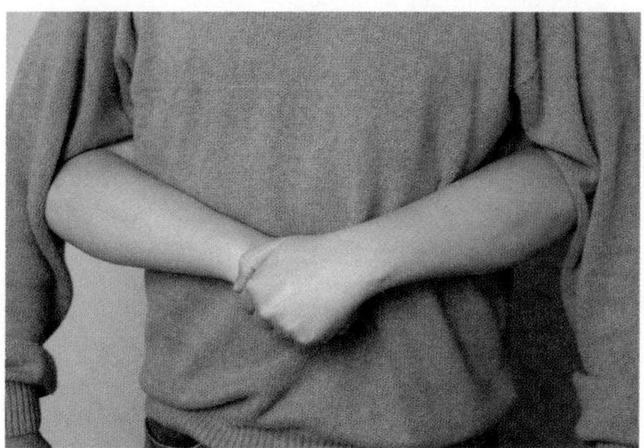

FIGURE 9-7 Abdominal thrusts with the person standing.

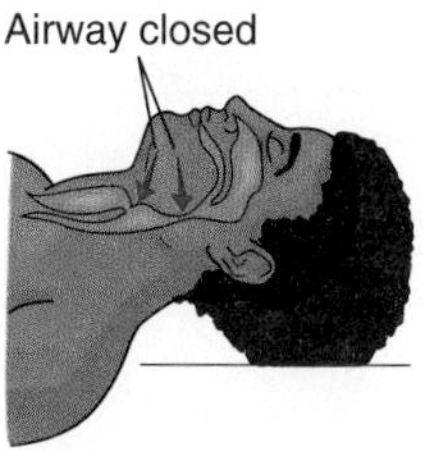

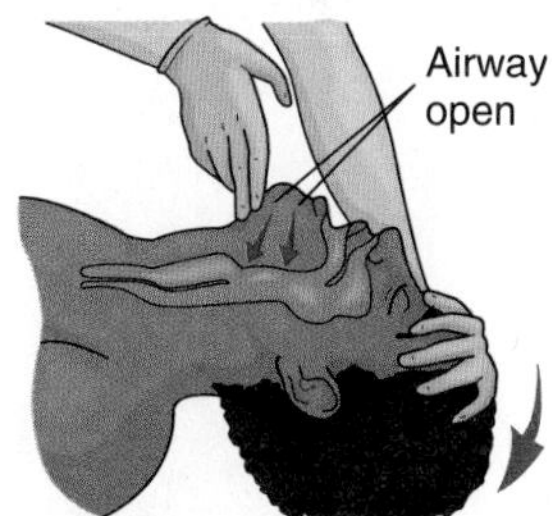

FIGURE 9-8 The head tilt–chin lift method opens the airway. One hand is on the person's forehead. Pressure is applied to lift the head back. The chin is lifted with the fingers of the other hand.

Self-Administered Abdominal Thrusts. You may choke when by yourself. Perform abdominal thrusts to relieve the obstructed airway.

1 Make a fist with 1 hand.
2 Place the thumb side of the fist above your navel and below the lower end of the sternum.
3 Grasp your fist with your other hand.
4 Press inward and upward quickly.
5 Press the upper abdomen against a hard surface if the thrust did not relieve the obstruction. Use the back of a chair, a table, or a railing.
6 Use as many thrusts as needed.

PREVENTING EQUIPMENT ACCIDENTS

All equipment is unsafe if broken, not used correctly, or not working properly. This includes hospital beds. Inspect all equipment before use. Check all items for cracks, chips, and sharp or rough edges. They can cause cuts, stabs, or scratches. Follow the Bloodborne Pathogen Standard (Chapter 12). Also follow the safety measures in Box 9-3.

See *Promoting Safety and Comfort: Preventing Equipment Accidents.*

PROMOTING SAFETY AND COMFORT

Preventing Equipment Accidents

Safety

Beds, chairs, wheelchairs, stretchers, toilets, commodes, and other equipment usually have a weight capacity of 250 to 350 pounds. Bariatric patients and residents can weigh from 250 pounds to over 1000 pounds. Bariatric equipment is labeled with:

- "EC" for "expanded capacity"
- The weight limit suggested by the manufacturer

Do not use the item if the person's weight is greater than the weight capacity. Follow the nurse's directions and the care plan.

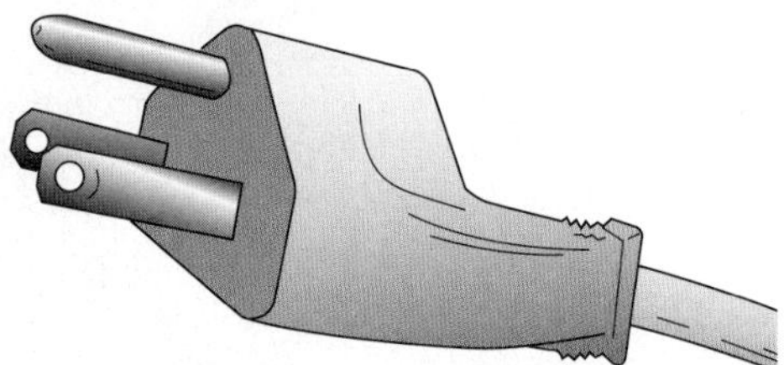

FIGURE 9-9 A 3-prong plug.

BOX 9-3 Preventing Equipment Accidents

General Safety

- Follow agency policies and procedures.
- Follow the manufacturer's instructions. Use equipment correctly.
- Read all caution and warning labels.
- Do not use an unfamiliar item. Ask for training. Also ask a nurse to supervise you the first time you use the item.
- Use an item only for its intended purpose.
- Make sure the item works before you begin.
- Make sure you have all needed equipment. For example, you need to plug in an item. There must be an outlet.
- Show a broken or damaged item to the nurse. Follow the nurse's instructions and agency policies for discarding items or sending them for repair.
- Do not try to repair broken or damaged items.
- Do not use broken or damaged items.

Electrical Safety

- Check cords and equipment for damage. Make sure they are in good repair.
- Use 3-pronged plugs on all electrical devices (Fig. 9-9).
- Avoid using extension cords. If you need one, use it for only 1 device. This prevents over-loading a circuit.
- Do not use power strips for care equipment.
- Do not cover any cord with rugs, carpets, linens, or other materials. Do not run cords under rugs.
- Connect a power cord directly to a wall outlet. Do not connect a bed power cord to an extension cord or outlet strip.
- Do not use electrical items owned by the person until they are safety checked. The maintenance staff does this.
- Keep electrical items away from water.
- Keep work areas clean and dry. Wipe up spills right away.
- Do not touch electrical items if you are wet, your hands are wet, or you are standing in water.
- Do not put a finger or any item into an outlet.
- Turn off equipment before unplugging it. Sparks occur when electrical items are unplugged while turned on.
- Hold on to the plug (not the cord) when removing it from an outlet.
- Do not give showers or tub baths during storms. Lightning can travel through pipes.
- Do not use electrical items or phones during storms.
- Do not use water to put out an electrical fire. If possible, turn off or unplug the item.
- Do not touch a person who is having an electrical shock. If possible, turn off or unplug the item. Call for help at once.
- Keep cords away from heating vents and other heat sources.
- Turn off the device when done using the item.
- Unplug all devices when not in use.

Electrical Equipment

Electrical items must work properly and be in good repair. Frayed cords (Fig. 9-10, *A*) and over-loaded electrical outlets (Fig. 9-10, *B*) can cause fires, burns, and electrical shocks. *Electrical shock* is *when electrical current passes through the body*. It can burn the skin, muscles, nerves, and other tissues. It can affect the heart and cause death.

Warning signs of a faulty electrical item include:

- Shocks
- Loss of power or a power surge
- Dimming or flickering lights
- Sparks
- Sizzling or buzzing sounds
- Burning odor
- Loose plugs

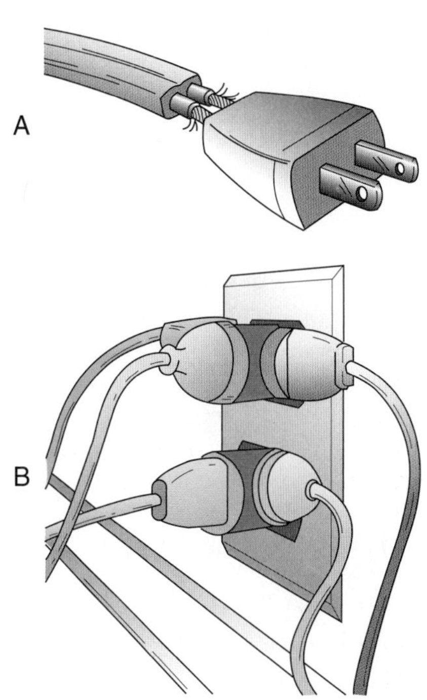

FIGURE 9-10 **A,** A frayed electrical cord. **B,** An over-loaded electrical outlet.

WHEELCHAIR AND STRETCHER SAFETY

Some people use wheelchairs (Fig. 9-11). You use the hand grips/push handles to push the wheelchair. Stretchers are used to transport persons who cannot use wheelchairs.

Follow the safety measures in Box 9-4 when using wheelchairs and stretchers. The person can fall from the wheelchair or stretcher. Or the person can fall during transfers to and from the wheelchair or stretcher.

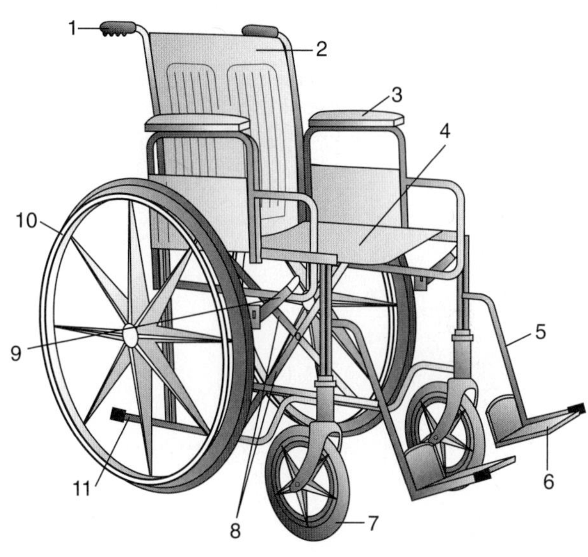

FIGURE 9-11 Parts of a wheelchair.

BOX 9-4 Wheelchair and Stretcher Safety

Wheelchair Safety

- Check the wheel locks (brakes). Make sure you can lock and unlock them.
- Check for flat or loose tires. A wheel lock will not work on a flat or loose tire.
- Make sure wheel spokes are intact. Damaged, broken, or loose spokes can interfere with moving the wheelchair or locking the wheels.
- Make sure the casters point forward. This keeps the wheelchair balanced and stable.
- Position the person's feet on the footplates.
- Make sure the person's feet are on the footplates before moving the chair. The person's feet must not touch or drag on the floor when the chair is moving.

Wheelchair Safety—cont'd

- Push the chair forward when transporting the person. Do not pull the chair backward unless going through a doorway or down a steep ramp or incline.
- Follow the care plan and agency policy for the number of staff needed to transport the person. As many as 4 staff members may be needed. This depends on:
  - The person's weight
  - If the person is cooperative
  - If the wheelchair is powered
- Lock both wheels before you transfer a person to or from the wheelchair.

Continued

BOX 9-4 Wheelchair and Stretcher Safety—cont'd

Wheelchair Safety—cont'd

- Follow the care plan for keeping the wheels locked when not moving the wheelchair. Locking the wheels prevents the chair from moving if the person wants to move to or from the chair. (Locking the wheelchair may be viewed as a restraint. See Chapter 11.)
- Do not let the person stand on the footplates.
- Do not let the footplates fall back onto the person's legs.
- Make sure the person has needed wheelchair accessories—safety belt, pouch, tray, lap-board, cushion.
- Remove the armrests (if removable) when the person transfers to the bed, toilet, commode, tub, or car (Chapter 14).
- Swing front rigging out of the way for transfers to and from the wheelchair. Some front riggings detach for transfers.
- Clean the wheelchair according to agency policy.
- Ask a nurse or physical therapist to show you how to propel wheelchairs up steps and ramps and over curbs.
- Follow the safety measures to prevent equipment accidents (p. 104).

Stretcher Safety

- Ask 2 or more co-workers to help you transfer the person to or from the stretcher.
- Lock the stretcher wheels before the transfer.
- Fasten the safety straps when the person is properly positioned on the stretcher.
- Follow the care plan and agency policy for the number of staff needed to transport the person. As many as 4 staff members may be needed. This depends on:
    - The person's weight
    - If the person is cooperative
- Raise the side rails. Keep them up during the transport.
- Make sure the person's arms, hands, legs, and feet do not dangle through the side rail bars.
- Stand at the head of the stretcher. Your co-worker stands at the foot of the stretcher.
- Move the stretcher feet first (Fig. 9-12).
- Do not leave the person alone.
- Follow the safety measures to prevent equipment accidents (p. 104).

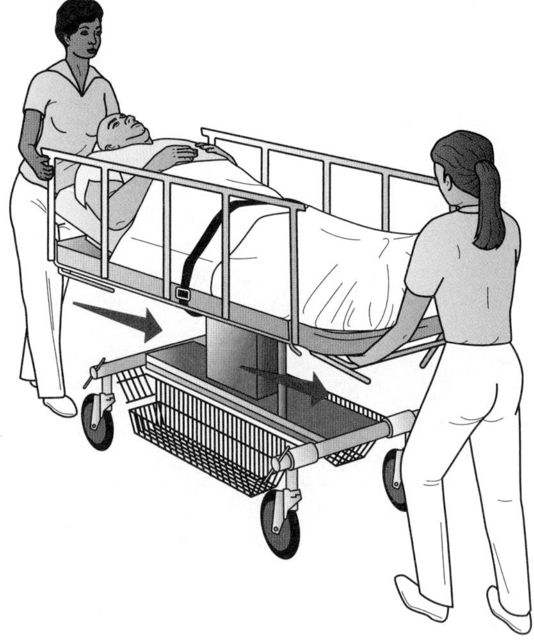

FIGURE 9-12 The stretcher is moved feet first.

HANDLING HAZARDOUS SUBSTANCES

A ***hazardous substance*** *is any chemical in the workplace that can cause harm.* *Physical hazards* can cause fires or explosions. *Health hazards* are chemicals that can cause health problems. Hazardous substances include:

- Drugs used in cancer therapy (chemotherapy, anticancer drugs)
- Anesthesia gases
- Gases used to sterilize equipment
- Oxygen
- Disinfectants and cleaning agents
- Radiation used for x-rays and cancer treatments
- Mercury (found in thermometers and blood pressure devices)

Your agency provides hazardous substance training. It also provides eyewash and total body wash stations in appropriate areas.

Labeling

Hazardous substance containers must have manufacturer warning labels (Fig. 9-13). Warning labels identify:

- Physical and health hazards. Health hazards include the organs affected and potential health problems.
- Precaution measures. For example: "Do not use near open flame." Or: "Avoid skin contact."
- What personal protective equipment to wear—gown, mask, gloves, goggles, and so on.
- How to use the substance safely.
- Storage and disposal information.

If a warning label is removed or damaged, do not use the substance. Show the container to the nurse and explain the problem. Do not leave the container unattended.

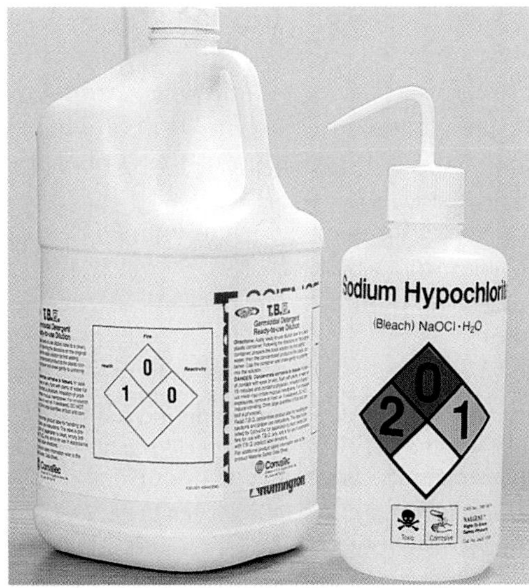

FIGURE 9-13 Warning labels on hazardous substances.

FOCUS ON SURVEYS

Disasters

The Centers for Medicare & Medicaid Services (CMS) requires that all staff be trained in emergency procedures. There may be unannounced disaster drills during a survey. They are done to test staff efficiency, knowledge, and response should a disaster occur.

A surveyor may ask you:

- About fire safety. See "Fire Safety." This includes:
  - What to do if a fire alarm goes off.
  - What to do if you find a fire in a person's room.
  - Where to find fire alarms and fire extinguishers.
  - How to use a fire extinguisher.
- What to do if a resident is missing. See "Elopement" on p. 109.

Material Safety Data Sheets

Every hazardous substance has a material safety data sheet (MSDS). It gives detailed information about the substance. Check the MSDS before using a hazardous substance, cleaning up a leak or spill, or disposing of the substance. Tell the nurse about a leak or spill right away. Do not leave a leak or spill unattended.

DISASTERS

A ***disaster*** *is a sudden catastrophic event. People are injured and killed. Property is destroyed.* Natural disasters include tornadoes, hurricanes, blizzards, earthquakes, volcanic eruptions, floods, and some fires. Human-made disasters include auto, bus, train, and airplane accidents. They also include fires, bombings, nuclear power plant accidents, gas or chemical leaks, explosions, and wars.

Communities, fire and police departments, and health care agencies have disaster plans. They include procedures to deal with people needing treatment. A disaster may damage the agency. The disaster plan includes evacuation procedures.

See *Focus on Surveys: Disasters.*

Bomb Threats

Follow agency procedures if a bomb threat is made or if you find an item that looks or sounds strange. Bomb threats can be sent by phone, mail, e-mail, messenger, or other means. Or the person can leave a bomb in the agency. If you see a stranger in the agency, tell the nurse at once. You cannot be too safe.

Fire Safety

Faulty electrical equipment and wiring, over-loaded electrical circuits, and smoking are major causes of fires. The health team must prevent fires and act quickly during a fire. See Box 9-5.

BOX 9-5 Fire Prevention Measures

- Follow the safety measures for oxygen use (p. 108).
- Follow the safety measures to prevent equipment accidents (p. 104).
- Follow the safety measures to prevent burns (p. 100).
- Smoke only where allowed to do so.
- Empty ashtrays only when sure that all ashes, cigars, cigarettes, and other smoking materials are out.
- Empty ashtrays into a metal container partially filled with sand or water. Do not empty ashtrays into plastic containers or wastebaskets lined with paper or plastic bags.
- Provide ashtrays for persons who are allowed to smoke.
- Supervise persons who smoke. This is very important for persons who are confused, disoriented, or sedated.
- Keep matches, lighters, and flammable liquids and materials away from confused or disoriented persons.
- Light matches carefully.
  - Be alert for sparks when lighting a match. The sparks can ignite material that can burn.
  - Keep your hair, clothing, and anything that will burn away from the match and flame.
- Do not leave cooking unattended on stoves, in ovens, or in microwave ovens.
- Store flammable liquids outside in their original containers. Follow the manufacturer's instructions.
- Do not smoke or light matches or lighters around flammable liquids or materials.

Fire and the Use of Oxygen. Three things are needed for a fire.

- A spark or flame
- A material that will burn
- Oxygen

Air has some oxygen. However, some people need extra oxygen (Chapter 26). Safety measures are needed where oxygen is used and stored.

- NO SMOKING signs are placed on the door and near the bed.
- The person and visitors cannot smoke in the room.
- Smoking materials (cigarettes, cigars, and pipes), matches, and lighters are removed from the room.
- Safety measures to prevent equipment accidents are followed (see Box 9-3).
- Wool blankets and synthetic fabrics that cause static electricity are removed from the person's room.
- The person wears a cotton gown or pajamas.
- Lit candles, incense, and other open flames are not allowed.
- Materials that ignite easily are removed from the room. They include oil, grease, nail polish remover, and so on.

See *Focus on Communication: Fire and the Use of Oxygen.*

What to Do During a Fire. Know your agency's procedures for fire emergencies. This includes evacuation procedures. Know where to find fire alarms, fire extinguishers, and emergency exits. Fire drills are held to practice emergency fire procedures. Remember the word *RACE* (Fig. 9-14).

- *R*—for *rescue.* Rescue persons in immediate danger. Move them to a safe place.
- *A*—for *alarm.* Sound the nearest fire alarm. Notify the operator.
- *C*—for *confine.* Close doors and windows to confine the fire. Turn off oxygen or electrical items used in the general area of the fire.
- *E*—for *extinguish.* Use a fire extinguisher on a small fire that has not spread to a larger area.

Clear equipment from all normal and emergency exits. *Do not use elevators if there is a fire.*

Using a Fire Extinguisher. Different extinguishers are used for different kinds of fires.

- Oil and grease fires
- Electrical fires
- Paper and wood fires

A general procedure for using a fire extinguisher follows. See procedure: *Using a Fire Extinguisher.*

FOCUS ON COMMUNICATION

Fire and the Use of Oxygen

You may have to remind a patient, resident, or visitor not to smoke inside the agency. You can simply say:

- "Mrs. Murphy, this is a smoke-free area. Here is an ashtray to put out your cigarette. If you want to smoke, I'll be happy to show you the smoking area outside."
- "Mr. Garcia, please don't smoke inside the center. We have a smoking area outside the back entrance on hallway 2. I'll be happy to show you the way."

Tell the nurse what happened and what you said and did. The nurse may need to speak with the person about not smoking.

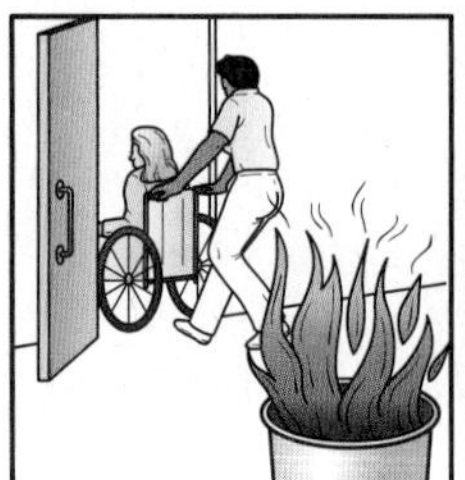
Rescue

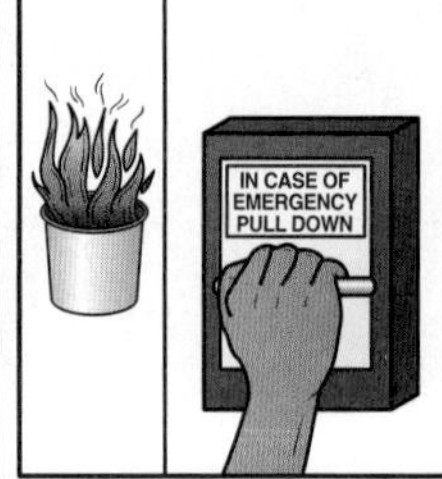

Alarm

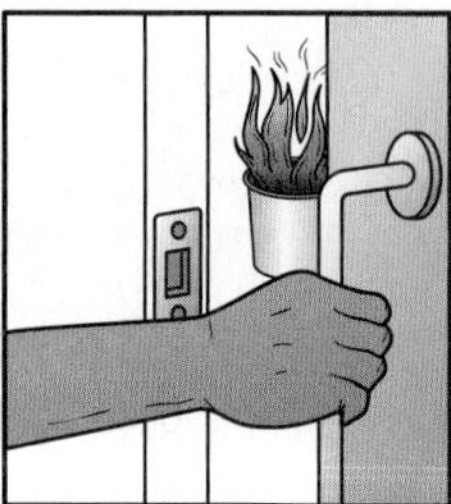
Confine

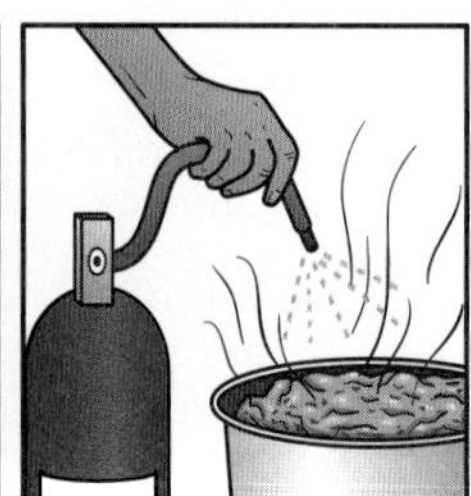
Extinguish

FIGURE 9-14 During a fire, remember RACE: Rescue, Alarm, Confine, Extinguish.

Using a Fire Extinguisher

PROCEDURE

1 Pull the fire alarm.
2 Get the nearest fire extinguisher.
3 Carry it upright.
4 Take it to the fire.
5 Follow the word *PASS.*
  a *P*—for *pull the safety pin* (Fig. 9-15, *A*). This unlocks the handle.
  b *A*—for *aim low* (Fig. 9-15, *B*). Direct the hose or nozzle at the base of the fire. Do not try to spray the tops of the flames.
  c *S*—for *squeeze the lever* (Fig. 9-15, *C*). Squeeze or push down on the lever, handle, or button to start the stream. Release the lever, handle, or button to stop the stream.
  d *S*—for *sweep back and forth* (Fig. 9-15, *D*). Sweep the stream back and forth (side to side) at the base of the fire.

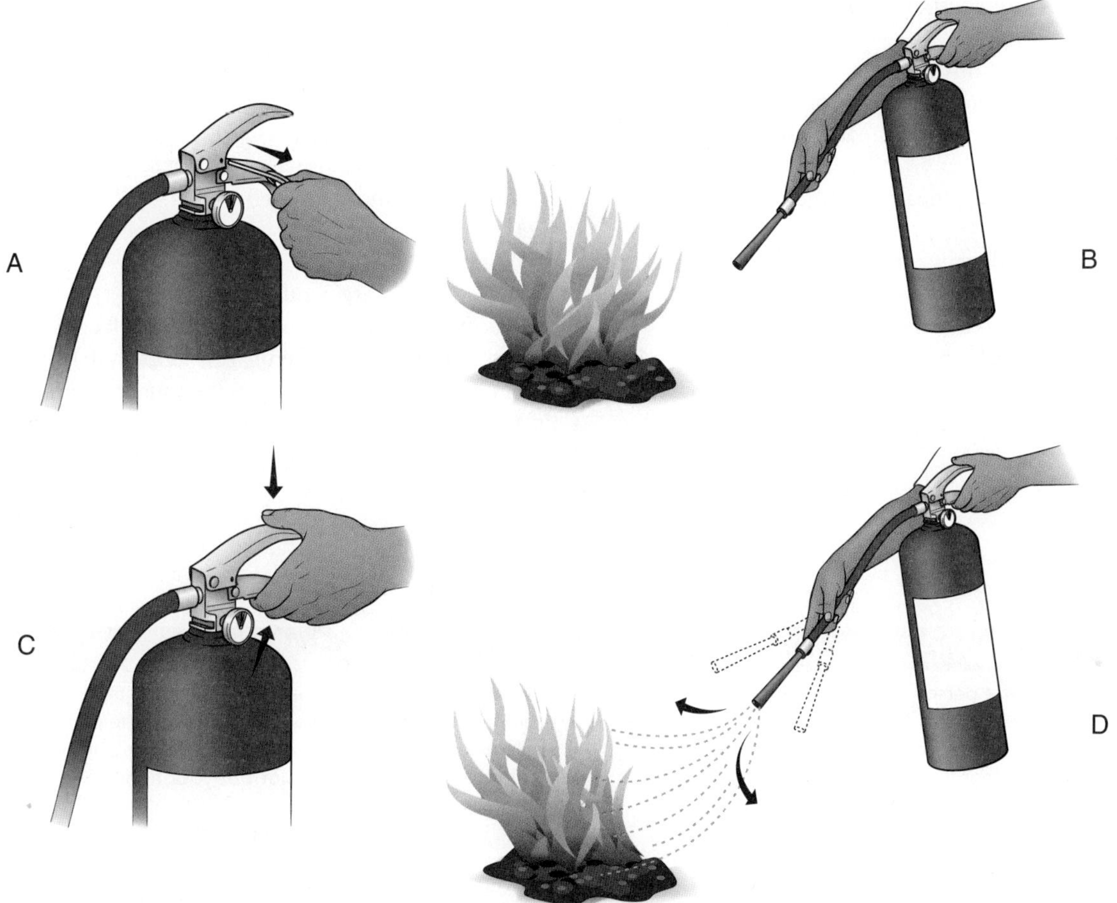

FIGURE 9-15 Using a fire extinguisher. **A,** *Pull* the safety pin. **B,** *Aim* the hose at the base of the fire. **C,** *Squeeze* the top handle down. **D,** *Sweep* back and forth.

Elopement

The CMS requires that an agency's disaster plan address elopement. *Elopement* is when a patient or resident leaves the agency without staff knowledge. The person who leaves a safe setting is at risk for many dangers. Heat or cold exposure, dehydration, drowning, and being struck by a car or truck are examples.

The agency must:

- Identify persons at risk for elopement.
- Monitor and supervise persons at risk.
- Address elopement in the person's care plan.
- Have a plan to find a missing patient or resident.

WORKPLACE VIOLENCE

Workplace violence *is violent acts (including assault or threat of assault) directed toward persons at work or while on duty.* It includes:

- Murders
- Beatings, stabbings, and shootings
- Rapes and sexual assaults
- Use of weapons—firearms, bombs, knives, and so on
- Kidnapping
- Robbery
- Threats—obscene phone calls; threatening oral, written, or body language; and harassment of any nature (being followed, sworn at, or shouted at)

Assaults occur in health care settings. Nurses and nursing assistants are at risk. They have the most contact with patients, residents, and visitors. Risk factors include:

- People with weapons.
- Police holds—persons arrested or convicted of crimes.
- Acutely disturbed and violent persons seeking health care.
- Alcohol and drug abuse.
- Mentally ill persons who do not take needed drugs, do not have follow-up care, and are not in hospitals unless they are an immediate threat to themselves or others.
- Pharmacies have drugs and are a target for robberies.
- Gang members and substance abusers are patients, residents, or visitors.
- Upset, agitated, and disturbed family and visitors.
- Long waits for emergency care or other services.
- Being alone with the person during care or transport to areas.
- Low staff levels during meals, emergencies, and at night.
- Poor lighting in hallways, rooms, parking lots, and other areas.
- Lack of training in recognizing and managing potentially violent situations.

The Occupational Safety and Health Administration (OSHA) has guidelines for violence prevention programs. Work-site hazards are identified. Prevention measures are developed and followed. Also, staff receive safety and health training. Box 9-6 has some measures to deal with agitated or aggressive persons.

RISK MANAGEMENT

Risk management involves identifying and controlling risks and safety hazards affecting the agency. The intent is to:

- Protect everyone in the agency—patients, residents, visitors, and staff.
- Protect agency property from harm or danger.
- Protect the person's valuables.
- Prevent accidents and injuries.

Risk management deals with these and other safety issues.

- Accident and fire prevention
- Negligence and malpractice
- Abuse
- Workplace violence
- Federal and state requirements

Risk managers look for patterns and trends in incident reports, complaints (patients, residents, staff), and accident and injury investigations. Unsafe situations are corrected. Procedure changes and training recommendations are made as needed.

BOX 9-6 Dealing With Agitated or Aggressive Persons

- Stand away from the person. Judge the length of the person's arms and legs. Stand far enough away so that the person cannot hit or kick you.
- Stand close to the door. Do not become trapped in the room.
- Be aware of items in the room that can be used as weapons. Move away from such objects. Examples include vases, phones, radios, letter openers, paper weights, and belts.
- Know where to find panic buttons, call lights, alarms, closed-circuit monitors, and other security devices.
- Keep your hands free.
- Stay calm. Talk to the person in a calm matter. Do not raise your voice or argue, scold, or interrupt the person.
- Be aware of your body language. Do not point a finger or glare at the person. Do not put your hands on your hips.
- Do not touch the person.
- Tell the person that you will get the nurse to speak to him or her.
- Leave the room as soon as you can. Make sure the person is safe.
- Tell the nurse or security officer about the matter at once. Report items in the room that can be used as weapons.
- Complete an incident report according to agency policy.

Color-Coded Wristbands

Color-coded wristbands promote the person's safety and prevent harm. They quickly communicate an alert or warning (Fig. 9-16). The type of alert is printed on the band. The printing is useful in dim lighting and for persons who are color blind. These colors are common.

- Red—for an "allergy alert." Red is a warning to "stop." A red wristband warns of allergies to food, drugs, treatment supplies such as tape or latex gloves, dust, plants, grass, and so on. Allergies are not listed on the wristband.
- Yellow—for a "fall risk." Yellow implies "caution." Yellow wristbands are used for persons with a history of falls. Or they are used for persons at risk for falls because of dizziness, balance problems, confusion, and so on.
- Purple—for a "Do Not Resuscitate" (DNR) order. See Chapter 32.

Some agencies have colors for other alerts. For example, pink is for a "limb alert." This means that an arm or leg is not used for blood pressure measurements, blood draws, or intravenous infusions. To safely use color-coded wristbands:

- Know the wristband colors used in your agency. Colors may vary among agencies.
- Check the care plan and your assignment sheet when you see a color-coded wristband. You need to know the reason for the wristband and the care measures needed. Ask the nurse if you have questions.
- Do not confuse "social cause" bands with your agency's color-coded wristbands. "Live Strong" is an example.
- Check for wristbands on persons transferred from another agency. That agency may use different colors. Or the meanings may differ from those in your agency. The nurse needs to remove wristbands from another agency.
- Tell the nurse if you think a person needs a color-coded wristband.

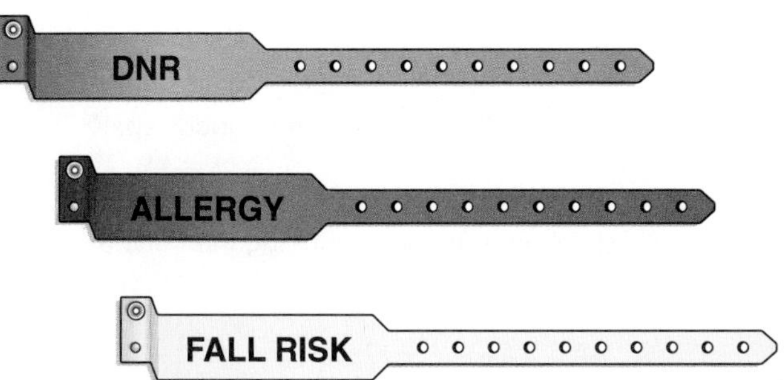

FIGURE 9-16 Color-coded wristbands. The alert is printed on the band.

Personal Belongings

The person's belongings must be kept safe. Often they are sent home with the family. A personal belongings list is completed. Each item is listed and described. The staff member and the person sign the completed list.

A valuables envelope is used for jewelry and money. Each jewelry item is listed and described on the envelope. Describe what you see. For example, describe a ring as having a white stone with 6 prongs in a yellow setting. Do not assume the stone is a diamond in a gold setting. For valuables:

- Count money with the person.
- Put money and each jewelry item in the envelope. Have the person watch. Seal and sign the envelope like a personal belongings list.
- Give the envelope to the nurse. The nurse takes it to the safe or sends it home with the family.

Dentures, eyeglasses, hearing aids, watches, some jewelry, radios, wireless phones, computers, and other electronic devices are kept at the bedside. Items kept at the bedside are listed in the person's record. Some people keep money for newspapers and personal items. The amount kept is noted in the person's record.

In nursing centers, clothing and shoes are labeled with the person's name. So are other items brought from home.

Reporting Incidents

An *incident* is *any event that has harmed or could harm a patient, resident, visitor, or staff member.* This includes:

- Accidents involving patients, residents, visitors, or staff.
- Errors in care. This includes giving the wrong care, giving care to the wrong person, or not giving care.
- Broken or lost items owned by the person. Dentures, hearing aids, and eyeglasses are examples.
- Lost money or clothing.
- Hazardous substance incidents.
- Workplace violence incidents.

Report accidents and errors at once. An *incident report* is completed as soon as possible. Incident reports are reviewed by risk management and a committee of health care workers. They look for patterns and trends in accidents or errors. For example, are falls occurring on the same shift and on the same unit? Are lost or missing items being reported on the same shift or same unit? Are residents being injured on the same shift or same unit? There may be new policies and procedures to prevent future incidents.

FOCUS ON PRIDE

The Person, Family, and Yourself

Personal and Professional Responsibility

Some persons are at risk for choking. Persons with developmental disabilities, young children, and older persons are examples. Safety measures must be taken to avoid harm.

You can help prevent such incidents. Know which persons are at risk for choking. Ask the nurse or check the care plan. Monitor those persons closely. Check that they have the right diet. See Chapter 20 for more precautions.

Rights and Respect

Patients and residents have the right to the care and security of personal items. Treat the person's items with respect. The items may not have value to you but are important to the person. Label a person's belongings with his or her name. Put valuables in a secure place until a family member can take them home. Follow agency policies for charting and storing personal items.

Protect yourself and the agency from being accused of stealing. Do not go through a person's belongings without consent. Sometimes the nurse wants a person's items inspected for safety reasons. If so, make sure the nurse and the person or legal representative are present. Do not search on your own. The nurse charts the details of the search in the person's record.

Independence and Social Interaction

Older persons are at increased risk for injury. Many cannot do things they used to do. They still may try. To promote safety:

- Know who you need to protect.
- Know common safety hazards and the causes of accidents.
- Practice safety measures to prevent accidents and injuries.
- Respect the desire of older persons to maintain independence. Listen to them. Discuss letting them try a task with help. Let them do as much as they safely can. Kindly communicate safety limits.

Delegation and Teamwork

Personal safety practices protect yourself and co-workers. Work as a team to ensure the safety of all staff arriving at and leaving the agency.

- Wait for a person finishing work a few minutes late. Ask if you can help the person.
- Walk with others to and from the parking area.
- Walk in well-lit areas at night.
- Do not leave the parking area until all of your co-workers are safely in their vehicles.
- Offer to call security escort services for a co-worker going to a different location. For example, a person is walking to a bus stop.

Take pride in caring about the safety of all team members.

Ethics and Laws

Accidents happen. Errors occur. No matter how much you try, mistakes are made. Do not lie or try to hide the incident. This is wrong. You must:

- Be honest.
- Tell the nurse.
- Fill out an incident report.

Incident reports are used to improve systems and promote safety, not for punishment. Information gained signals areas for improvement. Processes may be changed to make mistakes more difficult. Or they are changed to make it easier to do the right thing.

Always do your best to give safe care. When errors or accidents happen, take responsibility. Be accountable. Take pride in doing the right thing by honest reporting.

REVIEW QUESTIONS

Circle the BEST answer.

1 Which is safe?
 a Needing eyeglasses
 b Hearing problems
 c Memory problems
 d Oriented to person, time, and place

2 A person in a coma
 a Has suffered an electrical shock
 b Has dementia
 c Is unaware of surroundings
 d Has stopped breathing

3 To identify a person, you
 a Call the person by name
 b Ask the person his or her name
 c Compare information on the ID bracelet against your assignment sheet
 d Ask both roommates their names

4 To prevent burns
 a Keep smoking materials at the person's bedside
 b Pour hot liquids near a person
 c Turn on hot water first
 d Check water temperature before the person enters the shower

5 Which can cause suffocation?
 a Reporting loose teeth or dentures
 b Using electrical items that are in good repair
 c Cutting food into small, bite-sized pieces
 d Restraints

6 The *most* common cause of choking in adults is
 a A loose denture
 b Meat
 c Marbles
 d Candy

7 If severe airway obstruction occurs, the person usually
  a Clutches at the throat
  b Can speak, cough, and breathe
  c Is calm
  d Has a seizure

8 These statements are about relieving FBAO. Which is *false?*
  a Abdominal thrusts can be self-administered.
  b A person is pregnant. Give abdominal thrusts.
  c Injuries can occur from abdominal or chest thrusts.
  d CPR is started if the responsive victim loses consciousness.

9 You need to shave a new resident. Before using the person's electric shaver
  a You need to inspect it
  b The maintenance staff must do a safety check
  c You need to check for a frayed cord
  d You need an extension cord

10 You are using electrical equipment. Which measure is *not* safe?
  a Following the manufacturer's instructions
  b Keeping electrical items away from water and spills
  c Pulling on the cord to remove a plug from an outlet
  d Turning off electrical items after using them

11 A person uses a wheelchair. Which measure is *not* safe?
  a The wheels are locked for transfers.
  b The chair is pulled backward to transport the person.
  c The feet are positioned on the footplates.
  d The casters point forward.

12 To use a stretcher safely
  a Unlock the wheels for transfers to and from the stretcher
  b Fasten the safety straps
  c Lower the side rails during a transport
  d Move the stretcher head first

13 You spilled a hazardous substance. You should
  a Follow the instructions on the material safety data sheet
  b Cover the spill and go tell the nurse
  c Wipe up the spill with paper towels
  d Leave the spill for housekeeping

14 The fire alarm sounds. The following are done *except*
  a Turning off oxygen
  b Using elevators
  c Closing doors and windows
  d Moving residents to a safe place

15 You work in a nursing center. What should you do for a severe weather alert?
  a Take cover.
  b Follow the center's disaster plan.
  c Make sure your family is safe.
  d Pull the fire alarm.

16 A person is agitated and aggressive. Which is *not* safe?
  a Standing away from the person
  b Standing close to the door
  c Using touch to show you care
  d Talking to the person without raising your voice

17 A person has a yellow wristband. You should
  a Monitor the person closely for falls
  b Avoid wearing latex gloves
  c Use the person's right arm for checking blood pressures
  d Remove the wristband

18 You see a color-coded wristband. You should
  a Read the wristband for special instructions or care measures
  b Ask the person what it means
  c Check your assignment sheet and the person's care plan
  d Remove the wristband when the risk is no longer present

19 A resident brought a radio from home. To prevent property loss
  a Send the item home with the family
  b Label the item with the person's name
  c Put the item in a safe
  d Use a wheelchair pouch for the item

20 You gave a person the wrong treatment. Which is *true?*
  a Report the error at the end of the shift.
  b Take action only if the person was injured.
  c You are guilty of negligence.
  d You must complete an incident report.

Answers to these questions are on p. 504.

FOCUS ON **PRACTICE**

Problem Solving

You are assisting Mr. Park with feeding. He begins to cough loudly. He can speak a few words. You hear wheezing between breaths. What do you do? Mr. Park is suddenly unable to cough, speak, or breathe. What do you do?

CHAPTER

10 Assisting With Fall Prevention

OBJECTIVES

- Define the key terms listed in this chapter.
- Identify the causes and risk factors for falls.
- Describe the safety measures that prevent falls.
- Explain how to use bed rails safely.
- Explain the purpose of hand rails and grab bars.
- Explain how to use wheel locks safely.
- Describe how to use transfer/gait belts.
- Explain how to help the person who is falling.
- Perform the procedures described in this chapter.
- Explain how to promote PRIDE in the person, the family, and yourself.

KEY TERMS

bed rail A device that serves as a guard or barrier along the side of the bed; side rail

gait belt See "transfer belt"

transfer belt A device used to support a person who is unsteady or disabled; gait belt

The risk of falling increases with age. Persons older than 65 years are at risk. Falls are a leading cause of injuries and deaths among older persons. A history of falls increases the risk of falling again. Falls are the most common accidents in nursing centers.

See *Focus on Surveys: Assisting With Fall Prevention.*

FOCUS ON SURVEYS

Assisting With Fall Prevention

The Centers for Medicare & Medicaid Services defines a *fall* as:

- Unintentionally coming to rest on the ground, floor, or other lower level. Force, such as being pushed, was not involved.
- When a person loses his or her balance and would have fallen if staff did not act to prevent the fall.
- When a person is found on the floor unless matters suggest otherwise.

The survey team will observe:

- For the fall risk factors described in this chapter.
- For hazards described in this chapter and in Chapter 9.
- For safety measures to prevent falls.
- For the safe repair and use of bed rails, hand rails and grab bars, and wheel locks.
- For the use of assistive devices. Canes, walkers, and transfer/gait belts are examples.
- For safe transfer (Chapter 14) and ambulation (Chapter 23) procedures.
- If call lights are answered promptly.
- If the person's care needs are addressed.
- If the person's care plan is followed.

The survey team may interview you about identifying hazards (Chapter 9) and preventing falls.

CAUSES AND RISK FACTORS FOR FALLS

Most falls occur:

- In patient and resident rooms and in bathrooms.
- Within the first 72 hours of admission to a hospital or nursing center.
- During the night and after meals.
- During shift changes. Staff are busy going off and coming on duty. Confusion can occur about who gives care and answers call lights.

The accident risk factors described in Chapter 9 can lead to falls. The problems listed in Box 10-1 increase a person's risk of falling.

BOX 10-1 Fall Risk Factors

Care Setting

- Care equipment: IV (intravenous) poles, drainage tubes and bags, and others
- Cluttered floors
- Furniture out-of-place
- Lighting: poor
- Restraint use
- Setting: new, strange, and unfamiliar
- Throw rugs
- Wet and slippery floors, bathtubs, and showers
- Wheelchairs, walkers, canes, and crutches: improper use or fit

The Person

- Alcohol: over-use
- Balance problems
- Blood pressure: low or high
- Confusion
- Depression
- Disorientation
- Dizziness; dizziness on standing
- Drug side effects
  - Low blood pressure when standing or sitting
  - Drowsiness
  - Fainting
  - Dizziness
  - Coordination: poor
  - Unsteadiness
  - Urination: frequent
  - Diarrhea
  - Confusion and disorientation
- Elimination: special needs—incontinence (urinary, fecal), frequency, urgency, urinating at night *(nocturia)*
- Falls: history of
- Foot problems
- Gait: unsteady
- Joint pain and stiffness
- Judgment: poor
- Light-headedness
- Memory problems
- Mobility: impaired
- Muscle weakness
- Reaction time: slow
- Shoes that fit poorly
- Sleep problems
- Vision problems
- Weakness

FALL PREVENTION

Agencies have fall prevention programs. The measures listed in Box 10-2, p. 116 are part of such programs and the person's care plan. The care plan also lists measures for the person's risk factors.

See *Focus on Communication: Fall Prevention.*

See *Promoting Safety and Comfort: Fall Prevention.*

Text continued on p. 118

FOCUS ON COMMUNICATION

Fall Prevention

Often falls occur when the person tries to get needed items. The person has to reach too far and falls out of bed or from a chair. Or the person tries to get up without help. Prevent falls by asking the person these questions.

- "What things would you like near you?"
- "Can I move this closer to you?"
- "Can you reach the call light?"
- "Can you reach your cane?" (Walker and wheelchair are other examples.)
- "Do you need to use the bathroom now?"
- "Is there anything else you need before I leave the room?"

PROMOTING SAFETY AND COMFORT

Fall Prevention

Safety

Some people are visually impaired. Besides the measures in Box 10-2, p. 116, other safety measures are needed to protect them from falling. See Chapter 28.

BOX 10-2 Safety Measures to Prevent Falls

Basic Needs
- Fluid needs are met.
- Eyeglasses and hearing aids are worn as needed. Reading glasses are not worn when up and about.
- Tasks are explained before and while performing them.
- Help is given with elimination needs. Assist the person to the bathroom. Or provide the bedpan, urinal, or commode.
- The bedpan, urinal, or commode is kept within easy reach if the person can use the device without help.
- A warm drink, soft lights, or a back massage is used to calm the person who is agitated.
- Barriers are used to prevent wandering (Fig. 10-1).
- The person is properly positioned when in bed, a chair, or a wheelchair. Use pillows, wedge pads, seats, or other positioning devices as the nurse and care plan direct (Chapter 13).
- Correct procedures and equipment are used for transfers (Chapter 14). Follow the care plan.
- The person is involved in meaningful activities.
- Exercise programs are followed. They help improve balance, strength, walking, and physical function.

Bathrooms and Shower/Tub Rooms
- Tubs and showers have non-slip surfaces or non-slip bath mats.
- Grab bars (safety bars) are in showers (p. 118). They also are by tubs and toilets.
- Bathrooms have grab bars.
- The person uses grab bars in bathrooms and shower/tub rooms.
- Shower chairs are used (Chapter 16).
- Safety measures for tub baths and showers are followed (Chapter 16).

Floors
- Carpeting (if used) is wall-to-wall or tacked down.
- Scatter, area, and throw rugs are not used.
- Floor covers are 1 color. Bold designs can cause dizziness in older persons.
- Floors have non-glare, non-slip surfaces.
- Non-skid wax is used on hardwood, tiled, or linoleum floors.
- Loose floor boards and tiles are reported. So are frayed rugs and carpets.
- Floors and stairs are free of clutter, cords, and other items that can cause tripping.
- Floors are free of spills. Wipe up spills at once. Put a WET FLOOR sign by the wet area.
- Floors are free of excess furniture and equipment.
- Electrical and extension cords are out of the way. This includes power strips.
- Equipment and supplies are kept on 1 side of the hallway.

Furniture
- Furniture is placed for easy movement.
- Furniture is kept in place. It is not re-arranged.
- Chairs have armrests. Armrests give support when standing or sitting.
- A phone, lamp, and personal belongings are within the person's reach.

Beds and Other Equipment
- The bed is at the correct height for the person.
- The bed is in the lowest horizontal position, except when giving bedside care. The distance from the bed to the floor is reduced if the person falls or gets out of bed.
- Bed rails (p. 118) are used according to the care plan.
- A mattress, special mat, or floor cushion is placed on the floor beside the bed (Fig. 10-2). This reduces the chance of injury if the person falls or gets out of bed.
- Wheelchairs, walkers, canes, and crutches fit properly. They are in good repair. Another person's equipment is not used.
- Crutches, canes, and walkers have non-skid tips.
- Wheelchair and stretcher safety is followed (Chapter 9).
- Wheel locks on beds (p. 119), wheelchairs, and stretchers are in working order.
- Bed and wheelchair or stretcher wheels are locked for transfers.
- Linens are checked for sharp objects and for the person's property (dentures, eyeglasses, hearing aids, and so on).

Lighting
- Rooms, hallways, and stairways have good lighting. So do bathrooms and shower/tub rooms.
- Light switches (including those in bathrooms) are within reach and easy to find.
- Night-lights are in bedrooms, hallways, and bathrooms.

Shoes and Clothing
- Non-skid footwear is worn. Socks, bedroom slippers, and long shoelaces are avoided.
- Shoes fit well. They should not slip up and down on the person's feet. All shoelaces and straps are fastened.
- Clothing fits properly. Clothing is not loose. It does not drag on the floor. Belts are tied or secured in place.

Call Lights and Alarms
- The person is taught how to use the call light (Chapter 15).
- The call light is always within the person's reach. This includes when sitting in the chair, on the commode, and in the bathroom and shower/tub room.
- The person is asked to call for assistance when help is needed.
  - When getting out of bed or a chair
  - With walking
  - With getting to or from the bathroom or commode
  - With getting on or off the bedpan
- Call lights are answered promptly. The person may need help right away. He or she may not wait for help.
- Bed, chair, door, floor mat, and belt alarms are used. They sense when the person tries to get up, get out of bed, or open a door (Fig. 10-3).
- Alarms are responded to at once.

Other
- Color-coded alerts are used to warn of a fall risk. Yellow is the common color for a fall alert. Besides wristbands (Chapter 9), some agencies also use color-coded blankets, non-skid footwear, socks, and magnets or stickers to place on room doors.
- The person is checked often. This may be every 15 minutes or as required by the care plan. Careful and frequent observation is important.
- Frequent checks are made on persons with poor judgment or memory. This may be every 15 minutes or as required by the care plan.

BOX 10-2 Safety Measures to Prevent Falls—cont'd

Other—cont'd

- Persons at risk for falling are close to the nurses' station.
- Hand rails (p. 118) are on both sides of stairs and hallways.
- The person uses hand rails when walking or using stairs.
- Family and friends are asked to visit during busy times. Meal times and shift changes are examples. They are also asked to visit during the evening and night shifts.
- Companions are provided. Sitters, companions, or volunteers are with the person.
- Non-slip strips are on the floor next to the bed and in the bathroom. They are intact.

Other—cont'd

- Caution is used when turning corners, entering corridor intersections, and going through doors. You could injure a person coming from the other direction.
- Pull (do not push) wheelchairs, stretchers, carts, and other wheeled equipment through doorways. This allows you to lead the way and to see where you are going.
- A safety check is made of the room after visitors leave. (See the inside of the front cover.) They may have lowered a bed rail, removed a call light, or moved a walker out of reach. Or they may have brought an item that could harm the person.

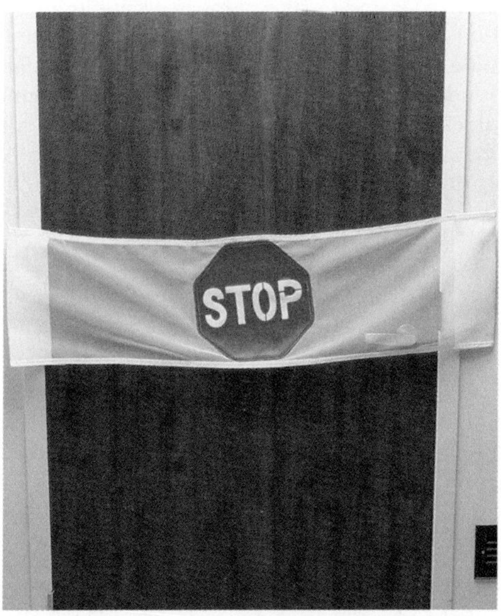

FIGURE 10-1 Barriers are used to prevent wandering.

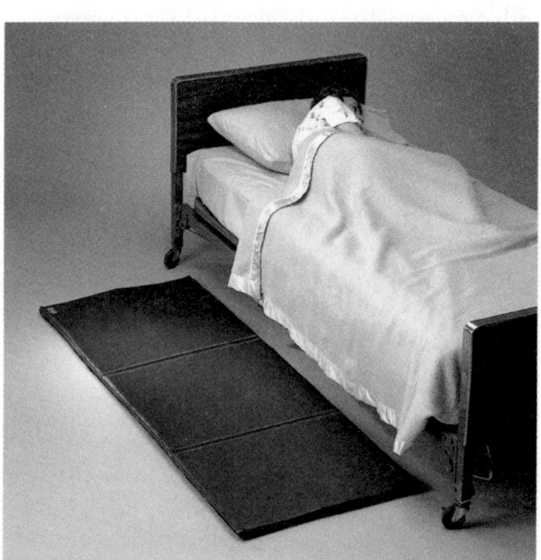

FIGURE 10-2 Floor cushion.

A

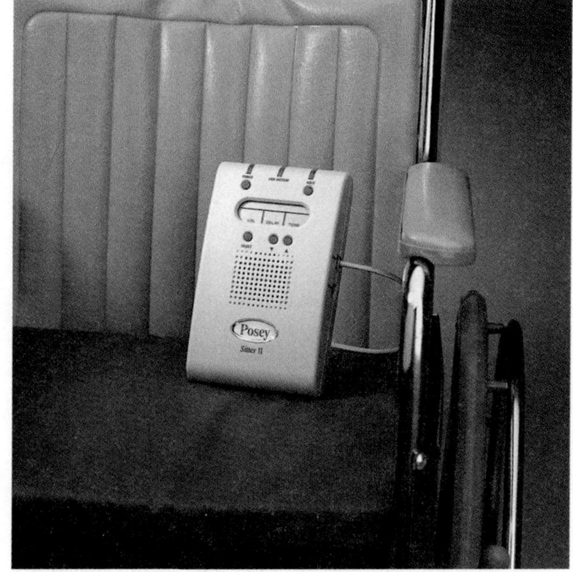

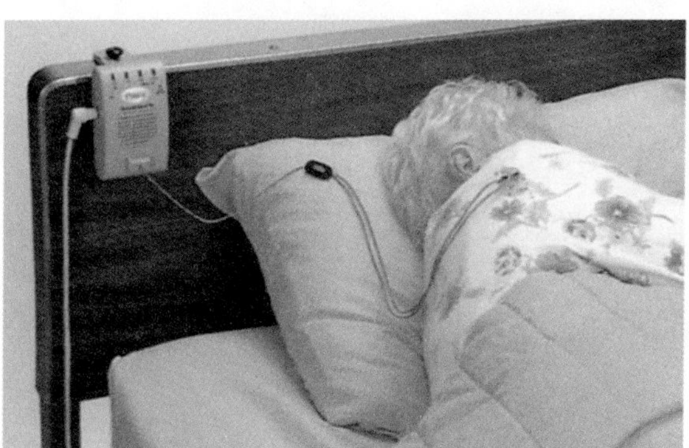

B

FIGURE 10-3 Alarms. **A,** Chair alarm. **B,** Bed alarm.

Bed Rails

A ***bed rail*** *(side rail) is a device that serves as a guard or barrier along the side of the bed.* Bed rails are raised and lowered (Fig. 10-4). They lock in place with levers, latches, or buttons. Bed rails are half, three-quarters (¾), or the full length of the bed. When half-length rails are used, each side may have 2 rails. One is for the upper part of the bed, the other for the lower part.

The nurse and the care plan tell you when to raise bed rails. They are needed by persons who are unconscious or sedated with drugs. Some confused or disoriented people need them. If a person needs bed rails, keep them up at all times except when giving bedside nursing care.

Bed rails present hazards. The person can fall when trying to climb over them, or the person cannot get out of bed or use the bathroom. *Entrapment* is a risk (Chapter 15). That is, the person can get caught, trapped, entangled, or strangled.

Bed rails are considered restraints (Chapter 11) if:
- The person cannot get out of bed.
- The person cannot lower them without help.

Bed rails cannot be used unless needed to treat a person's medical symptoms. They must be in the person's best interests. Some people feel safer with bed rails up. Others use them to change positions in bed. The person or legal representative must give consent for raised bed rails. The need for bed rails is carefully noted in the person's medical record and care plan.

The procedures in this book include using bed rails. This helps you learn how to use them correctly. The nurse, the care plan, and your assignment sheet tell you which people use bed rails. If a person does not use them, omit the "raise bed rails" and "lower bed rails" steps.

Check the person often. Report to the nurse that you checked the person. If you are allowed to chart, record when you checked the person and your observations.

See *Promoting Safety and Comfort: Bed Rails.*

PROMOTING SAFETY AND COMFORT

Bed Rails

Safety

You raise the bed to give care. Follow these safety measures to prevent the person from falling.
- *For a person who uses bed rails:* Always raise the far bed rail if you are working alone. Raise both bed rails if you need to leave the bedside for any reason.
- *For a person who does not use bed rails:* Ask a co-worker to help you. The co-worker stands on the far side of the bed. This protects the person from falling.
- Never leave the person alone when the bed is raised.
- Always lower the bed to a comfortable and safe level for the person when you are done giving care. Follow the care plan.

Comfort

The person has to reach over raised bed rails for items on the bedside stand and over-bed table (Chapter 15). Such items include the water mug with straw, tissues, phone, and TV and light controls. Adjust the over-bed table so it is within the person's reach. Ask if the person wants other items nearby. Place them on the over-bed table too. Always make sure needed items, including the call light, are within the person's reach.

Hand Rails and Grab Bars

Hand rails are in hallways and stairways (Fig. 10-5). They give support to persons who are weak or unsteady when walking.

Grab bars are in bathrooms and in shower/tub rooms (Fig. 10-6). They provide support for sitting down or getting up from a toilet. They also are used for getting in and out of the shower or tub.

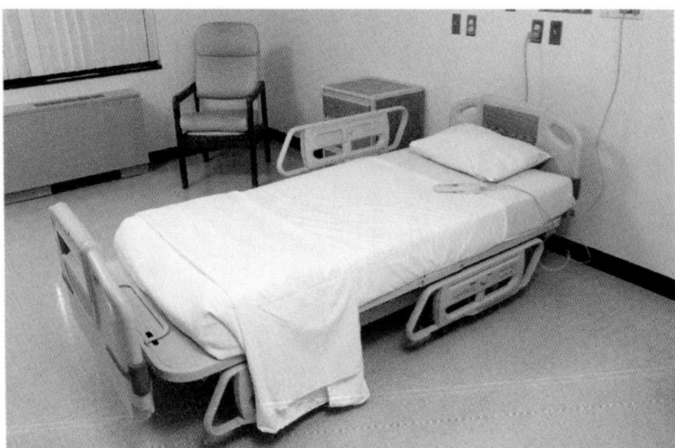

FIGURE 10-4 Bed rails. The far bed rail is raised. The near bed rail is lowered.

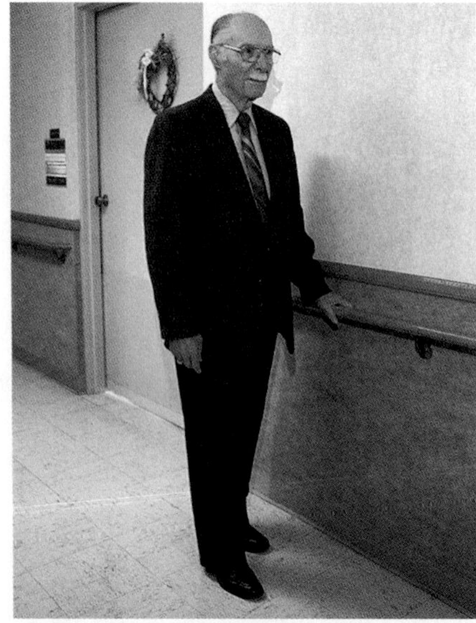

FIGURE 10-5 Hand rails provide support when walking.

Wheel Locks

Bed legs have wheels. They let the bed move easily. Wheels have locks to prevent the bed from moving (Fig. 10-7). Wheels are locked at all times except when moving the bed. Make sure bed wheels are locked:

- When giving bedside care
- When you transfer a person to and from the bed

Wheelchair and stretcher wheels also are locked during transfers (Chapter 14). You or the person can be injured if the bed, wheelchair, or stretcher moves.

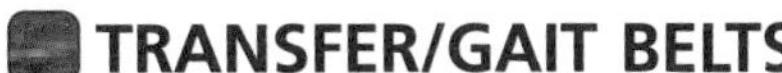

TRANSFER/GAIT BELTS

A ***transfer belt (gait belt)*** *is a device used to support a person who is unsteady or disabled* (Fig. 10-8). It helps prevent falls and injuries. When used to transfer a person (Chapter 14), it is called a *transfer belt.* When used to help a person walk, it is called a *gait belt.*

The belt goes around the person's waist. Grasp under the belt to support the person during the transfer or when assisting the person to walk.

See *Focus on Communication: Transfer/Gait Belts.*

See *Promoting Safety and Comfort: Transfer/Gait Belts,* p. 120.

See procedure: *Applying a Transfer/Gait Belt,* p. 120.

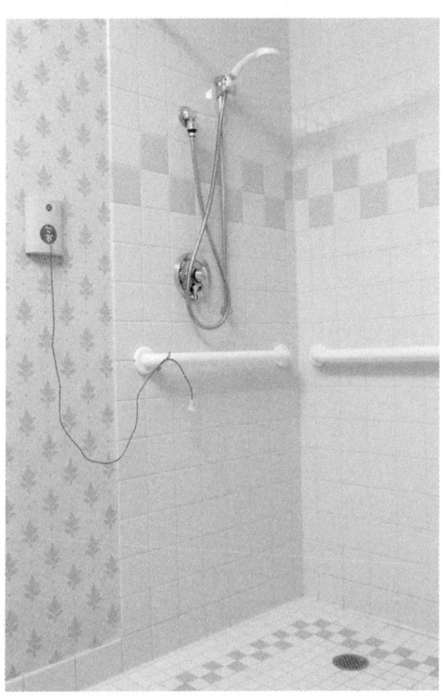

FIGURE 10-6 Grab bars in a shower.

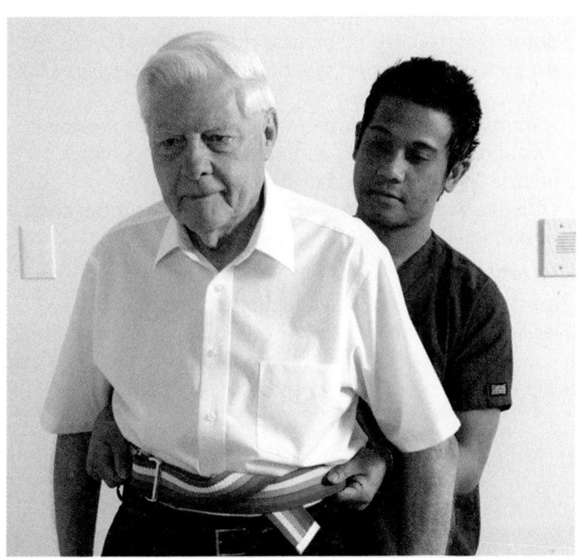

FIGURE 10-8 Transfer/gait belt. The belt buckle is positioned off-center. The buckle is not over the spine. Excess strap is tucked into the belt. The nursing assistant grasps the belt from underneath.

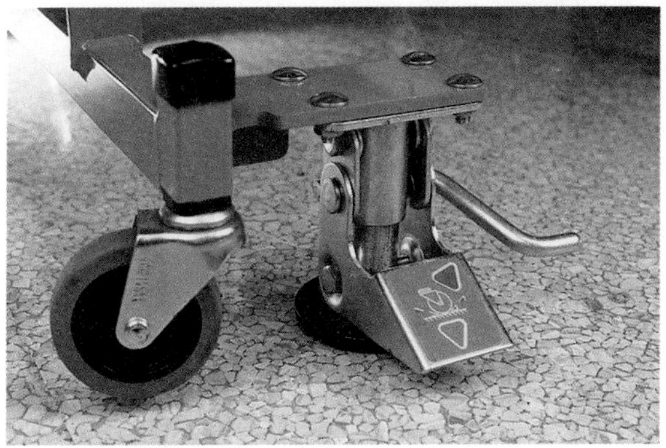

FIGURE 10-7 Lock on a bed wheel.

FOCUS ON COMMUNICATION

Transfer/Gait Belts

When applying a transfer/gait belt, ask the person about his or her comfort. You can say: "How does that feel? Is the belt too loose? Is it too tight?" Adjust the belt as needed for the person's comfort and safety.

PROMOTING SAFETY AND COMFORT

Transfer/Gait Belts

Safety

Transfer/gait belts are routinely used in nursing centers. If the person needs help, a belt is required. To use one safely, always follow the manufacturer's instructions.

Some transfer/gait belts have a quick-release buckle (Fig. 10-9). Position the quick-release buckle at the person's back where he or she cannot reach it. This prevents the person from releasing the buckle during the procedure. Injury could result if the buckle is released.

Do not leave excess strap dangling. Tuck the excess strap into the belt (see Fig. 10-8).

Remove the belt after the procedure. Do not leave the person alone while he or she is wearing a transfer/gait belt.

Using a transfer/gait belt is unsafe for some persons. The belt could cause pressure or rub against care equipment. Check with the nurse and the care plan before using a transfer/gait belt if the person has:

- An ostomy—colostomy or ileostomy (Chapter 19)
- A gastrostomy tube (Chapter 20)
- Chronic obstructive pulmonary disease (Chapter 28)
- An abdominal or chest wound, incision, or drainage tube
- Monitoring equipment
- A *hernia* (part of an organ that protrudes or projects through an opening in a muscle wall. Hernias often involve a loop of bowel or the stomach.)
- Other conditions or care equipment involving the chest or abdomen

Comfort

A transfer/gait belt is always applied over clothing. It is never applied over bare skin. Also, it is applied under the breasts. Breasts must not be caught under the belt. The belt buckle is never positioned over the person's spine.

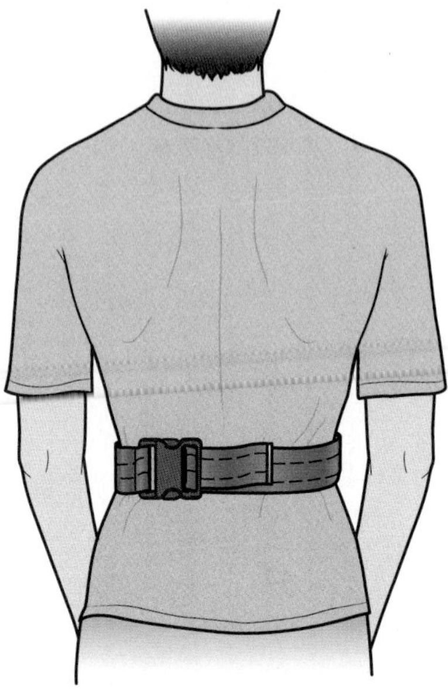

FIGURE 10-9 A transfer/gait belt with a quick-release buckle. The quick-release buckle is positioned off-center at the back.

Applying a Transfer/Gait Belt

QUALITY OF LIFE

- Knock before entering the person's room.
- Address the person by name.
- Introduce yourself by name and title.
- Explain the procedure before starting and during the procedure.
- Protect the person's rights during the procedure.
- Handle the person gently during the procedure.

PROCEDURE

1. See *Promoting Safety and Comfort: Transfer/Gait Belts.*
2. Practice hand hygiene.
3. Identify the person. Check the identification (ID) bracelet against the assignment sheet. Also call the person by name.
4. Provide for privacy.
5. Assist the person to a sitting position.
6. Apply the belt.
   a. Hold the belt by the buckle.
   b. Wrap the belt around the person's waist. Apply the belt over clothing. Do not apply it over bare skin.
   c. Insert the belt's metal tip into the buckle. Pass the belt through the side with the teeth first (Fig. 10-10, *A*).
   d. Bring the belt tip across the front of the buckle. Insert the tip through the buckle's smooth side (Fig. 10-10, *B*).
7. Tighten the belt so it is snug. It should not cause discomfort or impair breathing. You should be able to slide your open, flat hand under the belt. Ask the person about his or her comfort.
8. Make sure that a woman's breasts are not caught under the belt.
9. Place the buckle off-center in the front or off-center in the back for the person's comfort (Fig. 10-10, *C*). (A quick-release buckle is positioned at the person's back.) The buckle is not over the spine.
10. Tuck any excess strap into the belt (see Fig. 10-10, *C*).

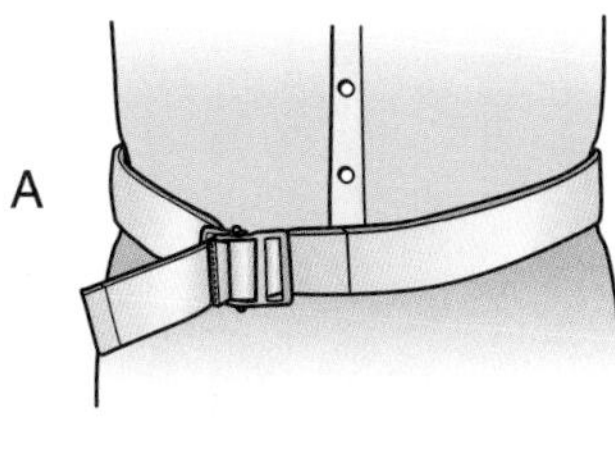

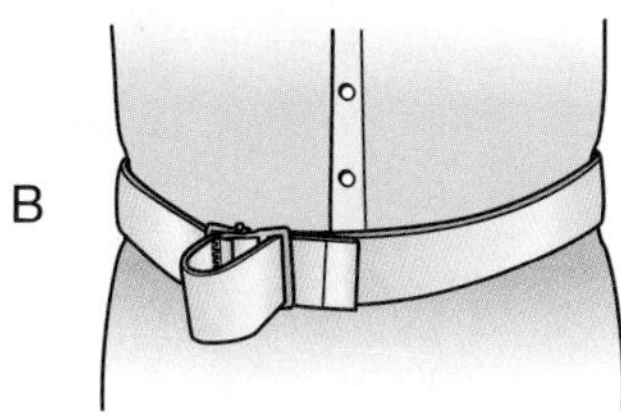

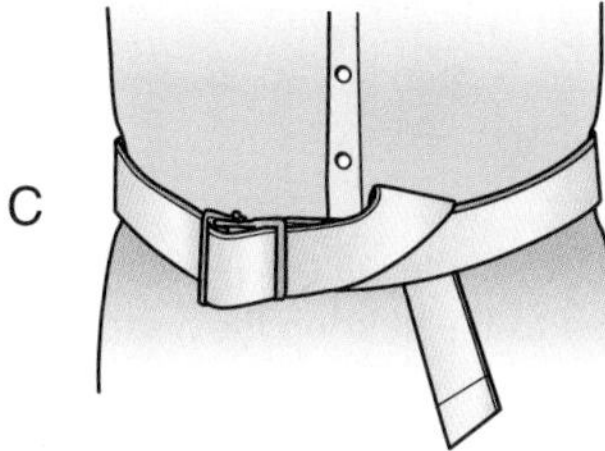

FIGURE 10-10 Applying a transfer/gait belt at the waist. **A,** The belt is inserted into the buckle. The belt goes through the side with the teeth first. **B,** The belt is inserted into the buckle's smooth side. **C,** The buckle is in the front. Excess strap is tucked into the belt.

THE FALLING PERSON

A person may start to fall when standing or walking. See the risk factors for falls (see Box 10-1).

Do not try to prevent the fall. You could injure yourself and the person while twisting and straining to prevent the fall. Head, wrist, arm, hip, knee, and back injuries could occur.

If a person starts to fall, ease him or her to the floor. This lets you control the direction of the fall. You can also protect the person's head. Do not let the person move or get up before the nurse checks for injuries.

If you find a person on the floor, do not move the person. Stay with the person and call for the nurse.

See *Focus on Older Persons: The Falling Person.*

See procedure: *Helping the Falling Person.*

FOCUS ON OLDER PERSONS

The Falling Person

Some older persons are confused. A confused person may not understand why you do not want him or her to move or get up after a fall. Forcing a person not to move may injure the person and you. You may need to let the person move for his or her safety and your own. Never use force to hold a person down. Stay calm and protect the person from injury. Talk to the person in a quiet, soothing voice. Call for help.

Helping the Falling Person

PROCEDURE

1 Stand behind the person with your feet apart. Keep your back straight.
2 Bring the person close to your body as fast as possible (Fig. 10-11, *A*, p. 122). Use the transfer/gait belt. Or wrap your arms around the person's waist. If necessary, you can also hold the person under the arms.
3 Move your leg so the person's buttocks rest on it (Fig. 10-11, *B*, p. 122). Move the leg near the person.
4 Lower the person to the floor. The person slides down your leg to the floor (Fig. 10-11 *C*, p. 122). Bend at your hips and knees as you lower the person.
5 Call a nurse to check the person. Stay with the person.
6 Help the nurse return the person to bed. Ask other staff to help if needed.

POST-PROCEDURE

7 Provide for comfort. (See the inside of the front cover.)
8 Place the call light within reach.
9 Raise or lower bed rails. Follow the care plan.
10 Complete a safety check of the room. (See the inside of the front cover.)
11 Practice hand hygiene.
12 Report and record the following.
   - How the fall occurred
   - How far the person walked
   - How activity was tolerated before the fall
   - Complaints before the fall
   - How much help the person needed while walking
13 Complete an incident report (Chapter 9).

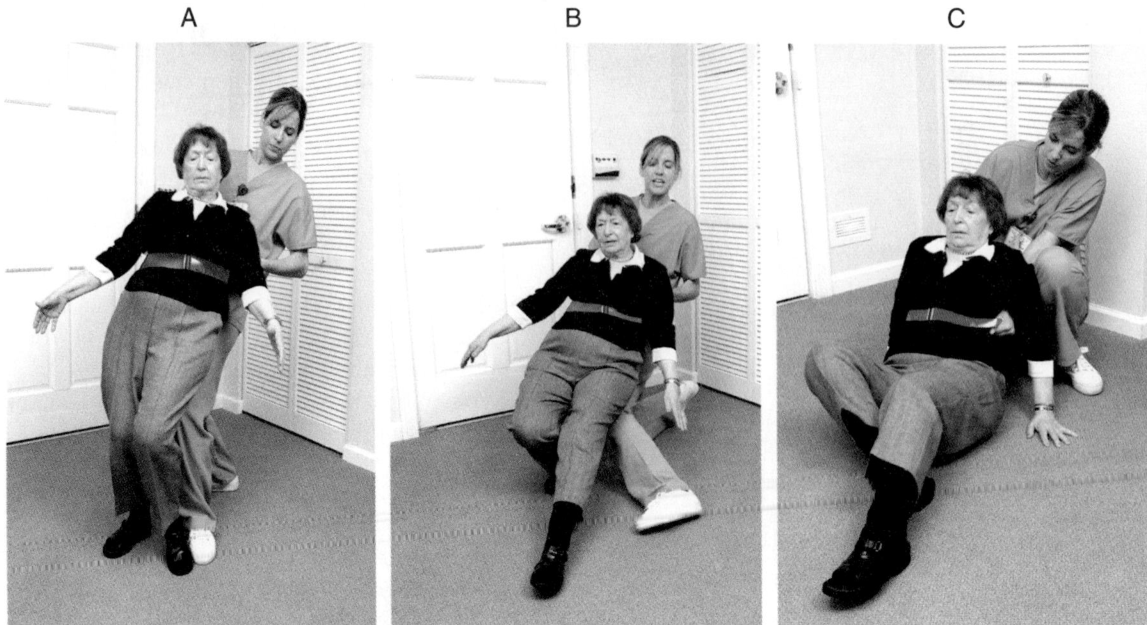

FIGURE 10-11 The falling person. **A,** The falling person is supported with the gait belt. **B,** The person's buttocks rest on the nursing assistant's leg. **C,** The person is eased to the floor on the nursing assistant's leg.

FOCUS ON PRIDE

The Person, Family, and Yourself

Personal and Professional Responsibility

Each person is unique. Some persons need other measures for safe care. For example, a person who is obese starts to fall. There is little that you can do. For the person's safety and yours:

- Do *not* follow the procedure: *Helping the Falling Person* (p. 121).
- Move any items out of the way that could cause injury. Do so as quickly as possible.
- Try to protect the person's head. Protect the person's head from striking the floor, equipment, or other objects.
- Call for the nurse at once. Stay with the person.
- Assist the health team as needed to return the person to bed.

You are responsible for providing safe care. Plan ahead and be prepared. Adjust to meet the person's specific needs.

Rights and Respect

Safety and security are not only rights, but basic needs (Chapter 6). Fear of falling does not make a person feel safe. Before moving a person, explain what you are going to do and what he or she needs to do. Also give step-by-step instructions as you progress. Do not move the person without telling him or her first. Good communication promotes comfort. It supports the person's right to safety and security. See Chapter 14 for how to safely move and transfer the person.

Independence and Social Interaction

Some people feel that safety devices limit independence. For example, Ms. Mills does not like having bed rails up. She says: "I feel trapped. Do these have to be up?" Ms. Mills has fallen out of bed at night. The care plan includes having bed rails up while she is in bed.

Listen to the person's concerns. Kindly explain the reason for the safety device. If the person still refuses, tell the nurse. Do not let the person talk you out of performing a safety measure or using a safety device. Safety is always a priority.

Delegation and Teamwork

Helping co-workers is an important part of teamwork. However, you may not be familiar with a person and his or her care plan. You must promote safety. Communication is essential. When assisting with the transfer of a co-worker's patient or resident, you must have certain information. Ask the nurse or co-worker:

- Is the person at risk for falls?
- Is the person weak? Can he or she bear weight?
- Are there activity limits?
- How many staff are needed for the transfer?
- Are assistive devices needed? A cane, transfer belt, wheelchair, and walker are examples.
- Is other equipment needed? Oxygen and braces are examples.

Ethics and Laws

Safety measures can be time consuming. Perhaps you cannot find a transfer belt. Or you need to get a walker. Or you must put on the person's shoes. Resist the urge to take short cuts. Take the time to:

- Find and use assistive devices.
- Put proper footwear on the person.
- Raise or lower the bed and bed rails as appropriate.
- Lock wheels on beds, stretchers, and wheelchairs.
- Ask others to help if needed.

Safe care includes taking measures to prevent falls. See Box 10-2. Hurrying is never an acceptable excuse for causing harm. Take time for safety. Take pride in doing the right thing by providing safe care.

REVIEW QUESTIONS

Circle the BEST answer.

1 Most falls occur in
- **a** Patient and resident rooms and bathrooms
- **b** Dining rooms
- **c** Lounges
- **d** Hallways

2 Which person has the *lowest* risk of falls?
- **a** A 75-year-old with confusion
- **b** A 68-year-old with a history of falls
- **c** A 60-year-old with a hearing aid
- **d** An 80-year-old with urinary incontinence

3 A person's care plan includes fall prevention measures. Which should you question?
- **a** Assist with elimination needs.
- **b** Keep phone, lamp, and TV controls within reach.
- **c** Check the person every 2 hours.
- **d** Complete a safety check after visitors leave the room.

4 You observe the following in the person's room. Which is *not* safe?
- **a** The lamp cord is by the chair.
- **b** The chair has armrests.
- **c** The night-light works.
- **d** The bed is in a low position.

5 You note the following after a person got dressed. Which is safe?
- **a** Pant cuffs are dragging on the floor.
- **b** The person is wearing non-skid shoes.
- **c** The belt is not fastened.
- **d** The shirt is too big.

6 A co-worker is helping Mr. Polk today. His chair alarm goes off. What should you do?
- **a** Find your co-worker.
- **b** Tell the nurse.
- **c** Assist Mr. Polk.
- **d** Wait for someone to respond to the alarm.

7 To help prevent falls, you need to report
- **a** Equipment and supplies being on 1 side of the hallway
- **b** A floor cushion beside the bed
- **c** A co-worker pulling a wheelchair through a doorway
- **d** Clutter on stairways

8 Bed rails are used
- **a** When you think they are needed
- **b** When the bed is raised
- **c** According to the care plan
- **d** To support persons who are weak or unsteady

9 You are going to transfer a person from the bed to a chair. Bed wheels must be locked.
- **a** True
- **b** False

10 A transfer/gait belt is applied
- **a** To the skin
- **b** Over clothing at the waist
- **c** Over the breasts
- **d** Under the robe

11 To safely use a transfer/gait belt, you must
- **a** Follow the manufacturer's instructions
- **b** Be able to slide a closed fist under the belt
- **c** Leave the belt on if the person is left alone
- **d** Position the buckle over the person's spine

12 You apply a transfer/gait belt. What should you do with the excess strap?
- **a** Cut it off.
- **b** Wrap it around the person's waist.
- **c** Tuck it into the belt.
- **d** Let it dangle.

13 A person starts to fall. Your *first* action is to
- **a** Try to prevent the fall
- **b** Call for help
- **c** Bring the person close to your body as fast as possible
- **d** Lower the person to the floor

14 You found a person lying on the floor. What should you do?
- **a** Call for the nurse.
- **b** Help the person back to bed.
- **c** Apply a transfer belt.
- **d** Lock the bed wheels.

Answers to these questions are on p. 504.

FOCUS ON **PRACTICE**

Problem Solving

You are assisting a resident in the bathroom. The resident is not to be left alone while in the bathroom. You hear another resident's chair alarm sound in the hallway outside the door. What will you do?

CHAPTER

11 Restraint Alternatives and Safe Restraint Use

OBJECTIVES

- Define the key terms and key abbreviations listed in this chapter.
- Describe the purpose of restraints.
- Identify restraint alternatives.
- Identify the risk factors related to restraint use.
- Explain the legal aspects of restraint use.
- Explain how to use restraints safely.
- Perform the procedure described in this chapter.
- Explain how to promote PRIDE in the person, the family, and yourself.

KEY TERMS

chemical restraint Any drug used for discipline or convenience and not required to treat medical symptoms
enabler A device that limits freedom of movement but is used to promote independence, comfort, or safety
freedom of movement Any change in place or position of the body or any part of the body that the person is able to control
medical symptom An indication or characteristic of a physical or psychological condition
physical restraint Any manual method or physical or mechanical device, material, or equipment attached to or near the person's body that he or she cannot remove easily and that restricts freedom of movement or normal access to one's body
remove easily The manual method, device, material, or equipment used to restrain the person that can be removed intentionally by the person in the same manner it was applied by the staff

KEY ABBREVIATIONS

CMS Centers for Medicare & Medicaid Services
FDA Food and Drug Administration
OBRA Omnibus Budget Reconciliation Act of 1987
TJC The Joint Commission

Chapters 9 and 10 have many safety measures. However, some persons need extra protection. They may present dangers to themselves or others (including staff).

The Centers for Medicare & Medicaid Services (CMS) has rules for using restraints. Like the Omnibus Budget Reconciliation Act of 1987 (OBRA), CMS rules protect the person's rights and safety. This includes the right to be free from restraint. Restraints may be used only to treat a medical symptom or for the immediate physical safety of the person or others. Restraints may be used only when less restrictive measures fail to protect the person or others. They must be discontinued as soon as possible.

The CMS uses these terms.

- ***Physical restraint****—any manual method or physical or mechanical device, material, or equipment attached to or near the person's body that he or she cannot remove easily and that restricts freedom of movement or normal access to one's body.*
- ***Chemical restraint****—any drug used for discipline or convenience and not required to treat medical symptoms.* The drug or dosage is not a standard treatment for the person's condition.
- ***Freedom of movement****—any change in place or position of the body or any part of the body that the person is able to control.*
- ***Remove easily****—the manual method, device, material, or equipment used to restrain the person that can be removed intentionally by the person in the same manner it was applied by the staff.* For example, the person can put bed rails down, untie a knot, or unclasp a buckle.

HISTORY OF RESTRAINT USE

Restraints were once used to *prevent* falls. Research shows that restraints *cause* falls. Falls occur when persons try to get free of the restraints. Injuries are more serious from falls in restrained persons than in those not restrained.

Restraints also were used to prevent wandering or interfering with treatment. They were often used for confusion, poor judgment, or behavior problems. Older persons were restrained more often than younger persons were. Restraints were viewed as necessary devices to protect a person. However, they can cause serious harm, even death. See "Risks From Restraint Use" on p. 127.

Besides the CMS, the Food and Drug Administration (FDA), state agencies, and The Joint Commission (TJC—an accrediting agency) have guidelines for restraint use. They do not forbid restraint use. *They require considering or trying all other appropriate alternatives first.*

Every agency has policies and procedures about restraints. They include identifying persons at risk for harm, harmful behaviors, restraint alternatives, and proper restraint use. Staff training is required.

RESTRAINT ALTERNATIVES

Often there are causes and reasons for harmful behaviors. Knowing and treating the cause can prevent restraint use. The nurse tries to find out what the behavior means.

- Is the person in pain, ill, or injured?
- Is the person short of breath? Are cells getting enough oxygen (Chapter 26)?
- Is the person afraid in a new setting?
- Does the person need to use the bathroom?
- Is clothing or a dressing (Chapter 24) tight or causing other discomfort?
- Is the person's position uncomfortable?
- Are body fluids, secretions, or excretions causing skin irritation?
- Is the person too hot or too cold? Hungry or thirsty?
- What are the person's life-long habits at this time of day?
- Does the person have problems communicating?
- Is the person seeing, hearing, or feeling things that are not real (Chapter 29)?
- Is the person confused or disoriented (Chapter 30)?
- Are drugs causing the behaviors?

Restraint alternatives for the person are identified (Box 11-1). They become part of the care plan. The care plan is changed as needed. Restraint alternatives may not protect the person. The doctor may need to order restraints.

BOX 11-1 Alternatives to Restraint Use

Physical Needs

- Life-long habits and routines are in the care plan. For example, showers before breakfast; reads in the bathroom; walks outside before lunch; watches TV after lunch.
- Pillows, wedge cushions, and posture and positioning devices are used.
- Food, fluid, hygiene, and elimination needs are met.
- The bedpan, urinal, or commode is within the person's reach.
- Back massages are given.
- A calm, quiet setting is provided.
- Exercise programs are provided.
- Outdoor time is planned for nice weather.
- Furniture meets the person's needs (lower bed, reclining chair, rocking chair).
- Observations and visits are made at least every 15 minutes. Or as often as noted in the care plan.
- The person is moved to a room close to the nurses' station.
- Light is adjusted to meet the person's needs and preferences.
- Staff assignments are consistent.
- Sleep is not interrupted.
- Noise levels are reduced.

Safety and Security Needs

- The call light is within reach.
- Call lights are answered promptly.
- The person wanders in safe areas.
- All staff are aware of persons who tend to wander. This includes staff in housekeeping, maintenance, the business office, dietary, and so on.

Safety and Security Needs—cont'd

- Knob guards are used on doors.
- Falls and injuries from falls are prevented (Chapter 10).
  - Padded hip protectors are worn under clothing (Fig. 11-1, p. 126).
  - Floor cushions are placed next to beds (Chapter 10).
  - Roll guards are attached to the bed frame (Fig. 11-2, p. 126).
- Warning devices are used on beds, chairs, and doors.
- Walls and furniture corners are padded.
- Procedures and care measures are explained.
- Frequent explanations are given about equipment or devices.
- Confused persons are oriented to person, time, and place. Calendars and clocks are provided.

Love, Belonging, and Self-Esteem Needs

- Diversion is provided—TV, videos, music, games, relaxation, tapes, and so on.
- Family and friends make videos of themselves for the person to watch.
- Videos are made of visits with family and friends for the person to watch.
- Time is spent in supervised areas (dining room, lounge, by the nurses' station).
- Family, friends, and volunteers visit.
- The person has companions or sitters.
- Time is spent with the person.
- Extra time is spent with a person who is restless.
- Reminiscing is done with the person.
- The person does jobs or tasks he or she consents to.

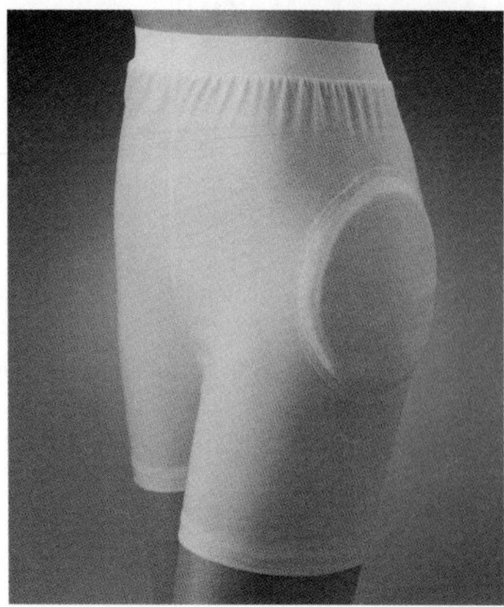

FIGURE 11-1 Hip protector.

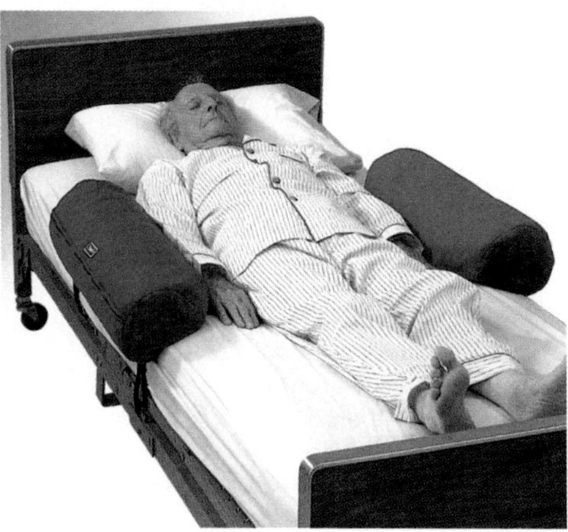

FIGURE 11-2 Roll guard.

SAFE RESTRAINT USE

Restraints can cause serious injury and even death. CMS, OBRA, FDA, and TJC guidelines are followed. So are state laws. They are part of the agency's policies and procedures for restraint use.

Restraints are not used to discipline a person. They are not used for staff convenience. *Discipline* is any action that punishes or penalizes a person. *Convenience* is any action that:

- Controls or manages the person's behavior.
- Requires less effort by the agency.
- Is not in the person's best interests.

Restraints are used only when necessary to treat medical symptoms. A ***medical symptom*** *is an indication or characteristic of a physical or psychological condition.* Symptoms may relate to physical, emotional, or behavioral problems. Sometimes restraints are needed to protect the person or others. That is, a person may have violent or aggressive behaviors that are harmful to self or others.

See *Focus on Surveys: Safe Restraint Use.*

Physical and Chemical Restraints

According to the CMS, *physical restraints* include these points.

- May be any manual method, physical or mechanical device, material, or equipment.
- Are attached to or next to the person's body.
- Cannot be easily removed by the person.
- Restrict freedom of movement or normal access to one's body.

FOCUS ON SURVEYS

Safe Restraint Use

Agencies must have a policy about restraint use. Surveyors will try to learn if restraints were used for:

- Discipline or staff convenience
- Only a certain time for the person's well-being

Surveyors will review medical records and interview staff. Some questions will focus on:

- The medical symptoms leading to restraint use. Could they be reversed or reduced?
- The cause of the medical symptoms. Were they caused by failure to:
  - Meet the person's needs?
  - Provide rehabilitation?
  - Provide meaningful activities?
  - Change the person's setting for safety?
- If restraint alternatives were used.
- If the least restrictive restraints were used.
- If restraints were used for a short time.

Physical restraints are applied to the chest, waist, elbows, wrists, hands, or ankles. They confine the person to a bed or chair. Or they prevent movement of a body part. Some furniture or barriers also prevent freedom of movement.

- A device used with a chair that the person cannot remove easily. The device prevents the person from rising. Trays, tables, bars, and belts are examples (Fig. 11-3).
- Any chair that prevents the person from rising.
- Any bed or chair placed so close to the wall that the person cannot get out of the bed or chair.
- Bed rails (Chapter 10) that prevent the person from getting out of bed. For example, 4 half-length bed rails are raised. They are restraints if the person cannot lower them.
- Tucking in or using Velcro to hold a sheet, fabric, or clothing so tightly that freedom of movement is restricted.

Drugs or drug dosages are *chemical restraints* if they:

- Control behavior or restrict movement.
- Are not standard treatment for the person's condition.

Drugs cannot be used for discipline or staff convenience. They cannot be used if they affect physical or mental function.

Sometimes drugs can help persons who are confused or disoriented. They may be anxious, agitated, or aggressive. The doctor may order drugs to control these behaviors. The drugs should not make the person sleepy and unable to function at his or her highest level.

Enablers. An *enabler is a device that limits freedom of movement but is used to promote independence, comfort, or safety.* Some devices are restraints and enablers. When the person can easily remove the device and it helps the person function, it is an enabler. For example:

- A chair or wheelchair with a lap-top tray is used for meals, writing, and so on (see Fig. 11-3). The chair is an enabler. If used to limit freedom of movement, the chair is a restraint.
- A person chooses to have raised bed rails. The bed rails are used to move in bed and to prevent falling out of bed. The bed rails are enablers, not restraints.

Risks From Restraint Use

Box 11-2 lists the risks from restraints. Injuries can occur as the person tries to get free of the restraint. Injuries also can occur from using the wrong restraint, applying it wrong, or keeping it on too long. Cuts, bruises, and fractures are common. *The most serious risk is death from strangulation.*

Restraints are medical devices. The Safe Medical Devices Act applies if a restraint causes illness, injury, or death. Also, the CMS requires the reporting of any death that occurs:

- While a person is in a restraint.
- Within 24 hours after a restraint was removed.
- Within 1 week after a restraint was removed. This is done if the restraint may have contributed directly or indirectly to the person's death.

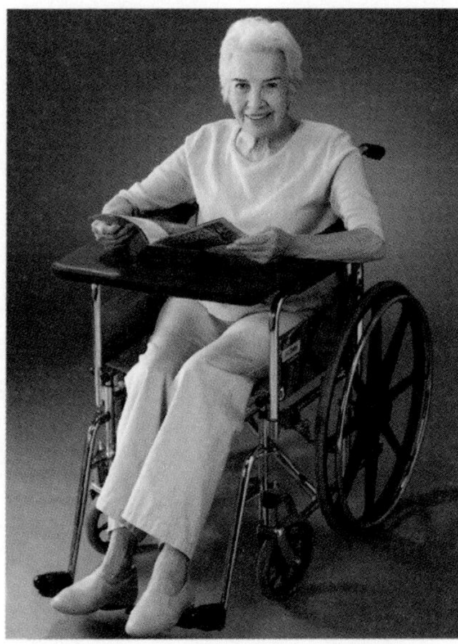

FIGURE 11-3 This lap-top tray is a restraint alternative. It is a restraint when used to prevent freedom of movement.

BOX 11-2 Risks From Restraint Use

- Constipation
- Contractures (Chapter 23)
- Cuts and bruises
- Decline in physical function (ability to walk, muscle condition)
- Dehydration
- Falls
- Fractures
- Head trauma
- Incontinence (Chapters 18 and 19)
- Infections: pneumonia and urinary tract
- Nerve injuries
- Pressure ulcers (Chapter 25)
- Social and mental health problems: agitation, anger, delirium, depression, loss of dignity, embarrassment and humiliation, mistrust, loss of self-respect, reduced social contact, withdrawal
- Strangulation

Legal Aspects

Laws applying to restraint use are followed. Remember:

- *Restraints must protect the person.* They are not used for staff convenience or to discipline a person. Using restraints is not easier than properly supervising and observing the person. A restrained person requires more staff time for care, supervision, and observation.
- *A doctor's order is required.* The doctor gives the reason for the restraint, what body part to restrain, what to use, and how long to use it. This information is on the care plan and your assignment sheet. In an emergency, the nurse can decide to apply restraints before getting a doctor's order.
- *The least restrictive method is used.* It allows the greatest amount of movement or body access possible. Some restraints attach to the person's body and to a fixed (non-movable) object. They restrict freedom of movement or body access. Vest, jacket, ankle, wrist, hand, and some belt restraints are examples. Other restraints are near but not directly attached to the person's body (bed rails or wedge cushions). They do not totally restrict freedom of movement and are less restrictive.
- *Restraints are used only after other measures fail to protect the person* (see Box 11-1). Some people can harm themselves or others. The care plan must include measures to protect the person and prevent harm to others. Many fall prevention measures are restraint alternatives (Chapter 10).
- *Unnecessary restraint is false imprisonment* (Chapter 3). You must clearly understand the reason for the restraint and its risks. If not, politely ask about its use. If you apply an unneeded restraint, you could face false imprisonment charges.
- *Informed consent is required.* The person must understand the reason for the restraint. The person is told how the restraint will help the planned medical treatment. The person is told about the risks of restraint use. If the person cannot give consent, his or her legal representative is given the information. Consent must be given before a restraint can be used. The doctor or nurse provides needed information and obtains the consent.

  See *Focus on Communication: Legal Aspects.*

FOCUS ON COMMUNICATION

Legal Aspects

You may not know the reason for a restraint. If so, politely ask the nurse why it is needed. For example:

- "Why does Mr. Reed need a restraint?"
- "I don't understand. Why did the doctor order a restraint?"

Safety Guidelines

The restrained person must be kept safe. Follow the safety measures in Box 11-3. Also remember these key points.

- *Observe for increased confusion and agitation.* Restraints can increase confusion and agitation. People are aware of restricted movements. They may try to get out of the restraint or struggle to pull at it. Some restrained persons beg others to free or to help release them. These behaviors often are viewed as signs of confusion. Not understanding what is happening to them can increase confusion. Restrained persons need repeated explanations and reassurance. Spending time with them has a calming effect.
- *Protect the person's quality of life.* Restraints are used for as short a time as possible. The care plan must show how to reduce restraint use. The person's needs are met with as little restraint as possible. You must meet physical, emotional, and social needs. Visit with the person and explain the reason for the restraint.
- *Follow the manufacturer's instructions.* They explain how to safely apply and secure the restraint. The restraint must be snug and firm, but not tight. Tight restraints affect circulation and breathing. The person must be comfortable and able to move the restrained part to a limited and safe extent. You could be negligent if you do not apply or secure a restraint properly.
- *Apply restraints with enough help to protect the person and staff from injury.* Persons in immediate danger of harming themselves or others are restrained quickly. Combative and agitated people can hurt themselves and the staff when restraints are applied. Enough staff members are needed to complete the task safely and quickly.
- *Observe the person at least every 15 minutes or as often as noted in the care plan.* Restraints are dangerous. Injuries and deaths can result from improper restraint use and poor observation. Prevent complications. Breathing and circulation problems are examples.
- *Remove or release the restraint, re-position the person, and meet basic needs at least every 2 hours. Or do so as often as noted on the care plan.*
  - Remove or release the restraint for at least 10 minutes.
  - Provide for food, fluid, comfort, safety, hygiene, and elimination needs. Also give skin care.
  - Perform range-of-motion exercises or help the person walk (Chapter 23). Follow the care plan.

  See *Focus on Communication: Safety Guidelines.*

Text continued on p. 133

FOCUS ON COMMUNICATION

Safety Guidelines

Restraints can increase confusion. Remind the person of the reason for the restraint and to call for help when it is needed. Repeat the following as often as needed.

- "Dr. Monroe ordered this restraint so you don't hurt yourself. If you need to get up, please call for help. I'll check on you every 15 minutes. Other staff will check on you too."
- "How does the restraint feel? Is it too tight? Is it too loose?"
- "Please put your call light on. I want to make sure that you can reach and use it with the restraint on."
- "Please call for help right away if you are having problems breathing."
- "Please call for help right away if the restraint is too tight."
- "Please call for help right away if you feel pain in your fingers or hands. Also call for me if you feel numbness or tingling."

BOX 11-3 Safety Measures for Using Restraints

Before Applying Restraints

- Do not use sheets, towels, tape, rope, straps, bandages, Velcro, or other items to restrain a person.
- Apply a restraint only after being instructed about its proper use.
- Demonstrate proper application of the restraint before applying it.
- Use the restraint noted in the care plan. Use the correct size. Small restraints are tight. They cause discomfort and agitation. They also restrict breathing and circulation. Strangulation is a risk from big or loose restraints.
- Use only restraints that have manufacturer instructions and warning labels.
  - Read the warning labels. Note the front and back of the restraint.
  - Follow the instructions. Some restraints are safe for bed, chair, and wheelchair use. Others are used only with certain equipment.
- Use intact restraints.
  - Look for broken stitches, tears, cuts, or frayed fabric or straps.
  - Look for missing or loose buckles, locks, hooks, loops, or straps or other damage. The restraint must hold securely.
- Test zippers, buckles, locks, hooks, loops, and other fasteners. The device must fasten securely.
- Do not use a restraint near a fire, a flame, or smoking materials.

Applying Restraints

- Follow agency policies and procedures.
- Do not use a restraint to:
  - Position a person on a toilet.
  - Position a person on furniture that does not allow for correct application.
- Position the person in good alignment before applying the restraint (Chapter 13).
  - Semi-Fowler's position (Chapter 15) is usually preferred for a vest, jacket, or belt restraint.
  - When in a chair, position the person so the hips are well to the back of the chair.
- Pad bony areas and the skin as instructed by the nurse. This prevents pressure and injury from the restraint.

Applying Restraints—cont'd

- Follow the manufacturer's instructions. A restraint applied wrong or backwards may cause serious injury or death. Death may occur from suffocation or strangulation.
  - For a vest restraint, the "V" neck is in front (Fig. 11-4, p. 130).
  - For a jacket restraint, the opening is in the back.
  - For a belt restraint when in a chair—Apply the restraint at a 45-degree angle over the thighs (Fig. 11-5, p. 130).
- Do not criss-cross straps in the back unless required by the manufacturer's instructions (Fig. 11-6, p. 131). Straps may loosen when the person moves and cause serious injury.
- Secure restraints according to agency policy. The policy should follow the manufacturer's instructions and allow for quick release in an emergency. Quick-release buckles or airline-type buckles are used (Fig. 11-7, p. 131). So are quick-release ties (Fig. 11-8, p. 131).
- Secure straps out of the person's reach.
- Leave 1 to 2 inches of slack in the straps if directed to do so by the nurse. This allows some movement of the part.
- Secure the restraint to the movable part of the bed frame (Fig. 11-9, p. 131). The restraint will not tighten or loosen when the head or foot of the bed is raised or lowered. For chairs, secure straps under the seat of the wheelchair or chair (Fig. 11-10, p. 131).
- Check for snugness after applying the restraint. The restraint should be snug but allow some movement of the restrained part. Follow the manufacturer's instructions. For example:
  - *If applied to the chest or waist*—Make sure the person can breathe easily. A flat hand should slide between the restraint and the person's body (Fig. 11-11, p. 132). Check with the nurse if you have very small or very large hands. Small or large hands could cause the restraint to be too tight or too loose.
  - *For wrist and mitt restraints*—You should be able to slide 1 finger under the restraint. Check with the nurse if you have very small or very large fingers. Small or large fingers could cause the restraint to be too tight or too loose.

Continued

BOX 11-3 Safety Measures for Using Restraints—cont'd

Applying Restraints—cont'd

- Make sure that the straps:
  - Cannot tighten, loosen, slip, or cause too much slack.
  - Will not slide in any direction. If straps slide, they change the restraint's position. The person can get suspended off the mattress or chair (Figs. 11-12, p. 132 and 11-13, p. 132). Strangulation can result.
- Never secure restraints to the bed rails. The person can reach bed rails to release knots or buckles. Also, injury to the person is likely when raising or lowering bed rails.
- Use bed rail covers or gap protectors as instructed by the nurse (Fig. 11-14, p. 132). They prevent entrapment between the bed rails or the bed rail bars (see Fig. 11-12). Entrapment can occur between:
  - The bars of a bed rail
  - The space between half-length (split) bed rails
  - The bed rail and mattress
  - The head-board or foot-board and mattress

After Applying Restraints

- Keep full bed rails up when using a vest, jacket, or belt restraint. Also use bed rail covers or gap protectors. Otherwise the person could fall off the bed and strangle on the restraint. Or the person can get caught between half-length bed rails.
- Do not use back cushions when a person is restrained in a chair. If the cushion moves out of place, slack occurs in the straps. Strangulation is a risk if the person slides forward or down from the extra slack.
- Do not cover the person with a sheet, blanket, bedspread, or other covering. The restraint must be in plain view at all times.
- Check the person at least every 15 minutes for safety, comfort, and signs of injury.
- Monitor persons in the supine (back-lying) position constantly. Aspiration is a great risk if vomiting occurs (Chapter 20). Call for the nurse at once.

After Applying Restraints—cont'd

- Check the person's circulation at least every 15 minutes.
  - *For mitt, wrist, or ankle restraints*—You should feel a pulse at a pulse site below the restraint. Fingers or toes should be warm and pink. Tell the nurse at once if:
    - You cannot feel a pulse.
    - Fingers or toes are cold, pale, or blue in color.
    - The person complains of pain, numbness, or tingling in the restrained part.
    - The skin is red or damaged.
  - *For a belt, jacket, or vest restraint*—The person should be able to breathe easily. Also check the position of the restraint, especially in the front and back.
- Keep scissors in your pocket. In an emergency, cutting the tie may be faster than untying a knot. Never leave scissors where the person can reach them. Make sure the person cannot reach the scissors in your pocket.
- Remove or release the restraint and re-position the person every 2 hours or as often as noted in the care plan. The restraint is removed or released for at least 10 minutes. Meet the person's basic needs. You need to:
  - Measure vital signs.
  - Meet elimination needs.
  - Offer food and fluids.
  - Meet hygiene needs.
  - Give skin care.
  - Perform range-of-motion exercises or help the person walk. Follow the care plan.
  - Provide for physical and emotional comfort. (See the inside of the front cover.)
- Keep the call light within the person's reach. Chart that this was done.
- Complete a safety check before leaving the room. (See the inside of the front cover.)
- Report to the nurse every time that you checked the person and removed or released the restraint. Report your observations and the care given. Follow agency policy for recording.

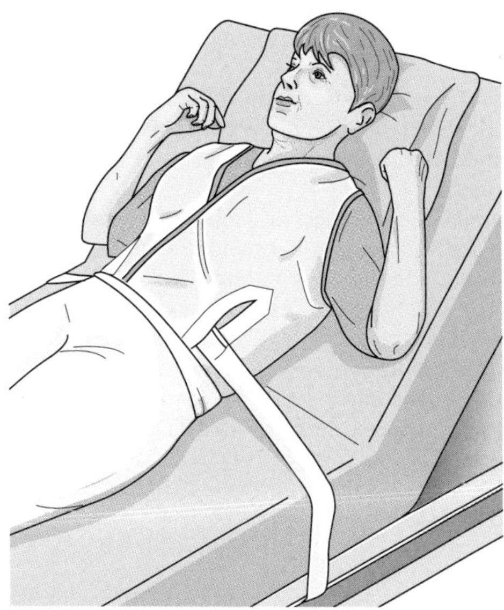

FIGURE 11-4 The vest restraint criss-crosses in front. The "V" neck is in front. (NOTE: The bed rails are raised after the restraint is applied.)

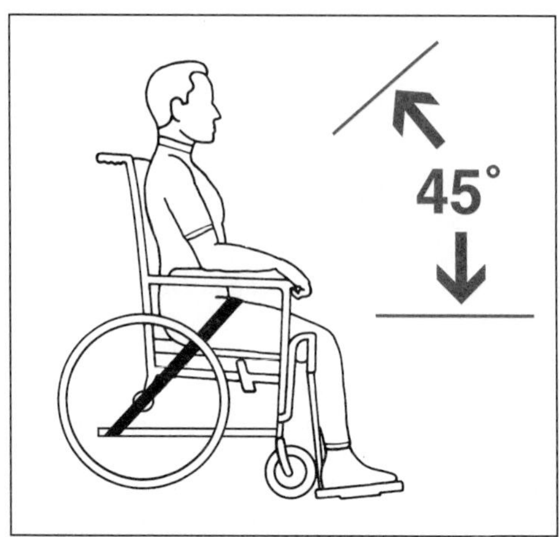

FIGURE 11-5 The belt restraint is at a 45-degree angle over the thighs.

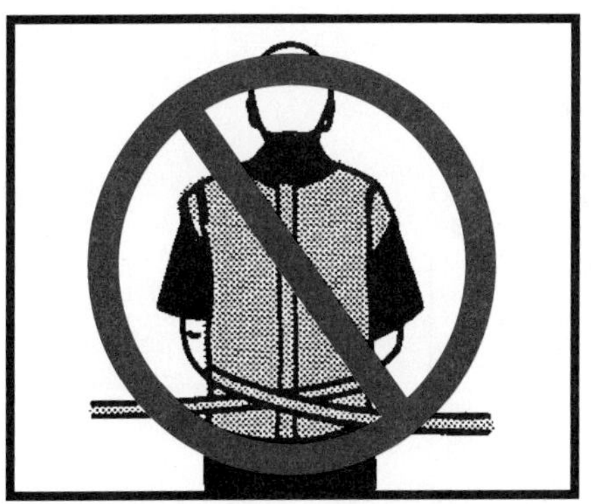

FIGURE 11-6 Never criss-cross vest or jacket straps in the back.

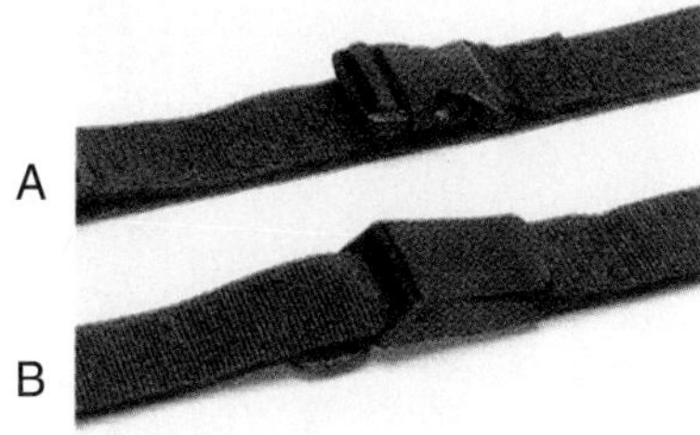

FIGURE 11-7 **A,** Quick-release buckle. **B,** Airline-type buckle.

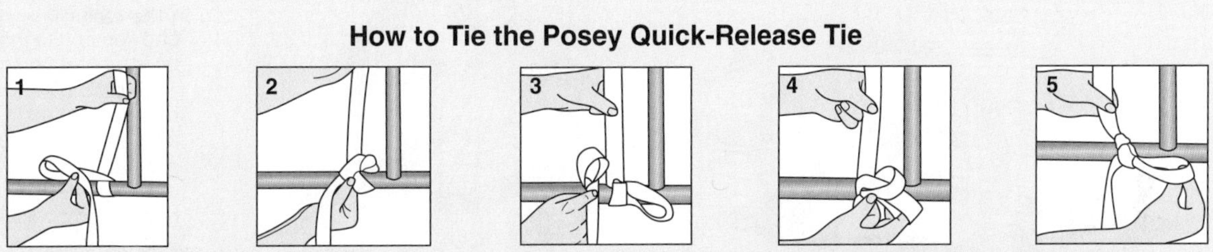

FIGURE 11-8 The Posey quick-release tie.

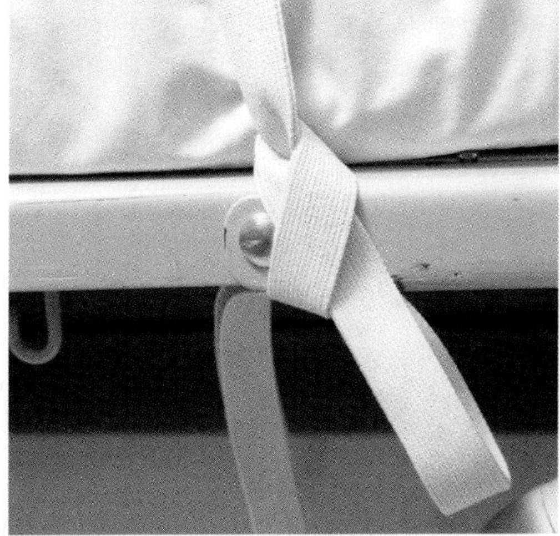

FIGURE 11-9 The restraint is secured to the movable part of the bed frame.

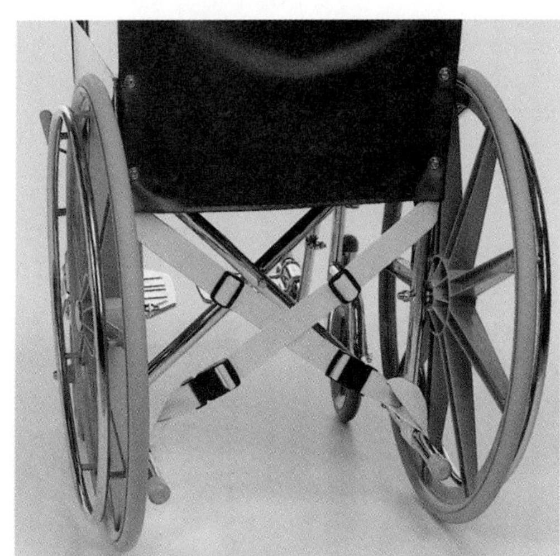

FIGURE 11-10 The restraint straps are secured to the wheelchair frame.

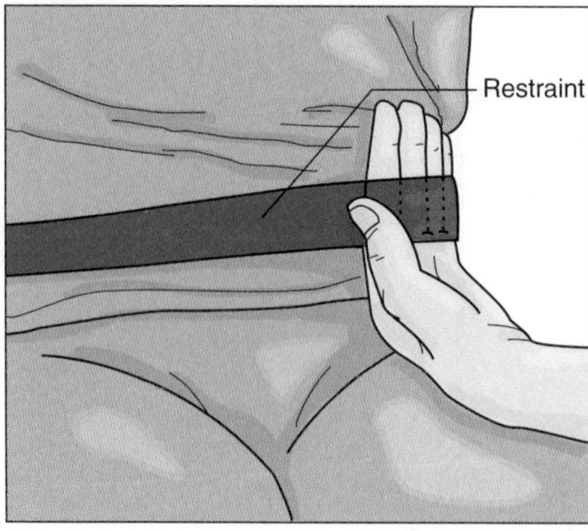

FIGURE 11-11 A flat hand slides between the restraint and the person.

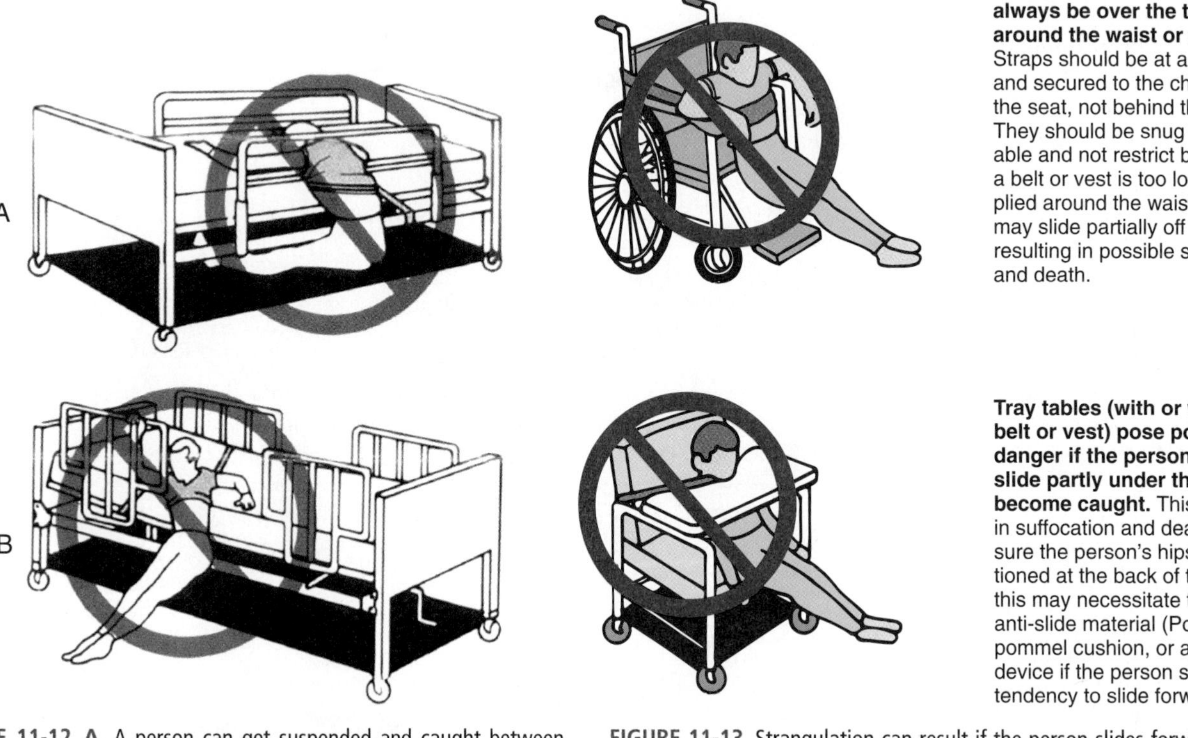

FIGURE 11-12 **A,** A person can get suspended and caught between bed rail bars. **B,** The person can get suspended and caught between half-length bed rails.

FIGURE 11-13 Strangulation can result if the person slides forward or down because of extra slack in the restraint.

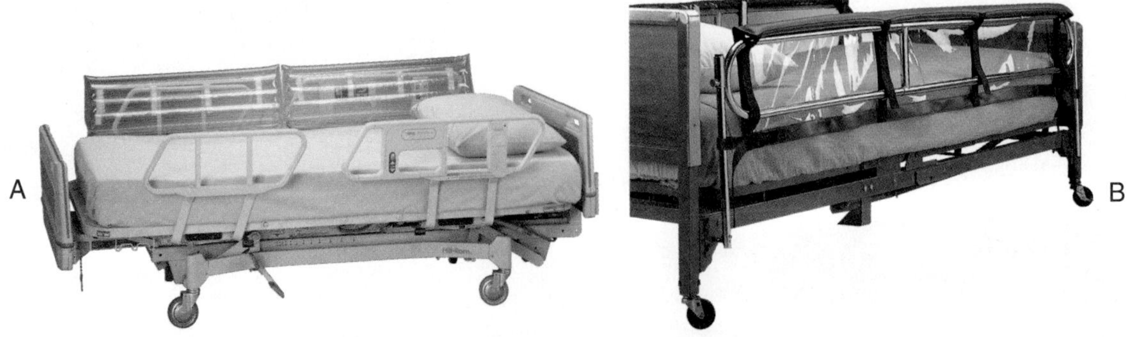

FIGURE 11-14 **A,** Bed rail protector. **B,** Guard-rail pads.

Reporting and Recording

Restraint information is recorded in the person's medical record. If you apply restraints or care for a restrained person, report and record:

- The type of restraint applied.
- The body part or parts restrained.
- The reason for the application.
- Safety measures taken (for example, bed rails padded and up, call light within reach).
- The time you applied the restraint.
- The time you removed or released the restraint and for how long.
- The person's vital signs.
- The care given when the restraint was removed and for how long.
- Skin color and condition.
- Condition of the limbs.
- The pulse felt in the restrained part.
- Changes in the person's behavior.
- Complaints of difficulty breathing; discomfort; a tight restraint; or pain, numbness, or tingling in the restrained part. Report these complaints at once.

Applying Restraints

Restraints are made of cloth or leather. Cloth restraints (soft restraints) are mitts, belts, straps, jackets, and vests. They are applied to the wrists, ankles, hands, waist, and chest. Leather restraints are applied to the wrists and ankles. Leather restraints are used for extreme agitation and combativeness.

Wrist Restraints. Wrist restraints (limb holders) limit arm movement (Fig. 11-15). They may be used when the person:

- Is at risk for pulling out tubes used for life-saving treatment (intravenous [IV] infusion, feeding tube).
- Is at risk for pulling at devices used to monitor vital signs.
- Scratches at, pulls at, or peels the skin, a wound, or a dressing. This can damage the skin or the wound.

Mitt Restraints. Hands are placed in mitt restraints. They prevent finger use. They allow hand, wrist, and arm movements. They have the same purpose as wrist restraints. Most mitts are padded (Fig. 11-16).

Belt Restraints. A belt restraint (Fig. 11-17, p. 134) may be used when injuries from falls are risks or for positioning during a medical treatment. The person cannot get out of bed or out of a chair. However, a roll belt allows the person to turn from side to side or sit up in bed.

The belt is applied around the waist and secured to the bed or chair (lap belt). It is applied over a garment. The person can release the quick-release type. It is less restrictive than those that only staff can release.

Vest Restraints and Jacket Restraints. Vest and jacket restraints are applied to the chest. They have the same purpose as belt restraints. The person cannot turn in bed or get out of a chair.

A jacket restraint is applied with the opening in the back. For a vest restraint, the "V neck" is in front and the vest crosses in the front (see Fig. 11-4). Vest and jacket restraints are never worn backward. Strangulation or other injuries are risks if the person slides down in the bed or chair. The restraint is always applied over a garment. *(Note: The straps of vest and jacket restraints cross in the front. A vest or jacket restraint may have a positioning slot in the back* [Fig. 11-18, p. 134]. *Criss-cross straps following the manufacturer's instructions.)*

Vest and jacket restraints have life-threatening risks. Death can occur from strangulation. If caught in the restraint, it can become so tight that the person's chest cannot expand to inhale air. The person quickly suffocates and dies. Correct application is critical. You are advised to only assist the nurse in applying them. The nurse should assume full responsibility for applying a vest or jacket restraint.

See *Focus on Communication: Applying Restraints,* p. 134.
See *Focus on Older Persons: Applying Restraints,* p. 134.
See *Delegation Guidelines: Applying Restraints,* p. 134.
See *Promoting Safety and Comfort: Applying Restraints,* p. 135.
See procedure: *Applying Restraints,* p. 135.

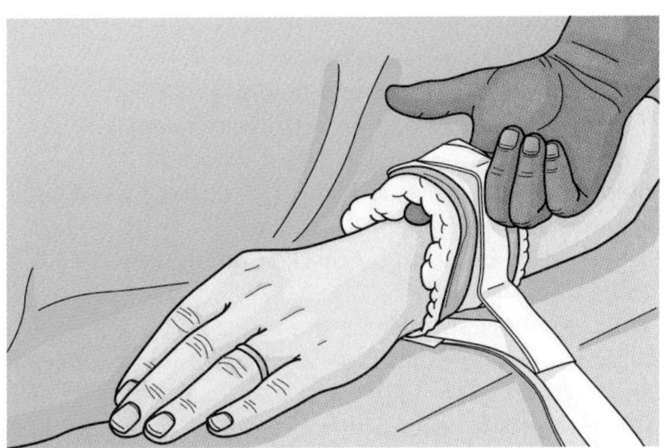

FIGURE 11-15 Wrist restraint. The soft part is toward the skin. Note that 1 finger fits between the restraint and the wrist.

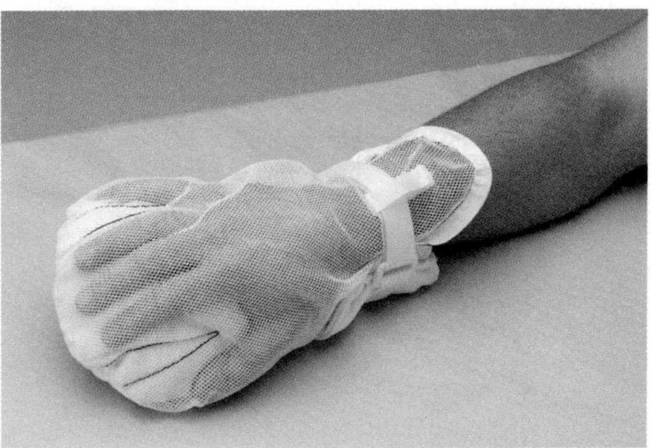

FIGURE 11-16 Mitt restraint.

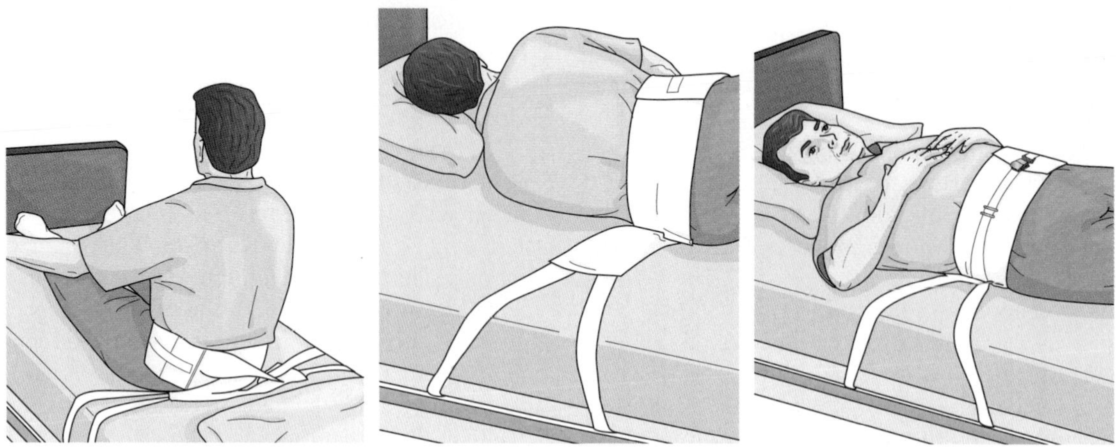

FIGURE 11-17 Belt restraint. (NOTE: The bed rails are raised after the restraint is applied.)

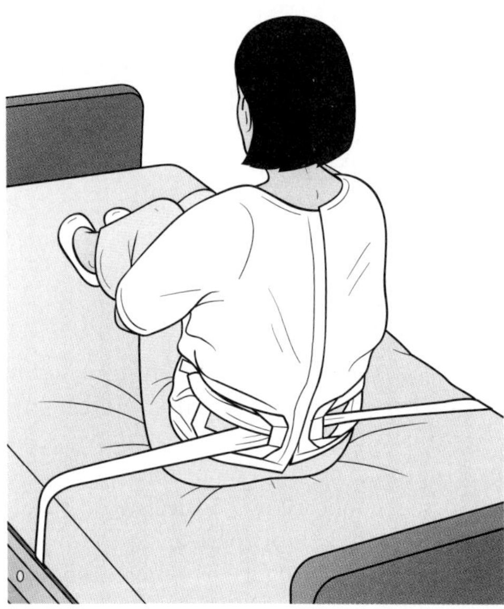

FIGURE 11-18 Jacket restraint. (NOTE: The bed rails are raised after the restraint is applied.)

FOCUS ON COMMUNICATION

Applying Restraints

If you do not know how to apply a certain restraint, do not do so. Ask the nurse to show you the correct way. You can say: "I've never applied a restraint like this before. Would you please show me how and then watch me apply it?" Then thank the nurse for helping you.

When applying a restraint, explain to the person what you are going to do. Then tell the person what you are doing step-by-step. Always check for safety and comfort. You can ask: "How does the restraint feel? Is it too tight? Is it too loose?"

Make sure the person can communicate with you after you leave the room. Place the call light in reach. Make sure the person can use it with the restraint on. Remind the person to call if uncomfortable or if anything is needed.

FOCUS ON OLDER PERSONS

Applying Restraints

Restraints may increase confusion and agitation in persons with dementia. They do not understand what you are doing. They may resist your efforts to apply a restraint. They may actively try to get free from the restraint. Serious injury and death are risks.

Never use force to apply a restraint. If a person is confused or agitated, ask a co-worker to help apply the restraint. Report problems to the nurse at once.

DELEGATION GUIDELINES

Applying Restraints

Before applying a restraint, you need this information from the nurse and the care plan.

- Why the doctor ordered the restraint
- What type and size to use
- Where to apply the restraint
- How to safely apply the restraint (Have the nurse show you how to apply it. Then show correct application back to the nurse.)
- How to correctly position the person
- What bony areas to pad and how to pad them
- If bed rail covers or gap protectors are needed
- If bed rails are up or down
- How low to keep the bed
- What special equipment is needed
- If the person needs to be checked more often than every 15 minutes
- When to apply and release the restraint
- What observations to report and record (see "Reporting and Recording," p. 133)
- When to report observations
- What patient or resident concerns to report at once

PROMOTING SAFETY AND COMFORT

Applying Restraints

Safety

Restraints can cause serious harm, even death. Always follow the manufacturer's instructions. The instructions for one restraint may not apply to another. Also, the manufacturer may have instructions for applying restraints on persons who are agitated.

Never use force. Ask a co-worker to help if a person is confused and agitated. Report problems to the nurse at once.

Check the person at least every 15 minutes or more often as instructed by the nurse and the care plan. Make sure the call light is within reach. Ask the person to use the call light at the first sign of problems or discomfort.

Never use a restraint as a seat belt in a car or other vehicle.

Mitt Restraints

Mitt restraints prevent finger use. Often they are not secured to the bed or chair. Therefore, the person can raise the mitt to his or her mouth. Observe the person closely to make sure that he or she does not:

- Use the teeth to remove or damage the device.
- Ingest any mitt material.

Persons with mitt restraints may be able to walk about. Falls are a risk. Practice safety measures to prevent falls (Chapter 10).

Safety—cont'd

Belt, Vest, and Jacket Restraints

If a belt, vest, or jacket restraint is ordered, monitor the person to make sure that he or she cannot:

- Slide forward or down in the chair or bed and become suspended or entrapped.
- Fall off the chair or mattress and become suspended or entrapped.

Comfort

The person's comfort is always important when restraints are used. Restraints limit movement. This affects position changes and reaching needed items. Position the person in good alignment before applying a restraint (Chapter 13). Also make sure the person can reach needed items—call light, water, tissues, phone, bed controls, and so on.

Applying Restraints

QUALITY OF LIFE

- Knock before entering the person's room.
- Address the person by name.
- Introduce yourself by name and title.
- Explain the procedure before starting and during the procedure.
- Protect the person's rights during the procedure.
- Handle the person gently during the procedure.

PRE-PROCEDURE

1 Follow *Delegation Guidelines: Applying Restraints.* See *Promoting Safety and Comfort: Applying Restraints.*

2 Collect the following as instructed by the nurse.
- Correct type and size of restraint
- Padding for skin and bony areas
- Bed rail pads or gap protectors (if needed)

3 Practice hand hygiene.

4 Identify the person. Check the ID (identification) bracelet against the assignment sheet. Also call the person by name.

5 Provide for privacy.

PROCEDURE

6 Position the person for comfort and good alignment.

7 Put the bed rail pads or gap protectors (if needed) on the bed if the person is in bed. Follow the manufacturer's instructions.

8 Pad bony areas. Follow the nurse's instructions and the care plan.

9 Read the manufacturer's instructions. Note the front and back of the restraint.

10 *For wrist restraints:*
- a Apply the restraint following the manufacturer's instructions. Place the soft or foam part toward the skin.
- b Secure the restraint so it is snug but not tight. Make sure you can slide 1 finger under the restraint (see Fig. 11-15). Follow the manufacturer's instructions. Adjust the straps if the restraint is too loose or too tight. Check for snugness again.
- c Secure the straps to the movable part of the bed frame out of the person's reach. Use the buckle or a quick-release tie.
- d Repeat steps 10, a–c for the other wrist.

Continued

Applying Restraints—cont'd

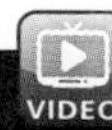

PROCEDURE—cont'd

11 *For mitt restraints:*
   a Clean and dry the person's hands.
   b Insert the person's hand into the restraint with the palm down. Follow the manufacturer's instructions.
   c Secure the restraint to the bed if directed to do so. Secure the straps to the movable part of the bed frame out of the person's reach. Use the buckle or a quick-release tie.
   d Check for snugness. Slide 1 finger between the restraint and the wrist. Follow the manufacturer's instructions. Adjust the straps if the restraint is too loose or too tight. Check for snugness again.
   e Repeat steps 11, b–d for the other hand.

12 *For a belt restraint:*
   a Assist the person to a sitting position.
   b Apply the restraint. Follow the manufacturer's instructions.
   c Remove wrinkles or creases from the front and back of the restraint.
   d Bring the ties through the slots in the belt.
   e Position the straps at a 45-degree angle between the wheelchair seat and sides (see Fig. 11-5). If in bed, help the person lie down.
   f Make sure the person is comfortable and in good alignment.
   g Secure the straps to the movable part of the bed frame. Use the buckle or a quick-release tie. The buckle or tie is out of the person's reach. For a wheelchair, criss-cross and secure the straps as in Figure 11-10.
   h Check for snugness. Slide an open hand between the restraint and the person. Adjust the restraint if it is too loose or too tight. Check for snugness again.

13 *For a vest restraint:*
   a Assist the person to a sitting position. If in a wheelchair:
      1 Position him or her as far back in the wheelchair as possible.
      2 Make sure the buttocks are against the chair back.
   b Apply the restraint. Follow the manufacturer's instructions. The "V" part of the vest crosses in front.
   c Bring the straps through the slots.
   d Remove wrinkles in the front and back.
   e Position the straps at a 45-degree angle between the wheelchair seat and sides. If in bed, help the person lie down.
   f Make sure the person is comfortable and in good alignment.
   g Secure the straps to the movable part of the bed frame at waist level. Use the buckle or a quick-release tie. The buckle or tie is out of the person's reach. For a wheelchair, criss-cross and secure the straps as in Figure 11-10.
   h Check for snugness. Slide an open hand between the restraint and the person. Adjust the restraint if it is too loose or too tight. Check for snugness again.

14 *For a jacket restraint:*
   a Assist the person to a sitting position. If in a wheelchair:
      1 Position him or her as far back in the wheelchair as possible.
      2 Make sure the buttocks are against the chair back.
   b Apply the restraint. Follow the manufacturer's instructions. The jacket opening goes in the back.
   c Close the back with the zipper, ties, or hook and loop closures.
   d Make sure the side seams are under the arms. Remove wrinkles in the front and back.
   e Position the straps at a 45-degree angle between the wheelchair seat and sides. If in bed, help the person lie down.
   f Make sure the person is comfortable and in good alignment.
   g Secure the straps to the movable part of the bed frame at waist level. Use the buckle or quick-release tie. The buckle or tie is out of the person's reach. For a wheelchair, criss-cross and secure the straps as in Figure 11-10.
   h Check for snugness. Slide an open hand between the restraint and the person. Adjust the restraint if it is too loose or too tight. Check for snugness again.

POST-PROCEDURE

15 Position the person as the nurse directs.
16 Provide for comfort. (See the inside of the front cover.)
17 Place the call light within the person's reach.
18 Raise or lower bed rails. Follow the care plan and the manufacturer's instructions for the restraint.
19 Unscreen the person.
20 Complete a safety check of the room. (See the inside of the front cover.)
21 Practice hand hygiene.
22 Check the person and the restraint at least every 15 minutes. Report and record your observations.
   a For wrist or mitt restraints: check the pulse, color, and temperature of the restrained parts.
   b For a vest, jacket, or belt restraint: check the person's breathing. *Call for the nurse at once if the person is not breathing or is having problems breathing.* Make sure the restraint is properly positioned in the front and back.
23 Do the following at least every 2 hours for at least 10 minutes.
   a Remove or release the restraint.
   b Measure vital signs.
   c Re-position the person.
   d Meet food, fluid, hygiene, and elimination needs.
   e Give skin care.
   f Perform range-of-motion exercises or help the person walk. Follow the care plan.
   g Provide for physical and emotional comfort. (See the inside of the front cover.)
   h Re-apply the restraint.
24 Complete a safety check of the room. (See the inside of the front cover.)
25 Practice hand hygiene.
26 Report and record your observations and the care given.

FOCUS ON PRIDE

The Person, Family, and Yourself

Personal and Professional Responsibility

Restraints have many risks. See Box 11-2. Therefore restraint use brings many responsibilities. You must:

- Monitor the person for safety.
- Apply the restraint properly.
- Promote comfort.
- Supervise the person closely.
- Meet basic needs.
- Report any concerns to the nurse.

If you do not know how to apply a restraint, do not do so. Ask the nurse to show you. To use restraints safely and responsibly, follow the guidelines in Box 11-3.

Rights and Respect

Every person has the right to freedom from restraint. Restraints are used only as a last resort to protect the person or others from harm. Other methods must be tried before restraints are used. You may be asked to assist with an alternative method (see Box 11-1). Make a genuine effort. Be honest. Do not tell the nurse you tried if you really did not. Do your best to allow the person the right to freedom from restraint.

Independence and Social Interaction

All restraints limit movement. Independence is restricted. To promote independence when restraints are used:

- Place the call light within reach at all times. Make sure the person can use it. Tell the person to signal for you if anything is needed. Answer the call light and meet the person's needs promptly.
- Keep needed items within reach. This is most important with restraints that allow hand and arm use. Belt, vest, and jacket restraints are examples.
- Check the person at least every 15 minutes.
- Remove or release the restraint at least every 2 hours.
- Meet food, fluid, hygiene, and elimination needs.
- Assist the person with walks or range-of-motion exercises.
- Allow choice. For example, let the person choose where to walk or what to eat and drink.
- Let the person do as much for himself or herself as safely possible.

Personal choice and freedom of movement promote independence, dignity, and self-esteem. Provide care that gives restrained persons the independence they deserve.

Delegation and Teamwork

Care conferences are held to meet the person's safety needs. The health team reviews and updates the person's care plan. Every attempt is made to protect the person without using restraints.

You are an important member of the team. Your input has value. Share your observations and ideas. For example, Mrs. Garner does not try to get out of her chair when she looks through her photo albums or reads a book. You share this with the team. They include diversion activities in her care plan.

Ethics and Laws

Imagine the following.

- Your nose itches. But your hands are restrained. You cannot scratch your nose.
- You need to use the bathroom. Your arms and legs are restrained. You cannot get up. You cannot reach your call light. You soil yourself with urine or a bowel movement.
- Your phone is ringing. You cannot answer it.
- You are wearing mitt restraints. You cannot reach your eyeglasses or put them on. You cannot see who is coming into and going out of your room. And you cannot speak because of a stroke.
- You are uncomfortable. You have a vest restraint. You cannot move or turn in bed.
- You are thirsty. Your hands and arms are restrained. You cannot reach the water mug.
- You hear the fire alarm. You have on a restraint. You cannot get up to move to a safe place. You must wait until someone rescues you.

What would you do? Would you calmly lie or sit there? Would you try to get free from the restraint? Would you yell for help? Would the staff think that you are uncomfortable? Or would they think that you are agitated and uncooperative? Would you feel angry, embarrassed, or humiliated?

Ethics deals with how others are treated. Restraints lessen the person's dignity and freedom. A person should not be treated in this way. That is why restraints are a last resort. Put yourself in the person's situation. Then you can better understand how the person feels. Treat the person like you would want to be treated—with kindness, caring, respect, and dignity.

REVIEW QUESTIONS

Circle* T *if the statement is TRUE or* F *if it is FALSE.

1 **T F** Restraint alternatives fail to protect a person. You can apply a restraint.

2 **T F** A restraint restricts a person's freedom of movement.

3 **T F** Some drugs are restraints.

4 **T F** Restraints can be used for staff convenience.

5 **T F** A device is a restraint only if it is attached to the person's body.

6 **T F** Bed rails are restraints if the person cannot lower them.

7 **T F** Restraints are used only for a person's specific medical symptom.

8 **T F** Unnecessary restraint is false imprisonment.

9 **T F** You can apply restraints when you think they are needed.

10 **T F** You can use a vest restraint to position a person on the toilet.

11 **T F** Restraints are removed or released at least every 2 hours.

12 **T F** Restraints are tied to bed rails.

13 **T F** Wrist restraints are used to prevent falls.

14 **T F** A vest restraint crosses in front.

15 **T F** Bed rails are left down when a vest restraint is used.

Circle the BEST answer.

16 Which is *not* a restraint alternative?
- **a** Positioning the person's chair close to the wall
- **b** Answering the call light promptly
- **c** Taking the person outside in nice weather
- **d** Padding walls and corners of furniture

17 Physical restraints
- **a** Can be removed easily by the person
- **b** Are not allowed by OBRA
- **c** Require a doctor's order
- **d** Are safer than chemical restraints

18 The following can occur because of restraints. Which is the *most* serious?
- **a** Fractures
- **b** Strangulation
- **c** Pressure ulcers
- **d** Urinary tract infections

19 A belt restraint is applied to a person in bed. Where should you secure the straps?
- **a** To the bed rails
- **b** To the head-board
- **c** To the movable part of the bed frame
- **d** To the foot-board

20 A person has a restraint. You should check the person and the position of the restraint at least every
- **a** 15 minutes
- **b** 30 minutes
- **c** Hour
- **d** 2 hours

21 A person has mitt restraints. Which will you report to the nurse at once?
- **a** The hands are clean, warm, and dry.
- **b** The person has numbness in the hands.
- **c** You removed the restraints for 10 minutes.
- **d** You felt a pulse in both arms.

22 The doctor ordered mitt restraints for a person. You need the following information from the nurse *except*
- **a** What size to use
- **b** What other equipment is needed
- **c** What drugs the person is taking
- **d** When to apply and release the restraints

23 A person has a vest restraint. It is not too tight or too loose if you can slide
- **a** A fist between the vest and the person
- **b** 1 finger between the vest and the person
- **c** An open hand between the vest and the person
- **d** 2 fingers between the vest and the person

24 The correct way to apply any restraint is to follow the
- **a** Nurse's directions
- **b** Doctor's orders
- **c** Care plan
- **d** Manufacturer's instructions

Answers to these questions are on p. 504.

FOCUS ON PRACTICE

Problem Solving

Mrs. Lopez has confusion and weakness in her legs. She uses a wheelchair and often tries to get up without help. What are some alternatives to restraints that may be tried? If a restraint is needed, how will you provide for her basic needs?

CHAPTER 12

Preventing Infection

OBJECTIVES

- Define the key terms and key abbreviations listed in this chapter.
- Identify what microbes need to live and grow.
- List the signs and symptoms of infection.
- Explain the chain of infection.
- Describe healthcare-associated infections and the persons at risk.
- Describe the principles of medical asepsis.
- Explain how to care for equipment and supplies.
- Describe disinfection and sterilization methods.
- Describe Standard Precautions and Transmission-Based Precautions.
- Explain the Bloodborne Pathogen Standard.
- Perform the procedures described in this chapter.
- Explain how to promote PRIDE in the person, the family, and yourself.

KEY TERMS

antibiotic A drug that kills certain pathogens
asepsis Being free of disease-producing microbes
biohazardous waste Items contaminated with blood, body fluids, secretions, or excretions; *bio* means *life,* and *hazardous* means *dangerous* or *harmful*
carrier A human or animal that is a reservoir for microbes but does not develop the infection
clean technique See "medical asepsis"
communicable disease A disease caused by pathogens that spread easily; a contagious disease
contagious disease See "communicable disease"
contamination The process of becoming unclean
disinfection The process of destroying pathogens
healthcare-associated infection (HAI) An infection that develops in a person cared for in any setting where health care is given; the infection is related to receiving health care
infection A disease state resulting from the invasion and growth of microbes in the body
infection control Practices and procedures that prevent the spread of infection
medical asepsis Practices used to remove or destroy pathogens and to prevent their spread from 1 person or place to another person or place; clean technique
microbe See "microorganism"
microorganism A small *(micro)* living thing *(organism)* seen only with a microscope; microbe
non-pathogen A microbe that does not usually cause an infection
pathogen A microbe that is harmful and can cause an infection
sterile The absence of *all* microbes—pathogens and non-pathogens
sterilization The process of destroying *all* microbes

KEY ABBREVIATIONS

AIIR	Airborne infection isolation room
CDC	Centers for Disease Control and Prevention
HAI	Healthcare-associated infection
HBV	Hepatitis B virus
HIV	Human immunodeficiency virus
MDRO	Multidrug-resistant organism
MRSA	Methicillin-resistant *Staphylococcus aureus*
OPIM	Other potentially infectious materials
OSHA	Occupational Safety and Health Administration
PPE	Personal protective equipment
SARS	Severe acute respiratory syndrome
TB	Tuberculosis
VRE	Vancomycin-resistant *Enterococci*

An ***infection*** *is a disease state resulting from the invasion and growth of microbes in the body.* Infection is a major safety and health hazard. Minor infections cause short illnesses. A serious infection can cause death. Older and disabled persons are at risk. The health team follows certain *practices and procedures to prevent the spread of infection **(infection control)**.* The goal is to protect patients, residents, visitors, and staff from infection.

MICROORGANISMS

A ***microorganism (microbe)*** *is a small (micro) living thing (organism). It is seen only with a microscope.* Microbes are everywhere—mouth, nose, respiratory tract, stomach, and intestines. They are on the skin and in the air, soil, water, and food. They are on animals, clothing, and furniture.

*Microbes that are harmful and can cause infections are called **pathogens**. **Non-pathogens** are microbes that do not usually cause an infection.*

Requirements of Microbes

Microbes need a *reservoir (host)*. The reservoir is the place where the microbe lives and grows. People, plants, animals, the soil, food, and water are examples. Microbes need *water* and *nourishment* from the reservoir. Most need *oxygen* to live. A *warm* and *dark* environment is needed. Most grow best at body temperature. They are destroyed by heat and light.

Multidrug-Resistant Organisms

Multidrug-resistant organisms (MDROs) are microbes that can resist the effects of antibiotics. ***Antibiotics*** *are drugs that kill certain pathogens.* Some pathogens can change their structures. This makes them harder to kill. They can live in the presence of antibiotics. Therefore the infections they cause are hard to treat.

MDROs are caused by prescribing antibiotics when not needed (over-prescribing). Not taking antibiotics for the length of time prescribed is another cause. Common MDROs are:

- *Methicillin-resistant* Staphylococcus aureus *(MRSA)*. *Staphylococcus aureus* ("staph") is a bacterium normally found in the nose and on the skin. MRSA is resistant to antibiotics often used for "staph" infections. MRSA can cause pneumonia and serious wound and bloodstream infections.
- *Vancomycin-resistant* Enterococci *(VRE)*. *Enterococcus* is a bacterium normally found in the intestines and in feces. It can be transmitted to others by contaminated hands, toilet seats, care equipment, and other items that the hands touch. When not in their natural site (the intestines), enterococci can cause urinary tract, wound, pelvic, and other infections. Enterococci resistant to the antibiotic vancomycin are called vancomycin-resistant *Enterococci* (VRE).

INFECTION

A *local infection* is in a body part. A *systemic infection* involves the whole body. (*Systemic* means *entire.*) The person has some or all of the signs and symptoms listed in Box 12-1.

See *Focus on Older Persons: Infection.*

See *Focus on Surveys: Infection.*

BOX 12-1 Signs and Symptoms of Infection

- Fever (elevated body temperature)
- Chills
- Pulse rate: increased
- Respiratory rate: increased
- Pain or tenderness
- Fatigue and loss of energy
- Appetite: loss of *(anorexia)*
- Nausea
- Vomiting
- Diarrhea
- Rash
- Sores on mucous membranes
- Redness and swelling of a body part
- Discharge or drainage from the infected area
- Heat or warmth in a body part
- Limited use of a body part
- Headache
- Muscle aches
- Joint pain
- Confusion

FOCUS ON OLDER PERSONS

Infection

The immune system protects the body from disease and infection (Chapter 7). Changes occur in this system with aging. Therefore older persons are at risk for infection.

An older person may not show the signs and symptoms of infection listed in Box 12-1. The person may have only a slight fever or no fever at all. Redness and swelling may be slight. The person may not complain of pain. Confusion and delirium may occur (Chapter 30).

An infection can become life-threatening before the older person has obvious signs and symptoms. Report minor changes in the person's behavior or condition at once.

Healing takes longer in older persons. Therefore an infection can prolong the rehabilitation process. Independence and quality of life are affected.

FOCUS ON SURVEYS

Infection

Infection control practices are a major focus of surveys. You may be asked:

- What do you do when you observe signs and symptoms of an infection?
- Who do you tell when you observe signs and symptoms of an infection?

The Chain of Infection

The chain of infection (Fig. 12-1) begins with a *source*—a pathogen. It must have a *reservoir* where it can grow and multiply. Humans, animals, and objects are reservoirs. A ***carrier*** *is a human or animal that is a reservoir for microbes but does not develop the infection.* Carriers can pass pathogens to others. To leave the reservoir, the pathogen needs a *portal of exit.* Exits are the respiratory, gastro-intestinal (GI), urinary, and reproductive tracts; breaks in the skin; and blood.

After leaving the reservoir, the pathogen must be *transmitted* to another host (Fig. 12-2). The pathogen enters the body through a *portal of entry*. Portals of entry and exit are the same. A *susceptible host* is needed for the microbe to grow and multiply.

Susceptible Hosts. Susceptible hosts are at risk for infection. They include persons who:

- Are very young or who are older.
- Are ill.
- Were exposed to the pathogen.
- Do not follow practices to prevent infection.
- Are burn patients. When burns destroy the skin, the wound is a portal of entry for microbes.
- Are transplant patients. A *transplant* involves transferring an organ or tissue from 1 person to another person or from 1 body part to another body part. The body's normal immune response is to attack (reject) the new organ or tissue. Therefore, drugs are given to prevent rejection. Such drugs suppress (prevent) the immune system from producing the antibodies needed to fight infection.
- Are chemotherapy patients (Chapter 28). Some types of chemotherapy affect the bone marrow's ability to produce white blood cells (WBCs). WBCs are needed to fight infection.

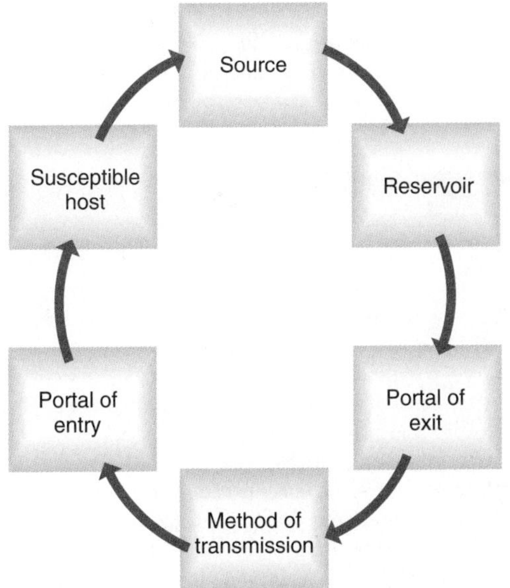

FIGURE 12-1 The chain of infection.

The human body can protect itself from infections. The ability to resist infection relates to age, nutrition, stress, fatigue, and health. Drugs, disease, and injury also are factors.

Healthcare-Associated Infection

A ***healthcare-associated infection (HAI)*** *is an infection that develops in a person cared for in any setting where health care is given. The infection is related to receiving health care.* HAIs also are called nosocomial infections. (*Nosocomial* comes from the Greek word for *hospital.*)

HAIs are caused by microbes normally found in the body. Or they are caused by microbes transmitted to the person from other sources. For example, *Escherichia coli* is normally in the colon and feces. *E. coli* can enter the urinary system from poor wiping after bowel movements. With poor hand washing, the hands can spread *E. coli* to any body part, thing, or person the hands touch.

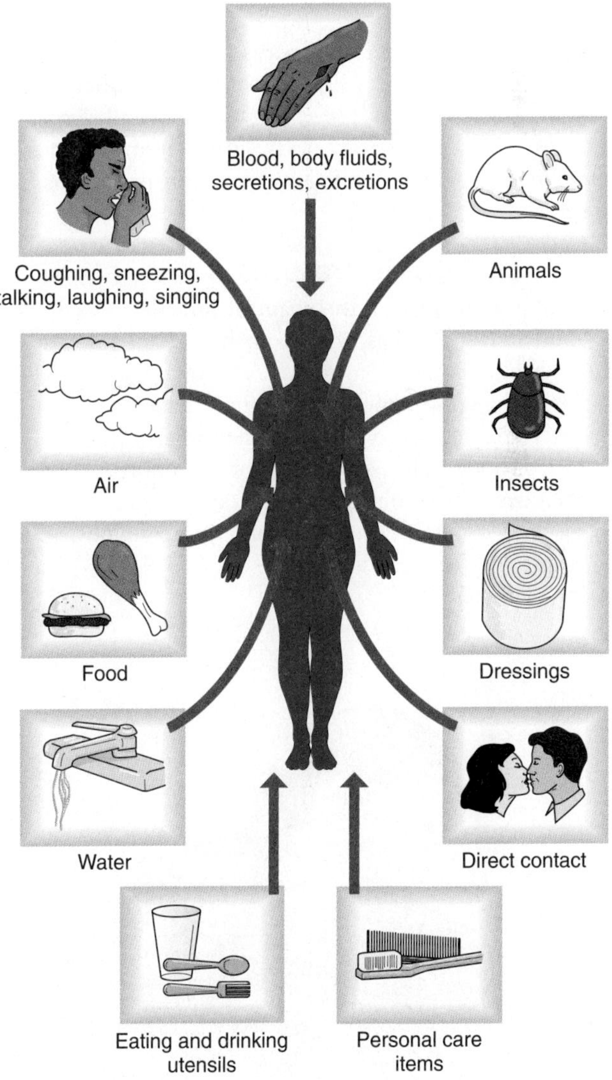

FIGURE 12-2 Methods of transmitting microbes.

Microbes can enter the body through care equipment and supplies. Such items must be free of microbes. Staff can transfer microbes from 1 person to another and from themselves to others. Common sites for HAIs are:

- The urinary system
- The respiratory system
- Wounds
- The bloodstream

The health team must prevent infection by following:

- Medical asepsis. This includes hand hygiene.
- Standard Precautions, p. 148.
- Transmission-Based Precautions, p. 148.
- The Bloodborne Pathogen Standard, p. 157.

MEDICAL ASEPSIS

***Asepsis** is being free of disease-producing microbes.* Microbes are everywhere. Measures are needed to achieve asepsis. ***Medical asepsis (clean technique)** is the practices used to:*

- *Remove or destroy pathogens.* The number of pathogens is reduced.
- *Prevent pathogens from spreading from 1 person or place to another person or place.*

***Contamination** is the process of becoming unclean.* In medical asepsis, an item or area is *clean* when it is free of pathogens. The item or area is *contaminated* when pathogens are present. ***Sterile** means the absence of* all *microbes—pathogens and non-pathogens.* A *sterile* item or area is *contaminated* when pathogens or non-pathogens are present.

Common Aseptic Practices

Aseptic practices break the chain of infection. To prevent the spread of microbes, wash your hands:

- After elimination.
- After changing tampons or sanitary pads.
- After contact with your own or another person's blood, body fluids, secretions, or excretions. This includes saliva, vomitus, urine, feces, vaginal discharge, mucus, semen, wound drainage, pus, and respiratory secretions.
- After coughing, sneezing, or blowing your nose.
- Before and after handling, preparing, or eating food.
- After smoking.

Also do the following.

- Provide all persons with their own linens and personal care items.
- Cover your nose and mouth when coughing, sneezing, or blowing your nose. If without tissues, cough or sneeze into your upper arm (Fig. 12-3). Do not cough or sneeze into your hands.
- Bathe, wash hair, and brush your teeth regularly.
- Wash fruits and raw vegetables before eating or serving them.
- Wash cooking and eating utensils with soap and water after use.

See *Focus on Older Persons: Common Aseptic Practices.*

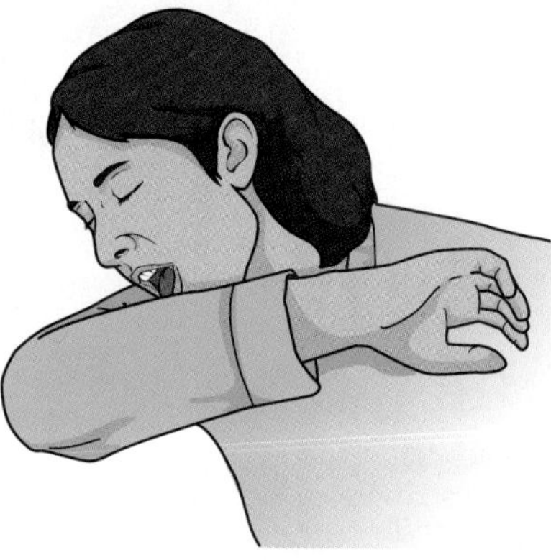

FIGURE 12-3 Sneezing into the upper arm.

Hand Hygiene

Hand hygiene is the easiest and most important way to prevent the spread of infection. You use your hands for almost everything. They are easily contaminated. They can spread microbes to other persons or items. *Practice hand hygiene before and after giving care.* See Box 12-2 for the rules of hand hygiene.

See *Focus on Surveys: Hand Hygiene.*

See *Promoting Safety and Comfort: Hand Hygiene.*

See procedure: *Hand Washing,* p. 145.

See procedure: *Using an Alcohol-Based Hand Rub,* p. 145.

Text continued on p. 146

FOCUS ON OLDER PERSONS

Common Aseptic Practices

Persons with dementia do not understand aseptic practices. The staff must protect them from infection. Assist them with hand washing:

- After elimination
- After coughing, sneezing, or blowing the nose
- Before or after they eat or handle food
- Any time their hands are soiled

Check and clean their hands and fingernails often. They may not or cannot tell you when soiling occurs.

FOCUS ON SURVEYS

Hand Hygiene

Hand hygiene is a focus of surveys. A surveyor may:

- Observe you washing your hands or using an alcohol-based hand rub according to agency policy.
- Observe if you practice hand hygiene:
  - After each direct patient or resident contact
  - Before and after all procedures
  - After removing gloves
  - When entering or leaving the room of a person on Transmission-Based Precautions (p. 148)
- Ask you questions about:
  - When you should wash your hands
  - When you can use an alcohol-based hand rub

BOX 12-2 Rules of Hand Hygiene

- Wash your hands (with soap and water) at these times.
  - When they are visibly dirty or soiled with blood, body fluids, secretions, or excretions
  - Before eating and after using a restroom
  - If exposure to the anthrax spore is suspected or proven
  - If an alcohol-based hand rub is not available
- Use an alcohol-based hand rub to practice hand hygiene if your hands are not visibly soiled. Follow this rule.
  - Before direct contact with a person.
  - After contact with the person's intact skin. After taking a pulse or blood pressure are examples.
  - After contact with body fluids or excretions, mucous membranes, non-intact skin, and wound dressings if hands are not visibly soiled.
  - When moving from a contaminated body site to a clean body site.
  - After contact with items in the person's care setting.
  - After removing gloves.
- Follow these rules for washing your hands with soap and water. See procedure: *Hand Washing,* p. 145.
  - Wash your hands under warm running water. Do not use hot water.
  - Stand away from the sink. Do not let your hands, body, or uniform touch the sink. The sink is contaminated. See Figure 12-4.
  - Do not touch the inside of the sink at any time.
  - Keep your hands and forearms lower than your elbows. Your hands are dirtier than your elbows and forearms. If you hold your hands and forearms up, dirty water runs from your hands to your elbows. Those areas become contaminated.
  - Rub your palms together (Fig. 12-5, p. 144) and interlace your fingers (Fig. 12-6, p. 144) to work up a good lather. The rubbing action helps remove microbes and dirt.
  - Pay attention to areas often missed during hand washing—thumbs, knuckles, sides of the hands, little fingers, and under the nails.
  - Clean fingernails by rubbing the fingertips against your palms (Fig. 12-7, p. 144).
  - Use a nail file or orangewood stick to clean under fingernails (Fig. 12-8, p. 144). Microbes grow easily under the fingernails.
  - Wash your hands for at least 15 to 20 seconds. Wash longer if they are dirty or soiled with blood, body fluids, secretions, or excretions. Use your judgment and follow agency policy.
  - Use clean, dry paper towels to dry your hands.
  - Dry your hands starting at the fingertips. Work up to your forearms. You will dry the cleanest area first.
  - Use a clean, dry paper towel for each faucet to turn the water off (Fig. 12-9, p. 144). Faucets are contaminated. The paper towels prevent you from contaminating your clean hands.
- Follow these rules when decontaminating your hands with an alcohol-based hand rub. See procedure: *Using an Alcohol-Based Hand Rub,* p. 145.
  - Apply the product to the palm of 1 hand. Follow the manufacturer's instructions for the amount to use.
  - Rub your hands together.
  - Cover all surfaces of your hands and fingers.
  - Continue rubbing your hands together until your hands are dry.
- Apply hand lotion or cream after hand hygiene. This prevents the skin from chapping and drying. Skin breaks can occur in chapped and dry skin. Skin breaks are portals of entry for microbes.

Modified from Centers for Disease Control and Prevention: Guidelines for hand hygiene in health-care settings, Morbidity and Mortality Weekly Report *51 (RR-16), 2002.*

PROMOTING SAFETY AND COMFORT

Hand Hygiene

Safety

Your hands can pick up microbes from a person, place, or thing. Your hands transfer them to other people, places, or things. That is why hand hygiene is so very important. Always practice hand hygiene before and after giving care.

Comfort

You will practice hand hygiene often during your shift. Hand lotions and hand creams help prevent chapping and dry skin. Apply hand lotion or cream as needed. Use an agency-approved lotion or cream.

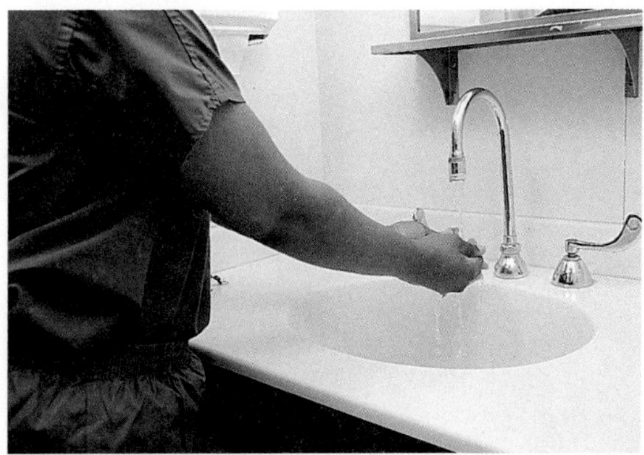

FIGURE 12-4 The uniform does not touch the sink. Soap and water are within reach. Hands are lower than the elbows. Hands do not touch the inside of the sink.

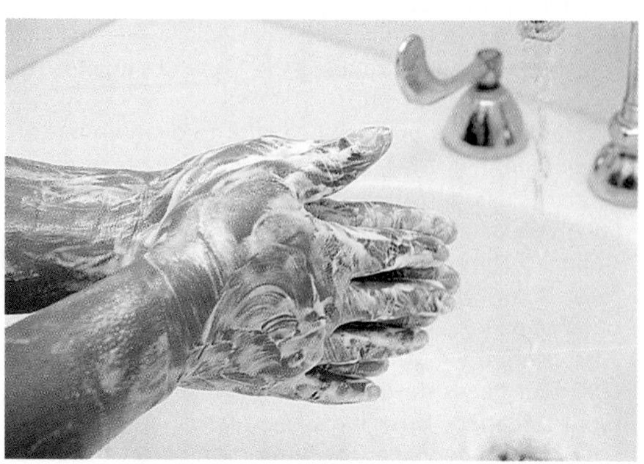

FIGURE 12-5 The palms are rubbed together to work up a good lather.

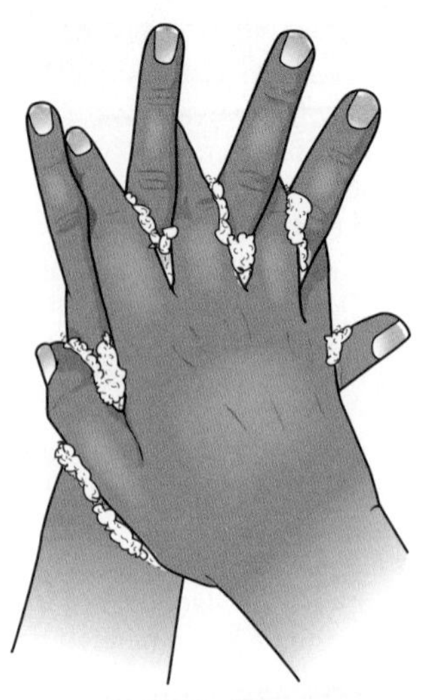

FIGURE 12-6 The fingers are interlaced to clean between the fingers.

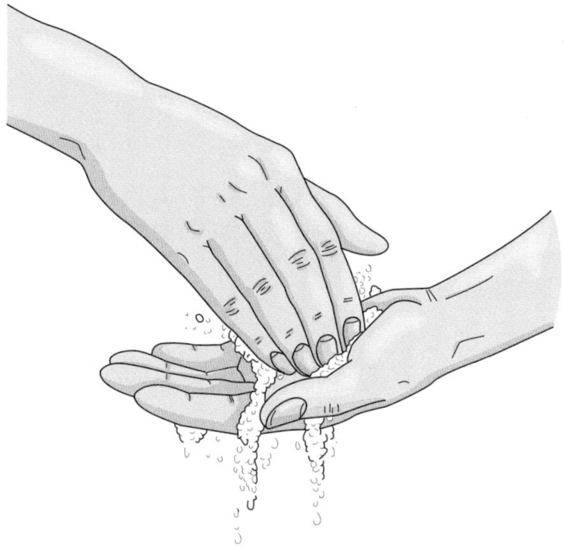

FIGURE 12-7 The fingertips are rubbed against the palms to clean under the fingernails.

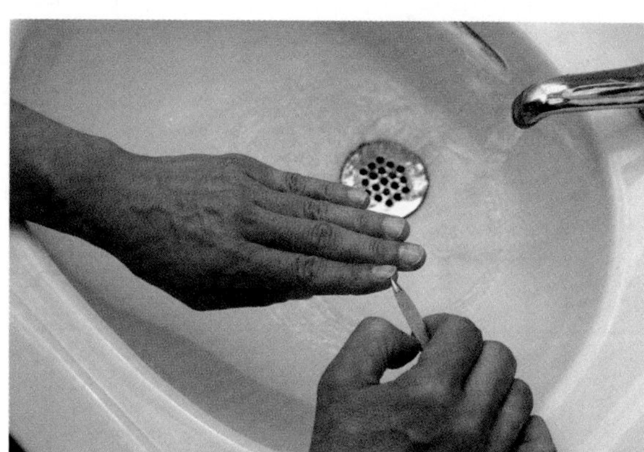

FIGURE 12-8 A nail file is used to clean under the fingernails.

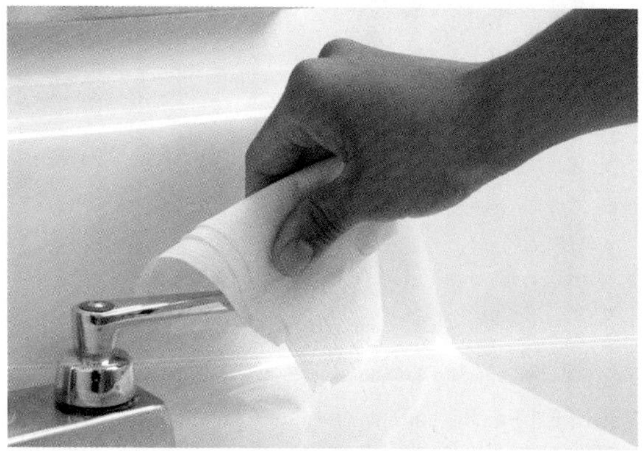

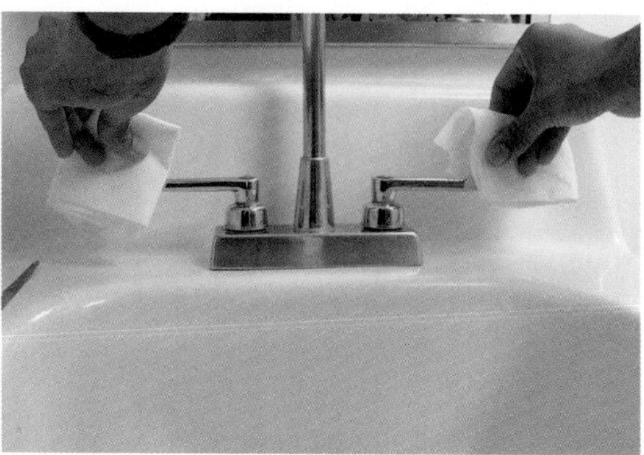

FIGURE 12-9 A paper towel is used to turn off each faucet.

Hand Washing

PROCEDURE

1 See *Promoting Safety and Comfort: Hand Hygiene,* p. 143.
2 Make sure you have soap, paper towels, an orangewood stick or nail file, and a wastebasket. Collect missing items.
3 Push your watch up your arm 4 to 5 inches. If uniform sleeves are long, push them up too.
4 Stand away from the sink so your clothes do not touch the sink. Stand so the soap and faucet are easy to reach (see Fig. 12-4). Do not touch the inside of the sink at any time.
5 Turn on and adjust the water until it feels warm.
6 Wet your wrists and hands. Keep your hands lower than your elbows. Be sure to wet the area 3 to 4 inches above your wrists.
7 Apply about 1 teaspoon of soap to your hands.
8 Rub your palms together and interlace your fingers to work up a good lather (see Fig. 12-5). Lather your wrists, hands, and fingers. Keep your hands lower than your elbows. This step should last at least 15 to 20 seconds.
9 Wash each hand and wrist thoroughly. Clean the back of your fingers and between your fingers (see Fig. 12-6).
10 Clean the fingernails. Rub your fingertips against your palms (see Fig. 12-7).
11 Clean under the fingernails with a nail file or orangewood stick (see Fig. 12-8). Do this for the first hand washing of the day and when your hands are highly soiled.
12 Rinse your wrists, hands, and fingers well. Water flows from above the wrists to your fingertips.
13 Repeat steps 7 through 12, if needed.
14 Dry your wrists and hands with clean, dry paper towels. Pat dry starting at your fingertips.
15 Discard the paper towels into the wastebasket.
16 Turn off faucets with clean, dry paper towels. This prevents contamination of your hands (see Fig. 12-9). Use a clean paper towel for each faucet. Or use knee or foot controls to turn off the faucet.
17 Discard the paper towels into the wastebasket.

Using an Alcohol-Based Hand Rub

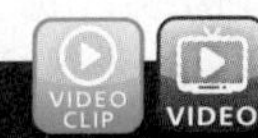

PROCEDURE

1 See *Promoting Safety and Comfort: Hand Hygiene,* p. 143.
2 Apply a palmful of an alcohol-based hand rub into a cupped hand (Fig. 12-10, *A*).
3 Rub your palms together (Fig. 12-10, *B*).
4 Rub the palm of 1 hand over the back of the other (Fig. 12-10, *C*). Do the same for the other hand.
5 Rub your palms together with your fingers interlaced (Fig. 12-10, *D*).
6 Interlock your fingers as in Figure 12-10, *E*. Rub your fingers back and forth.
7 Rub the thumb of 1 hand in the palm of the other (Fig. 12-10, *F*). Do the same for the other thumb.
8 Rub the fingers of 1 hand into the palm of the other hand (Fig. 12-10, *G*). Use a circular motion. Do the same for the fingers of the other hand.
9 Continue rubbing your hands until they are dry.

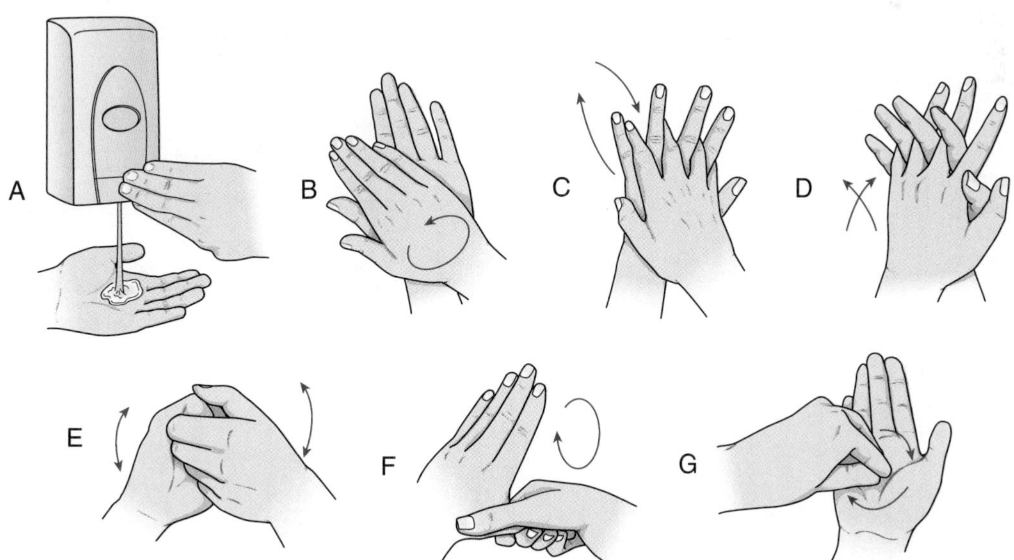

FIGURE 12-10 Using an alcohol-based hand rub. **A,** A palmful of an alcohol-based hand rub is applied into a cupped hand. **B,** The palms are rubbed together. **C,** The palm of 1 hand is rubbed over the back of the other. **D,** The palms are rubbed together with the fingers interlaced. **E,** The fingers are interlocked and the fingers rubbed back and forth. **F,** The thumb of 1 hand is rubbed in the palm of the other. **G,** The fingers of 1 hand are rubbed into the palm of the other hand with circular motions.

Supplies and Equipment

Most health care supplies and equipment are disposable. They help prevent the spread of infection. You discard single-use items after 1 use. A person uses multi-use items many times. They include bedpans, urinals, wash basins, and water mugs. Label such items with the person's room and bed number. Do not "borrow" them for another person.

Non-disposable items are cleaned and then disinfected. Then they are sterilized.

Cleaning. Cleaning reduces the number of microbes present. It also removes organic matter such as blood, body fluids, secretions, and excretions. To clean equipment:

- Wear personal protective equipment (PPE) when cleaning items contaminated with blood, body fluids, secretions, or excretions. PPE includes gloves, a mask, a gown, and goggles or a face shield.
- Work from *clean* to *dirty* areas. If you work from a *dirty* to a *clean* area, the *clean* area becomes contaminated *(dirty)*.
- Rinse the item to remove organic matter. Use cold water. Heat makes organic matter thick, sticky, and hard to remove.
- Wash the item with soap and hot water.
- Scrub thoroughly. Use a brush if necessary.
- Rinse the item in warm water.
- Dry the item.
- Disinfect or sterilize the item.
- Disinfect equipment and the sink used in the cleaning procedure.
- Discard PPE.
- Practice hand hygiene.

Disinfection. *Disinfection is the process of destroying pathogens. Chemical disinfectants* are used to clean surfaces. Counters, tubs, and showers are examples. They also are used to clean re-usable items. Such items include:

- Blood pressure cuffs
- Commodes and metal bedpans
- Wheelchairs and stretchers
- Furniture

See *Promoting Safety and Comfort: Disinfection.*

PROMOTING SAFETY AND COMFORT

Disinfection

Safety

Chemical disinfectants can burn and irritate the skin. Wear utility gloves or rubber household gloves to prevent skin irritation. These gloves are waterproof. Do not wear disposable gloves.

Some chemical disinfectants have special measures for use and storage. Check the material safety data sheet (MSDS). See Chapter 9.

Sterilization. *Sterilization is the process of destroying* all *microbes (non-pathogens and pathogens).* Very high temperatures are used. Heat destroys microbes.

Boiling water, radiation, liquid or gas chemicals, dry heat, and *steam under pressure* are sterilization methods. An *autoclave* (Fig. 12-11) is a pressure steam sterilizer. Glass, surgical items, and metal objects are autoclaved. High temperatures destroy plastic and rubber items. They are not autoclaved.

Other Aseptic Measures

Hand hygiene, cleaning, disinfection, and sterilization are important aseptic measures. So are the measures listed in Box 12-3.

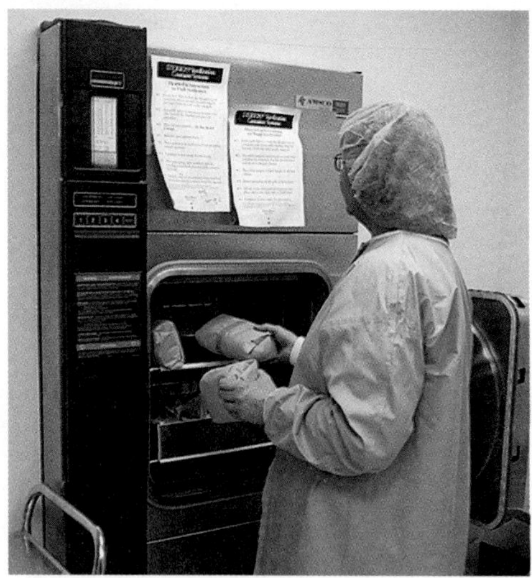

FIGURE 12-11 An autoclave.

BOX 12-3 Aseptic Measures

Controlling Reservoirs (Hosts—You or the Person)

- Provide for the person's hygiene needs (Chapter 16).
- Wash contaminated areas with soap and water. Feces, urine, and blood can contain microbes. So can body fluids, secretions, and excretions.
- Use leak-proof plastic bags for soiled tissues, linens, and other items.
- Keep tables, counters, wheelchair trays, and other surfaces clean and dry.
- Label bottles with the person's name and the date the bottle was opened.
- Keep bottles and fluid containers tightly capped or covered.
- Keep drainage containers below the drainage site (Chapters 18 and 24).
- Empty drainage containers and dispose of drainage following agency policy. Usually drainage containers are emptied every shift. Follow the nurse's directions if you need to empty them more often.

Controlling Portals of Exit

- Cover your nose and mouth when coughing or sneezing.
- Provide the person with tissues for coughing or sneezing.
- Wear PPE as needed (p. 148).

Controlling Transmission

- Provide all persons with their own personal care equipment. This includes wash basins, bedpans, urinals, commodes, and eating and drinking utensils.
- Do not take equipment from 1 person's room to use for another person. Even if un-used, do not take the item from 1 room to another.
- Hold equipment and linens away from your uniform (Fig. 12-12).
- Practice hand hygiene. See Box 12-2.
- Assist the person with hand washing.
  - Before and after eating
  - After elimination
  - After changing tampons, sanitary napkins, or other personal hygiene products
  - After contact with blood, body fluids, secretions, or excretions
- Prevent dust movement. Do not shake linens or equipment. Use a damp cloth for dusting.

Controlling Transmission—cont'd

- Clean from the cleanest area to the dirtiest. This prevents soiling a clean area.
- Clean away from your body. Do not dust, brush, or wipe toward yourself. Otherwise you transmit microbes to your skin, hair, and clothing.
- Flush urine and feces down the toilet. Avoid splatters and splashes.
- Pour contaminated liquids directly into sinks or toilets. Avoid splashing onto other areas.
- Do not sit on the person's bed or chair. You will pick up microbes. You will transfer them to the next surface that you sit on.
- Do not use items that are on the floor. The floor is contaminated.
- Follow the agency's disinfection procedures to clean:
  - Tubs, showers, and shower chairs after each use
  - Bedpans, urinals, and commodes after each use
- Report pests—ants, spiders, mice, and so on.

Controlling Portals of Entry

- Provide for good skin care (Chapter 16). This promotes intact skin.
- Provide for good oral hygiene (Chapter 16). This promotes intact mucous membranes.
- Protect the skin from injury.
  - Do not let the person lie on tubes or other items.
  - Make sure linens are dry and wrinkle-free (Chapter 15).
  - Turn and re-position the person as directed by the nurse and care plan (Chapters 13 and 14).
- Assist with or clean the genital area after elimination. (See "Perineal Care" in Chapter 16.) Wipe and clean from the urethra (the cleanest area) to the rectum (the dirtiest area). This helps prevent urinary tract infections.
- Make sure drainage tubes are properly connected. This prevents microbes from entering the drainage system.

Protecting the Susceptible Host

- Follow the care plan to meet hygiene needs. This protects the skin and mucous membranes.
- Follow the care plan to meet nutrition and fluid needs (Chapter 20). This helps prevent infection.
- Assist with deep-breathing and coughing exercises as directed (Chapter 26). This helps prevent respiratory infections.

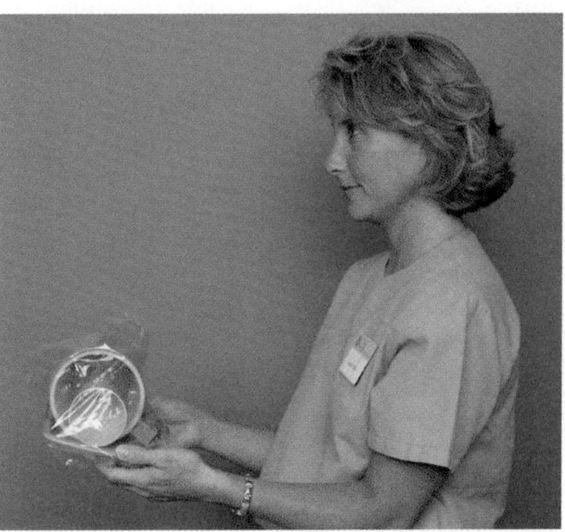

FIGURE 12-12 Hold equipment away from your uniform.

ISOLATION PRECAUTIONS

Blood, body fluids, secretions, and excretions can transmit pathogens. Sometimes barriers are needed to keep pathogens within a certain area. Usually the area is the person's room. This requires isolation precautions.

The *Guidelines for Isolation Precautions: Preventing Transmission of Infectious Agents in Healthcare Settings 2007* is followed. This is a guideline of the Centers for Disease Control and Prevention (CDC). Isolation precautions prevent the spread of **communicable diseases (contagious diseases)**. *They are diseases caused by pathogens that spread easily.*

Isolation precautions are based on *clean* and *dirty*. *Clean* areas or objects have no pathogens. They are not contaminated or *dirty*. *Dirty* areas or objects are contaminated with pathogens. If a *clean* area or object has contact with something *dirty*, the clean area or object is now dirty. *Clean* and *dirty* also depend on how the pathogen is spread.

The CDC guideline has 2 tiers of precautions.

- Standard Precautions
- Transmission-Based Precautions

Standard Precautions

Standard Precautions (Box 12-4):

- Reduce the risk of spreading pathogens.
- Reduce the risk of spreading known and unknown infections.

Standard Precautions are used for all persons whenever care is given. They prevent the spread of infection from:

- Blood.
- All body fluids, secretions, and excretions (except sweat) even if blood is not visible. Sweat is not known to spread infection.
- Non-intact skin (skin with open breaks).
- Mucous membranes.

Transmission-Based Precautions

Some infections require Transmission-Based Precautions (Box 12-5, p. 150). They are commonly called "isolation precautions." Isolation precautions involve wearing PPE—gloves, a gown, a mask, and goggles or a face shield. You must understand how certain infections are spread (see Fig. 12-2). This helps you understand the 3 types of Transmission-Based Precautions.

Removing linens, trash, and equipment from the room may require double-bagging (p. 156). Follow agency procedures to collect specimens and transport persons. Agency policies may differ from those in this text. The rules in Box 12-6, p. 151 are a guide for giving safe care when using isolation precautions.

See *Focus on Communication: Transmission-Based Precautions*, p. 151.

See *Focus on Surveys: Transmission-Based Precautions*, p. 151.

See *Delegation Guidelines: Transmission-Based Precautions*, p. 151.

See *Promoting Safety and Comfort: Transmission-Based Precautions*, p. 151.

Text continued on p. 153

BOX 12-4 Standard Precautions

Hand Hygiene

- Follow the rules for hand hygiene. See Box 12-2.
- Touch surfaces close to the person only when necessary. This prevents contamination of clean hands from environmental surfaces. It also prevents the transmission of pathogens from contaminated hands to other surfaces.
- Do not wear fake nails or nail extenders if you will have contact with persons at risk for infection or other adverse outcomes. (NOTE: Some agencies do not allow fake nails or nail extenders.)

Personal Protective Equipment (PPE)

- Wear PPE when contact with blood or body fluids is likely.
- Do not contaminate your clothing or skin when removing PPE.
- Remove and discard PPE before leaving the person's room or care setting.

Modified from Siegel JD, Rhinehart E, Jackson M, Chiarello L, and the Healthcare Infection Control Practices Advisory Committee: Guideline for isolation precautions: preventing transmission of infectious agents in healthcare settings 2007, *Atlanta, 2007, Centers for Disease Control and Prevention.*

BOX 12-4 Standard Precautions—cont'd

Gloves

- Wear gloves when contact with the following is likely.
  - Blood
  - Potentially infectious materials (body fluids, secretions, and excretions are examples)
  - Mucous membranes
  - Non-intact skin
  - Skin that may be contaminated (for example, a person is incontinent of feces or urine)
- Wear gloves that fit and are appropriate for the task.
  - Wear disposable gloves to provide direct care to the person.
  - Wear disposable gloves or utility gloves for cleaning equipment or care settings.
- Remove gloves after contact with:
  - The person
  - The person's care setting
  - Equipment used in the person's care or other care equipment
- Remove gloves after contact with a person and before going to another person.
- Do not wash gloves for re-use with different persons.
- Change gloves during care if your hands will move from a contaminated body site to a clean body site.

Gowns

- Wear a gown appropriate to the task.
- Wear a gown to protect your skin and clothing when contact with blood, body fluids, secretions, or excretions is likely.
- Wear a gown for direct contact if the person has uncontained secretions or excretions.
- Remove the gown and perform hand hygiene before leaving the person's room or care setting.
- Do not re-use gowns, even for repeat contacts with the same person.

Mouth, Nose, and Eye Protection

- Wear PPE—masks, goggles, face shields—for procedures and tasks that are likely to cause splashes and sprays of blood, body fluids, secretions, and excretions.
- Wear PPE—masks, goggles, face shields—appropriate for the procedure or task.
- Wear gloves, a gown, and 1 of the following for procedures that are likely to cause sprays of respiratory secretions.
  - A face shield that fully covers the front and sides of the face
  - A mask with attached shield
  - A mask and goggles

Respiratory Hygiene/Cough Etiquette

- Instruct persons with respiratory symptoms to:
  - Cover the nose and mouth when coughing or sneezing.
  - Use tissues to contain respiratory secretions.
  - Dispose of used tissues in the nearest waste container.
  - Perform hand hygiene after contact with respiratory secretions.
- Provide visitors with masks according to agency policy.

Care Equipment

- Wear appropriate PPE to handle care equipment that is visibly soiled with blood, body fluids, secretions, or excretions.
- Wear appropriate PPE to handle care equipment that may have been in contact with blood, body fluids, secretions, or excretions.
- Remove organic material before disinfection and sterilization procedures. Follow agency policy for using cleaning agents.

Care of the Environment

- Follow agency policies and procedures to clean and maintain surfaces. Environmental surfaces and care equipment are examples. Surfaces near the person may need frequent cleaning and maintenance—door knobs, bed rails, over-bed tables, toilet surfaces and areas, and so on.
- Follow agency policy to clean and disinfect multi-use electronic equipment. This includes:
  - Items used by patients and residents
  - Items used to give care
  - Mobile devices that are moved in and out of patient or resident rooms
- Follow these rules for children's toys. This includes toys in agency waiting areas.
  - Select toys that are easy to clean and disinfect.
  - Do not allow the use of stuffed, furry toys if they will be shared.
  - Clean and disinfect large stationary toys (for example, climbing equipment) at least weekly and whenever visibly soiled.
  - Rinse toys with water after disinfection if they may be mouthed by children. Or wash them in a dishwasher.
  - Clean and disinfect a toy immediately when it needs cleaning. Or store the toy in a labeled container away from toys that are clean and ready for use.

Textiles and Laundry

- Handle used textiles and fabrics (linens) with minimum agitation. This prevents contamination of air, surfaces, and other persons.

Worker Safety

- Protect yourself and others from exposure to bloodborne pathogens. This includes handling needles and other sharps. Follow federal and state standards and guidelines. See the Bloodborne Pathogen Standard (p. 157).
- Use a mouthpiece, resuscitation bag, or other ventilation device during resuscitation to prevent contact with the person's mouth and oral secretions. See Chapter 31.

Patient or Resident Placement

- A private room is preferred if the person is at risk for transmitting the infection to others.
- Follow the nurse's directions if a private room is not available.

BOX 12-5 Transmission-Based Precautions

Contact Precautions

- Used for persons with known or suspected infections or conditions that increase the risk of contact transmission.
- Patient or resident placement:
    - A single room is preferred.
    - Do the following if a room is shared with another person not infected with the same agent.
        - Keep the privacy curtain between the beds closed.
        - Change the PPE and practice hand hygiene between contact with persons in the same room. Do so regardless of whether 1 or both persons are on Contact Precautions.
- Gloves:
    - Don gloves upon entering the person's room.
    - Wear gloves to touch the person's intact skin.
    - Wear gloves to touch surfaces or items near the person.
- Gown:
    - Wear a gown when clothing may have direct contact with the person.
    - Wear a gown when contact is likely with surfaces or equipment near the person.
    - Don the gown upon entering the person's room.
    - Remove the gown and practice hand hygiene before leaving the person's room.
    - Make sure your clothing and skin do not touch potentially contaminated surfaces after removing the gown.
- Patient or resident transport:
    - Limit transport and movement of the person outside of the room to medically-necessary purposes.
    - Cover the infected area of the person's body.
    - Remove and discard contaminated PPE and practice hand hygiene before transporting the person.
    - Don clean PPE to handle the person at the transport destination.
- Care equipment:
    - Follow Standard Precautions.
    - Use disposable equipment when possible. If possible, leave non-disposable equipment in the person's room.
    - Clean and disinfect non-disposable and multi-use equipment before use on another person.

Droplet Precautions

- Used for persons known or suspected to be infected with pathogens transmitted by respiratory droplets. Such droplets come from coughing, sneezing, or talking.
- Patient or resident placement:
    - A single room is preferred.
    - Do the following if a room is shared with another person not infected with the same agent.
        - Keep the privacy curtain between the beds closed.
        - Change PPE and practice hand hygiene between contact with persons in the same room. Do so regardless of whether 1 or both persons are on Droplet Precautions.
- Personal protective equipment:
    - Don a mask upon entering the person's room.
- Patient or resident transport:
    - Limit transport and movement of the person outside of the room to medically-necessary purposes.
    - Have the person wear a mask.
    - Instruct the person to follow Respiratory Hygiene/Cough Etiquette (see Box 12-4).
    - No mask is required for staff transporting the person.

Airborne Precautions

- Used for persons known or suspected to be infected with pathogens transmitted person-to-person by the airborne route. Tuberculosis (TB) (Chapter 28), measles, chicken pox, smallpox, and severe acute respiratory syndrome (SARS) are examples.
- The person is placed in an airborne infection isolation room (AIIR). If not available, the person is transferred to an agency with an AIIR. An AIIR is a private (single person) room with a private bathroom. AIIR practices include:
    - All persons entering the room wear a TB respirator.
    - The room door is kept closed except when someone enters or leaves the room.
    - Treatments and procedures are done in the room.
    - The person wears a mask during transport.
- Staff susceptible to the infection are restricted from entering the room. This is if immune staff members are available.
- Personal protective equipment:
    - An approved respirator is worn on entering the room or home of a person with TB.
    - Respiratory protection is recommended for all staff when caring for persons with smallpox.
- Patient or resident transport:
    - Limit transport and movement of the person outside of the room to medically-necessary purposes.
    - Have the person wear a surgical mask.
    - Instruct the person to follow Respiratory Hygiene/Cough Etiquette (see Box 12-4).
    - Cover skin lesions infected with the microbe.
    - No mask or respirator is required for staff transporting the person.

Modified from Siegel JD, Rhinehart E, Jackson M, Chiarello L, and the Healthcare Infection Control Practices Advisory Committee: Guideline for isolation precautions: preventing transmission of infectious agents in healthcare settings 2007, *Atlanta, 2007, Centers for Disease Control and Prevention.*

BOX 12-6 Rules for Isolation Precautions

- Collect all needed items before entering the room.
- Do not contaminate equipment and supplies. Floors are contaminated. So is any object on the floor or that falls to the floor.
- Clean floors with mops wetted with a disinfectant solution. Floor dust is contaminated.
- Prevent drafts. Drafts can carry some microbes in the air.
- Use paper towels to handle contaminated items.
- Remove items from the room in leak-proof plastic bags.
- Double-bag items if the outside of the bag is or can be contaminated (p. 156).
- Follow agency policy to remove and transport disposable and re-usable items.
- Return re-usable dishes, drinking vessels, eating utensils, and trays to the food service (dietary) department. Discard disposable dishes, drinking vessels, eating utensils, and trays in the waste container in the person's room.
- Do not touch your hair, nose, mouth, eyes, or other body parts.
- Do not touch any clean area or object if your hands are contaminated.
- Wash your hands if they are visibly dirty or contaminated with blood, body fluids, secretions, or excretions.
- Place clean items on paper towels.
- Do not shake linens.
- Use paper towels to turn faucets on and off.
- Use a paper towel to open the door to the person's room. Discard it after use.
- Tell the nurse if you have any cuts, open skin areas, a sore throat, vomiting, or diarrhea.

FOCUS ON COMMUNICATION

Transmission-Based Precautions

Visitors may need to wear PPE to be with a person needing isolation precautions. Visitors may ask why if they do not understand the need for PPE. Some visitors ignore signs or requests to wear PPE. You must communicate with the person and visitors about PPE. You can politely say:

- "Your visitors will need to wear a gown and gloves while in your room."
- "Please wear this mask. It is our policy to protect you, your family member, and others."

Tell the nurse if the person or visitors have more questions. Also tell the nurse if someone refuses to follow isolation precautions.

You may see health team members not wearing PPE when needed. Remind the person that PPE is needed. Offer to get the person PPE. For example, you can say:

- "You need a mask when caring for Mrs. Stayton. I will get you one."
- "Here are gloves and a gown. You need to wear them in Mr. Parker's room."

Be polite. Tell the nurse if the person refuses.

FOCUS ON SURVEYS

Transmission-Based Precautions

When a person requires Transmission-Based Precautions, surveyors will observe if staff:

- Wash their hands correctly and at appropriate times.
- Change gloves after providing personal care.
- Don, wear, and dispose of PPE correctly.

DELEGATION GUIDELINES

Transmission-Based Precautions

If a person needs isolation precautions, review the type with the nurse. Also check with the nurse and care plan about:

- What PPE to use
- What special safety measures are needed

PROMOTING SAFETY AND COMFORT

Transmission-Based Precautions

Safety

Preventing the spread of infection is important. Isolation precautions protect everyone—patients, residents, visitors, staff, and you. If you are careless, everyone's safety is at risk.

The PPE needed depends on tasks, procedures, care measures, and isolation precautions. Sometimes only gloves are needed. The nurse tells you if other PPE is needed.

Gloves are always worn when gowns are worn. Sometimes other PPE is needed when gowns are worn. PPE is donned and removed in the following order.

- Donning PPE (Fig. 12-13, *A*, p. 152):
  - Gown
  - Mask or respirator
  - Eyewear (goggles or face shield)
  - Gloves
- Removing PPE (removed at the doorway before leaving the person's room) (Fig. 12-13, *B*, p. 152):
  - Gloves
  - Goggles or face shield
  - Gown
  - Mask or respirator

(NOTE: Some state competency tests require hand hygiene after removing each item of PPE. And some states use a different order for donning and removing PPE. Follow the procedures used in your state and agency.)

A

SEQUENCE FOR DONNING PERSONAL PROTECTIVE EQUIPMENT (PPE)

The type of PPE used will vary based on the level of precautions required; e.g., Standard and Contact, Droplet or Airborne Infection Isolation.

1. GOWN
- Fully cover torso from neck to knees, arms to end of wrists, and wrap around the back
- Fasten in back of neck and waist

2. MASK OR RESPIRATOR
- Secure ties or elastic bands at middle of head and neck
- Fit flexible band to nose bridge
- Fit snug to face and below chin
- Fit-check respirator

3. GOGGLES OR FACE SHIELD
- Place over face and eyes and adjust to fit

4. GLOVES
- Extend to cover wrist of isolation gown

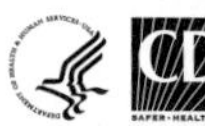

SECUENCIA PARA PONERSE EL EQUIPO DE PROTECCIÓN PERSONAL (PPE)

El tipo de PPE que se debe utilizar depende del nivel de precaución que sea necesario; por ejemplo, equipo Estándar y de Contacto o de Aislamiento de infecciones transportadas por gotas o por aire.

1. BATA
- *Cubra con la bata todo el torso desde el cuello hasta las rodillas, los brazos hasta la muñeca y dóblela alrededor de la espalda*
- *Átesela por detrás a la altura del cuello y la cintura*

2. MÁSCARA O RESPIRADOR
- *Asegúrese los cordones o la banda elástica en la mitad de la cabeza y en el cuello*
- *Ajústese la banda flexible en el puente de la nariz*
- *Acomódesela en la cara y por debajo del mentón*
- *Verifique el ajuste del respirador*

3. GAFAS PROTECTORAS O CARETAS
- *Colóquesela sobre la cara y los ojos y ajústela*

4. GUANTES
- *Extienda los guantes para que cubran la parte del puño en la bata de aislamiento*

USE SAFE WORK PRACTICES TO PROTECT YOURSELF AND LIMIT THE SPREAD OF CONTAMINATION
- Keep hands away from face
- Limit surfaces touched
- Change gloves when torn or heavily contaminated
- Perform hand hygiene

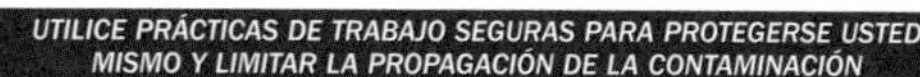

UTILICE PRÁCTICAS DE TRABAJO SEGURAS PARA PROTEGERSE USTED MISMO Y LIMITAR LA PROPAGACIÓN DE LA CONTAMINACIÓN
- *Mantenga las manos alejadas de la cara*
- *Limite el contacto con superficies*
- *Cambie los guantes si se rompen o están demasiado contaminados*
- *Realice la higiene de las manos*

B

SEQUENCE FOR REMOVING PERSONAL PROTECTIVE EQUIPMENT (PPE)

Except for respirator, remove PPE at doorway or in anteroom. Remove respirator after leaving patient room and closing door.

1. GLOVES
- Outside of gloves is contaminated!
- Grasp outside of glove with opposite gloved hand; peel off
- Hold removed glove in gloved hand
- Slide fingers of ungloved hand under remaining glove at wrist
- Peel glove off over first glove
- Discard gloves in waste container

2. GOGGLES OR FACE SHIELD
- Outside of goggles or face shield is contaminated!
- To remove, handle by head band or ear pieces
- Place in designated receptacle for reprocessing or in waste container

3. GOWN
- Gown front and sleeves are contaminated!
- Unfasten ties
- Pull away from neck and shoulders, touching inside of gown only
- Turn gown inside out
- Fold or roll into a bundle and discard

4. MASK OR RESPIRATOR
- Front of mask/respirator is contaminated — DO NOT TOUCH!
- Grasp bottom, then top ties or elastics and remove
- Discard in waste container

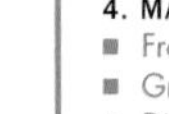

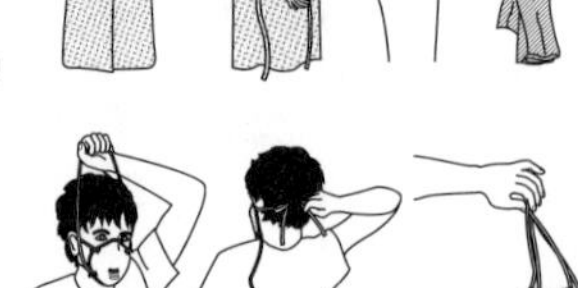

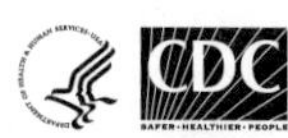

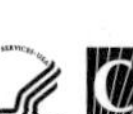

SECUENCIA PARA QUITARSE EL EQUIPO DE PROTECCIÓN PERSONAL (PPE)

Con la excepción del respirador, quítese el PPE en la entrada de la puerta o en la antesala. Quítese el respirador después de salir de la habitación del paciente y de cerrar la puerta.

1. GUANTES
- *¡El exterior de los guantes está contaminado!*
- *Agarre la parte exterior del guante con la mano opuesta en la que todavía tiene puesto el guante y quíteselo*
- *Sostenga el guante que se quitó con la mano enguantada*
- *Deslice los dedos de la mano sin guante por debajo del otro guante que no se ha quitado todavía a la altura de la muñeca*
- *Quítese el guante de manera que acabe cubriendo el primer guante*
- *Arroje los guantes en el recipiente de deshechos*

2. GAFAS PROTECTORAS O CARETA
- *¡El exterior de las gafas protectoras o de la careta está contaminado!*
- *Para quitárselas, tómelas por la parte de la banda de la cabeza o de las piezas de las orejas*
- *Colóquelas en el recipiente designado para reprocesar materiales o de materiales de deshecho*

3. BATA
- *¡La parte delantera de la bata y las mangas están contaminadas!*
- *Desate los cordones*
- *Tocando solamente el interior de la bata, pásela por encima del cuello y de los hombros*
- *Voltee la bata al revés*
- *Dóblela o enróllela y deséchela*

4. MÁSCARA O RESPIRADOR
- *La parte delantera de la máscara o respirador está contaminada — ¡NO LA TOQUE!*
- *Primero agarre la parte de abajo, luego los cordones o banda elástica de arriba y por último quítese la máscara o respirador*
- *Arrójela en el recipiente de deshechos*

PERFORM HAND HYGIENE IMMEDIATELY AFTER REMOVING ALL PPE

EFECTÚE LA HIGIENE DE LAS MANOS INMEDIATAMENTE DESPUÉS DE QUITARSE CUALQUIER EQUIPO DE PROTECCIÓN PERSONAL

FIGURE 12-13 A, Donning personal protective equipment. **B,** Removing personal protective equipment.

Gloves. Small skin breaks on the hands and fingers are common. Gloves act as a barrier. They protect:

- You from pathogens in the person's blood, body fluids, secretions, and excretions
- The person from microbes on your hands

Wear gloves whenever contact with blood, body fluids, secretions, excretions, mucous membranes, or non-intact skin is likely. Contact may be direct. Or contact may be with items or surfaces contaminated with blood, body fluids, secretions, or excretions.

Wearing gloves is the most common protective measure for Standard Precautions and Transmission-Based Precautions. When using gloves:

- Consider the outside of gloves as contaminated.
- Apply to dry hands. Gloves are easier to put on dry hands.
- Do not tear gloves when putting them on. Carelessness, long fingernails, and rings can tear gloves. Blood, body fluids, secretions, and excretions can enter the glove through the tear. This contaminates your hand.
- Apply a new pair for every person.
- Remove and discard torn, cut, or punctured gloves at once. Practice hand hygiene. Then put on a new pair.
- Wear gloves once. Discard them after use.
- Put on clean gloves just before touching mucous membranes or non-intact skin.
- Put on new gloves when gloves become contaminated with blood, body fluids, secretions, or excretions. A task may require more than 1 pair of gloves.
- Change gloves when moving from a contaminated body site to a clean body site.
- Change gloves when touching portable computer keyboards or other mobile equipment that is transported from room to room.
- Put on gloves last when they are worn with other PPE.
- Make sure gloves cover your wrists. If you wear a gown, gloves cover the cuffs (Fig. 12-14).
- Remove gloves so the inside part is on the outside. The inside is *clean.*
- Practice hand hygiene after removing gloves.

See *Promoting Safety and Comfort: Gloves.*
See procedure: *Removing Gloves,* p. 154.

Gowns. Gowns prevent the spread of microbes. They protect your clothes and body from contact with blood, body fluids, secretions, and excretions. They also protect against splashes and sprays.

Gowns must completely cover you from your neck to your knees. The long sleeves have tight cuffs. The gown opens at the back. It is tied at the neck and waist. The gown front and sleeves are considered *contaminated.*

Gowns are used once. A wet gown is contaminated. Remove it and put on a dry one. Discard gowns after use.

See procedure: *Donning and Removing a Gown,* p. 154.

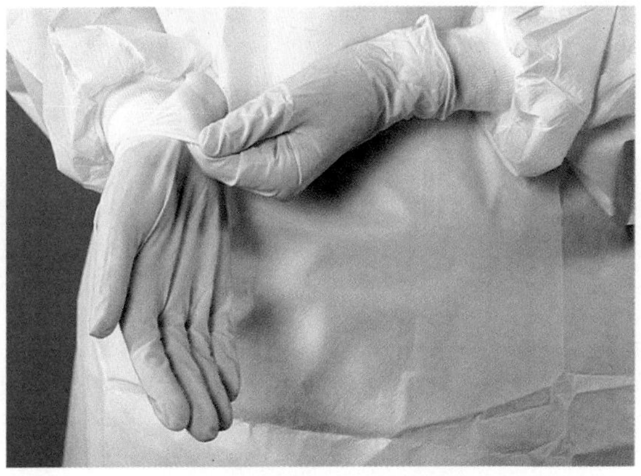

FIGURE 12-14 The gloves cover the gown cuffs.

PROMOTING SAFETY AND COMFORT

Gloves

Safety

No special method is needed to put on non-sterile gloves. To remove gloves, see procedure: *Removing Gloves,* p. 154.

Some gloves are made of latex (a rubber product). Latex allergies can cause skin rashes. Difficulty breathing and shock are more serious problems. Report skin rashes and breathing problems to the nurse at once.

You may have a latex allergy. Some patients and residents are allergic to latex. This is noted on the care plan and your assignment sheet. Latex-free gloves are worn for latex allergies.

Comfort

Gloves are needed when contact with blood, body fluids, secretions, excretions, mucous membranes, or non-intact skin is likely. Gloves are not needed when such contact is not likely. Back massages and brushing hair are examples. To reduce exposure to latex, wear gloves only when needed.

Removing Gloves

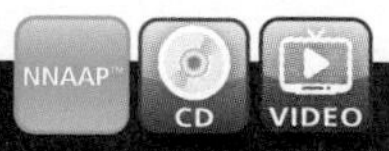

PROCEDURE

1 See *Promoting Safety and Comfort: Gloves*, p. 153.
2 Make sure that glove touches only glove.
3 Grasp a glove at the palm (Fig. 12-15, *A*). Grasp it on the outside.
4 Pull the glove down over your hand so it is inside out (Fig. 12-15, *B*).
5 Hold the removed glove with your other gloved hand.
6 Reach inside the other glove. Use the first 2 fingers of the ungloved hand (Fig. 12-15, *C*).
7 Pull the glove down (inside out) over your hand and the other glove (Fig. 12-15, *D*).
8 Discard the gloves. Follow agency policy.
9 Practice hand hygiene.

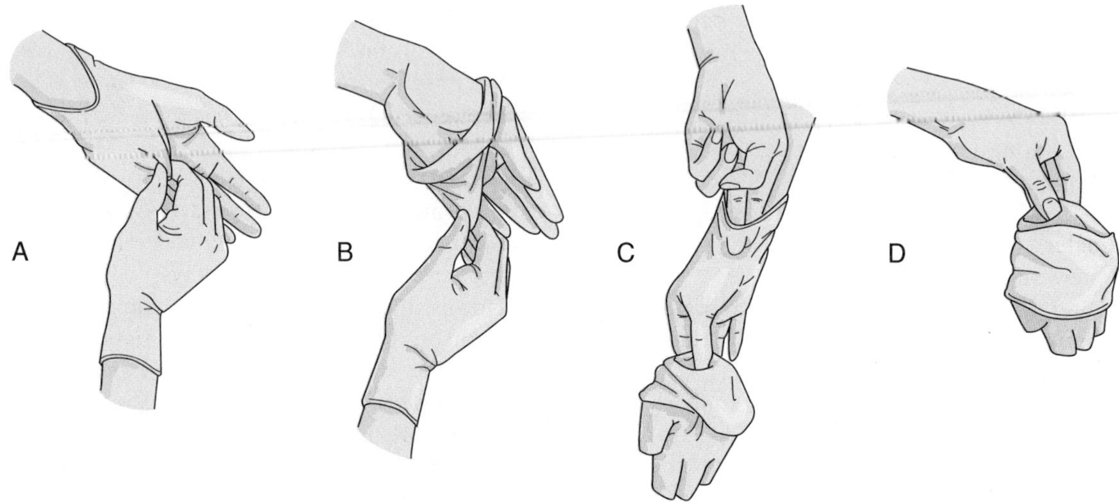

FIGURE 12-15 Removing gloves. **A,** Grasp the glove at the palm. **B,** Pull the glove down over the hand. The glove is inside out. **C,** Insert the fingers of the ungloved hand inside the other glove. **D,** Pull the glove down and over the other hand and glove. The glove is inside out.

Donning and Removing a Gown

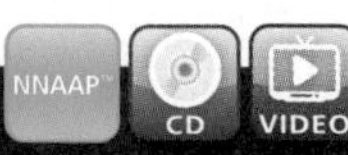

PROCEDURE

1 Remove your watch and all jewelry.
2 Roll up uniform sleeves.
3 Practice hand hygiene.
4 Hold a clean gown out in front of you. Let it unfold. Do not shake the gown.
5 Put your hands and arms through the sleeves (see Fig. 12-13, *A*).
6 Make sure the gown covers you from your neck to your knees. It must cover your arms to the end of your wrists.
7 Tie the strings at the back of the neck (see Fig. 12-13, *A*).
8 Overlap the back of the gown. Make sure it covers your uniform. The gown should be snug, not loose.
9 Tie the waist strings. Tie them at the back or the side. Do not tie them in front.
10 Put on other PPE.
  a Mask or respirator (if needed).
  b Goggles or face shield (if needed).
  c Gloves. Make sure gloves cover the gown cuffs.
11 Provide care.
12 Remove and discard the gloves.
13 Remove and discard the goggles or face shield if worn.
14 Remove the gown. Do not touch the outside of the gown.
  a Untie the neck and waist strings (see Fig. 12-13, *B*).
  b Pull the gown down from each shoulder toward the same hand (see Fig. 12-13, *B*).
  c Turn the gown inside out as it is removed. Hold it at the inside shoulder seams, and bring your hands together (Fig. 12-16).
15 Hold and roll up the gown away from you (see Fig. 12-13, *B*). Keep it inside out. Do not let the gown touch the floor.
16 Discard the gown.
17 Remove and discard the mask if worn.
18 Practice hand hygiene.

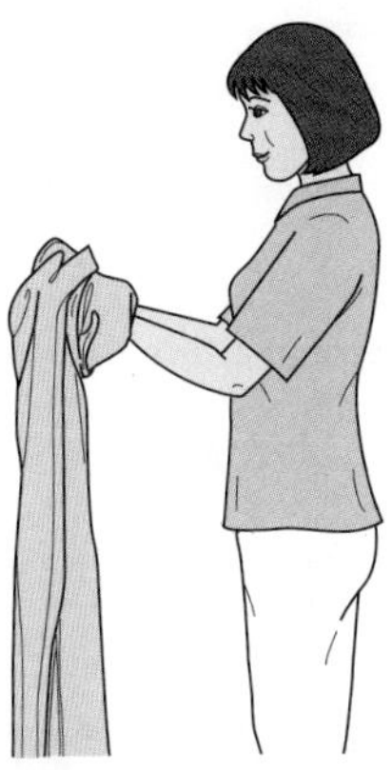

FIGURE 12-16 The gown is turned inside out as it is removed.

Masks and Respiratory Protection. You wear masks:

- For protection from contact with infectious materials from the person. Respiratory secretions and sprays of blood or body fluids are examples.
- When assisting with sterile procedures. This protects the person from infectious agents carried in your mouth or nose.

A wet or moist mask is contaminated. Breathing can cause masks to become wet or moist. Apply a new mask when contamination occurs.

A mask fits snugly over your nose and mouth. Practice hand hygiene before putting on a mask. To remove a mask, touch only the ties or the elastic bands. The front of the mask is contaminated.

See procedure: *Donning and Removing a Mask*.

Donning and Removing a Mask

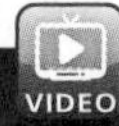

PROCEDURE

1 Practice hand hygiene.
2 Put on a gown if required.
3 Pick up a mask by its upper ties. Do not touch the part that will cover your face.
4 Place the mask over your nose and mouth (Fig. 12-17, *A*).
5 Place the upper strings above your ears. Tie them at the back in the middle of your head (Fig. 12-17, *B*).
6 Tie the lower strings at the back of your neck (Fig. 12-17, *C*). The lower part of the mask is under your chin.
7 Pinch the metal band around your nose. The top of the mask must be snug over your nose. If you wear eyeglasses, the mask must be snug under the bottom of the eyeglasses.
8 Make sure the mask is snug over your face and under your chin.
9 Put on goggles or a face shield if needed and if not part of the mask.
10 Put on gloves.
11 Provide care. Avoid coughing, sneezing, and unnecessary talking.
12 Change the mask if it becomes wet or contaminated.
13 Remove and discard the gloves. Remove and discard the goggles or face shield and gown if worn.
14 Remove the mask (see Fig.12-13, *B*).
  a Untie the lower strings of the mask.
  b Untie the top strings.
  c Hold the top strings. Remove the mask.
15 Discard the mask.
16 Practice hand hygiene.

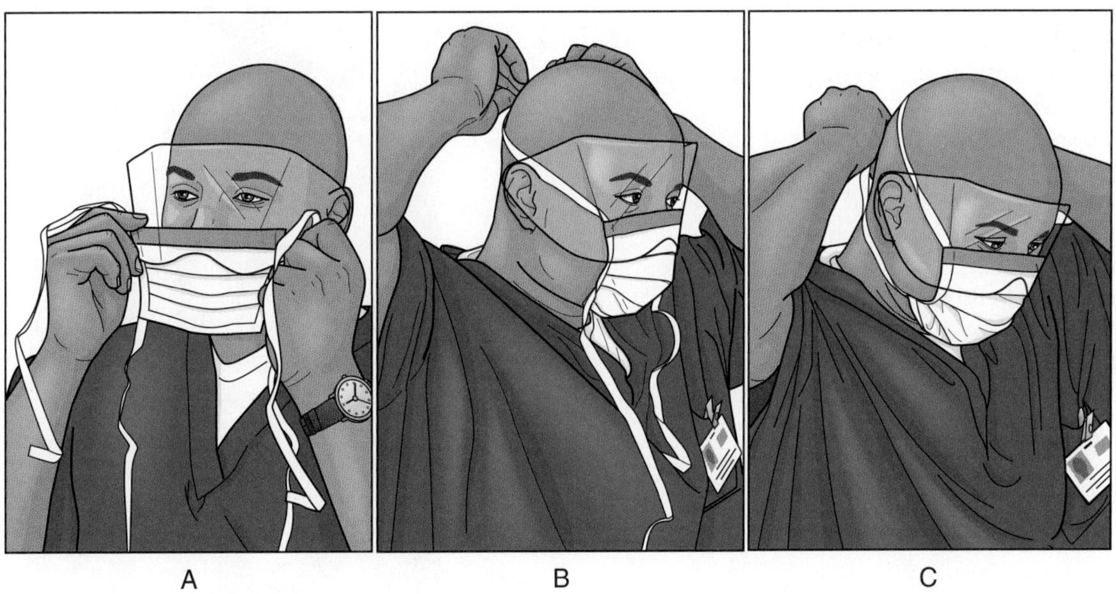

FIGURE 12-17 Donning and removing a mask. NOTE: The mask has a face shield. **A,** The mask covers the nose and mouth. **B,** Upper strings are tied at the back of the head. **C,** Lower strings are tied at the back of the neck.

Goggles and Face Shields. Goggles and face shields protect your eyes, mouth, and nose from splashing or spraying of blood, body fluids, secretions, and excretions (see Fig. 12-17). Splashes and sprays can occur when you give care, clean items, or dispose of fluids.

The front (outside) of goggles or a face shield is contaminated. The headband, ties, or ear-pieces used to secure the device are clean. Use them to remove the device after hand hygiene. They are safe to touch with bare hands.

Discard disposable goggles or face shields after use. Re-usable eyewear is cleaned before re-use. It is washed with soap and water. Then a disinfectant is used.

See *Promoting Safety and Comfort: Goggles and Face Shields.*

Bagging Items. Contaminated items are bagged for removal from the person's room. Leak-proof plastic bags are used. They have the *BIOHAZARD* symbol (Fig. 12-18). ***Biohazardous waste*** *is items contaminated with blood, body fluids, secretions, or excretions.* (*Bio* means *life*. *Hazardous* means *dangerous* or *harmful*.)

Bag and transport linens following agency policy. Laundry bags with contaminated linen need a *BIOHAZARD* symbol. Melt-away bags dissolve in hot water. Once soiled linen is bagged, no one needs to handle it. Do not over-fill the bag. Tie the bag securely. Then place it in a laundry hamper lined with a biohazard plastic bag.

Trash is placed in a container labeled with the *BIOHAZARD* symbol. Follow agency policy for bagging and transporting trash, equipment, and supplies.

Usually 1 bag is needed. Double-bagging involves 2 bags. Double-bagging is needed if the outside of the bag is wet, soiled, or may be contaminated. For double-bagging:

- Two workers are needed. A co-worker stands outside the doorway. You are in the room.
- Seal the *dirty* bag in the room.
- Have your co-worker make a wide cuff on a *clean* bag and hold it wide open.
- Place the *dirty* bag into the *clean* bag (Fig. 12-19). Do not touch the outside of the *clean* bag.
- Ask your co-worker to seal and label the *clean* bag. It is labeled with the *BIOHAZARD* symbol.
- Ask your co-worker to take the bag to the appropriate area for disposal, disinfection, or sterilization.

Collecting Specimens. Blood, body fluids, secretions, and excretions often require laboratory testing (Chapter 22). Specimens are transported to the laboratory in biohazard specimen bags. Follow agency procedures to collect and transport a specimen when a person is on Transmission-Based Precautions.

PROMOTING SAFETY AND COMFORT

Goggles and Face Shields

Safety

Eyeglasses and contact lenses do not provide eye protection. If you wear eyeglasses, use a face shield that fits over your glasses with minimal gaps.

Goggles do not provide splash or spray protection to other parts of your face.

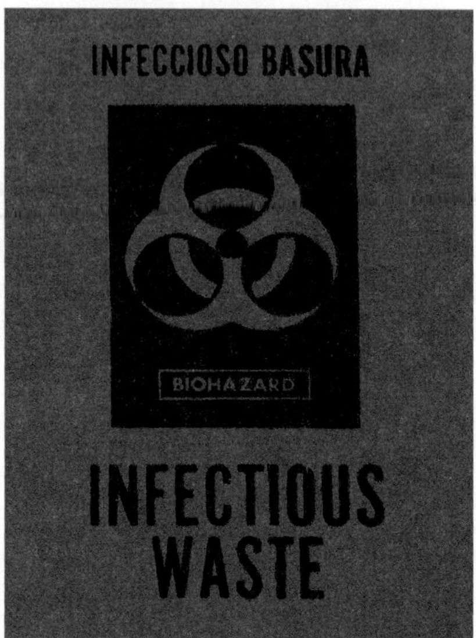

FIGURE 12-18 *BIOHAZARD* symbol.

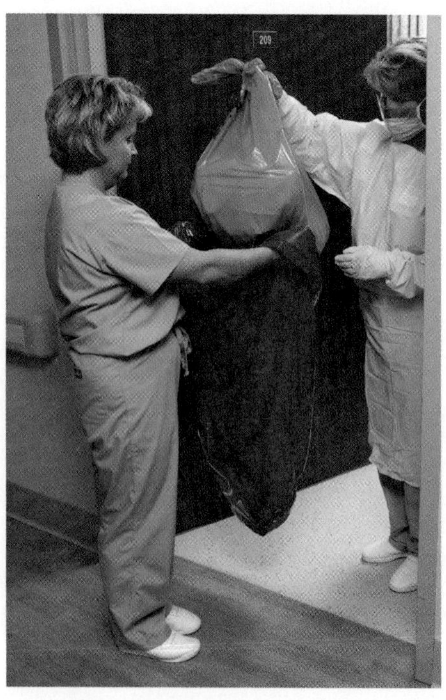

FIGURE 12-19 Double-bagging. One nursing assistant is in the room by the doorway. The other is outside the doorway. The *dirty* bag is placed inside the *clean* bag.

Transporting Persons. Persons on Transmission-Based Precautions usually do not leave their rooms. Sometimes they go to other areas for treatments or tests.

Transport procedures vary among agencies. Some require transport by bed. This prevents contaminating wheelchairs and stretchers. Others use wheelchairs and stretchers. Follow agency procedures for a safe transport when a person is on Transmission-Based Precautions.

Meeting Basic Needs

The person has love, belonging, and self-esteem needs. Often they are unmet when Transmission-Based Precautions are used. Visitors and staff may avoid the person. Putting on PPE takes extra effort before entering the room. Some are not sure what they can touch. They may fear getting the disease.

The person may feel lonely, unwanted, and rejected. The person knows the disease can be spread to others. He or she may feel dirty and undesirable. Without intending to, visitors and staff can make the person feel ashamed and guilty for having a contagious disease.

You can help meet love, belonging, and self-esteem needs. To help the person:

- Remember that the pathogen is undesirable, not the person.
- Treat the person with respect, kindness, and dignity.
- Provide newspapers, magazines, books, and other reading matter.
- Provide hobby materials if possible.
- Place a clock in the room.
- Suggest that the person call family and friends.
- Provide a current TV guide.
- Plan your work so you can stay to visit with the person.
- Say "hello" from the doorway often.

Items brought into the person's room become contaminated. Disinfect or discard them according to agency policy.

See *Focus on Communication: Meeting Basic Needs.*

See *Focus on Older Persons: Meeting Basic Needs.*

FOCUS ON COMMUNICATION

Meeting Basic Needs

Some questions or statements can make the person feel dirty or ashamed. Be careful what you say. For example, do not say:

- "How did you get that?"
- "What were you doing?"
- "I'm afraid to touch you."
- "Don't breathe on me."

Always treat the person with respect, kindness, and dignity.

BLOODBORNE PATHOGEN STANDARD

The Bloodborne Pathogen Standard protects against the human immunodeficiency virus (HIV) and the hepatitis B virus (HBV) (Chapter 28). It is a regulation of the Occupational Safety and Health Administration (OSHA).

Found in the blood, HIV and HBV are bloodborne pathogens. They exit the body through blood. They are spread to others by blood and other potentially infectious materials (OPIM). OPIM are contaminated with blood or with a body fluid that may contain blood. This includes semen, vaginal secretions, and saliva. OPIM also includes needles, suction equipment, soiled linens, dressings, and other care items.

Staff at risk for exposure to blood or OPIM receive free training. It occurs upon employment and yearly. Training is also done for new or changed tasks involving exposure to bloodborne pathogens.

Hepatitis B Vaccination

Hepatitis B is a liver disease caused by HBV. HBV is spread by the blood and sexual contact.

The hepatitis B vaccine produces immunity against hepatitis B. *Immunity* means that a person has protection against a certain disease. He or she will not get the disease.

A *vaccination* involves giving a vaccine to produce immunity against an infectious disease. A *vaccine* contains dead or weakened microbes. You can receive the hepatitis B vaccination within 10 working days of being hired. The agency pays for it. You can refuse the vaccination. If so, you must sign a statement refusing the vaccine. You can have the vaccination at a later date.

FOCUS ON OLDER PERSONS

Meeting Basic Needs

Some older persons have poor vision. Let them see your face before you put on a mask, goggles, or a face shield. State your name and explain what you are going to do. Then put on PPE.

Persons with dementia do not understand the need for isolation precautions. Masks, gowns, goggles, and face shields may increase confusion and cause fear and agitation. These measures can help.

- Let the person see your face before putting on PPE.
- Tell the person who you are and what you need to do.
- Use a calm, soothing voice.
- Do not hurry the person.
- Use touch to reassure the person.
- Follow the care plan and the nurse's instructions for other measures to help the person.
- Report signs of increased confusion or behavior changes.

Engineering and Work Practice Controls

Engineering controls reduce employee exposure in the workplace. *Work practice controls* also reduce exposure risks. All tasks involving blood or OPIM are done in ways to limit splatters, splashes, and sprays. Producing droplets also is avoided. OSHA requires these work practice controls.

- Do not eat, drink, smoke, apply cosmetics or lip balm, or handle contact lenses in areas of exposure.
- Do not store food or drinks where blood or OPIM are kept.
- Practice hand hygiene after removing gloves.
- Wash hands as soon as possible after skin contact with blood or OPIM.
- Never re-cap, bend, or remove needles by hand. Use mechanical means (forceps) or a 1-handed method.
- Never shear or break needles.
- Discard needles and sharp instruments (such as razors) in containers that are closable, puncture-resistant, and leak-proof. Containers are color-coded in red and have the *BIOHAZARD* symbol. Containers must be upright and not allowed to over-fill.

Personal Protective Equipment (PPE)

This includes gloves, goggles, face shields, masks, laboratory coats, gowns, shoe covers, and surgical caps. Blood or OPIM must not pass through them. They protect your clothes, undergarments, skin, eyes, mouth, and hair.

PPE is free to staff. OSHA requires these measures for PPE.

- Remove PPE before leaving the work area.
- Remove PPE when a garment becomes contaminated.
- Place used PPE in marked areas or containers when being stored, washed, decontaminated, or discarded.
- Wear gloves when you expect contact with blood or OPIM.
- Wear gloves when handling or touching contaminated items or surfaces.
- Replace worn, punctured, or contaminated gloves.
- Never wash or decontaminate disposable gloves for re-use.
- Discard utility gloves with signs of cracking, peeling, tearing, or puncturing. Utility gloves are decontaminated for re-use if the process will not ruin them.

Equipment

Contaminated equipment is cleaned and decontaminated. Decontaminate work surfaces with a proper disinfectant.

- Upon completing tasks
- At once when there is obvious contamination
- After any spill of blood or OPIM
- At the end of your work shift when surfaces became contaminated since the last cleaning

Use a brush and dustpan or tongs to clean up broken glass. Never pick up broken glass with your hands, not even with gloves. Discard broken glass into a puncture-resistant container.

Laundry

OSHA requires these measures for contaminated laundry.

- Handle it as little as possible.
- Wear gloves or other needed PPE.
- Bag contaminated laundry where it is used.
- Mark laundry bags or containers with the *BIOHAZARD* symbol for laundry sent off-site.
- Place wet, contaminated laundry in leak-proof containers before transport. The containers are color-coded in red or have the *BIOHAZARD* symbol.

See *Focus on Surveys: Laundry.*

Exposure Incidents

An *exposure incident* is any eye, mouth, other mucous membrane, non-intact skin, or parenteral contact with blood or OPIM. *Parenteral* means piercing the mucous membranes or the skin. Piercing occurs by needle-sticks, human bites, cuts, and abrasions.

Report exposure incidents at once. Medical evaluation, follow-up, and required tests are free. Your blood is tested for HIV and HBV. If you refuse testing, the blood sample is kept for at least 90 days. Testing is done later if you change your mind.

You are told of any medical conditions that may need treatment. You receive a written opinion of the medical evaluation within 15 days after its completion.

The *source individual* is the person whose blood or body fluids are the source of an exposure incident. His or her blood is tested for HIV or HBV. The agency informs you about laws affecting the source's identity and test results.

FOCUS ON SURVEYS

Laundry

Surveyors will observe how staff handle, store, process, and transport linen. For example:

- Are linens handled in a way that prevents exposure of urine or feces?
- Do staff handle linens in a way that prevents the spread of infection?
- Do staff handle linens according to agency policies and procedures?
- Are linens stored and transported properly?

FOCUS ON PRIDE

The Person, Family, and Yourself

Personal and Professional Responsibility
Observing for signs and symptoms of infection is an important part of your role. Some persons are at greater risk than others. Burn, transplant, and chemotherapy patients are examples. Some persons do not respond to infection as expected. For example, an older person is confused with no other signs or symptoms. Report even small changes.

Rights and Respect
Caring for persons needing Transmission-Based Precautions can be a challenge. You need extra time to apply and remove PPE and clean equipment used in the room. You must plan carefully to gather supplies before entering the room. If you forget an item, you must wait for help or remove and re-apply PPE. You may feel frustrated.

The person must not feel that he or she is a burden. The person deserves the same kindness and respect you give others. You must:

- Watch your verbal and nonverbal communication (Chapter 6).
- Avoid complaining.
- Practice good teamwork and time management.
- Tell the nurse if you feel overwhelmed.

Independence and Social Interaction
Patients and residents often cannot perform hygiene measures they would normally do independently. Hand hygiene is an example. Ask patients and residents often if they would like to wash their hands. Assist them with hand washing before and after eating, after elimination, after coughing or sneezing, and any time their hands are dirty. Hand hygiene is important for you and for patients and residents. Always promote hand hygiene to protect the person and others.

Delegation and Teamwork
Caring for persons needing isolation precautions requires teamwork. Once in the room, staff cannot easily leave the room to answer call lights or obtain needed items. Willingly help your co-workers. Bring needed items to the room. Also, answer call lights for your co-workers. Report what you did and what you observed. Likewise, ask co-workers to help you. Ask politely and say "thank you." Good teamwork promotes positive working relationships and quality care. Take pride in working as a team.

Ethics and Laws
Your role in preventing the spread of infection is important. Your actions affect the person's risk for infection. Follow the guidelines in this chapter. Practice good hand hygiene before and after giving care. Follow Standard Precautions, Transmission-Based Precautions, and the Bloodborne Pathogen Standard.

When assisting with or performing a procedure, remove items that become contaminated. If necessary, stop and get new supplies. Do not use a contaminated item. You may be alone. Be honest with yourself. Be responsible. Do the right thing, even if other staff are not present. Take pride in providing care that prevents the spread of infection.

REVIEW QUESTIONS

Circle* T *if the statement is TRUE or* F *if it is FALSE.

1 **T F** A pathogen can cause an infection.

2 **T F** Confusion can be a sign of infection.

3 **T F** An item is sterile if non-pathogens are present.

4 **T F** You hold your hands and forearms up during hand washing.

5 **T F** Un-used items in the person's room are used for another person.

6 **T F** A person received the hepatitis B vaccine. The person will develop the disease.

7 **T F** Hand hygiene helps prevent healthcare-associated infections.

Circle the BEST answer.

8 Which area is *best* for a pathogen to live and grow?
 a A cold and wet area
 b A warm and dark area
 c A hot and bright area
 d A dry area without oxygen

9 You suspect infection when a person has
 a A bruise
 b A fever, pain, and redness in a body part
 c Warm, dry, and intact skin
 d A bleeding wound

10 To control a portal of exit
 a Cover the mouth and nose when coughing
 b Position drainage containers above the drainage site
 c Clean the genital area from the rectum to the urethra
 d Leave an open wound uncovered

11 Your hands are soiled with blood. What should you do?
 a Wash your hands with soap and water.
 b Use an alcohol-based hand rub.
 c Rinse your hands.
 d Tell the nurse.

12 You move from a contaminated body site to a clean body site. Your hands are not visibly soiled. What should you do?
 a Change your gloves.
 b Practice hand hygiene.
 c Rinse your hands.
 d Continue care without hand hygiene.

13 To use an alcohol-based hand rub correctly
 a Wash your hands before applying the hand rub
 b Rinse your hands after applying the hand rub
 c Rub the product only on the palms of your hands
 d Rub your hands together until your hands are dry

14 When cleaning equipment
 a Rinse the item in hot water before cleaning
 b Wash the item with soap and cold water
 c Use a brush if necessary
 d Work from dirty to clean areas

15 Standard Precautions
 a Are used for all persons
 b Prevent the spread of pathogens through the air
 c Require gowns, masks, gloves, and goggles
 d Require a doctor's order

16 A mask
 a Can be re-used
 b Is clean on the outside
 c Is contaminated when moist
 d Should fit loosely for breathing

17 To use PPE correctly
 a Never change gloves in the person's room
 b Tie a gown's waist strings in front
 c Don gloves first when applying PPE
 d Apply new PPE for each person

18 Which task requires gloves?
 a Applying wrist restraints
 b Giving a back massage
 c Providing denture care
 d Moving the person up in bed

19 Contaminated surfaces are cleaned at the following times *except*
 a After completing a task
 b When there is obvious contamination
 c After blood is spilled
 d After removing gloves

20 According to the Bloodborne Pathogen Standard, you should
 a Practice hand hygiene after removing gloves
 b Discard a used razor in a wastebasket
 c Tell the nurse about exposure to blood before washing your hands
 d Re-cap used needles by hand

Answers to these questions are on p. 504.

FOCUS ON PRACTICE

Problem Solving

A nurse enters the room of a person who requires Contact Precautions. The nurse is not wearing PPE. What do you do? What PPE is needed? What precautions are needed upon entering and leaving the room and while in the room?

Body Mechanics

CHAPTER 13

OBJECTIVES

- Define the key terms and key abbreviations listed in this chapter.
- Explain the purpose and rules of body mechanics.
- Explain how ergonomics can prevent work-related injuries.
- Identify the causes, signs, and symptoms of back injuries.
- Position persons in the basic bed positions and in a chair.
- Explain how to promote PRIDE in the person, the family, and yourself.

KEY TERMS

base of support The area on which an object rests
body alignment The way the head, trunk, arms, and legs are aligned with one another; posture
body mechanics Using the body in an efficient and careful way
dorsal recumbent position The back-lying or supine position
ergonomics The science of designing a job to fit the worker
Fowler's position A semi-sitting position; the head of the bed is raised between 45 and 60 degrees
lateral position The person lies on 1 side or the other; side-lying position
posture See "body alignment"
prone position Lying on the abdomen with the head turned to 1 side
semi-prone side position See "Sims' position"
side-lying position See "lateral position"
Sims' position A left side-lying position in which the upper leg (right leg) is sharply flexed so it is not on the lower leg (left leg) and the lower arm (left arm) is behind the person; semi-prone side position
supine position The back-lying or dorsal recumbent position

KEY ABBREVIATIONS

MSD Musculo-skeletal disorder
OSHA Occupational Safety and Health Administration

Body mechanics means using the body in an efficient and careful way. It involves good posture, balance, and using your strongest and largest muscles for work. Fatigue, muscle strain, and injury can result from the improper use and positioning of the body during activity or rest.

PRINCIPLES OF BODY MECHANICS

Body alignment (posture) is the way the head, trunk, arms, and legs are aligned with one another. Good alignment lets the body move and function with strength and efficiency. Standing, sitting, and lying down require good alignment.

Base of support is the area on which an object rests. A good base of support is needed for balance (Fig. 13-1, p. 162). When standing, your feet are your base of support. Stand with your feet apart for a wider base of support and more balance.

Your strongest and largest muscles are in the shoulders, upper arms, hips, and thighs. Use these muscles to handle and move persons and heavy objects. Otherwise, you place strain and exertion on the smaller and weaker muscles. This causes fatigue and injury. *Back injuries are a major risk.* For good body mechanics:

- Bend your knees and squat to lift a heavy object (Fig. 13-2, p. 162). Do not bend from your waist. Bending from your waist places strain on small back muscles.
- Hold items close to your body and base of support (see Fig. 13-2). This involves upper arm and shoulder muscles. Holding objects away from your body places strain on small muscles in your lower arms.

All activities require good body mechanics. Follow the rules in Box 13-1, p. 162.

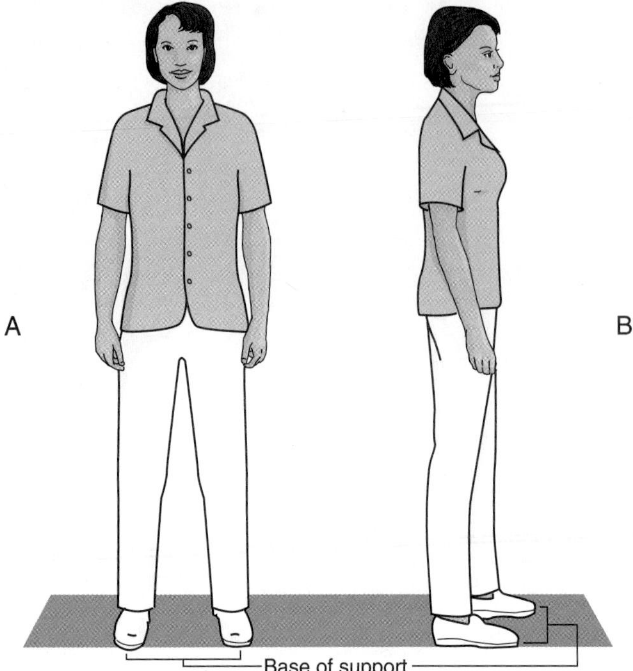

FIGURE 13-1 A, Anterior (front) view of an adult in good body alignment. The feet are apart for a wide base of support. **B,** Lateral (side) view of an adult with good posture and alignment.

BOX 13-1 Body Mechanics

- Keep your body in good alignment with a wide base of support.
- Use an upright posture. Bend your legs. Do not bend your back.
- Use the stronger and larger muscles in your shoulders, upper arms, thighs, and hips.
- Keep objects close to your body to lift, move, or carry them (see Fig. 13-2).
- Avoid unnecessary bending and reaching. Raise the bed and over-bed table to waist level.
- Face your work area. This prevents unnecessary twisting.
- Push, slide, or pull heavy objects when you can rather than lifting them. Pushing is easier than pulling.
- Widen your base of support to push or pull. Move your front leg forward when pushing. Move your rear leg back when pulling (Fig. 13-3).
- Use both hands and arms to lift, move, or carry objects.
- Turn your whole body to change direction instead of twisting your body.
- Work with smooth, even movements. Avoid sudden or jerky motions.
- Do not lean over a person to give care.
- *Get help from a co-worker to move heavy objects. Do not lift or move them by yourself.*
- Bend your hips and knees to lift heavy objects from the floor (see Fig. 13-2). Straighten your back as the object reaches thigh level. Your leg and thigh muscles work to raise the item off the floor and to waist level.
- Do not lift objects higher than chest level. Do not lift above your shoulders. Use a step stool or ladder to reach an object higher than chest level.

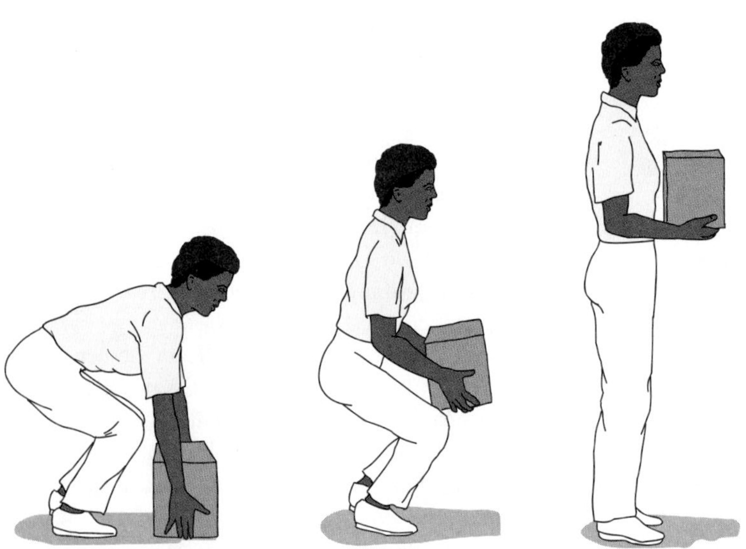

FIGURE 13-2 Picking up a box using good body mechanics.

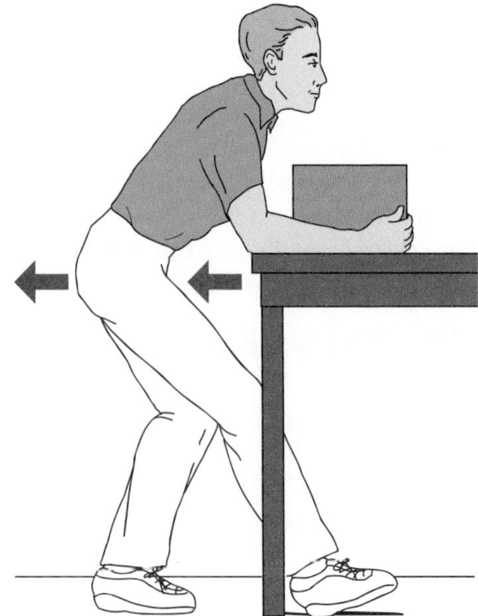

FIGURE 13-3 Move your rear leg back when pulling an item.

ERGONOMICS

***Ergonomics** is the science of designing a job to fit the worker.* (*Ergo* means *work. Nomos* means *law.*) It involves changing the task, work station, equipment, and tools to help reduce stress on the worker's body. The goal is to prevent a serious, painful, and disabling work-related musculo-skeletal disorder (MSD).

Work-Related MSDs

MSDs are injuries and disorders of the muscles, tendons, ligaments, joints, and cartilage. They can involve the nervous system. The arms and back are often affected. So are the hands, fingers, neck, wrists, legs, and shoulders. MSDs can develop slowly over weeks, months, and years. Or they can occur from 1 event. Pain, numbness, tingling, stiff joints, difficulty moving, and muscle loss can occur. So can paralysis.

Early signs and symptoms include pain, limited joint movement, or soft tissue swelling. Always report a work-related injury as soon as possible. Early attention can help prevent the problem from becoming worse. In later stages, the problem can become more serious and harder and more costly to treat.

The Occupational Safety and Health Administration (OSHA) has identified risk factors for MSDs. An MSD is more likely if risk factors are combined. For example, a task involves both force and repeating actions.

- *Force*—the amount of physical effort needed for a task. Lifting or transferring heavy persons, preventing falls, and sudden motions are examples.
- *Repeating action*—doing the same motion or series of motions often or continually. Re-positioning persons and transfers to and from beds, chairs, and commodes without adequate rest breaks are examples.
- *Awkward postures*—assuming positions that place stress on the body. Examples are reaching above shoulder height, kneeling, squatting, leaning over a bed, bending, or twisting the torso while lifting.
- *Heavy lifting*—manually lifting people who cannot move themselves.

See *Promoting Safety and Comfort: Ergonomics.*

PROMOTING SAFETY AND COMFORT

Ergonomics

Safety

Back injuries can occur from repeated activities or from 1 event. Use good body mechanics to protect yourself from injury. Do not work alone. Avoid lifting when possible. Have a co-worker help you handle, move, or transfer a person. Follow the rules in Box 13-1. Signs and symptoms of a back injury include:

- Pain when trying to assume a normal posture
- Decreased mobility
- Pain when standing or rising from a seated position

POSITIONING THE PERSON

The person must always be properly positioned. Regular position changes and good alignment promote comfort and well-being. Breathing is easier. Circulation is promoted. Pressure ulcers (Chapter 25) and contractures (Chapter 23) are prevented. A *contracture* is the lack of joint mobility caused by abnormal shortening of a muscle.

Whether in bed or chair, the person is re-positioned at least every 2 hours. Some people are re-positioned more often. Follow the nurse's instructions and the care plan. To safely position a person:

- Use good body mechanics.
- Ask a co-worker to help you if needed.
- Explain the procedure to the person.
- Be gentle when moving the person.
- Provide for privacy.
- Use pillows as directed by the nurse for support and alignment.
- Provide for comfort after positioning. (See the inside of the front cover.)
- Place the call light and needed items within reach after positioning.
- Complete a safety check before leaving the room. (See the inside of the front cover.)

See *Focus on Communication: Positioning the Person.*

See *Delegation Guidelines: Positioning the Person*, p. 164.

See *Promoting Safety and Comfort: Positioning the Person*, p. 164.

FOCUS ON COMMUNICATION

Positioning the Person

Moving can be painful. Some older persons have painful joints. Pain is common after surgery or an injury. Avoid causing pain when positioning the person. Tell the person what you are going to do before and during the procedure. Move the person slowly and gently. Give the person time to tell you if a movement is painful. Make sure the person is comfortable. You can say:

- "Am I hurting you?"
- "Please tell me if I'm moving you too fast."
- "Please tell me if you feel pain or discomfort."
- "Do you need a pillow adjusted?"
- "Are you comfortable?"
- "How can I help make you more comfortable?"

DELEGATION GUIDELINES

Positioning the Person

Many delegated tasks involve positioning and re-positioning. You need this information from the nurse and the care plan:

- Position or positioning limits ordered by the doctor
- How often to turn and re-position the person
- How many staff members need to help you
- What assist devices to use (Chapter 14)
- What skin care measures to perform (Chapter 16)
- What range-of-motion exercises to perform (Chapter 23)
- Where to place pillows
- What positioning devices are needed and how to use them (Chapter 23)
- What observations to report and record
- When to report observations
- What patient or resident concerns to report at once

PROMOTING SAFETY AND COMFORT

Positioning the Person

Safety

Pressure ulcers (Chapter 25) are serious threats from lying or sitting too long in 1 place. Wet, soiled, and wrinkled linens are other causes. When you re-position a person, make sure linens are clean, dry, and wrinkle-free. Change or straighten linens as needed.

Contractures can develop from staying in 1 position too long (Chapter 23). Re-positioning, exercise, and activity help prevent contractures.

Comfort

Pillows and positioning devices support body parts and keep the person in good alignment. This promotes comfort. Place pillows and positioning devices as directed by the nurse and the care plan.

Older persons may have limited range of motion in their necks. Usually the prone and Sims' positions are not comfortable for them. Check with the nurse before placing any older person in the prone or Sims' position.

Fowler's Position

***Fowler's position** is a semi-sitting position. The head of the bed is raised between 45 and 60 degrees* (Fig. 13-4). The knees may be slightly elevated. For good alignment:

- The spine is straight.
- The head is supported with a small pillow.
- The arms are supported with pillows.

The nurse may have you place small pillows under the lower back, thighs, and ankles. Persons with heart and respiratory disorders usually breathe easier in Fowler's position.

Supine Position

The ***supine position (dorsal recumbent position)** is the back-lying position* (Fig. 13-5). For good alignment:

- The bed is flat.
- The head and shoulders are supported on a pillow.
- Arms and hands are at the sides. You can support the arms with regular pillows. Or you can support the hands on small pillows with the palms down.

The nurse may have you place a folded or rolled towel under the lower back and a small pillow under the thighs. A pillow under the lower legs lifts the heels off of the bed. This prevents them from rubbing on the sheets.

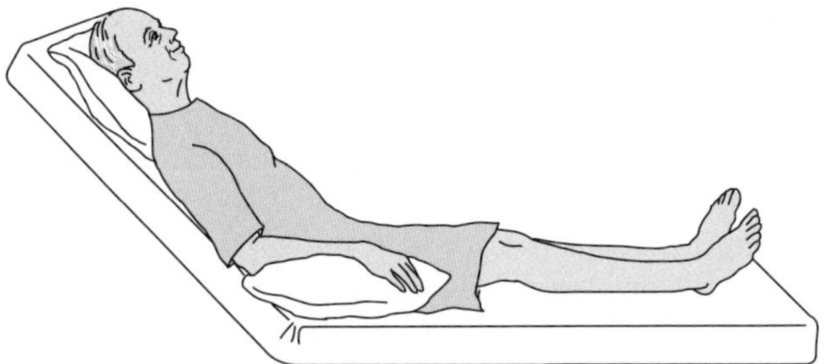

FIGURE 13-4 Fowler's position.

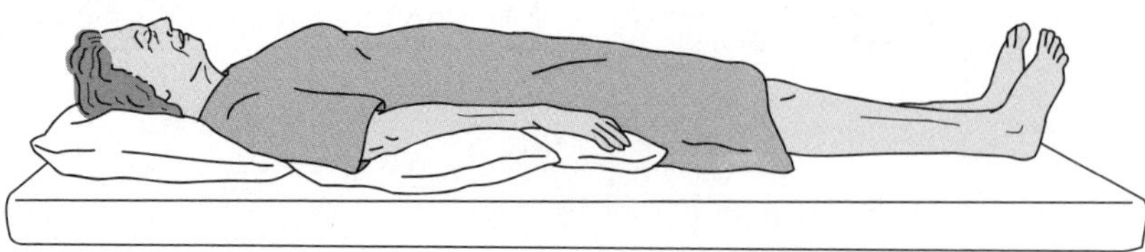

FIGURE 13-5 Supine position.

Prone Position

In the ***prone position,*** *the person lies on the abdomen with the head turned to 1 side.* For good alignment:

- The bed is flat.
- Small pillows are placed under the head, abdomen, and lower legs (Fig. 13-6).
- Arms are flexed at the elbows with the hands near the head.

You also can position a person with the feet hanging over the end of the mattress (Fig. 13-7). A pillow is not needed under the feet.

Lateral Position

In the ***lateral position (side-lying position),*** *the person lies on 1 side or the other* (Fig. 13-8).

- The bed is flat.
- A pillow is under the head and neck.
- The upper leg is in front of the lower leg. (The nurse may ask you to position the upper leg behind the lower leg, not on top of it.)
- The ankle, upper leg, and thigh are supported with pillows.
- A small pillow is positioned against the person's back. The person rolls back against the pillow so that his or her back is at a 45-degree angle with the mattress.
- A small pillow is under the upper hand and arm.

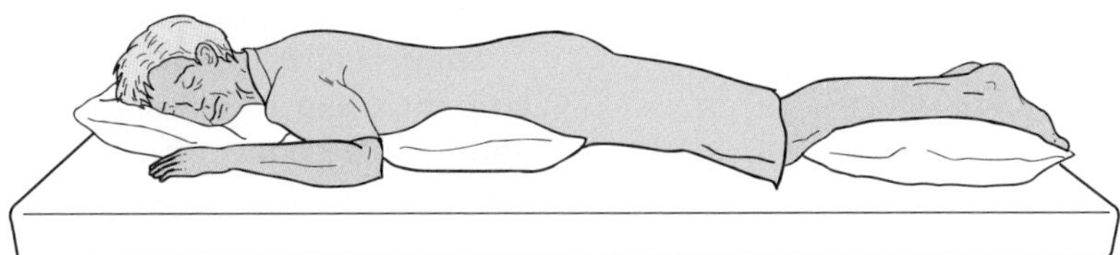

FIGURE 13-6 Prone position.

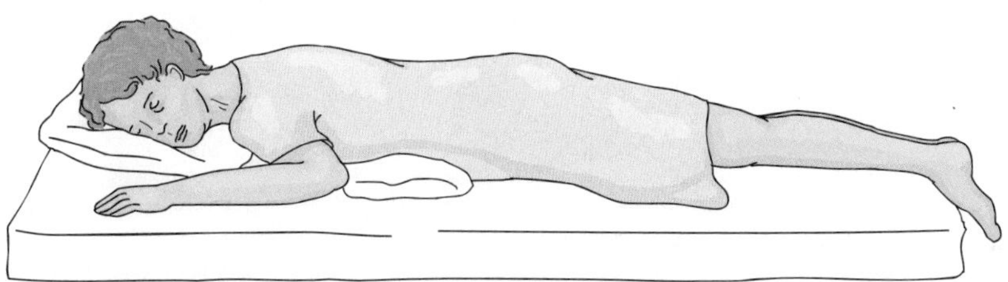

FIGURE 13-7 Prone position with the feet hanging over the edge of the mattress.

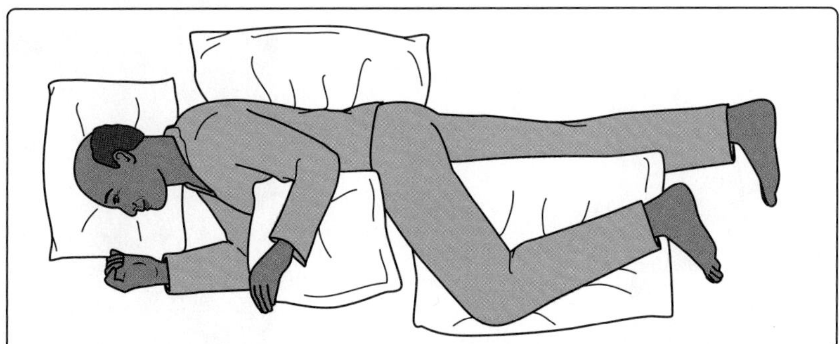

FIGURE 13-8 Lateral position.

Sims' Position

The ***Sims' position (semi-prone side position)*** *is a left side-lying position. The upper leg (right leg) is sharply flexed so it is not on the lower leg (left leg). The lower arm (left arm) is behind the person* (Fig. 13-9). For good alignment:

- The bed is flat.
- A pillow is under the person's head and shoulder.
- The upper leg (right leg) is supported with a pillow.
- A pillow is under the upper arm (right arm) and hand (right hand).

Chair Position

Persons who sit in chairs must hold their upper bodies and heads erect. If not, poor alignment results. For good alignment:

- The person's back and buttocks are against the back of the chair.
- Feet are flat on the floor or wheelchair footplates. Never leave feet unsupported.
- Backs of the knees and calves are slightly away from the edge of the seat (Fig. 13-10).

The nurse may have you put a small pillow between the person's lower back and the chair. This supports the lower back. *Remember, a pillow is not used behind the back if restraints are used* (Chapter 11).

Paralyzed arms are supported on pillows. Some persons have positioners (Fig. 13-11). Ask the nurse about their proper use. The nurse may have you position the wrists at a slight upward angle.

Some people require postural supports if they cannot keep their upper bodies erect (Fig. 13-12). Postural supports help keep them in good alignment. The health team selects the best product for the person's needs. The person's safety, dignity, and function are considered.

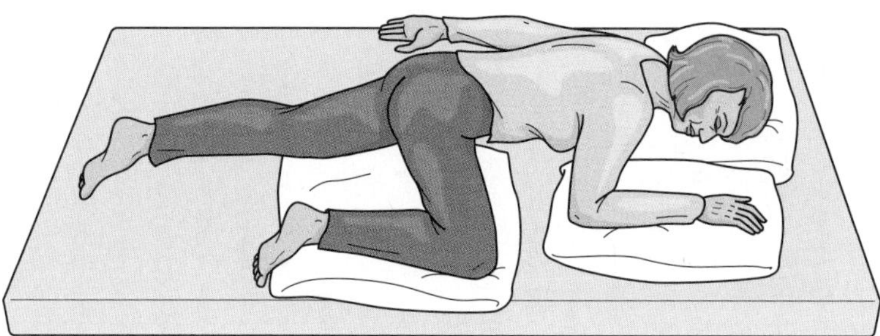

FIGURE 13-9 Sims' position.

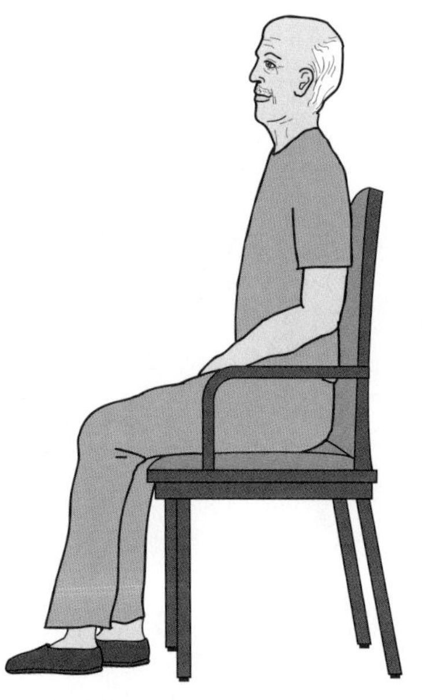

FIGURE 13-10 Chair position.

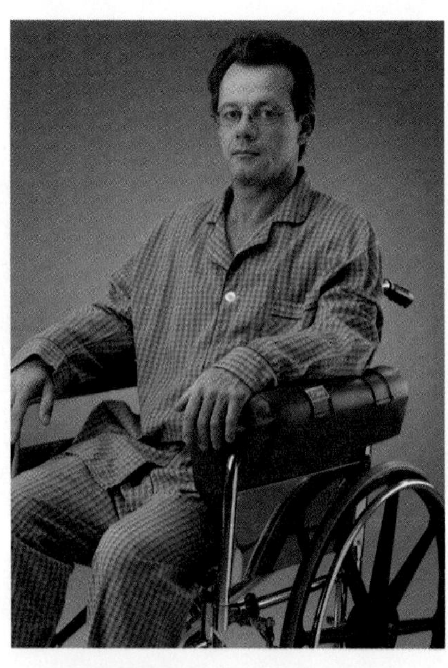

FIGURE 13-11 Elevated armrest.

A

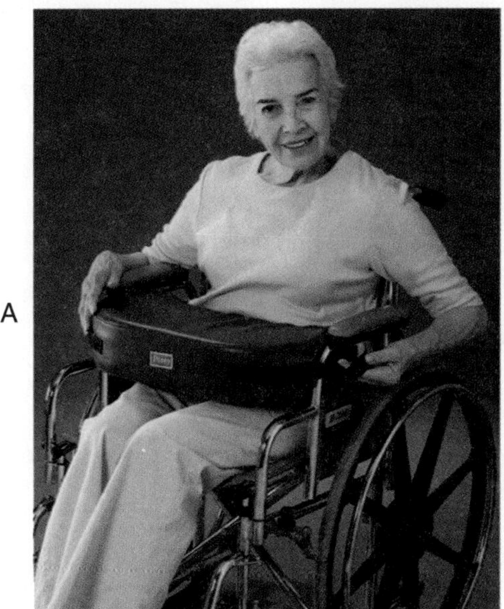

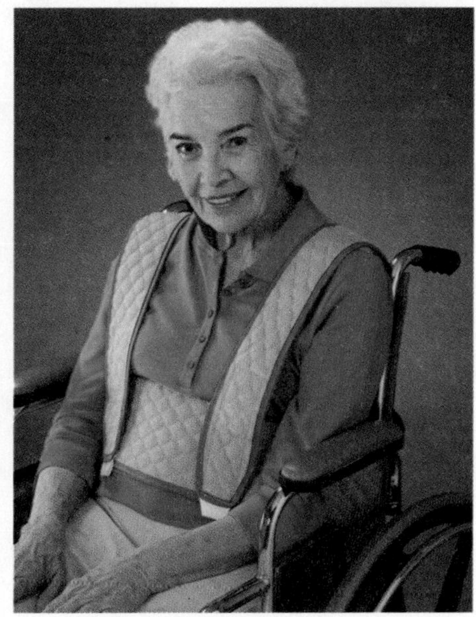

B

FIGURE 13-12 Postural supports. **A,** Posey Hugger. **B,** Torso support.

FOCUS ON PRIDE

The Person, Family, and Yourself

Personal and Professional Responsibility

Moving persons causes strain on your body. Injuries can occur. Some factors increase your risk for injury. For example:

- Poor physical condition—lacking the strength or endurance to perform tasks
- Fatigue
- Poor posture when sitting or standing
- Poor body mechanics when lifting, pushing, pulling, or carrying objects
- Repeated lifting of patients and residents or repeated lifting of awkward items or equipment
- Twisting or bending to lift
- Maintaining a bent posture
- Reaching over raised bed rails
- Lifting or moving an object or person alone

Protect yourself from injury. Avoid the factors listed above. Follow the rules for body mechanics in Box 13-1. Use good judgment to re-position and transfer patients and residents (Chapter 14). Ask for help when needed. Take responsibility for protecting yourself from harm.

Rights and Respect

OSHA requires a safe work setting. You have the right to ask employers about safety plans to reduce your risk of injury. Ask about training or orientation programs that focus on body mechanics, safe handling of persons, and workplace hazards. Know and follow agency procedures to report problems.

Independence and Social Interaction

Remaining independent to the extent possible promotes dignity, self-esteem, and pride. Let the person choose bed or chair positioning as allowed by the nurse and the care plan. Let the person help as much as safely possible. Talk with the person while moving him or her. Ask what he or she prefers. Doing so promotes comfort, independence, and social interaction.

Delegation and Teamwork

Moving and positioning are safer when done by 2 or more workers. This is very important for bariatric persons. You may need 3, 4, or more co-workers to safely move such persons. Or special equipment may be needed. Follow the person's care plan.

Never try to move a person without enough help. You can harm yourself, your co-workers, and the person. Work as a team to protect yourself and others from injury.

Ethics and Laws

Proper body mechanics help prevent injuries that could affect health and function. Failure to move and position the person correctly places the person at risk. For example:

- A person is left slumped in a chair for 3 hours. The person develops a pressure ulcer.
- A person is not re-positioned according to the care plan. The person's contracture worsens.
- A person is moved without enough help. The move is rough. The person is injured.

You must provide care in a manner that maintains or improves each person's quality of life, health, and safety. It is the right thing to do.

REVIEW QUESTIONS

Circle the BEST answer.

1 Good body mechanics involve
   a Having an upright posture
   b Having a narrow base of support
   c Using the muscles in the back and lower arms
   d Lifting a heavy object alone

2 Good alignment means
   a The area on which an object rests
   b Having the head, trunk, arms, and legs aligned with one another
   c Using muscles, tendons, ligaments, and joints correctly
   d The back-lying or supine position

3 Which action shows poor body mechanics?
   a Holding an object close to your body
   b Facing the direction you are working to prevent twisting
   c Leaning over a raised bed rail to give care
   d Using both hands and arms to lift an object

4 You need to move a large chair in a resident's room. You should
   a Push or slide the chair
   b Lift and carry the chair
   c Ask the nurse to move the chair for you
   d Pull the chair using quick jerking motions

5 The purpose of ergonomics is to
   a Reduce stress on the worker's body
   b Safely position a person
   c Promote quality of life
   d Use good body mechanics

6 Risk factors for MSDs include the following *except*
   a Repeating actions
   b Awkward postures
   c Bending your hips and knees
   d Force

7 You position a resident in the lateral position. Where do you place the call light?
   a At the head or foot of the bed
   b On either side of the bed
   c On the side of the bed facing the person's back side
   d On the side of the bed facing the person's front side

8 Patients and residents are re-positioned at least every
   a 15 minutes
   b 30 minutes
   c 2 hours
   d 3 hours

9 The back-lying position is called
   a Fowler's position
   b The supine position
   c The lateral position
   d Sims' position

10 For Fowler's position
   a The bed is flat
   b The head of the bed is raised 45 to 60 degrees
   c The person's head is turned to 1 side
   d The person's feet hang over the edge of the mattress

11 A pillow is placed against the person's back in
   a Fowler's position
   b The prone position
   c The lateral position
   d Sims' position

12 When in a chair, the person's feet
   a Must be flat on the floor
   b Are positioned on footplates
   c Dangle
   d Are positioned on pillows

Answers to these questions are on p. 504.

FOCUS ON PRACTICE

Problem Solving

You are giving Mr. Boyd a complete bed bath. He is in the supine position. He begins having trouble breathing. What do you do? What position will help him breathe easier? When will you tell the nurse? What will you report?

CHAPTER 14

Assisting With Moving and Transfers

OBJECTIVES

- Define the key terms and key abbreviations listed in this chapter.
- Identify comfort and safety measures for moving and transferring the person.
- Explain how to prevent work-related injuries when moving and transferring persons.
- Describe 5 levels of dependence.
- Identify the delegation information needed before moving and transferring the person.
- Perform the procedures described in this chapter.
- Explain how to promote PRIDE in the person, the family, and yourself.

KEY TERMS

friction The rubbing of 1 surface against another

logrolling Turning the person as a unit, in alignment, with 1 motion

shearing When skin sticks to a surface while muscles slide in the direction the body is moving

transfer How a person moves to and from surfaces—bed, chair, wheelchair, toilet, or standing position

KEY ABBREVIATIONS

ID Identification

OSHA Occupational Safety and Health Administration

You will turn and re-position persons often. You move them in bed. You assist with transfers. A *transfer is how a person moves to and from surfaces—bed, chair, wheelchair, toilet, or standing position.* You must use your body correctly to protect yourself and the person from injury.

See *Focus on Communication: Assisting With Moving and Transfers.*

See *Promoting Safety and Comfort: Assisting With Moving and Transfers,* p. 170.

FOCUS ON COMMUNICATION

Assisting With Moving and Transfers

Moving and transfers can be painful after an injury or surgery. Many older persons have painful joints. Provide for comfort and avoid causing pain. You can say:

- "Am I hurting you?"
- "Please tell me when you feel pain or discomfort."
- "Do you need a pillow adjusted?"
- "Are you comfortable?"
- "How can I make you more comfortable?"

Before any move or transfer, explain the procedure. Tell the person what you and your co-workers will do. Also explain what the person needs to do. Do so as you begin the procedure. Also, remind the person just before the move.

The procedures in this chapter explain how to move the person "on the count of 3." Staff move the person at the same time. The person is moved smoothly. One co-worker leads by counting. Decide who will count before the move. Be sure the person and staff know who is leading and what to do. You can say:

We will move you up in bed. I will count "1, 2, 3." When I say "3," you need to push against the bed with your feet and pull up on the trapeze. We will help move your body.

PROMOTING SAFETY AND COMFORT

Assisting With Moving and Transfers

Safety

Many older persons have fragile bones and joints. To prevent injuries:

- Follow the rules of body mechanics (Chapter 13).
- Always have help to move a person.
- Move the person carefully to prevent injury or pain.
- Keep the person in good alignment.
- Position the person in good alignment after the procedure.
- Make sure the face, nose, and mouth are not obstructed by a pillow or other device.

Comfort

To promote mental comfort when moving or transferring the person:

- Explain what you are going to do and how the person can help.
- Screen and cover the person to protect the right to privacy.

To promote physical comfort:

- Keep the person in good alignment.
- Do not let the person's head hit the head-board when he or she is moved up in bed. If the person can be without a pillow, place it upright against the head-board.
- Use pillows to position the person as directed by the nurse and the care plan. If a pillow is allowed under the person's head, position it under the head and shoulders.
- Use other positioning devices as directed by the nurse and the care plan.

PREVENTING WORK-RELATED INJURIES

You must prevent work-related injuries during moving and transfer procedures. Follow the rules in Box 14-1. The Occupational Safety and Health Administration (OSHA) recommends:

- Minimizing manual lifting in all cases.
- Eliminating manual lifting when possible.

To safely move and transfer the person, the nurse and health team determine:

- The person's dependence level. See Box 14-2, p. 172.
- The amount of help needed and the number of staff needed.
- What procedure to use.
- The equipment needed.

See *Focus on Older Persons: Preventing Work-Related Injuries*, p. 173.

See *Delegation Guidelines: Preventing Work-Related Injuries*, p. 173.

See *Promoting Safety and Comfort: Preventing Work-Related Injuries*, p. 173.

BOX 14-1 Preventing Work-Related Injuries

General Guidelines

- Practice good body mechanics (Chapter 13).
- Wear shoes with good traction. Avoid shoes with worn-down soles.
- Use assist equipment and devices when possible. Follow the care plan.
- Get help from other staff. The nurse and care plan tell you the number of staff needed for a task.
- Plan and prepare for the task. For example, know what equipment is needed, where to place chairs or wheelchairs, and what side of the bed to work on.
- Schedule harder tasks early in your shift.
- Balance lighter and harder tasks. Plan so you complete a lighter task after a harder one.
- Lock bed wheels and wheelchair or stretcher wheels.

General Guidelines—cont'd

- Tell the person how he or she can help. Give clear, simple instructions. Give the person time to respond.
- Do not hold or grab the person under the underarms.
- Do not let the person hold or grasp you around your neck.

Manual Lifting

- Use good mechanics.
  - Stand with good posture. Keep your back straight.
  - Bend your legs, not your back.
  - Use your legs to do the work.
  - Face the person.
  - Do not twist or turn. Pick up your feet, and pivot your whole body in the direction of the move.

Modified from Cal/OSHA: A back injury prevention guide for health care providers, *Sacramento, Calif, 1997, Author; and referenced in Occupational Safety and Health Administration:* Ergonomics: guidelines for nursing homes, *Washington, DC, 2009, Author.*

BOX 14-1 Preventing Work-Related Injuries—cont'd

Manual Lifting—cont'd

- Keep what you are moving close to you—the person, equipment, or supplies.
- Move the person toward you, not away from you.
- Use slides and lateral transfers instead of manual lifting.
- Use a wide, balanced base of support. Stand with 1 foot slightly ahead of the other.
- Lower the person slowly by bending your legs. Do not bend your back. Return to an erect position as soon as possible.
- Use smooth, even movements. Avoid jerking movements.
- Lift on the "count of 3" when lifting with others. Everyone lifts at the same time.

Lateral Transfers

- Position surfaces close to each other (bed and stretcher).
- Adjust surfaces to about waist height. Do 1 of the following as directed by the nurse and care plan.
  - Adjust the surfaces to the same level.
  - Adjust the receiving surface so it is slightly lower (about 1/2 inch) than the surface the person is on. This allows the use of gravity. For example: for a bed to stretcher transfer, the stretcher surface is lower than the bed.
- Lower bed rails and stretcher side rails.
- Use drawsheets (Chapter 15), turning pads (p. 176), or large waterproof pads (Chapter 15). Other friction-reducing devices include sliding boards, slide sheets, and low-friction mattress covers.
- Get a good hand-hold. Roll up drawsheets, turning pads, and large waterproof pads. Or use assist devices with handles.
- Kneel on the bed or stretcher. This prevents extended reaches and bending your back.
- Have staff on both sides of the bed or other surface. Move the person on the "count of 3." Use a smooth, push-pull motion. Do not reach across the person.

Transfer Belts

- Keep the person as close to you as possible.
- Avoid bending, reaching, or twisting to:
  - Apply or remove a belt.
  - Lower the person to the chair, bed, toilet, or floor.
  - Help the person walk.
- Use a gentle rocking motion to help the person stand. The rocking motion gives strength and force as you pull the person to the standing position.
- See Chapter 10.

Stand and Pivot Transfers

- Use assist devices as directed. Follow the care plan.
- Use a transfer belt with handles.
- Keep your feet at least shoulder-width apart.
- Lower the bed so the person can place his or her feet on the floor.
- Plan the transfer so the person's strong side moves first.
- Get the person close to the edge of the bed or the chair. Ask the person to lean forward as he or she stands.
- Block the person's weak leg with your legs or knees. If the position is awkward:
  - Use a transfer belt with handles.
  - Straddle your legs around the person's weak leg.
- Bend your legs. Do not bend your back.
- Pivot with your feet to turn.
- Use a gentle rocking motion to help the person stand. The rocking motion gives strength and force as you pull the person to the standing position.

Lifting or Moving the Person in Bed

- Adjust the height of the bed, stretcher, or other surface to waist level.
- Lower the bed rail or the stretcher side rail.
- Work on the side where the person will be closest to you.
- Place equipment or other items close to you at waist level.
- Use drawsheets, turning pads, large waterproof pads, or slide sheets.

Transporting the Person and Equipment

- Push, do not pull.
- Keep the load close to your body.
- Use an upright posture.
- Push with your whole body, not just your arms.
- Move down the center of the hallway. This helps avoid collisions.
- Watch out for door handles and high floor thresholds. These can cause abrupt stops.

Transferring the Person From the Floor

- Use a mechanical lift if possible (p. 191). If not, place a sling, blanket, drawsheet, cot, or other assist device under the person as directed by the nurse.
- Position at least 2 staff members on each side of the person. More staff is needed if the person is large.
- Bend your knees, not your back. Do not twist.
- Roll the person onto his or her side to position the assist device. Do not reach across the person.
- Lower the hoist (for a mechanical lift) to attach the sling. The hoist is low enough to easily attach the sling.
- Do the following for a manual lift.
  - Kneel on 1 knee.
  - Grasp the blanket, drawsheet, cot, or other device.
  - Lift smoothly with your legs as you stand on the "count of 3." Do not bend your back.

BOX 14-2 Levels of Dependence

Level 4: Total Dependence. The person cannot help with the transfer. Staff perform the task or procedure.
- The person is lifted and transferred with a full-sling mechanical lift (Fig. 14-1).

Level 3: Extensive Assistance. The person can bear some weight, can sit up with help, and may be able to pivot to transfer.
- The person is lifted and transferred with a mechanical lift—full-sling mechanical lift or stand-assist lift (Fig. 14-2).

Level 2: Limited Assistance. The person is highly involved in the moving or transfer procedure. Some help is needed moving the legs. The person can stand (bear weight). The person has upper body strength and can sit up. He or she can pivot transfer.
- Stand-assist devices may be needed. Some attach to the bed or chair (Fig. 14-3). Others include walkers (Chapter 23) and transfer belts with handles (Chapter 10).
- Sliding boards are useful for transfers to and from beds and chairs (Fig. 14-4).

Level 1: Supervision. The staff need to look after, encourage, or remind the person what to do.
- The devices for Level 2 may be needed.

Level 0: Independent. The person walks without help. Sometimes the person needs limited assistance.
- Mechanical assistance is not normally required for transfers, lifting, or re-positioning.

Modified from Ergonomics Technical Advisory Group: Patient care ergonomics resource guide: safe patient handling and movement, revised August 31, 2005, Patient Safety Center of Inquiry (Tampa, Fla), Veterans Health Administration, and Department of Defense.

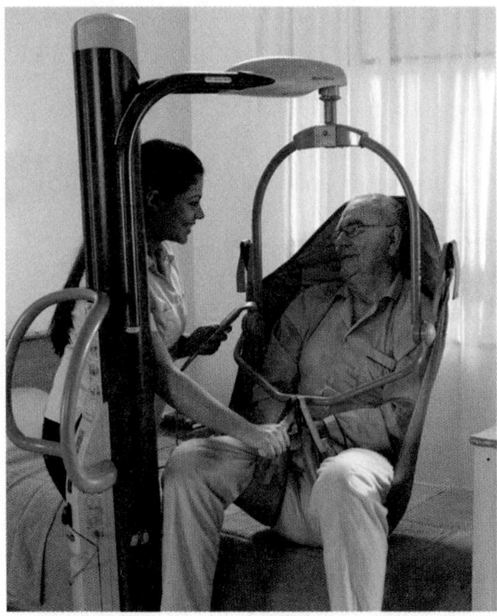

FIGURE 14-1 Full-sling mechanical lift.

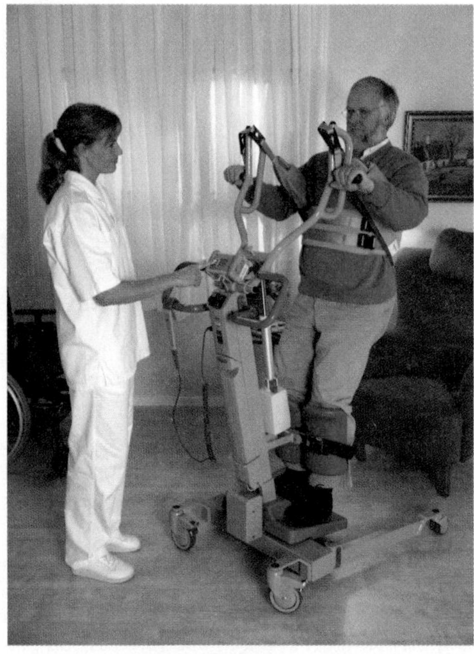

FIGURE 14-2 Stand-assist lift.

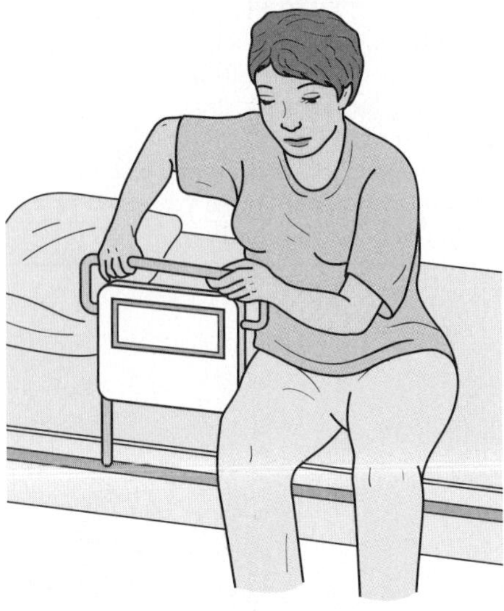

FIGURE 14-3 Stand-assist bed attachment.

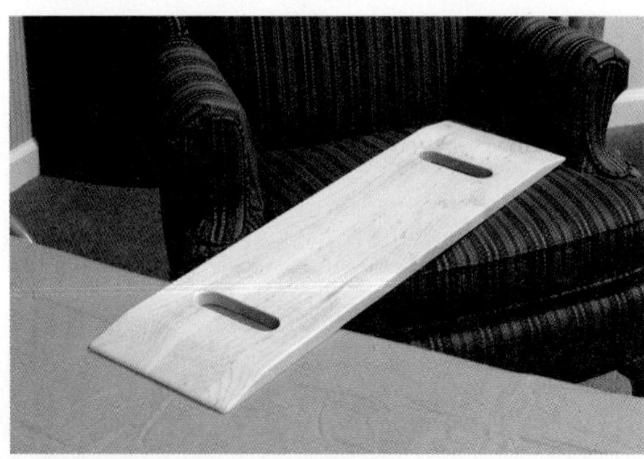

FIGURE 14-4 Sliding board for transferring to and from surfaces.

FOCUS ON OLDER PERSONS

Preventing Work-Related Injuries

Persons with dementia may not understand what you are doing. They may resist your moving and transfer efforts. The person may shout at you, grab you, or try to hit you. Always have a co-worker help you. Do not force the person. The person's care plan has measures for safe care. For example:

- Proceed slowly.
- Use a calm, pleasant voice.
- Divert the person's attention. For example, let the person hold a washcloth or other soft object. This helps distract the person and keeps the hands busy.

Tell the nurse at once if you have problems moving or transferring the person.

DELEGATION GUIDELINES

Preventing Work-Related Injuries

Many tasks involve moving and transferring persons. Before doing so, you need this information from the nurse and the care plan.

- The person's height and weight.
- The person's dependence level (see Box 14-2).
- The person's physical abilities. Can the person sit up, stand up, or walk without help? Does the person have strength in his or her arms?
- If the person has a weak side. If yes, which side?
- If the person has a medical condition that increases the risk of injury? Dizziness, confusion, hearing or vision problems, recent surgery, and fragile skin are examples.
- Any doctor's orders for moving or transferring the person.
- The person's ability to follow directions.
- If behavior problems are likely. Combative, agitated, uncooperative, and unpredictable behaviors are examples.
- The amount of assistance needed.
- The number of staff needed to complete the task safely.
- What procedure to use.
- What equipment to use.

PROMOTING SAFETY AND COMFORT

Preventing Work-Related Injuries

Safety

Decide how to move the person before starting the procedure. Ask needed staff to help before you begin. Also plan how to protect drainage tubes or containers connected to the person.

Beds are raised to move persons in bed (Chapter 15). This reduces bending and reaching. You must:

- Use the bed correctly.
- Protect the person from falling when the bed is raised.
- Follow the rules of body mechanics (Chapter 13).

PROTECTING THE SKIN

Protect the person's skin during moving and transfer procedures. Friction and shearing injure the skin. Both cause infection and pressure ulcers (Chapter 25).

- ***Friction*** *is the rubbing of 1 surface against another.* When moved in bed, the person's skin rubs against the sheet.
- ***Shearing*** *is when the skin sticks to a surface while muscles slide in the direction the body is moving* (Fig. 14-5). It occurs when the person slides down in bed or is moved in bed.

To reduce friction and shearing when moving the person in bed:

- Roll the person.
- Use friction-reducing devices. Such devices include a lift sheet (turning sheet). A cotton drawsheet (Chapter 15) serves as a lift sheet (turning sheet). Turning pads, large waterproof pads (Chapter 15), and slide sheets (p. 176) are other friction-reducing devices.

See *Focus on Older Persons: Protecting the Skin*, p. 174.
See *Focus on Surveys: Protecting the Skin*, p. 174.

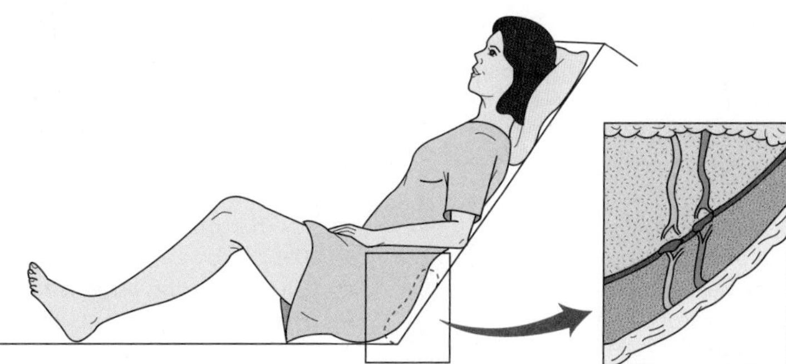

FIGURE 14-5 Shearing. When the head of the bed is raised to a sitting position, skin on the buttocks stays in place. However, internal structures move forward as the person slides down in bed. This pinches the skin between the mattress and the hip bones.

FOCUS ON OLDER PERSONS

Protecting the Skin

Older persons are at great risk for shearing. Their fragile skin is easily torn. Protect the skin from injury.

Ask a co-worker to help you move older persons. Use a friction-reducing device. Move older persons carefully and gently.

Persons with dementia may try to resist your efforts. Do not force the person. Work slowly. Use a calm voice. Divert the person's attention if necessary.

MOVING PERSONS IN BED

Some persons can move and turn in bed. Others need help from at least 1 person. Those who are weak, unconscious, paralyzed, or in casts need help. Sometimes 2 or 3 people or a mechanical lift is needed.

- *Level 4: Total Dependence*—a mechanical lift or friction-reducing device and at least 2 staff members
- *Level 3: Extensive Assistance*—a mechanical lift or friction-reducing device and at least 2 staff members
- *The person weighs less than 200 pounds*—2 to 3 staff members and a friction-reducing device
- *The person weighs more than 200 pounds*—at least 3 staff members and a friction-reducing device

  See *Delegation Guidelines: Moving Persons in Bed.*

DELEGATION GUIDELINES

Moving Persons in Bed

Before moving a person in bed, you need this information from the nurse and the care plan.

- What procedure to use
- The number of staff needed to safely move the person
- Position limits and restrictions
- How far you can lower the head of the bed
- Any limits in the person's ability to move or be re-positioned
- What pillows you can remove before moving the person
- What equipment is needed—trapeze, lift sheet, slide sheet, mechanical lift
- How to position the person
- If the person uses bed rails
- What observations to report and record:
  - Who helped you with the procedure
  - How much help the person needed
  - How the person tolerated the procedure
  - How you positioned the person
  - Complaints of pain or discomfort
- When to report observations
- What patient or resident concerns to report at once

FOCUS ON SURVEYS

Protecting the Skin

Shearing and friction can easily damage the skin. Surveyors will observe the measures taken by staff to prevent or reduce shearing and friction during transfers and re-positioning.

Moving the Person Up in Bed

When the head of the bed is raised, it is easy to slide down toward the middle and foot of the bed (Fig. 14-6). You move the person up in bed for good alignment and comfort.

You can sometimes move light-weight adults up in bed alone if they assist using a trapeze. However, it is best done with help and an assist device (p. 176). For heavy, weak, and older persons, 2 or more staff members are needed. Always protect the person and yourself from injury.

See *Promoting Safety and Comfort: Moving the Person Up in Bed.*

See procedure: *Moving the Person Up in Bed.*

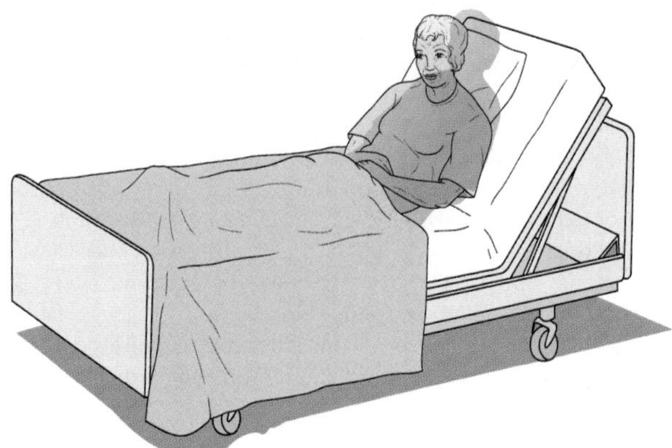

FIGURE 14-6 A person in poor alignment after sliding down in bed.

PROMOTING SAFETY AND COMFORT

Moving the Person Up in Bed

Safety

This procedure is best done with at least 2 staff members. Use an assist device as directed by the nurse and the care plan. Ask any questions before you begin the procedure.

Perform the procedure alone *only if:*

- The person is small in size.
- The person can follow directions.
- The person can assist with much of the moving.
- The person uses a trapeze.
- The person can push against the mattress with his or her feet.
- The nurse says it is safe to do so.
- You are comfortable doing so.

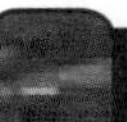

Moving the Person Up in Bed

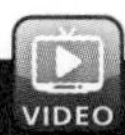

QUALITY OF LIFE

- Knock before entering the person's room.
- Address the person by name.
- Introduce yourself by name and title.
- Explain the procedure before starting and during the procedure.
- Protect the person's rights during the procedure.
- Handle the person gently during the procedure.

PRE-PROCEDURE

1 Follow *Delegation Guidelines:*
  a *Preventing Work-Related Injuries,* p. 173
  b *Moving Persons in Bed*
  See *Promoting Safety and Comfort:*
  a *Assisting With Moving and Transfers,* p. 170
  b *Preventing Work-Related Injuries,* p. 173
  c *Moving the Person Up in Bed*
2 Ask a co-worker to help you.
3 Practice hand hygiene.
4 Identify the person. Check the ID (identification) bracelet against the assignment sheet. Also call the person by name.
5 Provide for privacy.
6 Lock the bed wheels.
7 Raise the bed for body mechanics. Bed rails are up if used.

PROCEDURE

8 Lower the head of the bed to a level appropriate for the person. It is as flat as possible.
9 Stand on 1 side of the bed. Your co-worker stands on the other side.
10 Lower the bed rails if up.
11 Remove pillows as directed by the nurse. Place a pillow against the head-board if the person can be without it.
12 Stand with a wide base of support. Point the foot near the head of the bed toward the head of the bed. Face the head of the bed.
13 Bend your hips and knees. Keep your back straight.
14 Place 1 arm under the person's shoulder and 1 arm under the thighs. Your co-worker does the same. Grasp each other's forearms (Fig. 14-7).
15 Ask the person to grasp the trapeze.
16 Have the person flex both knees.
17 Explain that:
  a You will count "1, 2, 3."
  b The move will be on "3."
  c On "3," the person pushes against the bed with the feet if able. And the person pulls up with the trapeze.
18 Move the person to the head of the bed on the count of "3." Shift your weight from your rear leg to your front leg (see Fig. 14-7). Your co-worker does the same.
19 Repeat steps 12 through 18 if necessary.

POST-PROCEDURE

20 Put the pillow under the person's head and shoulders.
21 Position the person in good alignment. Raise the head of the bed to a level appropriate for the person.
22 Provide for comfort. (See the inside of the front cover.)
23 Place the call light and other needed items within reach.
24 Lower the bed to a safe and comfortable level appropriate for the person. Follow the care plan.
25 Raise or lower bed rails. Follow the care plan.
26 Unscreen the person.
27 Complete a safety check of the room. (See the inside of the front cover.)
28 Practice hand hygiene.
29 Report and record your observations.

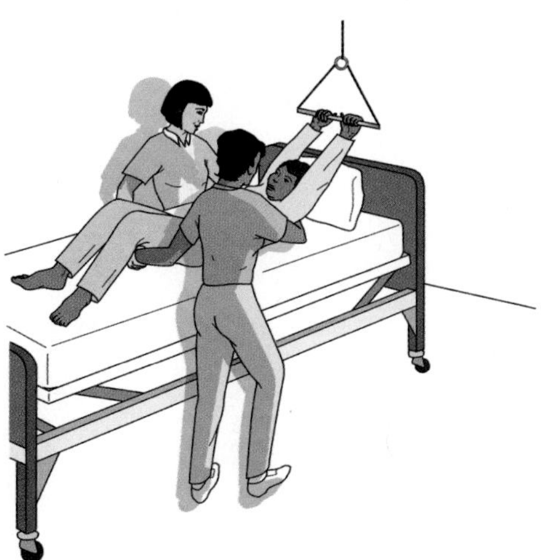

FIGURE 14-7 A person is moved up in bed by 2 nursing assistants. Each has 1 arm under the person's shoulders and the other under the thighs. They have locked arms under the person. The person grasps the trapeze and flexes the knees. The nursing assistants shift their weight from the rear leg to the front leg as the person is moved up in bed.

Moving the Person Up in Bed With an Assist Device

You use assist devices to move some persons up in bed. Such assist devices include a drawsheet (lift sheet), flat sheet folded in half, turning pad (Fig. 14-8), slide sheet (Fig. 14-9), and large waterproof pad. With these devices, the person is moved more evenly. And shearing and friction are reduced.

Place the device under the person from the head to above the knees or lower. At least 2 staff members are needed. This procedure is used for most patients and residents. It is used:

- Following the guidelines for "Moving Persons in Bed," p. 174
- For persons recovering from spinal cord surgery or spinal cord injuries
- For older persons

See *Promoting Safety and Comfort: Moving the Person Up in Bed With an Assist Device.*

See procedure: *Moving the Person Up in Bed With an Assist Device.*

PROMOTING SAFETY AND COMFORT

Moving the Person Up in Bed With an Assist Device

Safety

Not all waterproof pads are used as assist devices. Disposable, single-use underpads are not strong enough to hold the person's weight during the move. Re-usable underpads are stronger. For safety, the underpad must:

- Be strong enough to support the person's weight.
- Extend from under the person's head to above the knees or lower.
- Be wide enough for you and other staff to get a firm grip for the lift.

Ask the nurse if the person's underpad is safe as an assist device.

To use a slide sheet, place it under the person. See procedure: *Making an Occupied Bed* in Chapter 15 for this step. After the procedure, remove the slide sheet. Otherwise the person is in danger of sliding down in bed or off the bed.

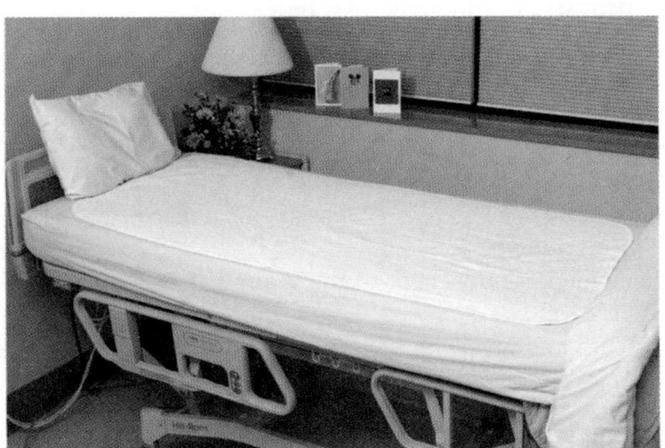

FIGURE 14-8 Turning pad.

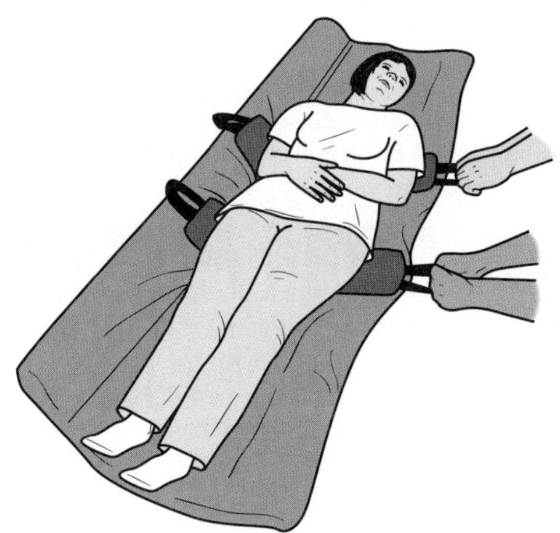

FIGURE 14-9 Slide sheet.

Moving the Person Up in Bed With an Assist Device

QUALITY OF LIFE

- Knock before entering the person's room.
- Address the person by name.
- Introduce yourself by name and title.
- Explain the procedure before starting and during the procedure.
- Protect the person's rights during the procedure.
- Handle the person gently during the procedure.

PRE-PROCEDURE

1 Follow *Delegation Guidelines:*
   a *Preventing Work-Related Injuries,* p. 173
   b *Moving Persons in Bed,* p. 174
   See *Promoting Safety and Comfort:*
   a *Assisting With Moving and Transfers,* p. 170
   b *Preventing Work-Related Injuries,* p. 173
   c *Moving the Person Up in Bed,* p. 174
   d *Moving the Person Up in Bed With an Assist Device*

2 Ask a co-worker to help you.
3 Practice hand hygiene.
4 Identify the person. Check the ID bracelet against the assignment sheet. Also call the person by name.
5 Provide for privacy.
6 Lock the bed wheels.
7 Raise the bed for body mechanics. Bed rails are up if used.

PROCEDURE

8 Lower the head of the bed to a level appropriate for the person. It is as flat as possible.
9 Stand on 1 side of the bed. Your co-worker stands on the other side.
10 Lower the bed rails if up.
11 Remove pillows as directed by the nurse. Place a pillow against the head-board if the person can be without it.
12 Stand with a wide base of support. Point the foot near the head of the bed toward the head of the bed. Face the head of the bed.
13 Roll the sides of the assist device up close to the person. (NOTE: Omit this step if the device has handles.)
14 Grasp the rolled-up assist device firmly near the person's shoulders and hips (Fig. 14-10). Or grasp it by the handles. Support the head.
15 Bend your hips and knees.
16 Move the person up in bed on the count of "3." Shift your weight from your rear leg to your front leg.
17 Repeat steps 12 through 16 if necessary.
18 Unroll the assist device. (NOTE: Omit this step if the device has handles.) Remove the slide sheet if used.

POST-PROCEDURE

19 Put the pillow under the person's head and shoulders.
20 Position the person in good alignment. Raise the head of the bed to a level appropriate for the person.
21 Provide for comfort. (See the inside of the front cover.)
22 Place the call light and other needed items within reach.
23 Lower the bed to a safe and comfortable level appropriate for the person. Follow the care plan.
24 Raise or lower bed rails. Follow the care plan.
25 Unscreen the person.
26 Complete a safety check of the room. (See the inside of the front cover.)
27 Practice hand hygiene.
28 Report and record your observations.

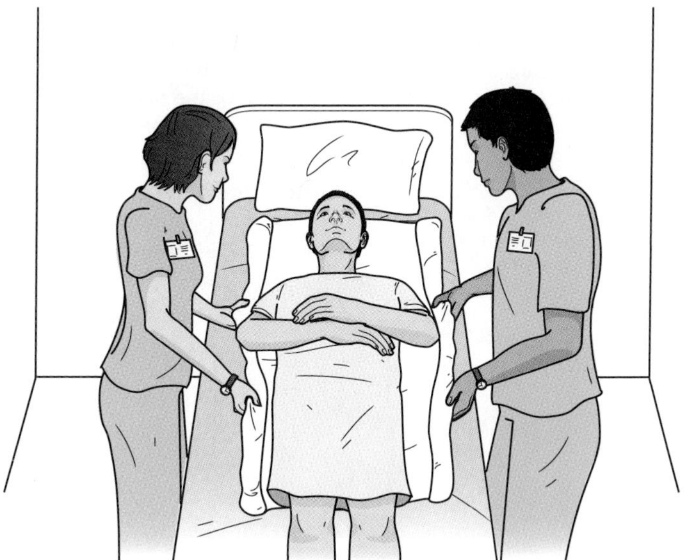

FIGURE 14-10 A drawsheet is used to move the person up in bed. It extends from the person's head to above the knees. Rolled close to the person, the drawsheet is held near the shoulders and hips.

Moving the Person to the Side of the Bed

Re-positioning and care procedures require moving the person to the side of the bed. Move the person to the side of the bed before turning. Otherwise, after turning, the person lies on the side of the bed—not in the middle.

Sometimes you have to reach over the person. During a bed bath is an example. You reach less if the person is near you.

In one method, the person is moved in segments (Fig. 14-11). Sometimes you can do this alone. With at least 1 co-worker, use a mechanical lift (p. 191) or an assist device:

- Following the guidelines for "Moving Persons in Bed," p. 174
- For older persons
- For persons with arthritis
- For persons recovering from spinal cord injures or surgeries

Assist devices for this procedure include a drawsheet (lift sheet), flat sheet folded in half, turning pad, slide sheet, and large waterproof pad. An assist device helps prevent pain and skin damage and injury to the bones, joints, and spinal cord.

See *Promoting Safety and Comfort: Moving the Person to the Side of the Bed.*

See procedure: *Moving the Person to the Side of the Bed.*

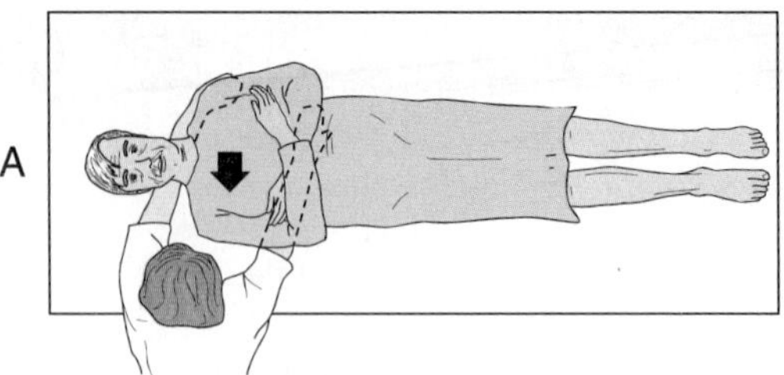

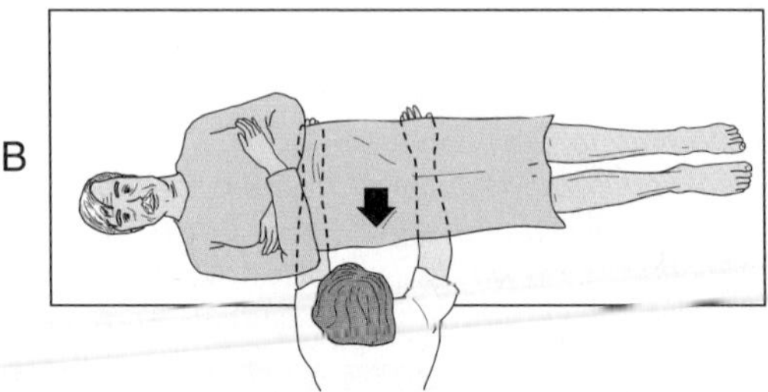

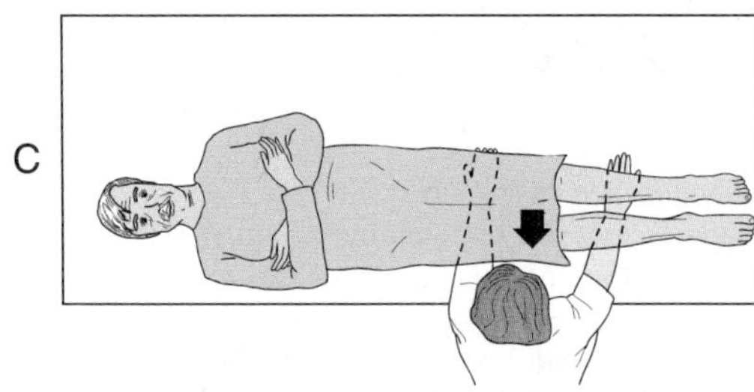

FIGURE 14-11 Moving the person to the side of the bed in segments. **A,** The upper part of the body is moved. **B,** The lower part of the body is moved. **C,** The legs and feet are moved.

PROMOTING SAFETY AND COMFORT

Moving the Person to the Side of the Bed

Safety

Use the method and equipment that are best for the person. Get this information from the nurse and the care plan for tasks that involve moving the person to the side of the bed. Such tasks include re-positioning, bedmaking, and bathing.

The wrong method could cause serious injury. This is very important for persons who are older, have arthritis, or have spinal cord involvement.

To use an assist device, you need at least 1 co-worker to help you. Depending on the person's size, 3 staff members may be needed.

Safety—cont'd

To use a slide sheet, place it under the person. After moving the person in bed, remove the device.

To move the person in segments, move the person toward you, not away from you. This helps protect you from injury.

Comfort

After moving the person to the side of the bed, move the pillow too. Position the pillow correctly. It should be under the person's head and shoulders.

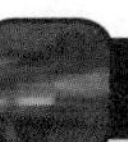

Moving the Person to the Side of the Bed

QUALITY OF LIFE

- Knock before entering the person's room.
- Address the person by name.
- Introduce yourself by name and title.
- Explain the procedure before starting and during the procedure.
- Protect the person's rights during the procedure.
- Handle the person gently during the procedure.

PRE-PROCEDURE

1 Follow *Delegation Guidelines:*
  a *Preventing Work-Related Injuries,* p. 173
  b *Moving Persons in Bed,* p. 174
  See *Promoting Safety and Comfort:*
  a *Assisting With Moving and Transfers,* p. 170
  b *Preventing Work-Related Injuries,* p. 173
  c *Moving the Person to the Side of the Bed*
2 Ask 1 or 2 co-workers to help you if using an assist device.
3 Practice hand hygiene.
4 Identify the person. Check the ID bracelet against the assignment sheet. Also call the person by name.
5 Provide for privacy.
6 Lock the bed wheels.
7 Raise the bed for body mechanics. Bed rails are up if used.

PROCEDURE

8 Lower the head of the bed to a level appropriate for the person. It is as flat as possible.
9 Stand on the side of the bed to which you will move the person.
10 Lower the bed rail near you if bed rails are used. (Both bed rails are lowered for step 15.)
11 Remove pillows as directed by the nurse.
12 Cross the person's arms over the person's chest.
13 Stand with your feet about 12 inches apart. One foot is in front of the other. Flex your knees.
14 *Method 1—Moving the person in segments:*
  a Place your arm under the person's neck and shoulders. Grasp the far shoulder.
  b Place your other arm under the mid-back.
  c Move the upper part of the person's body toward you. Rock backward and shift your weight to your rear leg (see Fig. 14-11, *A*).
  d Place 1 arm under the person's waist and 1 under the thighs.
  e Rock backward to move the lower part of the person toward you (see Fig. 14-11, *B*).
  f Repeat the procedure for the legs and feet (see Fig. 14-11, *C*). Your arms should be under the person's thighs and calves.
15 *Method 2—Moving the person with a drawsheet:*
  a Roll up the drawsheet close to the person (see Fig. 14-10).
  b Grasp the rolled-up drawsheet near the person's shoulders and hips. Your co-worker does the same. Support the person's head.
  c Rock backward on the count of "3" moving the person toward you. Your co-worker rocks backward slightly and then forward toward you while keeping the arms straight.
  d Unroll the drawsheet. Remove any wrinkles.

POST-PROCEDURE

16 Position the person in good alignment.
17 Provide for comfort. (See the inside of the front cover.)
18 Place the call light and other needed items within reach.
19 Lower the bed to a safe and comfortable level appropriate for the person. Follow the care plan.
20 Raise or lower bed rails. Follow the care plan.
21 Unscreen the person.
22 Complete a safety check of the room. (See the inside of the front cover.)
23 Practice hand hygiene.
24 Report and record your observations.

TURNING PERSONS

Turning persons onto their sides helps prevent complications from bedrest (Chapter 23). Certain procedures and care measures also require the side-lying position.

Many older persons have arthritis in their spines, hips, and knees. Less painful, logrolling (p. 182) is preferred for turning these persons.

See *Delegation Guidelines: Turning Persons.*

See *Promoting Safety and Comfort: Turning Persons.*

See procedure: *Turning and Re-Positioning the Person.*

DELEGATION GUIDELINES

Turning Persons

Before turning and re-positioning a person, you need this information from the nurse and the care plan.

- The person's dependency level (see Box 14-2)
- How much help the person needs
- The number of staff needed for safety
- The person's comfort level and what body parts are painful
- Which procedure to use
- What assist device to use
- What supportive devices to use for positioning (Chapter 23)
- Where to place pillows
- What observations to report and record:
  - Who helped you with the procedure
  - How much help the person needed
  - How the person tolerated the procedure
  - How you positioned the person
  - Complaints of pain or discomfort
- When to report observations
- What patient or resident concerns to report at once

PROMOTING SAFETY AND COMFORT

Turning Persons

Safety

Use good body mechanics to turn a person in bed (Chapter 13). Follow the rules in Box 14-1.

The person must be in good alignment. This helps prevent musculo-skeletal injuries, skin breakdown, and pressure ulcers.

Do not turn a person away from you with the far bed rail down. Raise the bed rail on the side near you. Then go to the other side of the bed. Lower the bed rail if up. Turn the person toward you.

Comfort

After turning, position the person in good alignment. Use pillows as directed to support the person in the side-lying position (Chapter 13). Make sure the person's face, nose, and mouth are not obstructed by a pillow or other device.

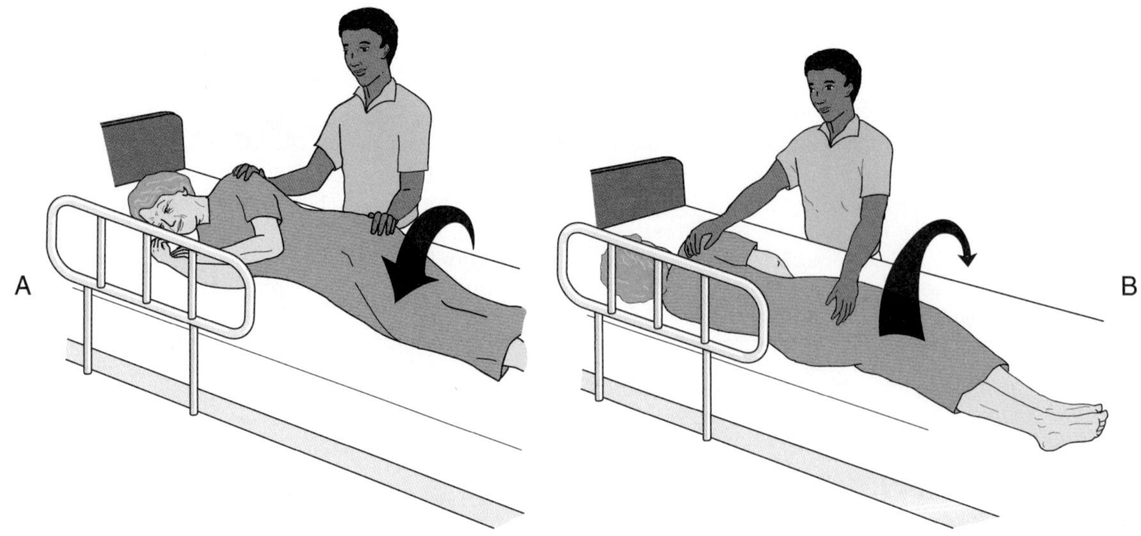

FIGURE 14-12 Turning the person. **A,** Turning the person away from you. **B,** Turning the person toward you. (NOTE: Non-standard bed rails are used to show positioning and hand placement.)

Turning and Re-Positioning the Person

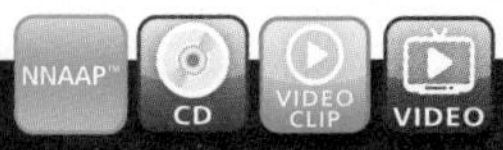

QUALITY OF LIFE

- Knock before entering the person's room.
- Address the person by name.
- Introduce yourself by name and title.
- Explain the procedure before starting and during the procedure.
- Protect the person's rights during the procedure.
- Handle the person gently during the procedure.

PRE-PROCEDURE

1 Follow *Delegation Guidelines:*
   a *Preventing Work-Related Injuries,* p. 173
   b *Moving Persons in Bed,* p. 174
   c *Turning Persons*
   See *Promoting Safety and Comfort:*
   a *Assisting With Moving and Transfers,* p. 170
   b *Preventing Work-Related Injuries,* p. 173
   c *Moving the Person to the Side of the Bed,* p. 178
   d *Turning Persons*
2 Practice hand hygiene.
3 Identify the person. Check the ID bracelet against the assignment sheet. Also call the person by name.
4 Provide for privacy.
5 Lock the bed wheels.
6 Raise the bed for body mechanics. Bed rails are up if used.

PROCEDURE

7 Lower the head of the bed to a level appropriate for the person. It is as flat as possible.
8 Stand on the side of the bed opposite to where you will turn the person.
9 Lower the bed rail.
10 Move the person to the side near you. (See procedure: *Moving the Person to the Side of the Bed,* p. 179.)
11 Cross the person's arms over the person's chest. Cross the leg near you over the far leg.
12 *Turning the person away from you:*
   a Stand with a wide base of support. Flex the knees.
   b Place 1 hand on the person's shoulder. Place the other on the hip near you.
   c Roll the person gently away from you toward the raised bed rail (Fig. 14-12, *A*).
   d Shift your weight from your rear leg to your front leg.
13 *Turning the person toward you:*
   a Raise the bed rail.
   b Go to the other side of the bed. Lower the bed rail.
   c Stand with a wide base of support. Flex your knees.
   d Place 1 hand on the person's shoulder. Place the other on the far hip.
   e Pull the person toward you gently (Fig. 14-12, *B*).
14 Position the person. Follow the nurse's directions and the care plan. The following are common.
   a Place a pillow under the head and neck.
   b Adjust the shoulder. The person should not be lying on an arm.
   c Place a small pillow under the upper hand and arm.
   d Position a pillow against the back.
   e Flex the upper knee. Position the upper leg in front of the lower leg.
   f Support the upper leg and thigh on pillows. Make sure the ankle is supported.

POST-PROCEDURE

15 Provide for comfort. (See the inside of the front cover.)
16 Place the call light and other needed items within reach.
17 Lower the bed to a safe and comfortable level appropriate for the person. Follow the care plan.
18 Raise or lower bed rails. Follow the care plan.
19 Unscreen the person.
20 Complete a safety check of the room. (See the inside of the front cover.)
21 Practice hand hygiene.
22 Report and record your observations.

Logrolling

Logrolling is turning the person as a unit, in alignment, with 1 motion. The spine is kept straight. The procedure is used to turn:

- Older persons with arthritic spines or knees.
- Persons recovering from hip fractures.
- Persons with spinal cord injuries. The spine is kept straight at all times after a spinal cord injury.
- Persons recovering from spinal cord surgery. The spine is kept straight at all times after spinal cord surgery.

See *Promoting Safety and Comfort: Logrolling.*
See procedure: *Logrolling the Person.*

PROMOTING SAFETY AND COMFORT

Logrolling

Safety

For logrolling, 2 or 3 staff members are needed. If the person is tall or heavy, 3 are needed. Sometimes you use an assist device—drawsheet, turning pad, large waterproof pad, slide sheet.

After spinal cord injury or surgery, the spine and neck are kept straight. The nurse holds the neck during moving or re-positioning. The nurse tells you what to do step-by-step. Assist the nurse as directed.

Comfort

After spinal cord injury or surgery, usually a pillow is not allowed under the head and neck. Follow the nurse's directions and the care plan to position the person and use pillows.

A

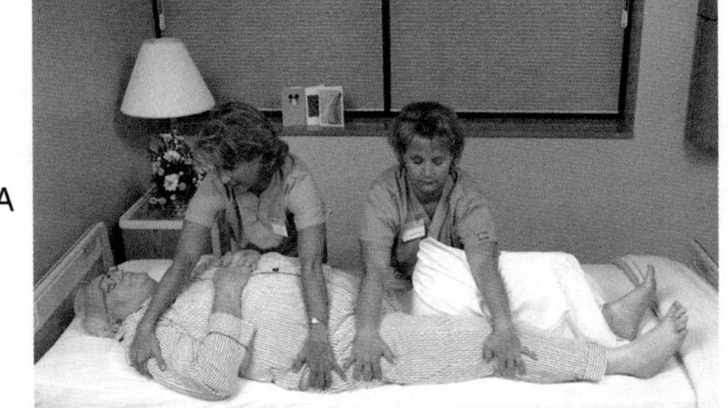

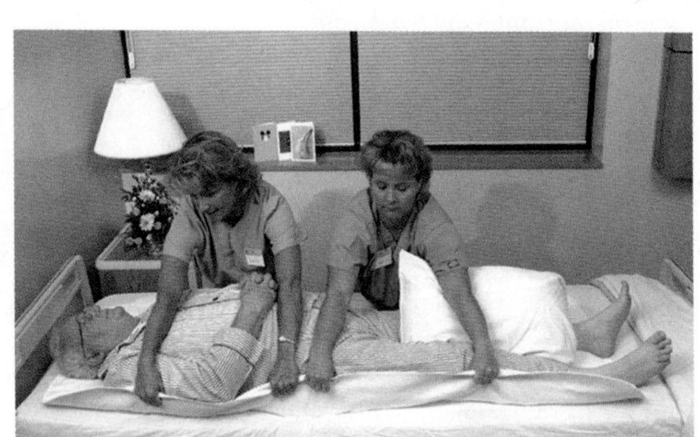

B

FIGURE 14-13 Logrolling. **A,** A pillow is between the person's legs. The arms are crossed on the chest. The person is on the far side of the bed. The person is turned as a unit. **B,** The assist device is used to logroll the person.

Logrolling the Person

QUALITY OF LIFE

- Knock before entering the person's room.
- Address the person by name.
- Introduce yourself by name and title.
- Explain the procedure before starting and during the procedure.
- Protect the person's rights during the procedure.
- Handle the person gently during the procedure.

PRE-PROCEDURE

1 Follow *Delegation Guidelines:*
  a *Preventing Work-Related Injuries,* p. 173
  b *Moving Persons in Bed,* p. 174
  c *Turning Persons,* p. 180
  See *Promoting Safety and Comfort:*
  a *Assisting With Moving and Transfers,* p. 170
  b *Preventing Work-Related Injuries,* p. 173
  c *Turning Persons,* p. 180
  d *Logrolling*
2 Ask a co-worker to help you.
3 Practice hand hygiene.
4 Identify the person. Check the ID bracelet against the assignment sheet. Also call the person by name.
5 Provide for privacy.
6 Lock the bed wheels.
7 Raise the bed for body mechanics. Bed rails are up if used.

PROCEDURE

8 Make sure the bed is flat.
9 Stand on the side opposite to which you will turn the person. Your co-worker stands on the other side.
10 Lower the bed rails if used.
11 Move the person as a unit to the side of the bed near you. Use the assist device. (If the person has a spinal cord injury, assist the nurse as directed.)
12 Place the person's arms across the chest. Place a pillow between the knees.
13 Raise the bed rail if used.
14 Go to the other side.
15 Stand near the shoulders and chest. Your co-worker stands near the hips and thighs.
16 Stand with a wide base of support. One foot is in front of the other.
17 Ask the person to hold his or her body rigid.
18 Roll the person toward you (Fig. 14-13, *A*). Or use the assist device (Fig. 14-13, *B*). Turn the person as a unit.
19 Position the person in good alignment. Use pillows as directed by the nurse and care plan. The following are common (unless the spinal cord is involved).
  a Place a pillow under the head and neck if allowed.
  b Adjust the shoulder. The person should not be lying on an arm.
  c Place a small pillow under the upper hand and arm.
  d Position a pillow against the back.
  e Flex the upper knee. Position the upper leg in front of the lower leg.
  f Support the upper leg and thigh on pillows. Make sure the ankle is supported.

POST-PROCEDURE

20 Provide for comfort. (See the inside of the front cover.)
21 Place the call light and other needed items within reach.
22 Lower the bed to a safe and comfortable level appropriate for the person. Follow the care plan.
23 Raise or lower bed rails. Follow the care plan.
24 Unscreen the person.
25 Complete a safety check of the room. (See the inside of the front cover.)
26 Practice hand hygiene.
27 Report and record your observations.

SITTING ON THE SIDE OF THE BED (DANGLING)

Patients and residents sit on the side of the bed *(dangle)* for many reasons. They may become dizzy or faint when getting out of bed too fast. They may need to sit on the side of the bed for 1 to 5 minutes before walking or transferring. Or activity may increase in stages—bedrest, to dangling, to sitting in a chair, and then to walking. This is common after surgery.

While dangling the legs, the person coughs and deep breathes. He or she moves the legs back and forth in circles. This stimulates circulation.

Two staff members may be needed. Persons with balance and coordination problems need support. If dizziness or fainting occurs, lay the person down.

See *Focus on Older Persons: Dangling.*

See *Delegation Guidelines: Dangling,* p. 184.

See *Promoting Safety and Comfort: Dangling,* p. 184.

See procedure: *Sitting on the Side of the Bed (Dangling),* p. 185.

Text continued on p. 186

FOCUS ON OLDER PERSONS

Dangling

Older persons may have circulatory changes. They may become dizzy or faint when getting up too fast. Let them sit on the side of the bed for a few minutes before a transfer or walking.

DELEGATION GUIDELINES

Dangling

The nurse may ask you to help a person sit on the side of the bed. The procedure is part of other tasks—assisting the person to stand, transferring from bed to chair, partial bath, and others. Before the dangling procedure, you need this information from the nurse and the care plan.

- Areas of weakness. For example, if the arms are weak, the person cannot hold on to the side of the mattress for support. If the left side is weak, turn the person onto the stronger right side. The person uses the right arm to help move from the lying to sitting position.
- The person's dependence level (see Box 14-2).
- The amount of help the person needs.
- If you need a co-worker to help you.
- If the bed is raised or in a low position safe and comfortable for the person.
- How long the person needs to sit on the side of the bed.
- What exercises are to be done while dangling.
    - Range-of-motion exercises (Chapter 23)
    - Deep-breathing and coughing exercises (Chapter 26)
- If the person will walk or transfer to a chair after dangling. If yes, the bed is in a low position safe and comfortable for the person.
- What observations to report and record:
    - Pulse and respiratory rates (Chapter 21)
    - Pale or bluish skin color *(cyanosis)*
    - Complaints of dizziness, light-headedness, or difficulty breathing
    - Who helped you with the procedure
    - How well the activity was tolerated
    - How long the person dangled
    - The amount of help needed
    - Other observations and complaints
- When to report observations.
- What patient or resident concerns to report at once.

PROMOTING SAFETY AND COMFORT

Dangling

Safety

The procedure is not used for persons with:

- Level 4: Total Dependence
- Level 3: Extensive Assistance

Sitting and balance problems can occur after illness, injury, surgery, and bedrest. Some disabilities affect sitting and balance. Support the person who is sitting on the side of the bed. Have a co-worker help you. This protects the person from falling and other injuries.

Comfort

Provide for warmth during the dangling procedure. Help the person put on a robe. Or cover the person's shoulders and back with a bath blanket.

The person may want to perform hygiene measures while sitting on the side of the bed. Oral hygiene and washing the face and hands are examples. These measures are refreshing and stimulate circulation. Follow the nurse's directions and the care plan.

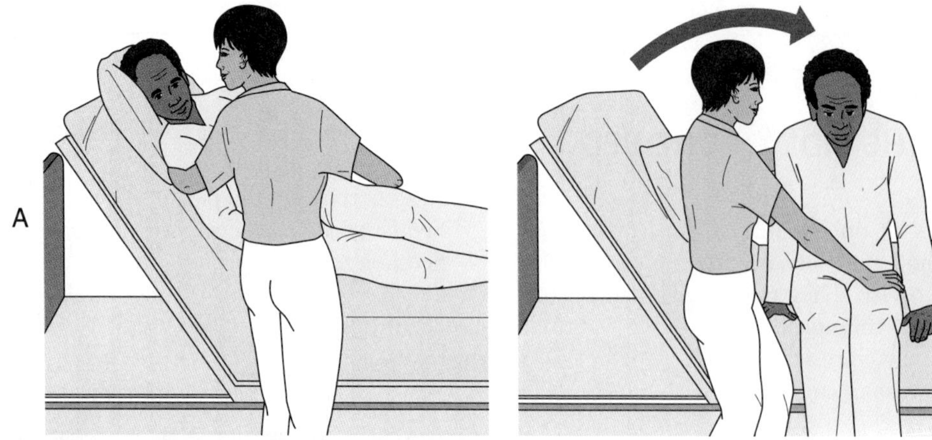

FIGURE 14-14 Helping the person sit on the side of the bed. **A,** The person's shoulders and thighs are supported. **B,** The person sits upright as the legs and feet are pulled over the edge of the bed.

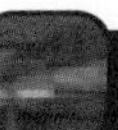

Sitting on the Side of the Bed (Dangling)

QUALITY OF LIFE

- Knock before entering the person's room.
- Address the person by name.
- Introduce yourself by name and title.
- Explain the procedure before starting and during the procedure.
- Protect the person's rights during the procedure.
- Handle the person gently during the procedure.

PRE-PROCEDURE

1 Follow *Delegation Guidelines:*
   a *Preventing Work-Related Injuries,* p. 173
   b *Dangling*
   See *Promoting Safety and Comfort:*
   a *Assisting With Moving and Transfers,* p. 170
   b *Preventing Work-Related Injuries,* p. 173
   c *Dangling*
2 Ask a co-worker to help you.
3 Practice hand hygiene.
4 Identify the person. Check the ID bracelet against the assignment sheet. Also call the person by name.
5 Provide for privacy.
6 Decide which side of the bed to use.
7 Move furniture to provide moving space.
8 Lock the bed wheels.
9 Raise the bed for body mechanics. Bed rails are up if used.

PROCEDURE

10 Lower the bed rail if up.
11 Position the person in a side-lying position facing you. The person lies on the strong side.
12 Raise the head of the bed to a sitting position.
13 Stand by the person's hips. Face the foot of the bed.
14 Stand with your feet apart. The foot near the head of the bed is in front of the other foot.
15 Slide 1 arm under the person's neck and shoulders. Grasp the far shoulder. Place your other hand over the thighs near the knees (Fig. 14-14, *A*).
16 Pivot toward the foot of the bed while moving the person's legs and feet over the side of the bed. As the legs go over the edge of the mattress, the trunk is upright (Fig. 14-14, *B*).
17 Ask the person to hold on to the edge of the mattress. This supports the person in the sitting position. If possible, raise a half-length bed rail (on the person's strong side) for the person to grasp. Have your co-worker support the person at all times.
18 Do not leave the person alone. Provide support at all times.
19 Check the person's condition.
   a Ask how the person feels. Ask if the person feels dizzy or light-headed.
   b Check the pulse and respirations.
   c Check for difficulty breathing.
   d Note if the skin is pale or bluish in color *(cyanosis).*
20 Reverse the procedure to return the person to bed. (Or prepare the person to walk or for a transfer to a chair or wheelchair. Lower the bed to a safe and comfortable level. The person's feet are flat on the floor. Support the person at all times.)
21 Lower the head of the bed after the person returns to bed. Lower the raised bed rail. Help him or her move to the center of the bed.
22 Position the person in good alignment.

POST-PROCEDURE

23 Provide for comfort. (See the inside of the front cover.)
24 Place the call light and other needed items within reach.
25 Lower the bed to a safe and comfortable level appropriate for the person. Follow the care plan.
26 Raise or lower bed rails. Follow the care plan.
27 Return furniture to its proper place.
28 Unscreen the person
29 Complete a safety check of the room. (See the inside of the front cover.)
30 Practice hand hygiene.
31 Report and record your observations.

TRANSFERRING PERSONS

Patients and residents are moved to and from beds, chairs, wheelchairs, shower chairs, commodes, toilets, and stretchers. The amount of help needed and the method used vary with the person's dependency level (see Box 14-2).

Arrange the room to allow enough space for a safe transfer. Correctly place the chair, wheelchair, or other device. Follow the rules for body mechanics (Chapter 13). Also see Box 14-1.

See *Delegation Guidelines: Transferring Persons.*

See *Promoting Safety and Comfort: Transferring Persons.*

DELEGATION GUIDELINES

Transferring Persons

Before a transfer, you need this information from the nurse and the care plan

- What procedure to use.
- The person's dependency level (see Box 14-2).
- The amount of help the person needs.
- What equipment to use—transfer belt, wheelchair, mechanical assist device, positioning devices, wheelchair cushion, bed or chair alarm, and so on.
- The person's height and weight.
- The number of staff needed.
- Areas of weakness. For example, if the arms are weak, the person cannot hold on to the mattress for support. If the left side is weak, he or she gets out of bed on the stronger right side. The person uses the right arm to help move from the lying to sitting position.
- What observations to report and record:
  - Pulse rate before and after the transfer (Chapter 21)
  - Complaints of dizziness, pain, discomfort, difficulty breathing, weakness, or fatigue
  - The amount of help needed to transfer the person
  - Who helped you with the procedure
  - How the person helped with the procedure
  - How you positioned the person
- When to report observations.
- What patient or resident concerns to report at once.

PROMOTING SAFETY AND COMFORT

Transferring Persons

Safety

The person wears non-skid footwear for transfers. Such footwear protects the person from falls. Slipping and sliding are prevented. Tie shoelaces securely. Otherwise the person can trip and fall.

Long gowns and robes can cause falls. Avoid robes with long ties. The person can trip and fall.

Lock bed and wheelchair wheels and wheels on other devices. This prevents the bed and the device from moving during the transfer. Otherwise, the person can fall. You also are at risk for injury.

Comfort

After the transfer, position the person in good alignment. Place needed items within reach.

Transfer Belts

Transfer belts (gait belts) are discussed in Chapter 10. They are used to:

- Support patients and residents during transfers.
- Re-position persons in chairs and wheelchairs (p. 195).

Wider belts have padded handles. They are easier to grip and allow better control should the person fall.

See *Promoting Safety and Comfort: Transfer Belts.*

PROMOTING SAFETY AND COMFORT

Transfer Belts

Safety

To use a transfer belt safely, always follow the manufacturer's instructions. Follow these safety measures.

- Position the belt buckle where the person cannot reach and release it.
- Check for snugness by sliding an open, flat hand under the belt. Ask it if feels too loose or too tight.
- Do not leave excess strap dangling. Tuck the excess strap into the belt.
- Grasp the belt from underneath. If the belt has handles, grasp the belt by the handles.
- Remove the belt after the procedure. Do not leave the person alone while he or she is wearing the belt.

See Chapter 10 for how to apply and use a transfer belt safely.

Comfort

A transfer belt is always applied over clothing. It is never applied over bare skin. Also, it is applied under the breasts. Breasts must not be caught under the belt. The belt buckle is never positioned over the person's spine.

Bed to Chair or Wheelchair Transfers

Safety is important for chair, wheelchair, commode, and shower chair transfers. Help the person out of bed on his or her strong side. If the left side is weak and the right side is strong, get the person out of bed on the right side. In transferring, the strong side moves first. It pulls the weaker side along. Transfers from the weak side are awkward and unsafe.

Some persons are able to stand and pivot. To *pivot* means *to turn*. A stand and pivot transfer is used if:

- The person's legs are strong enough to bear some or all of his or her weight.
- The person is cooperative and can follow directions.
- The person can assist with the transfer.

See *Focus on Surveys: Bed to Chair or Wheelchair Transfers.*

See *Promoting Safety and Comfort: Bed to Chair or Wheelchair Transfers.*

See procedure: *Transferring the Person to a Chair or Wheelchair.*

Text continued on p. 190

FOCUS ON SURVEYS

Bed to Chair or Wheelchair Transfers

Agencies must ensure that nursing assistants can safely perform the skills needed for safe care. Surveyors will observe how nursing assistants function. One of the skills they will focus on is transferring a person from the bed to a wheelchair.

PROMOTING SAFETY AND COMFORT

Bed to Chair or Wheelchair Transfers

Safety

The chair, wheelchair, or other device must support the person's weight. The number of staff needed depends on the person's abilities, condition, and size. Sometimes you will use a mechanical lift (p. 191).

The person must not put his or her arms around your neck. Otherwise the person can pull you forward or cause you to lose your balance. Neck, back, and other injuries are possible.

If not using a mechanical lift, a transfer belt is used for chair or wheelchair transfers. It is safer for the person and you. Putting your arms around the person and grasping the shoulder blades is another method. It can cause the person discomfort. And it can be stressful for you. Use this method only if instructed to do so by the nurse and the care plan.

Bed and wheelchair wheels are locked for a safe transfer. After the transfer, unlock the wheelchair wheels to position the chair as the person prefers. After positioning the chair, lock the wheels or keep them unlocked according to the care plan. Locked wheels may be viewed as restraints if the person cannot unlock them to move the wheelchair (Chapter 11). However, falls and other injuries are risks if the person tries to stand when the wheels are unlocked.

Comfort

Most wheelchairs and bedside chairs have vinyl seats and backs. Vinyl holds body heat. The person becomes warm and perspires more. If the nurse allows, cover the back and seat with a folded bath blanket. This increases the person's comfort.

Some people have wheelchair cushions or positioning devices. Ask the nurse how to use and place the devices. Also follow the manufacturer's instructions.

Transferring the Person to a Chair or Wheelchair

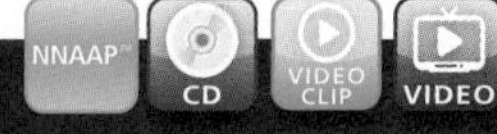

QUALITY OF LIFE

- Knock before entering the person's room.
- Address the person by name.
- Introduce yourself by name and title.
- Explain the procedure before starting and during the procedure.
- Protect the person's rights during the procedure.
- Handle the person gently during the procedure.

PRE-PROCEDURE

1 Follow *Delegation Guidelines:*
   a *Preventing Work-Related Injuries,* p. 173
   b *Transferring Persons*
   See *Promoting Safety and Comfort:*
   a *Assisting With Moving and Transfers,* p. 170
   b *Preventing Work-Related Injuries,* p. 173
   c *Transferring Persons*
   d *Transfer Belts*
   e *Bed to Chair or Wheelchair Transfers*
2 Collect:
   - Wheelchair or arm chair
   - Bath blanket
   - Lap blanket (if used)
   - Robe and non-skid footwear
   - Paper or sheet
   - Transfer belt (if needed)
   - Seat cushion (if needed)
3 Practice hand hygiene.
4 Identify the person. Check the ID bracelet against the assignment sheet. Also call the person by name.
5 Provide for privacy.
6 Decide which side of the bed to use. Move furniture for a safe transfer.

Continued

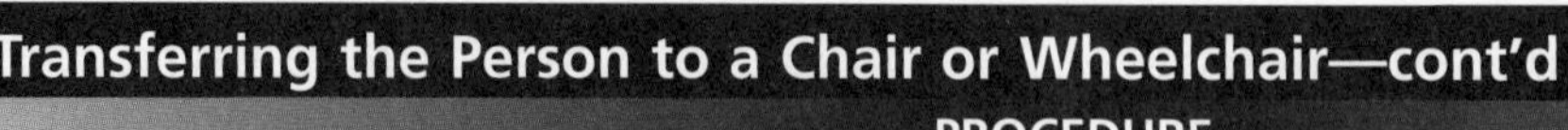

Transferring the Person to a Chair or Wheelchair—cont'd

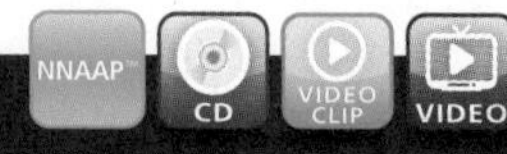

PROCEDURE

7 Raise the wheelchair footplates. Remove or swing front rigging out of the way if possible. Position the chair or wheelchair near the bed on the person's strong side.
  a If at the head of the bed, it faces the foot of the bed.
  b If at the foot of the bed, it faces the head of the bed.
  c The armrest almost touches the bed.
8 Place a folded bath blanket or cushion on the seat (if needed).
9 Lock the wheelchair wheels.
10 Fan-fold top linens to the foot of the bed.
11 Place the paper or sheet under the person's feet. (This protects linens from footwear.) Put footwear on the person.
12 Lower the bed to a safe and comfortable level. Lock the bed wheels.
13 Help the person sit on the side of the bed (p. 183). His or her feet must be flat on the floor.
14 Help the person put on a robe.
15 Apply the transfer belt if needed (Chapter 10). It is applied at the waist over clothing.
16 *Method 1: Using a transfer belt:*
  a Stand in front of the person.
  b Have the person hold on to the mattress.
  c Make sure the person's feet are flat on the floor.
  d Have the person lean forward.
  e Grasp the transfer belt at each side. Grasp the handles or grasp the belt from underneath. See Chapter 10.
  f Prevent the person from sliding or falling. Do 1 of the following.
    1 Brace your knees against the person's knees (Fig. 14-15). Block his or her feet with your feet.
    2 Use the knee and foot of 1 leg to block the person's weak leg or foot. Place your other foot slightly behind you for balance.
    3 Straddle your legs around the person's weak leg.
  g Explain the following.
    1 You will count "1, 2, 3."
    2 The move will be on "3."
    3 On "3," the person pushes down on the mattress and stands.
  h Ask the person to push down on the mattress and to stand on the count of "3." Pull the person to a standing position as you straighten your knees (Fig. 14-16).
17 *Method 2: No transfer belt:* (NOTE: Use this method only if directed by the nurse and the care plan.)
  a Follow steps 16, a–c.
  b Place your hands under the person's arms. Your hands are around the person's shoulder blades (Fig. 14-17).
  c Have the person lean forward.
  d Prevent the person from sliding or falling. Do 1 of the following.
    1 Brace your knees against the person's knees. Block his or her feet with your feet.
    2 Use the knee and foot of 1 leg to block the person's weak leg or foot. Place your other foot slightly behind you for balance.
    3 Straddle your legs around the person's weak leg
  e Explain the "count of 3." See step 16, g.
  f Ask the person to push down on the mattress and to stand on the count of "3." Pull the person up into a standing position as you straighten your knees.
18 Support the person in the standing position. Hold the transfer belt, or keep your hands around the person's shoulder blades. Continue to prevent the person from sliding or falling.
19 Turn the person so he or she can grasp the far arm of the chair or wheelchair. The legs will touch the edge of the seat (Fig. 14-18).
20 Continue to turn the person until the other armrest is grasped.
21 Lower him or her into the chair or wheelchair as you bend your hips and knees. To assist, the person leans forward and bends the elbows and knees (Fig. 14-19).
22 Make sure the hips are to the back of the seat. Position the person in good alignment.
23 Attach the wheelchair front rigging. Position the person's feet on the footplates.
24 Cover the person's lap and legs with a lap blanket (if used). Keep the blanket off the floor and the wheels.
25 Remove the transfer belt if used.
26 Position the chair as the person prefers. Lock the wheelchair wheels according to the care plan.

POST-PROCEDURE

27 Provide for comfort. (See the inside of the front cover.)
28 Place the call light and other needed items within reach.
29 Unscreen the person.
30 Complete a safety check of the room. (See the inside of the front cover.)
31 Practice hand hygiene.
32 Report and record your observations.
33 See procedure: *Transferring the Person From a Chair or Wheelchair to Bed* (p. 190) to return the person to bed.

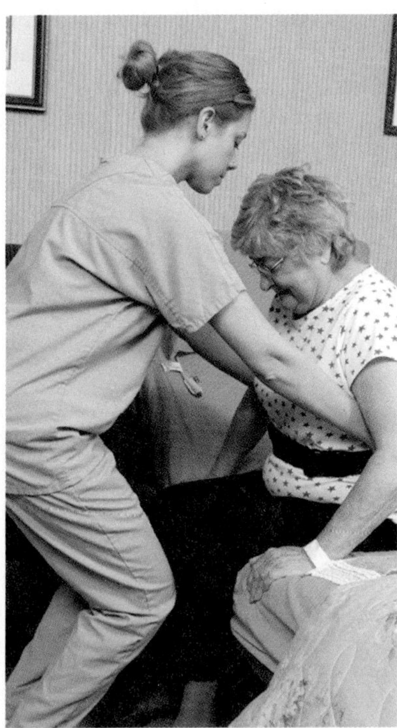

FIGURE 14-15 The person's feet and knees are blocked by the nursing assistant's feet and knees. This prevents the person from sliding or falling.

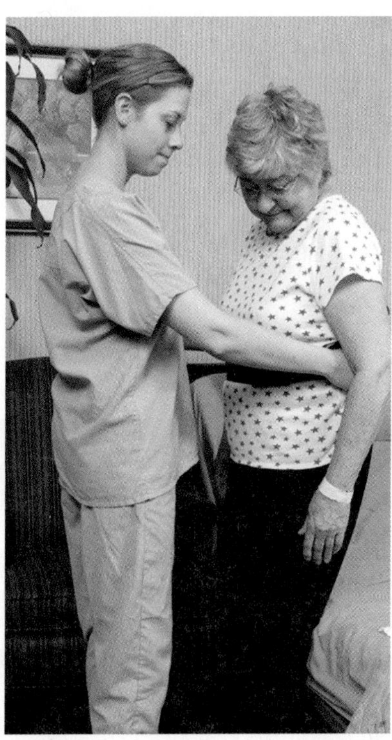

FIGURE 14-16 The person is pulled up to a standing position and supported by holding the transfer belt.

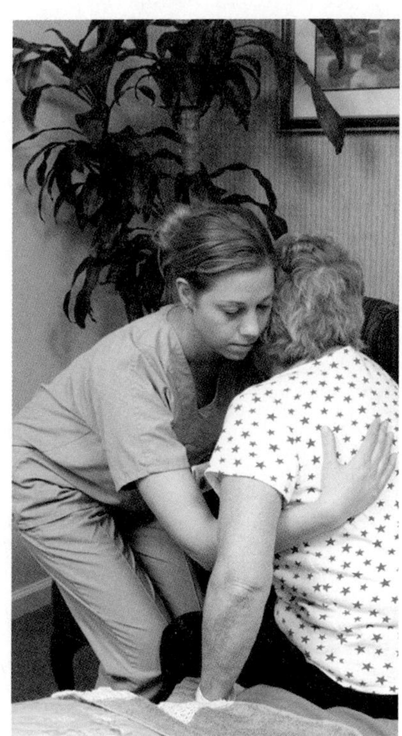

FIGURE 14-17 The person is being prepared to stand. The hands are placed under the person's arms and around the shoulder blades.

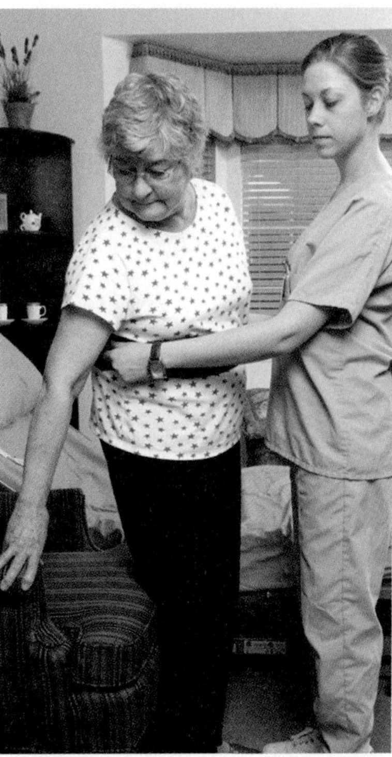

FIGURE 14-18 The person is supported as he or she grasps the far arm of the chair. The legs are against the chair.

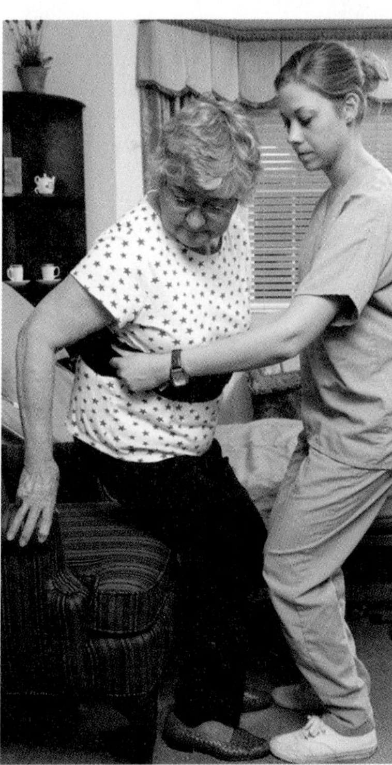

FIGURE 14-19 The person holds the armrests, leans forward, and bends the elbows and knees while being lowered into the chair.

Chair or Wheelchair to Bed Transfers

Chair or wheelchair to bed transfers have the same rules as bed to chair transfers. If the person is weak on 1 side, transfer the person so that the strong side moves first. Or position the chair or wheelchair so the person's strong side is near the bed. The strong side moves first.

For example, Mrs. Lee's right side is weak. Her left side is strong. For a bed to chair transfer, the chair was on the left side of the bed. Her left side (strong side) moved first. Now you will transfer Mrs. Lee back to bed. With the chair on the left side of the bed, her weak right side is near the bed. Moving the weak side first is not safe. Move the chair to the other side of the bed or turn the chair around. Mrs. Lee's stronger left side will be near the bed. The stronger side moves first for a safe transfer.

See procedure: *Transferring the Person From a Chair or Wheelchair to Bed.*

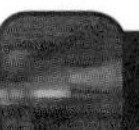

Transferring the Person From a Chair or Wheelchair to Bed

QUALITY OF LIFE

- Knock before entering the person's room.
- Address the person by name.
- Introduce yourself by name and title.
- Explain the procedure before starting and during the procedure.
- Protect the person's rights during the procedure.
- Handle the person gently during the procedure.

PRE-PROCEDURE

1 Follow *Delegation Guidelines:*
  a *Preventing Work-Related Injuries,* p. 173
  b *Transferring Persons,* p. 186
  See *Promoting Safety and Comfort:*
  a *Assisting With Moving and Transfers,* p. 170
  b *Preventing Work-Related Injuries,* p. 173
  c *Transferring Persons,* p. 186
  d *Transfer Belts,* p. 186
  e *Bed to Chair or Wheelchair Transfers,* p. 187
2 Collect a transfer belt if needed.
3 Practice hand hygiene.
4 Identify the person. Check the ID bracelet against the assignment sheet. Also call the person by name.
5 Provide for privacy.

PROCEDURE

6 Move furniture for moving space.
7 Raise the head of the bed to a sitting position. Lower the bed to a safe and comfortable level. When the person transfers to the bed, his or her feet must be flat on the floor when sitting on the side of the bed.
8 Move the call light so it is on the strong side when the person is in bed.
9 Position the chair or wheelchair so the person's strong side is next to the bed (Fig. 14-20). Have a co-worker help you if necessary.
10 Lock the wheelchair and bed wheels.
11 Remove and fold the lap blanket (if used).
12 Remove the person's feet from the footplates. Raise the footplates. Remove or swing front rigging out of the way. Put non-skid footwear on the person if needed.
13 Apply the transfer belt if needed.
14 Make sure the person's feet are flat on the floor.
15 Stand in front of the person.
16 Have the person hold on to the armrests. (If the nurse directs you to do so, place your arms under the person's arms. Your hands are around the shoulder blades.)
17 Have the person lean forward.
18 Grasp the transfer belt on each side if using it. Grasp the handles or grasp the belt from underneath.
19 Prevent the person from sliding or falling. Do 1 of the following.
  a Brace your knees against the person's knees. Block his or her feet with your feet.
  b Use the knee and foot of 1 leg to block the person's weak leg or foot. Place your other foot slightly behind you for balance.
  c Straddle your legs around the person's weak leg.
20 Explain the count of "3." (See procedure: *Transferring the Person to a Chair or Wheelchair,* p. 188.)
21 Ask the person to push down on the armrests on the count of "3." Pull the person into a standing position as you straighten your knees.
22 Support the person in the standing position. Hold the transfer belt, or keep your hands around the person's shoulder blades. Continue to prevent the person from sliding or falling.
23 Turn the person so he or she can reach the edge of the mattress. The legs will touch the mattress.
24 Continue to turn the person until he or she can reach the mattress with both hands.
25 Lower him or her onto the bed as you bend your hips and knees. To assist, the person leans forward and bends the elbows and knees.
26 Remove the transfer belt.
27 Remove the robe and footwear.
28 Help the person lie down.

Transferring the Person From a Chair or Wheelchair to Bed—cont'd

POST-PROCEDURE

29 Provide for comfort. (See the inside of the front cover.)
30 Place the call light and other needed items within reach.
31 Raise or lower bed rails. Follow the care plan.
32 Arrange furniture to meet the person's needs.
33 Unscreen the person.
34 Complete a safety check of the room. (See the inside of the front cover.)
35 Practice hand hygiene.
36 Report and record your observations.

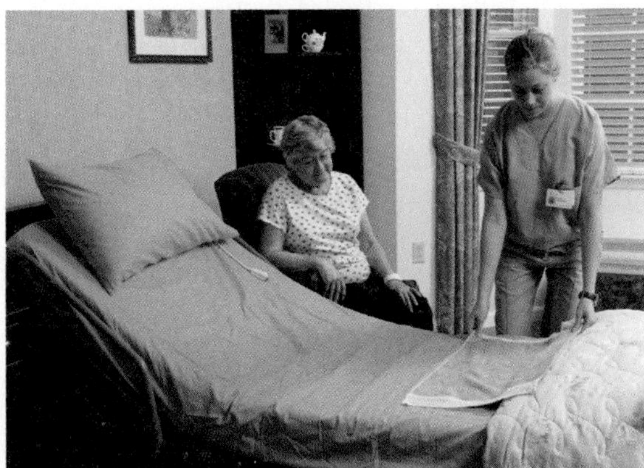

FIGURE 14-20 The chair is positioned so the person's strong side is near the bed.

Mechanical Lifts

Persons who cannot help themselves are transferred with mechanical lifts (Fig. 14-21). So are persons too heavy for the staff to transfer. Use the lift for transfers to and from beds, chairs, wheelchairs, stretchers, tubs, shower chairs, toilets, commodes, whirlpools, or vehicles.

There are manual, battery-operated, and electric lifts. Some lifts are mounted on the ceiling.

Slings. The sling used depends on the person's size, condition, and other needs. Slings are padded, unpadded, or made of mesh.

- *Standard full sling*—for normal transfers.
- *Extended length sling*—for persons with extra large thighs.
- *Bathing sling*—to transfer the person directly from the bed or chair into a bathtub. The sling is left in place and attached to the lift during the bath.
- *Toileting sling*—the sling bottom is open. Each person has his or her own toileting sling.
- *Amputee sling*—for the person who has had both legs amputated.
- *Bariatric sling*—for use with a bariatric lift.

Follow agency policy and the manufacturer's instructions for washing slings.

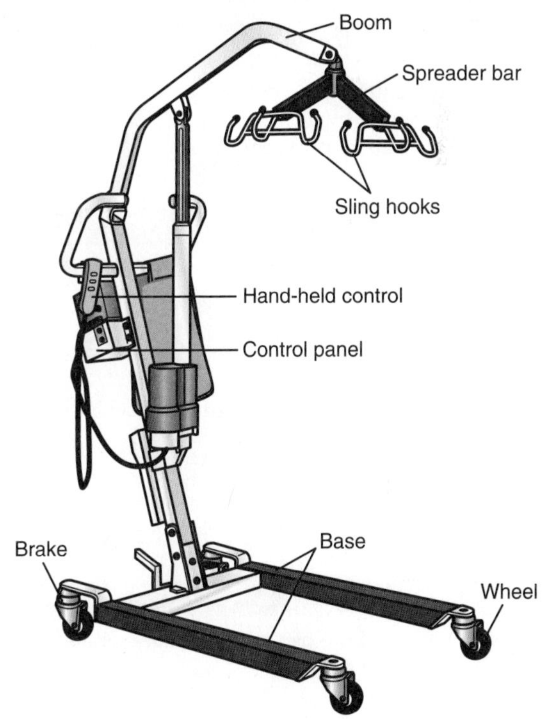

FIGURE 14-21 Parts of a mechanical lift.

Using a Mechanical Lift. Before using a lift:
- You must be trained in its use.
- It must work.
- The sling, straps, hooks, and chains must be in good repair.
- The person's weight must not exceed the lift's capacity.
- At least 2 staff members are needed.

There are different types of mechanical lifts. Always follow the manufacturer's instructions. The following procedure is used as a guide.

See *Delegation Guidelines: Using a Mechanical Lift.*

See *Promoting Safety and Comfort: Using a Mechanical Lift.*

See procedure: *Transferring the Person Using a Mechanical Lift.*

DELEGATION GUIDELINES

Using a Mechanical Lift

Before using a mechanical lift, you need this information from the nurse and the care plan.
- The person's dependency level (see Box 14-2)
- What lift to use
- What sling to use (p. 191)—standard, extended length, bathing, toileting, amputee, bariatric
- If a padded, unpadded, or mesh sling is needed
- What size sling to use
- The number of staff needed to perform the task safely

PROMOTING SAFETY AND COMFORT

Using a Mechanical Lift

Safety

Always follow the manufacturer's instructions. Knowing how to use one lift does not mean that you know how to use others.

If you have questions, ask the nurse. If you have not used a certain lift before, ask for needed training. Ask the nurse to help you until you are comfortable using the lift.

Mechanical lifts must be in good working order. Tell the nurse when a lift needs repair or is not working properly.

Some mechanical lifts are battery-powered. Batteries must be well-charged. Follow the manufacturer's instructions and agency policy.

Comfort

The person is lifted up and off the bed or chair. Falling is a common fear. To promote mental comfort, always explain the procedure before you begin. Also show the person how the lift works.

Transferring the Person Using a Mechanical Lift

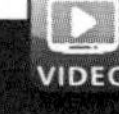

QUALITY OF LIFE

- Knock before entering the person's room.
- Address the person by name.
- Introduce yourself by name and title.
- Explain the procedure before starting and during the procedure.
- Protect the person's rights during the procedure.
- Handle the person gently during the procedure.

PRE-PROCEDURE

1 Follow *Delegation Guidelines:*
  a *Preventing Work-Related Injuries,* p. 173
  b *Transferring Persons,* p. 186
  c *Using a Mechanical Lift*
  See *Promoting Safety and Comfort:*
  a *Assisting With Moving and Transfers,* p. 170
  b *Preventing Work-Related Injuries,* p. 173
  c *Transferring Persons,* p. 186
  d *Using a Mechanical Lift*
2 Ask a co-worker to help you.
3 Collect:
  - Mechanical lift and sling
  - Arm chair or wheelchair
  - Footwear
  - Bath blanket or cushion
  - Lap blanket (if used)
4 Practice hand hygiene.
5 Identify the person. Check the ID bracelet against the assignment sheet. Also call the person by name.
6 Provide for privacy.
7 Raise the bed for body mechanics. Bed rails are up if used.

PROCEDURE

8 Lower the head of the bed to a level appropriate for the person. It is as flat as possible.
9 Stand on 1 side of the bed. Your co-worker stands on the other side.
10 Lower the bed rails if up. Lock the bed wheels.
11 Center the sling under the person (Fig. 14-22, *A*). To position the sling, turn the person from side-to-side as if making an occupied bed (Chapter 15). Follow the manufacturer's instructions to position the sling.
12 Position the person in the semi-Fowler's position (Chapter 15).

Transferring the Person Using a Mechanical Lift—cont'd

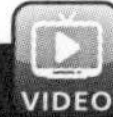

PROCEDURE—cont'd

13 Place the chair at the head of the bed. It is even with the head-board and about 1 foot away from the bed. Place a folded bath blanket or cushion in the chair.
14 Lower the bed so it is level with the chair.
15 Raise the lift to position it over the person.
16 Position the lift over the person (Fig. 14-22, *B*).
17 Lock the lift wheels.
18 Attach the sling to the sling hooks (Fig. 14-22, *C*).
19 Raise the head of the bed to a comfortable level for the person.
20 Cross the person's arms over the chest.
21 Raise the lift until the person and sling are free of the bed (Fig. 14-22, *D*).
22 Have your co-worker support the person's legs as you move the lift and the person away from the bed (Fig. 14-22, *E*).
23 Position the lift so the person's back is toward the chair.
24 Position the chair so you can lower the person into it.
25 Lower the person into the chair. Guide the person into the chair (Fig. 14-22, *F*).
26 Lower the lift to unhook the sling. Remove the sling from under the person unless otherwise indicated.
27 Put footwear on the person. Position the person's feet on the wheelchair footplates.
28 Cover the person's lap and legs with a lap blanket (if used). Keep it off the floor and wheels.
29 Position the chair as the person prefers. Lock the wheelchair wheels according to the care plan.

POST-PROCEDURE

30 Provide for comfort. (See the inside of the front cover.)
31 Place the call light and other needed items within reach.
32 Unscreen the person.
33 Complete a safety check of the room. (See the inside of the front cover.)
34 Practice hand hygiene.
35 Report and record your observations.
36 Reverse the procedure to return the person to bed.

A
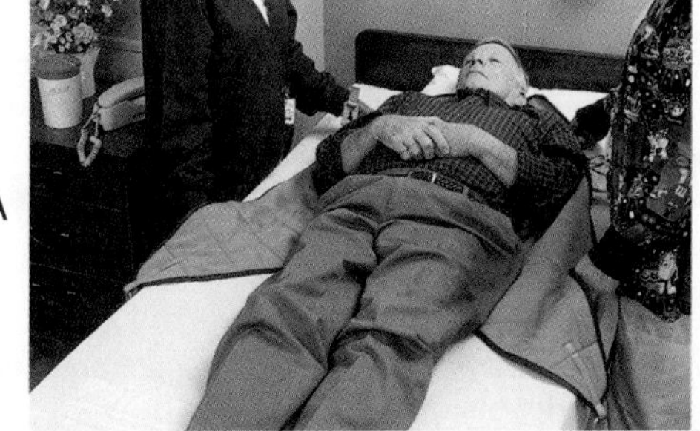
B
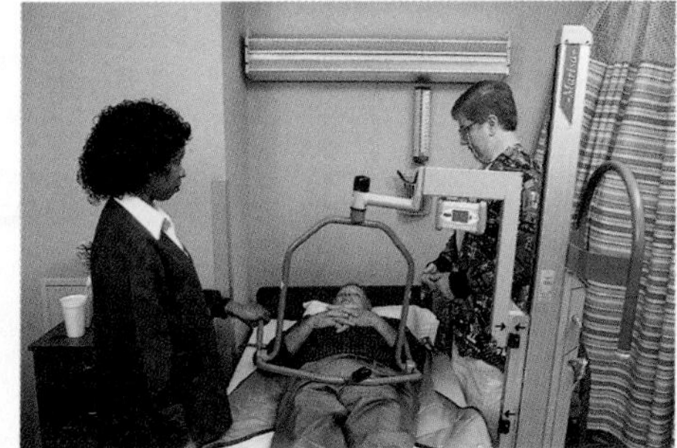
C
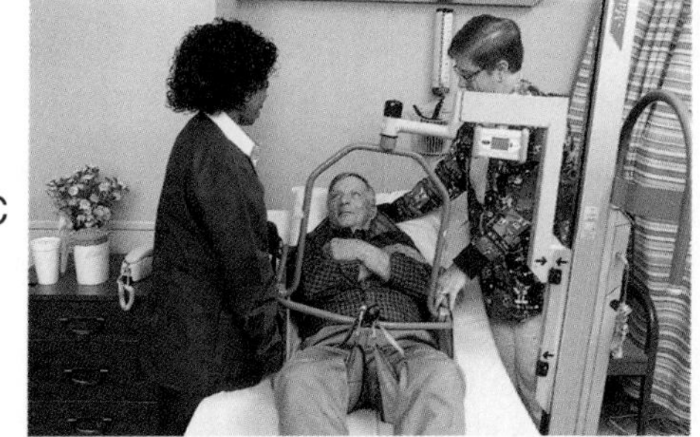
D
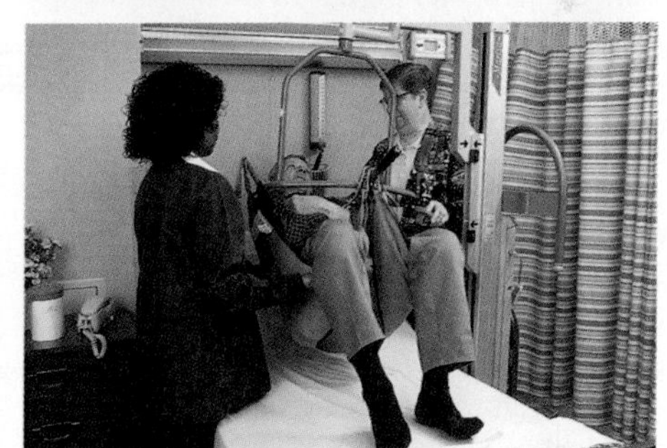
E
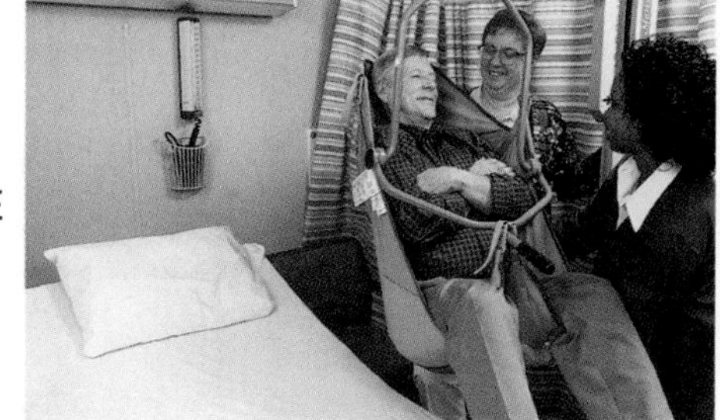
F
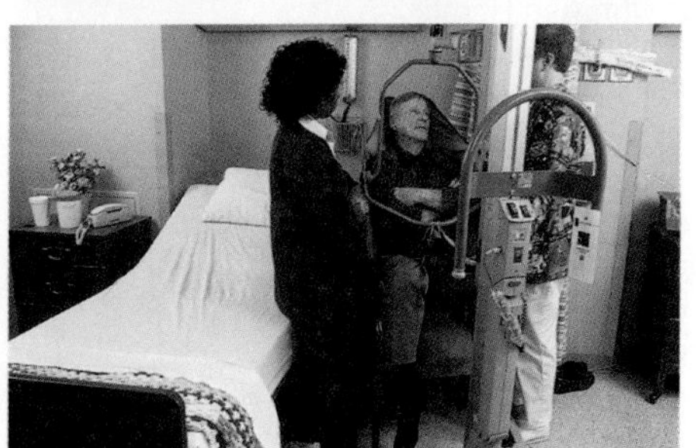

FIGURE 14-22 Using a mechanical lift. **A,** The sling is positioned under the person. **B,** The lift is over the person. **C,** The sling is attached to the spreader bar. **D,** The lift is raised until the sling and person are off of the bed. **E,** The person's legs are supported as the person and lift are moved away from the bed. **F,** The person is guided into a chair.

Transferring the Person To and From the Toilet

Using the bathroom for elimination promotes dignity, self-esteem, and independence. It also is more private than using a bedpan, urinal, or bedside commode. However, getting to the toilet is hard for persons who use wheelchairs. Bathrooms are often small. There is little room for you or a wheelchair. Therefore transfers with wheelchairs and toilets are often hard. Falls and work-related injuries are risks.

Sometimes mechanical lifts are used for toilet transfers. The following procedure can be used if the person can stand and pivot from the wheelchair to the toilet.

See *Promoting Safety and Comfort: Transferring the Person To and From the Toilet.*

See procedure: *Transferring the Person To and From the Toilet.*

PROMOTING SAFETY AND COMFORT

Transferring the Person To and From the Toilet

Safety

Make sure the person has a raised toilet seat. The toilet seat and wheelchair are at the same level.

Check the grab bars by the toilet. If loose, tell the nurse. Do not transfer the person to the toilet if grab bars are not secure.

Follow Standard Precautions and the Bloodborne Pathogen Standard. Wear gloves if the person is incontinent of urine or feces or if contact with urine or feces is likely.

Transferring the Person To and From the Toilet

QUALITY OF LIFE

- Knock before entering the person's room.
- Address the person by name.
- Introduce yourself by name and title.
- Explain the procedure before starting and during the procedure.
- Protect the person's rights during the procedure.
- Handle the person gently during the procedure.

PRE-PROCEDURE

1 Follow *Delegation Guidelines:*
  a *Preventing Work-Related Injuries,* p. 173
  b *Transferring Persons,* p. 186
  See *Promoting Safety and Comfort:*
  a *Assisting With Moving and Transfers,* p. 170
  b *Preventing Work-Related Injuries,* p. 173
  c *Transferring Persons,* p. 186
  d *Transfer Belts,* p. 186
  e *Bed to Chair or Wheelchair Transfers,* p. 187
  f *Transferring the Person To and From the Toilet*
2 Practice hand hygiene.

PROCEDURE

3 Put non-skid footwear on the person.
4 Position the wheelchair next to the toilet if there is enough room. If not, position the chair at a right angle (90-degree angle) to the toilet (Fig. 14-23). It is best if the person's strong side is near the toilet.
5 Lock the wheelchair wheels.
6 Raise the footplates. Remove or swing front rigging out of the way.
7 Apply the transfer belt.
8 Help the person unfasten clothing.
9 Use the transfer belt to help the person stand and turn to the toilet. (See procedure: *Transferring the Person to a Chair or Wheelchair,* p. 187.) The person uses the grab bars to turn to the toilet.
10 Support the person with the transfer belt while he or she lowers clothing. Or have the person hold on to the grab bars for support. Lower the person's clothing.
11 Use the transfer belt to lower the person onto the toilet seat. Check for proper positioning on the toilet.
12 Remove the transfer belt.
13 Tell the person you will stay nearby. Remind the person to use the call light or call for you when help is needed. Stay with the person if required by the care plan.
14 Close the bathroom door for privacy.
15 Stay near the bathroom. Complete other tasks in the person's room. Check on the person every 5 minutes.
16 Knock on the bathroom door when the person calls for you.
17 Help with wiping, perineal care (Chapter 16), flushing, and hand washing as needed. Wear gloves and practice hand hygiene after removing the gloves.
18 Apply the transfer belt.
19 Use the transfer belt to help the person stand.
20 Help the person raise and secure clothing.
21 Use the transfer belt to transfer the person to the wheelchair. (See procedure: *Transferring the Person to a Chair or Wheelchair,* p. 187.)
22 Make sure the person's buttocks are to the back of the seat. Position the person in good alignment.
23 Position the person's feet on the footplates.
24 Remove the transfer belt.
25 Cover the person's lap and legs with a lap blanket (if used). Keep the blanket off the floor and wheels.
26 Position the chair as the person prefers. Lock the wheelchair wheels according to the care plan.

Transferring the Person To and From the Toilet—cont'd

POST-PROCEDURE

27 Provide for comfort. (See the inside of the front cover.)
28 Place the call light and other needed items within reach.
29 Unscreen the person.
30 Complete a safety check of the room. (See the inside of the front cover.)
31 Practice hand hygiene.
32 Report and record your observations.

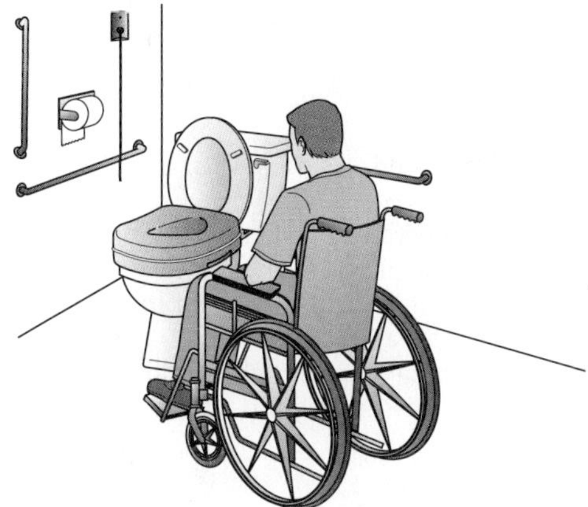

FIGURE 14-23 The wheelchair is placed at a right angle (90-degree angle) to the toilet.

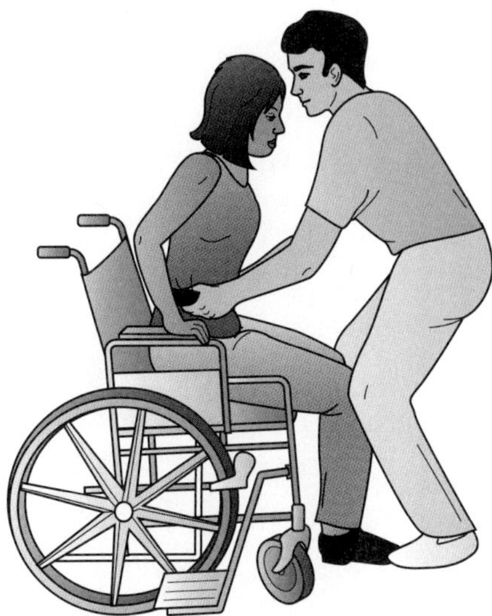

FIGURE 14-24 Re-positioning the person in a wheelchair. A transfer belt is used to move the person to the back of the chair.

RE-POSITIONING IN A CHAIR OR WHEELCHAIR

The person can slide down in a chair. For good alignment and safety, the person's back and buttocks must be against the back of the chair.

Some persons can help with re-positioning. If the person cannot help, use a mechanical lift. Follow the nurse's directions and the care plan for the best way to re-position a person in a chair or wheelchair. *Do not pull the person from behind the chair or wheelchair.*

If the person's chair reclines:

1 Ask a co-worker to help you.
2 Lock the wheels.
3 Recline the chair.
4 Position a friction-reducing device (drawsheet or slide sheet) under the person.
5 Use the device to move the person up. See procedure: *Moving the Person Up in Bed With an Assist Device,* p. 177.

Use this method if the person is alert and cooperative. The person must be able to follow directions. And the person must have the strength to help.

1 Lock the wheelchair wheels.
2 Remove or swing front rigging out of the way.
3 Position the person's feet flat on the floor.
4 Apply a transfer belt.
5 Position the person's arms on the armrests.
6 Stand in front of the person. Block his or her knees and feet with your knees and feet.
7 Grasp the transfer belt on each side while the person leans forward.
8 Ask the person to push with his or her feet and arms on the count of "3."
9 Move the person back into the chair on the count of "3" as the person pushes with his or her feet and arms (Fig. 14-24).
10 Remove the transfer belt.

FOCUS ON PRIDE

The Person, Family, and Yourself

Personal and Professional Responsibility

Take the time to explain what you will do before starting a procedure. Then explain what you are doing step-by-step. This promotes comfort. When giving directions:

- Speak slowly and clearly.
- Talk loudly enough for the person to hear you.
- Give directions calmly and kindly. Do not yell at or insult the person.
- Face the person and use eye contact when possible.
- Give 1 direction at a time.
- Repeat directions as needed.

Rights and Respect

When moving or transferring a person, remember to respect privacy. Close privacy curtains, doors, and window coverings. Properly cover the person. For example, a person wears a gown that opens in the back. Apply a robe or another gown to cover the person's backside. Use a covering that is safe for transfers.

Independence and Social Interaction

Persons who need help moving and transferring have limited independence. They cannot turn or move in bed alone, sit up in a chair alone, or go to the bathroom alone. The person may feel embarrassed or helpless.

To promote pride and independence:

- Focus on the person's abilities.
- Encourage the person.
- Let the person help as much as safely possible.
- Tell the person when you notice even small improvements. This can improve self-esteem.

Delegation and Teamwork

You may need help transferring a person. Your co-workers are busy. You have a choice. Do you ask for help? Or do you try to move the person alone?

Never be afraid to ask for help. You are not bothering a co-worker by asking for help. Ask politely and say "thank you." Also, willingly help others when asked. If you cannot stop what you are doing, tell your co-worker when you can help. Then help the person when you said that you would. Work as a team to ensure the person's safety and to protect yourself and others from injury.

Ethics and Laws

You must move and transfer persons safely. Otherwise injuries can result. To avoid injury:

- Move a person with enough help.
- Position the chair or wheelchair close to the bed.
- Use the proper equipment such as a transfer belt or mechanical lift.
- Do not pull on the person's clothing or arm, underarm, or other body part.
- Do not use broken or damaged equipment.
- Do not exceed equipment weight limits.

You learned the right way to move and transfer persons. The *right* way is not always the *easy* way. Choose to give care the *right* way. Take pride in providing care in a way that prevents harm and promotes comfort and safety.

REVIEW QUESTIONS

Circle the BEST answer.

1 Lift sheets and drawsheets are used to
  a Remove shearing
  b Reduce friction
  c Promote ergonomics
  d Improve posture

2 To protect the person's skin when moving in bed
  a Roll the person
  b Slide the person
  c Move the mattress
  d Use a transfer belt

3 To protect the person's rights during a transfer
  a Allow the person to transfer without shoes
  b Perform the procedure alone
  c Ask the person what procedure to use
  d Close the privacy curtain

4 When moving persons in bed
  a The nurse tells you how to position the person
  b You decide which procedure to use
  c Bed rails are used at all times
  d 3 workers are needed to complete the task safely

5 As an assist device, a drawsheet is placed so that it
  a Covers the person's body
  b Extends from the mid-back to mid-thigh level
  c Is under the head to above the knees
  d Covers the entire mattress

6 Before turning a person onto his or her side, you
  a Move the person to the middle of the bed
  b Move the person to the side of the bed
  c Raise the head of the bed
  d Position pillows for comfort

7 A patient with a spinal cord injury is turned with
  a The logrolling procedure
  b A transfer belt
  c A mechanical lift
  d A pillow under the head and neck

8 To assist with dangling, you need to know
  a If a transfer belt is needed
  b Where to position pillows
  c If a mechanical lift is needed
  d Which side is stronger

9 For chair and wheelchair transfers, the person must
  a Wear non-skid footwear
  b Have the bed rails up
  c Use a mechanical lift
  d Have a drawsheet or other assist device

10 A stand and pivot transfer is unsafe for a person who
  a Is hard of hearing but able to follow directions
  b Can bear some weight with the legs
  c Is confused and combative
  d Uses a wheelchair

11 When transferring the person to bed, a chair, or a wheelchair
  a The strong side moves first
  b The weak side moves first
  c Pillows are used for support
  d The transfer belt is removed

12 When using a mechanical lift
  a Position the lift on the person's strong side
  b Compare the person's weight to the lift's weight limit
  c Collect a sling, battery, and transfer belt
  d Allow the person to control the lift

13 To safely transfer a person with a mechanical lift, at least
  a 1 worker is needed
  b 2 workers are needed
  c 3 workers are needed
  d 4 workers are needed

14 When transferring a person from a wheelchair to a toilet
  a Position the wheelchair facing the toilet
  b Remove the transfer belt when lowering clothing
  c Tell the person to hold on to the towel bar for support
  d Lock the wheelchair wheels

15 You need to re-position a person in a wheelchair. Which is safe?
  a Pulling the person from behind the wheelchair
  b Using a transfer belt for a weak and confused person
  c Using a friction-reducing device and the help of a co-worker
  d Keeping the wheelchair wheels unlocked

Answers to these questions are on p. 504.

FOCUS ON **PRACTICE**

Problem Solving

A resident yells that she needs to go to the bathroom right away. She is at risk for falls and needs the help of 2 staff members to transfer safely. All other staff are busy. The resident is trying to get up on her own. What do you do?

CHAPTER

15 Assisting With Comfort

OBJECTIVES

- Define the key terms and key abbreviations listed in this chapter.
- Explain how to maintain the person's unit.
- Describe how to control temperature, odors, noise, and lighting for the person's comfort.
- Describe the basic bed positions.
- Identify the 7 hospital bed system entrapment zones.
- Identify the persons at risk for entrapment.
- Explain how to use the furniture and equipment in the person's unit.
- Describe 4 ways to make beds.
- Explain how to properly handle linens.
- Explain how to assist the nurse with pain relief.
- Explain the purposes of a back massage.
- Explain how to assist the nurse with promoting sleep.
- Perform the procedures described in this chapter.
- Explain how to promote PRIDE in the person, the family, and yourself.

KEY TERMS

Fowler's position A semi-sitting position; the head of the bed is raised between 45 and 60 degrees
full visual privacy Having the means to be completely free from public view while in bed
high-Fowler's position A semi-sitting position; the head of the bed is raised 60 to 90 degrees
insomnia A chronic condition in which the person cannot sleep or stay asleep all night
pain To ache, hurt, or be sore
reverse Trendelenburg's position The head of the bed is raised and the foot of the bed is lowered
semi-Fowler's position The head of the bed is raised 30 degrees; or the head of the bed is raised 30 degrees and the knee portion is raised 15 degrees
sleep deprivation The amount and quality of sleep are decreased
sleepwalking The sleeping person leaves the bed and walks about
Trendelenburg's position The head of the bed is lowered and the foot of the bed is raised

KEY ABBREVIATIONS

CMS Centers for Medicare & Medicaid Services
F Fahrenheit
ID Identification

Comfort is a state of well-being. Many factors affect comfort. Sleep is promoted when the person is comfortable and pain free.

THE PERSON'S UNIT

The *person's unit* is the personal space, furniture, and equipment provided for the person by the agency (Fig. 15-1). The person's unit is designed to provide comfort, safety, and privacy. In nursing centers, resident units also are as personal and home-like as possible. Always treat the person's unit with respect.

Designed for 1 person, a private patient or resident room has 1 unit. Those designed for 2 people have 2 units. Some rooms have 3 or 4 units.

You need to keep the person's unit clean, neat, safe, and comfortable. See Box 15-1.

COMFORT

Age, illness, and activity affect comfort. So do temperature, ventilation, noise, odors, and lighting. These factors are controlled to meet the person's needs.

See *Focus on Communication: Comfort.*

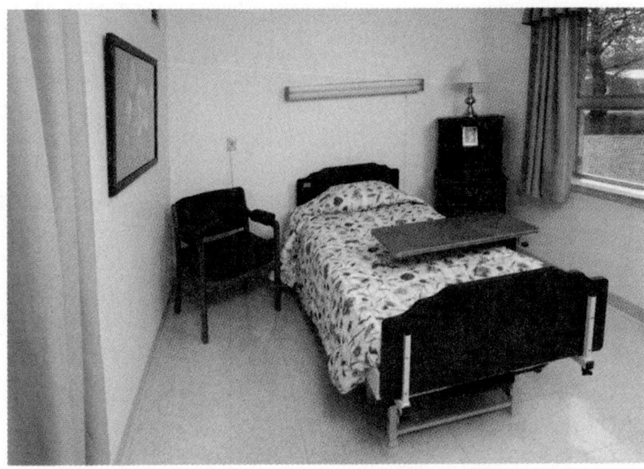

FIGURE 15-1 Furniture and equipment in a resident's unit.

BOX 15-1 Maintaining the Person's Unit

- Keep the call light within the person's reach at all times.
- Meet the needs of persons who cannot use the call system (p. 205).
- Make sure the person can reach the over-bed table (p. 205) and the bedside stand (p. 205).
- Arrange personal items as the person prefers. They are within easy reach.
- Place the phone and TV, bed, and light controls within the person's reach.
- Provide enough tissues and toilet paper.
- Adjust lighting, temperature, and ventilation for the person's comfort.
- Handle equipment carefully to prevent noise.
- Explain the causes of strange noises.
- Use room deodorizers according to agency policy.
- Empty wastebaskets at least once a day. In some agencies, they are emptied every shift. Always empty them when full.
- Respect the person's belongings. An item may not seem important to you. But even a scrap of paper can mean a great deal to the person.
- Do not throw away any items that belong to the person.
- Do not move furniture or the person's items. Persons with poor vision rely on memory or feel to find items.
- Straighten bed linens and towels as often as needed.
- Complete a safety check before leaving the room. (See the inside of the front cover.)

FOCUS ON COMMUNICATION

Comfort

What is comfortable for one person may not be for another. Ask about the person's comfort. You can say:

- "How is the temperature? Is it too hot or too cold?"
- "Is the noise level okay?"
- "Please let me know if you notice any bad odors."
- "How is the lighting? Is it too bright or too dark?"
- "Are you comfortable?"

Temperature and Ventilation

Most healthy people are comfortable when the temperature is 68°F (Fahrenheit) to 74°F. Persons who are older or ill may need higher temperatures for comfort. The Centers for Medicare & Medicaid Services (CMS) requires that nursing centers maintain a temperature of 71°F to 81°F.

To protect older and ill persons from cool areas and drafts:

- Have them wear the correct clothing.
- Have them wear enough clothing.
- Offer lap robes to those in chairs and wheelchairs. Lap robes cover the legs.
- Provide enough blankets for warmth.
- Cover them with bath blankets when giving care.
- Move them from drafty areas.

Odors

Odors occur in health care settings. Bowel movements and urine have embarrassing odors. So do draining wounds and vomitus. Body, breath, and smoking odors may offend others. To reduce odors:

- Empty, clean, and disinfect bedpans, urinals, commodes, and kidney basins promptly.
- Make sure toilets are flushed.
- Check incontinent persons often (Chapters 18 and 19).
- Clean persons who are wet or soiled from urine, feces, vomitus, or wound drainage.
- Change wet or soiled linens and clothing promptly.
- Keep laundry containers closed.
- Follow agency policy for wet or soiled linens and clothing.
- Dispose of incontinence and ostomy products promptly (Chapters 18 and 19).
- Provide good hygiene to prevent body and breath odors (Chapter 16).
- Use room deodorizers as needed and allowed by agency policy. Sometimes odors remain after removing the cause. Do not use sprays around persons with breathing problems. Ask the nurse if you are unsure.

Smoke odors present special problems. If you smoke, follow the agency's policy. Practice hand washing after smoking or handling smoking materials and before giving care. Give careful attention to your uniform, hair, and breath because of smoke odors.

Noise

According to the CMS, a "comfortable" sound level:
- Does not interfere with a person's hearing.
- Promotes privacy when privacy is desired.
- Allows the person to take part in social activities.

Common health care sounds may disturb some persons. Such sounds include:
- The clanging and clattering of equipment, dishes, and meal trays
- Loud voices, TVs, radios, music players, ringing phones, and so on
- Intercom systems and call lights
- Equipment or wheels needing repair or oil
- Cleaning and housekeeping equipment

To decrease noise levels:
- Control your voice.
- Handle equipment carefully.
- Keep equipment in good working order.
- Answer phones, call lights, and intercoms promptly.

See *Focus on Communication: Noise.*

See *Focus on Older Persons: Noise.*

See *Focus on Surveys: Noise.*

FOCUS ON COMMUNICATION
Noise

All staff must try to reduce noise. To reduce noise:
- Do not talk loudly in the hallways or nurses' station.
- Ask others to speak more softly. Ask politely.
- Avoid unnecessary conversation. Be professional. Do not discuss inappropriate topics at work. Others may overhear and become offended.

FOCUS ON OLDER PERSONS
Noise

Persons with dementia do not understand what is happening around them. Common, everyday sounds may disturb them. For example, a person may not know or understand the sound of a ringing phone. He or she may have an extreme reaction to the sound (Chapter 30). The reaction may be more severe at night. This is likely if the sound awakens the person suddenly. A dark, strange room can make the problem worse.

FOCUS ON SURVEYS
Noise

Surveyors will observe for comfortable sound levels. They will observe if:
- Background noises affect the person's ability to be heard or take part in activities.
- Staff have to raise their voices to be heard.
- Sound levels are comfortable in the evening and during the night.
- The intercom volume is too loud.

Do your best to decrease noise and provide comfortable sound levels.

Lighting

Good lighting is needed for safety and comfort. Glares, shadows, and dull lighting can cause falls, headaches, and eyestrain. A bright room is cheerful. Dim light is relaxing and restful.

Adjust lighting and window coverings to meet the person's changing needs. The over-bed light can provide soft, medium, or bright lighting. Keep light controls within the person's reach. This protects the right to personal choice.

See *Focus on Older Persons: Lighting.*

FOCUS ON OLDER PERSONS
Lighting

For persons with dementia, lighting is adjusted to help control agitated and aggressive behaviors. Soft, non-glare lights are relaxing. They can decrease agitation. Bright lighting lets the person see surroundings more clearly. This may improve orientation.

ROOM FURNITURE AND EQUIPMENT

Rooms are furnished and equipped to meet basic needs. The right to privacy is considered.

The Bed

Beds have electrical or manual controls. Beds are raised horizontally to give care. A low horizontal position lets the person get out of bed with ease. The head and foot of the bed are flat or raised varying degrees.

Electric beds are common. Controls are on a side panel, bed rail, or the foot-board. Some controls are hand-held devices (Fig. 15-2). Patients and residents are taught to use the controls safely. They are warned not to raise the bed to the high position or to adjust the bed to harmful positions. They are told of any position limits or restrictions.

Manual beds have cranks at the foot of the bed (Fig. 15-3). Pull the cranks up for use. Keep them down at all other times. Cranks in the "up" position are safety hazards. Anyone walking past may bump into them.

See *Promoting Safety and Comfort: The Bed.*

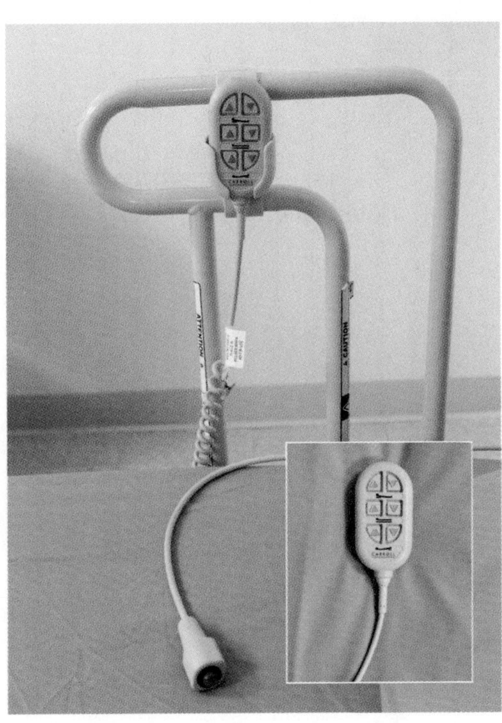

FIGURE 15-2 A hand-held bed control (see inset) can be attached to the bed rail.

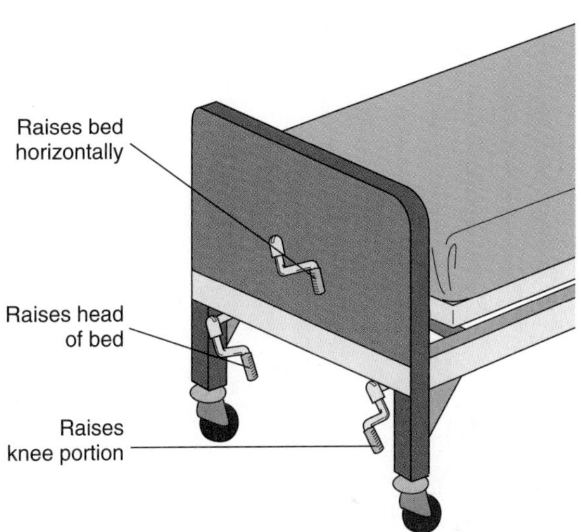

FIGURE 15-3 Manually operated bed.

PROMOTING SAFETY AND COMFORT

The Bed

Safety

The staff can lock most electric beds into any position. The person cannot adjust the bed to unsafe positions. Beds are locked for persons restricted to certain positions. They may be locked for persons with confusion or dementia.

Beds have bed rails and wheels (Chapter 9). Bed wheels are locked at all times except when moving the bed. They must be locked to:

- Give bedside care.
- Transfer the person to and from the bed. The person can be injured if the bed moves. So can you.

Use bed rails as the nurse and care plan direct. Otherwise the person could suffer injury or harm.

Comfort

Some persons spend a lot of time in bed. Adjust the bed to meet the person's needs. Tell the nurse if the person complains about the bed or mattress.

Bed Positions. There are 6 basic bed positions.

- *Flat* is the usual sleeping position.
- ***Fowler's position*** *is a semi-sitting position. The head of the bed is raised between 45 and 60 degrees* (Fig. 15-4). See Chapter 13.
- ***High-Fowler's position*** *is a semi-sitting position. The head of the bed is raised 60 to 90 degrees* (Fig. 15-5).
- ***Semi-Fowler's position*** *means the head of the bed is raised 30 degrees* (Fig. 15-6). Some agencies define semi-Fowler's position as when the *head of the bed is raised 30 degrees and the knee portion is raised 15 degrees.* Know the definition used by your agency.
- ***Trendelenburg's position*** *means the head of the bed is lowered and the foot of the bed is raised* (Fig. 15-7). A doctor orders this position. Blocks are placed under the bed legs at the foot of the bed. Or the bed frame is tilted.
- ***Reverse Trendelenburg's position*** *means the head of the bed is raised and the foot of the bed is lowered* (Fig. 15-8). A doctor orders this position. Blocks are placed under the bed legs at the head of the bed. Or the bed frame is tilted.

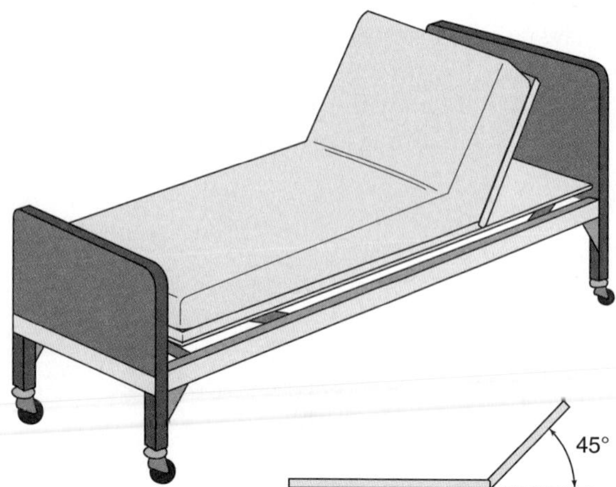

FIGURE 15-4 Fowler's position.

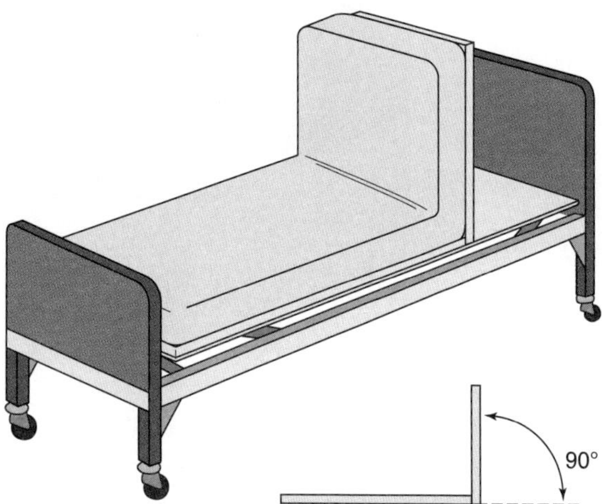

FIGURE 15-5 High-Fowler's position.

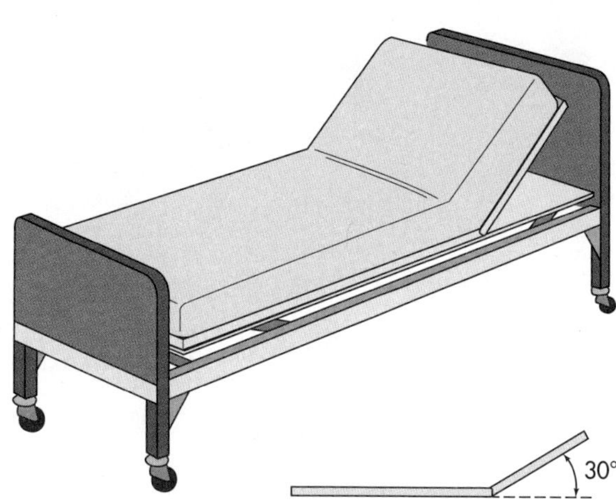

FIGURE 15-6 Semi-Fowler's position.

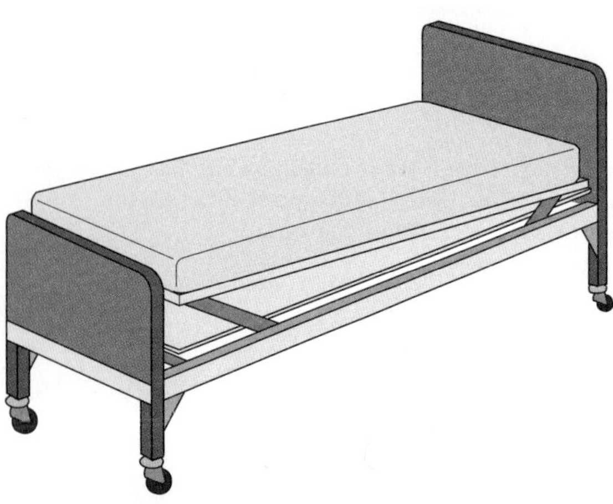
FIGURE 15-7 Trendelenburg's position.

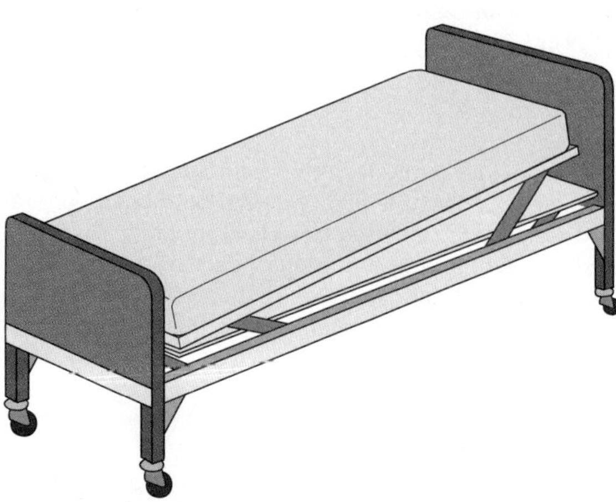
FIGURE 15-8 Reverse Trendelenburg's position.

Bed Safety. Bed safety involves the *hospital bed system*—the bed frame and its parts. The parts include the mattress, bed rails, head-board and foot-board, and bed attachments.

Hospital bed systems have 7 entrapment zones (Figs. 15-9 and 15-10, p. 204). *Entrapment* means that the person can get caught, trapped, or entangled in spaces created by the bed rails, the mattress, the bed frame, the head-board, or the foot-board. Head, neck, and chest entrapment can cause serious injuries and death. Arm and leg entrapment also can occur. Persons at greatest risk:

- Are older.
- Are frail.
- Are confused or disoriented.
- Are restless.
- Have uncontrolled body movements.
- Have poor muscle control.
- Are small in size.
- Are restrained (Chapter 11).

Always check the person for entrapment. If a person is caught, trapped, or entangled in the bed or any of its parts, try to release the person. Also call for the nurse at once.

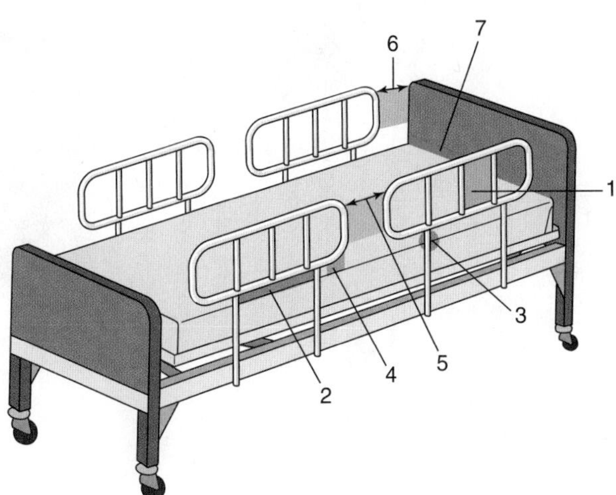

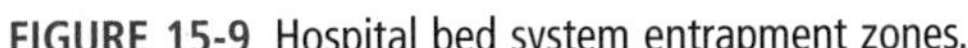

FIGURE 15-9 Hospital bed system entrapment zones.

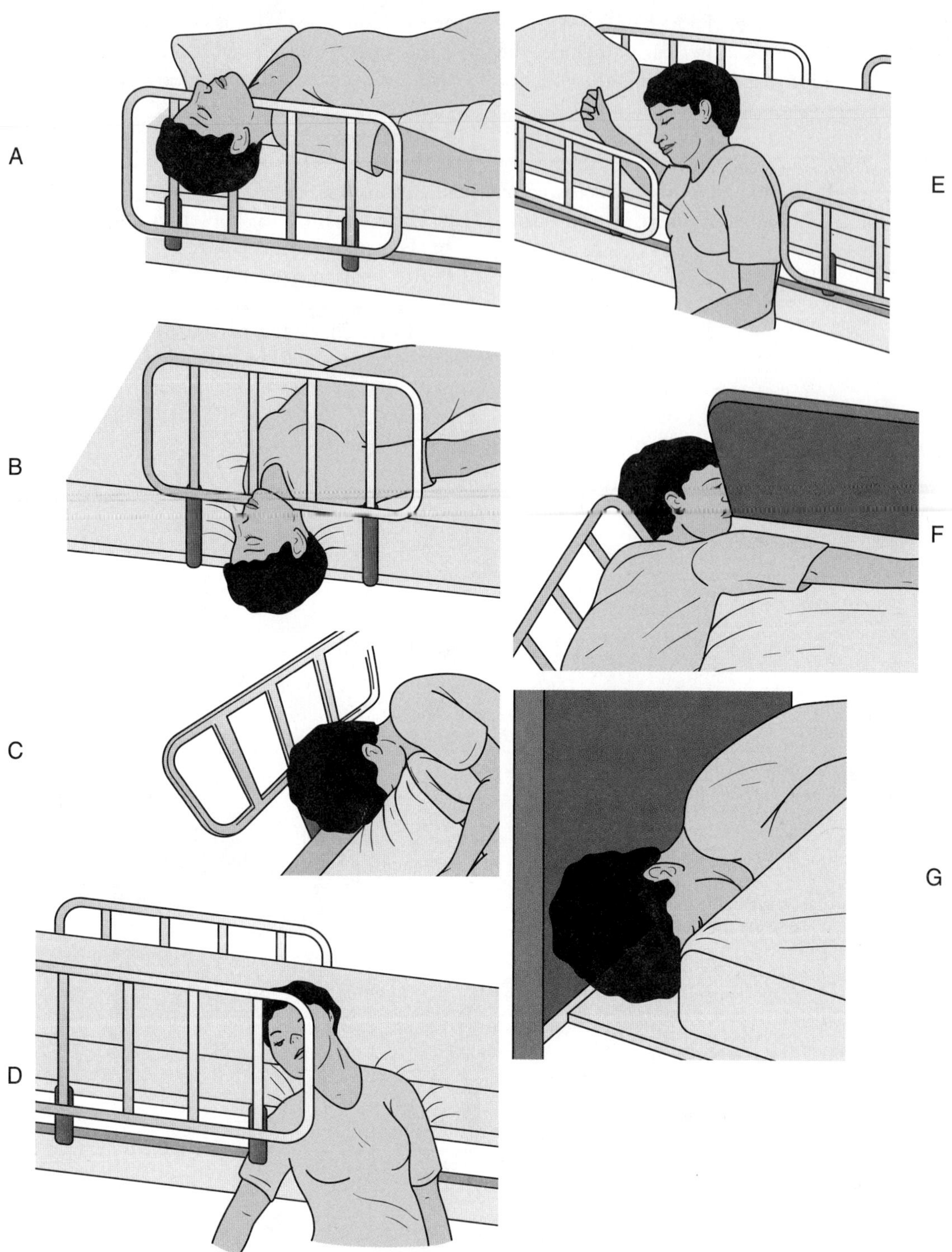

FIGURE 15-10 Hospital bed system entrapment zones. **A,** *Zone 1:* Within the bed rail. **B,** *Zone 2:* Between the top of the compressed mattress and the bottom of the bed rail and between the rail supports. **C,** *Zone 3:* Between the bed rail and the mattress. **D,** *Zone 4:* Between the top of the compressed mattress and the bottom of the bed rail and at the end of the bed rail. **E,** *Zone 5:* Between the split bed rails. **F,** *Zone 6:* Between the end of the bed rail and the side edge of the head-board or foot-board. **G,** *Zone 7:* Between the head-board or foot-board and the end of the mattress.

The Over-Bed Table

The over-bed table (see Fig. 15-1) is moved over the bed by sliding the base under the bed. The table is raised or lowered for bed or chair use. Use the handle or lever to adjust table height. The table is used for meals, writing, reading, and other activities.

The nursing team uses the over-bed table as a work area. Place only clean and sterile items on the table. Never place bedpans, urinals, or soiled linen on the over-bed table. Clean the table after use as a work surface. Also clean it before serving meal trays.

The Bedside Stand

By the bed, the bedside stand has a top drawer and a lower cabinet with shelves or drawers (Fig. 15-11). The top drawer is used for small items—money, eyeglasses, books, and so on.

The top shelf or middle drawer is used for the wash basin. The wash basin holds personal care items—soap and soap dish, powder, lotion, deodorant, towels, washcloth, bath blanket, and sleepwear. An emesis basin or kidney basin (shaped like a kidney) holds oral hygiene items. The kidney basin is stored in the top drawer, middle drawer, or on the top shelf. The bedpan and its cover, the urinal, and toilet paper are stored on the lower shelf or in the bottom drawer.

The stand top is often used for tissues and other personal items. A clock, photos, phone, flowers, cards, and gifts are examples.

Place only clean and sterile items on the bedside stand. Never place bedpans, urinals, or soiled linen on the top of the stand. Clean the bedside stand after use as a work surface.

Chairs

The person's unit has at least 1 chair. It must be comfortable, sturdy, and not move or tip during transfers. The person should be able to get in and out of the chair with ease. Nursing center residents may bring chairs from home.

Privacy Curtains

Each person has the right to ***full visual privacy***—*having the means to be completely free from public view while in bed.* The privacy curtain is pulled around the bed to provide privacy. *Always pull the curtain completely around the bed before giving care.*

Privacy curtains do not block sounds or voices. Others in the room can hear sounds or talking behind the curtain.

The Call System

The call system lets the person signal for help. The call light is at the end of a long cord (Fig. 15-12). It attaches to the bed or chair. (See p. 207 for call lights in bathrooms and shower and tub rooms.) *Always keep the call light within the person's reach—in the room, bathroom, and shower or tub room.*

To get help, the person presses a button at the end of the call light. The call light connects to a light above the room door. The call light also connects to a computer, light panel, or intercom system at the nurses' station (Fig. 15-13, p. 206). These tell the staff that the person needs help.

An intercom system lets the staff talk with the person from the nurses' station. The person tells what is needed. Then the light is turned off at the station. Hard-of-hearing persons may have problems with an intercom. Be careful when using an intercom. Remember confidentiality. Persons nearby can hear what you and the person say.

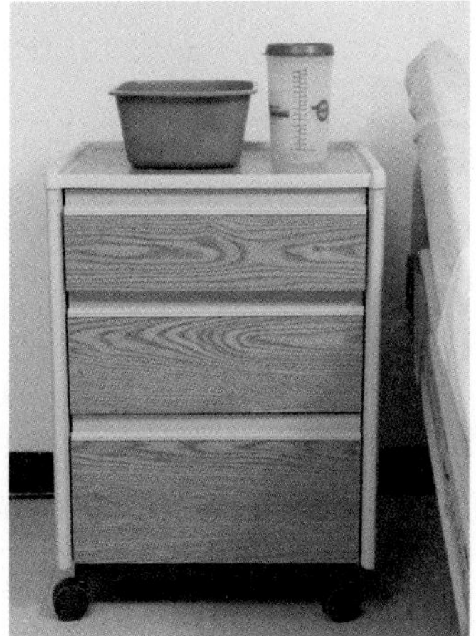

FIGURE 15-11 The bedside stand.

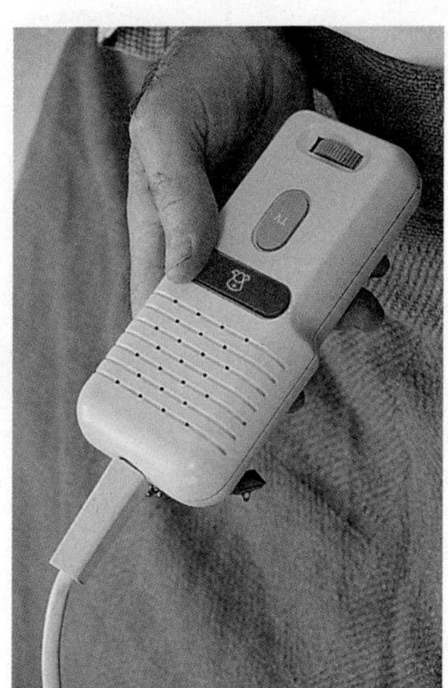

FIGURE 15-12 The call light. The call light button is pressed when help is needed.

Some call lights are turned on by tapping with a hand or fist (Fig. 15-14). They are useful for persons with limited hand movement.

Some people cannot use call lights. Examples are persons who are confused or in a coma. The care plan lists special communication measures. Check these persons often. Make sure their needs are met.

See *Focus on Communication: The Call System.*

See *Promoting Safety and Comfort: The Call System.*

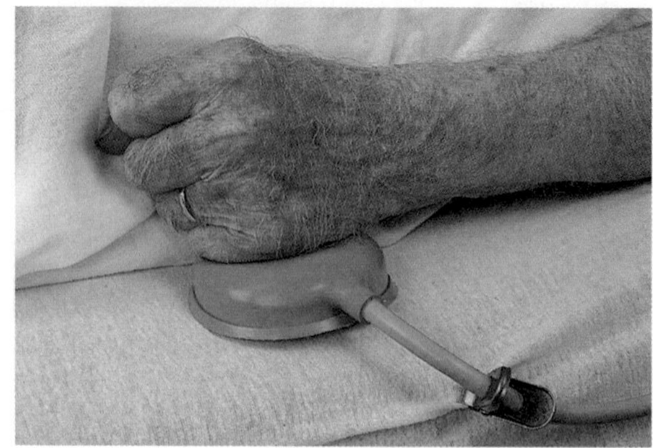

FIGURE 15-14 Call light for a person with limited hand movement.

A

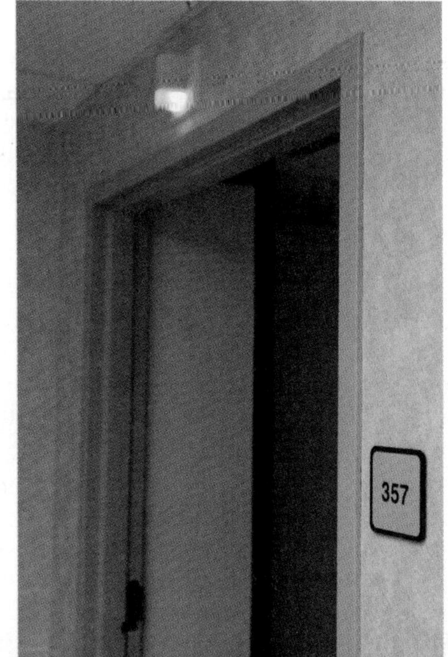

B

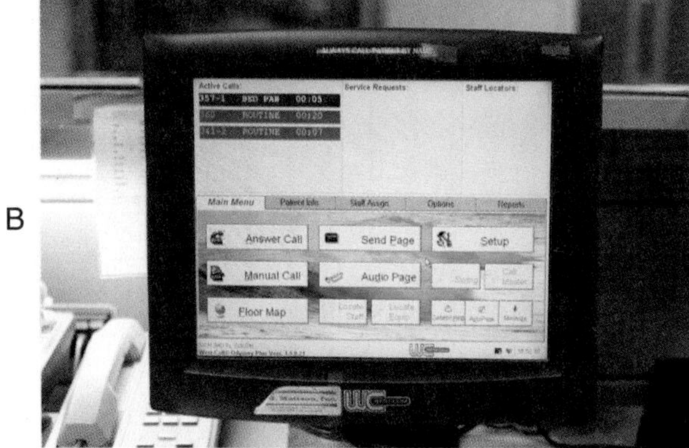

FIGURE 15-13 A, Light above the room door. With this system, the color signals the type of help needed using the hand-held call light—red for a nurse, green for pain, yellow for elimination needs. **B,** Computer monitor at the nurses' station.

FOCUS ON COMMUNICATION

The Call System

You will answer call lights for co-workers. You may not know their patients and residents and they may not know you. To promote quality of life and safe care, you can say:

- "My name is Kate Hines. I'm a nursing assistant. How can I help you?"
- "Mrs. Janz, I'll need to check your care plan before I bring you more salt. I'll be right back, but is there anything else I can do before I leave?"
- "Mr. Duncan, I'll be happy to take your meal tray. I'll tell your nursing assistant what you ate."
- "Mrs. Palmer, do you use the bathroom or the bedpan?"

Sometimes patients and residents signal for help often. Do not delay in meeting their needs. Never take call lights away from them. This is not safe. Avoid statements that make a person feel as if he or she is a burden. For example, do not say:

- "I just helped you to the bathroom. Can't you wait?"
- "I was just in your room. What do you want now?"

Do not discourage the person from asking for help. The person may try to do something alone. This could cause injury. Tell the nurse. Your co-workers can help you meet the person's needs.

PROMOTING SAFETY AND COMFORT

The Call System

Safety

Each patient and resident has a call light. When in their rooms, using the toilet, or in a bathing area, they must be able to call for help. To promote safety, you must:

- Keep the call light within the person's reach. Even if the person cannot use the call light, keep it within reach for use by visitors and staff. They may need to call for help.
- Place the call light on the person's strong side.
- Remind the person to use the call light when help is needed.
- Answer call lights promptly. For example, the person may have an urgent need to use the bathroom. Helping promptly prevents embarrassing problems. You also help prevent infection, skin breakdown, pressure ulcers, and falls.
- Answer bathroom and shower or tub room call lights at once.

The Bathroom

A toilet, sink, call system, and mirror are standard equipment in bathrooms. Some bathrooms have showers.

Grab bars are by the toilet for safety. The person uses them for support to get on and off the toilet. Some bathrooms have higher toilets or raised toilet seats. They make wheelchair transfers easier and are helpful for persons with joint problems.

Towel racks, toilet paper, soap, paper towel dispenser, and a wastebasket are in the bathroom. They are within the person's reach.

Usually the call light is a button or pull cord next to the toilet. The bathroom call light flashes red above the room door and at the nurses' station. To alert the staff, the sound at the nurses' station is different from room call lights. Someone must respond at once when a person needs help in the bathroom.

Closet and Drawer Space

Closet and drawer space are provided. The CMS requires that nursing centers provide each person with closet space with shelves and a clothes rack. Hanging clothes must be within the person's reach. The person has free access to items in the closet.

Sometimes people hoard items—napkins, straws, food, sugar, salt, pepper, and so on. Hoarding can cause safety or health risks. The staff can inspect a person's closet or drawers if hoarding is suspected. The person is informed of the inspection. He or she is present when it takes place.

See *Promoting Safety and Comfort: Closet and Drawer Space.*

PROMOTING SAFETY AND COMFORT

Closet and Drawer Space

Safety

Items in closets and drawers are the person's property. You must have the person's permission to open closets or drawers.

The nurse may ask you to inspect a person's closet, drawers, or personal items. If so, the person must be present. Also have a co-worker with you. Your co-worker is a witness to what you are doing. This protects you if the person claims that something was stolen or damaged.

Other Equipment

Many agencies furnish rooms with other equipment. A TV, radio, and clock provide comfort and relaxation. Many rooms have phones, a computer, and Internet access.

See *Promoting Safety and Comfort: Other Equipment.*

PROMOTING SAFETY AND COMFORT

Other Equipment

Safety

Nursing center residents are allowed personal choice in arranging items. The choices must be safe and not cause falls or other accidents. You may have to help the person choose the best place for personal items.

Comfort

Nursing center residents have left their homes. Each had furniture, appliances, a bathroom, and many belongings and treasures. Now the person lives in a new place. He or she probably has a roommate. Leaving one's home is a hard part of growing old with poor health. The person's unit should be as home-like as possible.

Residents may bring some furniture and personal items from home. A chair, footstool, lamp, and small table are often allowed. They can bring photos, religious items, and books. Some have plants to care for.

The center is now the person's home. Help the person feel safe, secure, and comfortable. A home-like setting is important for quality of life.

BEDMAKING

Beds are made every day. Clean, dry, and wrinkle-free linens:

- Promote comfort.
- Prevent skin breakdown.
- Prevent pressure ulcers (Chapter 25).

Beds are usually made in the morning after baths. Or they are made while the person is in the shower, up in the chair, or out of the room. To keep beds neat and clean:

- Change linens when they are wet, soiled, or damp.
- Straighten linens when loose or wrinkled and at bedtime.
- Check for and remove food and crumbs after meals and snacks.
- Check linens for dentures, eyeglasses, hearing aids, sharp objects, and other items.
- Follow Standard Precautions and the Bloodborne Pathogen Standard. Contact with blood, body fluids, secretions, or excretions is likely.

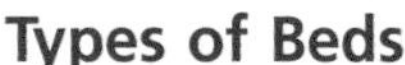

Types of Beds

Beds are made in these ways.

- A *closed bed* is not in use. Top linens are not folded back (Fig. 15-15). The bed is ready for a new patient or resident. In nursing centers, closed beds are made for residents who are up during the day.
- An *open bed* is in use. Top linens are fan-folded back. A closed bed becomes an open bed by fan-folding back the top linens (Fig. 15-16).
- An *occupied bed* is made with the person in it (Fig. 15-17).
- A *surgical bed* is made to transfer a person from a stretcher to bed (Fig. 15-18). This includes an ambulance stretcher.

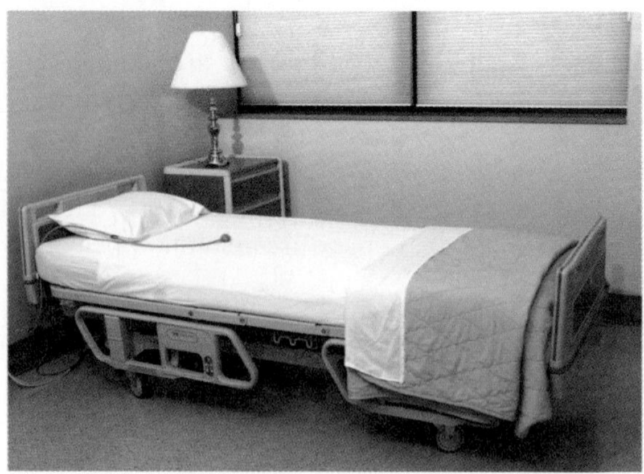

FIGURE 15-16 Open bed. Top linens are fan-folded to the foot of the bed.

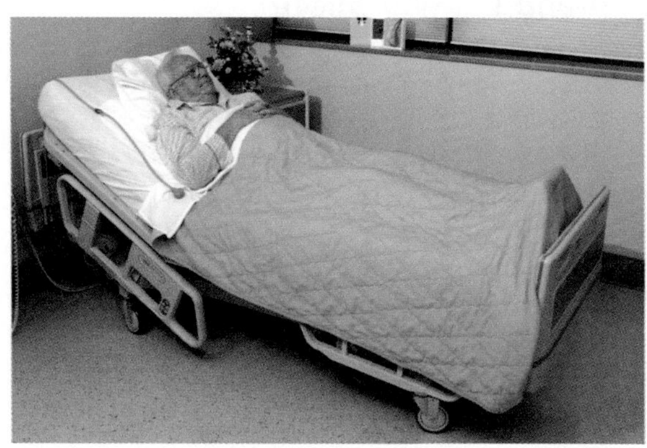

FIGURE 15-17 Occupied bed.

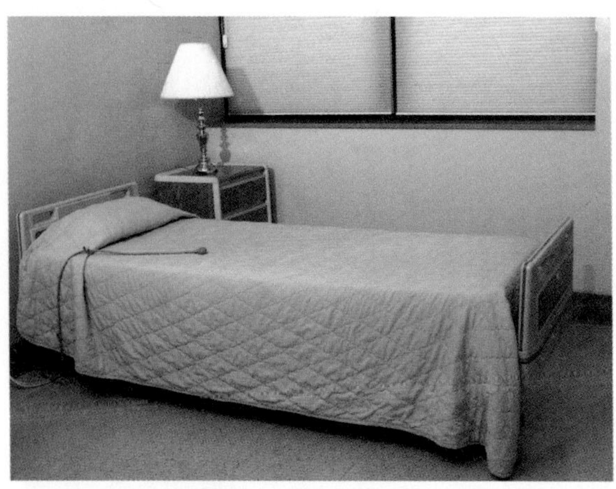

FIGURE 15-15 Closed bed.

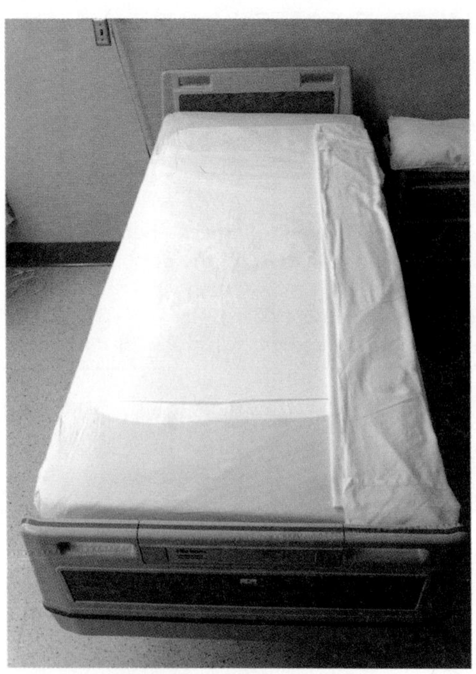

FIGURE 15-18 Surgical bed.

Linens

Collect linens in the order you will use them. Doing so makes it easy to remember what you need.

- Mattress pad (if needed)
- Bottom sheet (flat or fitted)
- Waterproof drawsheet or waterproof pad (if needed)
- Cotton drawsheet (if needed)
- Top sheet
- Blanket
- Bedspread
- Pillowcase(s)
- Bath towel(s)
- Hand towel
- Washcloth
- Gown or pajamas
- Bath blanket

Use 1 arm to hold the linens. Use your other hand to pick them up. The first item is at the bottom of the stack. (The mattress pad is at the bottom. The bath blanket is on top.) To get the mattress pad on top, place your arm over the bath blanket. Then turn the stack over onto the arm on the bath blanket (Fig. 15-19). The arm that held the linens is now free. Place the clean linen on a clean surface.

Remove dirty linen 1 piece at a time. Roll each piece away from you. The side that touched the person is inside the roll and away from you (Fig. 15-20). Discard each piece into a laundry bag.

In hospitals, top and bottom sheets, the cotton drawsheet, and pillowcases are changed daily. If still clean, the mattress pad, waterproof drawsheet, blanket, and bedspread are re-used for the same person.

In nursing centers, linens are not changed every day. A complete linen change is usually done on the person's shower day. This may be once or twice a week. Pillowcases, top and bottom sheets, and drawsheets (if used) may be changed twice a week.

Linens are not re-used if soiled, wet, or wrinkled. Wet, damp, or soiled linens are changed right away. Wear gloves and follow Standard Precautions and the Bloodborne Pathogen Standard.

See *Focus on Surveys: Linens.*

A

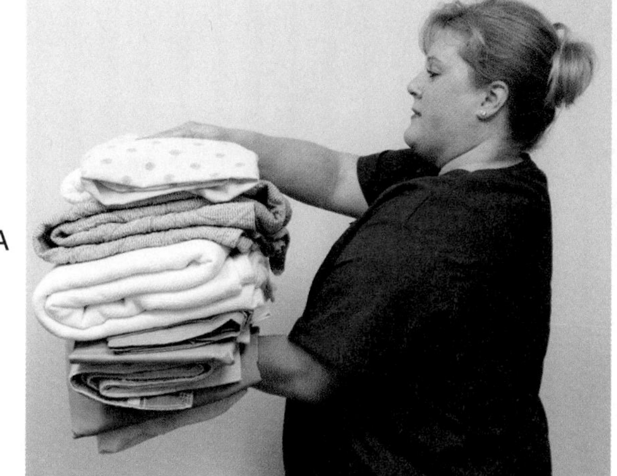

B

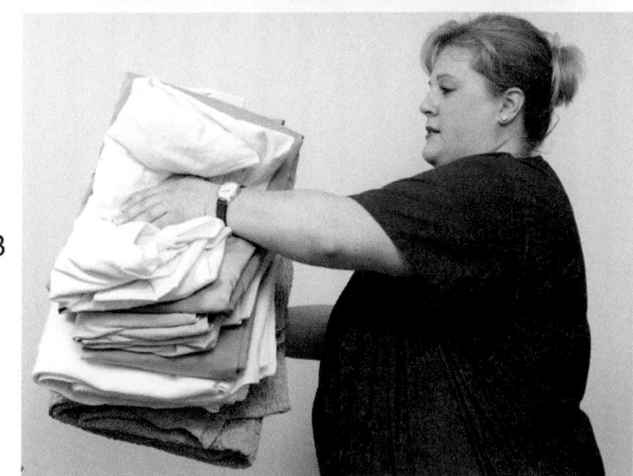

FIGURE 15-19 Collecting linens. Linens are held away from the body and uniform. **A,** The arm is placed over the top of the stack of linens. **B,** The stack of linens is turned onto the arm.

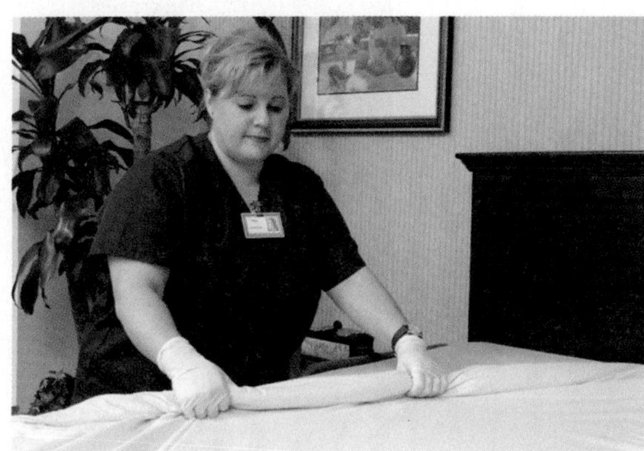

FIGURE 15-20 Roll dirty linen away from you.

FOCUS ON SURVEYS

Linens

Linens may contain blood, body fluids, secretions, or excretions. They may contain microbes. You must help prevent and control the spread of infection. Surveyors will observe:

- How you transport linens.
- If you practice hand hygiene after handling soiled or used linens.
- If you double-bag linen when the outside of the laundry bag is visibly contaminated or wet.
- If you bag contaminated linen where it is used. The person's room and the shower room are examples.

Drawsheets and Waterproof Pads. Drawsheets and waterproof pads absorb moisture and protect the skin. A *drawsheet* is a small sheet placed over the middle of the bottom sheet.

- A *cotton drawsheet* is made of cotton. It helps keep the mattress and bottom linens clean.
- A *waterproof drawsheet* is a drawsheet made of plastic, rubber, or absorbent material. It protects the mattress and bottom linens from dampness and soiling. Some are rubber or plastic on 1 side—the waterproof side. The waterproof side is placed down, away from the person. The other side is cotton. It is placed up, toward the person. Other waterproof drawsheets are disposable. They are discarded when wet, soiled, or wrinkled.

The cotton drawsheet protects the person from contact with plastic or rubber and absorbs moisture. Plastic and rubber retain heat. Waterproof drawsheets are hard to keep tight and wrinkle-free. Discomfort and skin breakdown may occur.

Many agencies use incontinence products (Chapter 18) to keep the person and linens dry. Waterproof pads or disposable bed protectors are also used (Fig. 15-21).

Cotton drawsheets are often used without waterproof drawsheets. Plastic-covered mattresses cause some persons to perspire. This causes discomfort. A cotton drawsheet reduces heat retention and absorbs moisture. Cotton drawsheets are often used as assist devices to move and transfer persons in bed (Chapter 14). If used as an assist device, leave the sides untucked if allowed by agency policy.

The procedures that follow include waterproof and cotton drawsheets. This is so you learn how to use them. Ask the nurse what is used in your agency. Follow the care plan and the nurse's directions.

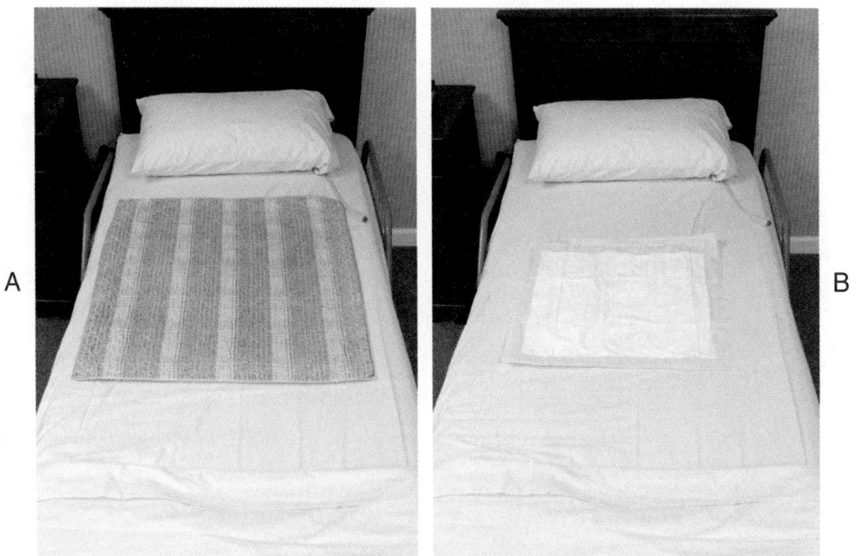

FIGURE 15-21 **A,** Waterproof pad. **B,** Disposable bed protector.

Making Beds

When making beds, follow the rules in Box 15-2.
See *Delegation Guidelines: Making Beds.*
See *Promoting Safety and Comfort: Making Beds.*

The Closed Bed. Closed beds are made for:

- New patients and residents. The bed is made after the bed frame and mattress are cleaned and disinfected. Clean linens are needed for the entire bed.
- For persons who are up for most or all of the day. Top linens are folded back at bedtime. Clean linens are used as needed.

See procedure: *Making a Closed Bed,* p. 212.

Text continued on p. 216

BOX 15-2 Rules for Bedmaking

- Use good body mechanics at all times (Chapter 13).
- Follow the rules in Chapter 14 to safely move and transfer the person.
- Follow the rules of medical asepsis.
- Follow Standard Precautions and the Bloodborne Pathogen Standard.
- Practice hand hygiene before handling clean linen.
- Bring enough linen to the person's room. Do not bring extra linen.
- Bring only the linens that you will need. You cannot use extra linen for another person.
- Place clean linen on a clean surface. Use the bedside chair, over-bed table, or bedside stand. Place a barrier (towel, paper towel) between the clean surface and the linen if required by agency policy.
- Do not use extra linen in the person's room for another resident. Extra linen is considered contaminated. Put it with the dirty laundry.
- Do not use torn or frayed linen.
- Never shake linens. Shaking spreads microbes.
- Hold linens away from your body and uniform. Do not let dirty or clean linen touch your uniform. Your uniform is considered "dirty."
- Wear gloves to remove linen. Linens may contain blood, body fluids, secretions, or excretions. Practice hand hygiene after removing the gloves.
- Never put dirty linens on the floor or on clean linens. Follow agency policy for dirty linen.
- Keep bottom linens tucked in and wrinkle-free.
- Cover a waterproof drawsheet with a cotton drawsheet. Plastic or rubber must not touch the person's body.
- Straighten and tighten loose sheets, blankets, and bedspreads as needed.
- Make as much of 1 side of the bed as possible before going to the other side. This saves time and energy.
- Change wet, damp, or soiled linens right away.

DELEGATION GUIDELINES

Making Beds

Before making a bed, you need this information from the nurse and the care plan.

- What type of bed to make—closed, open, occupied, or surgical.
- If you need to use a cotton drawsheet.
- If you need to use a waterproof drawsheet, waterproof pad, or incontinence product.
- If the person uses bed rails.
- The person's treatment, therapy, and activity schedule. For example, Mr. Smith needs a treatment in bed. Change linens after the treatment. Change Mrs. Chapman's bed while she is in physical therapy.
- Position restrictions or limits in the person's movement or activity.
- How to position the person and the positioning devices needed.
- If the bed needs to be locked into a certain position (p. 201).
- When to report observations.
- What patient or resident concerns to report at once.

PROMOTING SAFETY AND COMFORT

Making Beds

Safety

You need to raise the bed for body mechanics. The bed also must be flat. If the bed is locked, unlock it. Then adjust the bed. Return the bed to the correct position when you are done. Then lock the bed.

Wear gloves to remove linen. Also follow other aspects of Standard Precautions and the Bloodborne Pathogen Standard. Linens may contain blood, body fluids, secretions, or excretions.

After making a bed, lower the bed to the correct level for the person. Follow the care plan. For an occupied bed, raise or lower bed rails according to the care plan.

Comfort

For an occupied bed, cover the person with a bath blanket before removing the top sheet. Do not leave the person uncovered. The bath blanket provides warmth and privacy.

Adjust the person's pillow as needed during the procedure. After the procedure, position the person as directed by the nurse and the care plan. Always make sure linens are straight and wrinkle-free.

Making a Closed Bed

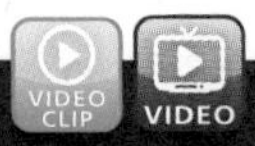

QUALITY OF LIFE

- Knock before entering the person's room.
- Address the person by name.
- Introduce yourself by name and title.
- Explain the procedure before starting and during the procedure.
- Protect the person's rights during the procedure.
- Handle the person gently during the procedure.

PRE-PROCEDURE

1 Follow *Delegation Guidelines: Making Beds,* p. 211. See *Promoting Safety and Comfort: Making Beds,* p. 211.
2 Practice hand hygiene.
3 Collect clean linen and other supplies.
   - Mattress pad (if needed)
   - Bottom sheet (flat sheet or fitted sheet)
   - Waterproof drawsheet or waterproof pad (if needed)
   - Cotton drawsheet (if needed)
   - Top sheet
   - Blanket
   - Bedspread
   - A pillowcase for each pillow
   - Bath towel
   - Hand towel
   - Washcloth
   - Gown or pajamas
   - Bath blanket
   - Gloves
   - Laundry bag
   - Paper towels (as a barrier for clean linens)
4 Place linen on a clean surface. Use the paper towels as a barrier between the clean surface and clean linen if required by agency policy.
5 Raise the bed for body mechanics. Bed rails are down.

PROCEDURE

6 Put on the gloves.
7 Remove linen. Roll each piece away from you. Place each piece in a laundry bag. (NOTE: Discard the incontinence product, disposable bed protector, and disposable drawsheet in the trash. Do not put them in the laundry bag.)
8 Clean the bed frame and mattress (if this is your job).
9 Remove and discard the gloves. Practice hand hygiene.
10 Move the mattress to the head of the bed.
11 Put the mattress pad on the mattress. It is even with the top of the mattress.
12 Place the bottom sheet on the mattress pad (Fig. 15-22). Unfold it length-wise. Place the center crease in the middle of the bed. If using a flat sheet:
   a Position the lower edge even with the bottom of the mattress.
   b Place the large hem at the top and the small hem at the bottom.
   c Face hem-stitching downward away from the person.
13 Open the sheet. Fan-fold it to the other side of the bed (Fig. 15-23).
14 Tuck the corners of a fitted sheet over the mattress at the top and then foot of the bed. For a flat sheet, tuck the top of the sheet under the mattress. The sheet is tight and smooth.
15 Make a mitered corner at the top if using a flat sheet (Fig. 15-24, p. 214).
16 *If using a cotton drawsheet:*
   a Place the drawsheet on the bed. It is in the middle of the mattress.
   b Open the drawsheet. Fan-fold it to the other side of the bed.
   c Tuck the drawsheet under the mattress.
17 *If using a waterproof pad,* place the waterproof pad on the bed. It is in the middle of the mattress. See Fig. 15-21, *A*.
18 *If using waterproof and cotton drawsheets:*
   a Place the waterproof drawsheet on the bed. It is in the middle of the mattress.
   b Open the waterproof drawsheet. Fan-fold it to the other side of the bed.
   c Place a cotton drawsheet over the waterproof drawsheet. It covers the entire waterproof drawsheet (Fig. 15-25, p. 214).
   d Open the cotton drawsheet. Fan-fold it to the other side of the bed.
   e Tuck both drawsheets under the mattress. Or tuck each in separately.
19 Go to the other side of the bed.
20 Miter the top corner of the flat bottom sheet.
21 Pull the bottom sheet tight so there are no wrinkles. Tuck in the sheet.
22 Pull the drawsheets tight so there are no wrinkles (Fig. 15-26, p. 215). Tuck in the drawsheets.
23 Go to the other side of the bed.
24 Put the top sheet on the bed.
   a Unfold it length-wise. Place the center crease in the middle.
   b Place the large hem even with the top of the mattress.
   c Open the sheet. Fan-fold it to the other side.
   d Face hem-stitching outward, away from the person.
   e Do not tuck the bottom in yet.
   f Never tuck top linens in on the sides.
25 Place the blanket on the bed.
   a Unfold it so the center crease is in the middle.
   b Put the upper hem about 6 to 8 inches from the top of the mattress.
   c Open the blanket. Fan-fold it to the other side.
   d If steps 31 and 32 are not done, turn the top sheet down over the blanket. Hem-stitching is down, away from the person.

Making a Closed Bed—cont'd

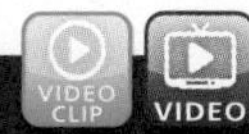

PROCEDURE—cont'd

26 Place the bedspread on the bed.
  a Unfold it so the center crease is in the middle.
  b Place the upper hem even with the top of the mattress.
  c Open and fan-fold the bedspread to the other side.
  d Make sure the bedspread facing the door is even. It covers all top linens.

27 Tuck in top linens together at the foot of the bed so they are smooth and tight. Make a mitered corner.

28 Go to the other side.

29 Straighten all top linen. Work from the head of the bed to the foot.

30 Tuck in top linens together at the foot of the bed. Make a mitered corner.

31 Turn the top hem of the bedspread under the blanket to form a cuff (Fig. 15-27, p. 215).

32 Turn the top sheet down over the bedspread. Hem-stitching is down. (Steps 31 and 32 are not done in some agencies. The bedspread covers the pillow. If so, tuck the bedspread under the pillow.)

33 Put the pillowcase on the pillow as in Figure 15-28, p. 215 or Figure 15-29, p. 215. Fold extra material under the pillow at the open end of the pillowcase.

34 Place the pillow on the bed. The open end of the pillowcase is away from the door. The seam is toward the head of the bed.

POST-PROCEDURE

35 Provide for comfort. (See the inside of the front cover.) NOTE: Omit this step if the bed is prepared for a new patient or resident.

36 Attach the call light to the bed. Or place it within the person's reach.

37 Lower the bed to a safe and comfortable level for the person. Follow the care plan. Lock the bed wheels.

38 Put the towels, washcloth, gown or pajamas, and bath blanket in the bedside stand.

39 Complete a safety check of the room. (See the inside of the front cover.)

40 Follow agency policy for dirty linen.

41 Practice hand hygiene.

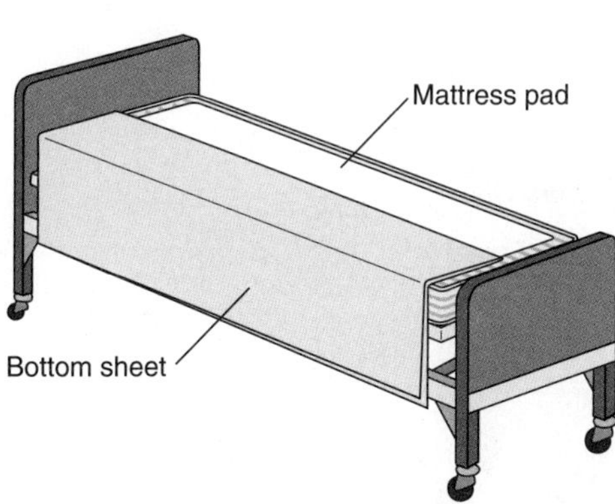

FIGURE 15-22 A flat bottom sheet is on the bed with the center crease in the middle. The lower edge of the sheet is even with the bottom of the mattress.

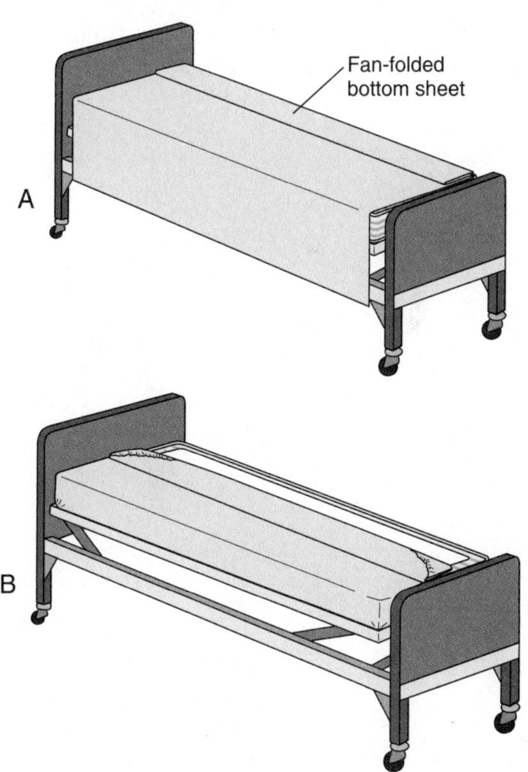

FIGURE 15-23 **A,** The flat bottom sheet is fan-folded to the other side of the bed. **B,** A fitted sheet is on the bed with the center crease in the middle.

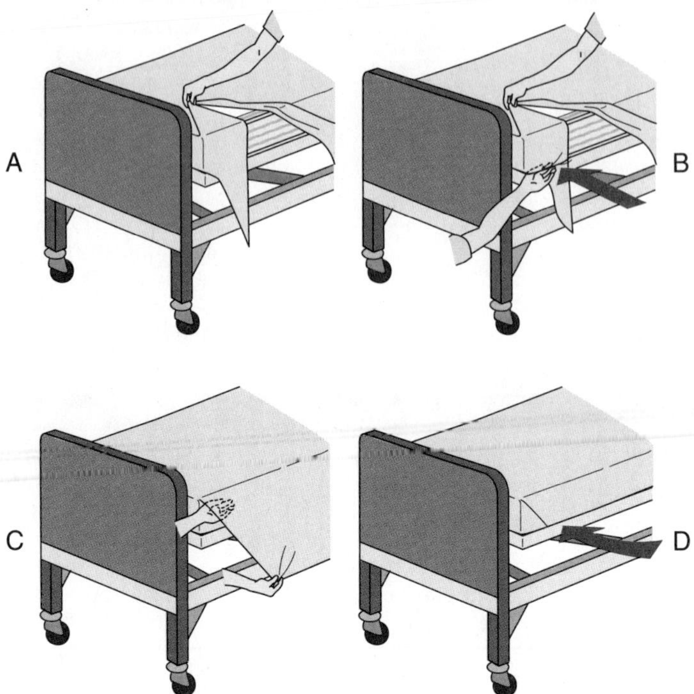

FIGURE 15-24 Making a mitered corner. **A,** The flat bottom sheet is tucked under the mattress at the head of the bed. The side of the sheet is raised onto the mattress. **B,** The remaining portion of the sheet is tucked under the mattress. **C,** The raised portion of the sheet is brought off the mattress. **D,** The entire side of the sheet is tucked under the mattress.

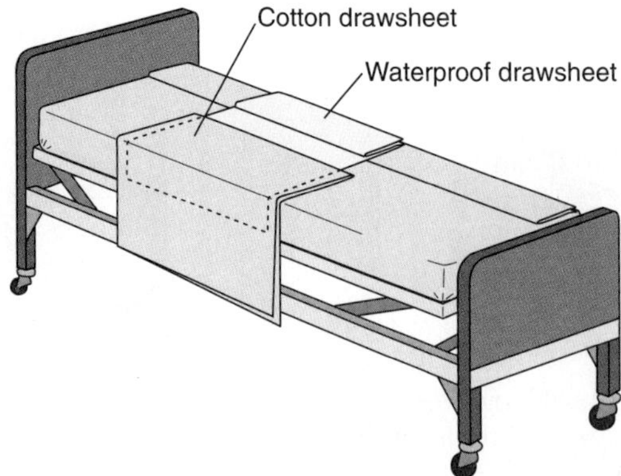

FIGURE 15-25 A cotton drawsheet is over the waterproof drawsheet. The cotton drawsheet completely covers the waterproof drawsheet.

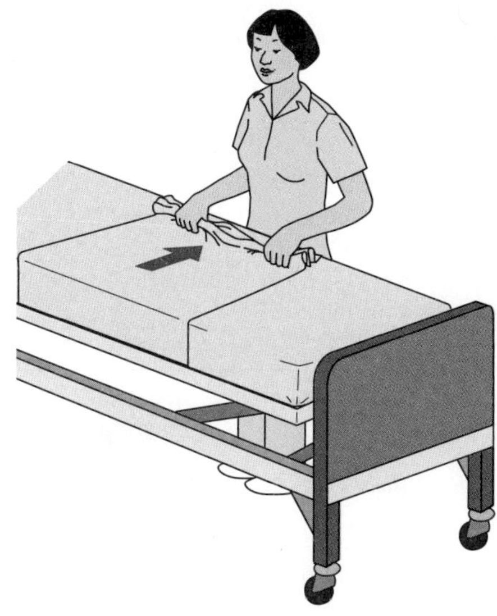

FIGURE 15-26 The drawsheet is pulled tight to remove wrinkles.

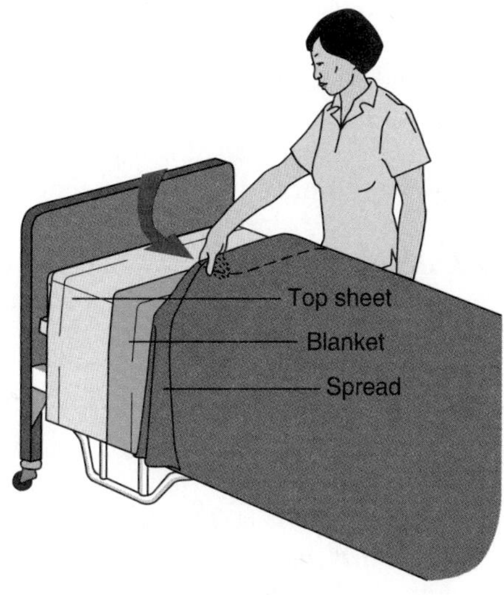

FIGURE 15-27 The top hem of the bedspread is turned under the top hem of the blanket to make a cuff.

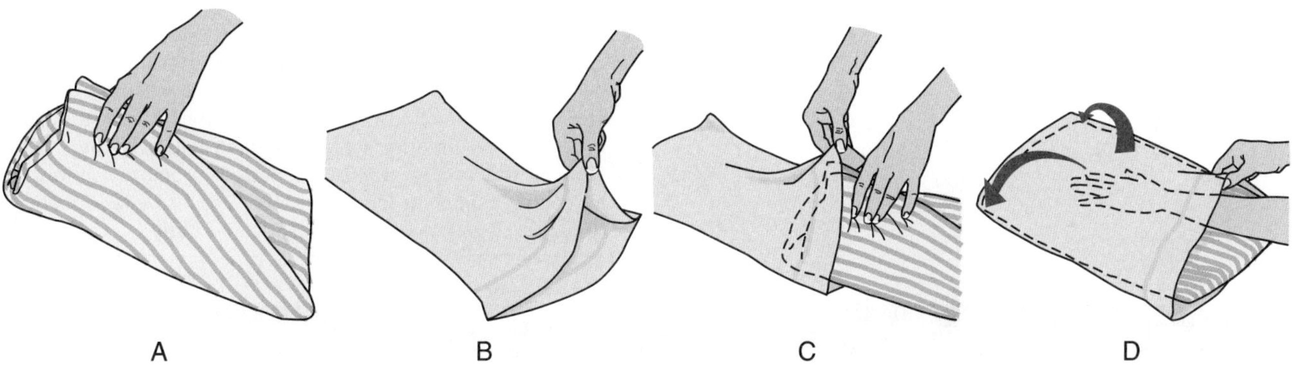

FIGURE 15-28 Putting a pillowcase on a pillow. **A,** Grasp the corners of the pillow at the seam end and form a "V" with the pillow. **B,** Open the pillowcase with your free hand. **C,** Guide the "V" end of the pillow into the pillowcase. **D,** Let the "V" end of the pillow fall into the corners of the pillowcase.

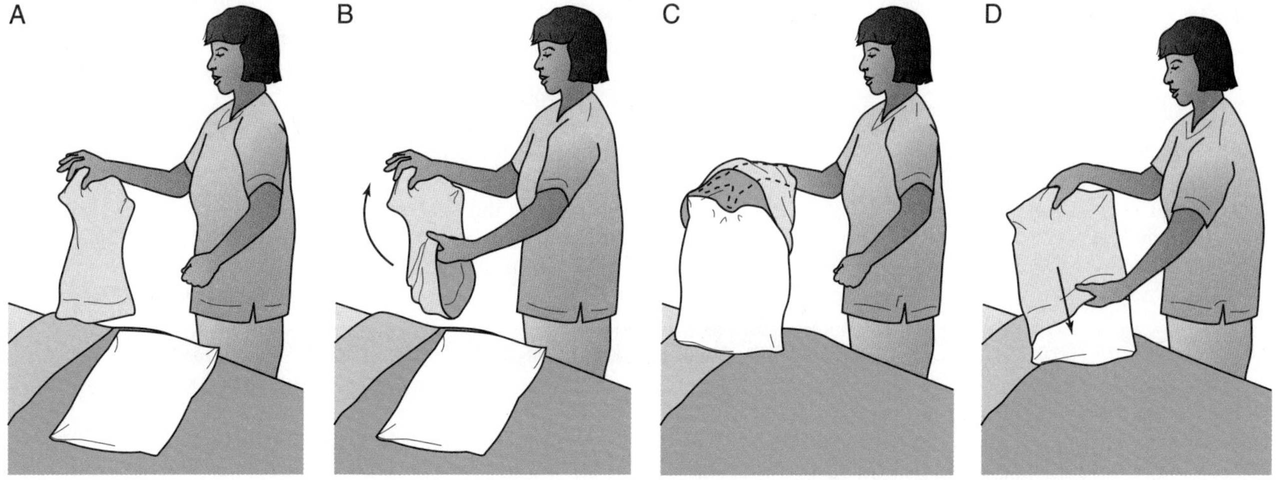

FIGURE 15-29 Putting a pillowcase on a pillow. **A,** Grasp the closed end of the pillowcase. **B,** Using your other hand, gather up the pillowcase. The pillowcase should cover your hand holding the closed end. **C,** Grasp the pillow with the hand covered by the pillowcase. **D,** Pull the pillowcase down over the pillow with your other hand.

The Open Bed. A closed bed becomes an open bed by fan-folding back the top linen. The open bed lets the person get into bed with ease. Make this bed for:

- Newly admitted persons arriving by wheelchair
- Persons who are getting ready for bed
- Persons who are out of bed for a short time

The Occupied Bed. You make an occupied bed when the person stays in bed. Keep the person in good alignment. Follow restrictions or limits in the person's movement or position.

Explain each procedure step to the person before it is done. This is important even if the person cannot respond or is in a coma.

See *Focus on Communication: The Occupied Bed.*

See *Promoting Safety and Comfort: The Occupied Bed.*

See procedure: *Making an Occupied Bed.*

FOCUS ON COMMUNICATION

The Occupied Bed

After making an occupied bed, make sure the person is comfortable. You can ask:

- "Are you comfortable?"
- "How can I make you more comfortable?"
- "Are you warm enough?"
- "Do you feel any creases or wrinkles?"
- "Can I adjust your pillow?"

After making the bed, thank the person for cooperating.

PROMOTING SAFETY AND COMFORT

The Occupied Bed

Safety

The person lies on 1 side of the bed and then the other. Protect the person from falling out of bed. If bed rails are used, the far bed rail is up. If bed rails are not used, have a co-worker help you. You work on 1 side of the bed. Your co-worker works on the other.

Comfort

For an occupied bed, the person lies on 1 side. You tuck dirty bottom linens under the person. Then you put clean linens on the bed. These, too, are tucked under the person. The tucked linens create a "bump" in the middle of the bed. To make the other side, the person rolls over the "bump" to the other side of the bed. To promote comfort, make the "bump" as low as possible. Do this by fan-folding dirty and clean bottom linens neatly and flatly.

Making an Occupied Bed

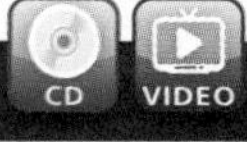

QUALITY OF LIFE

- Knock before entering the person's room.
- Address the person by name.
- Introduce yourself by name and title.
- Explain the procedure before starting and during the procedure.
- Protect the person's rights during the procedure.
- Handle the person gently during the procedure.

PROCEDURE

1 Follow *Delegation Guidelines: Making Beds,* p. 211. See *Promoting Safety and Comfort:*
  a *Making Beds,* p. 211
  b *The Occupied Bed*
2 Practice hand hygiene.
3 Collect the following.
  - Gloves
  - Laundry bag
  - Clean linen (see procedure: *Making a Closed Bed,* p. 212)
  - Paper towels (as a barrier for clean linen)
4 Place linen on a clean surface. Place the paper towels between the clean surface and the clean linen if a barrier is required by agency policy.
5 Identify the person. Check the ID (identification) bracelet against the assignment sheet. Also call the person by name.
6 Provide for privacy.
7 Remove the call light.
8 Raise the bed for body mechanics. Bed rails are up if used. Bed wheels are locked.
9 Lower the head of the bed. It is as flat as possible.

PROCEDURE

10 Practice hand hygiene. Put on gloves.
11 Loosen top linens at the foot of the bed.
12 Lower the bed rail near you if up.
13 Fold and remove the bedspread (Fig. 15-30, p. 218). Fold and remove the blanket the same way. Place each over the chair.
14 Cover the person with a bath blanket. Use the one in the bedside stand.
  a Unfold the bath blanket over the top sheet.
  b Ask the person to hold the bath blanket. If he or she cannot, tuck the top part under the person's shoulders.
  c Grasp the top sheet under the bath blanket at the shoulders. Bring the sheet down toward the foot of the bed. Remove the sheet from under the blanket (Fig. 15-31, p. 218).

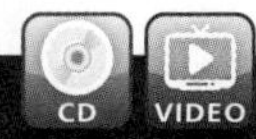

Making an Occupied Bed—cont'd

PROCEDURE—cont'd

15 Position the person on the side of the bed away from you. Adjust the pillow for comfort.
16 Loosen bottom linens from the head to the foot of the bed.
17 Fan-fold bottom linens 1 at a time toward the person. Start with the item on top (Fig. 15-32, p. 218). If re-using the mattress pad, do not fan-fold it.
18 Remove and discard the gloves. Practice hand hygiene. Put on clean gloves.
19 Place a clean mattress pad on the bed. Unfold it length-wise. The center crease is in the middle. Fan-fold the top part toward the person. If re-using the mattress pad, straighten and smooth any wrinkles.
20 Place the bottom sheet on the mattress pad. Hem-stitching is away from the person. Unfold the sheet so the crease is in the middle. If using a flat sheet, the small hem is even with the bottom of the mattress. Fan-fold the top part toward the person.
21 Tuck the corners of a fitted sheet over the mattress. If using a flat sheet, make a mitered corner at the head of the bed. Tuck the sheet under the mattress from the head to the foot.
22 *If using a cotton drawsheet:*
  a Place the drawsheet on the bed. It is in the middle of the mattress.
  b Open the drawsheet. Fan-fold it toward the person.
  c Tuck in excess fabric.
23 *If using a waterproof pad:*
  a Place the waterproof pad on the bed. It is in the middle of the mattress.
  b Fan-fold it toward the person.
24 *If re-using the waterproof drawsheet:*
  a Pull the drawsheet toward you over the bottom sheet.
  b Tuck excess material under the mattress.
  c Place the cotton drawsheet over the waterproof drawsheet. It covers the entire waterproof drawsheet. Fan-fold the top part toward the person. Tuck in excess fabric.
25 *If using a clean waterproof drawsheet* (Fig. 15-33, p. 219):
  a Place the waterproof drawsheet on the bed. It is in the middle of the mattress.
  b Fan-fold the top part toward the person.
  c Tuck in excess material.
  d Place the cotton drawsheet over the waterproof drawsheet. It covers the entire waterproof drawsheet. Fan-fold the top part toward the person. Tuck in excess fabric.
26 Explain to the person that he or she will roll over a "bump." Assure the person that he or she will not fall.
27 Help the person turn to the other side. Adjust the pillow for comfort.
28 Raise the bed rail. Go to the other side, and lower the bed rail.
29 Loosen bottom linens. Remove 1 piece at a time. Place each piece in the laundry bag. (NOTE: Discard the disposable bed protector, incontinence product, and disposable drawsheet in the trash. Do not put them in the laundry bag.)
30 Remove and discard the gloves. Practice hand hygiene.
31 Straighten and smooth the mattress pad.
32 Pull the clean bottom sheet toward you. Tuck the corners of a fitted sheet over the mattress. If using a flat sheet, make a mitered corner at the top. Tuck the sheet under the mattress from the head to the foot of the bed.
33 Pull the drawsheets tightly toward you. Tuck in the drawsheets.
34 Position the person supine in the center of the bed. Adjust the pillow for comfort.
35 Put the top sheet on the bed. Unfold it length-wise. The crease is in the middle. The large hem is even with the top of the mattress. Hem-stitching is on the outside.
36 Ask the person to hold the top sheet so you can remove the bath blanket. Or tuck the top sheet under the person's shoulders. Remove and discard the bath blanket.
37 Place the blanket on the bed. Unfold it so the crease is in the middle and it covers the person. The upper hem is 6 to 8 inches from the top of the mattress.
38 Place the bedspread on the bed. Unfold it so the center crease is in the middle and it covers the person. The top hem is even with the mattress top.
39 Turn the top hem of the bedspread under the blanket to make a cuff.
40 Bring the top sheet down over the bedspread to form a cuff.
41 Go to the foot of the bed.
42 Make a toe pleat. Make a 2-inch pleat across the foot of the bed. The pleat is about 6 to 8 inches from the foot of the bed.
43 Lift the mattress corner with 1 arm. Tuck all top linens under the mattress. Make a mitered corner.
44 Raise the bed rail. Go to the other side, and lower the bed rail.
45 Straighten and smooth top linens.
46 Tuck all top linens under the mattress. Make a mitered corner.
47 Change each pillowcase.

POST-PROCEDURE

48 Provide for comfort. (See the inside of the front cover.)
49 Place the call light within reach.
50 Lower the bed to a safe and comfortable level for the person. Follow the care plan. The bed wheels are locked.
51 Raise or lower bed rails. Follow the care plan.
52 Put the clean towels, washcloth, gown or pajamas, and bath blanket in the bedside stand.
53 Unscreen the person.
54 Complete a safety check of the room. (See the inside of the front cover.)
55 Follow agency policy for dirty linen.
56 Practice hand hygiene.

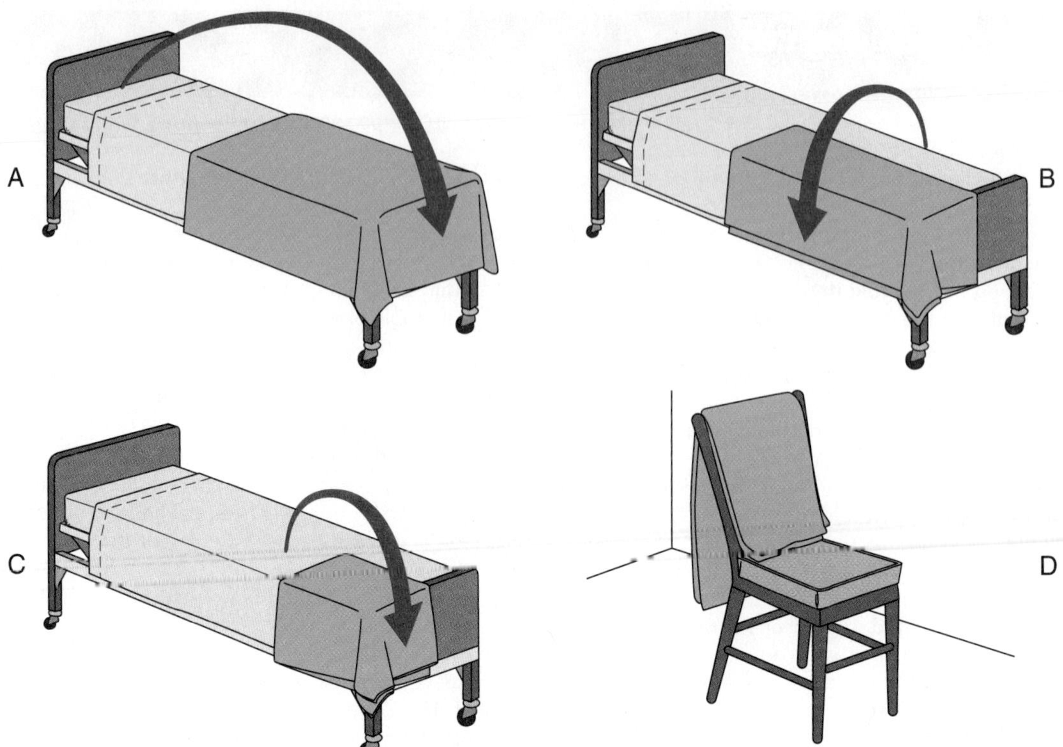

FIGURE 15-30 Folding linen for re-use. **A,** Fold the top edge of the bedspread down to the bottom edge. **B,** Fold the bedspread from the far side of the bed to the near side. **C,** Fold the top edge of the bedspread down to the bottom edge again. **D,** Place the folded bedspread over the back of the chair.

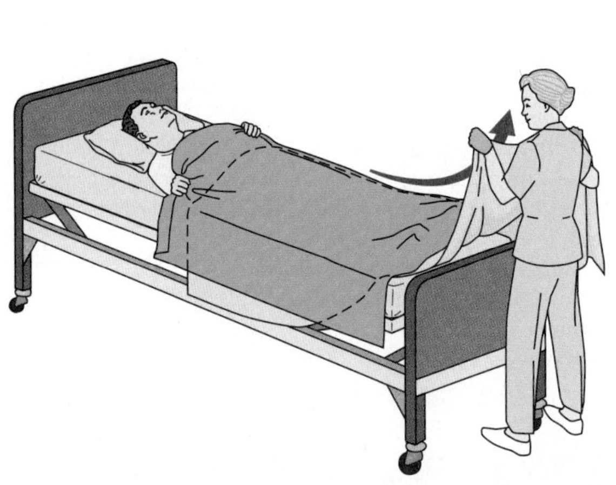

FIGURE 15-31 The person holds on to the bath blanket. The top sheet is removed from under the bath blanket. (NOTE: Bed rails are used according to the care plan.)

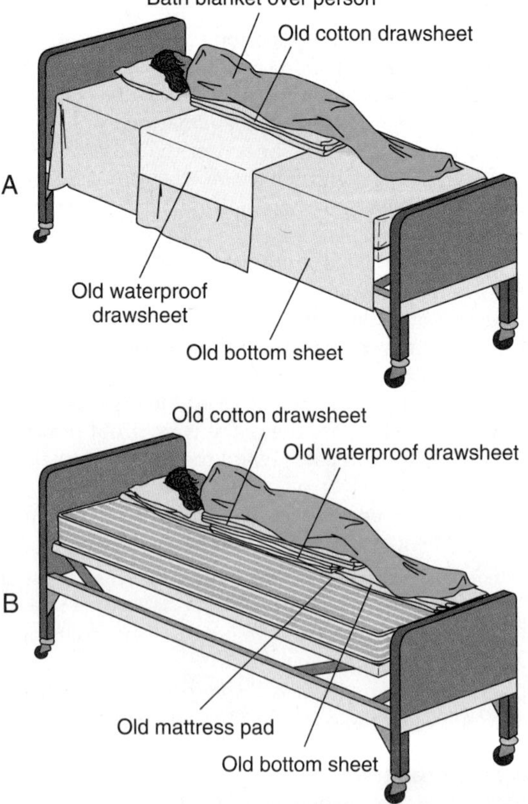

FIGURE 15-32 **A,** The cotton drawsheet is fan-folded and tucked under the person. **B,** All bottom linens are tucked under the person. (NOTE: Bed rails are used according to the care plan.)

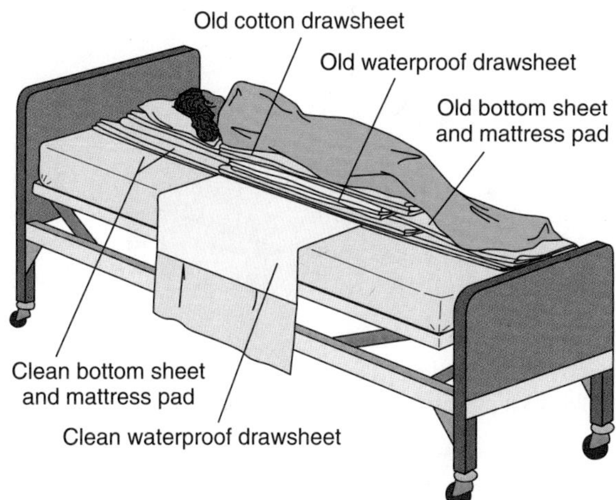

FIGURE 15-33 A clean bottom sheet and waterproof drawsheet are on the bed with both fan-folded and tucked under the person. (NOTE: Bed rails are used according to the care plan.)

The Surgical Bed. The surgical bed also is called a *recovery bed* or *post-operative bed.* Top linens are folded to transfer the person from a stretcher to the bed. These beds are made for persons:

- Returning to their rooms from surgery. A complete linen change is needed.
- Who arrive at the agency by ambulance. A complete linen change is needed if the person:
  - Is a new patient or resident.
  - Is returning to the nursing center from the hospital.
- Who go by stretcher to treatment or therapy areas. A complete linen change is not needed.
- Using portable tubs (Chapter 16). Because of bathing, a complete linen change is needed.

  See *Promoting Safety and Comfort: The Surgical Bed.*
  See procedure: *Making a Surgical Bed.*

PROMOTING SAFETY AND COMFORT
The Surgical Bed

Safety

Follow the rules for stretcher safety (Chapter 9). After the transfer, lower the bed to a safe and comfortable level for the person. Follow the care plan. Lock the bed wheels. Raise or lower bed rails according to the care plan.

Making a Surgical Bed

PROCEDURE

1 Follow *Delegation Guidelines: Making Beds,* p. 211. See *Promoting Safety and Comfort:*
   a *Making Beds,* p. 211
   b *The Surgical Bed*
2 Practice hand hygiene.
3 Collect the following.
   - Clean linen (see procedure: *Making a Closed Bed,* p. 212)
   - Gloves
   - Laundry bag
   - Equipment requested by the nurse
   - Paper towels (as a barrier for clean linen)
4 Place linen on a clean surface. Place the paper towels between the clean surface and clean linen if a barrier is required by agency policy.
5 Remove the call light.
6 Raise the bed for body mechanics.
7 Remove all linen from the bed. Wear gloves. Practice hand hygiene after removing and discarding them.
8 Make a closed bed (see procedure: *Making a Closed Bed,* p. 212). Do not tuck top linens under the mattress.
9 Fold all top linens at the foot of the bed back onto the bed. The fold is even with the edge of the mattress (Fig. 15-34, *A*, p. 220).
10 Know on which side of the bed the stretcher will be placed. Fan-fold linen length-wise to the other side of the bed (Fig. 15-34, *B*, p. 220).
11 Put a pillowcase on each pillow.
12 Place the pillow(s) on a clean surface.
13 Leave the bed in its highest position.
14 Leave both bed rails down.
15 Put the clean towels, washcloth, gown or pajamas, and bath blanket in the bedside stand.
16 Move furniture away from the bed. Allow room for the stretcher and the staff.
17 Do not attach the call light to the bed.
18 Complete a safety check of the room. (See the inside of the front cover.)
19 Follow agency policy for soiled linen.
20 Practice hand hygiene.

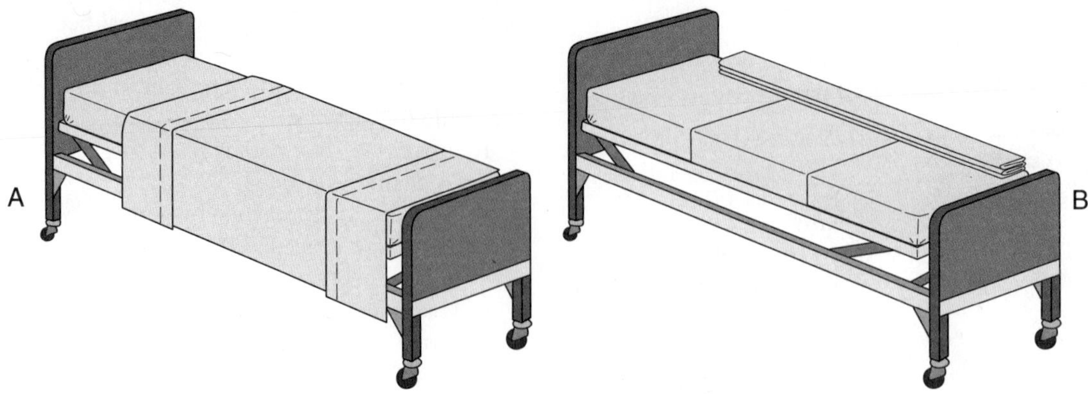

FIGURE 15-34 Surgical bed. **A,** The bottom of the top linens is folded back onto the bed. The fold is even with the bottom edge of the mattress. **B,** Top linens are fan-folded length-wise to the side of the bed.

ASSISTING WITH PAIN RELIEF

Pain means to ache, hurt, or be sore. Pain is subjective (Chapter 5). That is, you cannot see, hear, touch, or smell pain or discomfort. You must rely on what the person says.

The nurse uses the nursing process to promote comfort and relieve pain. The types, signs, and symptoms of pain are described in Chapter 21. Report the person's complaints and your observations. The person's care plan may include the measures in Box 15-3.

See *Focus on Communication: Pain.*

See *Focus on Surveys: Pain.*

FOCUS ON COMMUNICATION

Pain

Communicating with persons about pain promotes comfort. You can say:

- "I want you to be comfortable. Please tell me if you are having any pain."
- "I will tell the nurse about your pain."

If a person complains of pain, the person has pain. You must rely on what the person tells you. Promptly report any complaints of pain to the nurse.

BOX 15-3 Promoting Comfort and Relieving Pain

- Position the person in good alignment. Use pillows for support.
- Keep bed linens tight and wrinkle-free.
- Make sure the person is not lying on tubes.
- Assist with elimination needs.
- Provide blankets for warmth and to prevent chilling.
- Use correct moving and turning procedures.
- Wait 30 minutes after pain-relief drugs are given before giving care or starting activities.
- Give a back massage (p. 222).
- Provide soft music to distract the person.
- Talk softly and gently.
- Use touch to provide comfort.
- Allow family and friends at the bedside as requested by the person.
- Avoid sudden or jarring movements of the bed or chair.
- Handle the person gently.
- Practice safety measures if the person takes strong pain-relief drugs or sedatives.
  - Keep the bed in the low position.
  - Raise bed rails as directed. Follow the care plan.
  - Check on the person every 10 to 15 minutes.
  - Provide help when the person needs to get up and when he or she is up and about.
- Apply warm or cold applications as directed by the nurse (Chapter 24).
- Provide a calm, quiet, and dim setting.

FOCUS ON SURVEYS

Pain

Pain interferes with the person's well-being. Pain affects function, mobility, mood, sleep, and quality of life. The agency must:

- Recognize when a person has pain.
- Identify when pain might occur.
- Evaluate pain and its causes.
- Manage or prevent pain.

You may be the first person to notice signs and symptoms of pain. You must be able to recognize a change in the person's behavior and function. And you must report such changes to the nurse. You also assist the nurse in providing pain-relief measures. Therefore a surveyor may ask you questions about pain. For example:

- What are the signs and symptoms of pain? (See Chapter 21.)
- How do you ask a person to rate the intensity of pain? (See Chapter 21.)
- What factors can cause pain or make it worse?
- When and how do you report observations about pain?
- How do you assist the nurse with pain-relief measures?

Factors Affecting Pain

Many factors affect reactions to pain.

- *Past experience.* The severity of pain, its cause, how long it lasted, and if relief occurred all affect the current response to pain. Knowing what to expect can help or hinder how the person handles pain. Some people have not had pain. When it occurs, pain can cause fear and anxiety. They can make pain worse.
- *Anxiety.* Anxiety relates to feelings of fear, dread, worry, and concern. The person is uneasy and tense. Pain and anxiety are related. Pain can cause anxiety. Anxiety increases how much pain is felt. Reducing anxiety helps lessen pain.
- *Rest and sleep.* Pain seems worse when tired and unable to rest or sleep. The person tends to focus on pain at these times.
- *Personal and family duties.* Often pain is ignored when there are children to care for. Some people go to work with pain. Others deny pain if fearing a serious illness. The illness can interfere with a job; going to school; or caring for children, a partner, or ill parents.
- *The value or meaning of pain.* To some people, pain is a sign of weakness. It may mean a serious illness and the need for painful tests and treatments. Sometimes pain gives pleasure. The pain of childbirth is one example. For some persons, pain is used to avoid certain people or things. Some people like doting and pampering by others. The person values and wants such attention.
- *Support from others.* Dealing with pain is often easier when family and friends offer comfort and support. The use of touch by a valued person is very comforting. Just being nearby also helps. Some people do not have caring family or friends. Dealing with pain alone can increase anxiety.
- *Culture.* Culture affects pain responses. Non–English-speaking persons may have problems describing pain in English. The agency uses interpreters to communicate with the person. See *Caring About Culture: Pain Reactions.*
- *Illness.* Some diseases cause decreased pain sensations. Central nervous system disorders are examples. The person may not feel pain. Or it may not feel severe.
- *Age.* See *Focus on Older Persons: Factors Affecting Pain.*

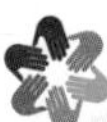

CARING ABOUT CULTURE

Pain Reactions

People of *Mexico* and the *Philippines* may appear stoic in reaction to pain. In the *Philippines,* pain is viewed as the will of God. It is believed that God will give strength to bear the pain.

In *Vietnam,* pain may be severe before pain relief measures are requested. The people of *India* accept pain quietly. They accept pain-relief measures.

In *China,* showing emotion is a weakness of character. Therefore pain is often suppressed.

From D'Avanzo CE, Geissler EM: Pocket guide to cultural health assessment, *ed 4, St Louis, 2008, Mosby.*

FOCUS ON OLDER PERSONS

Factors Affecting Pain

Older persons may have decreased pain sensations. They may not feel pain or it may not feel severe.

Some older persons have many painful health problems. Chronic pain may mask new pain. Older persons may ignore or deny new pain. They may think it relates to a known health problem. Older persons often deny or ignore pain because of what it may mean.

Thinking and reasoning are affected in some older persons. Some cannot tell you about pain. Changes in usual behavior may signal pain. Increased confusion, grimacing, restlessness, and loss of appetite are examples. A person who normally moans and groans may become quiet and withdrawn. A person who is friendly and outgoing may become agitated and aggressive. One who is nonverbal and quiet may become restless and cry easily.

Always report changes in the person's behavior. All persons have the right to correct pain management. The nurse does a pain assessment when behavior changes.

The Back Massage

The back massage (back rub) can promote comfort and help relieve pain. It relaxes muscles and stimulates circulation. A good time to give back massages is after re-positioning. You also give them after baths and showers and with evening care. Back massages last 3 to 5 minutes. Observe the skin before the massage. Look for breaks in the skin, bruises, reddened areas, and other signs of skin breakdown.

Lotion reduces friction during the massage. Warm the lotion before applying it. Do 1 of the following.

- Rub some lotion between your hands.
- Place the bottle in the bath water.
- Hold the bottle under warm water.

Use firm strokes. Always keep your hands in contact with the person's skin. After the massage, apply lotion to the elbows, knees, and heels. This keeps the skin soft. These bony areas are at risk for skin breakdown.

See *Delegation Guidelines: The Back Massage.*

See Promoting Safety and Comfort: The Back Massage.

See procedure: *Giving a Back Massage.*

DELEGATION GUIDELINES

The Back Massage

Before giving a back massage, you need this information from the nurse and the care plan.

- If the person can have a back massage (see *Promoting Safety and Comfort: The Back Massage*)
- How to position the person
- If the person has position limits
- When to give a back massage
- If the person needs back massages often for comfort and to relax
- What observations to report and record:
    - Breaks in the skin
    - Bruising
    - Reddened areas
    - Signs of skin breakdown
- When to report observations
- What patient or resident concerns to report at once

PROMOTING SAFETY AND COMFORT

The Back Massage

Safety

Back massages can harm persons with certain heart diseases, back injuries and surgeries, skin diseases, and lung disorders. Check with the nurse and the care plan before giving back massages.

Do not massage reddened bony areas. Reddened areas signal skin breakdown and pressure ulcers. Massage can lead to more tissue damage.

Wear gloves if the person's skin is not intact. Do not massage areas where skin is not intact. Always follow Standard Precautions and the Bloodborne Pathogen Standard.

Comfort

The prone position is best for a massage. The side-lying position is often used. Older and disabled persons usually find the side-lying position more comfortable.

Giving a Back Massage

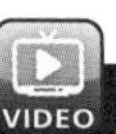

QUALITY OF LIFE

- Knock before entering the person's room.
- Address the person by name.
- Introduce yourself by name and title.
- Explain the procedure before starting and during the procedure.
- Protect the person's rights during the procedure.
- Handle the person gently during the procedure.

PRE-PROCEDURE

1 Follow *Delegation Guidelines: The Back Massage.* See *Promoting Safety and Comfort: The Back Massage.*

2 Practice hand hygiene.

3 Identify the person. Check the ID bracelet against the assignment sheet. Also call the person by name.

4 Collect the following.
- Bath blanket
- Bath towel
- Lotion

5 Provide for privacy.

6 Raise the bed for body mechanics. Bed rails are up if used.

Giving a Back Massage—cont'd

VIDEO

PROCEDURE

7 Lower the bed rail near you if up.
8 Position the person in the prone or side-lying position. The back is toward you.
9 Expose the back, shoulders, and upper arms. Cover the rest of the body with the bath blanket.
10 Lay the towel on the bed along the back. Do this if the person is in a side-lying position.
11 Warm the lotion.
12 Explain that the lotion may feel cool and wet.
13 Apply lotion to the lower back area.
14 Stroke up from the lower back to the shoulders. Then stroke down over the upper arms. Stroke up the upper arms, across the shoulders, and down the back (Fig. 15-35). Use firm strokes. Keep your hands in contact with the person's skin.
15 Repeat step 14 for at least 3 minutes.
16 Knead the back (Fig. 15-36).
  a Grasp the skin between your thumb and fingers.
  b Knead half of the back. Start at the lower back and move up to the shoulder. Then knead down from the shoulder to the lower back.
  c Repeat on the other half of the back.
17 Apply lotion to bony areas. Use circular motions with the tips of your index and middle fingers. (Do not massage reddened bony areas.)
18 Use fast movements to stimulate. Use slow movements to relax the person.
19 Stroke with long, firm movements to end the massage. Tell the person when you are finishing.
20 Straighten and secure clothing or sleepwear.
21 Cover the person. Remove the towel and bath blanket.

POST-PROCEDURE

22 Provide for comfort. (See the inside of the front cover.)
23 Place the call light within reach.
24 Lower the bed to a safe and comfortable level for the person. Follow the care plan.
25 Raise or lower bed rails. Follow the care plan.
26 Return lotion to its proper place.
27 Unscreen the person.
28 Complete a safety check of the room. (See the inside of the front cover.)
29 Follow agency policy for dirty linen.
30 Practice hand hygiene.
31 Report and record your observations.

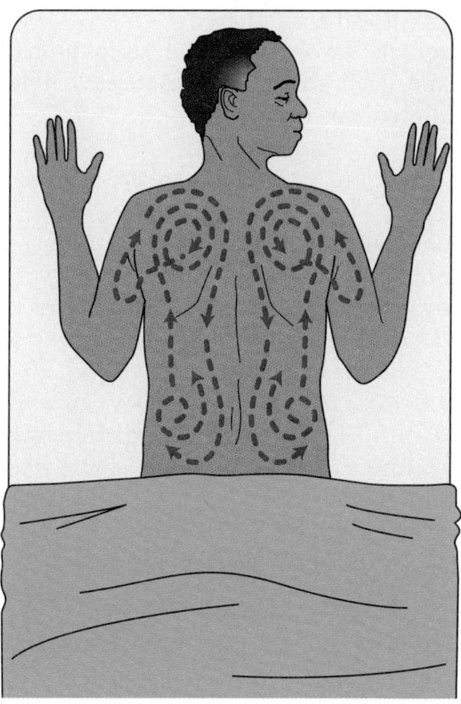

FIGURE 15-35 The person lies in the prone position for a back massage. Stroke upward from the lower back to the shoulders, down over the upper arms, back up the upper arms, across the shoulders, and down to the lower back.

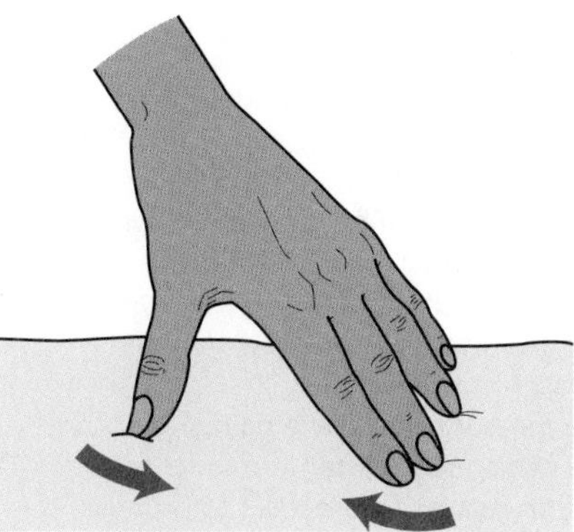

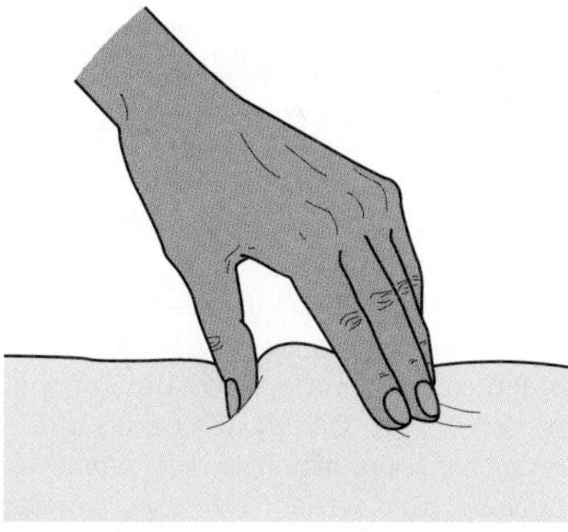

FIGURE 15-36 Kneading is done by picking up tissue between the thumb and fingers.

SLEEP

Sleep is a basic need. The mind and body rest. The body saves energy. Body functions slow. Vital signs (temperature, pulse, respirations, and blood pressure) are lower than when awake. Tissue healing and repair occur. Sleep lowers stress, tension, and anxiety. It refreshes and renews the person. The person regains energy and mental alertness. The person thinks and functions better after sleep.

The nurse uses the nursing process to promote sleep. Report your observations about how the person slept. The person's care plan may include the measures in Box 15-4.

See *Focus on Older Persons: Promoting Sleep.*

BOX 15-4 Promoting Sleep

- Plan care for uninterrupted rest.
- Avoid physical activity before bedtime.
- Encourage the person to avoid business or family matters before bedtime.
- Allow a flexible bedtime. Bedtime is when the person is tired, not a certain time.
- Let the person take a warm bath or shower.
- Provide a bedtime snack.
- Avoid caffeine (coffee, tea, colas, chocolate) and alcoholic beverages.
- Have the person void before going to bed.
- Make sure incontinent persons are clean and dry.
- Follow bedtime routines. Hygiene, elimination, and prayer are examples.
- Have the person wear loose-fitting sleepwear.
- Provide for warmth (blankets, socks) for those who tend to be cold.
- Reduce noise.
- Darken the room—close window coverings and the privacy curtain. Shut off or dim lights.
- Dim lights in hallways and the nursing unit.
- Make sure linens are clean, dry, and wrinkle-free.
- Position the person in good alignment and in a comfortable position.
- Support body parts as ordered.
- Give a back massage.
- Provide measures to relieve pain.
- Let the person read, listen to music, or watch TV.
- Assist with relaxation exercises as ordered.
- Sit and talk with the person.

FOCUS ON OLDER PERSONS

Promoting Sleep

Older persons have less energy than younger people. They may nap during the day. You need to let the person sleep. Plan care to allow uninterrupted naps.

Sleep problems are common in persons with Alzheimer's disease and other dementias. Night wandering is common. Restlessness and confusion often increase at night. This increases the risk of falls. Quietly and calmly directing the person to his or her room may help. Night-time wandering in a safe and supervised setting is the best approach for some persons. The measures listed in Box 15-4 are tried. Follow the care plan.

Factors Affecting Sleep

Many factors affect the amount and quality of sleep.

- *Illness.* Illness increases the need for sleep. However, pain, nausea, vomiting, coughing, difficulty breathing, diarrhea, frequent voiding, and itching can interfere with sleep. So can treatments and therapies. Often the person is awakened for treatments or drugs. Care devices can cause uncomfortable positions. Fear, anxiety, and worry also affect sleep.
- *Nutrition.* Foods with caffeine (chocolate, coffee, tea, or colas) prevent sleep. Caffeine is a stimulant. The protein *tryptophan* tends to help sleep. It is found in protein sources—milk, cheese, red meat, fish, poultry, and peanuts.
- *Exercise.* Exercise causes the release of substances into the bloodstream that stimulate the body. Exercise is avoided 2 hours before bedtime.
- *Environment.* People adjust to their usual sleep settings. They get used to the bed, pillows, noises, lighting, and a sleeping partner. Any change in the usual setting can affect sleep.
- *Drugs and other substances.* Sleeping pills promote sleep. Drugs for anxiety, depression, and pain may cause sleep. Alcohol interferes with sleep. Some drugs contain caffeine. The side effects of some drugs cause frequent voiding and nightmares.
- *Emotional problems.* Fear, worry, depression, and anxiety affect sleep. People may have problems falling asleep or they awaken often. Some have problems getting back to sleep.

Sleep Disorders

Sleep disorders involve repeated sleep problems. The amount and quality of sleep are affected. Physical and behavioral problems may result.

- ***Insomnia*** *is a chronic condition in which the person cannot sleep or stay asleep all night.* There are 3 forms of insomnia.
  - Cannot fall asleep
  - Cannot stay asleep
  - Early awakening and cannot fall back asleep
- ***Sleep deprivation*** *means the amount and quality of sleep are decreased.* Sleep is interrupted.
- ***Sleepwalking*** *is when the sleeping person leaves the bed and walks about.* The person is not aware of sleepwalking and has no memory of the event on awakening. The event lasts 3 to 4 minutes or longer. Protect the person from injury. Falling is a risk. Guide sleepwalkers back to bed. They startle easily. Awaken them gently.

FOCUS ON PRIDE

The Person, Family, and Yourself

Personal and Professional Responsibility

Loud talking and laughter in hallways and at the nurses' station can disturb patients, residents, and visitors. They may think the staff is not working. Or they may think the staff is talking about or laughing at them. Some find this irritating and upsetting. They become anxious, uncomfortable, or angry.

Reducing noise requires cooperation from all staff. It is not your responsibility alone. But you can help. Do your part to reduce noise. Politely remind others to speak softly. Take pride in providing patients and residents with a quiet and comfortable setting.

Rights and Respect

Nursing center residents have the right to make their settings as home-like as possible. Residents often bring bedspreads, blankets, quilts, and so on from home. The items have meaning and value. For example, Mr. Baker wants his afghan on his bed at night. His wife made it years ago. Mr. Baker moved into the nursing center after his wife died. The sight and smell of the afghan remind him of his wife and home.

Protect personal items from loss and damage. Handle the person's belongings with care and respect.

Independence and Social Interaction

Allow personal choice when possible. What is best for you may not be best for the person. For example, you planned to make Mrs. Beck's bed and straighten her room after breakfast. However, her family comes to visit then. Mrs. Beck wants her bed made during breakfast.

Ask about the person's preferences. Consider such preferences when planning your day and managing your time. The more choices are allowed, the greater the person's sense of control and independence.

Delegation and Teamwork

Agencies have different ways of handling dirty linen. Some have containers in each room. Others have carts in the hallways. The carts are emptied each shift or as needed. Some agencies have a room where dirty linen is placed. Others have chutes.

When handling dirty linen:

- Wear gloves.
- Follow agency policy for dirty linen.
- Do not over-fill the bag or container. The person emptying the bag or cart may be injured.
- Work as a team. Some units assign a person to empty linen containers. Linen must not over-flow carts. If you see a full cart, empty it. Do so without complaining. The person assigned the task may be busy. If no one is assigned the task, work together to complete it.
- Clean up after yourself. If you fill a cart, empty it. If you place an item in a cart that will cause an odor, empty it.
- Place dirty linen in the correct location. Do not place dirty linen in a room or cart where it does not belong. If chutes are used, use the correct chute. Other chutes in the area may be for trash.

Ethics and Laws

This chapter focused on how objects and surroundings in the person's unit affect comfort and well-being. You are a part of that setting. You must help the person feel safe, secure, and comfortable.

Your words and actions are heard and seen by others. Bad conduct reduces quality of care and reflects poorly on you. You can lose your job and the ability to work as a nursing assistant. Always provide care in a way that promotes the person's comfort, safety, and quality of life.

REVIEW QUESTIONS

Circle* T *if the statement is TRUE or* F *if it is FALSE.

1 **T F** You can adjust the person's room temperature for your comfort.
2 **T F** The call light is placed on the person's strong side.
3 **T F** You can look through a person's closet and drawers.
4 **T F** Changes in usual behavior may signal pain.
5 **T F** Culture affects how a person reacts to pain.
6 **T F** A back massage relaxes muscles and stimulates circulation.

Circle the BEST answer.

7 To protect a person from drafts
- **a** Adjust the room temperature to 70°F
- **b** Provide a bath blanket when making an occupied bed
- **c** Dress the person in light-weight clothing
- **d** Position the person near a fan

8 To prevent odors
- **a** Place flowers in the room
- **b** Empty commodes at the end of your shift
- **c** Keep laundry containers open
- **d** Clean persons who are wet or soiled

9 To control noise
- **a** Answer phones after the third ring
- **b** Use the intercom system when possible
- **c** Handle equipment carefully
- **d** Talk with others in the hallway

10 The head of the bed is raised 30 degrees. This is called
- **a** Fowler's position
- **b** Semi-Fowler's position
- **c** Trendelenburg's position
- **d** Reverse Trendelenburg's position

11 Bed safety involves
- **a** Monitoring older and confused persons closely for entrapment
- **b** Removing the entrapment zones from the bed
- **c** Leaving the bed in the highest horizontal position
- **d** Restraining persons at risk for entrapment

12 The over-bed table is *not* used
- **a** For eating
- **b** As a working surface
- **c** For the urinal
- **d** For writing

13 Which must be done *first?*
- **a** Give a back massage.
- **b** Make a closed bed.
- **c** Answer a bathroom call light.
- **d** Take a blanket to a person.

14 When handling linens
- **a** Put dirty linens on the floor
- **b** Take extra linen to another person's room
- **c** Shake linens to unfold them
- **d** Hold linens away from your body and uniform

15 A resident is out of the bed most of the day. You should make
- **a** A closed bed
- **b** An open bed
- **c** An occupied bed
- **d** A surgical bed

16 When using a waterproof drawsheet
- **a** Waterproof pads are needed
- **b** A cotton drawsheet must completely cover the waterproof drawsheet
- **c** The person's consent is needed
- **d** The plastic or rubber is in contact with the person's skin

17 When making an occupied bed
- **a** Explain that the person will roll over a "bump" of linens
- **b** Wear the same gloves throughout the procedure
- **c** Lower the far bed rail if working alone
- **d** Fan-fold top linens to the foot of the bed

18 The nurse gave a drug for pain relief. When should you give scheduled care?
- **a** Before the nurse gives the drug
- **b** Right after the nurse gives the drug
- **c** 30 minutes after the nurse gives the drug
- **d** When you have time

19 Dementia can cause the person to
- **a** Sleep better at night
- **b** Have extreme reactions to common sounds
- **c** Feel more relaxed in a dark room
- **d** Be less confused at night

20 To promote sleep
- **a** Have the person void before bedtime
- **b** Keep lights on in the room
- **c** Have the person walk before bedtime
- **d** Avoid reading or listening to music before bedtime

21 A person has insomnia. These measures for sleep are in the person's care plan. Which should you question?
- **a** Let the person choose the bedtime.
- **b** Provide hot tea at bedtime.
- **c** Position the person in good alignment.
- **d** Follow the person's bedtime rituals.

22 When giving a back massage
- **a** Massage for 15 to 20 minutes
- **b** Position the person in Fowler's position
- **c** Massage reddened areas
- **d** Warm the lotion before applying it

Answers to these questions are on p. 504.

FOCUS ON **PRACTICE**

Problem Solving

A resident uses his call light often. Some needs are urgent. Others are not. Since your shift began, he has called for help 15 times. You just left his room and are helping another resident with her bedtime routine. His call light signals. What do you do?

The resident uses his call light more often at night, after family visits, and when he is not checked on regularly. How might sharing this information with the nurse be helpful in care planning?

CHAPTER 16

Assisting With Hygiene

OBJECTIVES

- Define the key terms and key abbreviations listed in this chapter.
- Explain why personal hygiene is important.
- Identify the observations to report and record when assisting with hygiene.
- Describe the care given before and after breakfast, after lunch, and in the evening.
- Explain the purposes of oral hygiene.
- Describe safety measures when giving mouth care to unconscious persons.
- Explain how to care for dentures.
- Describe the rules for bathing.
- Identify safety measures for tub baths and showers.
- Explain the purposes of perineal care.
- Perform the procedures described in this chapter.
- Explain how to promote PRIDE in the person, the family, and yourself.

KEY TERMS

aspiration Breathing fluid, food, vomitus, or an object into the lungs
circumcised The fold of skin (foreskin) covering the glans of the penis was surgically removed
denture An artificial tooth or a set of artificial teeth
oral hygiene Mouth care
perineal care Cleaning the genital and anal areas; pericare
uncircumcised The person has foreskin covering the head of the penis

KEY ABBREVIATIONS

C Centigrade
F Fahrenheit
ID Identification

The skin is the body's first line of defense against disease. Intact skin prevents microbes from entering the body and causing an infection. Likewise, mucous membranes of the mouth, genital area, and anus must be clean and intact. Besides cleansing, good hygiene prevents body and breath odors. It is relaxing and increases circulation.

Culture and personal choice affect hygiene. (See *Caring About Culture: Personal Hygiene*.) The person's preferences are part of the care plan.

See *Focus on Communication: Assisting With Hygiene*, p. 228.

See *Focus on Older Persons: Assisting With Hygiene*, p. 228.

See *Promoting Safety and Comfort: Assisting With Hygiene*, p. 228.

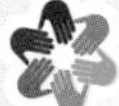

CARING ABOUT CULTURE

Personal Hygiene

Personal hygiene is very important to *East Indian Hindus.* Their religion requires at least 1 bath a day. Some believe bathing after a meal is harmful. Another belief is that a cold bath prevents a blood disease. Some believe that eye injuries can occur if bath water is too hot. Hot water can be added to cold water. However, cold water is not added to hot water. After bathing, the body is carefully dried with a towel.

From Giger JN: Transcultural nursing: assessment and intervention, *ed 6, St Louis, 2013, Mosby.*

FOCUS ON COMMUNICATION

Assisting With Hygiene

During hygiene procedures, make sure that the person is warm enough. You can ask:

- "Is the water warm enough? Is it too hot? Is it too cold?"
- "Are you warm enough?"
- "Do you need another bath blanket?"
- "Is the water starting to cool?"
- "Is the room warm enough?"

FOCUS ON OLDER PERSONS

Assisting With Hygiene

Some older persons resist your efforts to assist with hygiene. Illness, disability, dementia, and personal choice are common reasons. Follow the care plan to meet the person's needs. Also see Chapter 30.

Bending and reaching are hard for older and disabled persons. Some have weak hand grips. They cannot hold soap or a washcloth. Adaptive devices for hygiene promote independence (Chapter 27). Let the person do as much for himself or herself as safely possible.

PROMOTING SAFETY AND COMFORT

Assisting With Hygiene

Safety

Personal hygiene measures often involve exposing and touching private areas—breasts, perineum, rectum. Sexual abuse has occurred in health care settings. The person may feel threatened or may be being abused. He or she needs to call for help. Keep the call light within the person's reach at all times. And always act in a professional manner.

BOX 16-1 Daily Care

Before Breakfast (Early Morning Care or AM Care)

- Prepare persons for breakfast or morning tests.
- Assist with elimination.
- Clean incontinent persons.
- Change wet or soiled linens and garments.
- Assist with face and hand washing and oral hygiene.
- Assist with dressing and hair care.
- Position patients and residents for breakfast—dining room, bedside chair, or in bed.
- Make beds and straighten units.

After Breakfast (Morning Care)

- Assist with elimination.
- Clean incontinent persons.
- Change wet or soiled linens and garments.
- Assist with face and hand washing, oral hygiene, bathing, back massage, and perineal care.
- Assist with hair care, shaving, dressing, and undressing.
- Assist with range-of-motion exercises and ambulation.
- Make beds and straighten rooms.

Afternoon Care

- Prepare persons for naps, visitors, or activity programs.
- Assist with elimination.
- Clean incontinent persons.
- Change wet or soiled linens and garments.
- Assist with face and hand washing, oral hygiene, and hair care.
- Assist with range-of-motion exercises and ambulation.
- Straighten beds and units.

Evening Care (PM Care)

- Prepare persons for sleep.
- Assist with elimination.
- Clean incontinent persons.
- Change wet or soiled linens and garments.
- Assist with face and hand washing, oral hygiene, and back massages.
- Help persons change into sleepwear.
- Straighten beds and units.

DAILY CARE

Most people have hygiene routines and habits. For example, teeth are brushed and the face and hands washed after sleep. These and other hygiene measures are often done before and after meals and at bedtime.

You give routine care during the day and evening (Box 16-1). You also assist with hygiene whenever it is needed. Always protect the right to privacy and to personal choice.

ORAL HYGIENE

Oral hygiene *(mouth care):*

- Keeps the mouth and teeth clean.
- Prevents mouth odors and infections.
- Increases comfort.
- Makes food taste better.
- Reduces the risk for *cavities (dental caries)* and *periodontal disease (gum disease, pyorrhea).*

The nurse assesses the person's need for mouth care. Illness, disease, and some drugs often cause:

- A bad taste in the mouth.
- A whitish coating in the mouth and on the tongue.
- Redness and swelling in the mouth and on the tongue.
- Dry mouth. Dry mouth also is common from oxygen, smoking, decreased fluid intake, and anxiety.

See *Delegation Guidelines: Oral Hygiene.*

See *Promoting Safety and Comfort: Oral Hygiene.*

DELEGATION GUIDELINES

Oral Hygiene

To assist with oral hygiene, you need this information from the nurse and the care plan.

- The type of oral hygiene to give:
  - *Brushing and Flossing the Person's Teeth*
  - *Providing Mouth Care for the Unconscious Person,* p. 232
  - *Providing Denture Care,* p. 233
- If flossing is needed.
- What cleaning agent and equipment to use.
- If you apply lubricant to the lips. If yes, what lubricant to use.
- How often to give oral hygiene.
- How much help the person needs.
- What observations to report and record:
  - Dry, cracked, swollen, or blistered lips
  - Mouth or breath odor
  - Redness, swelling, irritation, sores, or white patches in the mouth or on the tongue
  - Bleeding, swelling, or redness of the gums
  - Loose teeth
  - Rough, sharp, or chipped areas on dentures
- When to report observations.
- What patient or resident concerns to report at once.

PROMOTING SAFETY AND COMFORT

Oral Hygiene

Safety

Follow Standard Precautions and the Bloodborne Pathogen Standard. You may have contact with the person's mucous membranes. Gums may bleed during mouth care. Also, the mouth has many microbes. Pathogens spread through sexual contact may be in the mouths of some persons.

Comfort

Assist with oral hygiene after sleep, after meals, and at bedtime. Many people practice oral hygiene before meals. Some persons need mouth care every 2 hours or more often. Always follow the care plan.

Brushing and Flossing Teeth

Oral hygiene involves brushing and flossing teeth. Flossing removes food from between the teeth. It also removes *plaque* (a thin film that sticks to teeth) and *tartar* (hardened plaque). Plaque and tartar cause periodontal disease.

Usually done after brushing, flossing can be done at other times. Some people floss after meals. If done once a day, bedtime is the best time to floss. You need to floss for persons who cannot do so themselves.

Some people need help gathering and setting up oral hygiene equipment. You perform oral hygiene for persons who:

- Are very weak.
- Cannot move or use their arms.
- Are too confused to brush their teeth.

See procedure: *Brushing and Flossing the Person's Teeth.*

Brushing and Flossing the Person's Teeth

NNAAP™ CD VIDEO CLIP VIDEO

QUALITY OF LIFE

- Knock before entering the person's room.
- Address the person by name.
- Introduce yourself by name and title.
- Explain the procedure before starting and during the procedure.
- Protect the person's rights during the procedure.
- Handle the person gently during the procedure.

PRE-PROCEDURE

1 Follow *Delegation Guidelines: Oral Hygiene*. See *Promoting Safety and Comfort: Oral Hygiene.*
2 Practice hand hygiene.
3 Collect the following.
- Toothbrush with soft bristles
- Toothpaste
- Mouthwash (or solution noted on the care plan)
- Dental floss (if used)
- Water cup with cool water
- Straw
- Kidney basin
- Hand towel
- Paper towels
- Gloves

4 Place the paper towels on the over-bed table. Arrange items on top of them.
5 Identify the person. Check the ID (identification) bracelet against the assignment sheet. Also call the person by name.
6 Provide for privacy.
7 Raise the bed for body mechanics. Bed rails are up if used.

Continued

Brushing and Flossing the Person's Teeth—cont'd

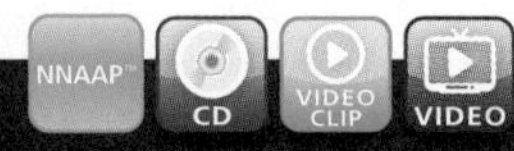

PROCEDURE

8 Lower the bed rail near you if up.
9 Assist the person to a sitting position or to a side-lying position near you. (NOTE: Some state competency tests require that the person is at a 75- to 90-degree angle.)
10 Place the towel across the person's chest.
11 Adjust the over-bed table so you can reach it with ease.
12 Practice hand hygiene. Put on the gloves.
13 Hold the toothbrush over the kidney basis. Pour some water over the brush.
14 Apply toothpaste to the toothbrush.
15 Brush the teeth gently (Fig. 16-1).
16 Brush the tongue gently.
17 Let the person rinse the mouth with water. Hold the kidney basin under the person's chin (Fig. 16-2). Repeat this step as needed.
18 Floss the person's teeth (optional).
  a Break off an 18-inch piece of dental floss from the dispenser.
  b Hold the floss between the middle fingers of each hand (Fig. 16-3, *A*).
  c Stretch the floss with your thumbs.
  d Start at the upper back tooth on the right side. Work around to the left side.
  e Move the floss gently up and down between the teeth (Fig. 16-3, *B*). Move the floss up and down against the side of the tooth. Work from the top of the crown to the gum line.
  f Move to a new section of floss after every second tooth.
  g Floss the lower teeth. Use up and down motions as for the upper teeth. Start on the right side. Work around to the left side.
19 Let the person use mouthwash or other solution. Hold the kidney basin under the chin.
20 Wipe the person's mouth. Remove the towel.
21 Remove and discard the gloves. Practice hand hygiene.

POST-PROCEDURE

22 Provide for comfort. (See the inside of the front cover.)
23 Place the call light within reach.
24 Lower the bed to a safe and comfortable level appropriate for the person. Follow the care plan.
25 Raise or lower bed rails. Follow the care plan.
26 Rinse the toothbrush. Clean, rinse, and dry equipment. Return the toothbrush and equipment to their proper place. Wear gloves.
27 Wipe off the over-bed table with the paper towels. Discard the paper towels.
28 Unscreen the person.
29 Complete a safety check of the room. (See the inside of the front cover.)
30 Follow agency policy for dirty linen.
31 Remove and discard the gloves. Practice hand hygiene.
32 Report and record your observations.

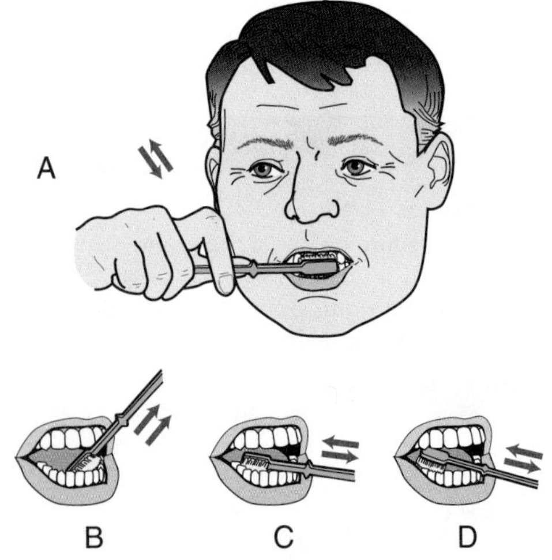

FIGURE 16-1 Brushing teeth. **A,** The brush is held at a 45-degree angle to the gums. Teeth are brushed with short strokes. **B,** The brush is at a 45-degree angle against the inside of the front teeth. Teeth are brushed from the gum to the crown of the tooth with short strokes. **C,** The brush is held horizontally against the inner surfaces of the teeth. The teeth are brushed back and forth. **D,** The brush is positioned on the chewing surfaces of the teeth. The teeth are brushed back and forth.

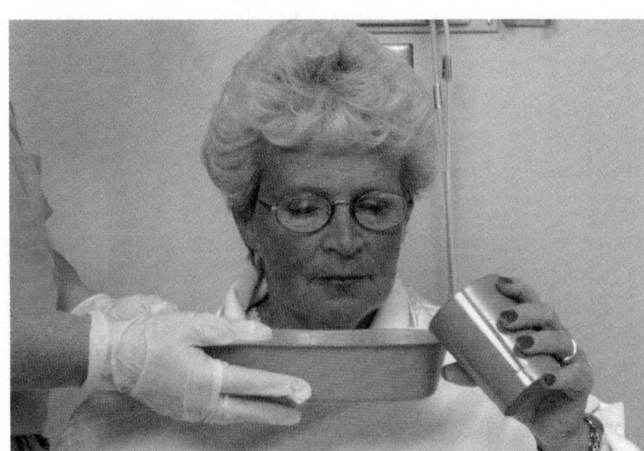

FIGURE 16-2 The kidney basin is held under the person's chin.

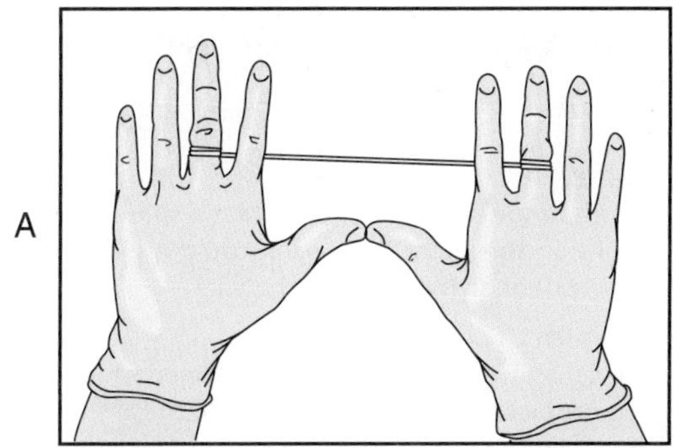

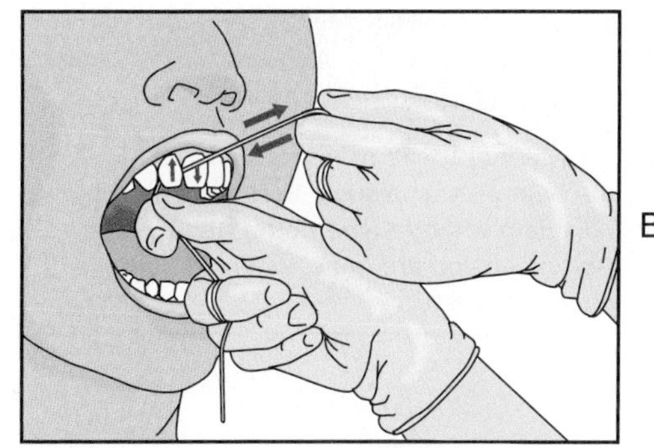

FIGURE 16-3 Flossing. **A,** Floss is wrapped around the middle fingers. **B,** Floss is moved in up-and-down motions between the teeth. Floss is moved up and down from the crown to the gum line.

Mouth Care for the Unconscious Person

Unconscious persons cannot eat or drink. Some breathe with their mouths open. Many receive oxygen. These factors cause mouth dryness. They also cause crusting on the tongue and mucous membranes. Oral hygiene keeps the mouth clean and moist. It also helps prevent infection.

The care plan tells you what cleaning agent to use. Use sponge swabs to apply the cleaning agent. Apply a lubricant (check the care plan) to the lips after cleaning. It prevents cracking of the lips.

Unconscious persons usually cannot swallow. Protect them from choking and aspiration. ***Aspiration** is breathing fluid, food, vomitus, or an object into the lungs.* It can cause pneumonia and death. To prevent aspiration:

- Position the person on 1 side with the head turned well to the side (Fig. 16-4). In this position, excess fluid runs out of the mouth.
- Use only a small amount of fluid to clean the mouth.
- Do not insert dentures. Dentures are not worn when the person is unconscious.

Keep the person's mouth open with a padded tongue blade (Fig. 16-5). Do not use your fingers. The person can bite down on them. The bite breaks the skin and creates a portal of entry for microbes. Infection is a risk.

Mouth care is given at least every 2 hours. Follow the nurse's directions and the care plan.

See *Focus on Communication: Mouth Care for the Unconscious Person*, p. 232.

See *Promoting Safety and Comfort: Mouth Care for the Unconscious Person*, p. 232.

See procedure: *Providing Mouth Care for the Unconscious Person*, p. 232.

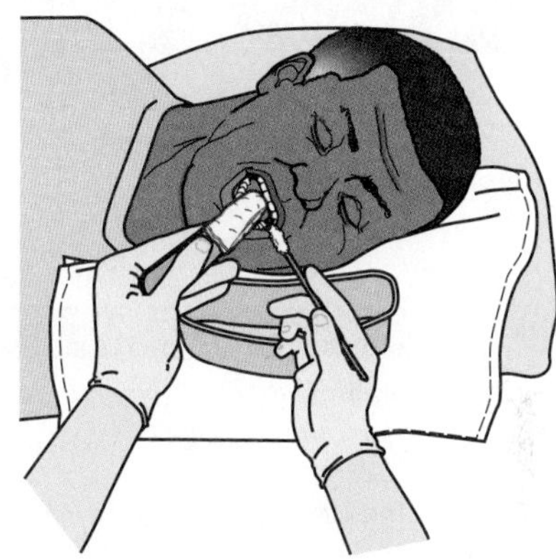

FIGURE 16-4 The unconscious person's head is turned well to the side to prevent aspiration. A padded tongue blade is used to keep the mouth open while cleaning the mouth with swabs.

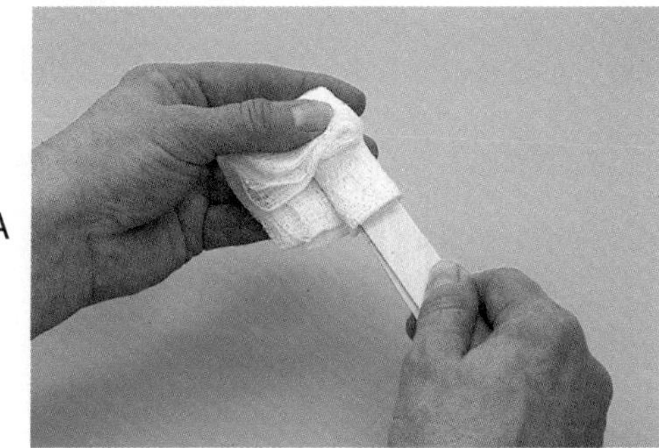

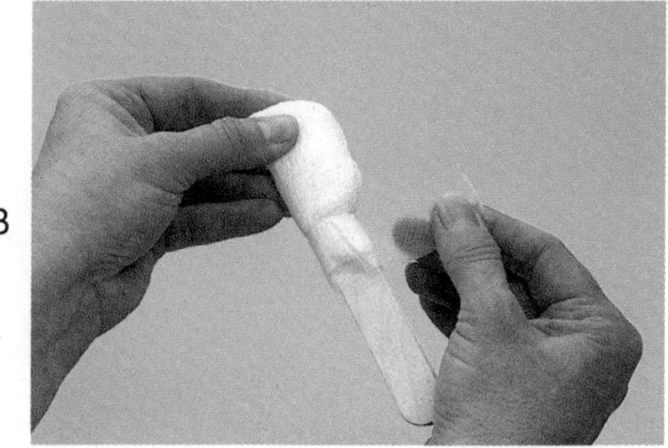

FIGURE 16-5 Making a padded tongue blade. **A,** Place 2 wooden tongue blades together. Wrap gauze around the top half. **B,** Tape the gauze in place.

FOCUS ON COMMUNICATION

Mouth Care for the Unconscious Person

Unconscious persons cannot speak or respond to you. However, some can hear. Always assume that unconscious persons can hear. Explain what you are doing step-by-step. Also, tell the person when you are done, when you are leaving, and when you will return.

PROMOTING SAFETY AND COMFORT

Mouth Care for the Unconscious Person

Safety

Use sponge swabs with care. Make sure the sponge pad is tight on the stick. The person could aspirate or choke on the sponge if it comes off the stick.

Comfort

Unconscious persons are re-positioned at least every 2 hours. To promote comfort, combine mouth care with skin care, re-positioning, and other comfort measures.

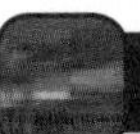

Providing Mouth Care for the Unconscious Person

QUALITY OF LIFE

- Knock before entering the person's room.
- Address the person by name.
- Introduce yourself by name and title.
- Explain the procedure before starting and during the procedure.
- Protect the person's rights during the procedure.
- Handle the person gently during the procedure.

PRE-PROCEDURE

1 Follow *Delegation Guidelines: Oral Hygiene,* p. 229. See *Promoting Safety and Comfort:*
   a *Oral Hygiene,* p. 229
   b *Mouth Care for the Unconscious Person*
2 Practice hand hygiene.
3 Collect the following.
   - Cleaning agent (check the care plan)
   - Sponge swabs
   - Padded tongue blade
   - Water cup with cool water
   - Hand towel
   - Kidney basin
   - Lip lubricant
   - Paper towels
   - Gloves
4 Place the paper towels on the over-bed table. Arrange items on top of them.
5 Identify the person. Check the ID bracelet against the assignment sheet. Also call the person by name.
6 Provide for privacy.
7 Raise the bed for body mechanics. Bed rails are up if used.

PROCEDURE

8 Lower the bed rail near you.
9 Position the person in a side-lying position near you. Turn his or her head well to the side.
10 Put on the gloves.
11 Place the towel under the person's face.
12 Place the kidney basin under the chin.
13 Separate the upper and lower teeth. Use the padded tongue blade. Be gentle. Never use force. If you have problems, ask the nurse for help.
14 Clean the mouth using sponge swabs moistened with the cleaning agent (see Fig. 16-4).
   a Clean the chewing and inner surfaces of the teeth.
   b Clean the gums and outer surfaces of the teeth.
   c Swab the roof of the mouth, inside of the cheek, and the lips.
   d Swab the tongue.
   e Moisten a clean swab. Swab the mouth to rinse.
   f Place used swabs in the kidney basin.
15 Remove the kidney basin and supplies.
16 Wipe the person's mouth. Remove the towel.
17 Apply lubricant to the lips.
18 Remove and discard the gloves. Practice hand hygiene.

POST-PROCEDURE

19 Provide for comfort. (See the inside of the front cover.)
20 Place the call light within reach.
21 Lower the bed to a level safe and comfortable for the person. Follow the care plan.
22 Raise or lower bed rails. Follow the care plan.
23 Clean, rinse, dry, and return equipment to its proper place. Discard disposable items. (Wear gloves.)
24 Wipe off the over-bed table with paper towels. Discard the paper towels.
25 Unscreen the person.
26 Complete a safety check of the room. (See the inside of the front cover.)
27 Tell the person that you are leaving the room. Tell him or her when you will return.
28 Follow agency policy for dirty linen.
29 Remove and discard the gloves. Practice hand hygiene.
30 Report and record your observations.

Denture Care

A *denture is an artificial tooth or a set of artificial teeth* (Fig. 16-6). Often called "false teeth," dentures replace missing teeth. Mouth care is given and dentures cleaned as often as natural teeth. Dentures are slippery when wet. They easily break or chip if dropped onto a hard surface (floors, sinks, counters). Hold them firmly when removing or inserting them. During cleaning, firmly hold them over a basin of water lined with a towel. This prevents them from falling onto a hard surface.

Use only denture cleaning products. Otherwise, you could damage dentures. To use a cleaning agent, follow the manufacturer's instructions. They tell how to use the cleaning agent and what water temperature to use.

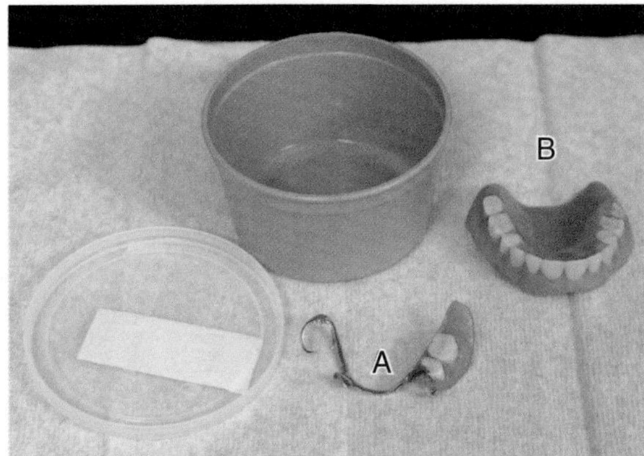

FIGURE 16-6 Dentures. **A,** Partial denture. **B,** Full denture.

Hot water causes dentures to lose their shape (warp). If not worn after cleaning, store dentures in a container with cool or warm water or a denture soaking solution. Otherwise they can dry out and warp.

Dentures are usually removed at bedtime. Some people do not wear their dentures. Others wear dentures for eating and remove them after meals. Remind them not to wrap dentures in tissues or napkins. Otherwise, they are easily discarded.

See *Promoting Safety and Comfort: Denture Care.*

See procedure: *Providing Denture Care.*

PROMOTING SAFETY AND COMFORT

Denture Care

Safety

Dentures are the person's property. They are costly. Handle them very carefully. Label dentures with the person's name and room and bed number. Report lost or damaged dentures at once. Losing or damaging dentures is negligent conduct.

Never carry dentures in your hands. Always use a denture cup or kidney basin. You could easily drop the dentures as you move to and from the bedside and bathroom.

Comfort

Many people do not like being seen without their dentures. Privacy is important. Allow privacy when the person cleans dentures. If you clean dentures, return them to the person as quickly as possible.

Persons with dentures may have some natural teeth. They need to brush and floss the natural teeth. See procedure: *Brushing and Flossing the Person's Teeth,* p. 229.

Providing Denture Care

NNAAP CD VIDEO CLIP VIDEO

QUALITY OF LIFE

- Knock before entering the person's room.
- Address the person by name.
- Introduce yourself by name and title.
- Explain the procedure before starting and during the procedure.
- Protect the person's rights during the procedure.
- Handle the person gently during the procedure.

PRE-PROCEDURE

1 Follow *Delegation Guidelines: Oral Hygiene,* p. 229. See *Promoting Safety and Comfort:*
   a *Oral Hygiene,* p. 229
   b *Denture Care*
2 Practice hand hygiene.
3 Collect the following.
   - Denture brush or toothbrush (for cleaning dentures)
   - Denture cup labeled with the person's name and room and bed number
   - Denture cleaning agent
   - Soft-bristled toothbrush or sponge swabs (for oral hygiene)
   - Toothpaste
   - Water cup with cool water
   - Straw
   - Mouthwash (or other noted solution)
   - Kidney basin
   - 2 hand towels
   - Gauze squares
   - Paper towels
   - Gloves
4 Place the paper towels on the over-bed table. Arrange items on top of them.
5 Identify the person. Check the ID bracelet against the assignment sheet. Also call the person by name.
6 Provide for privacy.
7 Raise the bed for body mechanics.

Continued

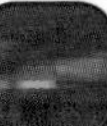

Providing Denture Care—cont'd

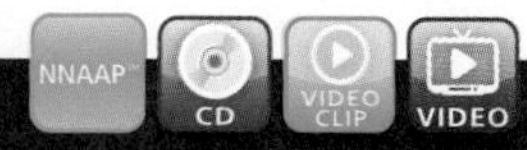

PROCEDURE

8 Lower the bed rail near you if up.
9 Practice hand hygiene. Put on the gloves.
10 Place a towel over the person's chest.
11 Ask the person to remove the dentures. Carefully place them in the kidney basin.
12 Remove the dentures if the person cannot do so. Use gauze squares for a good grip on the slippery dentures.
  a Grasp the upper denture with your thumb and index finger (Fig. 16-7). Move it up and down slightly to break the seal. Gently remove the denture. Place it in the kidney basin.
  b Grasp and remove the lower denture with your thumb and index finger. Turn it slightly, and lift it out of the person's mouth. Place it in the kidney basin.
13 Follow the care plan for raising bed rails.
14 Take the kidney basin, denture cup, denture brush, and denture cleaning agent to the sink.
15 Line the bottom of the sink with a towel. Fill the sink half-way with water.
16 Rinse each denture under cool or warm running water. Follow agency policy for water temperature.
17 Return dentures to the kidney basin or denture cup.
18 Apply the denture cleaning agent to the brush.
19 Brush the dentures as in Figure 16-8. Brush the inner, outer, and chewing surfaces.
20 Rinse the dentures under running water. Use warm or cool water as directed by the cleaning agent manufacturer.
21 Rinse the denture cup and lid. Place dentures in the denture cup. Cover the dentures with cool or warm water. Follow agency policy for water temperature.
22 Clean the kidney basin.
23 Take the denture cup and kidney basin to the over-bed table.
24 Lower the bed rail if up.
25 Position the person for oral hygiene.
26 Clean the person's gums and tongue. Use toothpaste and the toothbrush (or sponge swabs).
27 Have the person use mouthwash (or noted solution). Hold the kidney basin under the chin.
28 Ask the person to insert the dentures. Insert them if the person cannot.
  a Hold the upper denture firmly with your thumb and index finger. Raise the upper lip with the other hand. Insert the denture. Gently press on the denture with your index finger to make sure it is in place.
  b Hold the lower denture with your thumb and index finger. Pull the lower lip down slightly. Insert the denture. Gently press down on it to make sure it is in place.
29 Place the denture cup in the top drawer of the bedside stand if the dentures are not worn. The dentures must be in water or in a denture soaking solution.
30 Wipe the person's mouth. Remove the towel.
31 Remove and discard the gloves. Practice hand hygiene.

POST-PROCEDURE

32 Assist with hand washing.
33 Provide for comfort. (See the inside of the front cover.)
34 Place the call light within reach.
35 Lower the bed to a safe and comfortable level appropriate for the person. Follow the care plan.
36 Raise or lower bed rails. Follow the care plan.
37 Remove the towel from the sink. Drain the sink.
38 Rinse the brushes. Clean, rinse, and dry equipment. Return the brushes and equipment to their proper place. Discard disposable items. Wear gloves for this step.
39 Wipe off the over-bed table with paper towels. Discard the paper towels.
40 Unscreen the person.
41 Complete a safety check of the room. (See the inside of the front cover.)
42 Follow agency policy for dirty linen.
43 Remove and discard the gloves. Practice hand hygiene.
44 Report and record your observations.

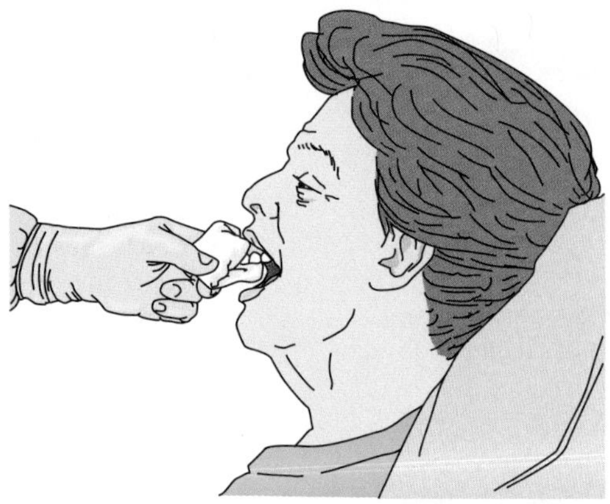

FIGURE 16-7 Remove the upper denture by grasping it with the thumb and index finger of 1 hand. Use a piece of gauze to grasp the slippery denture.

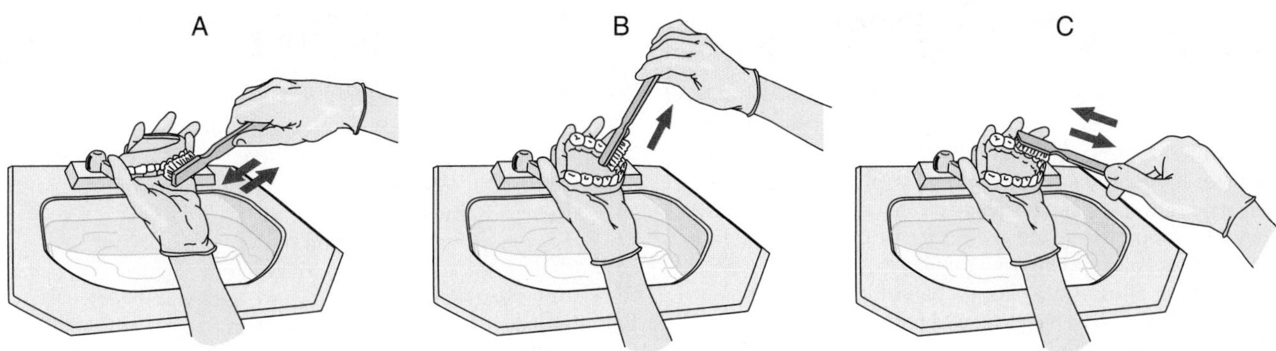

FIGURE 16-8 Cleaning dentures. **A,** Brush the outer surfaces of the denture with back-and-forth motions. (Note that the denture is held over the sink. The sink is lined with a towel and filled half-way with water.) **B,** Position the brush vertically to clean the inner surfaces of the denture. Use upward strokes. **C,** Brush the chewing surfaces with back-and-forth motions.

BATHING

Bathing cleans the skin. It also cleans the mucous membranes of the genital and anal areas. Microbes, dead skin, perspiration, and excess oils are removed. A bath is refreshing and relaxing. Circulation is stimulated and body parts exercised. Observations are made, and you have time to talk to the person.

Complete or partial baths, tub baths, or showers are given. The method depends on the person's condition, self-care abilities, and personal choice. In hospitals, bathing is common after breakfast. In nursing centers, bathing usually occurs after breakfast or the evening meal. The person's choice of bath time is respected whenever possible.

Bathing frequency is a personal matter. Some people bathe daily. Others bathe 1 or 2 times a week. Personal choice, weather, activity, and illness affect bathing. Other illnesses and dry skin may limit bathing to every 2 or 3 days.

The rules for bed baths, showers, and tub baths are listed in Box 16-2.

See *Focus on Communication: Assisting With Hygiene,* p. 228.

See *Focus on Older Persons: Bathing,* p. 236.

See *Delegation Guidelines: Bathing,* p. 236.

See *Promoting Safety and Comfort: Bathing,* p. 237.

BOX 16-2 Rules for Bathing

- Follow the care plan for bathing method and skin care products.
- Allow personal choice when possible.
- Follow Standard Precautions and the Bloodborne Pathogen Standard (Chapter 12).
- Collect needed items before starting the procedure.
- Remove hearing aids before bathing. Water will damage hearing aids.
- Provide for privacy. Screen the person. Close doors and window coverings—drapes, shades, blinds, shutters, and so on.
- Assist with elimination. Bathing stimulates the need to urinate. Comfort and relaxation increase if urination needs are met.
- Cover the person for warmth and privacy.
- Reduce drafts. Close doors and windows.
- Protect the person from falling.
- Use good body mechanics at all times.
- Follow the rules to safely move and transfer the person (Chapter 14).
- Know what water temperature to use. See *Delegation Guidelines: Bathing,* p. 236.
- Keep bar soap in the soap dish between latherings. This prevents soapy water. It also helps prevent slipping and falls in showers and tubs.
- Wash from the cleanest areas to the dirtiest areas.
- Encourage the person to help as much as is safely possible.
- Rinse the skin thoroughly. Remove all soap.
- Pat the skin dry to avoid irritating or breaking the skin. Do not rub the skin.
- Dry well under the breasts, between skin folds, in the perineal area, and between the toes.
- Bathe skin when urine or feces are present. This prevents skin breakdown and odors.

FOCUS ON OLDER PERSONS

Bathing

Bathing procedures can threaten persons with dementia. They do not understand what is happening or why. And they may fear harm or danger. Confusion can increase. Therefore, they may resist care and become agitated and combative. They may shout at you and cry out for help. You must be calm, patient, and soothing.

The nurse assesses the person's behaviors and routines. The person may be calmer and less confused or agitated during a certain time of day. Bathing is scheduled for the person's calm times. The nurse decides the best bathing procedure for the person.

The rules in Box 16-2 apply. The care plan also includes measures to help the person through the bath. For example:

- Use terms such as "cleaned up" or "washed" rather than "shower" or "bath."
- Complete pre-procedure activities. For example, ready supplies and linens. Make sure you have everything that you need.
- Provide for warmth. Prevent drafts. Have extra towels and a robe nearby.
- Play soft music to help the person relax.
- Provide for safety.
  - Use a hand-held shower nozzle.
  - Have the person use a shower chair or shower bench.
  - Do not use bath oil. It can make the tub or shower slippery. And it may cause a urinary tract infection.
  - Do not leave the person alone in the tub or shower.
- Draw bath water ahead of time. Test the water temperature. Add warm or cold water as needed.
- Tell the person what you are doing step-by-step. Use clear, simple statements.
- Let the person help as much as possible. For example, give the person a washcloth. Ask him or her to wash the arms. If the person does not know what to do, let the person hold the washcloth if safe to do so.
- Put a towel over the person's shoulder or lap (tub bath or shower). This helps the person feel less exposed.
- Do not rush the person.
- Use a calm, pleasant voice.
- Distract the person if needed.
- Calm the person.
- Handle the person gently.
- Try a partial bath if a shower or tub bath agitates the person.
- Try the bath later if the person continues to resist care.

Persons with dementia often respond well to a *towel bath.* An over-sized towel is used. It covers the body from the neck to the feet. The towel is wet with a cleansing solution—water, cleaning agent, and skin-softening agent. It also has a drying agent so the person's body dries fast. The nurse and care plan tell you when to use a towel bath. To give a towel bath, follow agency policy.

DELEGATION GUIDELINES

Bathing

To assist with bathing, you need this information from the nurse and the care plan.

- What bath to give—complete bed bath, partial bath, tub bath, or shower.
- How much help the person needs.
- The person's activity or position limits.
- What water temperature to use. Bath water cools rapidly. Heat is lost to the bath basin, over-bed table, washcloth, and your hands. Therefore water temperature for complete bed baths and partial baths is usually between 110°F and 115°F (Fahrenheit) (43.3°C and 46.1°C [centigrade]) for adults. Older persons have fragile skin. They need lower water temperatures.
- What skin care products to use and what the person prefers.
- What observations to report and record:
  - The color of the skin, lips, nail beds, and sclera (whites of the eyes)
  - If the skin appears pale, grayish, yellow (*jaundice*—Chapter 28), or bluish *(cyanotic)*
  - The location and description of rashes
  - Skin texture—smooth, rough, scaly, flaky, dry, moist
  - *Diaphoresis*—profuse (excessive) sweating
  - Bruises or open skin areas
  - Pale or reddened areas, particularly over bony parts
  - Drainage or bleeding from wounds or body openings
  - Swelling of the feet and legs
  - Corns or calluses on the feet
  - Skin temperature (cold, cool, warm, hot)
  - Complaints of pain or discomfort
- When to report observations.
- What patient or resident concerns to report at once.

The Complete Bed Bath

For a complete bed bath, you wash the person's entire body in bed. Bed baths are usually needed by persons who are:

- Unconscious
- Paralyzed
- In casts or traction
- Weak from illness or surgery

A bed bath is new to some people. Some are embarrassed to have their bodies seen. Some fear exposure. Explain how you give the bath. Also explain how you cover the body for privacy.

See procedure: *Giving a Complete Bed Bath.*

Text continued on p. 241

PROMOTING SAFETY AND COMFORT

Bathing

Safety

Hot water can burn the skin. Measure water temperature according to agency policy. If unsure if the water is too hot, ask the nurse to check it.

Protect the person from falls and other injuries. Practice the safety measures in Chapters 9 and 10. Also protect the person from drafts.

Apply powder with caution. Do not use powders near persons with respiratory disorders. Inhaling powder can irritate the airway and lungs. Before using powder, check with the nurse and the care plan. To safely apply powder:

- Turn away from the person.
- Sprinkle a small amount onto your hand or a cloth. Do not shake or sprinkle powder onto the person.
- Apply the powder in a thin layer.
- Make sure powder does not get on the floor. Powder is slippery and can cause falls.

You make beds after baths. After making the bed, lower the bed to a safe and comfortable level appropriate for the person. Follow the care plan. For an occupied bed, raise or lower bed rails according to the care plan. Make sure the bed wheels are locked.

Protect the person and yourself from infection. During baths and bedmaking, contact with blood, body fluids, secretions, or excretions is likely. Follow Standard Precautions and the Bloodborne Pathogen Standard.

Comfort

Before bathing, let the person meet elimination needs (Chapters 18 and 19). Bathing stimulates the need to urinate. Comfort is greater when the bladder is empty. Also bathing is not interrupted.

Oral hygiene is common during bathing routines. Some persons do so before bathing; others do so after. Allow personal choice and follow the person's care plan.

Provide for warmth. Cover the person with a bath blanket. Make sure the water is warm enough for the person. Cool water causes chilling.

If the person prefers, remove sleepwear after washing the eyes, face, ears, and neck. Removing sleepwear at this time helps the person feel less exposed and provides more mental comfort with the bath.

If the person is able, let him or her wash the genital area. This promotes privacy and helps prevent embarrassment. See "Perineal Care" on p. 245.

Giving a Complete Bed Bath

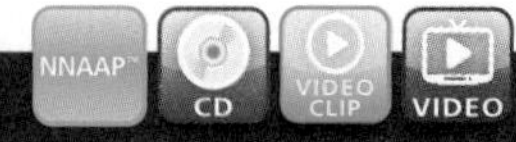

QUALITY OF LIFE

- Knock before entering the person's room.
- Address the person by name.
- Introduce yourself by name and title.
- Explain the procedure before starting and during the procedure.
- Protect the person's rights during the procedure.
- Handle the person gently during the procedure.

PRE-PROCEDURE

1 Follow *Delegation Guidelines: Bathing*. See *Promoting Safety and Comfort:*
  a *Assisting With Hygiene*, p. 228
  b *Bathing*
2 Practice hand hygiene.
3 Identify the person. Check the ID bracelet against the assignment sheet. Also call the person by name.
4 Collect clean linen (see procedure: *Making a Closed Bed* in Chapter 15). Place linen on a clean surface.
5 Collect the following.
  - Wash basin
  - Soap
  - Bath thermometer
  - Orangewood stick or nail file
  - Washcloth (and at least 4 washcloths for perineal care, p. 245)
  - 2 bath towels and 2 hand towels
  - Bath blanket
  - Clothing or sleepwear
  - Lotion
  - Powder
  - Deodorant or antiperspirant
  - Brush and comb
  - Other grooming items as requested
  - Paper towels
  - Gloves
6 Cover the over-bed table with paper towels. Arrange items on the over-bed table. Adjust the height as needed.
7 Provide for privacy.
8 Raise the bed for body mechanics. Bed rails are up if used.

Continued

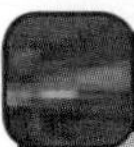

Giving a Complete Bed Bath—cont'd

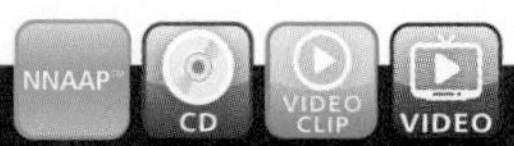

PROCEDURE

9 Practice hand hygiene. Put on gloves.
10 Remove the sleepwear. Do not expose the person. Follow agency policy for dirty sleepwear.
11 Cover the person with a bath blanket. Remove top linens (see procedure: *Making an Occupied Bed* in Chapter 15).
12 Lower the head of the bed. It is as flat as possible. The person has at least 1 pillow.
13 Fill the wash basin ⅔ (two-thirds) full with water. Follow the care plan for water temperature. Water temperature is usually 110°F to 115°F (43.3°C to 46.1°C) for adults. Measure water temperature. Use the bath thermometer. Or dip your elbow or inner wrist into the basin to test the water.
14 Lower the bed rail near you if up.
15 Ask the person to check the water temperature. Adjust the temperature if it is too hot or too cold. Raise the bed rail before leaving the bedside. Lower it when you return.
16 Place the basin on the over-bed table.
17 Place a hand towel over the person's chest.
18 Make a mitt with the washcloth (Fig. 16-9). Use a mitt for the entire bath.
19 Wash around the person's eyes with water. Do not use soap.
   a Clean the far eye. Gently wipe from the inner to the outer aspect of the eye with a corner of the mitt (Fig. 16-10).
   b Clean around the eye near you. Use a clean part of the washcloth for each stroke.
20 Ask the person if you should use soap to wash the face.
21 Wash the face, ears, and neck. Rinse and pat dry with the towel on the chest.
22 Help the person move to the side of the bed near you.
23 Expose the far arm. Place a bath towel length-wise under the arm. Apply soap to the washcloth.
24 Support the arm with your palm under the person's elbow. His or her forearm rests on your forearm.
25 Wash the arm, shoulder, and underarm. Use long, firm strokes (Fig. 16-11). Rinse and pat dry.
26 Place the basin on the towel. Put the person's hand into the water (Fig. 16-12). Wash it well. Clean under the fingernails with an orangewood stick or nail file.
27 Have the person exercise the hand and fingers.
28 Remove the basin. Dry the hand well. Cover the arm with the bath blanket.
29 Repeat steps 23 to 28 for the near arm.
30 Place a bath towel over the chest cross-wise. Hold the towel in place. Pull the bath blanket from under the towel to the waist. Apply soap to the washcloth.
31 Lift the towel slightly, and wash the chest (Fig. 16-13). Do not expose the person. Rinse and pat dry, especially under the breasts.
32 Move the towel length-wise over the chest and abdomen. Do not expose the person. Pull the bath blanket down to the pubic area. Apply soap to the washcloth.
33 Lift the towel slightly, and wash the abdomen (Fig. 16-14, p. 240). Rinse and pat dry.
34 Pull the bath blanket up to the shoulders. Cover both arms. Remove the towel.
35 Change soapy or cool water. Measure bath water temperature as in step 13. If bed rails are used, raise the bed rail near you before leaving the bedside. Lower it when you return.
36 Uncover the far leg. Do not expose the genital area. Place a towel length-wise under the foot and leg. Apply soap to a washcloth.
37 Bend the knee, and support the leg with your arm. Wash it with long, firm strokes. Rinse and pat dry.
38 Place the basin on the towel near the foot.
39 Lift the leg slightly. Slide the basin under the foot.
40 Place the foot in the basin (Fig. 16-15, p. 240). Use an orangewood stick or nail file to clean under the toenails if necessary. If the person cannot bend the knees:
   a Wash the foot. Carefully separate the toes. Rinse and pat dry.
   b Clean under the toenails with an orangewood stick or nail file if necessary.
41 Remove the basin. Dry the leg and foot. Apply lotion to the foot if directed by the nurse and care plan. Do not apply lotion between the toes. Cover the leg with the bath blanket. Remove the towel.
42 Repeat steps 36 to 41 for the near leg.
43 Change the water. Measure water temperature as in step 13. Raise the bed rail near you before leaving the bedside. Lower it when you return.
44 Turn the person onto the side away from you. The person is covered with the bath blanket.
45 Uncover the back and buttocks. Do not expose the person. Place a towel length-wise on the bed along the back. Apply soap to a washcloth.
46 Wash the back. Work from the back of the neck to the lower end of the buttocks. Use long, firm, continuous strokes (Fig. 16-16, p. 240). Rinse and dry well.
47 Turn the person onto his or her back.
48 Change water for perineal care (p. 245). See step 14 in procedure: *Giving Female Perineal Care* (p. 246) for water temperature. (Some state competency tests also require changing gloves and hand hygiene at this time.) Raise the bed rail near you before leaving the bedside. Lower it when you return.
49 Allow the person to perform perineal care if able. Provide perineal care if the person cannot do so (p. 245). At least 4 washcloths are used. (Practice hand hygiene and wear clean gloves for perineal care.)
50 Remove and discard the gloves. Practice hand hygiene.
51 Give a back massage (Chapter 15).
52 Apply deodorant or antiperspirant. Apply lotion and powder as requested. See *Promoting Safety and Comfort: Bathing,* p. 237.
53 Put clean garments on the person (Chapter 17).
54 Comb and brush the person's hair (Chapter 17).
55 Make the bed.

Giving a Complete Bed Bath—cont'd

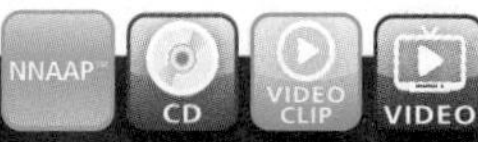

POST-PROCEDURE

56 Provide for comfort. (See the inside of the front cover.)
57 Place the call light within reach.
58 Lower the bed to a safe and comfortable level for the person. Follow the care plan.
59 Raise or lower bed rails. Follow the care plan.
60 Put on clean gloves.
61 Empty, clean, rinse, and dry the wash basin. Return it and other supplies to their proper place.
62 Wipe off the over-bed table with paper towels. Discard the paper towels.
63 Unscreen the person.
64 Complete a safety check of the room. (See the inside of the front cover.)
65 Follow agency policy for dirty linen.
66 Remove and discard the gloves. Practice hand hygiene.
67 Report and record your observations.

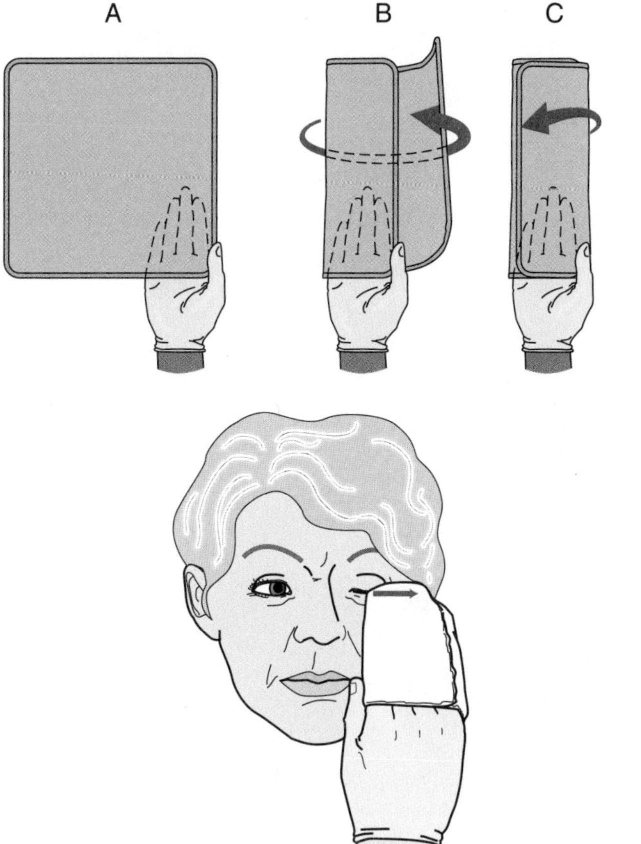

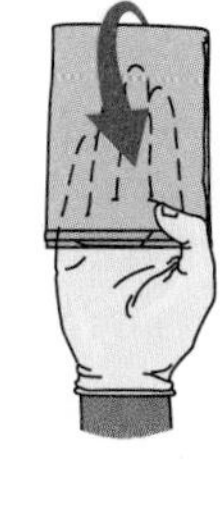

FIGURE 16-9 Making a mitted washcloth. **A,** Grasp the near side of the washcloth with your thumb. **B,** Bring the washcloth around and behind your hand. **C,** Fold the side of the washcloth over your palm as you grasp it with your thumb. **D,** Fold the top of the washcloth down and tuck it under next to your palm.

FIGURE 16-10 Wash the person's eyes with a mitted washcloth. Wipe from the inner to the outer aspect of the eye.

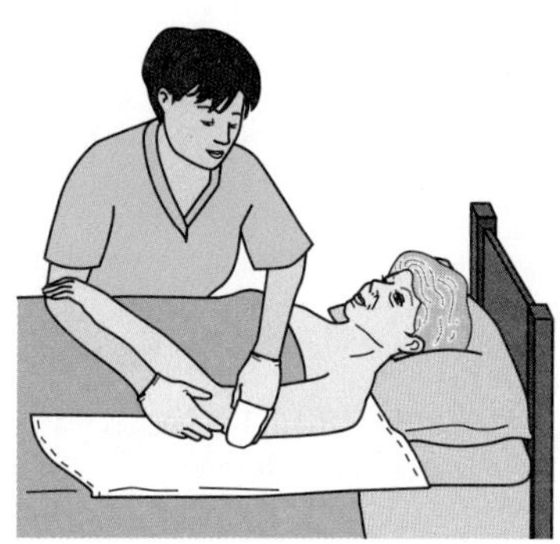

FIGURE 16-11 The person's arm is washed with firm, long strokes using a mitted washcloth.

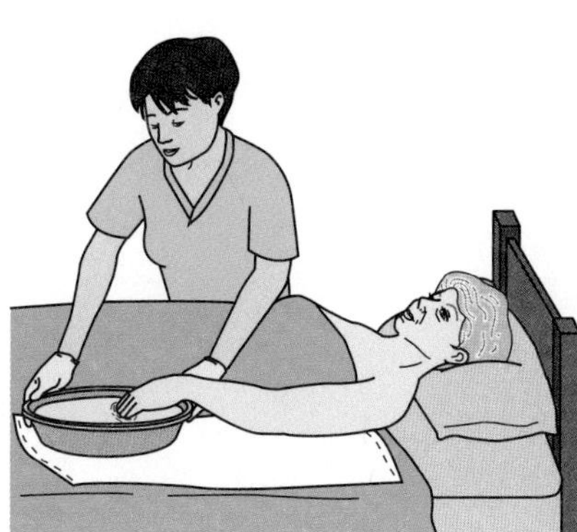

FIGURE 16-12 The person's hand is washed by placing the wash basin on the bed.

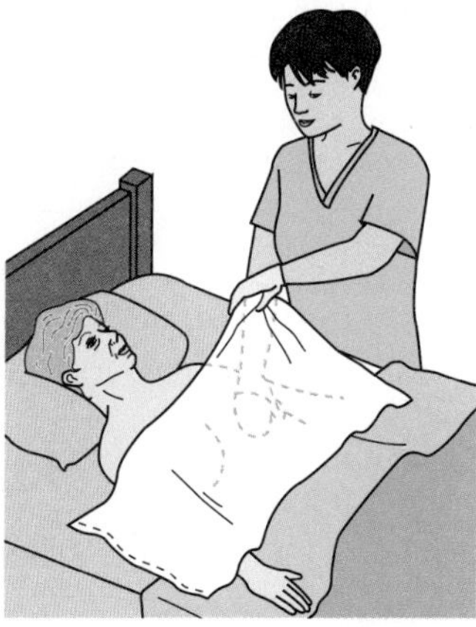

FIGURE 16-13 The person's breasts are not exposed during the bath. A bath towel is placed horizontally over the chest area. The towel is lifted slightly for reaching under to wash the breasts and chest.

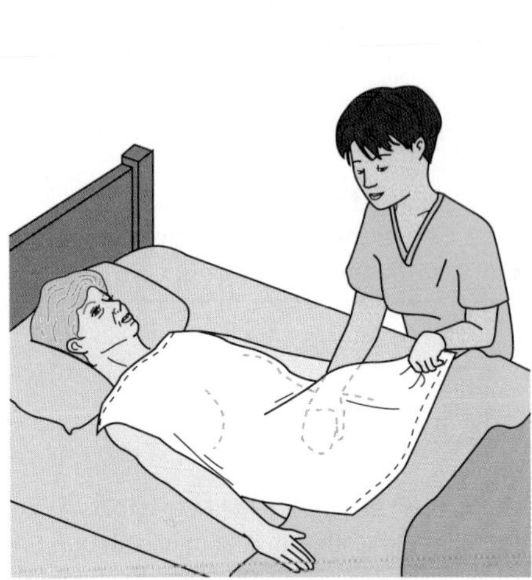

FIGURE 16-14 The bath towel is turned so that it is vertical to cover the breasts and abdomen. The towel is lifted slightly to bathe the abdomen. The bath blanket covers the pubic area.

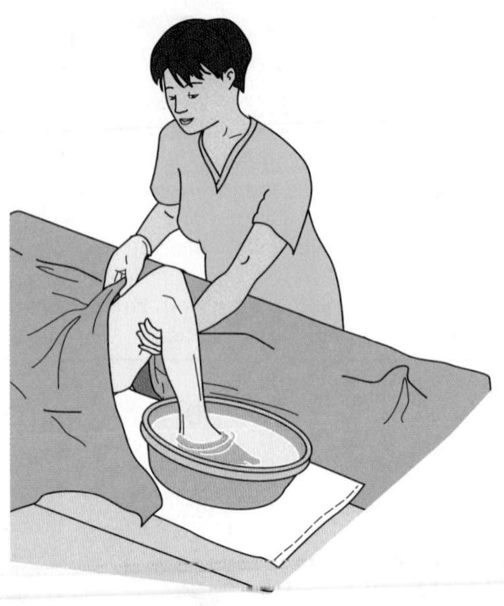

FIGURE 16-15 The foot is washed by placing it in the wash basin on the bed.

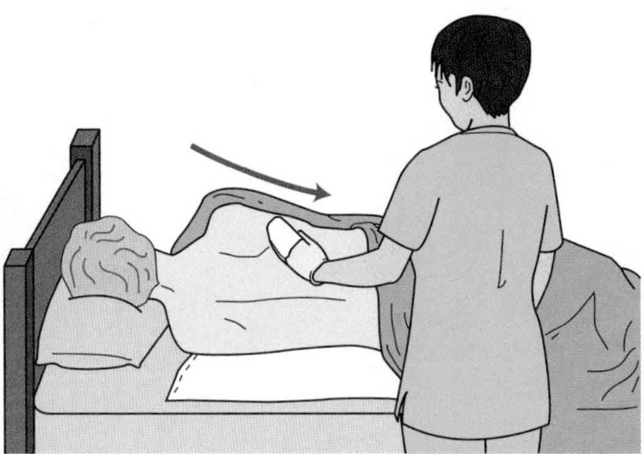

FIGURE 16-16 The back is washed with long, firm, continuous strokes. Note that the person is in a side-lying position. A towel is placed length-wise on the bed to protect the linens from water.

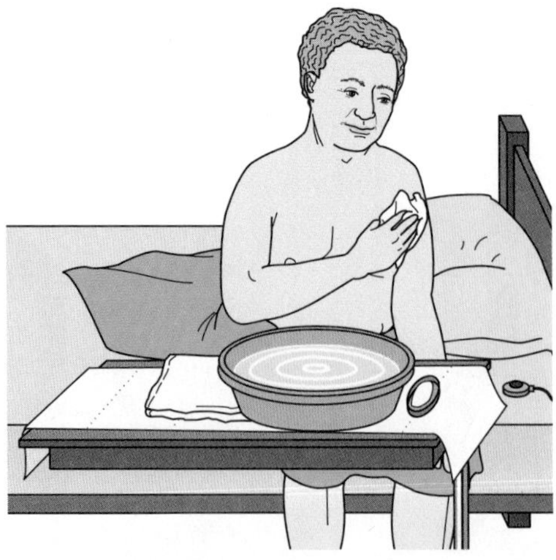

FIGURE 16-17 The person is bathing himself while sitting on the side of the bed. Needed equipment is within reach.

The Partial Bath

The *partial bath* involves bathing the face, hands, axillae (underarms), back, buttocks, and perineal area. Odors or discomfort occur if these areas are not clean. Some persons bathe themselves in bed or at the sink. You assist as needed. Most need help washing the back. You give partial baths to persons who cannot bathe themselves.

The rules for bathing apply (see Box 16-2). So do the complete bed bath considerations.

See procedure: *Assisting With the Partial Bath.*

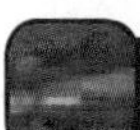

Assisting With the Partial Bath

VIDEO CLIP VIDEO

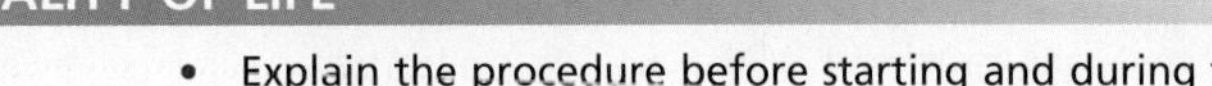

QUALITY OF LIFE

- Knock before entering the person's room.
- Address the person by name.
- Introduce yourself by name and title.
- Explain the procedure before starting and during the procedure.
- Protect the person's rights during the procedure.
- Handle the person gently during the procedure.

PRE-PROCEDURE

1 Follow *Delegation Guidelines: Bathing,* p. 236. See *Promoting Safety and Comfort:*
   a *Assisting With Hygiene,* p. 228
   b *Bathing,* p. 237

2 Follow steps 2 through 7 in procedure: *Giving a Complete Bed Bath,* p. 237.

PROCEDURE

3 Make sure the bed is in the low position.
4 Practice hand hygiene. Put on gloves.
5 Cover the person with a bath blanket. Remove top linens.
6 Fill the wash basin ⅔ (two-thirds) full with water. Water temperature is usually 110°F to 115°F (43.3°C to 46.1°C) or as directed by the nurse. Measure water temperature with the bath thermometer. Or dip your elbow or inner wrist into the basin to test the water.
7 Ask the person to check the water temperature. Adjust the water temperature if it is too hot or too cold.
8 Place the basin on the over-bed table.
9 Position the person in Fowler's position. Or assist him or her to sit at the bedside.
10 Adjust the over-bed table so the person can reach the basin and supplies.
11 Help the person undress. Provide for privacy and warmth with the bath blanket.
12 Ask the person to wash easy to reach body parts (Fig. 16-17, p. 240). Explain that you will wash the back and areas the person cannot reach.
13 Place the call light within reach. Ask the person to signal when help is needed or bathing is complete.
14 Remove and discard the gloves. Practice hand hygiene. Then leave the room.
15 Return when the call light is on. Knock before entering. Practice hand hygiene.
16 Change the bath water. Measure bath water temperature as in step 6.
17 Raise the bed for body mechanics. The far bed rail is up if used.
18 Ask what was washed. Put on gloves. Wash and dry areas the person could not reach. The face, hands, underarms, back, buttocks, and perineal area are washed for the partial bath.
19 Remove and discard the gloves. Practice hand hygiene.
20 Give a back massage (Chapter 15).
21 Apply lotion, powder, and deodorant or antiperspirant as requested.
22 Help the person put on clean garments.
23 Assist with hair care and other grooming needs.
24 Assist the person to a chair. (Lower the bed if the person transfers to a chair.) Or turn the person onto the side away from you.
25 Make the bed. (Raise the bed for body mechanics.)

POST-PROCEDURE

26 Provide for comfort. (See the inside of the front cover.)
27 Place the call light within reach.
28 Lower the bed to a safe and comfortable level appropriate for the person. Follow the care plan.
29 Raise or lower bed rails. Follow the care plan.
30 Put on clean gloves.
31 Empty, clean, rinse, and dry the wash basin. Return the basin and supplies to their proper place.
32 Wipe off the over-bed table with the paper towels. Discard the paper towels.
33 Unscreen the person.
34 Complete a safety check of the room. (See the inside of the front cover.)
35 Follow agency policy for dirty linen.
36 Remove and discard the gloves. Practice hand hygiene.
37 Report and record your observations.

Tub Baths and Showers

Some people like tub baths. Others like showers. Falls, burns, and chilling from water are risks. Safety is important (Box 16-3). The measures in Box 16-2 also apply. Follow the nurse's directions and the care plan.

Tub Baths. Tub baths are relaxing. A tub bath can make a person feel faint, weak, or tired. These are great risks for persons who were on bedrest. A tub bath lasts no longer than 20 minutes.

BOX 16-3 Tub Bath and Shower Safety

- Clean, disinfect, and dry the tub or shower before and after use.
- Dry the tub or shower room floor.
- Check hand rails, grab bars, hydraulic lifts, and other safety aids. They must be in working order.
- Place a bath mat in the tub or on the shower floor. This is not needed if there are non-skid strips or a non-skid surface.
- Cover the person for warmth and privacy. This includes during transport to and from the tub or shower room.
- Place needed items within reach.
- Place the call light within reach.
- Show the person how to use the call light in the tub or shower room.
- Have the person use grab bars when getting in and out of the tub. The person must not use towel bars for support.
- Turn cold water on first, then hot water. Turn hot water off first, then cold water.
- Know what water temperature to use. See *Delegation Guidelines: Tub Baths and Showers.*
- Adjust water temperature and pressure to prevent chilling or burns. Do this before the person gets into the shower. If a shower chair is used, position it first.
- Direct water away from the person while adjusting water temperature and pressure.
- Fill the tub before the person gets into it. If using a tub with a side entry door, follow the manufacturer's instructions.
- Measure water temperature. For showers and tub baths, use the digital display. Or you can use a bath thermometer for a tub bath.
- Keep the water spray directed toward the person during the shower. This helps keep him or her warm. (NOTE: Do not direct the water spray toward the person's face. This can frighten the person.)
- Keep bar soap in the soap dish between latherings. This reduces the risk of slipping and falls. It also prevents soapy tub water.
- Avoid using bath oils. They make tub and shower surfaces slippery.
- Do not leave weak or unsteady persons unattended.
- Stay within hearing distance if the person can be left alone. Wait outside the shower curtain or door. You must be nearby if the person calls for you or has an accident.
- Drain the tub before the person gets out of the tub. Turn off the shower before the person gets out of the shower. Cover him or her to provide privacy and prevent chilling.

To get in and out of the tub, the person may use:

- A tub with a side entry door (Fig. 16-18).
- Wheelchair or stretcher lift. The person is transferred to the tub room by wheelchair or stretcher. Then the device and person are lifted into the tub (Fig. 16-19).
- Mechanical lift (Chapter 14).

Whirlpool tubs have a cleansing action. You wash the upper body. Carefully wash under the breasts and between skin folds. Also wash the perineal area. Pat dry the person with towels after the bath.

Showers. Some people can stand to use a regular shower. They use the grab bars for support. Like tubs, showers have non-skid surfaces. If not, a bath mat is used. Never let weak or unsteady persons stand in the shower. They need to use:

- *Shower chairs.* Water drains through an opening (Fig. 16-20). You use the chair to transport the person to and from the shower. Lock the wheels during the shower to prevent the chair from moving.
- *Shower trolley (portable tub).* The person has a shower lying down (Fig. 16-21). You lower the sides to transfer the person from the bed to the trolley. Raise the side rails after the transfer. Then transport the person to the tub or shower room. Use the hand-held nozzle to give the shower.

Some shower rooms have 2 or more stations. Provide for privacy. The person has the right not to have his or her body seen by others. Properly screen and cover the person. Also close doors and the shower curtain.

See *Delegation Guidelines: Tub Baths and Showers.*

See *Promoting Safety and Comfort: Tub Baths and Showers.*

See procedure: *Assisting With a Tub Bath or Shower,* p. 244.

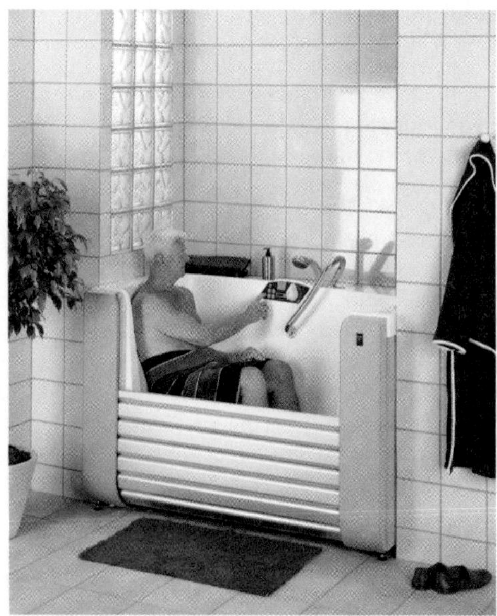

FIGURE 16-18 Tub with a side entry door.

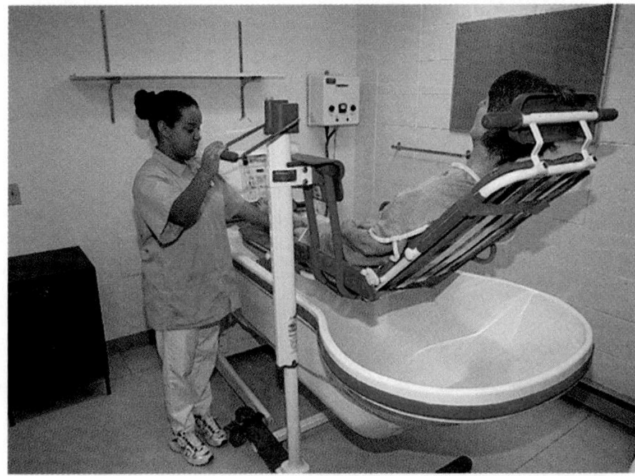

FIGURE 16-19 The stretcher and person are lowered into the tub.

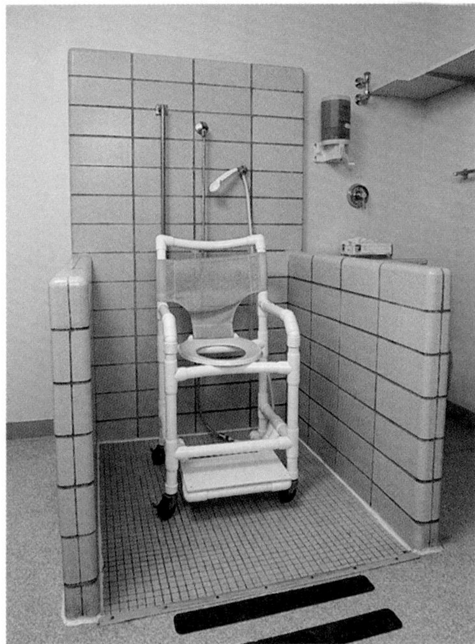

FIGURE 16-20 A shower chair in a shower stall.

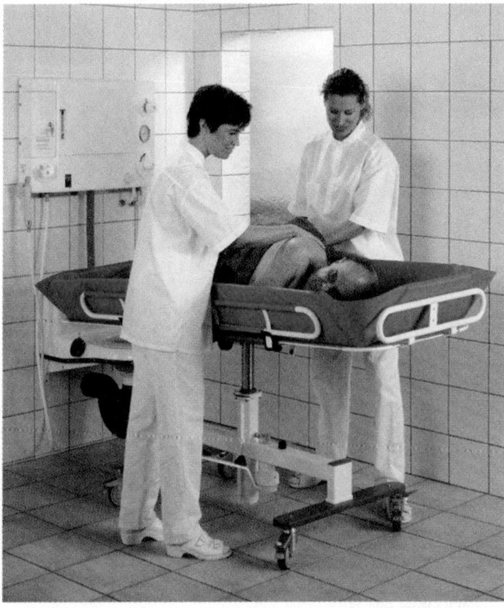

FIGURE 16-21 Shower trolley. The sides are lowered for transfers into and out of the trolley.

DELEGATION GUIDELINES

Tub Baths and Showers

Before assisting with a tub bath or shower, you need this information from the nurse and the care plan.

- If the person takes a tub bath or shower
- What water temperature to use (usually 105°F; 40.5°C)
- What equipment is needed—shower chair, shower trolley, and so on
- How much help the person needs
- If the person can bathe himself or herself
- What observations to report and record
  - Dizziness
  - Light-headedness
  - See *Delegation Guidelines: Bathing,* p. 236
- When to report observations
- What patient or resident concerns to report at once

PROMOTING SAFETY AND COMFORT

Tub Baths and Showers

Safety

Some persons are very weak. At least 2 staff are needed to safely assist them with tub baths and showers. If the person is heavy, 3 or more staff may be needed.

The person may use a tub with a side entry door, a shower chair, a shower trolley, or other device. Always follow the manufacturer's instructions.

Protect the person from falls, chilling, and burns. Follow the safety measures in Chapters 9 and 10. Remember to measure water temperature.

Clean, disinfect, and dry the tub or shower before and after use. This prevents the spread of microbes and infection.

Comfort

Warmth and privacy promote comfort during tub baths and showers. You need to:

- Make sure the tub or shower room is warm.
- Provide for privacy. Close the room door, screen the person, and close window coverings.
- Make sure water temperature is warm enough for the person.
- Have the person remove his or her clothing or robe and footwear just before getting into the tub or shower. Do not have the person exposed longer than necessary.
- Leave the room if the person can be left alone. Stay within hearing distance.

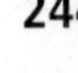
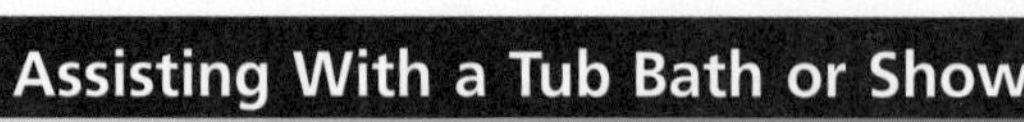

Assisting With a Tub Bath or Shower

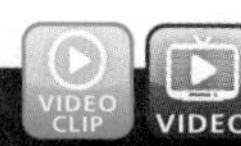

QUALITY OF LIFE

- Knock before entering the person's room.
- Address the person by name.
- Introduce yourself by name and title.
- Explain the procedure before starting and during the procedure.
- Protect the person's rights during the procedure.
- Handle the person gently during the procedure.

PRE-PROCEDURE

1 Follow *Delegation Guidelines:*
  a *Bathing,* p. 236
  b *Tub Baths and Showers,* p. 243
  See *Promoting Safety and Comfort:*
  a *Assisting With Hygiene,* p. 228
  b *Bathing,* p. 237
  c *Tub Baths and Showers,* p. 243
2 Reserve the tub or shower room.
3 Practice hand hygiene.
4 Identify the person. Check the ID bracelet against the assignment sheet. Also call the person by name.
5 Collect the following.
  - Washcloth and 2 bath towels
  - Bath blanket
  - Soap
  - Bath thermometer (for a tub bath)
  - Clothing or sleepwear
  - Grooming items as requested
  - Robe and non-skid footwear
  - Rubber bath mat if needed
  - Disposable bath mat
  - Gloves
  - Wheelchair, shower chair, and so on as needed

PROCEDURE

6 Place items in the tub or shower room. Use the space provided or a chair.
7 Clean, disinfect, and dry the tub or shower.
8 Place a rubber bath mat in the tub or on the shower floor. Do not block the drain.
9 Place the disposable bath mat on the floor in front of the tub or shower.
10 Put the OCCUPIED sign on the door.
11 Return to the person's room. Provide for privacy. Practice hand hygiene.
12 Help the person sit on the side of the bed.
13 Help the person put on a robe and non-skid footwear. Or the person can leave on clothing.
14 Assist or transport the person to the tub or shower room.
15 Have the person sit on a chair if he or she walked to the tub or shower room.
16 Provide for privacy.
17 *For a tub bath:*
  a Fill the tub half-way with warm water (usually 105°F; 40.5°C). Follow the care plan for water temperature.
  b Measure water temperature. Use the bath thermometer or check the digital display.
  c Ask the person to check the water temperature. Adjust the water temperature if it is too hot or too cold.
18 *For a shower:*
  a Turn on the shower.
  b Adjust water temperature and pressure. Check the digital display.
  c Ask the person to check the water temperature. Adjust the water temperature if it is too hot or too cold.
19 Help the person undress and remove footwear.
20 Help the person into the tub or shower. Position the shower chair and lock the wheels.
21 Assist with washing as necessary. Wear gloves.
22 Ask the person to use the call light when done or when help is needed. Remind the person that a tub bath lasts no longer than 20 minutes.
23 Place a towel across the chair.
24 Leave the room if the person can bathe alone. If not, stay in the room or nearby. Remove and discard the gloves and practice hand hygiene if you will leave the room.
25 Check the person at least every 5 minutes.
26 Return when the person signals for you. Knock before entering. Practice hand hygiene.
27 Turn off the shower, or drain the tub. Cover the person with the bath blanket while the tub drains.
28 Help the person out of the shower or tub and onto the chair.
29 Help the person dry off. Pat gently. Dry under the breasts, between skin folds, in the perineal area, and between the toes.
30 Assist with lotion and other grooming items as needed.
31 Help the person dress and put on footwear.
32 Help the person return to the room. Provide for privacy.
33 Assist the person to a chair or into bed.
34 Provide a back massage if the person returns to bed (Chapter 15).
35 Assist with hair care and other grooming needs.

POST-PROCEDURE

36 Provide for comfort. (See the inside of the front cover.)
37 Place the call light within reach.
38 Raise or lower bed rails. Follow the care plan.
39 Unscreen the person.
40 Complete a safety check of the room. (See the inside of the front cover.)
41 Clean, disinfect, and dry the tub or shower. Remove soiled linen. Wear gloves.
42 Discard disposable items. Put the UNOCCUPIED sign on the door. Return supplies to their proper place.
43 Follow agency policy for dirty linen.
44 Remove and discard the gloves. Practice hand hygiene.
45 Report and record your observations.

PERINEAL CARE

Perineal care *(pericare) involves cleaning the genital and anal areas.* These areas provide a warm, moist, and dark place for microbes to grow. Cleaning prevents infection and odors, and it promotes comfort.

Perineal care is done daily during the bath. It also is done when the area is soiled with urine or feces. Perineal care is very important for persons who:

- Have urinary catheters (Chapter 18).
- Have had rectal or genital surgery.
- Are menstruating (Chapter 7).
- Are incontinent of urine or feces (Chapters 18 and 19).
- Are uncircumcised (Fig. 16-22). Being ***circumcised*** *means that the fold of skin (foreskin) covering the glans of the penis was surgically removed.* Being ***uncircumcised*** *means that the person has foreskin covering the head of the penis.*

The person does perineal care if able. Otherwise, it is given by the nursing staff. This procedure embarrasses many people and staff, especially when it involves the other sex.

Perineal and *perineum* are not common terms. Most people understand *privates, private parts, crotch, genitals,* or *the area between your legs.* Use terms the person understands. The terms must be in good taste professionally.

Follow Standard Precautions, medical asepsis, and the Bloodborne Pathogen Standard. Work from the cleanest area to the dirtiest. This is commonly called from "front to back." The urethral area (the front) is the cleanest. The anal area (the back) is the dirtiest. Therefore clean from the urethra to the anal area. This prevents the spread of bacteria from the anal area to the vagina and urinary system.

The perineal area is delicate and easily injured. Use warm water, not hot. Use washcloths, towelettes, cotton balls, or swabs according to agency policy. Rinse thoroughly. Pat dry after rinsing. This reduces moisture and promotes comfort.

See *Focus on Communication: Perineal Care.*

See *Delegation Guidelines: Perineal Care.*

See *Promoting Safety and Comfort: Perineal Care,* p. 246.

See procedure: *Giving Female Perineal Care,* p. 246.

See procedure: *Giving Male Perineal Care,* p. 248.

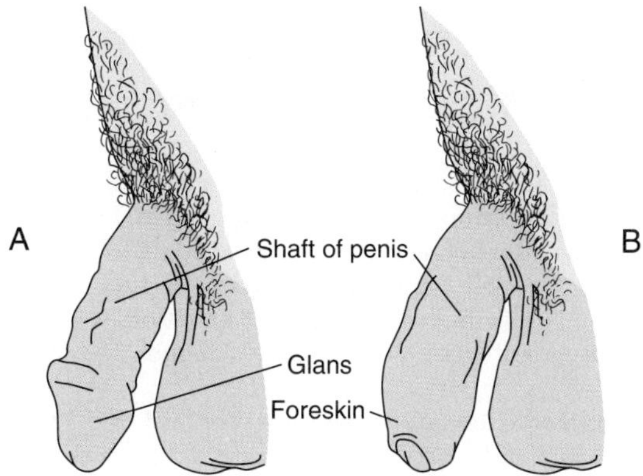

FIGURE 16-22 A, Circumcised male. **B,** Uncircumcised male.

FOCUS ON COMMUNICATION

Perineal Care

Talking to the person about perineal care may be difficult. You may be embarrassed. However, you must explain the procedure to the person.

When a person performs his or her own perineal care, you can say:

- "Mrs. Bell, I'll give you some privacy while you finish your bath. Can you reach everything you need? Please call for me if you need help. Here is your call light."
- "Mr. Baker, I'll give you time to finish your bath. Please wash your genital and rectal areas. Signal for me when you're done or need help."

If you provide perineal care for the person, you can say:

- "Mrs. Allan, next I'll clean between your legs. I'll keep you covered with the bath blanket. I'll tell you before I touch you. Please tell me if you feel any pain or discomfort."
- "Mr. Scott, I'll clean your private parts now. Please let me know if you feel any pain or discomfort."

DELEGATION GUIDELINES

Perineal Care

Before giving perineal care, you need this information from the nurse and the care plan.

- When to give perineal care.
- What terms the person understands—perineum, privates, private parts, crotch, area between the legs, and so on.
- How much help the person needs.
- What water temperature to use—usually 105°F to 109°F (40.5°C to 42.7°C). Water in a basin cools rapidly.
- What cleaning agent to use.
- Any position restrictions or limits.
- What observations to report and record:
  - Odors
  - Redness, swelling, discharge, bleeding, or irritation
  - Complaints of pain, burning, or other discomfort
  - Signs of urinary or fecal incontinence
- When to report observations.
- What patient or resident concerns to report at once.

PROMOTING SAFETY AND COMFORT

Perineal Care

Safety

Hot water can burn perineal tissues. To prevent burns, measure water temperature according to agency policy. If water seems too hot, ask the nurse to check it.

Protect yourself and the person from infection. Contact with blood, body fluids, secretions, or excretions is likely. Follow Standard Precautions and the Bloodborne Pathogen Standard.

Persons who are incontinent need perineal care. Protect the person and dry garments and linens from wet or soiled items. Remove the wet or soiled incontinence product, garments, and linen. Then apply clean, dry ones.

Comfort

If you provide perineal care, explain how you protect privacy. Always act in a professional manner.

Perineal care involves touching the genital and anal areas. The person may prefer that someone of the same sex provide this care. Or the person may fear sexual assault. Always obtain the person's consent before providing perineal care. For mental comfort, the person may want a family member or another staff member present to witness the procedure. Ask if he or she wants someone present and that person's name. Also keep the call light within the person's reach. If feeling threatened, the person needs to be able to call for help.

If the person is able, let him or her perform perineal care. This promotes privacy and helps prevent embarrassment. You need to:

1 Provide clean water. See step 14 in procedure: *Giving Female Perineal Care*.
2 Adjust the over-bed table so the person can reach the wash basin, soap, and towels with ease.
3 Make sure the person understands what to do.
4 Place the call light within reach. Ask the person to signal when finished.
5 Lower the bed to a safe and comfortable level appropriate for the person. Follow the care plan.
6 Remove and discard the gloves. Practice hand hygiene.
7 Leave the room.
8 Answer the call light promptly. Knock before entering the room.
9 Raise the bed for body mechanics.
10 Practice hand hygiene. Put on gloves.
11 Make sure the person has cleaned thoroughly.
12 Finish the bathing procedure.

Giving Female Perineal Care

NNAAP CD VIDEO CLIP VIDEO

QUALITY OF LIFE

- Knock before entering the person's room.
- Address the person by name.
- Introduce yourself by name and title.
- Explain the procedure before starting and during the procedure.
- Protect the person's rights during the procedure.
- Handle the person gently during the procedure.

PRE-PROCEDURE

1 Follow *Delegation Guidelines: Perineal Care,* p. 245. See *Promoting Safety and Comfort:*
   a *Assisting With Hygiene,* p. 228
   b *Perineal Care*
2 Practice hand hygiene.
3 Collect the following.
   - Soap or other cleaning agent as directed
   - At least 4 washcloths
   - Bath towel
   - Bath blanket
   - Bath thermometer
   - Wash basin
   - Waterproof pad
   - Gloves
   - Paper towels
4 Cover the over-bed table with paper towels. Arrange items on top of them.
5 Identify the person. Check the ID bracelet against the assignment sheet. Also call the person by name.
6 Provide for privacy.
7 Raise the bed for body mechanics. Bed rails are up if used.

PROCEDURE

8 Lower the bed rail near you if up.
9 Practice hand hygiene. Put on gloves.
10 Cover the person with a bath blanket. Move top linens to the foot of the bed.
11 Position the person on the back.
12 Drape the person as in Figure 16-23.
13 Raise the bed rail if used.
14 Fill the wash basin. Water temperature is usually 105°F to 109°F (40.5°C to 42.7°C). Follow the care plan for water temperature. Measure water temperature according to agency policy.
15 Ask the person to check the water temperature. Adjust the water temperature if it is too hot or too cold. Raise the bed rail before leaving the bedside. Lower it when you return.
16 Place the basin on the over-bed table.
17 Lower the bed rail if up.
18 Help the person flex her knees and spread her legs. Or help her spread her legs as much as possible with the knees straight.
19 Fold the corner of the bath blanket between her legs onto her abdomen.

Giving Female Perineal Care—cont'd

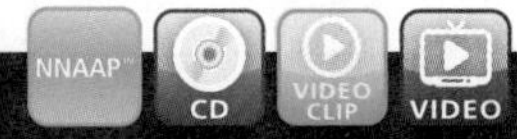

PROCEDURE—cont'd

20 Place a waterproof pad under her buttocks. Remove any wet or soiled incontinence products.
21 Remove and discard the gloves. Practice hand hygiene. Put on clean gloves.
22 Wet the washcloths.
23 Squeeze out excess water from a washcloth. Make a mitted washcloth. Apply soap.
24 Separate the labia. Clean downward from front to back with 1 stroke (Fig. 16-24).
25 Repeat steps 23 and 24 until the area is clean. Use a clean part of the washcloth for each stroke. Use more than 1 washcloth if needed.
26 Rinse the perineum with a clean washcloth. Separate the labia. Stroke downward from front to back. Repeat as necessary. Use a clean part of the washcloth for each stroke. Use more than 1 washcloth if needed.
27 Pat the area dry with the towel. Dry from front to back.
28 Fold the blanket back between her legs.
29 Help the person lower her legs and turn onto her side away from you.
30 Apply soap to a mitted washcloth.
31 Clean the rectal area. Clean from the vagina to the anus with 1 stroke (Fig. 16-25).
32 Repeat steps 30 and 31 until the area is clean. Use a clean part of the washcloth for each stroke. Use more than 1 washcloth if needed.
33 Rinse the rectal area with a washcloth. Stroke from the vagina to the anus. Repeat as necessary. Use a clean part of the washcloth for each stroke. Use more than 1 washcloth if needed.
34 Pat the area dry with the towel. Dry from front to back.
35 Remove the waterproof pad.
36 Remove and discard the gloves. Practice hand hygiene. Put on clean gloves.
37 Provide clean and dry linens and incontinence products as needed.

POST-PROCEDURE

38 Cover the person. Remove the bath blanket.
39 Provide for comfort. (See the inside of the front cover.)
40 Place the call light within reach.
41 Lower the bed to a safe and comfortable level appropriate for the person. Follow the care plan.
42 Raise or lower bed rails. Follow the care plan.
43 Empty, clean, rinse, and dry the wash basin.
44 Return the basin and supplies to their proper place.
45 Wipe off the over-bed table with the paper towels. Discard the paper towels.
46 Unscreen the person.
47 Complete a safety check of the room. (See the inside of the front cover.)
48 Follow agency policy for dirty linen.
49 Remove and discard the gloves. Practice hand hygiene.
50 Report and record your observations.

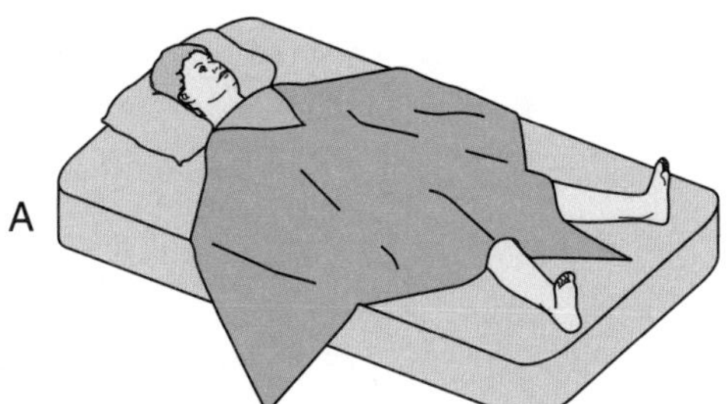

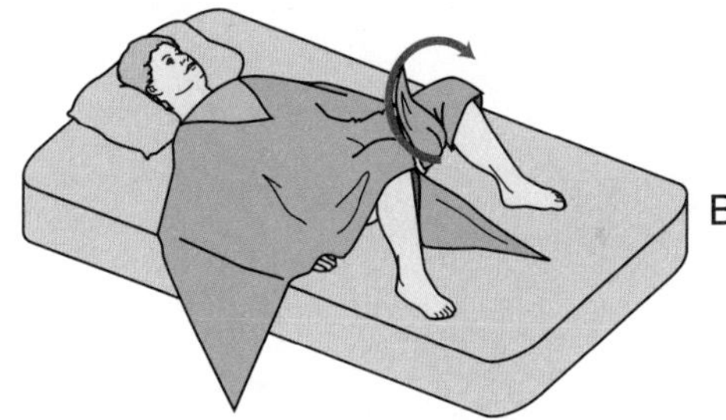

FIGURE 16-23 Draping for perineal care. **A,** Position the bath blanket like a diamond: 1 corner is at the neck, there is a corner at each side, and 1 corner is between the person's legs. **B,** Wrap the blanket around a leg by bringing the corner around the leg and over the top. Tuck the corner under the hip.

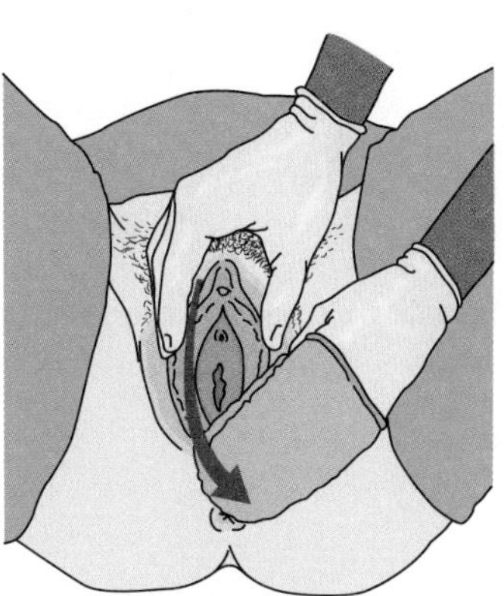

FIGURE 16-24 Separate the labia with 1 hand. Use a mitted washcloth to clean between the labia with downward strokes.

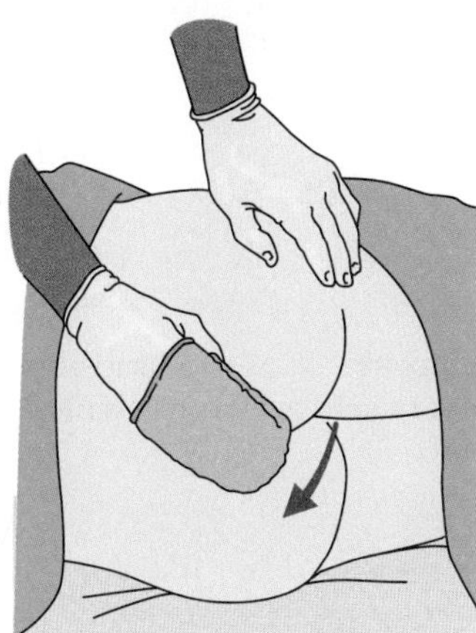

FIGURE 16-25 The rectal area is cleaned by wiping from the vagina to the anus. The side-lying position allows the anal area to be cleaned more thoroughly.

Giving Male Perineal Care

QUALITY OF LIFE

- Knock before entering the person's room.
- Address the person by name.
- Introduce yourself by name and title.
- Explain the procedure before starting and during the procedure.
- Protect the person's rights during the procedure.
- Handle the person gently during the procedure.

PROCEDURE

1. Follow steps 1 through 17 in procedure: *Giving Female Perineal Care,* p. 246. Drape the person as in Figure 16-23.
2. Fold the corner of the bath blanket between the legs onto his abdomen.
3. Place a waterproof pad under the buttocks. Remove any wet or soiled incontinence products.
4. Remove and discard the gloves. Practice hand hygiene. Put on clean gloves.
5. Retract the foreskin if the person is uncircumcised (Fig. 16-26).
6. Grasp the penis.
7. Clean the tip. Use a circular motion. Start at the meatus of the urethra and work outward (Fig. 16-27). Repeat as needed. Use a clean part of the washcloth each time.
8. Rinse the area with another washcloth. Use the same circular motion.
9. Return the foreskin to its natural position immediately after rinsing.
10. Clean the shaft of the penis. Use firm downward strokes. Rinse the area.
11. Help the person flex his knees and spread his legs. Or help him spread his legs as much as possible with his knees straight.
12. Clean the scrotum. Rinse well. Observe for redness and irritation of the skin folds.
13. Pat dry the penis and the scrotum. Use the towel.
14. Fold the bath blanket back between his legs.
15. Help him lower his legs and turn onto his side away from you.
16. Clean the rectal area (see procedure: *Giving Female Perineal Care,* p. 246). (NOTE: For males, clean from the scrotum to the anus.) Rinse and dry well.
17. Remove the waterproof pad.
18. Remove and discard the gloves. Practice hand hygiene. Put on clean gloves.
19. Provide clean and dry linens and incontinence products.
20. Follow steps 38 through 50 in procedure: *Giving Female Perineal Care,* p. 247.

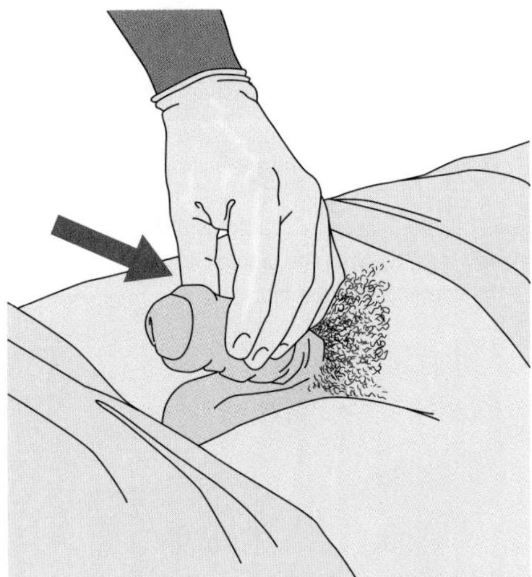

FIGURE 16-26 The foreskin of the uncircumcised male is pulled back for perineal care. It is returned to the normal position immediately after cleaning and rinsing.

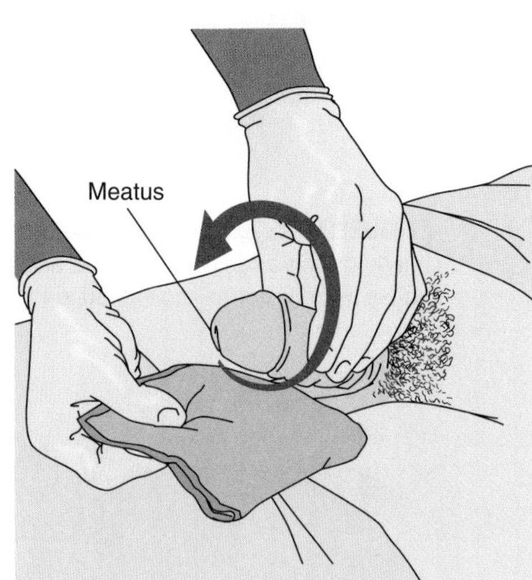

FIGURE 16-27 The penis is cleaned with circular motions starting at the meatus.

FOCUS ON PRIDE

The Person, Family, and Yourself

Personal and Professional Responsibility

Patients and residents depend on you for their hygiene needs. You are responsible for providing care to maintain or improve the person's quality of life, health, and safety. To do so:

- Follow the guidelines and procedures presented in this chapter.
- Focus on the "Quality of Life" section at the beginning of each procedure.
- View the person as an individual with unique needs. Ask about the person's needs and preferences.

Take pride in providing care that benefits the person's overall well-being.

Rights and Respect

Patients and residents have the right to choose schedules and routines based on their preferences. They also have the right to refuse care. Some persons refuse care because it does not meet their preferences. For example:

- A resident refuses a shower because she prefers a bath.
- A patient prefers to bathe at night, not in the morning.
- A male resident prefers to be bathed by a male nursing assistant but a female is caring for him today.

Refusal of care for these reasons does not mean the person refuses to be clean. The person may accept the care if his or her preferences are met. Tell the nurse of any refusal of care. Adjust as needed to provide care and respect the person's preferences.

Independence and Social Interaction

Hygiene is a very personal matter. Allow personal choice in such matters as bath time, products used, and what to wear. Encourage the person to do as much self-care as safely possible. Doing so promotes independence and improves self-esteem.

Delegation and Teamwork

Many agencies do not have tub and shower rooms for each person. You need to reserve the room and equipment for the person. Co-workers do the same.

Consider the needs of others. For example, you reserve the room from 0945 to 1030. Do your best to follow the schedule. Communicate if the schedule must change. Plan a new schedule with your co-workers.

Also make sure the room is clean and ready for the next person. Avoid the "someone else can do it" attitude. This shows poor teamwork and work ethics. Take pride in being a helpful and courteous member of the team.

Ethics and Laws

You will perform some tasks often. Bathing and other personal hygiene measures are examples. Over time, some staff become less careful with routine tasks. They may forget about dangers. They may be busy and not take time for safety measures. Or they think that nothing bad will happen. This is very unsafe.

Always be careful. Harm can result from routine care measures. Follow the safety measures in this chapter at all times.

REVIEW QUESTIONS

Circle* T *if the statement is TRUE or* F *if it is FALSE.

1 **T F** Hygiene is needed for comfort, safety, and health.
2 **T F** During evening care, you prepare the person for sleep.
3 **T F** You should place the upper denture in the sink while cleaning the lower denture.
4 **T F** A person has a partial denture. Natural teeth are brushed.
5 **T F** To wash the eye, wash from the outer to the inner aspect.
6 **T F** A tub bath lasts 30 minutes.
7 **T F** Weak persons may be left alone in the shower if they are sitting.
8 **T F** Perineal care helps prevent infection.
9 **T F** You must wear gloves for perineal care.
10 **T F** Foreskin is returned to its normal position immediately after rinsing.

Circle the BEST answer.

11 When assisting with daily care, you
- **a** Clean incontinent persons as often as needed
- **b** Give early morning care after breakfast
- **c** Follow your own routines and habits
- **d** Change soiled linens in the afternoon

12 You perform oral hygiene to
- **a** Prevent aspiration
- **b** Remove excess oils and perspiration
- **c** Prevent mouth odors and infection
- **d** Remove cavities

13 When performing oral hygiene
- **a** Clean dentures over a towel on the counter
- **b** Use a soft-bristled toothbrush
- **c** Floss once daily in the morning
- **d** Clean dentures in hot water

14 When providing mouth care for the unconscious person
- **a** Use a small amount of fluid to clean the mouth
- **b** Use your fingers to keep the mouth open
- **c** Position the person supine
- **d** Insert dentures after cleaning them

15 Which must you report to the nurse?
- **a** Clean skin
- **b** Moist and intact lips
- **c** A bruise on the arm
- **d** Food between the teeth

16 When bathing a person
- **a** Keep bar soap in the wash basin or tub
- **b** Wash from the dirtiest to the cleanest area
- **c** Assist with elimination after a bath
- **d** Rinse the skin well to remove all soap

17 To apply powder
- **a** Turn the person toward you
- **b** Sprinkle a small amount onto your hand
- **c** Apply a thick layer of powder
- **d** Shake the powder onto the person

18 When drying the person
- **a** Dry well between skin folds
- **b** Rub the skin dry
- **c** Avoid drying between the toes
- **d** Allow the person to air dry

19 Water for a complete bed bath is between
- **a** 100°F and 104°F
- **b** 105°F and 109°F
- **c** 110°F and 115°F
- **d** 120°F and 125°F

20 When assisting with a shower in a shower room
- **a** Direct the water spray at the person's face
- **b** Allow a weak person to stand if you provide support
- **c** Go to the person's room to make the bed during the shower
- **d** Clean and disinfect the shower before and after use

21 Water temperature for perineal care is between
- **a** 100°F and 104°F
- **b** 105°F and 109°F
- **c** 110°F and 115°F
- **d** 120°F and 125°F

22 These statements are about perineal care. Which is *true?*
- **a** Do not explain the procedure to avoid embarrassment.
- **b** The person does perineal care if able.
- **c** You use hot water for perineal care.
- **d** Draping the person is not needed.

Answers to these questions are on p. 504.

FOCUS ON **PRACTICE**

Problem Solving

You are a student in the clinical setting. You are helping a nursing assistant position and turn a resident during perineal care. The nursing assistant does not wear gloves, does not use a clean part of the washcloth or a new washcloth for each stroke, and wipes from back to front. What do you do?

CHAPTER

17

Assisting With Grooming

OBJECTIVES

- Define the key terms and key abbreviations listed in this chapter.
- Explain why grooming is important.
- Describe how to safely provide grooming measures—hair care, shaving, nail and foot care, and changing clothing and gowns.
- Perform the procedures described in this chapter.
- Explain how to promote PRIDE in the person, the family, and yourself.

KEY TERMS

alopecia Hair loss
dandruff Excessive amounts of dry, white flakes from the scalp
hirsutism Excessive body hair
lice See "pediculosis"
pediculosis Infestation with wingless insects; lice
scabies A skin disorder caused by the female mite—a very small spider-like organism

KEY ABBREVIATIONS

C	Centigrade
F	Fahrenheit
ID	Identification
IV	Intravenous

Hair care, shaving, nail and foot care, and clean garments prevent infection and promote comfort. They also affect love, belonging, and self-esteem needs.

As with hygiene, the person should perform grooming measures to the extent possible. This promotes independence and quality of life. The person may use adaptive devices for grooming (Chapter 27).

See *Focus on Surveys: Assisting With Grooming.*

FOCUS ON SURVEYS

Assisting With Grooming

Every person must be cared for in a way and in a setting that promotes dignity and respect. Grooming is one way to promote the person's self-esteem and self-worth. Therefore surveyors will observe if patients and residents:

- Are groomed as they wish to be groomed.
- Have their hair combed and styled.
- Have their beards shaved or trimmed.
- Are dressed in their own clothes.
- Are wearing the correct clothing for the time of day.
- Can reach grooming supplies.

HAIR CARE

Some people perform their own hair care. Many nursing centers have beauty and barber shops. You assist patients and residents to brush, comb, and shampoo hair according to the care plan. The nursing process reflects the person's culture, personal choice, skin and scalp conditions, health history, and self-care ability.

Skin and Scalp Conditions

Skin and scalp conditions include:

- ***Alopecia** means hair loss.* Hair loss may be complete or partial. Male pattern baldness occurs with aging. It results from heredity. Hair also thins in some women with aging. Cancer treatments (radiation therapy to the head and chemotherapy) often cause alopecia in persons of all ages.
- ***Hirsutism** is excessive body hair.* It can occur in men, women, and children. It results from heredity and abnormal amounts of male hormones.
- ***Dandruff** is the excessive amount of dry, white flakes from the scalp.* Itching is common. Sometimes eyebrows and ear canals are involved.
- ***Pediculosis (lice)** is the infestation with wingless insects.* See Figure 17-1. *Infestation* means being in or on a host. Lice attach their eggs *(nits)* to hair shafts. Nits are oval and yellow to white in color. After hatching, they bite the scalp or skin to feed on blood. Adult lice are tan to grayish white in color and about the size of a sesame seed. Lice bites cause severe itching in the affected area. Lice easily spread to others through clothing, head coverings, furniture, beds, towels, bed linen, sexual contact, and by sharing combs and brushes. Lice are treated with medicated shampoos, lotions, and creams specific for lice. Thorough bathing is needed. So is washing clothing and linens in hot water.
  - *Pediculosis capitis* ("head lice") is the infestation of the scalp *(capitis)* with lice.
  - *Pediculosis pubis* ("crabs") is the infestation of the pubic *(pubis)* hair with lice.
  - *Pediculosis corporis* is the infestation of the body *(corporis)* with lice.
- ***Scabies** is a skin disorder caused by the female mite—a very small spider-like organism* (Fig. 17-2). The female mite burrows into the skin and lays eggs. When the eggs hatch, the females produce more eggs. The person becomes infested with mites. The person has a rash and intense itching. Common sites are between the fingers, around the wrists, in the underarm areas, on the thighs, and in the genital area. Other sites include the breasts, waist, and buttocks. Highly contagious, scabies is transmitted to others by close contact. Special creams are used to kill the mites. The person's room is cleaned. Clothing and linens are washed in hot water.

See *Focus on Communication: Skin and Scalp Conditions.*

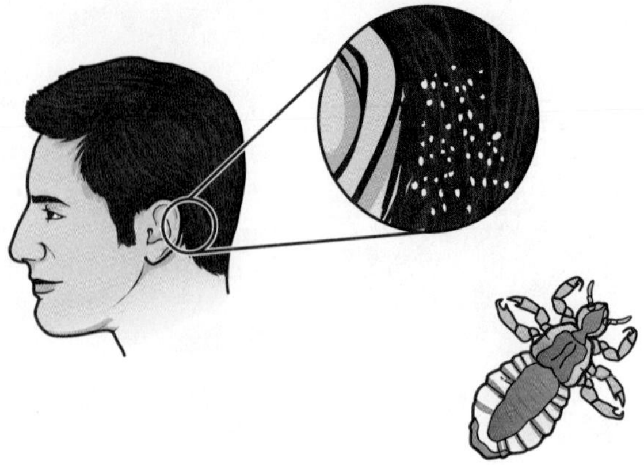

FIGURE 17-1 Head lice.

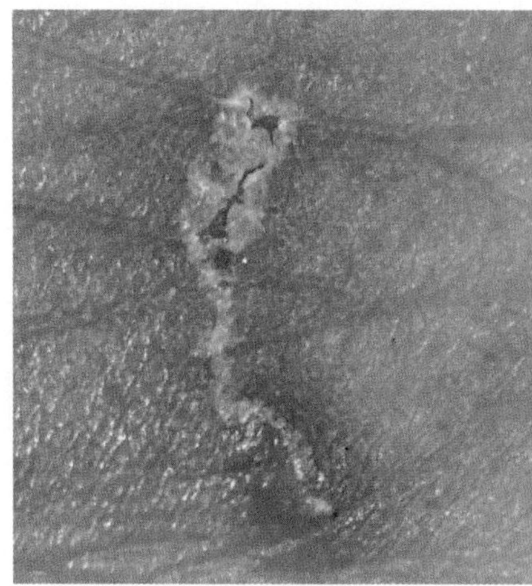

FIGURE 17-2 Scabies.

FOCUS ON COMMUNICATION

Skin and Scalp Conditions

Some skin or scalp conditions may alarm you. Be professional. Do not say things that may embarrass the person.

Report an abnormal skin or scalp condition. Describe what you saw as best as you can. For example:

- "I saw some small red dots on Mr. Martin's right underarm during his bath. Would you please take a look at them?"
- "I saw some small white specks in Mrs. Patel's hair. Would you please look at them before I wash her hair?"

Brushing and Combing Hair

Brushing and combing hair are part of early morning care, morning care, and afternoon care. Some people also do so at bedtime. Provide hair care when it is needed and before visitors arrive.

Encourage patients and residents to do their own hair care. Assist as needed. The person chooses how to brush, comb, and style hair.

Long hair easily mats and tangles. Daily brushing and combing prevent the problem. So does braiding. You need the person's consent to braid hair. *Never cut the person's hair.*

Special measures are needed for curly, coarse, and dry hair. The person may have certain hair care practices and products. They are part of the care plan. Also, let the person guide you when giving hair care.

See *Caring About Culture: Brushing and Combing Hair.*

See *Delegation Guidelines: Brushing and Combing Hair.*

See *Promoting Safety and Comfort: Brushing and Combing Hair.*

See procedure: *Brushing and Combing Hair.*

CARING ABOUT CULTURE

Brushing and Combing Hair

Styling hair in small braids is a common practice in some cultures. The braids are left intact for shampooing. To undo these braids, the nurse obtains the person's consent.

DELEGATION GUIDELINES

Brushing and Combing Hair

To brush and comb hair, you need this information from the nurse and the care plan.

- How much help the person needs
- What to do for matted or tangled hair
- What to do for curly, coarse, or dry hair
- What hair care products to use
- The person's preferences and routine hair care measures
- What observations to report and record:
  - Scalp sores
  - Flaking
  - Itching
  - Patches of hair loss
  - Hair falling out in patches
  - Very dry or very oily hair
  - Matted or tangled hair
  - The presence of nits or lice
    - Itching
    - Complaints of a tickling feeling or something moving in the hair
    - Irritability
    - Sores on the head or body caused by scratching
    - Rash
- When to report observations
- What patient or resident concerns to report at once

PROMOTING SAFETY AND COMFORT

Brushing and Combing Hair

Safety

Sharp brush bristles can injure the scalp. So can a comb with sharp or broken teeth. Report any concerns about the person's brush or comb.

Comfort

Place a towel across the person's back and shoulders to protect garments from falling hair. If the person is in bed, give hair care before changing linens and the pillowcase. If done after a linen change, place a towel across the pillow to collect falling hair.

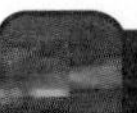

Brushing and Combing Hair

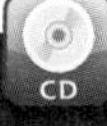

QUALITY OF LIFE

- Knock before entering the person's room.
- Address the person by name.
- Introduce yourself by name and title.
- Explain the procedure before starting and during the procedure.
- Protect the person's rights during the procedure.
- Handle the person gently during the procedure.

PRE-PROCEDURE

1. Follow *Delegation Guidelines: Brushing and Combing Hair.* See *Promoting Safety and Comfort: Brushing and Combing Hair.*
2. Practice hand hygiene.
3. Identify the person. Check the ID (identification) bracelet against the assignment sheet. Also call the person by name.
4. Ask the person how to style hair.
5. Collect the following.
   - Comb and brush
   - Bath towel
   - Other hair care items as requested
6. Arrange items on the bedside stand.
7. Provide for privacy.

Continued

Brushing and Combing Hair—cont'd

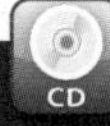

PROCEDURE

8 Lower the bed rail if up.
9 Position the person.
  a *In a chair*—Help the person to the chair. The person puts on a robe and non-skid footwear when up.
  b *In bed*—Raise the bed for body mechanics. Bed rails are up if used. Lower the bed rail near you. Assist the person to a semi-Fowler's position if allowed.
10 Place a towel across the person's back and shoulders or across the pillow.
11 Ask the person to remove eyeglasses. Put them in the eyeglass case. Put the case inside the bedside stand.
12 *Brush and comb hair that is not matted or tangled.*
  a Use the comb to part the hair.
    1 Part hair down the middle into 2 sides (Fig. 17-3, *A*).
    2 Divide 1 side into 2 smaller sections (Fig. 17-3, *B*).
  b Brush 1 of the small sections of hair. Start at the scalp and brush toward the hair ends (Fig. 17-4). Do the same for the other small section of hair.
  c Repeat step 12, a(2) and 12, b for the other side.
13 *Brush or comb matted or tangled hair.*
  a Take a small section of hair near the ends.
  b Comb or brush through to the hair ends.
  c Add small sections of hair as you work up to the scalp.
  d Comb or brush through each longer section to the hair ends.
14 Style the hair as the person prefers.
15 Remove the towel.
16 Let the person put on the eyeglasses.

POST-PROCEDURE

17 Provide for comfort. (See the inside of the front cover.)
18 Place the call light within reach.
19 Lower the bed to a safe and comfortable level appropriate for the person. Follow the care plan.
20 Raise or lower bed rails. Follow the care plan.
21 Clean and return hair care items to their proper place.
22 Unscreen the person.
23 Complete a safety check of the room. (See the inside of the front cover.)
24 Follow agency policy for dirty linen.
25 Practice hand hygiene.

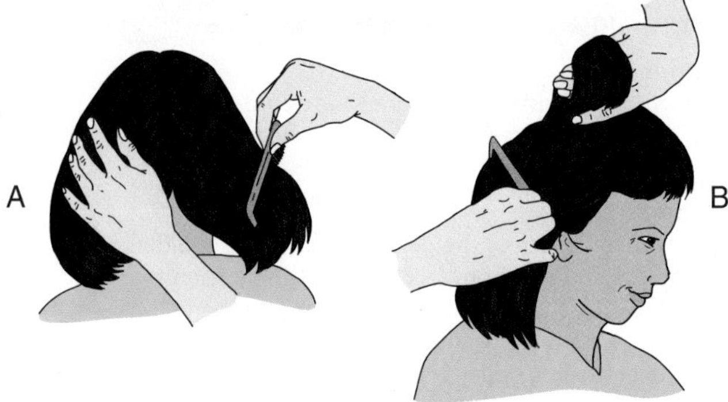

FIGURE 17-3 Part hair. **A,** Part hair down the middle. Divide it into 2 sides. **B,** Then part 1 side into 2 smaller sections.

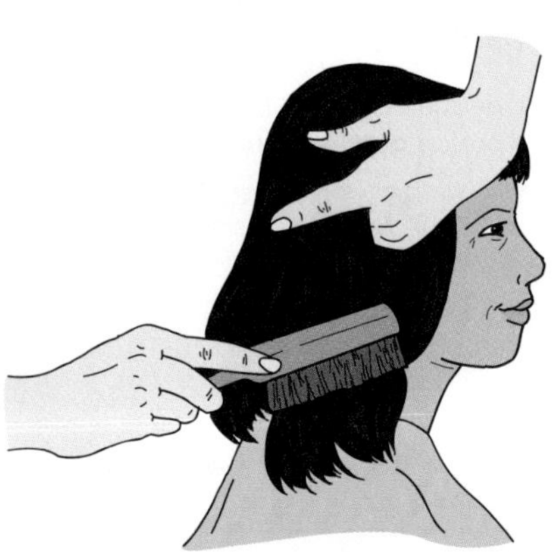

FIGURE 17-4 Brush hair by starting at the scalp. Brush down to the hair ends.

Shampooing

Many people shampoo 1, 2, or 3 times a week. Others shampoo every day. In nursing centers, shampooing is usually done on the person's bath or shower day. If done by a hairdresser or barber, do not shampoo the person's hair. Provide a shower cap for the bath or shower.

The shampoo method depends on the person's condition, safety factors, and personal choice. The nurse tells you what method to use.

- *Shampoo during the shower or tub bath.* The person shampoos in the shower. You use a hand-held nozzle for those using shower chairs or taking tub baths. You direct a spray of water at the hair.
- *Shampoo at the sink.* The person sits or lies facing away from the sink. A folded towel is placed over the sink edge to protect the neck. The person's head is tilted back over the edge of the sink (Fig. 17-5). You use a water pitcher or hand-held nozzle to wet and rinse the hair.
- *Shampoo in bed.* The person's head and shoulders are moved to the edge of the bed if possible. A shampoo tray placed under the head drains water into a basin placed on a chair by the bed (Fig. 17-6). You use a water pitcher to wet and rinse the hair.

Dry and style hair as quickly as possible after the shampoo. Women may want hair curled or rolled up before drying. Check with the nurse before doing so.

See *Focus on Older Persons: Shampooing.*
See *Delegation Guidelines: Shampooing.*
See *Promoting Safety and Comfort: Shampooing.*
See procedure: *Shampooing the Person's Hair*, p. 256.

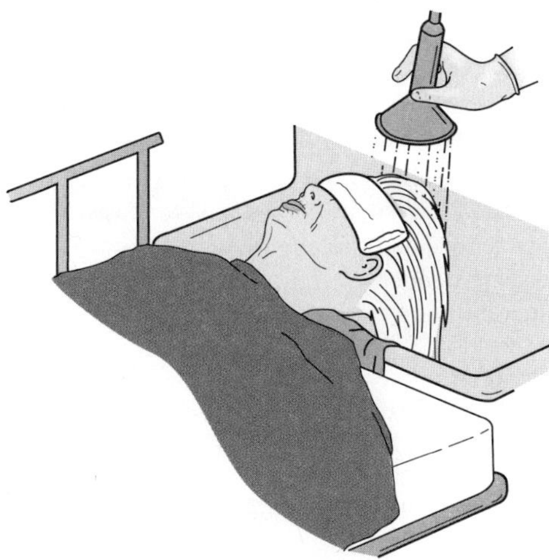

FIGURE 17-5 Shampooing at the sink. This person is on a stretcher in front of the sink.

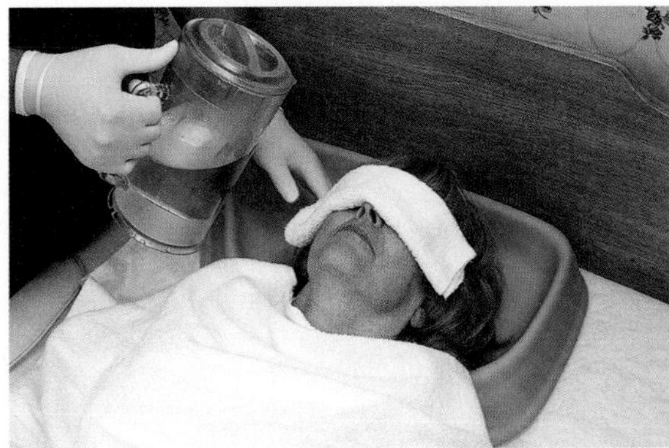

FIGURE 17-6 A shampoo tray is used for a person in bed. The tray is directed to the side of the bed so water drains into a collecting basin.

FOCUS ON OLDER PERSONS

Shampooing

Oil gland secretion decreases with aging. Therefore older persons have dry hair. They may shampoo less often than younger adults do.

DELEGATION GUIDELINES

Shampooing

To shampoo a person, you need this information from the nurse and the care plan.

- When to shampoo the person's hair
- What method to use
- What shampoo and conditioner to use
- The person's position restrictions or limits
- What water temperature to use—usually 105°F (Fahrenheit) (40.5°C [centigrade])
- If hair is curled or rolled up before drying
- What observations to report and record:
  - Scalp sores
  - Flaking
  - Itching
  - The presence of nits or lice
  - Patches of hair loss
  - Hair falling out in patches
  - Very dry or very oily hair
  - Matted or tangled hair
  - How the person tolerated the procedure
- When to report observations
- What patient or resident concerns to report at once

PROMOTING SAFETY AND COMFORT

Shampooing

Safety

Keep shampoo away from and out of the eyes. Have the person hold a washcloth over the eyes. To rinse, cup your hand at the person's forehead. This keeps soapy water from running down the person's forehead and into the eyes.

Remove hearing aids before shampooing. Water will damage hearing aids.

Return medicated products to the nurse. Never leave them at the bedside unless the nurse tells you to do so.

Wear gloves if the person has scalp sores. Follow Standard Precautions and the Bloodborne Pathogen Standard.

For a shampoo on a stretcher at a sink, follow the rules for stretcher use (Chapter 9). Lock the stretcher wheels and use the safety straps and side rails. The far side rail is raised during the procedure.

Some people shampoo themselves during a tub bath or shower. Place an extra towel, shampoo, and hair conditioner within the person's reach. Assist as needed.

Comfort

When shampooing during the tub bath or shower, the person tips his or her head back to keep shampoo and water out of the eyes. Support the back of the person's head with 1 hand. Shampoo with your other hand. Some persons cannot tip their heads back. They lean forward and hold a folded washcloth over the eyes. Support the forehead with 1 hand as you shampoo with the other. Make sure that the person can breathe easily.

Many people have limited range of motion in their necks. They are not shampooed at the sink or on a stretcher.

Shampooing the Person's Hair

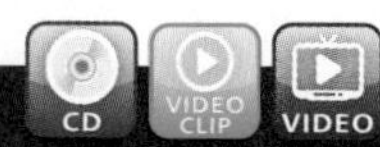

QUALITY OF LIFE

- Knock before entering the person's room.
- Address the person by name.
- Introduce yourself by name and title.
- Explain the procedure before starting and during the procedure.
- Protect the person's rights during the procedure.
- Handle the person gently during the procedure.

PRE-PROCEDURE

1 Follow *Delegation Guidelines: Shampooing,* p. 255. See *Promoting Safety and Comfort: Shampooing,* p. 255.
2 Practice hand hygiene.
3 Collect the following.
   - 2 bath towels
   - Washcloth
   - Shampoo
   - Hair conditioner (if requested)
   - Bath thermometer
   - Pitcher or hand-held nozzle (if needed)
   - Shampoo tray (if needed)
   - Basin or pan (if needed)
   - Waterproof pad (if needed)
   - Gloves (if needed)
   - Comb and brush
   - Hair dryer

4 Arrange items nearby.
5 Identify the person. Check the ID bracelet against the assignment sheet. Also call the person by name.
6 Provide for privacy.
7 Raise the bed for body mechanics for a shampoo in bed. Bed rails are up if used.
8 Practice hand hygiene.

PROCEDURE

9 Lower the bed rail near you if up.
10 Cover the person's chest with a bath towel.
11 Brush and comb the hair to remove snarls and tangles.
12 Position the person for the method used. To shampoo the person in bed:
   a Lower the head of the bed and remove the pillow.
   b Place the waterproof pad and shampoo tray under the head and shoulders.
   c Support the head and neck with a folded towel if necessary.

13 Raise the bed rail if used.
14 Obtain water. Water temperature is usually 105°F (40.5°C). Test water temperature according to agency policy. Also ask the person to check the water. Adjust the water temperature as needed. Raise the bed rail before leaving the bedside.
15 Lower the bed rail near you if up.
16 Put on gloves (if needed).
17 Ask the person to hold a washcloth over the eyes. It should not cover the nose and mouth. (NOTE: A damp washcloth is easier to hold. It will not slip. However, your agency may require a dry washcloth.)
18 Use the pitcher or nozzle to wet the hair.
19 Apply a small amount of shampoo.
20 Work up a lather with both hands. Start at the hairline. Work toward the back of the head.
21 Massage the scalp with your fingertips. Do not scratch the scalp with your fingernails.
22 Rinse the hair until the water runs clear.
23 Repeat steps 19 through 22.
24 Apply conditioner. Follow the container's directions.
25 Squeeze water from the person's hair.
26 Cover the hair with a bath towel.
27 Remove the shampoo tray, basin, and waterproof pad.
28 Dry the person's face with a towel. Use the towel on the person's chest.
29 Help the person raise the head if appropriate. For the person in bed, raise the head of the bed.
30 Rub the hair and scalp with the towel. Rub gently. Use the second towel if the first one is wet.
31 Comb the hair to remove snarls and tangles.
32 Dry and style hair as quickly as possible.
33 Remove and discard the gloves (if used). Practice hand hygiene.

POST-PROCEDURE

34 Provide for comfort. (See the inside of the front cover.)
35 Place the call light within reach.
36 Lower the bed to a safe and comfortable level appropriate for the person. Follow the care plan.
37 Raise or lower bed rails. Follow the care plan.
38 Unscreen the person.
39 Complete a safety check of the room. (See the inside of the front cover.)
40 Clean, rinse, dry, and return equipment to its proper place. Remember to clean the comb and brush. Discard disposable items.
41 Follow agency policy for dirty linen.
42 Practice hand hygiene.
43 Report and record your observations.

SHAVING

Many men shave for comfort and well-being. Many women shave their legs and underarms. Some women shave facial hair. Or they may use other hair removal methods—waxing, hair removal products, plucking, threading. See Box 17-1 for shaving rules.

Safety razors or electric shavers are used (Fig. 17-7). Patients and residents may have their own electric shavers. If the agency's shaver is used, clean it before and after use. To brush out whiskers, follow the manufacturer's instructions. Also follow agency policy for cleaning electric shavers.

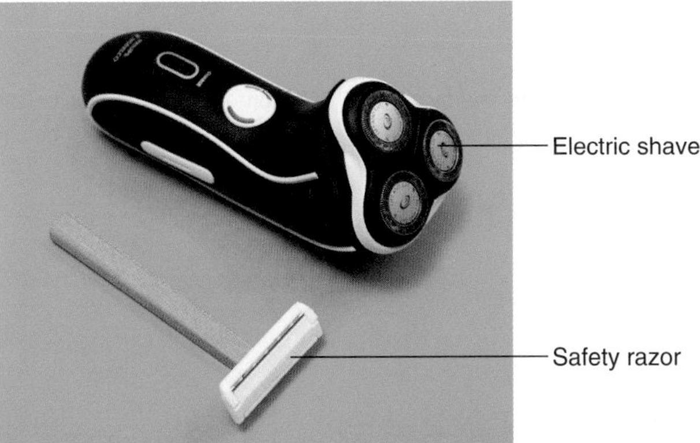

FIGURE 17-7 Electric shaver and safety razor.

Safety razors (blade razors) have razor blades. They can cause nicks and cuts. Do not use safety razors on persons who have healing problems or for those taking anticoagulant drugs. An *anticoagulant* is a drug that prevents or slows down *(anti)* blood clotting *(coagulate)*. Bleeding occurs easily and is hard to stop. A nick or cut can cause serious bleeding. Electric shavers are used instead.

Soften the beard before shaving. To do so, apply a moist, warm washcloth or towel for a few minutes. Then pat dry the face and apply talcum powder if using an electric shaver. For a safety razor, lather the face with soap and water or shaving cream.

See *Focus on Older Persons: Shaving.*

See *Delegation Guidelines: Shaving.*

See *Promoting Safety and Comfort: Shaving,* p. 258.

See procedure: *Shaving the Person's Face With a Safety Razor,* p. 258.

BOX 17-1 Rules for Shaving

- Use electric shavers for persons taking anticoagulant drugs. Never use safety razors.
- Protect bed linens. Place a towel under the part being shaved. Or place a towel across the person's chest and shoulders to protect clothing.
- Soften the beard before shaving. Apply a warm, moist washcloth or towel to the face for a few minutes.
- Encourage the person to do as much as safely possible.
- Hold the skin taut as needed.
- Shave in the correct direction.
  - *Shaving the face with a safety razor*—shave in the direction of hair growth.
  - *Shaving the underarms with a safety razor*—shave in the direction of hair growth.
  - *Shaving the legs with a safety razor*—shave up from the ankles. This is against hair growth.
  - *Using an electric shaver*—shave against the direction of hair growth. If using a rotary-type shaver, move the shaver in small circles over the face. (NOTE: Your state and agency may require shaving in the direction of hair growth. Follow the manufacturer's instructions and the rules in your state and agency.)
- Do not cut, nick, or irritate the skin.
- Rinse the skin thoroughly.
- Apply direct pressure to nicks or cuts (Chapter 31).
- Report nicks, cuts, or irritation to the nurse at once.

FOCUS ON OLDER PERSONS

Shaving

Older persons with wrinkled skin are at risk for nicks and cuts. Safety razors are not used to shave them or persons with dementia. Persons with dementia may not understand what you are doing. They may resist care and move suddenly. Serious nicks and cuts can occur. Use electric shavers for these persons.

DELEGATION GUIDELINES

Shaving

To shave a person, you need this information from the nurse and the care plan.

- What shaver to use—electric or safety
- If the person takes anticoagulant drugs
- When to shave the person
- What facial hair to shave
- If there are tender or sensitive areas on the person's face
- What observations to report and record:
  - Nicks (report at once)
  - Cuts (report at once)
  - Bleeding (report at once)
  - Irritation
- When to report observations
- What patient or resident concerns to report at once

PROMOTING SAFETY AND COMFORT

Shaving

Safety

Safety razors are very sharp. Protect the person and yourself from nicks and cuts. Prevent contact with blood. For an electric shaver, follow safety measures for electrical equipment (Chapter 9).

Rinse the safety razor often. Rinsing removes whiskers and lather. Then wipe the razor. To protect yourself from cuts:

- Place several thicknesses of tissues or paper towels on the over-bed table. Do not hold them in your hand.
- Wipe the razor on the tissues or paper towels.

Follow Standard Precautions and the Bloodborne Pathogen Standard. Discard used razor blades and disposable shavers in the sharps container. Do not re-cap the razor.

Comfort

In some men, the neck area below the jaw is tender and sensitive. Some electric shavers become very warm or hot while in use. The heat can irritate the skin. Shave tender areas first while the shaver is cool. Then move to other areas of the face.

Some people apply lotion or after-shave to the skin after shaving. Lotion softens the skin. After-shave closes skin pores. To soften the skin and open pores, apply heat before shaving.

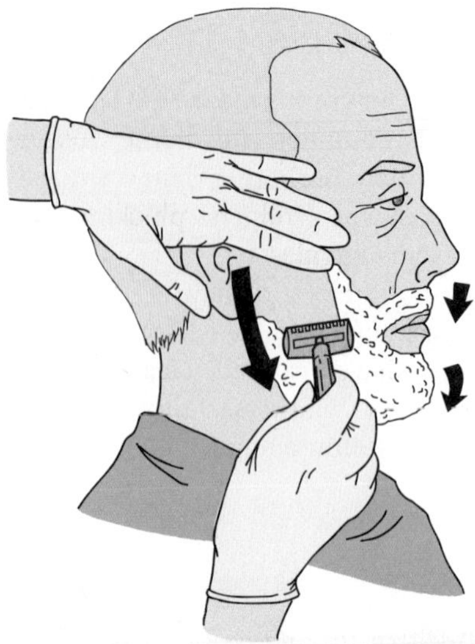

FIGURE 17-8 Shave the face in the direction of hair growth. Use long strokes on the larger areas of the face. Use short strokes around the chin and lips.

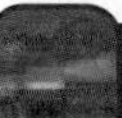

Shaving the Person's Face With a Safety Razor

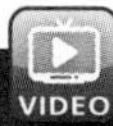

VIDEO

QUALITY OF LIFE

- Knock before entering the person's room.
- Address the person by name.
- Introduce yourself by name and title.
- Explain the procedure before starting and during the procedure.
- Protect the person's rights during the procedure.
- Handle the person gently during the procedure.

PRE-PROCEDURE

1 Follow *Delegation Guidelines: Shaving,* p. 257. See *Promoting Safety and Comfort: Shaving.*
2 Practice hand hygiene.
3 Collect the following.
   - Wash basin
   - Bath towel
   - Hand towel
   - Washcloth
   - Safety razor
   - Mirror
   - Shaving cream, soap, or lotion
   - Shaving brush
   - After-shave or lotion
   - Tissues or paper towels
   - Paper towels
   - Gloves
4 Arrange paper towels and supplies on the over-bed table.
5 Identify the person. Check the ID bracelet against the assignment sheet. Also call the person by name.
6 Provide for privacy.
7 Raise the bed for body mechanics. Bed rails are up if used.

Shaving the Person's Face With a Safety Razor—cont'd

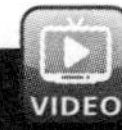

PROCEDURE

8 Fill the wash basin with warm water.
9 Place the basin on the over-bed table.
10 Lower the bed rail near you if up.
11 Practice hand hygiene. Put on gloves.
12 Assist the person to semi-Fowler's position if allowed or to the supine position.
13 Adjust lighting to clearly see the person's face.
14 Place the bath blanket over the person's chest and shoulders.
15 Adjust the over-bed table for easy reach.
16 Tighten the razor blade to the shaver if necessary.
17 Wash the person's face. Do not dry.
18 Wet the washcloth or towel. Wring it out.
19 Apply the washcloth or towel to the face for a few minutes.
20 Apply shaving cream with your hands. Or use a shaving brush to apply lather.
21 Hold the skin taut with 1 hand.
22 Shave in the direction of hair growth. Use shorter strokes around the chin and lips (Fig. 17-8).
23 Rinse the razor often. Wipe it with tissues or paper towels.
24 Apply direct pressure to any bleeding areas (Chapter 31).
25 Wash off any remaining shaving cream or soap. Pat dry with a towel.
26 Apply after-shave or lotion if requested. (If there are nicks or cuts, do not apply after-shave or lotion.)
27 Remove and discard the towel and gloves. Practice hand hygiene.

POST-PROCEDURE

28 Provide for comfort. (See the inside of the front cover.)
29 Place the call light within reach.
30 Lower the bed to a safe and comfortable level for the person. Follow the care plan.
31 Raise or lower bed rails. Follow the care plan.
32 Clean, rinse, dry, and return equipment and supplies to their proper place. Discard the razor blade or disposable razor into the sharps container. Discard other disposable items. Wear gloves.
33 Wipe off the over-bed table with paper towels. Discard the paper towels.
34 Unscreen the person.
35 Complete a safety check of the room. (See the inside of the front cover.)
36 Follow agency policy for dirty linen.
37 Remove and discard the gloves. Practice hand hygiene.
38 Report nicks, cuts, irritation, or bleeding to the nurse at once. Also report and record other observations.

Caring for Mustaches and Beards

Mustaches and beards need daily care. Food can collect in the whiskers. So can mouth and nose drainage. Daily washing and combing are needed. Ask the person how to groom his mustache or beard. *Never trim a mustache or beard without the person's consent.*

Shaving Legs and Underarms

Many women shave their legs and underarms. This practice varies among cultures.

To shave legs and underarms:

- Follow the rules in Box 17-1.
- Collect shaving items with bath items.
- Shave after bathing. The skin is soft at this time.
- Use soap and water, shaving cream, or lotion for the lather. Follow the care plan.
- Use the kidney basin to rinse the razor. Do not use bath water.

NAIL AND FOOT CARE

Nail and foot care prevents infection, injury, and odors. Hangnails, ingrown nails (nails that grow in at the side), and nails torn away from the skin cause skin breaks. These breaks are portals of entry for microbes. Long or broken nails can scratch the skin and snag clothing.

Dirty feet, socks, or stockings harbor microbes and cause odors. Shoes and socks provide a warm, moist environment for microbes to grow. Injuries occur from stubbing on toes, stepping on sharp objects, or being stepped on. Shoes that fit poorly cause blisters.

Poor circulation prolongs healing. Diabetes and vascular diseases are common causes of poor circulation. Infections or foot injuries are very serious for older persons and persons with circulatory disorders. Trimming and clipping toenails can easily cause injuries.

Nails are easier to trim and clean right after soaking or bathing. Use nail clippers to cut fingernails. *Never use scissors.* Use extreme caution to prevent damage to nearby tissues.

Some agencies do not let nursing assistants cut or trim toenails. Follow agency policy.

See *Delegation Guidelines: Nail and Foot Care.*

See *Promoting Safety and Comfort: Nail and Foot Care.*

See procedure: *Giving Nail and Foot Care.*

DELEGATION GUIDELINES

Nail and Foot Care

To give nail and foot care, you need this information from the nurse and the care plan.

- What water temperature to use
- How long to soak fingernails (usually 5 to 10 minutes)
- How long to soak feet (usually 15 to 20 minutes)
- What observations to report and record:
  - Dry, reddened, irritated, or callused areas
  - Breaks in the skin
  - Corns (Chapter 24) on top of and between the toes
  - Blisters
  - Very thick nails
  - Loose nails
- When to report observations
- What patient or resident concerns to report at once

PROMOTING SAFETY AND COMFORT

Nail and Foot Care

Safety

Remember, some states and agencies do not let nursing assistants cut and trim toenails. The nurse or podiatrist (foot *[pod]* doctor) cuts toenails and provides foot care for the following persons. *You do not cut or trim the toenails for persons who:*

- Have diabetes.
- Have poor circulation to the legs and feet.
- Take drugs that affect blood clotting.
- Have very thick nails or ingrown toenails.

Check between the toes for cracks and sores. These areas are often overlooked. If not treated, a serious infection could occur.

The feet are easily burned. Persons with decreased sensation or circulatory problems may not feel hot temperatures.

After soaking, apply lotion or petroleum jelly to the feet. This can cause slippery feet. Help the person put on non-skid footwear before you transfer the person or let the person walk.

Breaks in the skin and bleeding can occur. Follow Standard Precautions and the Bloodborne Pathogen Standard.

Comfort

Sometimes you just trim the fingernails. Sometimes you just give foot care. When you do both, the person sits at the over-bed table (Fig. 17-9). Provide for warmth and comfort.

Promote your own comfort during nail and foot care. Sit in front of the over-bed table to trim and clean fingernails. For foot care, rest the person's lower leg and foot on your lap. Or position the feet on the floor and kneel on the floor. Lay a towel across your lap or a bath mat on the floor to protect your uniform. Use good body mechanics. Always support the person's foot and ankle when giving foot care.

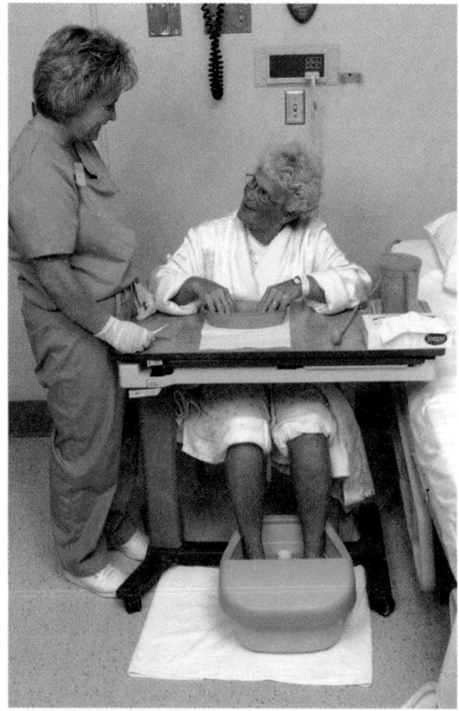

FIGURE 17-9 Nail and foot care. The feet soak in a whirlpool foot bath. The fingers soak in a kidney basin.

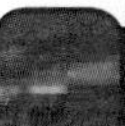

Giving Nail and Foot Care

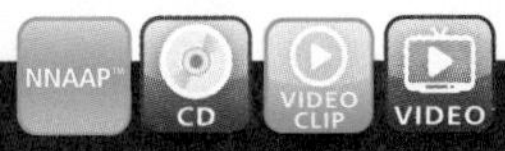

QUALITY OF LIFE

- Knock before entering the person's room.
- Address the person by name.
- Introduce yourself by name and title.
- Explain the procedure before starting and during the procedure.
- Protect the person's rights during the procedure.
- Handle the person gently during the procedure.

PRE-PROCEDURE

1 Follow *Delegation Guidelines: Nail and Foot Care*. See *Promoting Safety and Comfort: Nail and Foot Care.*
2 Practice hand hygiene.
3 Collect the following.
  - Wash basin or whirlpool foot bath
  - Soap
  - Bath thermometer
  - Bath towel
  - Hand towel
  - Washcloth
  - Kidney basin
  - Nail clippers
  - Orangewood stick
  - Emery board or nail file
  - Lotion for the hands
  - Lotion or petroleum jelly for the feet
  - Paper towels
  - Bath mat
  - Gloves
4 Arrange paper towels and other items on the over-bed table.
5 Identify the person. Check the ID bracelet against the assignment sheet. Also call the person by name.
6 Provide for privacy.
7 Assist the person to the bedside chair. Remove footwear and socks or stockings. Place the call light within reach.

PROCEDURE

8 Place the bath mat under the feet.
9 Fill the wash basin or whirlpool foot bath ⅔ (two-thirds) full with water. The nurse tells you what water temperature to use. (Measure water temperature with a bath thermometer. Or test it by dipping your elbow or inner wrist into the basin. Follow agency policy.) Also ask the person to check the water temperature. Adjust the water temperature as needed.
10 Place the basin or foot bath on the bath mat.
11 Put on gloves.
12 Help the person put his or her bare feet into the basin or foot bath. Both feet are completely covered by water.
13 Adjust the over-bed table in front of the person.
14 Fill the kidney basin ⅔ (two-thirds) full with water. See step 9 for water temperature.
15 Place the kidney basin on the over-bed table.
16 Place the person's fingers into the basin. Position the arms for comfort (see Fig. 17-9).
17 Let the fingers soak for 5 to 10 minutes. Let the feet soak for 15 to 20 minutes. Re-warm water as needed.
18 Remove the kidney basin.
19 Clean under the fingernails with the orangewood stick. Use a towel to wipe the orangewood stick after each nail.
20 Dry the hands and between the fingers thoroughly.
21 Clip fingernails straight across with the nail clippers (Fig. 17-10, p. 262).
22 Shape nails with an emery board or nail file. Nails are smooth with no rough edges. Check each nail for smoothness. File as needed.
23 Push cuticles back with the orangewood stick or a washcloth (Fig. 17-11, p. 262).
24 Apply lotion to the hands. Warm lotion before applying it.
25 Move the over-bed table to the side.
26 Lift a foot out of the water. Support the foot and ankle with 1 hand. With your other hand, wash the foot and between the toes with soap and a washcloth. Return the foot to the water for rinsing. Rinse well between the toes.
27 Repeat step 26 for the other foot.
28 Remove the feet from the basin or foot bath. Dry thoroughly, especially between the toes. Support the foot and ankle as needed.
29 Apply lotion or petroleum jelly to the tops, soles, and heels of the feet. Do not apply between the toes. Warm lotion or petroleum jelly before applying it. Remove excess lotion or petroleum jelly with a towel. Support the foot and ankle as needed.
30 Remove and discard the gloves. Practice hand hygiene.
31 Help the person put on non-skid footwear.

POST-PROCEDURE

32 Provide for comfort. (See the inside of the front cover.)
33 Place the call light within reach.
34 Raise or lower bed rails. Follow the care plan.
35 Clean, rinse, dry, and return equipment and supplies to their proper place. Discard disposable items. Wear gloves.
36 Unscreen the person.
37 Complete a safety check of the room. (See the inside of the front cover.)
38 Follow agency policy for dirty linen.
39 Remove and discard the gloves. Practice hand hygiene.
40 Report and record your observations.

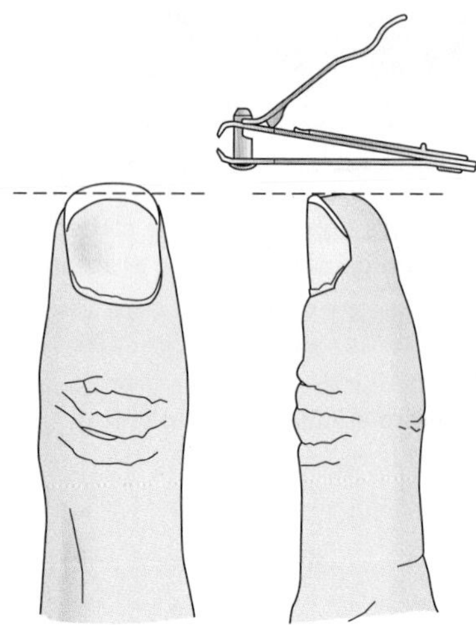

FIGURE 17-10 Clip fingernails straight across. Use a nail clipper.

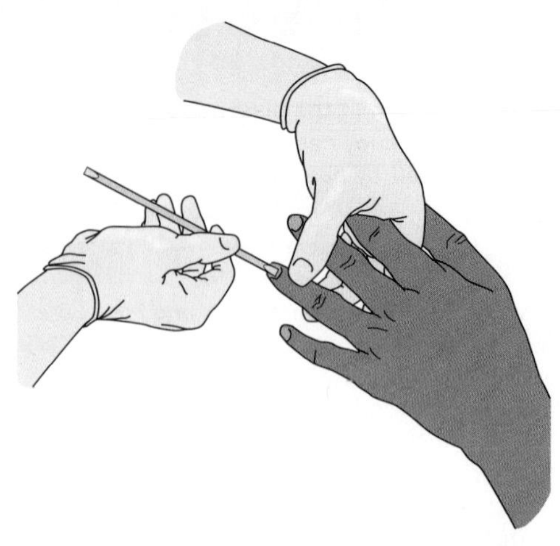

FIGURE 17-11 Push the cuticle back with an orangewood stick.

CHANGING GARMENTS

Most residents wear street clothes during the day and sleepwear at bedtime. Most patients wear gowns. Gowns are changed daily. Garments are also changed:

- After bathing
- On admission and discharge
- When wet or soiled

Dressing and Undressing

Some patients and residents dress and undress themselves. Others need help. Personal choice is a resident right. Let the person choose what to wear. When you assist with dressing and undressing, follow the rules in Box 17-2.

See *Focus on Communication: Dressing and Undressing.*

See *Focus on Older Persons: Dressing and Undressing.*

See *Delegation Guidelines: Dressing and Undressing.*

See *Promoting Safety and Comfort: Dressing and Undressing.*

See procedure: *Undressing the Person.*

See procedure: *Dressing the Person*, p. 266.

Text continued on p. 267

BOX 17-2 Rules for Dressing and Undressing

- Provide for privacy. Do not expose the person.
- Encourage the person to do as much as possible.
- Let the person choose what to wear. Have the person choose the right undergarments.
- Make sure garments and footwear are the correct size.
- Remove clothing from the strong or "good" side first. This is often called the *unaffected side.*
- Put clothing on the weak side first. This is often called the *affected side.*
- Support the arm or leg to remove or put on a garment.
- Move and handle the body gently. Do not force a joint beyond its range of motion or to the point of pain. See Chapter 23.

FOCUS ON COMMUNICATION

Dressing and Undressing

Allow for personal choice and independence when assisting with dressing and undressing. You can ask:

- "What would you like to wear today?"
- "There's a concert today in the lounge. Do you want to wear something special?"
- "Can I help you with those buttons?"
- "Would you like me to help you with that zipper?"

FOCUS ON OLDER PERSONS

Dressing and Undressing

Persons with dementia may not want to change clothes. Or they may not know how. For example, a person tries to put slacks on over his or her head. Or a person wears the wrong clothes for the season or weather. The Alzheimer's Disease Education and Referral Center (ADEAR) suggests the following.

- Try to assist with dressing at the same time each day. The person learns to expect dressing as a part of the daily routine.
- Let the person dress himself or herself to the extent possible. Allow extra time. Do not rush the person.
- Let the person choose from 2 or 3 outfits. If the person has a favorite outfit, the family may buy several of the same outfit. This makes dressing easier if the person insists on wearing the same thing.
- Choose comfortable clothes that are easy to get on and off. Garments with elastic waistbands and Velcro closures are examples. The person does not have to handle zippers, buttons, hooks, snaps, or other closures.
- Stack clothes in the order that they are put on. The person sees 1 item at a time. For example, underpants or undergarments are put on first. The item is on top of the stack.
- Give clear, simple, and step-by-step directions.

DELEGATION GUIDELINES

Dressing and Undressing

To assist with dressing and undressing, you need this information from the nurse and the care plan.

- How much help the person needs
- Which side is the person's strong side
- If the person needs to wear certain garments
- What observations to report and record:
  - How much help was given
  - How the person tolerated the procedure
  - Any complaints by the person
  - Any changes in the person's behavior
- When to report observations
- What patient or resident concerns to report at once

PROMOTING SAFETY AND COMFORT

Dressing and Undressing

Safety

When assisting with dressing and undressing, you turn the person from side to side. If the person uses bed rails, raise the far bed rail. If bed rails are not used, ask a co-worker to help turn and position the person. This protects the person from falling.

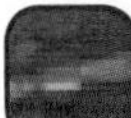

Undressing the Person

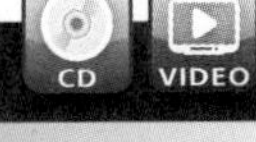

QUALITY OF LIFE

- Knock before entering the person's room.
- Address the person by name.
- Introduce yourself by name and title.
- Explain the procedure before starting and during the procedure.
- Protect the person's rights during the procedure.
- Handle the person gently during the procedure.

PRE-PROCEDURE

1 Follow *Delegation Guidelines: Dressing and Undressing*. See *Promoting Safety and Comfort: Dressing and Undressing*.
2 Ask a co-worker to help turn and position the person if needed.
3 Practice hand hygiene.
4 Collect a bath blanket and clothing as requested by the person.
5 Identify the person. Check the ID bracelet against the assignment sheet. Also call the person by name.
6 Provide for privacy.
7 Raise the bed for body mechanics. Bed rails are up if used.
8 Lower the bed rail on the person's weak side.
9 Position him or her supine.
10 Cover the person with a bath blanket. Fan-fold linens to the foot of the bed.

PROCEDURE

11 Remove garments that open in back.
  a Raise the head and shoulders. Or turn the person onto the side away from you.
  b Undo buttons, zippers, ties, or snaps.
  c Bring the sides of the garment to the sides of the person (Fig. 17-12, p. 264). If in a side-lying position, tuck the far side under the person. Fold the near side onto the chest (Fig. 17-13, p. 264).
  d Position the person supine.
  e Slide the garment off the shoulder on the strong side. Remove it from the arm (Fig. 17-14, p. 264).
  f Remove the garment from the weak side.
12 Remove garments that open in the front.
  a Undo buttons, zippers, ties, or snaps.
  b Slide the garment off the shoulder and arm on the strong side.
  c Assist the person to sit up or raise the head and shoulders. Bring the garment over to the weak side (Fig. 17-15, p. 264).
  d Lower the head and shoulders. Remove the garment from the weak side.
  e If you cannot raise the head and shoulders:
    1 Turn the person toward you. Tuck the removed part under the person.
    2 Turn him or her onto the side away from you.
    3 Pull the side of the garment out from under the person. Make sure he or she will not lie on it when supine.
    4 Return the person to the supine position.
    5 Remove the garment from the weak side.
13 Remove pullover garments.
  a Undo any buttons, zippers, ties, or snaps.
  b Remove the garment from the strong side.
  c Raise the head and shoulders. Or turn the person onto the side away from you. Bring the garment up to the person's neck (Fig. 17-16, p. 265).
  d Bring the garment over the person's head.
  e Remove the garment from the weak side.
  f Position the person in the supine position.

Continued

Undressing the Person—cont'd

CD VIDEO

PROCEDURE—cont'd

14 Remove pants or slacks.
- **a** Remove footwear and socks.
- **b** Position the person supine.
- **c** Undo buttons, zippers, ties, snaps, or buckles.
- **d** Remove the belt.
- **e** Ask the person to lift the buttocks off the bed. Slide the pants down over the hips and buttocks (Fig. 17-17). Have the person lower the hips and buttocks.
- **f** If the person cannot raise the hips off the bed:
  1. Turn the person toward you.
  2. Slide the pants off the hip and buttocks on the strong side (Fig. 17-18).
  3. Turn the person away from you.
  4. Slide the pants off the hip and buttocks on the weak side (Fig. 17-19).
- **g** Slide the pants down the legs and over the feet.

15 Dress the person. See procedure: *Dressing the Person,* p. 266.

POST-PROCEDURE

16 Provide for comfort. (See the inside of the front cover.)
17 Place the call light within reach.
18 Lower the bed to a safe and comfortable level appropriate for the person. Follow the care plan.
19 Raise or lower bed rails. Follow the care plan.
20 Unscreen the person.
21 Complete a safety check of the room. (See the inside of the front cover.)
22 Follow agency policy for soiled clothing.
23 Practice hand hygiene.
24 Report and record your observations.

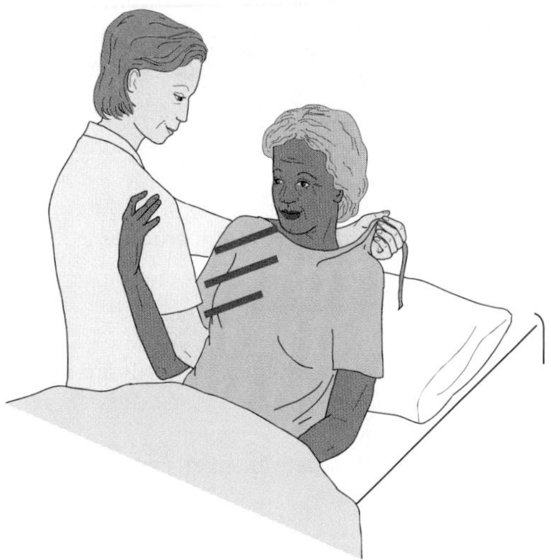

FIGURE 17-12 The sides of the garment are brought from the back to the sides of the person. (Note: *The "weak" side is indicated by slash marks.*)

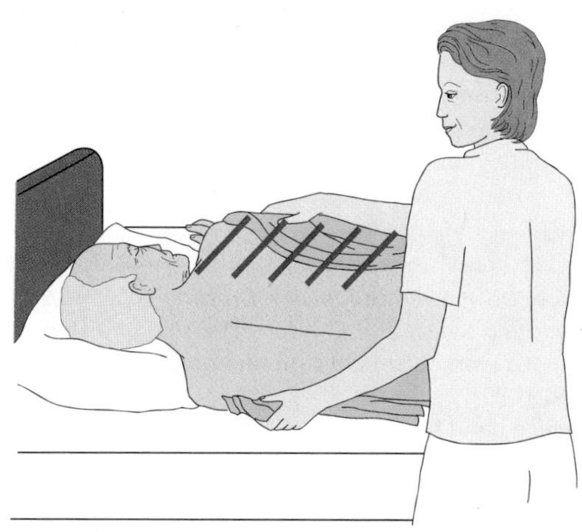

FIGURE 17-13 A garment that opens in the back is removed from the person in the side-lying position. The far side of the garment is tucked under the person. The near side is folded onto the person's chest. (Note: *The "weak" side is indicated by slash marks.*)

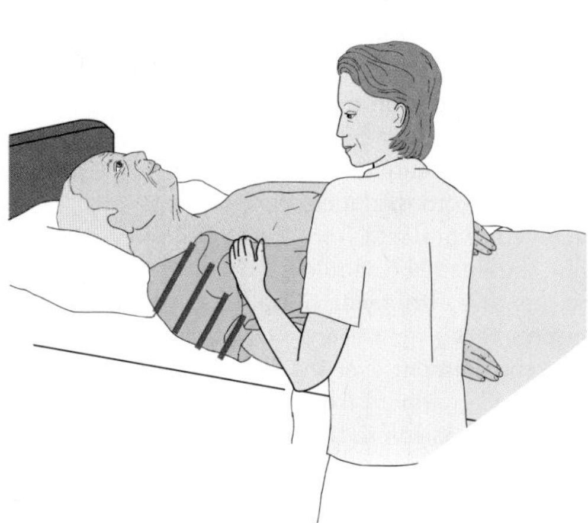

FIGURE 17-14 The garment is removed from the strong side first. (Note: *The "weak" side is indicated by slash marks.*)

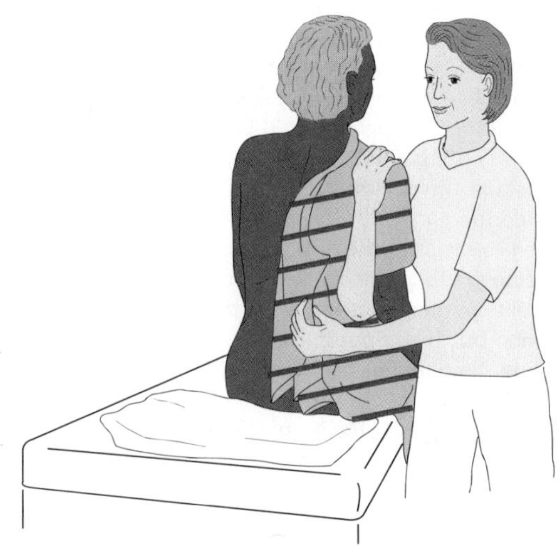

FIGURE 17-15 A front-opening garment is removed with the person's head and shoulders raised. The garment is removed from the strong side first. Then it is brought around the back to the weak side. (Note: *The "weak" side is indicated by slash marks.*)

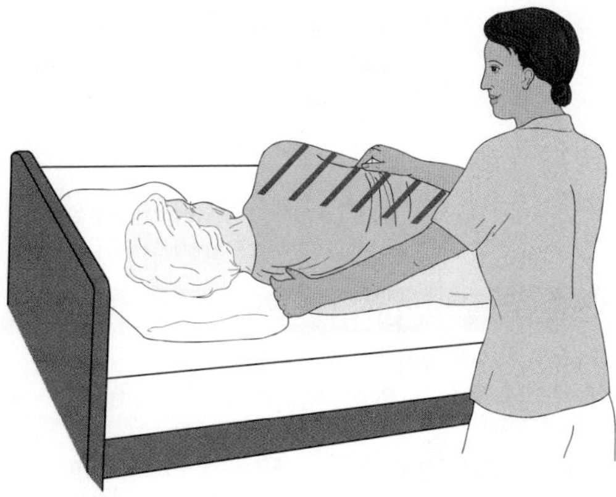

FIGURE 17-16 A pullover garment is removed from the strong side first. Then the garment is brought up to the person's neck so that it can be removed from the weak side. (Note: *The "weak" side is indicated by slash marks.*)

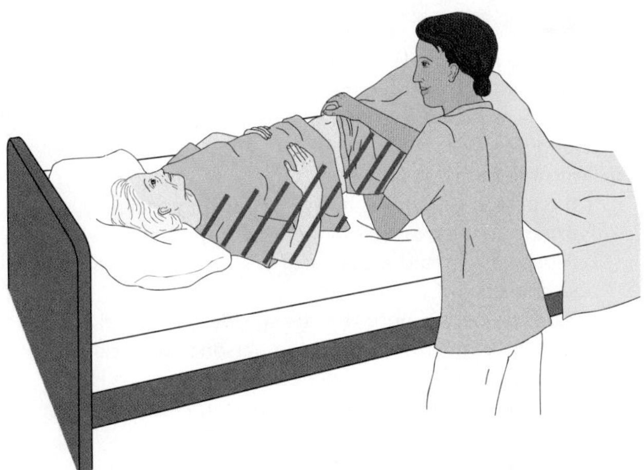

FIGURE 17-17 The person lifts the hips and buttocks to remove the pants. The pants are slid down over the hips and buttocks. (Note: *The "weak" side is indicated by slash marks.*)

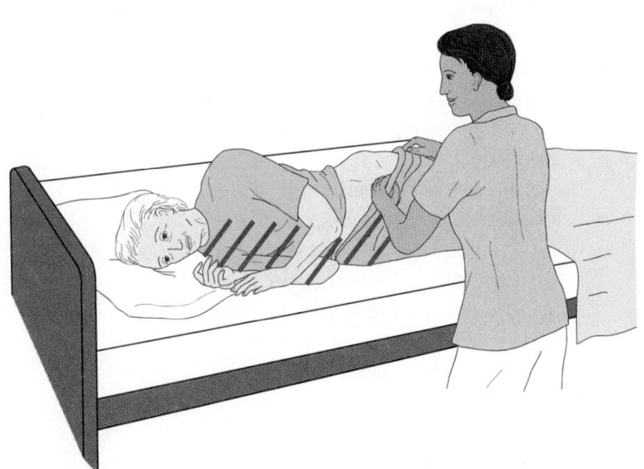

FIGURE 17-18 Pants are removed in the side-lying position. They are removed from the strong side first. They are slid over the hip and buttock. (Note: *The "weak" side is indicated by slash marks.*)

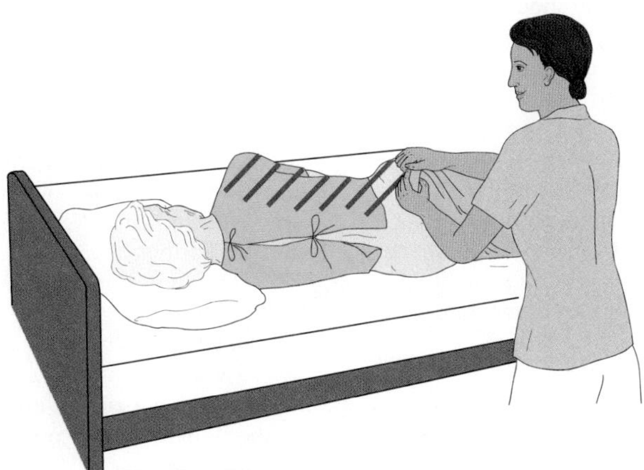

FIGURE 17-19 The person is turned onto the strong side. The pants are removed from the weak side. (Note: *The "weak" side is indicated by slash marks.*)

NNAAP CD VIDEO CLIP VIDEO

Dressing the Person

QUALITY OF LIFE

- Knock before entering the person's room.
- Address the person by name.
- Introduce yourself by name and title.
- Explain the procedure before starting and during the procedure.
- Protect the person's rights during the procedure.
- Handle the person gently during the procedure.

PRE-PROCEDURE

1 Follow *Delegation Guidelines: Dressing and Undressing,* p. 263. See *Promoting Safety and Comfort: Dressing and Undressing,* p. 263.
2 Ask a co-worker to help turn and position the person if needed.
3 Practice hand hygiene.
4 Ask the person what he or she would like to wear.
5 Get a bath blanket and clothing requested by the person.
6 Identify the person. Check the ID bracelet against the assignment sheet. Also call the person by name.
7 Provide for privacy.
8 Raise the bed for body mechanics. Bed rails are up if used.
9 Lower the bed rail near you if up.
10 Position the person supine.
11 Cover the person with a bath blanket. Fan-fold linens to the foot of the bed.
12 Undress the person. (See procedure: *Undressing the Person,* p. 263).

PROCEDURE

13 Put on garments that open in the back.
  a Slide the garment onto the arm and shoulder of the weak side.
  b Slide the garment onto the arm and shoulder of the strong side.
  c Raise the person's head and shoulders.
  d Bring the sides to the back.
  e If you cannot raise the person's head and shoulders:
    1 Turn the person toward you.
    2 Bring 1 side of the garment to the person's back (Fig. 17-20, *A*).
    3 Turn the person away from you.
    4 Bring the other side to the person's back (Fig. 17-20, *B*).
  f Fasten buttons, zippers, snaps, or other closures.
  g Position the person supine.
14 Put on garments that open in the front.
  a Slide the garment onto the arm and shoulder on the weak side.
  b Raise the head and shoulders. Bring the side of the garment around to the back. Lower the person down. Slide the garment onto the arm and shoulder of the strong arm.
  c If the person cannot raise the head and shoulders:
    1 Turn the person onto the strong side.
    2 Tuck the garment under him or her.
    3 Turn the person onto the weak side.
    4 Pull the garment out from under him or her.
    5 Turn the person back to the supine position.
    6 Slide the garment over the arm and shoulder of the strong arm.
  d Fasten buttons, zippers, ties, snaps, or other closures.
15 Put on pullover garments.
  a Position the person supine.
  b Slide the arm and shoulder of the garment onto the weak side.
  c Raise the person's head and shoulders.
  d Bring the neck of the garment over the head.
  e Slide the arm and shoulder of the garment onto the strong side.
  f Bring the garment down.
  g If the person cannot assume a semi-sitting position:
    1 Bring the neck of the garment over the head.
    2 Slide the arm and shoulder of the garment onto the strong side.
    3 Turn the person onto the strong side.
    4 Pull the garment down on the person's weak side.
    5 Turn the person onto the weak side.
    6 Pull the garment down on the person's strong side.
    7 Position the person supine.
16 Put on pants or slacks.
  a Slide the pants over the feet and up the legs.
  b Ask the person to raise the hips and buttocks off the bed.
  c Bring the pants up over the buttock and hip on the weak side.
  d Pull the pants over the buttock and hip on the strong side.
  e If the person cannot raise the hips and buttocks:
    1 Turn the person onto the strong side.
    2 Pull the pants over the buttock and hip on the weak side.
    3 Turn the person onto the weak side.
    4 Pull the pants over the buttock and hip on the strong side.
    5 Position the person supine.
  f Fasten buttons, zippers, ties, snaps, a belt buckle, or other closures.
17 Put socks and non-skid footwear on the person. Make sure socks are up all the way and smooth.
18 Help the person get out of bed. If the person will stay in bed, cover the person. Remove the bath blanket.

POST-PROCEDURE

19 Provide for comfort. (See the inside of the front cover.)
20 Place the call light within reach.
21 Lower the bed to a safe and comfortable level appropriate for the person. Follow the care plan.
22 Raise or lower bed rails. Follow the care plan.
23 Unscreen the person.
24 Complete a safety check of the room. (See the inside of the front cover.)
25 Follow agency policy for soiled clothing.
26 Practice hand hygiene.
27 Report and record your observations.

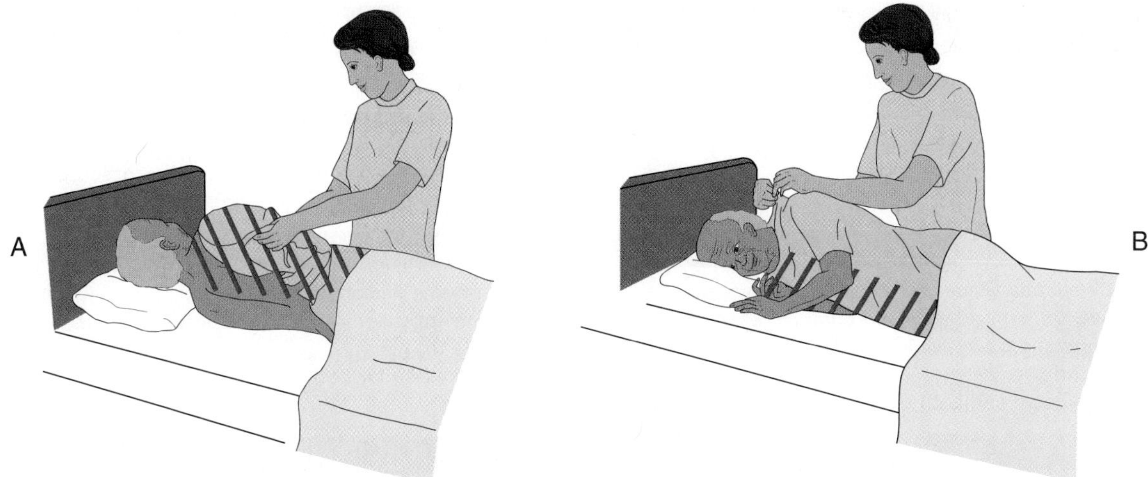

FIGURE 17-20 Dressing a person. **A,** The side-lying position can be used to put on garments that open in the back. Turn the person toward you after the garment is put on the arms. The side of the garment is brought to the person's back. **B,** Then turn the person away from you. The other side of the garment is brought to the back and fastened. (Note: *The "weak" side is indicated by slash marks.*)

Changing Patient Gowns

Many patients wear gowns. So do some nursing center residents. Gowns are usually worn for IV (intravenous) therapy (Chapter 20). Some agencies have special gowns for IV therapy. They open along the sleeve and close with ties, snaps, or Velcro. Sometimes standard gowns are used.

For injury or paralysis, remove the gown from the strong arm first. Support the weak arm while removing the gown. Put the clean gown on the weak arm first and then on the strong arm.

See *Delegation Guidelines: Changing Patient Gowns.*

See *Promoting Safety and Comfort: Changing Patient Gowns.*

See procedure: *Changing the Gown on the Person With an IV*, p. 268.

DELEGATION GUIDELINES

Changing Patient Gowns

Before changing a gown, you need this information from the nurse and the care plan.

- Which arm has the IV
- If the person has an IV pump (see *Promoting Safety and Comfort: Changing Patient Gowns*)

PROMOTING SAFETY AND COMFORT

Changing Patient Gowns

Safety

IV pumps control the *flow rate*—how fast fluid enters a vein. If the person has an IV pump and a standard gown, do not use the procedure on p. 268. The nurse handles the arm with the IV.

To change a gown, you must move the IV bag. Moving the IV bag can change the IV flow rate. Always ask the nurse to check the flow rate after you change a gown.

Do not disconnect or remove any part of the IV set-up.

Comfort

Some patient gowns tie at the upper back. The back and buttocks are exposed when the person stands. Cover the person for warmth and privacy. A robe may be used. Or a second gown can be worn backwards to cover the back and buttocks. Other gowns overlap in the back and tie at the side. They provide more privacy. Because they tie at the side, uncomfortable bows and knots at the back are avoided.

Changing the Gown on the Person With an IV

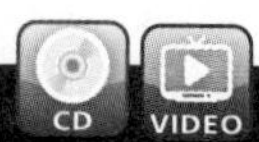

QUALITY OF LIFE

- Knock before entering the person's room.
- Address the person by name.
- Introduce yourself by name and title.
- Explain the procedure before starting and during the procedure.
- Protect the person's rights during the procedure.
- Handle the person gently during the procedure.

PRE-PROCEDURE

1 Follow *Delegation Guidelines: Changing Patient Gowns,* p. 267. See *Promoting Safety and Comfort: Changing Patient Gowns,* p. 267.
2 Practice hand hygiene.
3 Get a clean gown and bath blanket.
4 Identify the person. Check the ID bracelet against the assignment sheet. Also call the person by name.
5 Provide for privacy.
6 Raise the bed for body mechanics. Bed rails are up if used.

PROCEDURE

7 Lower the bed rail near you (if up).
8 Cover the person with the bath blanket. Fan-fold linens to the foot of the bed.
9 Untie the gown. Free parts that the person is lying on.
10 Remove the gown from the arm with *no IV.*
11 Gather up the sleeve of the arm *with the IV.* Slide it over the IV site and tubing. Remove the arm and hand from the sleeve (Fig. 17-21, *A*).
12 Keep the sleeve gathered. Slide your arm along the tubing to the bag (Fig. 17-21, *B*).
13 Remove the bag from the pole. Slide the bag and tubing through the sleeve (Fig. 17-21, *C*). Do not pull on the tubing. Keep the bag above the person.
14 Hang the IV bag on the pole.
15 Gather the sleeve of the clean gown that will go on the arm with the IV infusion.
16 Remove the bag from the pole. Slip the sleeve over the bag at the shoulder part of the gown (Fig. 17-21, *D*). Hang the bag.
17 Slide the gathered sleeve over the tubing, hand, arm, and IV site. Then slide it onto the shoulder.
18 Put the other side of the gown on the person. Fasten the gown.
19 Cover the person. Remove the bath blanket.

POST-PROCEDURE

20 Provide for comfort. (See the inside of the front cover.)
21 Place the call light within reach.
22 Lower the bed to a safe and comfortable level appropriate for the person. Follow the care plan.
23 Raise or lower bed rails. Follow the care plan.
24 Unscreen the person.
25 Complete a safety check of the room. (See the inside of the front cover.)
26 Follow agency policy for dirty linen.
27 Practice hand hygiene.
28 Ask the nurse to check the flow rate.
29 Report and record your observations.

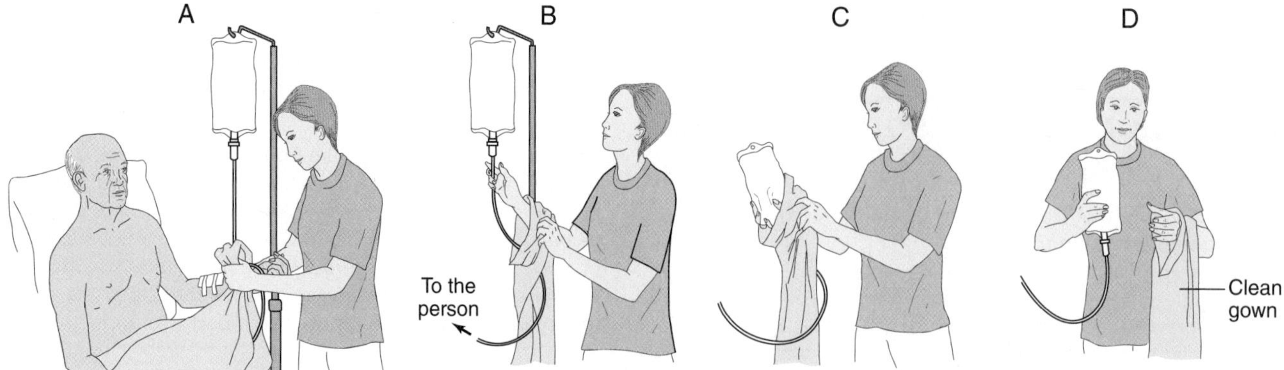

FIGURE 17-21 Changing a gown. **A,** The gown is removed from the arm with no IV. The sleeve on the arm with the IV is gathered up, slipped over the IV site and tubing, and removed from the arm and hand. **B,** The gathered sleeve is slipped along the IV tubing to the bag. **C,** The IV bag is removed from the pole and passed through the sleeve. **D,** The gathered sleeve of the clean gown is slipped over the IV bag at the shoulder part of the gown.

FOCUS ON PRIDE

The Person, Family, and Yourself

Personal and Professional Responsibility

Grooming promotes comfort. Self-esteem and body image improve when the person likes how he or she looks. Clean hair, nails, and garments all help mental well-being. So does a clean-shaven face or a well-groomed beard or mustache.

Your attitude is reflected in how you give care. To show that you value the person's self-esteem and comfort:

- Be pleasant. Talk with the person.
- Ask about the person's preferences. Allow personal choice.
- Avoid seeming rushed. Let the person know that you have time for him or her.
- Avoid thinking that care measures are tasks to be completed. You are caring for a *person.* Show that you care about the person's needs and feelings.
- Do a good job. Be thorough and careful.
- Clean up after yourself. Leave the person's setting neat and orderly.

Also, care for your own appearance. Patients, residents, and family members notice when others are not well groomed. If not groomed well, they may question the quality of care you provide. Have a professional appearance.

Rights and Respect

People have different grooming preferences. Ask what the person prefers. For example, ask what he or she would like to wear. Or ask how to style the person's hair. Follow the person's grooming routines when possible.

You may not like the person's hairstyle, clothing choices, or personal care products. Do not judge the person by your own standards or impose your choices on the person. Do not make the person feel badly about his or her choices. Respect the person's right to choose. Assist with grooming in a way that improves the person's self-esteem.

Independence and Social Interaction

Sometimes family members want to help with grooming. For example, they want to style the person's hair. Or they want to apply lotion to the person's hands and feet. With the person's permission, allow family members to assist with grooming as much as safely possible. This promotes social interaction. It also involves the family in the person's care.

Delegation and Teamwork

Grooming takes time. You, the person, the nurse, and other team members work together to plan and organize care. For example, Mr. Horn had a stroke. He needs help with grooming. He eats breakfast at 0800, has speech therapy at 0930, has physical therapy at 1030, and his wife visits at lunchtime. Mr. Horn prefers to comb his hair and shave after breakfast but before his wife visits. He also likes to rest before and after physical therapy. You plan to assist Mr. Horn with grooming after breakfast and before speech therapy.

Grooming is important. Do not neglect grooming because of a busy schedule. Plan to meet the person's needs at a time best for the person and the team.

Ethics and Laws

Patients and residents have the right to be free from mistreatment and restraint (Chapter 2). Never force a care measure on a person. If a person resists or refuses care, stop. Do not proceed. Politely ask the person for the reason. Tell the nurse. You, the nurse, and the person can discuss a solution.

Special care measures are needed for persons with confusion or dementia who resist care. See Chapter 30. Patience, kindness, and problem solving are needed. A co-worker or family member may need to give care. Or care is given at a different time. Provide care in a way that protects the person's rights and shows dignity and respect.

REVIEW QUESTIONS

Circle* T *if the statement is TRUE or* F *if it is FALSE.

1 **T F** Mr. Polk has a mustache. To promote comfort, you can shave his beard and mustache.

2 **T F** Clothing is removed from the strong side first.

3 **T F** The person chooses what to wear.

4 **T F** A person has poor circulation in the legs and feet. You can cut the person's toenails.

5 **T F** You can cut matted hair.

Circle the BEST answer.

6 A person with alopecia has
 a Excessive body hair
 b Dry, white flakes from the scalp
 c An infestation with lice
 d Hair loss

7 Which prevents hair from matting and tangling?
 a Bedrest
 b Daily brushing and combing
 c Daily shampooing
 d Cutting hair

8 A person's hair is *not* matted or tangled. When brushing hair, start at
 a The forehead and brush backward
 b The hair ends
 c The scalp
 d The back of the neck and brush forward

9 Brushing keeps the hair
 a Soft and shiny
 b Clean
 c Free of lice
 d Long

10 A person requests a shampoo. You should
 a Shampoo the hair during the person's shower
 b Shampoo hair at the sink
 c Shampoo the person in bed
 d Follow the care plan

11 When shaving a person's face with a safety razor
 a Discard the razor in the wastebasket when done
 b Shave against the direction of hair growth
 c Hold the skin taut
 d Shave when the skin is dry

12 A person is nicked during shaving. Your *first* action is to
 a Wash your hands
 b Apply direct pressure
 c Tell the nurse
 d Apply a bandage

13 Fingernails are cut with
 a An emery board
 b Scissors
 c A nail file
 d Nail clippers

14 Fingernails are trimmed
 a Before soaking
 b After soaking
 c Before trimming toenails
 d After trimming toenails

Answers to these questions are on p. 504.

FOCUS ON PRACTICE

Problem Solving

A resident with dementia has long fingernails. Some are broken and have rough edges. As you begin nail care, she resists. She swings her arms at you and yells. What do you do? Why is nail care important for this resident? How might you provide care safely?

Assisting With Urinary Elimination

CHAPTER 18

OBJECTIVES

- Define the key terms and key abbreviations listed in this chapter.
- Describe normal urine.
- Describe the rules for normal urination.
- Identify the observations to report to the nurse.
- Describe urinary incontinence and the care required.
- Explain why catheters are used.
- Explain how to care for persons with catheters.
- Describe the bladder training methods.
- Perform the procedures described in this chapter.
- Explain how to promote PRIDE in the person, the family, and yourself.

KEY TERMS

catheter A tube used to drain or inject fluid through a body opening
dysuria Painful or difficult *(dys)* urination *(uria)*
functional incontinence The person has bladder control but cannot use the toilet in time
hematuria Blood *(hemat)* in the urine *(uria)*
mixed incontinence The combination of stress incontinence and urge incontinence
nocturia Frequent urination *(uria)* at night *(noc)*
oliguria Scant amount *(olig)* of urine *(uria)*; less than 500 mL in 24 hours
overflow incontinence Small amounts of urine leak from a full bladder
polyuria Abnormally large amounts *(poly)* of urine *(uria)*
reflex incontinence Urine is lost at predictable intervals when the bladder is full
stress incontinence When urine leaks during exercise and certain movements that cause pressure on the bladder
transient incontinence Temporary or occasional incontinence that is reversed when the cause is treated
urge incontinence The loss of urine in response to a sudden, urgent need to void; the person cannot get to a toilet in time
urinary frequency Voiding at frequent intervals
urinary incontinence The involuntary loss or leakage of urine
urinary retention The inability to void
urinary urgency The need to void at once
urination The process of emptying urine from the bladder; voiding
voiding See "urination"

KEY ABBREVIATIONS

BM	Bowel movement
C	Centigrade
F	Fahrenheit
ID	Identification
IV	Intravenous
mL	Milliliter
UTI	Urinary tract infection

Eliminating waste is a physical need. The urinary system removes waste products from the blood. It also maintains the body's water balance.

See *Promoting Safety and Comfort: Assisting With Urinary Elimination.*

PROMOTING SAFETY AND COMFORT

Assisting With Urinary Elimination

Safety

Urinary elimination measures often involve exposing and touching private areas—the perineum and rectum. Sexual abuse has occurred in health care settings. The person may feel threatened or may be being abused. He or she needs to call for help. Keep the call light within the person's reach at all times. And always act in a professional manner.

Urine may contain blood and microbes. Microbes can live and grow in dirty bedpans, urinals, commodes, and urinary drainage bags. Follow Standard Precautions and the Bloodborne Pathogen Standard (Chapter 12) when handling urinary devices and their contents. This includes incontinence products. Thoroughly clean and disinfect bedpans, urinals, and commodes after use. Remember to practice hand hygiene.

NORMAL URINATION

The healthy adult produces about 1500 mL (milliliters) or 3 pints of urine a day. Many factors affect urine production. They include age, disease, the amount and kinds of fluid ingested, dietary salt, body temperature, perspiration (sweating), and some drugs. Some substances increase urine production—coffee, tea, alcohol, and some drugs. A diet high in salt causes the body to retain water. So do some drugs. When water is retained, less urine is produced.

Urination (voiding) *means the process of emptying urine from the bladder.* The amount of fluid intake, habits, and available toilet facilities affect frequency. So do activity, work, and illness. People usually void at bedtime, after sleep, and before meals. Some people void every 2 to 3 hours.

Some persons need help getting to the bathroom. Others use bedpans, urinals, or commodes. Follow the rules in Box 18-1 and the person's care plan.

See *Focus on Communication: Normal Urination.*

Observations

Normal urine is pale yellow, straw-colored, or amber (Fig. 18-1). It is clear with no particles. A faint odor is normal. Observe urine for color, clarity, odor, amount, particles, and blood.

Ask the nurse to observe urine that looks or smells abnormal. Report these problems.

- ***Dysuria****—painful or difficult* (dys) *urination* (uria)
- ***Hematuria****—blood* (hemat) *in the urine* (uria)
- ***Nocturia****—frequent urination* (uria) *at night* (noc)
- ***Oliguria****—scant amount* (olig) *of urine* (uria); *less than 500 mL in 24 hours*
- ***Polyuria****—abnormally large amounts* (poly) *of urine* (uria)
- ***Urinary frequency****—voiding at frequent intervals*
- ***Urinary incontinence****—the involuntary loss or leakage of urine*
- ***Urinary retention****—the inability to void*
- ***Urinary urgency****—the need to void at once*

BOX 18-1 Rules for Normal Urination

- Practice medical asepsis.
- Follow Standard Precautions and the Bloodborne Pathogen Standard.
- Provide fluids as the nurse and care plan direct.
- Follow the person's voiding routines and habits. Check with the nurse and the care plan.
- Help the person to the bathroom upon request. Or provide the commode, bedpan, or urinal. The need to void may be urgent.
- Help the person assume a normal position for voiding if possible. Women sit or squat. Men stand.
- Warm the bedpan or urinal.
- Cover the person for warmth and privacy.
- Provide for privacy. Pull the curtain around the bed, close room and bathroom doors, and close window coverings. Leave the room if the person can be alone.
- Tell the person that running water, flushing the toilet, or playing music can mask voiding sounds. Voiding with others close by embarrasses some people.
- Stay nearby if the person is weak or unsteady.
- Place the call light and toilet tissue within reach.
- Allow enough time. Do not rush the person.
- Promote relaxation. Some people like to read.
- Run water in a sink if the person cannot start the stream. Or place the person's fingers in warm water.
- Provide perineal care as needed (Chapter 16).
- Assist with hand washing after voiding. Provide a wash basin, soap, washcloth, and towel.
- Assist the person to the bathroom or offer the bedpan, urinal, or commode at regular times. Some people are embarrassed or are too weak to ask for help.

FOCUS ON COMMUNICATION

Normal Urination

Patients and residents may not use "voiding" or "urinating" terms. The person may not understand what you are saying. Do not ask: "Do you need to void?" or "Do you need to urinate?" Instead, ask these questions.

- "Do you need to use the bathroom?"
- "Do you need to use the bedpan (urinal)?"
- "Do you need to pass urine?"
- "Do you need to pass water?"
- "Do you need to pee?"

The word "pee" may offend some persons. Choose words the person understands and uses.

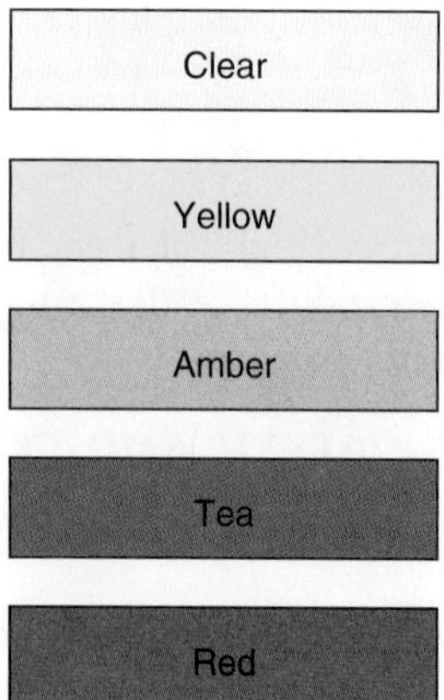

FIGURE 18-1 Color chart for urine.

Bedpans

Bedpans are used for persons who cannot be out of bed. Women use bedpans for voiding and bowel movements (BMs). Men use them for BMs.

The *standard bedpan* is shown in Figure 18-2. The wide rim is placed under the buttocks. A *fracture pan* has a thin rim. It is only about ½-inch deep at one end (see Fig. 18-2). The smaller end is placed under the buttocks (Fig. 18-3). Fracture pans are used:

- By persons with casts
- By persons in traction
- By persons with limited back motion
- After spinal cord injury or surgery
- After a hip fracture or hip replacement surgery

See *Delegation Guidelines: Bedpans.*
See *Promoting Safety and Comfort: Bedpans.*
See procedure: *Giving the Bedpan,* p. 274.

Text continued on p. 276

DELEGATION GUIDELINES

Bedpans

To assist with a bedpan, you need this information from the nurse and the care plan.

- What bedpan to use—standard bedpan or fracture pan
- Position or activity limits
- If you can leave the room or if you need to stay with the person
- If the nurse needs to observe the results before disposing of the contents
- What observations to report and record:
  - Urine color, clarity, and odor
  - Amount
  - Presence of particles
  - Blood in the urine
  - Cloudy urine
  - Complaints of urgency, burning, dysuria, or other problems
  - For bowel movements, see Chapter 19
- When to report observations
- What patient or resident concerns to report at once

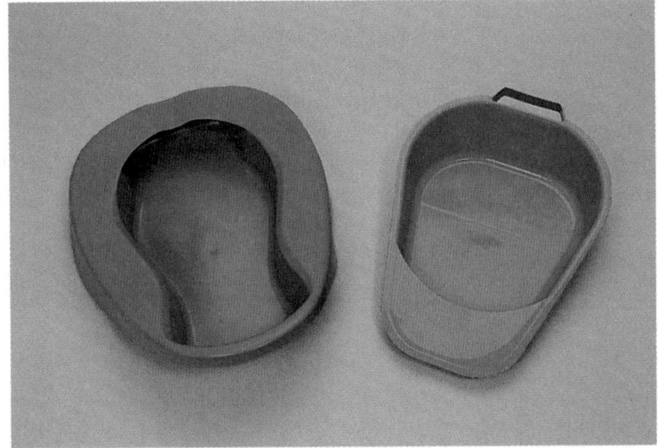

FIGURE 18-2 Standard bedpan *(left)* and the fracture pan *(right).*

PROMOTING SAFETY AND COMFORT

Bedpans

Safety

Remember to raise the bed as needed for good body mechanics. Lower the bed before leaving the room. Raise or lower the bed rails according to the care plan.

Comfort

Some older persons have fragile bones or painful joints. For them, fracture pans are more comfortable.

Most bedpans are made of plastic. Those made of metal are often cold. Warm them with warm water and then dry them before use.

The person must not sit on a bedpan for a long time. Bedpans are uncomfortable. And they can lead to pressure ulcers (Chapter 25).

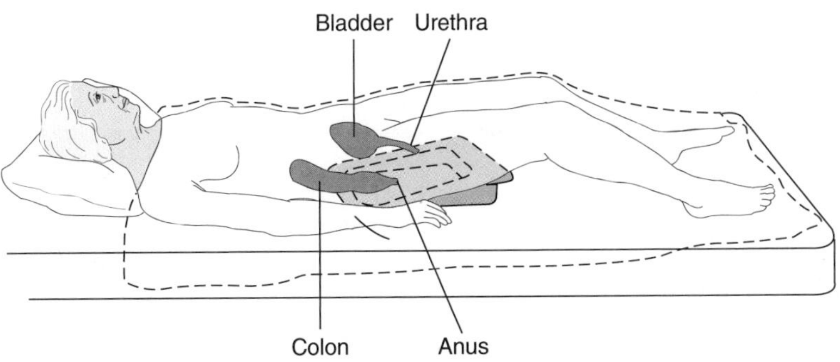

FIGURE 18-3 A person positioned on a fracture pan. The small end is under the buttocks.

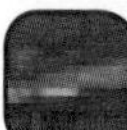

Giving the Bedpan

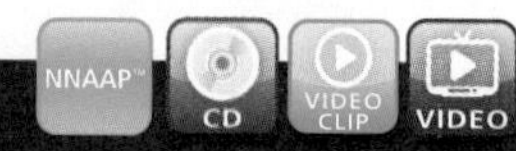

QUALITY OF LIFE

- Knock before entering the person's room.
- Address the person by name.
- Introduce yourself by name and title.
- Explain the procedure before starting and during the procedure.
- Protect the person's rights during the procedure.
- Handle the person gently during the procedure.

PRE-PROCEDURE

1 Follow *Delegation Guidelines: Bedpans,* p. 273. See *Promoting Safety and Comfort:*
   a *Assisting With Urinary Elimination,* p. 271
   b *Bedpans,* p. 273
2 Provide for privacy.
3 Practice hand hygiene.
4 Put on gloves.
5 Collect the following.
   - Bedpan
   - Bedpan cover
   - Toilet tissue
   - Waterproof pad (if required by agency policy)
6 Arrange equipment on the chair or bed.

PROCEDURE

7 Lower the bed rail near you.
8 Lower the head of the bed. Position the person supine. Or raise the head of the bed slightly for the person's comfort.
9 Fold the top linens and gown out of the way. Keep the lower body covered.
10 Ask the person to flex the knees and raise the buttocks by pushing against the mattress with his or her feet.
11 Slide your hand under the lower back. Help raise the buttocks. If using a waterproof pad, place it under the person's buttocks.
12 Slide the bedpan under the person (Fig. 18-4).
13 If the person cannot assist in getting on the bedpan:
   a Place the waterproof pad under the person's buttocks if using one.
   b Turn the person onto the side away from you.
   c Place the bedpan firmly against the buttocks (Fig. 18-5).
   d Hold the bedpan securely. Turn the person onto his or her back.
   e Make sure the bedpan is centered under the person.
14 Cover the person.
15 Raise the head of the bed so the person is in a sitting position (Fowler's position) if the person uses a standard bedpan. (NOTE: Some state competency tests require that you remove gloves and wash your hands before raising the head of the bed.)
16 Make sure the person is correctly positioned on the bedpan (Fig. 18-6).
17 Raise the bed rail if used.
18 Place the toilet tissue and call light within reach. (NOTE: Some state competency tests require that you ask the person to use hand wipes to clean the hands after wiping with toilet tissue.)
19 Ask the person to signal when done or when help is needed.
20 Remove and discard the gloves. Practice hand hygiene.
21 Leave the room and close the door.
22 Return when the person signals. Or check on the person every 5 minutes. Knock before entering.
23 Practice hand hygiene. Put on gloves.
24 Raise the bed for body mechanics. Lower the bed rail (if used) and lower the head of the bed.
25 Ask the person to raise the buttocks. Remove the bedpan. Or hold the bedpan and turn him or her onto the side away from you.
26 Clean the genital area if the person cannot do so. Clean from front (urethra) to back (anus) with toilet tissue. Use fresh tissue for each wipe. Provide perineal care if needed. Remove and discard the waterproof pad if using one.
27 Cover the bedpan. Take it to the bathroom. Raise the bed rail (if used) before leaving the bedside.
28 Note the color, amount, and character of urine or feces.
29 Empty the bedpan contents into the toilet and flush.
30 Rinse the bedpan. Pour the rinse into the toilet and flush.
31 Clean the bedpan with a disinfectant. Pour disinfectant into the toilet and flush.
32 Remove and discard soiled gloves. Practice hand hygiene and put on clean gloves.
33 Return the bedpan and clean cover to the bedside stand.
34 Help the person with hand washing. (Wear gloves for this step.)
35 Remove and discard the gloves. Practice hand hygiene.

POST-PROCEDURE

36 Provide for comfort. (See the inside of the front cover.)
37 Place the call light within reach.
38 Lower the bed to a comfortable and safe level appropriate for the person. Follow the care plan.
39 Raise or lower bed rails. Follow the care plan.
40 Unscreen the person.
41 Complete a safety check of the room. (See the inside of the front cover.)
42 Follow agency policy for soiled linen.
43 Practice hand hygiene.
44 Report and record your observations.

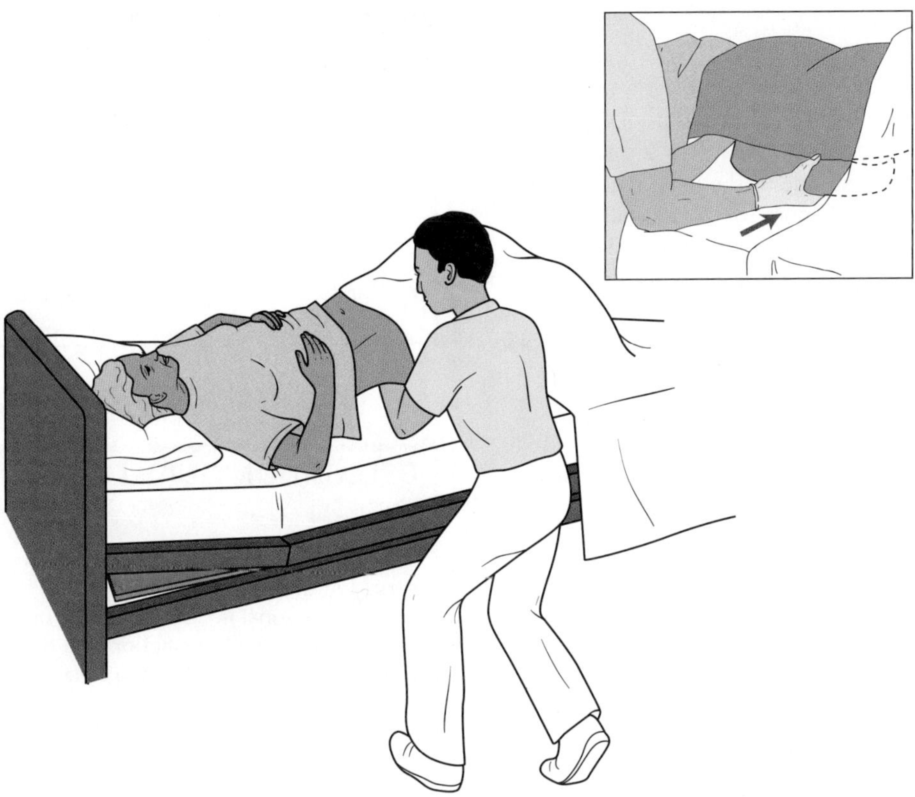

FIGURE 18-4 The person raises the buttocks off the bed with help. The bedpan is slid under the person.

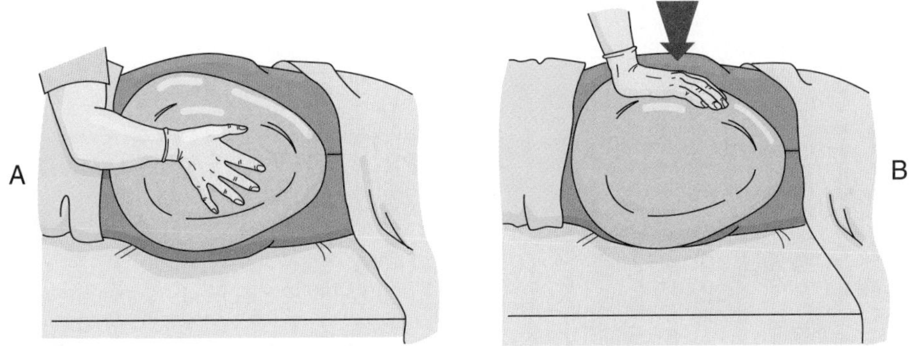

FIGURE 18-5 Giving a bedpan. **A,** Position the person on the side away from you. Place the bedpan firmly against the buttocks. **B,** Push downward on the bedpan and toward the person.

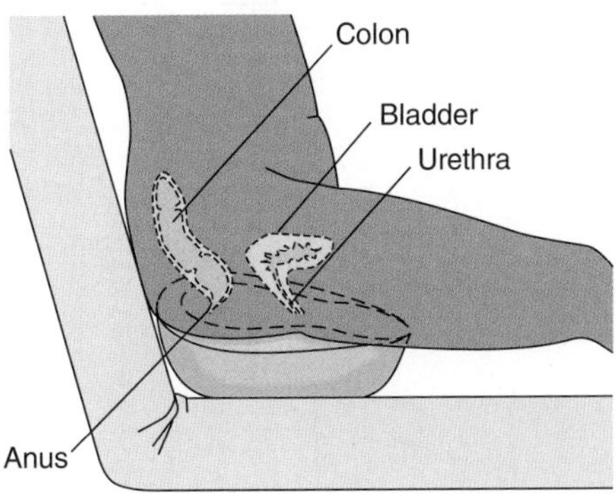

FIGURE 18-6 The person is positioned on the bedpan so the urethra and anus are directly over the opening.

Urinals

Men use urinals to void (Fig. 18-7). Plastic urinals have caps and hook-type handles. The urinal hooks to the bed rail within the man's reach. He stands to use the urinal if possible. Or he sits on the side of the bed or lies in bed to use it. Some men need support when standing. You may have to place and hold the urinal for some men.

After voiding, the urinal cap is closed. This prevents urine spills. Remind men to hang urinals on bed rails and to signal after using them. Remind them not to place urinals on over-bed tables and bedside stands. These surfaces must not be contaminated with urine.

Some beds may not have bed rails. Follow agency policy for where to place urinals.

See *Focus on Communication: Urinals.*

See *Delegation Guidelines: Urinals.*

See *Promoting Safety and Comfort: Urinals.*

See procedure: *Giving the Urinal.*

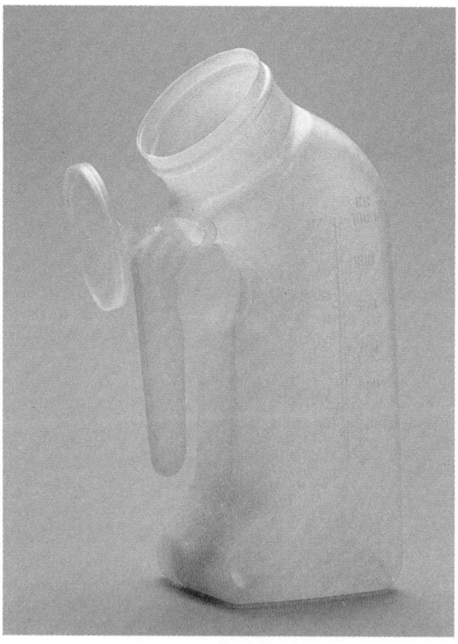

FIGURE 18-7 Male urinal.

FOCUS ON COMMUNICATION

Urinals

Some men cannot use a urinal on their own. You may need to assist them. You may need to stay with the person. For the person's comfort, explain why you must help him. You can say:

- "Mr. Turner, I'll help you use your urinal. I need to stay with you to make sure you don't fall."
- "Mr. Gomez, I'll help you place and remove your urinal so it doesn't spill."

DELEGATION GUIDELINES

Urinals

To assist with urinals, you need this information from the nurse and the care plan.

- How the urinal is used—standing, sitting, or lying in bed.
- If help is needed to place or hold the urinal.
- If the man needs support to stand. If yes, how many staff are needed.
- If you can leave the room or if you need to stay with the person.
- If the nurse needs to observe the urine before its disposal.
- What observations to report and record (see *Delegation Guidelines: Bedpans,* p. 273).
- When to report observations.
- What patient or resident concerns to report at once.

PROMOTING SAFETY AND COMFORT

Urinals

Safety

Empty urinals promptly to prevent odors and the spread of microbes. A filled urinal spills easily, causing hazards. Also, it is an unpleasant sight and a source of odor.

Comfort

You may have to place the urinal for some men. This means placing the penis in the urinal. This may embarrass both the person and you. Always act in a professional manner.

Giving the Urinal

VIDEO

QUALITY OF LIFE

- Knock before entering the person's room.
- Address the person by name.
- Introduce yourself by name and title.
- Explain the procedure before starting and during the procedure.
- Protect the person's rights during the procedure.
- Handle the person gently during the procedure.

PRE-PROCEDURE

1 Follow *Delegation Guidelines: Urinals.* See *Promoting Safety and Comfort:*
   a *Assisting With Urinary Elimination,* p. 271
   b *Urinals*
2 Provide for privacy.
3 Determine if the man will stand, sit, or lie in bed.
4 Practice hand hygiene.
5 Put on gloves.
6 Collect the following.
   - Urinal
   - Non-skid footwear if the man will stand to void

PROCEDURE

7 Give him the urinal if he is in bed. Remind him to tilt the bottom down to prevent spills.
8 If he will stand:
   a Help him sit on the side of the bed.
   b Put non-skid footwear on him.
   c Help him stand. Provide support if he is unsteady.
   d Give him the urinal.
9 Position the urinal if necessary. Place his penis in the urinal if he cannot do so.
10 Place the call light within reach. Ask him to signal when done or when he needs help.
11 Provide for privacy.
12 Remove and discard the gloves. Practice hand hygiene.
13 Leave the room and close the door.
14 Return when he signals for you. Or check on him every 5 minutes. Knock before entering.
15 Practice hand hygiene. Put on gloves.
16 Close the cap on the urinal. Take it to the bathroom.
17 Note the color, amount, and clarity of urine.
18 Empty the urinal into the toilet and flush.
19 Rinse the urinal with cold water. Pour rinse into the toilet and flush.
20 Clean the urinal with a disinfectant. Pour disinfectant into the toilet and flush.
21 Return the urinal to its proper place.
22 Remove and discard the soiled gloves. Practice hand hygiene and put on clean gloves.
23 Assist with hand washing.
24 Remove and discard the gloves. Practice hand hygiene.

POST-PROCEDURE

25 Provide for comfort. Pour disinfectant into the toilet. (See the inside of the front cover.)
26 Place the call light within reach.
27 Raise or lower bed rails. Follow the care plan.
28 Unscreen him.
29 Complete a safety check of the room. (See the inside of the front cover.)
30 Follow agency policy for soiled linen.
31 Practice hand hygiene.
32 Report and record your observations.

Commodes

A commode is a chair or wheelchair with an opening for a container (Fig. 18-8). Persons unable to walk to the bathroom often use commodes. The commode allows a normal position for elimination. The commode arms and back provide support and help prevent falls.

Some commodes are wheeled into bathrooms and placed over toilets. They are useful for persons who need support when sitting. The container is removed if the commode is used with the toilet. Wheels are locked after the commode is in position.

See *Delegation Guidelines: Commodes,* p. 278.
See *Promoting Safety and Comfort: Commodes,* p. 278.
See procedure: *Helping the Person to the Commode,* p. 278.

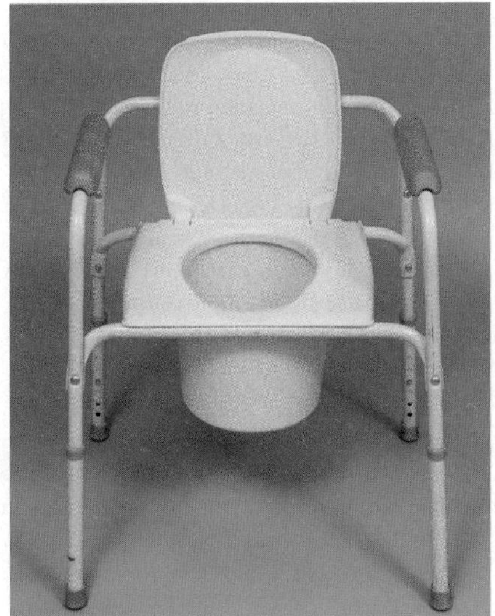

FIGURE 18-8 The commode has a toilet seat with a container. The container slides out from under the seat for emptying.

DELEGATION GUIDELINES

Commodes

You need this information from the nurse and care plan when assisting with commodes.

- If the commode is used at the bedside or over the toilet
- How much help the person needs
- If you can leave the room or if you need to stay with the person
- If the nurse needs to observe urine or BMs
- What observations to report and record (see *Delegation Guidelines: Bedpans,* p. 273)
- When to report observations
- What patient or resident concerns to report at once

PROMOTING SAFETY AND COMFORT

Commodes

Safety

For commode use, transfer the person from the bed, chair, or wheelchair to the commode. Practice safe transfer procedures (Chapter 14). Use the transfer belt and lock the wheels. Remove the transfer belt after the transfer. See "Transfer/Gait Belts" in Chapter 10.

Comfort

After the person transfers to the commode, cover his or her lap and legs with a bath blanket. This promotes warmth and privacy.

Helping the Person to the Commode

VIDEO

QUALITY OF LIFE

- Knock before entering the person's room.
- Address the person by name.
- Introduce yourself by name and title.
- Explain the procedure before starting and during the procedure.
- Protect the person's rights during the procedure.
- Handle the person gently during the procedure.

PRE-PROCEDURE

1 Follow *Delegation Guidelines: Commodes.* See *Promoting Safety and Comfort:*
   a *Assisting with Urinary Elimination,* p. 271
   b *Commodes*
2 Provide for privacy.
3 Practice hand hygiene.
4 Put on gloves.
5 Collect the following.
   - Commode
   - Toilet tissue
   - Bath blanket
   - Transfer belt
   - Robe and non-skid footwear

PROCEDURE

6 Bring the commode next to the bed.
7 Help the person sit on the side of the bed. Lower the bed rail if used.
8 Help him or her put on a robe and non-skid footwear.
9 Apply the transfer belt.
10 Assist the person to the commode. Use the transfer belt.
11 Remove the transfer belt. Cover the person with a bath blanket for warmth.
12 Place the toilet tissue and call light within reach.
13 Ask him or her to signal when done or when help is needed. (Stay with the person if necessary. Be respectful. Provide as much privacy as possible.)
14 Remove and discard the gloves. Practice hand hygiene.
15 Leave the room. Close the door.
16 Return when the person signals. Or check on the person every 5 minutes. Knock before entering.
17 Practice hand hygiene. Put on the gloves.
18 Help the person clean the genital area as needed. Remove and discard the gloves. Practice hand hygiene.
19 Apply the transfer belt. Help the person back to bed using the transfer belt. Remove the transfer belt, robe, and footwear. Raise the bed rail if used.
20 Put on clean gloves. Remove and cover the commode container.
21 Take the container to the bathroom.
22 Observe urine and feces for color, amount, and character.
23 Empty the contents into the toilet and flush.
24 Rinse the container. Pour the rinse into the toilet and flush.
25 Clean and disinfect the container. Pour disinfectant into the toilet and flush.
26 Return the container to the commode. Close the lid on the commode. Clean other parts of the commode if necessary.
27 Return supplies to their proper place.
28 Remove and discard the soiled gloves. Practice hand hygiene and put on clean gloves.
29 Assist with hand washing.
30 Remove and discard the gloves. Practice hand hygiene.

POST-PROCEDURE

31 Provide for comfort. (See the inside of the front cover.)
32 Place the call light within reach.
33 Raise or lower bed rails. Follow the care plan.
34 Unscreen the person.
35 Complete a safety check of the room. (See the inside of the front cover.)
36 Follow agency policy for dirty linen.
37 Practice hand hygiene.
38 Report and record your observations.

URINARY INCONTINENCE

Urinary incontinence is the involuntary loss or leakage of urine. It may be temporary or permanent. The basic types of incontinence are:

- ***Stress incontinence.*** *Urine leaks during exercise and certain movements that cause pressure on the bladder.* Urine loss is small (less than 50 mL). Often called *dribbling,* it occurs with laughing, sneezing, coughing, lifting, or other activities.
- ***Urge incontinence.*** *Urine is lost in response to a sudden, urgent need to void. The person cannot get to a toilet in time.* Urinary frequency, urinary urgency, and night-time voiding are common.
- ***Overflow incontinence.*** *Small amounts of urine leak from a full bladder.* The person feels like the bladder is not empty. The person only dribbles or has a weak urine stream.
- ***Functional incontinence.*** *The person has bladder control but cannot use the toilet in time.* Immobility, restraints, unanswered call lights, no call light within reach, and not knowing where to find the bathroom are causes. So is difficulty removing clothing. Confusion and disorientation are other causes.
- ***Reflex incontinence.*** *Urine is lost at predictable intervals when the bladder is full.* The person does not feel the need to void. Nervous system disorders and injuries are common causes.
- ***Mixed incontinence.*** *The person has a combination of stress incontinence and urge incontinence.* Many older women have this type.
- ***Transient incontinence.*** *This refers to temporary or occasional incontinence that is reversed when the cause is treated. Transient* means *for a short time.*

Sometimes incontinence results from intestinal, rectal, and reproductive system surgeries. It may result from a physical illness or drugs. Some causes can be reversed. Others cannot. If incontinence is a new problem, tell the nurse at once.

See *Focus on Older Persons: Urinary Incontinence.*

Managing Incontinence

The goals of incontinence management are to:

- Prevent urinary tract infections (UTIs).
- Restore as much normal bladder function as possible.

Incontinence is embarrassing. Garments are wet and odors develop. The person is uncomfortable. Skin irritation, infection, and pressure ulcers are risks. Falling is a risk when trying to get to the bathroom quickly. Pride, dignity, and self-esteem are affected. Social isolation, loss of independence, and depression are common. Quality of life suffers.

The person's care plan may include some of the measures listed in Box 18-2. *Good skin care and dry garments and linens are essential.* Promoting normal urinary elimination prevents incontinence in some people (see Box 18-1). Others need bladder training (p. 291). Sometimes catheters are needed (p. 283).

FOCUS ON OLDER PERSONS

Urinary Incontinence

While incontinence occurs in older persons, it is not a normal part of aging. However, older persons are at risk because of changes in the urinary tract, medical and surgical conditions, and drug therapy.

BOX 18-2 Nursing Measures for Urinary Incontinence

- Record the person's voidings—times and amount. This includes incontinent times and successful use of the toilet, commode, bedpan, or urinal.
- Answer call lights promptly. The need to void may be urgent.
- Promote normal urinary elimination (see Box 18-1).
- Promote normal bowel elimination (Chapter 19).
- Assist with elimination after sleep, before and after meals, and at bedtime.
- Follow the person's bladder training program (p. 291).
- Make sure the person has a clear pathway to the bathroom.
- Have the person wear easy-to-remove clothing. Incontinence can occur while dealing with buttons, zippers, other closures, and undergarments.
- Encourage the person to do pelvic muscle exercises as instructed by the nurse.
- Check the person often to make sure he or she is clean and dry.
- Help prevent UTIs.
    - Promote fluid intake as the nurse directs.
    - Have the person wear cotton underwear.
    - Keep the perineal area clean and dry.
- Decrease fluid intake at bedtime.
- Provide good skin care.
- Apply a barrier cream or moisturizer (cream, lotion, paste) as directed by the nurse. The cream prevents irritation and skin damage.
- Provide dry garments and linens.
- Observe for signs of skin breakdown (Chapters 24 and 25).
- Use incontinence products as the nurse directs. Follow the manufacturer's instructions.
- Do not leave urinals in place to catch urine in men who are incontinent.
- Keep the perineal area clean and dry (Chapter 16). Remember to:
    - Use soap and water or a no-rinse incontinence cleanser (perineal rinse). Follow the care plan. If using soap and water, use a safe and comfortable water temperature.
    - Follow Standard Precautions and the Bloodborne Pathogen Standard.
    - Protect the person and dry garments and linen from the wet incontinence product.
    - Expose only the perineal area.
    - Dry the perineal area and buttocks.
    - Remove wet incontinence products, garments, and linen. Apply clean, dry ones.

Incontinence is linked to abuse, mistreatment, and neglect. Frequent care is needed. The person may wet again right after skin care and changing wet garments and linens. Remember, incontinence is beyond the person's control. It is not something the person chooses to do. Be patient. The person's needs are great. If you become short-tempered, talk to the nurse at once. The person has the right to be free from abuse, mistreatment, and neglect. Kindness, empathy, understanding, and patience are needed.

See *Focus on Older Persons: Managing Incontinence.*

See *Focus on Surveys: Managing Incontinence.*

FOCUS ON SURVEYS

Managing Incontinence

Surveyors will observe how incontinence is prevented, improved, or managed. They will observe if staff:

- Follow the person's care plan.
- Keep call lights within reach and answer call lights promptly.
- Provide a clear path to the person's bathroom.
- Provide adequate lighting when the person needs to void.
- Assist with bedpans, urinals, and commodes as needed.
- Assist the person to the bathroom as needed.
- Respond appropriately when incontinence occurs.
- Protect the person's dignity when incontinence occurs.
- Check incontinent persons often.
- Change wet incontinence products and clothing promptly.
- Prevent prolonged exposure of the skin to urine.
- Provide hygiene measures to prevent skin breakdown.

FOCUS ON OLDER PERSONS

Managing Incontinence

Complications from incontinence pose serious problems for older persons. These include falls, pressure ulcers, and UTIs. Long hospital or long-term care stays are often necessary.

Persons with dementia may void in the wrong places. Trash cans, planters, heating vents, and closets are examples. Some persons remove incontinence products and throw them on the floor or in the toilet. Others resist staff efforts to keep them clean and dry.

You must provide safe care. The care plan lists needed measures. The care plan may include these measures recommended by the Alzheimer's Disease Education and Referral Center (ADEAR).

- Follow the person's bathroom routine. For example, take the person to the bathroom every 2 to 3 hours during the day. Do not wait for the person to ask.
- Observe for signs that signal the need to void. Restlessness and pulling at clothes are examples. Respond quickly.
- Stay calm when the person is incontinent. Re-assure the person if he or she becomes upset.
- Tell the nurse when the person is incontinent. Report the time, what the person was doing, and other observations. A pattern may emerge to the person's incontinence. If so, measures are planned to prevent the problem.
- Prevent episodes of incontinence during sleep. Limit the type and amount of fluids in the evening. Follow the care plan.
- Plan ahead if the person will leave the agency. Have the person wear clothing that is easy to remove. Pack incontinence products and an extra set of clothing. Know where to find restrooms.

You may need a co-worker's help to keep the person clean and dry. If you have questions, ask the nurse for help.

Remember, everyone has the right to privacy and safe care. They also have the right to be treated with dignity.

Applying Incontinence Products

Incontinence products help keep the person dry. They usually have 2 layers and a waterproof back. Fluid passes through the first layer. It is absorbed by the lower layer. Common incontinence products are shown in Figure 18-9. The nurse helps the person select products to meet his or her needs.

See *Focus on Communication: Applying Incontinence Products.*

See *Delegation Guidelines: Applying Incontinence Products.*

See *Promoting Safety and Comfort: Applying Incontinence Products.*

See procedure: *Applying an Incontinence Brief,* p. 282.

FOCUS ON COMMUNICATION

Applying Incontinence Products

Incontinence products are often called "adult diapers." The word "diaper" may offend the person or lower self-esteem. Instead, say: "brief," "pad," or "underwear." Some persons prefer the brand name of the product they use. Use a term that promotes dignity and self-esteem.

A
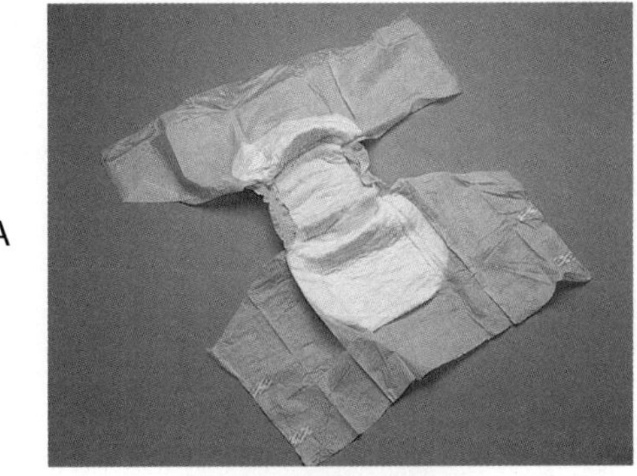

B
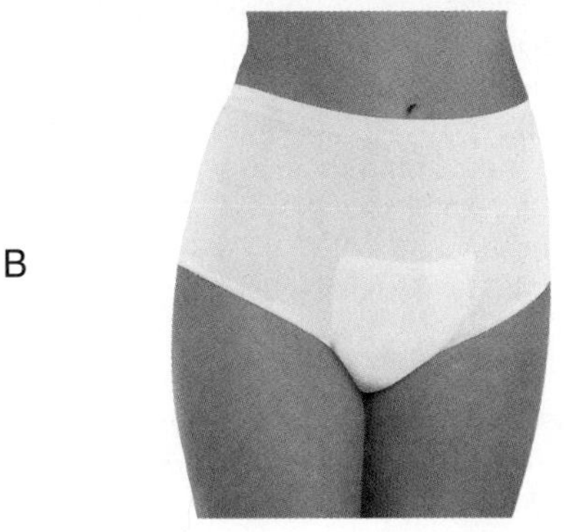

C
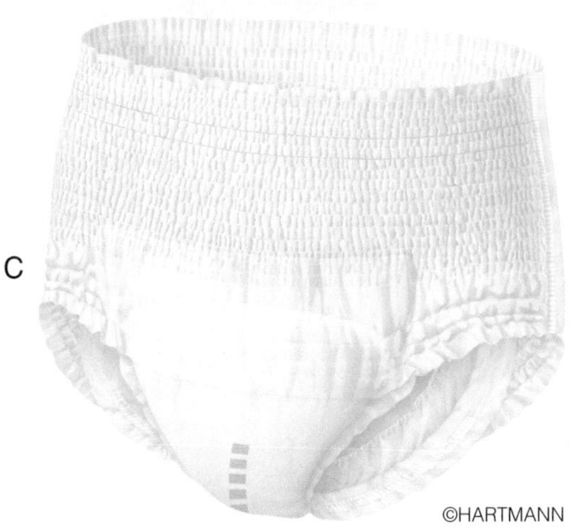

D
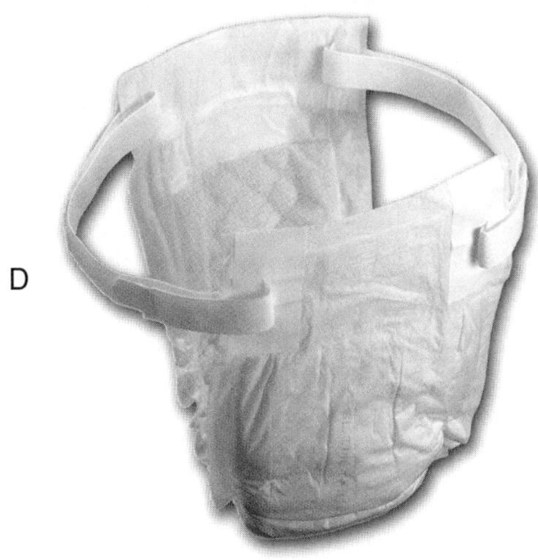

FIGURE 18-9 Disposable incontinence products. **A,** Complete incontinence brief. **B,** Pad and undergarment. **C,** Pull-on underwear. **D,** Belted undergarment.

DELEGATION GUIDELINES

Applying Incontinence Products

To apply an incontinence product, you need this information from the nurse and the care plan.

- What product to use.
- What size to use.
- If you need to apply a barrier cream. If yes, what cream to use.
- What observations to report and record:
  - Complaints of pain, burning, irritation, or the need to void
  - Signs and symptoms of skin breakdown: redness, irritation, blisters, and complaints of pain, burning, tingling, or itching
  - The amount of urine—small, moderate, large
  - Urine color
  - Blood in the urine
  - Leakage
  - A poor product fit
- When to report observations.
- What patient or resident concerns to report at once.

PROMOTING SAFETY AND COMFORT

Applying Incontinence Products

Safety

To safely apply an incontinence product, follow the manufacturer's instructions. The guidelines in Box 18-3 will help prevent:

- Leakage
- Skin irritation and blisters
- Tearing

Comfort

For the person's comfort, always use the correct size. If the product is too large, urine can leak. If too small, the product will cause discomfort from being too tight.

BOX 18-3 Applying Incontinence Products

- Follow the manufacturer's instructions.
- Use the correct size. The nurse measures the person's hips and thighs. The largest measurement is used for the correct size.
- Note the front and back of the product.
- Center the product in the perineal area.
- Position the man's penis downward.
- Check for proper placement. The product should be in the creases between the thighs and the perineal area (groin area). It should fit the shape of the body.
- Note the amount of urine (small, moderate, large). Also note how often you change the product. An extended wear product may be needed for large amounts of urine or diarrhea (Chapter 19).
- Do not let the plastic backing touch the person's skin.
- Provide perineal care after each incontinent episode.
- Do not use the product as a turning or lift sheet.

Applying an Incontinence Brief

QUALITY OF LIFE

- Knock before entering the person's room.
- Address the person by name.
- Introduce yourself by name and title.
- Explain the procedure before starting and during the procedure.
- Protect the person's rights during the procedure.
- Handle the person gently during the procedure.

PRE-PROCEDURE

1 Follow *Delegation Guidelines: Applying Incontinence Products,* p. 281. See *Promoting Safety and Comfort:*
  a *Assisting With Urinary Elimination,* p. 271
  b *Applying Incontinence Products,* p. 281
2 Practice hand hygiene.
3 Collect the following.
  - Incontinence brief
  - Barrier cream as directed by the nurse
  - Cleanser
  - Items for perineal care (Chapter 16)
  - Paper towels
  - Trash bag
  - Gloves
4 Cover the over-bed table with paper towels. Arrange items on top of them.
5 Identify the person. Check the ID (identification) bracelet against the assignment sheet. Also call the person by name.
6 Provide for privacy.
7 Fill the wash basin. Water temperature is usually 105°F to 109°F (Fahrenheit) (40.5°C to 42.7°C [centigrade]). Measure water temperature according to agency policy. Ask the person to check the water temperature. Adjust water temperature as needed.
8 Raise the bed for body mechanics. Bed rails are up if used.

PROCEDURE

9 Lower the head of the bed. The bed is as flat as possible.
10 Lower the bed rail near you if up.
11 Practice hand hygiene. Put on the gloves.
12 Cover the person with a bath blanket. Lower top linens to the foot of the bed.
13 Place a waterproof pad under the buttocks. Ask the person to raise the buttocks off the bed. Or turn the person from side to side.
14 Loosen the tabs on each side of the product.
15 Turn the person onto the side away from you.
16 Remove the product from front to back. Observe the urine as you roll the product up (Fig. 18-10, *A*).
17 Place the product in the trash bag. Set the bag aside.
18 Perform perineal care (Chapter 16) wearing clean gloves.
19 Open the new brief. Fold it in half length-wise along the center (Fig. 18-10, *B*).
20 Insert the product between the legs from front to back (Fig. 18-10, *C*).
21 Unfold and spread the back panel (Fig. 18-10, *D*).
22 Center the product in the perineal area.
23 Turn the person onto his or her back.
24 Unfold and spread the front panel. Provide a "cup" shape in the perineal area. For a man, position the penis downward.
25 Make sure the product is positioned high in the groin folds. This allows the product to fit the shape of the body.
26 Secure the product (Fig. 18-10, *E*).
  a Pull the lower tape tab forward on the side near you. Attach it at a slightly upward angle. Do the same for the other side.
  b Pull the upper tape tab forward on the side near you. Attach it in a horizontal manner. Do the same for the other side.
27 Smooth out all wrinkles and folds.
28 Remove and discard the gloves. Practice hand hygiene.

POST-PROCEDURE

29 Provide for comfort. (See the inside of the front cover.)
30 Place the call light within reach.
31 Lower the bed to a comfortable and safe level appropriate for the person. Follow the care plan.
32 Raise or lower bed rails. Follow the care plan.
33 Unscreen the person.
34 Practice hand hygiene. Put on clean gloves.
35 Estimate the amount of urine in the old product: small, moderate, large. Open the product to observe for urine color and blood.
36 Clean, rinse, dry, and return the wash basin and other equipment. Return items to their proper place.
37 Remove and discard the gloves. Practice hand hygiene.
38 Complete a safety check of the room. (See the inside of the front cover.)
39 Report and record your observations.

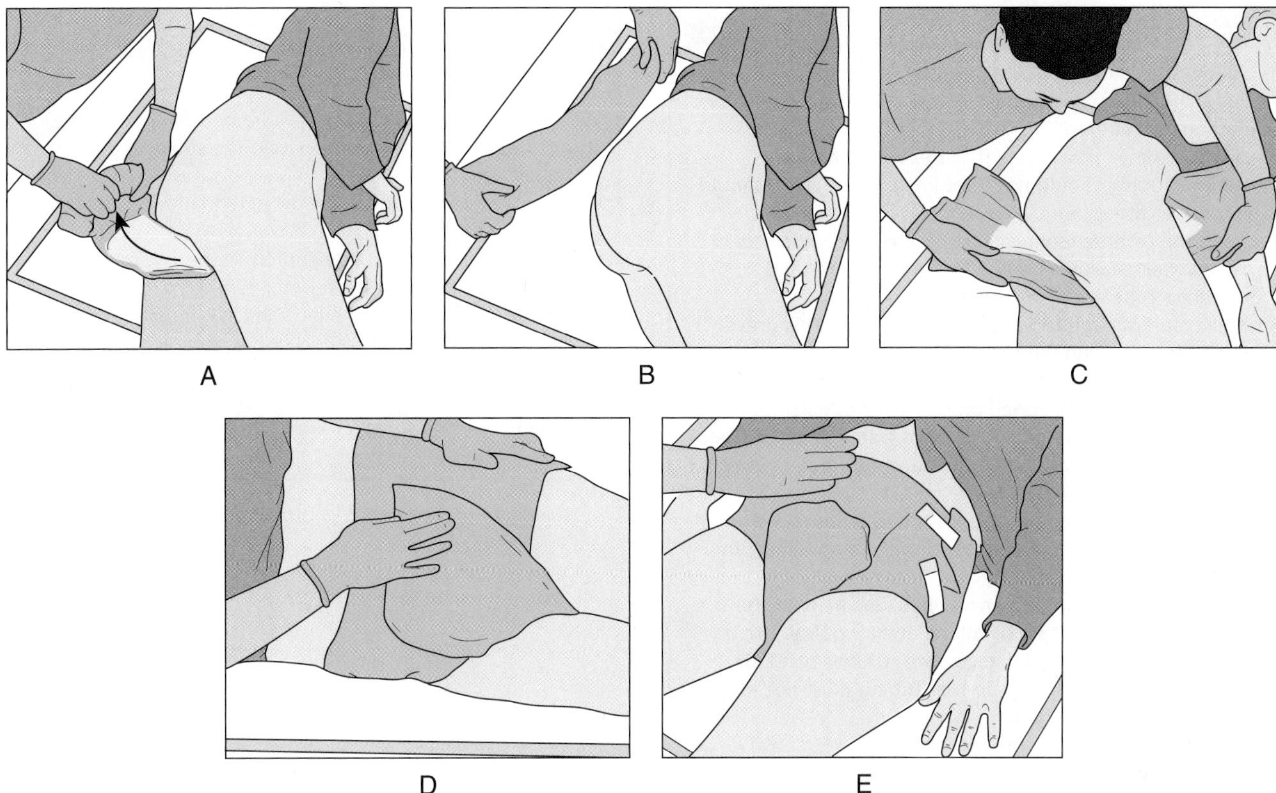

FIGURE 18-10 Applying an incontinence brief. **A,** The product is removed from front to back. **B,** The new product is opened length-wise. **C,** The product is inserted length-wise between the legs from front to back. **D,** The back panel is spread open. **E,** The lower tape tab is attached at a slightly upward angle. The upper tape tab is attached in a horizontal manner.

CATHETERS

A ***catheter*** *is a tube used to drain or inject fluid through a body opening.* Inserted through the urethra into the bladder, a urinary catheter drains urine. An *indwelling catheter* (*retention* or *Foley catheter*) is left in the bladder (Fig. 18-11). Urine drains constantly into a drainage bag. Tubing connects the catheter to the drainage bag.

Catheterization is the process of inserting a catheter. It is done by a doctor or nurse. With proper education and supervision, some states and agencies let nursing assistants insert and remove catheters.

Some people are too weak or disabled to use the bedpan, urinal, commode, or toilet. For them, catheters can promote comfort and prevent incontinence. Catheters can protect wounds and pressure ulcers from contact with urine. They also allow hourly urinary output measurements. However, they are a last resort for incontinence. Catheters do not treat the cause of incontinence.

Persons with catheters are at risk for UTIs. Follow the rules in Box 18-4, p. 284.

See *Focus on Surveys: Catheters*, p. 284.

See *Delegation Guidelines: Catheters*, p. 285.

See *Promoting Safety and Comfort: Catheters*, p. 285.

See procedure: *Giving Catheter Care*, p. 285.

Text continued on p. 287

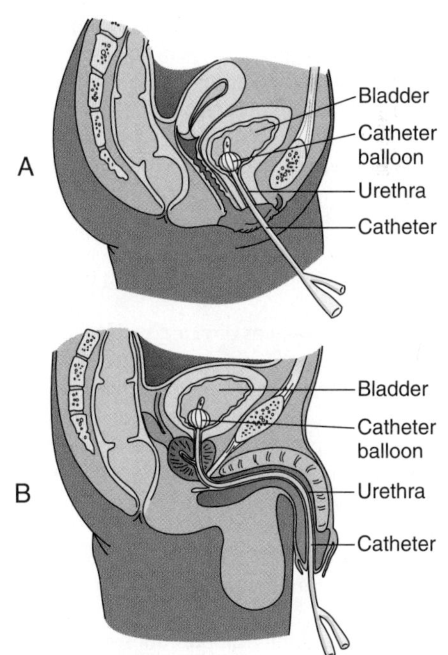

FIGURE 18-11 Indwelling catheter. **A,** Indwelling catheter is in the female bladder. The inflated balloon at the tip prevents the catheter from slipping out through the urethra. **B,** Indwelling catheter with the balloon inflated is in the male bladder.

BOX 18-4 Indwelling Catheter Care

- Follow the rules of medical asepsis.
- Follow Standard Precautions and the Bloodborne Pathogen Standard.
- Allow urine to flow freely through the catheter or tubing. Tubing should not have kinks. The person should not lie on the tubing.
- Keep the catheter connected to the drainage tubing. Follow the measures on p. 287 if the catheter and drainage tube are disconnected.
- Keep the drainage tube below the bladder. This prevents urine from flowing backward into the bladder.
- Move the bag to the other side of the bed when the person is turned and re-positioned on his or her other side.
- Attach the drainage bag to the bed frame, back of the chair, or lower part of the IV (intravenous) pole. *Never attach the drainage bag to the bed rail.* Otherwise it is higher than the bladder when the bed rail is raised.
- Do not let the drainage bag rest on the floor. This can contaminate the system.
- Coil the drainage tubing on the bed. Secure it to the bottom linens (Fig. 18-12). Follow agency policy. Use a clip, bed sheet clamp, tape, pin with rubber band, or other device as the nurse directs. Tubing must not loop below the drainage bag.
- Secure the catheter to the inner thigh (see Fig. 18-12). Or secure it to the man's abdomen. This prevents excess catheter movement and friction at the insertion site. Secure the catheter with a tube holder, tape, or other device as the nurse directs.
- Check for leaks. Check the site where the catheter connects to the drainage bag. Report any leaks to the nurse at once.
- Provide perineal care and catheter care according to the care plan—daily, twice a day, after BMs, or when vaginal discharge is present. (See procedure: *Giving Catheter Care.*)
- Empty the drainage bag at the end of the shift or as the nurse directs. Measure and record the amount of urine (see procedure: *Emptying a Urinary Drainage Bag,* p. 288). Report an increase or decrease in the amount of urine.
- Use a separate measuring container for each person. This prevents the spread of microbes from 1 person to another.
- Do not let the drain on the drainage bag touch any surface.
- Encourage fluid intake as directed by the nurse and the care plan.
- Report complaints at once—pain, burning, the need to void, or irritation. Also report the color, clarity, and odor of urine and the presence of particles or blood.
- Observe for signs and symptoms of a UTI. Report the following at once.
  - Fever.
  - Chills.
  - Flank pain or tenderness. The flank area is in the back between the ribs and the hip.
  - Change in the urine—blood, foul smell, particles, cloudiness, oliguria.
  - Change in mental or functional status—confusion, decreased appetite, falls, decreased activity, tiredness, and so on.
  - Urine leakage around the catheter.

FOCUS ON SURVEYS

Catheters

Surveys are done to determine if the person is receiving appropriate treatment and services. The surveyor may ask you questions about:

- Your understanding of the person's bladder management program
- Your training related to handling catheters, catheter tubing, drainage bags, catheter care, UTIs, catheter-related injuries, dislodgment, and skin breakdown
- What observations to report, when to report them, and to whom you should report observations

Answer questions the best you can. If you do not know an answer, tell the surveyor who you would ask or where you would find the answer.

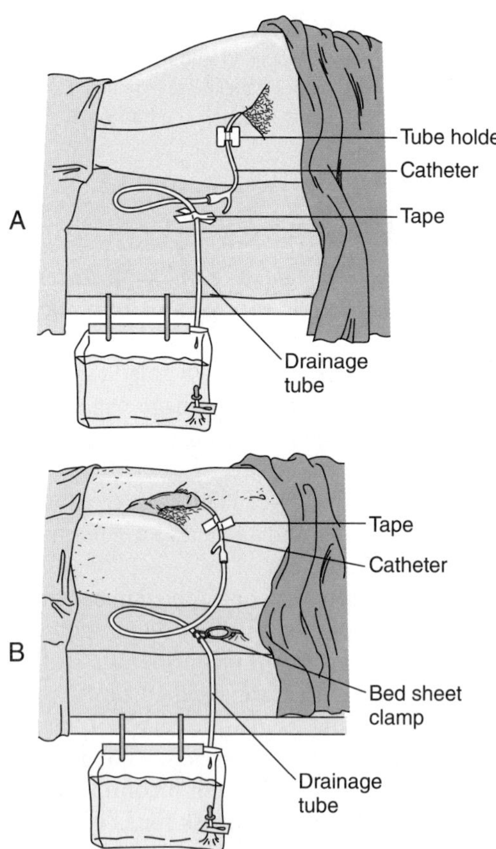

FIGURE 18-12 Securing catheters. **A,** The catheter is secured to the inner thigh with a tube holder. The drainage tube is coiled on the bed and secured to bottom linens with tape. **B,** The catheter is secured to the man's abdomen with tape. Drainage tubing is secured to bottom linens with a bed sheet clamp.

DELEGATION GUIDELINES

Catheters

The nurse may delegate catheter care to you. If so, you need this information from the nurse and the care plan.

- When to give catheter care—daily, twice a day, after BMs, or when vaginal discharge is present
- What water temperature to use for perineal care
- Where to secure the catheter—inner thigh or abdomen
- How to secure the catheter—tube holder, tape, or other device
- How to secure drainage tubing—clip, bed sheet clamp, tape, safety pin with rubber band, or other device
- What observations to report and record:
  - Complaints of pain, burning, irritation, or the need to void (report at once)
  - Crusting, abnormal drainage, or secretions
  - The color, clarity, and odor of urine
  - Particles in the urine
  - Blood in the urine
  - Cloudy urine
  - Urine leaking at the insertion site
  - Drainage system leaks
- When to report observations
- What patient or resident concerns to report at once

PROMOTING SAFETY AND COMFORT

Catheters

Safety

Use caution if using a safety pin and rubber band to secure the drainage tubing to the bottom linens.

- Check the safety pin and rubber band.
  - The safety pin must work properly. It must not be stretched out of shape.
  - The rubber band must be intact. It must not be frayed or over-stretched.
- Do not insert the pin through the catheter.
- Point the pin away from the person.

Comfort

The catheter must not pull at the insertion site. This causes discomfort and irritation. Hold the catheter securely during catheter care. Then properly secure the catheter. Make sure the tubing is not under the person. Besides obstructing urine flow, lying on the tubing is uncomfortable. It can also cause skin breakdown. To promote comfort, see Box 18-4.

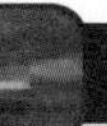

Giving Catheter Care

NNAAP™ CD VIDEO CLIP VIDEO

QUALITY OF LIFE

- Knock before entering the person's room.
- Address the person by name.
- Introduce yourself by name and title.
- Explain the procedure before starting and during the procedure.
- Protect the person's rights during the procedure.
- Handle the person gently during the procedure.

PRE-PROCEDURE

1 Follow *Delegation Guidelines:*
  a *Perineal Care* (Chapter 16)
  b *Catheters*
  See *Promoting Safety and Comfort:*
  a *Perineal Care* (Chapter 16)
  b *Assisting With Urinary Elimination,* p. 271
  c *Catheters*
2 Practice hand hygiene.
3 Collect the following.
  - Items for perineal care (Chapter 16)
  - Gloves
  - Bath blanket
4 Cover the over-bed table with paper towels. Arrange items on top of them.
5 Identify the person. Check the ID bracelet against the assignment sheet. Call the person by name.
6 Provide for privacy.
7 Fill the wash basin. Water temperature is usually 105°F to 109°F (40.5°C to 42.7°C). Measure water temperature according to agency policy. Ask the person to check the water temperature. Adjust water temperature as needed.
8 Raise the bed for body mechanics. Bed rails are up if used.
9 Lower the bed rail near you if up.

PROCEDURE

10 Practice hand hygiene. Put on the gloves.
11 Cover the person with a bath blanket. Fan-fold top linens to the foot of the bed.
12 Drape the person for perineal care (Chapter 16).
13 Fold back the bath blanket to expose the perineal area.
14 Ask the person to flex the knees and raise the buttocks off the bed. Place the waterproof pad under the buttocks. Have the person lower the buttocks.
15 Separate the labia (female). In an uncircumcised male, retract the foreskin (Chapter 16). Check for crusts, abnormal drainage, or secretions.
16 Give perineal care (Chapter 16) wearing clean gloves. Keep the foreskin of the uncircumcised male retracted until step 22.
17 Apply soap to a clean, wet washcloth.
18 Hold the catheter at the meatus. Do so for steps 19, 20, and 21.

Continued

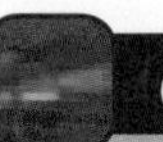

Giving Catheter Care—cont'd

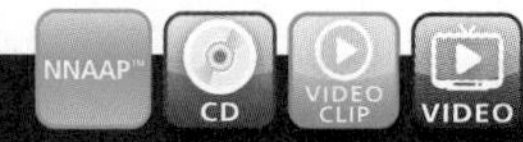

PROCEDURE—cont'd

19 Clean the catheter from the meatus down the catheter at least 4 inches (Fig. 18-13). Clean downward, away from the meatus with 1 stroke. Do not tug or pull on the catheter. Repeat as needed with a clean area of the washcloth. Use a clean washcloth if needed.
20 Rinse the catheter with a clean washcloth. Rinse from the meatus down the catheter at least 4 inches. Rinse downward, away from the meatus with 1 stroke. Do not tug or pull on the catheter. Repeat as needed with a clean area of the washcloth. Use a clean washcloth if needed.
21 Dry the catheter with a towel. Dry from the meatus down the catheter at least 4 inches. Do not tug or pull on the catheter.
22 Return the foreskin to its natural position.
23 Pat dry the perineal area. Dry from front to back.
24 Secure the catheter. Coil and secure tubing (see Fig. 18-12).
25 Remove the waterproof pad.
26 Cover the person. Remove the bath blanket.
27 Remove and discard the gloves. Practice hand hygiene.

POST-PROCEDURE

28 Provide for comfort. (See the inside of the front cover.)
29 Place the call light within reach.
30 Lower the bed to a comfortable and safe level appropriate for the person. Follow the care plan.
31 Raise or lower bed rails. Follow the care plan.
32 Clean, rinse, dry, and return equipment to its proper place. Discard disposable items. (Wear gloves for this step.)
33 Unscreen the person.
34 Complete a safety check of the room. (See the inside of the front cover.)
35 Follow agency policy for soiled linen.
36 Remove and discard the gloves. Practice hand hygiene.
37 Report and record your observations.

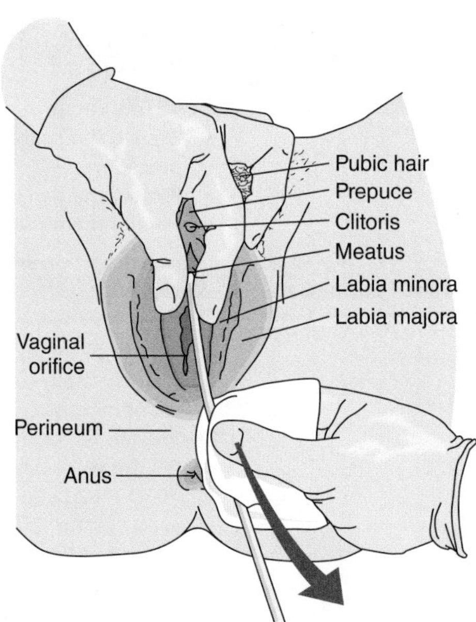

FIGURE 18-13 The catheter is cleaned starting at the meatus. At least 4 inches of the catheter are cleaned.

Drainage Systems

A closed drainage system is used for indwelling catheters. Only urine should enter the drainage bag. The urinary system is sterile. Infection can occur if microbes enter the drainage system. The microbes travel up the tubing or catheter into the bladder and kidneys. A UTI can threaten health and life.

There are 2 types of drainage bags. Follow the care measures for drainage systems in Box 18-5.

- *Leg bags* attach to the thigh or calf with elastic bands (p. 289). The bag holds less than 1000 mL of urine.
- *Standard drainage bags* usually hold at least 2000 mL of urine.

See *Delegation Guidelines: Drainage Systems.*
See *Promoting Safety and Comfort: Drainage Systems.*
See procedure: *Emptying a Urinary Drainage Bag*, p. 288.

BOX 18-5 Drainage Systems

- Hang the bag from the bed frame, chair, or wheelchair. It must not touch the floor.
- Keep the bag lower than the person's bladder (see Fig. 18-12). Microbes can grow in urine. If the drainage bag is higher than the bladder, urine can flow back into the bladder. A UTI can occur.
- *Do not hang the drainage bag on a bed rail.* When the bed rail is raised, the bag is higher than bladder level.
- Hold the bag lower than the bladder when the person walks.
- Tell the nurse at once if the drainage system becomes disconnected. Do not touch the ends of the catheter or tubing. Do the following.
  1. Practice hand hygiene. Put on gloves.
  2. Wipe the end of the tube with an antiseptic wipe.
  3. Wipe the end of the catheter with another antiseptic wipe.
  4. Do not put the ends down. Do not touch the ends after you clean them.
  5. Connect the tubing to the catheter.
  6. Discard the wipes into a biohazard bag.
  7. Remove the gloves. Practice hand hygiene.
- Change a leg bag to a standard drainage bag when the person is in bed. Prevent microbes from entering the system when you open the closed drainage system.
- Empty drainage bags and measure urine:
  - At the end of every shift
  - When changing from a leg bag to a standard drainage bag
  - When changing from a standard drainage bag to a leg bag
  - When the bag is becoming full

DELEGATION GUIDELINES

Drainage Systems

Delegated tasks may involve urinary drainage systems. If so, you need this information from the nurse and the care plan.

- When to empty the drainage bag
- If the person uses a leg bag
- When to switch a standard drainage bag and leg bag
- If you should clean or discard the drainage bag
- What observations to report and record:
  - The amount of urine measured
  - The color, clarity, and odor of urine
  - Particles in the urine
  - Blood in the urine
  - Cloudy urine
  - Complaints of pain, burning, irritation, or the need to urinate
  - Drainage system leaks
- When to report observations
- What patient or resident concerns to report at once

PROMOTING SAFETY AND COMFORT

Drainage Systems

Safety

Leg bags fill faster than standard drainage bags. Check leg bags often. Empty the leg bag if it is becoming half full. Measure, report, and record the amount of urine.

Comfort

Urine in a drainage bag embarrasses some people. Visitors can see the urine. To promote mental comfort, have visitors sit on the side away from the drainage bag. Sometimes you can empty the bag before visitors arrive. Make sure you measure, report, and record the amount of urine.

Some agencies have drainage bag holders. The drainage bag is placed inside the holder. Urine cannot be seen.

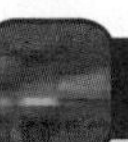

Emptying a Urinary Drainage Bag

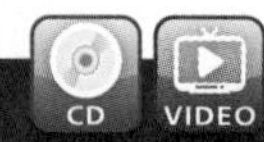

QUALITY OF LIFE

- Knock before entering the person's room.
- Address the person by name.
- Introduce yourself by name and title.
- Explain the procedure before starting and during the procedure.
- Protect the person's rights during the procedure.
- Handle the person gently during the procedure.

PRE-PROCEDURE

1 Follow *Delegation Guidelines: Drainage Systems,* p. 287. See *Promoting Safety and Comfort:*
  a *Assisting With Urinary Elimination,* p. 271
  b *Drainage Systems,* p. 287
2 Collect the following.
  - Graduate (measuring container)
  - Gloves
  - Paper towels
  - Antiseptic wipes
3 Practice hand hygiene.
4 Identify the person. Check the ID bracelet against the assignment sheet. Call the person by name.
5 Provide for privacy.

PROCEDURE

6 Put on the gloves.
7 Place a paper towel on the floor. Place the graduate on top of it.
8 Position the graduate under the collection bag.
9 Open the clamp on the drain.
10 Let all urine drain into the graduate. Do not let the drain touch the graduate (Fig. 18-14).
11 Clean the end of the drain with an antiseptic wipe.
12 Close and position the clamp (Fig. 18-15).
13 Measure urine. See procedure: *Measuring Intake and Output* in Chapter 21.
14 Remove and discard the paper towel.
15 Empty the contents of the graduate into the toilet and flush.
16 Rinse the graduate. Empty the rinse into the toilet and flush.
17 Clean and disinfect the graduate.
18 Return the graduate to its proper place.
19 Remove and discard the gloves. Practice hand hygiene.
20 Record the time and amount of urine on the intake and output (I&O) record (Chapter 21).

POST-PROCEDURE

21 Provide for comfort. (See the inside of the front cover.)
22 Place the call light within reach.
23 Unscreen the person.
24 Complete a safety check of the room. (See the inside of the front cover.)
25 Report and record the amount of urine and other observations.

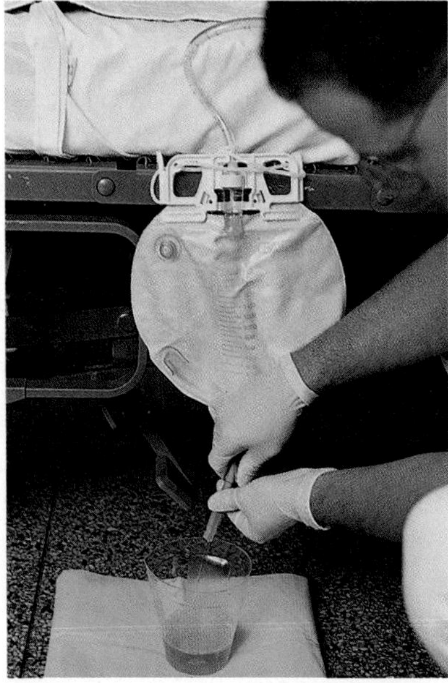

FIGURE 18-14 The clamp on the drainage bag is opened. The drain is directed into the graduate. The drain must not touch the inside of the graduate.

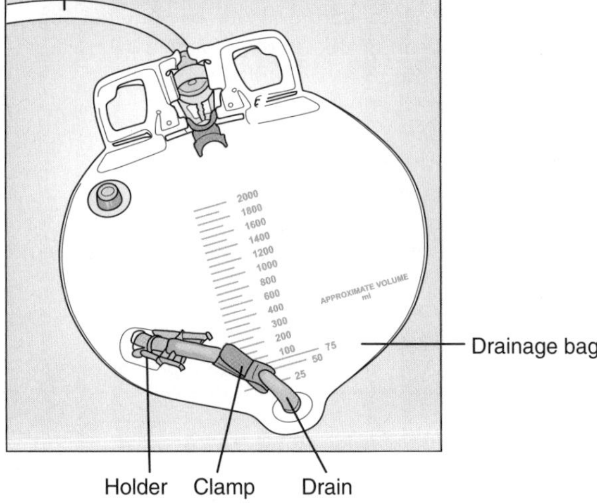

FIGURE 18-15 The clamp is closed and positioned in the holder on the drainage bag.

Condom Catheters

Condom catheters are common for incontinent men. They also are called *external catheters*, *Texas catheters*, and *urinary sheaths*. A condom catheter is a soft sheath that slides over the penis. Tubing connects the condom catheter to the drainage bag. Many men prefer leg bags (Fig. 18-16).

Condom catheters are changed daily after perineal care. To apply one, follow the manufacturer's instructions. Thoroughly wash the penis with soap and water. Then dry it before applying the catheter.

Some condom catheters are self-adhering. Adhesive inside the catheter adheres to the penis. Other catheters are secured with elastic tape. Use the elastic tape packaged with the catheter. This allows blood flow to the penis. *Only use elastic tape. Never use adhesive tape or other tape to secure catheters. They do not expand. Blood flow to the penis is cut off, injuring the penis.*

See *Delegation Guidelines: Condom Catheters.*

See *Promoting Safety and Comfort: Condom Catheters.*

See procedure: *Applying a Condom Catheter*, p. 290.

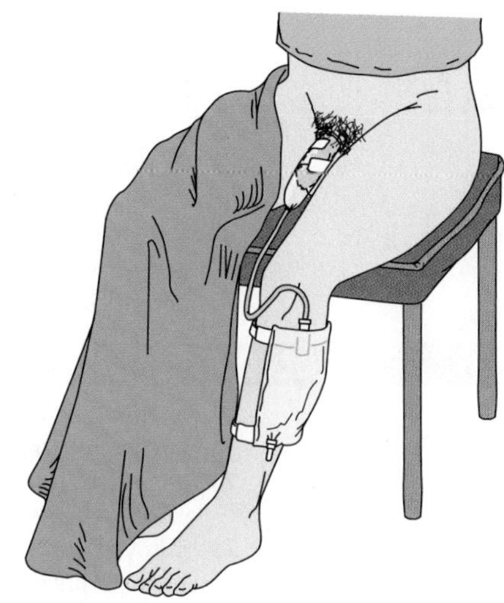

FIGURE 18-16 Condom catheter attached to a leg bag.

DELEGATION GUIDELINES

Condom Catheters

To remove or apply a condom catheter, you need this information from the nurse and the care plan.

- What size to use—small, medium, or large
- When to remove the catheter and apply a new one
- If a leg bag or standard drainage bag is used
- What water temperature to use for perineal care
- What observations to report and record:
  - Reddened or open areas on the penis
  - Swelling of the penis
  - Color, clarity, and odor of urine
  - Particles in the urine
  - Blood in the urine
  - Cloudy urine
- When to report observations
- What patient or resident concerns to report at once

PROMOTING SAFETY AND COMFORT

Condom Catheters

Safety

Do not apply a condom catheter if the penis is red, irritated, or shows signs of skin breakdown. Report your observations at once.

If you do not know how to use your agency's condom catheters, ask the nurse to show you the correct application. Then ask the nurse to observe you applying the catheter.

Blood must flow to the penis. If tape is needed, use the elastic tape packaged with the catheter. Apply it in a spiral.

Comfort

To apply a condom catheter, you need to touch and handle the penis. This can embarrass the man. Some men become sexually aroused. Always act in a professional manner. If necessary, allow the man privacy. Provide for safety and place the urinal within reach. Tell him when you will return and then leave the room. Or ask him to use the call light when ready for you to finish the procedure. Knock before entering the room again.

Applying a Condom Catheter

QUALITY OF LIFE

- Knock before entering the person's room.
- Address the person by name.
- Introduce yourself by name and title.
- Explain the procedure before starting and during the procedure.
- Protect the person's rights during the procedure.
- Handle the person gently during the procedure.

PRE-PROCEDURE

1 Follow *Delegation Guidelines:*
  a *Perineal Care* (Chapter 16)
  b *Condom Catheters,* p. 289
  See *Promoting Safety and Comfort:*
  a *Perineal Care* (Chapter 16)
  b *Assisting With Urinary Elimination,* p. 271
  c *Condom Catheters,* p. 289
2 Practice hand hygiene.
3 Collect the following.
  - Condom catheter
  - Elastic tape
  - Standard drainage bag or leg bag
  - Cap for the drainage bag
  - Bath basin
  - Soap
  - Towel and washcloths
  - Bath blanket
  - Gloves
  - Waterproof pad
  - Paper towels
4 Cover the over-bed table with paper towels. Arrange items on top of them.
5 Identify the person. Check the ID bracelet against the assignment sheet. Also call the person by name.
6 Provide for privacy.
7 Fill the wash basin. Water temperature is usually 105°F to 109°F (40.5°C to 42.7°C). Measure water temperature according to agency policy. Ask the person to check the water temperature. Adjust water temperature as needed.
8 Raise the bed for body mechanics. Bed rails are up if used.

PROCEDURE

9 Lower the bed rail near you if up.
10 Practice hand hygiene. Put on the gloves.
11 Cover the person with a bath blanket. Lower top linens to the knees.
12 Ask the person to raise his buttocks off the bed. Or turn him onto his side away from you.
13 Slide the waterproof pad under his buttocks.
14 Have the person lower his buttocks. Or turn him onto his back.
15 Secure the drainage bag to the bed frame. Or have a leg bag ready. Close the drain.
16 Expose the genital area.
17 Remove the condom catheter.
  a Remove the tape. Roll the sheath off the penis.
  b Disconnect the drainage tubing from the condom. Cap the drainage tube.
  c Discard the tape and condom.
18 Provide perineal care (Chapter 16) wearing clean gloves. Observe the penis for reddened areas, skin breakdown, and irritation.
19 Remove and discard the gloves. Practice hand hygiene. Put on clean gloves.
20 Remove the protective backing from the condom. This exposes the adhesive strip.
21 Hold the penis firmly. Roll the condom onto the penis. Leave a 1-inch space between the penis and the end of the catheter (Fig. 18-17).
22 Secure the condom.
  a *For a self-adhering condom:* press the condom to the penis.
  b *For a condom secured with elastic tape:* apply elastic tape in a spiral. See Figure 18-17. Do not apply tape completely around the penis.
23 Make sure the penis tip does not touch the condom. Make sure the condom is not twisted.
24 Connect the condom to the drainage tubing. Coil and secure excess tubing on the bed. Or attach a leg bag.
25 Remove the waterproof pad and gloves. Discard them. Practice hand hygiene.
26 Cover the person. Remove the bath blanket.

POST-PROCEDURE

27 Provide for comfort. (See the inside of the front cover.)
28 Place the call light within reach.
29 Lower the bed to a comfortable and safe level appropriate for the person. Follow the care plan.
30 Raise or lower bed rails. Follow the care plan.
31 Unscreen the person.
32 Practice hand hygiene. Put on clean gloves.
33 Measure and record the amount of urine in the bag. Clean or discard the collection bag.
34 Clean, rinse, dry, and return the wash basin and other equipment. Return items to their proper place.
35 Remove and discard the gloves. Practice hand hygiene.
36 Complete a safety check of the room. (See the inside of the front cover.)
37 Report and record your observations.

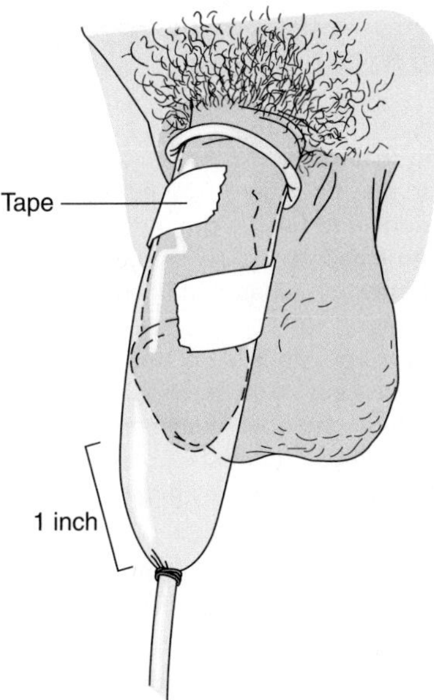

FIGURE 18-17 A condom catheter applied to the penis. A 1-inch space is between the penis and the end of the catheter. Elastic tape is applied in a spiral to secure the condom catheter to the penis.

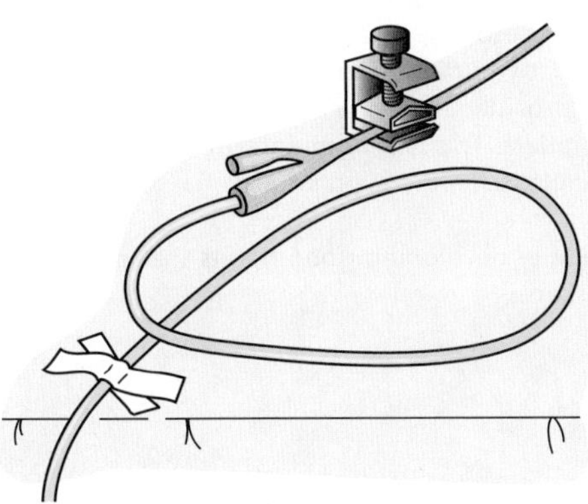

FIGURE 18-18 The clamped catheter prevents urine from draining out of the bladder. The clamp is applied directly to the catheter, not to the drainage tube.

BLADDER TRAINING

Bladder training may help with urinary incontinence. Some persons need bladder training after catheter removal. Control of urination is the goal. Bladder control promotes comfort and quality of life. It also increases self-esteem.

The person's care plan may include 1 of the following.

- *Bladder re-training (bladder rehabilitation).* The person needs to:
  - Resist or ignore the strong desire to urinate.
  - Postpone or delay voiding.
  - Urinate following a schedule rather than the urge to void.

  The time between voidings may increase as bladder re-training progresses.
- *Prompted voiding.* The person voids at scheduled times. The person is taught to:
  - Recognize when the bladder is full.
  - Recognize the need to void.
  - Ask for help.
  - Respond when prompted to void.
- *Habit training/scheduled voiding.* Voiding is scheduled at regular times to match the person's voiding habits. This is usually every 3 to 4 hours while awake. The person does not delay or resist voiding. Timed-voiding is based on the person's usual voiding patterns.
- *Catheter clamping.* The catheter is clamped to prevent urine flow from the bladder (Fig. 18-18). It is usually clamped for 1 hour at first. Over time, it is clamped for 3 to 4 hours. Urine drains when the catheter is unclamped. When the catheter is removed, voiding is encouraged every 3 to 4 hours or as directed by the nurse and the care plan.

FOCUS ON PRIDE

The Person, Family, and Yourself

Personal and Professional Responsibility

Some states allow nursing assistants to insert or remove urinary catheters. To safely insert or remove a catheter:

- The procedure must be allowed by your state and agency.
- The procedure must be in your job description.
- You must have the necessary education and training.
- You must know how to use the agency's supplies and equipment.
- A nurse must be available to answer questions and supervise you.

Rights and Respect

Illness, disease, and aging can affect the private act of voiding. Respect the person's right to privacy. Allow as much privacy as safely possible. Pull privacy curtains and close doors and window coverings. If you must stay in the room, allow as much privacy as possible. Stand just outside the bathroom door in case the person needs you. Or stand on the other side of the privacy curtain. The nurse helps you with ways to protect the person's privacy. Follow the nurse's directions and the care plan.

Empty urinals, bedpans, and commodes promptly. Urine-filled devices in the person's room do not respect the right to a neat and clean setting. They also may cause embarrassment. Do your best to promote comfort, dignity, and respect when assisting with elimination needs.

Independence and Social Interaction

Some persons can place bedpans and urinals themselves. Some can get on and off bedside commodes themselves. Others need some help but can be left alone to void. Let the person do as much as safely possible.

To safely promote independence, keep devices within reach for persons who use them without help. For persons who need some help, check on them often. Do not leave a person sitting on a bedpan, commode, or toilet for a long time. Discomfort, odors, and skin breakdown are likely. Also, the person may think you forgot about him or her. The person may try to get off the bedpan, commode, or toilet alone. Harm can result. Make sure the call light is within reach. Respond promptly when the person calls for you.

Delegation and Teamwork

The need to void may be urgent. The person may try to go to the bathroom alone and fall. Or the person is incontinent. The person is wet and embarrassed. He or she is at risk for skin breakdown and infection. Changing linens and garments requires extra work.

Answer call lights promptly. Also, answer call lights for co-workers. You like help when you are busy. So do your co-workers. If needed, ask how much help the person needs. Some persons can tell you themselves. Ask the nurse if you are unsure. Work as a team to meet elimination needs promptly.

Ethics and Laws

Negligence occurs when a staff member does not act in a reasonable and careful manner and the person or the person's property is harmed (Chapter 3). Although the error is not intentional, the negligent person is responsible. For example, you forget a patient is on a bedpan. Hours later, you remember. A pressure ulcer results.

To avoid this mistake:

- Be careful and focused when performing all procedures. Avoid distractions.
- Remind the person to press the call light if you do not return promptly.
- Report and record promptly. When you report, the nurse knows what you did. When you record, there is a record of the care provided.
- Use reminders. This is very important when you are busy. For example, set a timer on your watch or write yourself a note.

Take pride in developing good habits that promote safety and quality care.

REVIEW QUESTIONS

Circle the BEST answer.

1 Which must you report to the nurse?
- a Clear, amber urine
- b Urine with a faint odor
- c Cloudy urine with particles
- d Urine output of 1500 mL in 24 hours

2 Which prevents normal elimination?
- a Helping the person assume a normal position for voiding
- b Providing privacy
- c Helping the person to the bathroom as soon as requested
- d Staying with the person who uses a bedpan

3 Which definition is *correct?*
- a Dysuria means painful or difficult urination.
- b Oliguria means a large amount of urine.
- c Urinary retention means the need to void at once.
- d Urinary incontinence means the inability to void.

4 The person using a standard bedpan is in
- a Fowler's position
- b The supine position
- c The prone position
- d The side-lying position

5 After using the urinal, the man should
- a Put it on the bedside stand
- b Use the call light
- c Put it on the over-bed table
- d Empty it

6 After a person uses a commode, you should
- a Empty, clean, and disinfect the commode
- b Return the commode to the supply area
- c Get a new container
- d Get a new commode

7 Urinary incontinence
- a Is always permanent
- b Requires good skin care
- c Is treated with a catheter
- d Requires bladder training

8 Which is a cause of functional incontinence?
- a A nervous system disorder
- b Sneezing
- c Unanswered call light
- d UTI

9 When applying an incontinence product
- a Let the plastic backing touch the person's skin
- b Remove the old product from back to front
- c Apply the new product from front to back
- d Use the product to turn and position the person

10 A person has a catheter. Which is safe?
- a Keeping the drainage bag above the level of the bladder
- b Taping a leak at the connection site
- c Attaching the drainage bag to the bed rail
- d Removing a kink from the drainage tubing

11 A person has a catheter. Which is *correct?*
- a Report pain, burning, the need to void, or irritation at once.
- b Allow the tubing to hang below the drainage bag.
- c Empty the drainage bag once daily.
- d Use the same measuring container for all persons.

12 A person has a catheter. You are going to turn the person from the left to the right side. What should you do with the drainage bag?
- a Move it to the right side.
- b Keep it on the left side.
- c Hang it from an IV pole.
- d Remove the catheter and the drainage bag.

13 When giving catheter care
- a Clean from the drainage tube connection up the catheter at least 4 inches
- b Clean from the meatus down the catheter at least 4 inches
- c Pull on the catheter to make sure it is secure
- d Clamp the catheter to prevent leaking

14 For a condom catheter, you apply elastic tape
- a Completely around the penis
- b To the inner thigh
- c To the abdomen
- d In a spiral

15 The goal of bladder training is to
- a Remove the catheter
- b Clamp the catheter
- c Gain control of urination
- d Allow the person to walk to the bathroom

16 A person's care plan includes bladder training using habit training (scheduled voiding). You will
- a Remind the person to resist the urge to void
- b Tell the nurse when the person needs to void
- c Clamp the person's catheter for 3 to 4 hours at a time
- d Assist the person to void every 3 to 4 hours while awake

Answers to these questions are on p. 505.

FOCUS ON PRACTICE

Problem Solving

You assist a patient onto the commode. The person is unsteady and is not to be left alone. The person says: "I can't go with you standing here." What do you do? How will you provide privacy and safe care?

CHAPTER

19 Assisting With Bowel Elimination

OBJECTIVES

- Define the key terms and key abbreviations listed in this chapter.
- Describe normal defecation and the observations to report.
- Identify the factors affecting bowel elimination.
- Explain how to promote comfort and safety during defecation.
- Describe the common bowel elimination problems.
- Describe bowel training.
- Explain why enemas are given.
- Describe the common enema solutions.
- Describe the rules for giving enemas.
- Describe how to care for a person with an ostomy.
- Perform the procedures described in this chapter.
- Explain how to promote PRIDE in the person, the family, and yourself.

KEY TERMS

colostomy A surgically created opening *(stomy)* between the colon *(colo)* and abdominal wall

constipation The passage of a hard, dry stool

defecation The process of excreting feces from the rectum through the anus; a bowel movement

diarrhea The frequent passage of liquid stools

enema The introduction of fluid into the rectum and lower colon

fecal impaction The prolonged retention and buildup of feces in the rectum

fecal incontinence The inability to control the passage of feces and gas through the anus

feces The semi-solid mass of waste products in the colon that is expelled through the anus; also called a *stool*

flatulence The excessive formation of gas or air in the stomach and intestines

flatus Gas or air passed through the anus

ileostomy A surgically created opening *(stomy)* between the ileum (small intestine *[ileo]*) and the abdominal wall

ostomy A surgically created opening; see "colostomy" and "ileostomy"

stoma A surgically created opening seen through the abdominal wall; see "colostomy" and "ileostomy"

stool Excreted feces

suppository A cone-shaped, solid drug that is inserted into a body opening; it melts at body temperature

KEY ABBREVIATIONS

BM	Bowel movement
C	Centigrade
F	Fahrenheit
GI	Gastro-intestinal
ID	Identification
IV	Intravenous
mL	Milliliter
oz	Ounce
SSE	Soapsuds enema

Bowel elimination is a basic physical need. Wastes are excreted from the gastro-intestinal (GI) system (Chapter 7). You assist patients and residents in meeting elimination needs.

See *Delegation Guidelines: Assisting With Bowel Elimination.*

See *Promoting Safety and Comfort: Assisting With Bowel Elimination.*

DELEGATION GUIDELINES

Assisting With Bowel Elimination

Your state and agency may not allow you to perform the procedures in this chapter. Before performing a procedure, make sure that:

- Your state allows you to perform the procedure.
- The procedure is in your job description.
- You have the necessary education and training.
- You review the procedure with a nurse.
- A nurse is available to answer questions and to supervise you.

PROMOTING SAFETY AND COMFORT

Assisting With Bowel Elimination

Safety

Assisting with bowel elimination involves exposing and touching the rectum, a private area. And you may have to give perineal care. Sexual abuse has occurred in health care settings. The person may feel threatened or may be being abused. He or she needs to call for help. Keep the call light within the person's reach at all times. And always act in a professional manner.

Contact with feces is likely when assisting with bowel elimination. Feces contain microbes and may contain blood. Follow Standard Precautions and the Bloodborne Pathogen Standard (Chapter 12).

NORMAL BOWEL ELIMINATION

Some people have a bowel movement (BM) every day. Others have 1 every 2 to 3 days. Some people have 2 or 3 BMs a day. Many people have a BM after breakfast. Others do so in the evening.

To assist with bowel elimination, you need to know these terms.

- ***Defecation****—the process of excreting feces from the rectum through the anus; a bowel movement.*
- ***Feces****—the semi-solid mass of waste products in the colon that is expelled through the anus. It is also called a* stool.
- ***Stool****—excreted feces.*

Observations

Stools are normally brown. Bleeding in the stomach and small intestine causes black or tarry stools. Bleeding in the lower colon and rectum causes red-colored stools. So can some foods. Diseases and infection can cause clay-colored or white, pale, orange-colored, or green-colored stools and stools with mucus.

Stools are normally soft, formed, moist, and shaped like the rectum. They normally have an odor.

Carefully observe stools. Ask the nurse to observe abnormal stools. Observe and report the following.

- Color
- Amount
- Consistency
- Presence of blood or mucus
- Odor
- Shape and size
- Frequency of BMs
- Complaints of pain or discomfort

See *Focus on Communication: Observations.*

FOCUS ON COMMUNICATION

Observations

Many patients and residents tend to their own bowel elimination needs. However, information is still needed for the person's record and the nursing process. You may need to ask about the person's BMs. You can say:

- "Did you have a BM today?"
- "Please tell me about your BM."
- "When did you have a BM?"
- "What was the amount?"
- "Were the stools soft or hard?"
- "Were the stools formed or loose?"
- "What was the color?"
- "Did you have any bleeding, pain, or problems having a BM?"
- "Did you pass any gas?"
- "Do you need to pass more gas?"
- "Do you need help cleaning yourself?"

FACTORS AFFECTING BMs

These factors affect stool frequency, consistency, color, and odor. They are part of the nursing process to meet the person's elimination needs. Normal, regular elimination is the goal.

- *Privacy.* Lack of privacy can prevent a BM despite the urge. Odors and sounds are embarrassing. Some people ignore the urge when others are present.
- *Habits.* Many people have a BM after breakfast. Some drink a hot beverage, read, or take a walk. These activities are relaxing. A BM is easier when the person is relaxed, not tense.
- *Diet—high-fiber foods.* High-fiber foods leave a residue for needed bulk and prevent constipation. Fruits, vegetables, and whole-grain cereals and breads are high in fiber. Some people cannot chew these foods. They may not have teeth. Or dentures fit poorly. Some nursing centers add bran to cereal, prunes, or prune juice.
- *Diet—other foods.* Milk and milk products can cause constipation or diarrhea. Chocolate and other foods cause similar reactions. Spicy foods can cause frequent BMs or diarrhea. Gas-forming foods stimulate peristalsis, thus aiding BMs. Such foods include onions, beans, cabbage, cauliflower, radishes, and cucumbers.
- *Fluids.* Feces contain water. Stool consistency depends on the amount of water absorbed in the colon. Feces harden and dry when large amounts of water are absorbed or when fluid intake is poor. Hard, dry feces move slowly through the colon. Constipation can occur. Drinking 6 to 8 glasses of water daily promotes normal bowel elimination. Warm fluids—coffee, tea, hot cider, warm water—increase peristalsis.
- *Activity.* Exercise and activity maintain muscle tone and stimulate peristalsis.
- *Drugs.* Drugs can prevent constipation or control diarrhea. Other drugs have diarrhea or constipation as side effects.
- *Disability.* Some people cannot control BMs. They have a BM whenever feces enter the rectum. A bowel training program is needed (p. 298).
- *Aging.* Aging causes changes in the GI tract. Feces pass through the intestines at a slower rate. Constipation is a risk. Some older persons lose bowel control (see "Fecal Incontinence," p. 298).

Safety and Comfort

The care plan has measures to meet the person's elimination needs. It may involve diet, fluids, and exercise. Follow the measures in Box 19-1 to promote safety and comfort.

See *Focus on Communication: Safety and Comfort.*

BOX 19-1 Safety and Comfort During Bowel Elimination

- Follow Standard Precautions and the Bloodborne Pathogen Standard.
- Provide for privacy.
  - Ask visitors to leave the room.
  - Close doors, privacy curtains, and window coverings.
- Help the person to the toilet or commode. Or provide the bedpan upon request.
- Wheel the person into the bathroom on the commode if possible. This provides privacy. Remove the container if the commode is used with the toilet. Remember to lock the commode wheels.
- Warm the bedpan.
- Position the person in a normal sitting or squatting position.
- Cover the person for warmth and privacy.
- Allow enough time for a BM.
- Place the call light and toilet tissue within reach.
- Leave the room if the person can be alone. Check on the person every 5 minutes.
- Stay nearby if the person is weak or unsteady.
- Provide perineal care.
- Dispose of stools promptly. This reduces odors and prevents the spread of microbes.
- Assist the person with hand washing after elimination.
- Follow the care plan if the person has fecal incontinence. The care plan tells you when to assist with elimination.

FOCUS ON COMMUNICATION

Safety and Comfort

Odors and sounds often occur with BMs. You must control your verbal and nonverbal responses. Always be professional. Do not laugh at or make fun of another person. Your words and actions must promote comfort, dignity, and self-esteem.

COMMON PROBLEMS

Common problems include constipation, fecal impaction, diarrhea, fecal incontinence, and flatulence.

Constipation

***Constipation** is the passage of a hard, dry stool.* The person usually strains to have a BM. Stools are large or marble-sized. Large stools cause pain as they pass through the anus. Constipation occurs when feces move slowly through the bowel. This allows more time for water absorption. Common causes of constipation include:

- A low-fiber diet
- Ignoring the urge to have a BM
- Decreased fluid intake
- Inactivity
- Drugs
- Aging
- Certain diseases

Dietary changes, fluids, and activity prevent or relieve constipation. The doctor may order 1 or more of the following.

- Stool softeners—drugs that soften feces
- Laxatives—drugs that promote bowel elimination
- Suppositories (p. 298)
- Enemas (p. 298)

Fecal Impaction

*A **fecal impaction** is the prolonged retention and buildup of feces in the rectum.* Feces are hard or putty-like. Fecal impaction results if constipation is not relieved. The person cannot have a BM. More water is absorbed from the already hard feces. Liquid feces pass around the hardened fecal mass in the rectum. The liquid feces seep from the anus.

Signs and symptoms of fecal impaction include:

- Trying many times to have a BM
- Abdominal discomfort
- Abdominal distention (swelling)
- Nausea
- Cramping
- Rectal pain
- Poor appetite (especially older persons)
- Confusion (especially older persons)
- Fever (especially older persons)

Diarrhea

***Diarrhea** is the frequent passage of liquid stools.* Feces move through the intestines rapidly. This reduces the time for fluid absorption. The need for a BM is urgent. Some people cannot get to a bathroom in time. Abdominal cramping, nausea, and vomiting may occur.

Causes of diarrhea include infections, some drugs, irritating foods, and microbes in food and water. Diet and drugs are ordered to reduce peristalsis. You need to:

- Assist with elimination needs promptly.
- Dispose of stools promptly. This prevents odors and the spread of microbes.
- Give good skin care. Liquid stools irritate the skin. So does frequent wiping with toilet tissue. Skin breakdown and pressure ulcers are risks.
- Follow Standard Precautions and the Bloodborne Pathogen Standard when in contact with stools.

See *Focus on Older Persons: Diarrhea.*
See *Promoting Safety and Comfort: Diarrhea.*

FOCUS ON OLDER PERSONS

Diarrhea

Dehydration is the excessive loss of water from tissues. Older persons are at risk for dehydration. The amount of body water decreases with aging. Many diseases common in older persons affect body fluids. So do many drugs. Report diarrhea at once. Ask the nurse to observe the stool. Death is a risk when dehydration is not recognized and treated.

PROMOTING SAFETY AND COMFORT

Diarrhea

Safety

Clostridium difficile (C. difficile) is a microbe that causes diarrhea and intestinal infections. Commonly called *C. diff*, it can cause death. Persons at risk include those who are older, ill, or need prolonged use of antibiotics. Signs and symptoms include:

- Watery diarrhea
- Fever
- Loss of appetite
- Nausea
- Abdominal pain or tenderness

The microbe is found in feces. A person becomes infected by touching items or surfaces contaminated with feces and when touching the mouth or mucous membranes. You can spread the microbe if your contaminated hands or gloves:

- Touch a person.
- Contaminate surfaces.

You must practice good hand hygiene. Alcohol-based hand rubs are not effective against *C. difficile*. Wash your hands with soap and water. Follow Standard Precautions and Transmission-Based Precautions.

Fecal Incontinence

***Fecal incontinence** is the inability to control the passage of feces and gas through the anus.* Causes include:
- Intestinal diseases.
- Nervous system diseases and injuries.
- Fecal impaction or diarrhea.
- Some drugs.
- Aging.
- Mental health disorders or dementia (Chapters 29 and 30). The person may not recognize the need for or act of having a BM.
- Unanswered call lights.
- Not getting to the bathroom in time. The person may have mobility problems or he or she may walk slowly. Or the bathroom may be too far away or occupied by another person.
- Difficulty removing clothes.
- Not finding the bathroom in a new setting.

Fecal incontinence affects the person emotionally. Frustration, embarrassment, anger, and humiliation are common. The person may need:
- Bowel training
- Help with elimination after meals and every 2 to 3 hours
- Incontinence products to keep garments and linens clean
- Good skin care

See *Focus on Older Persons: Fecal Incontinence.*

Flatulence

Gas and air are normally in the stomach and intestines. They are expelled through the mouth (burping, belching, eructating) and anus. *Gas or air passed through the anus is called **flatus**. **Flatulence** is the excessive formation of gas or air in the stomach and intestines.* Causes include:
- Swallowing air while eating and drinking
- Bacterial action in the intestines
- Gas-forming foods (p. 296)
- Constipation
- Bowel and abdominal surgeries
- Drugs that decrease peristalsis

If flatus is not expelled, the intestines distend. That is, they swell or enlarge from the pressure of gases. Abdominal cramping or pain, shortness of breath, and a swollen abdomen occur. "Bloating" is a common complaint. Exercise, walking, moving in bed, and the left side-lying position often expel flatus. Doctors may order enemas and drugs to relieve flatulence.

FOCUS ON OLDER PERSONS
Fecal Incontinence

Persons with dementia may smear stools on themselves, furniture, and walls. Some are not aware of having BMs. Some resist care. Follow the person's care plan. The measures for urinary incontinence (Chapter 18) may be part of the care plan. Be patient. Ask for help from co-workers. Talk to the nurse if you have problems keeping the person clean.

BOWEL TRAINING

Bowel training has 2 goals.
- To gain control of BMs.
- To develop a regular pattern of elimination. Fecal impaction, constipation, and fecal incontinence are prevented.

Meals, especially breakfast, stimulate the urge for a BM. The person's usual time of day for BM is noted on the care plan. So is toilet, commode, or bedpan use. Offer help with elimination at the times noted. Factors that promote elimination are part of the care plan and bowel training program.

The doctor may order a suppository to stimulate a BM. *A **suppository** is a cone-shaped, solid drug that is inserted into a body opening. It melts at body temperature.* A nurse inserts a rectal suppository into the rectum (Fig. 19-1). A BM occurs about 30 minutes later.

ENEMAS

*An **enema** is the introduction of fluid into the rectum and lower colon.* Doctors order enemas to:
- Remove feces.
- Relieve constipation, fecal impaction, or flatulence.
- Clean the bowel of feces before certain surgeries and diagnostic procedures.

Safety and comfort measures for bowel elimination are practiced when giving enemas (see Box 19-1). So are the rules in Box 19-2.

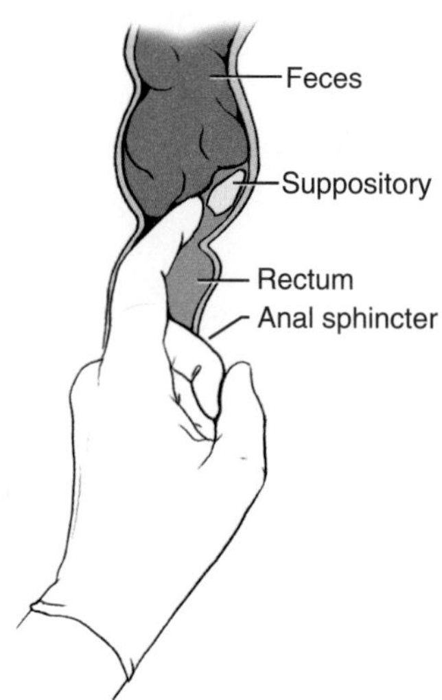

FIGURE 19-1 The suppository is inserted into the rectum.

The doctor orders the enema solution. The solution depends on the enema's purpose—for cleansing, constipation, fecal impaction, or flatulence.

- *Tap water enema*—is obtained from a faucet.
- *Saline enema*—a solution of salt and water. For adults, add 1 to 2 teaspoons of table salt to 500 to 1000 mL (milliliters) of tap water.
- *Soapsuds enema (SSE)*—for adults, add 3 to 5 mL of castile soap to 500 to 1000 mL of tap water.
- *Small-volume enema*—the adult size contains about 120 mL (4 ounces [oz]) of solution.
- *Oil-retention enema*—has mineral, olive, or cottonseed oil. The adult size contains about 120 mL (4 oz) of solution.

See *Delegation Guidelines: Enemas.*
See *Promoting Safety and Comfort: Enemas.*

BOX 19-2 Giving Enemas

- Have the person void first. This increases comfort during the enema procedure.
- Measure solution temperature with a bath thermometer. See *Delegation Guidelines: Enemas.*
- Position the person as the nurse directs. The Sims' position or the left side-lying position is preferred.
- Ask the nurse and check the procedure manual for how far to insert the enema tubing. It is usually inserted 2 to 4 inches in adults.
- Lubricate the enema tip before inserting it.
- Stop tube insertion if you feel resistance, the person complains of pain, or bleeding occurs.
- Ask the nurse how high to raise the enema bag. For adults, it is usually held 12 inches above the anus.
- Give the amount of solution ordered. Give the solution slowly. Usually it takes 10 to 15 minutes to give 750 to 1000 mL.
- Hold the enema tube in place while giving the solution.
- Ask the nurse how long the person should retain the solution. The length of time depends on the amount and type of solution.
- Make sure the bathroom will be vacant when the person needs to have a BM. Make sure that another person will not use the bathroom. If the person uses the bedpan or commode, have the device ready.
- Ask the nurse to observe the enema results.

DELEGATION GUIDELINES

Enemas

If giving an enema is delegated to you, make sure the conditions in *Delegation Guidelines: Assisting With Bowel Elimination* (p. 295) are met. If those conditions are met, you need this information from the nurse.

- What type of enema to give—cleansing, small-volume, or oil-retention
- What size enema tube to use
- What lubricant to use
- When to give the enema
- How many times to repeat the enema
- The amount of solution ordered—usually 500 to 1000 mL for a cleansing enema (for adults)
- How much castile soap to use for an SSE
- How much salt to use for a saline enema
- What the solution temperature should be—usually body temperature (98.6°F [Fahrenheit] or 37.0°C [centigrade]); sometimes warmer temperatures (105°F [40.5°C]) are used for adults
- How to position the person—Sims' or the left side-lying position
- How far to insert the enema tubing—usually 2 to 4 inches for adults
- How high to hold the solution container—usually 12 inches above the anus
- How fast to give the solution—750 to 1000 mL are usually given over 10 to 15 minutes
- How long the person should try to retain the solution
- What observations to report and record:
  - The amount of solution given
  - If you noted bleeding or resistance when inserting the tube
  - How long the person retained the enema solution
  - Color, amount, consistency, shape, and odor of stools
  - Complaints of cramping, pain, or discomfort
  - Complaints of nausea or weakness
  - How the person tolerated the procedure
- When to report observations
- What patient or resident concerns to report at once

PROMOTING SAFETY AND COMFORT

Enemas

Safety

Enemas are usually safe procedures. Many people give themselves enemas at home. However, enemas are dangerous for older persons and those with certain heart and kidney diseases.

Comfort

Before starting the procedure, make sure the bathroom is ready for the person's use. If the person will use the commode or bedpan, have the device ready. Always keep a bedpan nearby in case the person starts to expel the enema solution and stools. Mental comfort is promoted when the person knows the bathroom, commode, or bedpan is ready for use.

The person needs to retain the solution as long as possible. Make sure the person is comfortable in the Sims' or left side-lying position. When comfortable, it is easier to tolerate the procedure.

To prevent cramping:

- Use the correct water temperature. Cool water causes cramping.
- Give the solution slowly.

The Cleansing Enema

Cleansing enemas clean the bowel of feces and flatus. They relieve constipation and fecal impaction. They are needed before certain surgeries and diagnostic procedures. Cleansing enemas take effect in 10 to 20 minutes.

The doctor orders a tap water, saline, or soapsuds enema. The doctor may order *enemas until clear.* This means that enemas are given until the return solution is clear and free of stools. Ask the nurse how many enemas to give. Agency policy may allow repeating enemas 2 or 3 times.

See procedure: *Giving a Cleansing Enema.*

Giving a Cleansing Enema

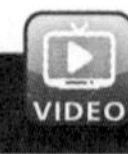

QUALITY OF LIFE

- Knock before entering the person's room.
- Address the person by name.
- Introduce yourself by name and title.
- Explain the procedure before starting and during the procedure.
- Protect the person's rights during the procedure.
- Handle the person gently during the procedure.

PRE-PROCEDURE

1 Follow *Delegation Guidelines:*
  a *Assisting With Bowel Elimination,* p. 295
  b *Enemas,* p. 299
  See *Promoting Safety and Comfort:*
  a *Assisting With Bowel Elimination,* p. 295
  b *Enemas,* p. 299
2 Practice hand hygiene.
3 Collect the following before going to the person's room.
  - Disposable enema kit as directed by the nurse (enema bag, tube, clamp, and waterproof pad)
  - Bath thermometer
  - Waterproof pad (if not in the enema kit)
  - Water-soluble lubricant
  - 3 to 5 mL (1 teaspoon) castile soap or 1 to 2 teaspoons of salt
  - IV (intravenous) pole
  - Gloves
4 Arrange items in the person's room and bathroom.
5 Practice hand hygiene.
6 Identify the person. Check the ID (identification) bracelet against the assignment sheet. Also call the person by name.
7 Put on gloves.
8 Collect the following.
  - Commode or bedpan and cover
  - Toilet tissue
  - Bath blanket
  - Robe and non-skid footwear
  - Paper towels
9 Remove and discard the gloves. Practice hand hygiene. Put on clean gloves.
10 Provide for privacy.
11 Raise the bed for body mechanics. Bed rails are up if used.

PROCEDURE

12 Lower the bed rail near you if up.
13 Cover the person with a bath blanket. Fan-fold top linens to the foot of the bed.
14 Position the IV pole so the enema bag is 12 inches above the anus. Or it is at the height directed by the nurse.
15 Raise the bed rail if used.
16 Prepare the enema.
  a Close the clamp on the tube.
  b Adjust water flow until it is lukewarm.
  c Fill the enema bag for the amount ordered.
  d Measure water temperature with the bath thermometer. The nurse tells you what water temperature to use.
  e Prepare the solution as directed by the nurse.
    1 *Tap water:* add nothing.
    2 *Saline enema:* add salt as directed.
    3 *SSE:* add castile soap as directed.
  f Stir the solution with the bath thermometer. Scoop off any suds (SSE).
  g Seal the bag.
  h Hang the bag on the IV pole.
17 Lower the bed rail near you if up.
18 Position the person in Sims' position or in a left side-lying position.
19 Place a waterproof pad under the buttocks.
20 Expose the anal area.
21 Place the bedpan behind the person.
22 Position the enema tube in the bedpan. Remove the cap from the tubing.
23 Open the clamp. Let solution flow through the tube to remove air. Clamp the tube.
24 Lubricate the tube 2 to 4 inches from the tip.
25 Separate the buttocks to see the anus.
26 Ask the person to take a deep breath through the mouth.
27 Insert the tube gently 2 to 4 inches into the adult's rectum (Fig. 19-2). Do this when the person is exhaling. Stop if the person complains of pain, you feel resistance, or bleeding occurs.
28 Check the amount of solution in the bag.
29 Unclamp the tube. Give the solution slowly (Fig. 19-3).
30 Ask the person to take slow deep breaths. This helps the person relax.

Giving a Cleansing Enema—cont'd

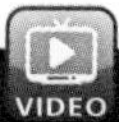

PROCEDURE—cont'd

31 Clamp the tube if the person needs to have a BM, has cramping, or starts to expel the solution. Also, clamp the tube if the person is sweating or complains of nausea or weakness. Unclamp when symptoms subside.
32 Give the amount of solution ordered. Stop if the person cannot tolerate the procedure.
33 Clamp the tube before it is empty. This prevents air from entering the bowel.
34 Hold toilet tissue around the tube and against the anus. Remove the tube.
35 Discard toilet tissue into the bedpan.
36 Wrap the tubing tip with paper towels. Place it inside the enema bag.
37 Assist the person to the bathroom or commode. The person wears a robe and non-skid footwear when up. The bed is at a low level that is comfortable and safe for the person. Or help the person onto the bedpan. Raise the head of the bed. Raise or lower bed rails according to the care plan.
38 Place the call light and toilet tissue within reach. Remind the person not to flush the toilet.
39 Discard disposable items.
40 Remove and discard the gloves. Practice hand hygiene.
41 Leave the room if the person can be left alone.
42 Return when the person signals. Or check on the person every 5 minutes. Knock before entering the room or bathroom.
43 Practice hand hygiene and put on gloves. Lower the bed rail if up.
44 Observe enema results for amount, color, consistency, shape, and odor. Call the nurse to observe the results.
45 Provide perineal care as needed.
46 Remove the waterproof pad.
47 Empty, rinse, clean, and disinfect equipment. Flush the toilet after the nurse observes the results.
48 Return equipment to its proper place.
49 Remove and discard the gloves. Practice hand hygiene.
50 Assist with hand washing. Wear gloves for this step. Practice hand hygiene after removing and discarding the gloves.
51 Cover the person. Remove the bath blanket.

POST-PROCEDURE

52 Provide for comfort. (See the inside of the front cover.)
53 Place the call light within reach.
54 Lower the bed to a comfortable and safe level appropriate for the person. Follow the care plan.
55 Raise or lower bed rails. Follow the care plan.
56 Unscreen the person.
57 Complete a safety check of the room. (See the inside of the front cover.)
58 Follow agency policy for dirty linen and used supplies.
59 Practice hand hygiene.
60 Report and record your observations.

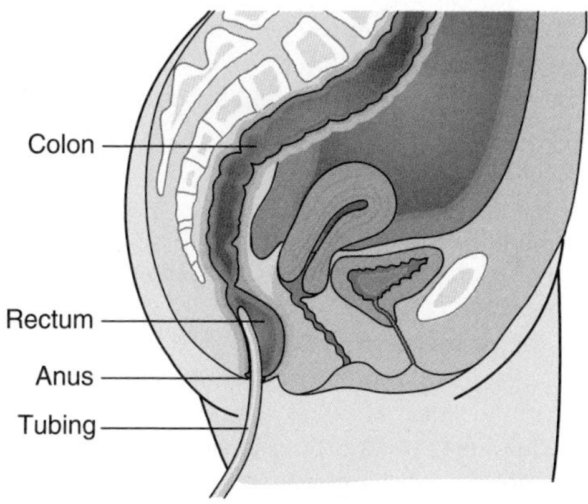

FIGURE 19-2 Enema tubing inserted into the adult rectum.

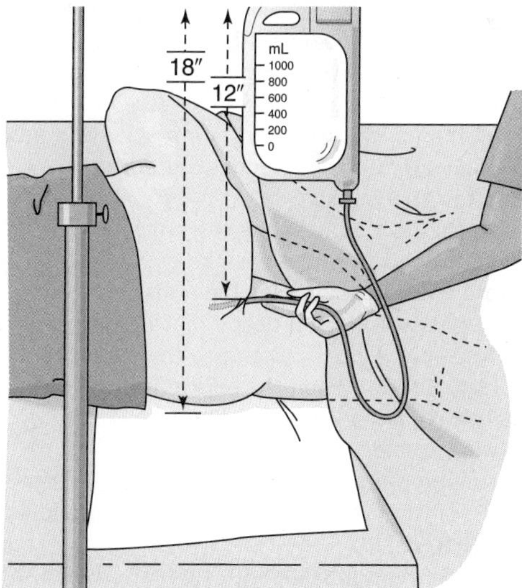

FIGURE 19-3 Giving an enema. The person is in Sims' position. The enema bag hangs from an IV pole. The bag is 12 inches above the anus and 18 inches above the mattress.

The Small-Volume Enema

Small-volume enemas irritate and distend the rectum. This causes a BM. They are often ordered for constipation or when the bowel does not need complete cleansing.

These enemas are ready to give. The solution is usually given at room temperature. To give the enema, squeeze and roll up the plastic container from the bottom. Do not release pressure on the bottle. Otherwise, solution is drawn from the rectum back into the bottle.

Urge the person to retain the solution until he or she needs to have a BM. This usually takes about 5 to 10 minutes. Staying in the Sims' or left side-lying position helps retain the enema.

See procedure: *Giving a Small-Volume Enema.*

Giving a Small-Volume Enema

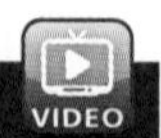

QUALITY OF LIFE

- Knock before entering the person's room.
- Address the person by name.
- Introduce yourself by name and title.
- Explain the procedure before starting and during the procedure.
- Protect the person's rights during the procedure.
- Handle the person gently during the procedure.

PRE-PROCEDURE

1 Follow *Delegation Guidelines:*
   a *Assisting With Bowel Elimination,* p. 295
   b *Enemas,* p. 299
   See *Promoting Safety and Comfort:*
   a *Assisting With Bowel Elimination,* p. 295
   b *Enemas,* p. 299
2 Practice hand hygiene.
3 Collect the following before going to the person's room.
   - Small-volume enema
   - Waterproof pad
   - Gloves
4 Arrange items in the person's room.
5 Practice hand hygiene.
6 Identify the person. Check the ID bracelet against the assignment sheet. Also call the person by name.
7 Put on gloves.
8 Collect the following.
   - Commode or bedpan
   - Toilet tissue
   - Robe and non-skid footwear
   - Bath blanket
9 Remove and discard the gloves. Practice hand hygiene. Put on clean gloves.
10 Provide for privacy.
11 Raise the bed for body mechanics. Bed rails are up if used.

PROCEDURE

12 Lower the bed rail near you if up.
13 Cover the person with a bath blanket. Fan-fold top linens to the foot of the bed.
14 Position the person in Sims' or a left side-lying position.
15 Place the waterproof pad under the buttocks.
16 Expose the anal area.
17 Position the bedpan near the person.
18 Remove the cap from the enema tip.
19 Separate the buttocks to see the anus.
20 Ask the person to take a deep breath through the mouth.
21 Insert the enema tip 2 inches into the adult's rectum (Fig. 19-4). Do this when the person is exhaling. Insert the tip gently. Stop if the person complains of pain, you feel resistance, or bleeding occurs.
22 Squeeze and roll up the container gently. Release pressure on the bottle after you remove the tip from the rectum.
23 Put the container into the box, tip first. Discard the container and box.
24 Assist the person to the bathroom or commode when he or she has the urge to have a BM. The person wears a robe and non-skid footwear when up. The bed is at a low level that is comfortable and safe for the person. Or help the person onto the bedpan, and raise the head of the bed. Raise or lower bed rails according to the care plan.
25 Place the call light and toilet tissue within reach. Remind the person not to flush the toilet.
26 Discard disposable items.
27 Remove and discard the gloves. Practice hand hygiene.
28 Leave the room if the person can be left alone.
29 Return when the person signals. Or check on the person every 5 minutes. Knock before entering the room or bathroom.
30 Practice hand hygiene. Put on gloves.
31 Lower the bed rail if up.
32 Observe enema results for amount, color, consistency, shape, and odor. Call the nurse to observe the results.
33 Provide perineal care as needed.
34 Remove the waterproof pad.
35 Empty, rinse, clean, and disinfect equipment. Flush the toilet after the nurse observes the results.
36 Return equipment to its proper place.
37 Remove and discard the gloves. Practice hand hygiene.
38 Assist with hand washing. Wear gloves for this step. Practice hand hygiene after removing and discarding the gloves.
39 Cover the person. Remove the bath blanket.

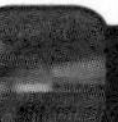

Giving a Small-Volume Enema—cont'd

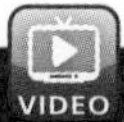

POST-PROCEDURE

40 Provide for comfort. (See the inside of the front cover.)
41 Place the call light within reach.
42 Lower the bed to a comfortable and safe level appropriate for the person. Follow the care plan.
43 Raise or lower bed rails. Follow the care plan.
44 Unscreen the person.
45 Complete a safety check of the room. (See the inside of the front cover.)
46 Follow agency policy for dirty linen and used supplies.
47 Practice hand hygiene.
48 Report and record your observations.

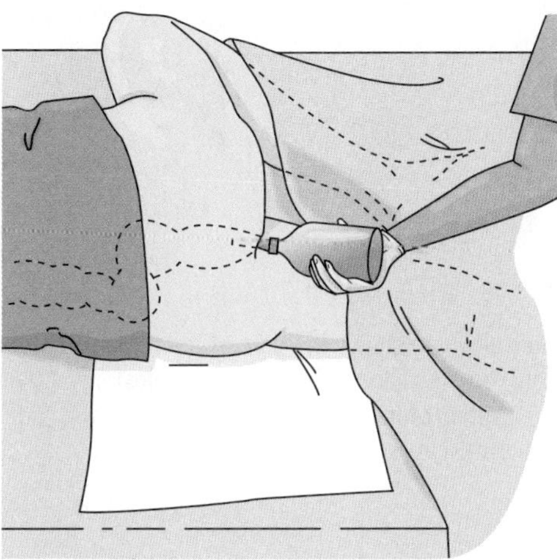

FIGURE 19-4 The small-volume enema tip is inserted 2 inches into the rectum.

The Oil-Retention Enema

Oil-retention enemas relieve constipation and fecal impaction. The oil is retained for 30 to 60 minutes or longer (1 to 3 hours). Retaining oil softens feces and lubricates the rectum. This lets feces pass with ease. Most oil-retention enemas are commercially prepared.

Giving an oil-retention enema is like giving a small-volume enema. After giving an oil-retention enema:

- Leave the person in the Sims' or left side-lying position. Cover the person for warmth.
- Urge the person to retain the enema for the time ordered.
- Place extra waterproof pads on the bed if needed.
- Check the person often while he or she retains the enema.

See *Promoting Safety and Comfort: The Oil-Retention Enema.*

PROMOTING SAFETY AND COMFORT

The Oil-Retention Enema

Safety

The oil-retention enema is retained for at least 30 to 60 minutes. Leave the room after giving the enema. Check on the person often. After checking on the person, tell him or her when you will return. Remind the person to signal for you if he or she needs help. Report any problems at once.

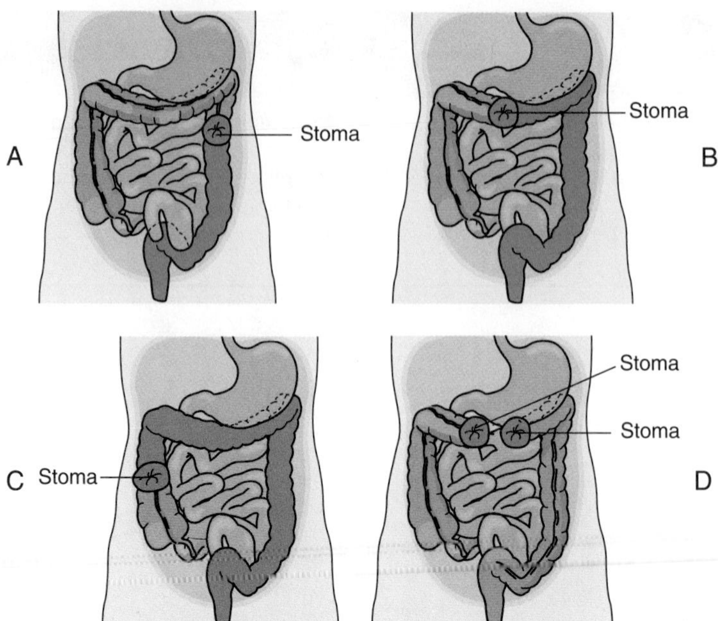

FIGURE 19-5 Colostomy sites. *Shading* shows the part of the bowel surgically removed. **A,** Sigmoid or descending colostomy. **B,** Transverse colostomy. **C,** Ascending colostomy. **D,** Double-barrel colostomy has 2 stomas. One allows for the excretion of feces. The other is for the introduction of drugs to help the bowel heal. This type is usually temporary.

THE PERSON WITH AN OSTOMY

Sometimes a part of the intestines is removed surgically. Cancer, bowel disease, and trauma (stab or bullet wounds) are common reasons. An ostomy is sometimes necessary. An ***ostomy*** *is a surgically created opening. The opening seen through the abdominal wall is called a* ***stoma.*** The person wears a pouch over the stoma to collect stools and flatus.

Colostomy

A ***colostomy*** *is a surgically created opening* (stomy) *between the colon* (colo) *and abdominal wall.* Part of the colon is brought out onto the abdominal wall, and a stoma is made. Feces and flatus pass through the stoma instead of the anus.

With a permanent colostomy, the diseased part of the colon is removed. A temporary colostomy gives the diseased or injured bowel time to heal. After healing, surgery is done to reconnect the bowel.

The colostomy site depends on the site of disease or injury (Fig. 19-5). Stool consistency—liquid to formed—depends on the colostomy site. The more colon remaining to absorb water, the more solid and formed the stool. If the colostomy is near the end of the colon, stools are formed.

Stools irritate the skin. Skin care prevents skin breakdown around the stoma. The skin is washed and dried. Then a skin barrier is applied around the stoma. It prevents stools from having contact with the skin. The skin barrier is part of the pouch or a separate device.

Ileostomy

An ***ileostomy*** *is a surgically created opening* (stomy) *between the ileum* (small intestine [ileo]) *and the abdominal wall.* Part of the ileum is brought out onto the abdominal wall, and a stoma is made. The entire colon is removed (Fig. 19-6).

Liquid stools drain constantly from an ileostomy. Water is not absorbed because the colon was removed. Feces in the small intestine contain digestive juices that are very irritating to the skin. The ileostomy pouch must fit well. Stools must not touch the skin. Good skin care is required.

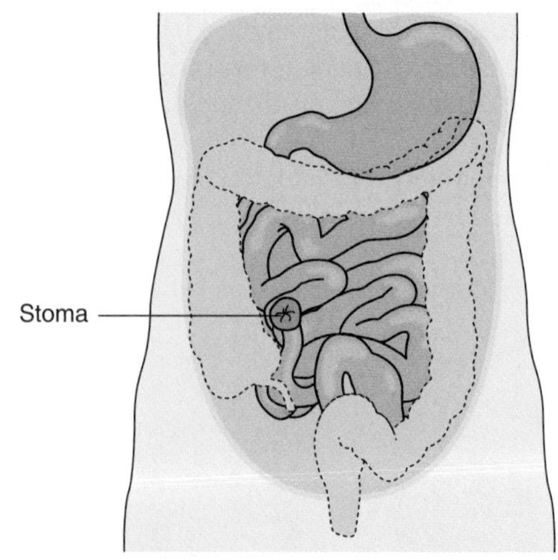

FIGURE 19-6 An ileostomy. The entire large intestine is surgically removed.

Ostomy Pouches

The pouch has an adhesive backing that is applied to the skin. Some pouches are secured to ostomy belts (Fig. 19-7).

Pouches have a drain at the bottom that closes with a clip, clamp, or wire closure. The drain is opened to empty the pouch when stools are present. It also is opened when it bulges with flatus. The drain is wiped with toilet tissue before it is closed.

The pouch is changed every 3 to 7 days and when it leaks. Frequent pouch changes can damage the skin.

Odors are prevented by:

- Performing good personal hygiene.
- Emptying the pouch.
- Avoiding gas-forming foods.
- Putting deodorants into the pouch. The nurse tells you what to use.

The person wears normal clothes. However, tight garments can prevent feces from entering the pouch. Also, bulging from stools and flatus can be seen with tight clothes.

Peristalsis increases after eating and drinking. After sleep, stomas are less likely to expel feces. If the person showers or bathes with the pouch off, it is best done before breakfast. Showers and baths are delayed for 1 to 2 hours after applying a new pouch. This gives adhesive time to seal to the skin.

Do not flush pouches down the toilet. Follow agency policy to dispose of them.

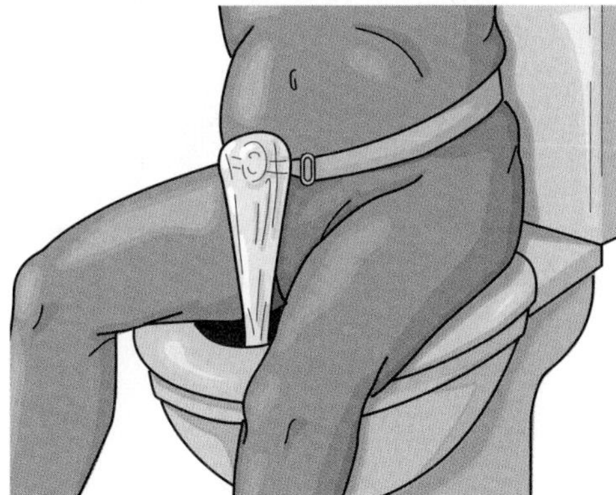

FIGURE 19-7 The ostomy pouch is secured to an ostomy belt. The pouch is emptied by directing it into the toilet and opening the end.

FOCUS ON PRIDE

The Person, Family, and Yourself

Personal and Professional Responsibility

The nurse may ask you to do a task that you have not done before. For example, you are asked to empty a colostomy bag. You must know what your state and agency allow. If not allowed, politely refuse the task. If allowed, ask the nurse for help. Never attempt a task that you are not comfortable doing. You can say: "I'm sorry, but I have never done that task before. I'm not comfortable doing it on my own. Would you please show me how?" To provide safe care, follow the limits of your role and tell the nurse about concerns.

Rights and Respect

Bowel elimination is usually private. Illness, disease, surgery, and aging can affect this private act. Some persons may feel embarrassed to have a BM in a strange setting. You can increase comfort by respecting the person's privacy. To promote comfort and privacy:

- Ask others to leave the room.
- Close doors, curtains, and window coverings.
- Turn on water or music to mask sounds.
- Cover the person.
- Allow the person enough time. Place the call light nearby and instruct the person to call if help is needed.
- Knock before entering the room. Tell the person who you are. Ask the person if you may enter before opening the door completely.
- Use an agency-approved spray for odors.

Independence and Social Interaction

Persons with ostomies manage their care if able. Some have had ostomies for a long time. They may have special routines or care measures. Do not react to things that seem odd to you. When assisting, ask what they prefer. Listen to their requests. Follow their choices in ostomy care. To promote independence, allow personal choice and control as much as safely possible.

Delegation and Teamwork

The need to have a BM may be urgent. Answer call lights promptly. Also help co-workers answer call lights. Listen closely for bathroom call lights. The sound at the nurses' station is different from call lights in rooms. Respond at once.

Do not leave a person sitting on a toilet, commode, or bedpan longer than needed. Avoid having the "that is not my patient (resident) attitude." Help your co-workers. Thank your co-workers for helping you. Take pride in working as a team to promptly meet elimination needs.

Ethics and Laws

All persons must be protected from abuse, mistreatment, and neglect. Examples include:

- Leaving a person sitting or lying in urine or feces.
- Leaving a person on a toilet, commode, or bedpan for a long time.
- Telling a person to void or have a BM in bed.

You will lose your job if found guilty of abuse, mistreatment, or neglect. The offense is noted on your registry. You cannot work in a nursing center or on a hospital's skilled care nursing unit. Other agencies may not hire you.

Protect yourself from being accused. Check on your patients and residents often. Be careful and focused. And always treat the person with dignity.

REVIEW QUESTIONS

Circle the BEST answer.

1 Which is *true?*
  a A person must have a BM every day.
  b Stools are normally brown, soft, and formed.
  c Diarrhea occurs when feces move slowly through the bowel.
  d Constipation occurs when feces move rapidly through the bowel.

2 Which should you ask the nurse to observe?
  a A black and tarry stool
  b The person's first BM of the day
  c Stool with an odor
  d Liquid stool from an ileostomy

3 The prolonged retention and buildup of feces in the rectum is called
  a Constipation
  b Fecal impaction
  c Diarrhea
  d Fecal incontinence

4 These measures promote normal BMs. Which is outside your role limits?
  a Give fluids according to the care plan.
  b Assist with activity according to the care plan.
  c Give drugs to control diarrhea.
  d Provide privacy during bowel elimination.

5 To promote comfort for bowel elimination
  a Close the door and privacy curtain
  b Help the person to a lying position
  c Allow visitors to stay in the room
  d Tell the person that you will return very soon

6 Bowel training is aimed at
  a Ostomy control
  b Preventing fecal impaction and constipation
  c Bowel control and regular elimination
  d Preventing bleeding

7 Which is used for a cleansing enema?
  a Mineral, olive, or cottonseed oil
  b Tap water, saline, or a soapsuds enema
  c A 120 mL bottle of solution
  d A suppository

8 When giving an enema
  a Use a cool solution
  b Place the person in the supine position
  c Have the person void after giving the enema
  d Give the solution slowly

9 In adults, the enema tube is inserted
  a 2 to 4 inches
  b 6 to 8 inches
  c 12 inches
  d Until you feel resistance

10 A small-volume enema is retained
  a For 2 minutes
  b At least 10 to 20 minutes
  c At least 30 to 60 minutes
  d Until the urge to have a BM is felt

11 Which care measure for an ostomy should you question?
  a Use deodorants in the pouch.
  b Perform good skin care around the stoma.
  c Change the pouch daily.
  d Apply a skin barrier around the stoma.

12 An ostomy pouch is usually emptied
  a Every 4 to 6 hours
  b When it is full
  c Every 3 to 7 days
  d When stools are present

Answers to these questions are on p. 505.

FOCUS ON PRACTICE

Problem Solving

A resident shares a bathroom with a roommate. You respond to the resident's call light. He says he needs to have a BM urgently. The bathroom is occupied. What do you do?

Assisting With Nutrition and Fluids

CHAPTER 20

OBJECTIVES

- Define the key terms and key abbreviations listed in this chapter.
- Explain the purpose and use of the MyPlate symbol.
- Describe the functions and sources of nutrients.
- Describe the factors that affect eating and nutrition.
- Describe OBRA requirements for serving food.
- Describe the special diets and between-meal snacks.
- Identify the signs, symptoms, and precautions for aspiration and regurgitation.
- Describe fluid requirements and the causes of dehydration.
- Explain how to assist with special fluid orders.
- Explain how to assist with food and fluid needs.
- Explain how to assist with calorie counts.
- Explain how to provide drinking water.
- Explain how to assist with enteral nutrition and IV therapy.
- Perform the procedures described in this chapter.
- Explain how to promote PRIDE in the person, the family, and yourself.

KEY TERMS

anorexia The loss of appetite
aspiration Breathing fluid, food, vomitus, or an object into the lungs
calorie The fuel or energy value of food
dehydration A decrease in the amount of water in body tissues
dysphagia Difficulty *(dys)* swallowing *(phagia)*
edema The swelling of body tissues with water
enteral nutrition Giving nutrients into the gastro-intestinal (GI) tract *(enteral)* through a feeding tube
flow rate The number of drops per minute *(gtt/min)* or milliliters per hour *(mL/hr)*
gavage The process of giving a tube feeding
intake The amount of fluid taken in
intravenous (IV) therapy Giving fluids through a needle or catheter into a vein; IV and IV infusion
nutrient A substance that is ingested, digested, absorbed, and used by the body
nutrition The processes involved in the ingestion, digestion, absorption, and use of food and fluids by the body
output The amount of fluid lost
regurgitation The backward flow of stomach contents into the mouth

KEY ABBREVIATIONS

GI	Gastro-intestinal
gtt	Drops
gtt/min	Drops per minute
ID	Identification
IV	Intravenous
mg	Milligram
mL	Milliliter
mL/hr	Milliliters per hour
NG	Naso-gastric
NPO	*Non per os;* nothing by mouth
OBRA	Omnibus Budget Reconciliation Act of 1987
oz	Ounce
RN	Registered nurse
USDA	United States Department of Agriculture

Food and water are physical needs necessary for life. The person's diet affects physical and mental well-being and function. A poor diet and poor eating habits:

- Increase the risk for disease and infection.
- Cause healing problems.
- Increase the risk for accidents and injuries.

See *Focus on Surveys: Assisting With Nutrition and Fluids.*

BASIC NUTRITION

Nutrition *is the processes involved in the ingestion, digestion, absorption, and use of food and fluids by the body.* Good nutrition is needed for growth, healing, and body functions. A ***nutrient*** *is a substance that is ingested, digested, absorbed, and used by the body.* Nutrients are grouped into fats, proteins, carbohydrates, vitamins, minerals, and water (p. 316).

Fats, proteins, and carbohydrates give the body fuel for energy. A ***calorie*** *is the fuel or energy value of food.*

- 1 gram of fat—9 calories
- 1 gram of protein—4 calories
- 1 gram of carbohydrate—4 calories

FOCUS ON SURVEYS

Assisting With Nutrition and Fluids

The health team must develop a care plan to meet the person's nutritional and fluid needs. Surveyors may ask you about the following. You will learn how to answer their questions as you study this chapter.

- How the person's food and fluid intake are observed and reported.
- How the person's eating ability is observed and reported.
- The measures taken to prevent or meet changes in the person's nutritional needs. Snacks and frequent meals are examples.
- The goals for nutrition in the person's care plan.

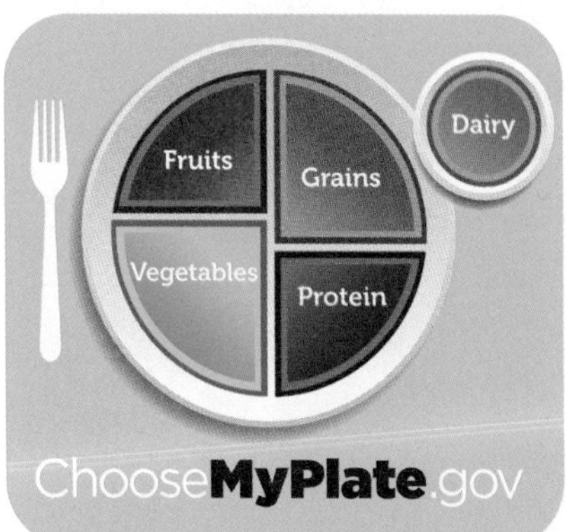

FIGURE 20-1 The MyPlate symbol.

MyPlate

The MyPlate symbol (Fig. 20-1) encourages healthy eating from 5 food groups. Issued by the United States Department of Agriculture (USDA), MyPlate is a nutrition guide that encourages physical activity (Box 20-1). MyPlate helps you make wise food choices by:

- Balancing calories
  - Eating less
  - Avoiding over-sized portions
- Increasing certain foods
  - Making half of your plate fruits and vegetables
  - Making at least half of your grains whole grains
  - Drinking fat-free or low-fat (1%) milk
- Reducing certain foods
  - Choosing low-sodium foods
  - Drinking water instead of sugary drinks

The amount needed from each food group depends on age, sex, and physical activity (Table 20-1). Activity should be moderate or vigorous (see Box 20-1). The USDA recommends that adults do at least 1 of the following.

- 2 hours and 30 minutes each week of moderate physical activity
- 1 hour and 15 minutes each week of vigorous physical activity

Physical activity at least 3 days a week is best. Each activity should be for at least 10 minutes at a time. Adults also should do strengthening activities at least 2 days a week. Push-ups, sit-ups, and weight-lifting are examples.

BOX 20-1 Physical Activities

Moderate Physical Activities

- Walking briskly (about 3½ miles per hour)
- Bicycling (less than 10 miles per hour)
- Gardening (raking, trimming bushes)
- Dancing
- Golf (walking and carrying clubs)
- Water aerobics
- Canoeing
- Tennis (doubles)

Vigorous Physical Activities

- Running and jogging (5 miles per hour)
- Walking very fast (4½ miles per hour)
- Bicycling (more than 10 miles per hour)
- Heavy yard work, such as chopping wood
- Swimming (freestyle laps)
- Aerobics
- Basketball (competitive)
- Tennis (singles)

From U.S. Department of Agriculture: What is physical activity? *June 4, 2011.*

Grains Group. Foods made from wheat, rice, oats, cornmeal, barley, or other cereal grains are grain products. Bread, pasta, oatmeal, breakfast cereals, tortillas, and grits are examples.

- *Whole grains* have the entire grain kernel. Whole-wheat flour, bulgar (cracked wheat), oatmeal, whole cornmeal, and brown rice are examples.
- *Refined grains* were processed to remove the grain kernel. They have a fine texture. White flour, white bread, and white rice are examples. They have less dietary fiber than whole grains.

Grains, especially whole grains, have these health benefits.

- Reduce the risk of heart disease
- May prevent constipation
- May help with weight management
- May prevent certain birth defects
- Contain these nutrients—dietary fiber, several B vitamins (thiamin, riboflavin, niacin, folate), and minerals (iron, magnesium, and selenium)

Vegetable Group. Vegetables can be eaten raw or cooked. They may be fresh, frozen, canned, dried, or juice. The 5 vegetable sub-groups are:

- *Dark green vegetables*—bok choy, broccoli, collard greens, dark green leafy lettuce, kale, mesclun, mustard greens, romaine lettuce, spinach, turnips, watercress
- *Red and orange vegetables*—acorn, butternut, and hubbard squashes; carrots; pumpkin; red peppers; sweet potatoes; tomatoes; tomato juice
- *Beans and peas*—black beans, black-eyed peas, garbanzo beans (chickpeas), kidney beans, lentils, navy beans, pinto beans, soybeans, split peas, and white beans
- *Starchy vegetables*—corn, green bananas, green peas, green lima beans, plantains, potatoes, taro, water chestnuts
- *Other vegetables*—artichokes, asparagus, bean sprouts, beets, Brussels sprouts, cabbage, cauliflower, celery, cucumbers, eggplant, green beans, green peppers, iceberg (head) lettuce, mushrooms, okra, onions, parsnips, turnips, wax beans, zucchini

Vegetables have these health benefits.

- May reduce the risk for stroke, heart disease, high blood pressure, cardiovascular diseases, and type 2 diabetes.
- May protect against certain cancers. Cancers of the mouth, stomach, and colon-rectum are examples.
- May reduce the risk of kidney stones.
- May reduce the risk of bone loss.
- May help lower calorie intake. Most vegetables are low in fat and calories.
- Contain no cholesterol. (*Cholesterol* is a soft, waxy substance. It is found in the bloodstream and all body cells. Dietary sources are from animal foods—egg yolks, meat, poultry, shellfish, milk, and milk products.)
- May prevent certain birth defects.
- Contain these nutrients—potassium, dietary fiber, folate (folic acid), vitamins A and C.

TABLE 20-1 MyPlate Serving Sizes

Group	Daily Servings	Serving Sizes
Grains	• Adult women: 5 to 6 ounces (oz); at least 3 oz from whole grains • Adult men: 6 to 8 oz; at least 3 to 4 oz from whole grains	• 1 oz = 1 slice bread • 1 oz = 1 cup breakfast cereal • 1 oz = ½ cup cooked rice, cereal, or pasta
Vegetables	• Adult women: 2 to 2½ cups • Adult men: 2½ to 3 cups	• 1 cup = 1 cup raw or cooked vegetables or vegetable juice • 1 cup = 2 cups raw leafy greens
Fruits	• Adult women: 1½ to 2 cups • Adult men: 2 cups	• 1 cup = 1 cup fruit • 1 cup = 1 cup fruit juice • 1 cup = ½ cup dried fruit
Dairy	• Adult women: 3 cups • Adult men: 3 cups	• 1 cup = 1 cup milk or yogurt • 1 cup = 1½ oz natural cheese • 1 cup = 2 oz processed cheese
Protein foods	• Adult women: 5 to 5½ oz • Adult men: 5½ to 6½ oz	• 1 oz = 1 oz lean meat, poultry, or fish • 1 oz = 1 egg • 1 oz = 1 tablespoon peanut butter • 1 oz = ¼ cup cooked dry beans • 1 oz = ½ oz nuts or seeds

Modified from U.S. Department of Agriculture: MyPlate, June 2011.

Fruit Group. Any fruit or 100% fruit juice counts as part of the fruit group. Fruits may be fresh, frozen, canned, or dried. Avoid fruits canned in syrup. Syrup contains added sugar. Choose fruits canned in 100% fruit juice or water.

Fruits have these health benefits.

- May reduce the risk for stroke, heart disease, high blood pressure, cardiovascular diseases, obesity, and type 2 diabetes.
- May protect against certain cancers. Cancers of the mouth, stomach, and colon-rectum are examples.
- May reduce the risk of kidney stones.
- May reduce the risk of bone loss.
- May help prevent constipation.
- May help lower calorie intake. Most fruits are low in fat and calories.
- Contain no cholesterol.
- Are low in sodium.
- May prevent certain birth defects.
- Contain these nutrients—potassium, dietary fiber, vitamin C, and folate (folic acid).

Dairy Group. All fluid milk products are part of the dairy group. So are many foods made from milk. Low-fat or fat-free choices are best. The milk group includes all fluid milk, yogurt, and cheese. (Cream, cream cheese, and butter are not in this group.)

Milk has these health benefits.

- Helps build and maintain bone mass throughout life. This may reduce the risk of osteoporosis.
- May reduce the risk of cardiovascular disease, type 2 diabetes, and high blood pressure.
- Contains these nutrients—calcium, potassium, and vitamin D.

Protein Foods Group. This group includes all foods made from meat, poultry, seafood, eggs, processed soy products, nuts, and seeds. Beans and peas are included in this group as well as the vegetable group.

When selecting foods from this group, remember:

- To choose lean or low-fat meat and poultry. Higher fat choices include regular ground beef (75% to 80% lean) and chicken with skin.
- Using fat for cooking increases the calories. Fried chicken and eggs fried in butter are examples.
- Salmon, trout, and herring are rich in substances that may reduce the risk of heart disease.
- Liver and other organ meats are high in cholesterol.
- Egg yolks are high in cholesterol. Egg whites are cholesterol-free.
- Processed meats have added sodium (salt). (See p. 314.)

Many proteins are high in fat and cholesterol. Heart disease is a major risk. However, this group provides nutrients needed for health and body maintenance.

- Protein
- B vitamins (niacin, thiamin, riboflavin, and B_6) and vitamin E
- Iron, zinc, and magnesium

Oils. Oils are fats that are liquid at room temperature. Vegetable oils for cooking are examples. They include canola oil, corn oil, and olive oil. Oils come from plants and fish. Because they have nutrients, the USDA includes oils in food patterns. However, *oils are not a food group.*

Adult women are allowed 5 to 6 teaspoons daily. Adult men are allowed 6 to 7 teaspoons daily. Some foods are high in oil—nuts, olives, some fish, and avocados.

When making oil choices, remember:

- Oils are high in calories.
- The best oil choices come from fish, nuts, and vegetables.
- Some foods are mainly oil. Mayonnaise, certain salad dressings, and soft margarine (tub or squeeze) are examples.
- Oils from plant sources do not contain cholesterol.
- *Solid fats* are solid at room temperature. Common solid fats include butter, milk fat, beef fat (tallow, suet), chicken fat, pork fat (lard), stick margarine, and shortening.
- Oils and solid fats have about 120 calories in each tablespoon.
- Enough oil is usually consumed daily from nuts, fish, cooking oil, and salad dressings.

Nutrients

No food or food group has every essential nutrient. A well-balanced diet ensures an adequate intake of essential nutrients.

- *Protein*—is the most important nutrient. It is needed for tissue growth and repair. Sources include meat, fish, poultry, eggs, milk and milk products, cereals, beans, peas, and nuts.
- *Carbohydrates*—provide energy and fiber for bowel elimination. They are found in fruits, vegetables, breads, cereals, and sugar. Fiber is not digested. It provides the bulky part of chyme for elimination.
- *Fats*—provide energy. They provide flavor and help the body use certain vitamins. Sources include meats, lard, butter, shortening, oils, milk, cheese, egg yolks, and nuts. Unneeded dietary fat is stored as body fat *(adipose tissue).*
- *Vitamins*—are needed for certain body functions. The body stores vitamins A, D, E, and K. Vitamin C and the B complex vitamins are not stored. They must be ingested daily. The lack of a certain vitamin results in illness.
- *Minerals*—are needed for bone and tooth formation, nerve and muscle function, fluid balance, and other body processes. Foods containing calcium help prevent musculo-skeletal changes.
- *Water*—is needed for all body processes (p. 316).

FACTORS AFFECTING EATING AND NUTRITION

Many factors affect eating and nutrition. Some begin in childhood and continue throughout life. Others develop later.

- *Culture.* Culture influences dietary practices, food choices, and food preparation. Frying, baking, smoking, or roasting food and eating raw food are cultural practices. So is using sauces, herbs, and spices. See *Caring About Culture: Food Practices.*
- *Religion.* Selecting, preparing, and eating food often involve religious practices. A person may follow all, some, or none of the dietary practices of his or her faith. Respect the person's religious practices.
- *Finances.* People with limited incomes often buy the cheaper carbohydrate foods. Their diets often lack protein and certain vitamins and minerals.
- *Appetite.* Appetite relates to the desire for food. *Loss of appetite* ***(anorexia)*** can occur. Causes include illness, drugs, anxiety, pain, and depression. Unpleasant sights, thoughts, and smells are other causes.
- *Personal choice.* Food likes and dislikes are influenced by foods served in the home. Usually food likes expand with age and social experiences.
- *Body reactions.* People usually avoid foods that cause allergic reactions. They also avoid foods that cause nausea, vomiting, diarrhea, indigestion, gas, or headaches.
- *Illness.* Appetite usually decreases during illness and recovery from injuries. However, nutritional needs increase. The body must fight infection, heal tissue, and replace lost blood cells. Nutrients lost through vomiting and diarrhea need replacement.
- *Drugs.* Drugs can cause loss of appetite, confusion, nausea, constipation, impaired taste, or changes in GI function. They can cause inflammation of the mouth, throat, esophagus, and stomach.
- *Chewing and swallowing problems.* Mouth, teeth, and gum problems can affect chewing. Examples include oral pain, dry or sore mouth, gum disease (Chapter 16), dental problems, and dentures that fit poorly. Stroke; pain; confusion; dry mouth; and diseases of the mouth, throat, and esophagus can affect swallowing. See "The Dysphagia Diet," on p. 315.
- *Disability.* Disease or injury can affect the hands, wrists, and arms. Assistive devices let the person eat independently. (See p. 312.)
- *Impaired cognitive function.* Impaired cognitive function may affect the person's ability to use eating utensils. And it may affect eating, chewing, and swallowing.
- *Age.* Many GI changes occur with aging.

See *Focus on Older Persons: Factors Affecting Eating and Nutrition.*

CARING ABOUT CULTURE

Food Practices

Rice, corn, and beans are protein sources in *Mexico.* In the *Philippines,* rice is a main food. And fish, vegetables, and native fruits are preferred. A diet high in sugar and animal fat is common in *Poland.* In *China,* a meal of rice with meat, fish, and vegetables is common. High sodium content is from the use of soy sauce and dried and preserved foods.

Eating beef is common in the *United States.* In *India,* Hindus do not eat beef.

Modified from D'Avanzo CE: Pocket guide to cultural health assessment, *ed 4, St Louis, 2008, Mosby.*

FOCUS ON OLDER PERSONS

Factors Affecting Eating and Nutrition

With aging, changes occur in the GI system.

- Taste and smell dull.
- Appetite decreases.
- Secretion of digestive juices decreases. Fried and fatty foods are hard to digest and may cause indigestion.

Some people must avoid high-fiber foods needed for bowel elimination. High-fiber foods are hard to chew and can irritate the intestines. Examples are apricots, celery, and fruits and vegetables with skins and seeds.

Foods providing soft bulk are often ordered for persons with chewing problems or constipation. These foods include whole-grain cereals and cooked fruits and vegetables.

Calorie needs are lower. Energy and activity levels are lower. Foods that contain calcium help prevent musculoskeletal changes. Protein is needed for tissue growth and repair. Because of cost, diets may lack high-protein foods.

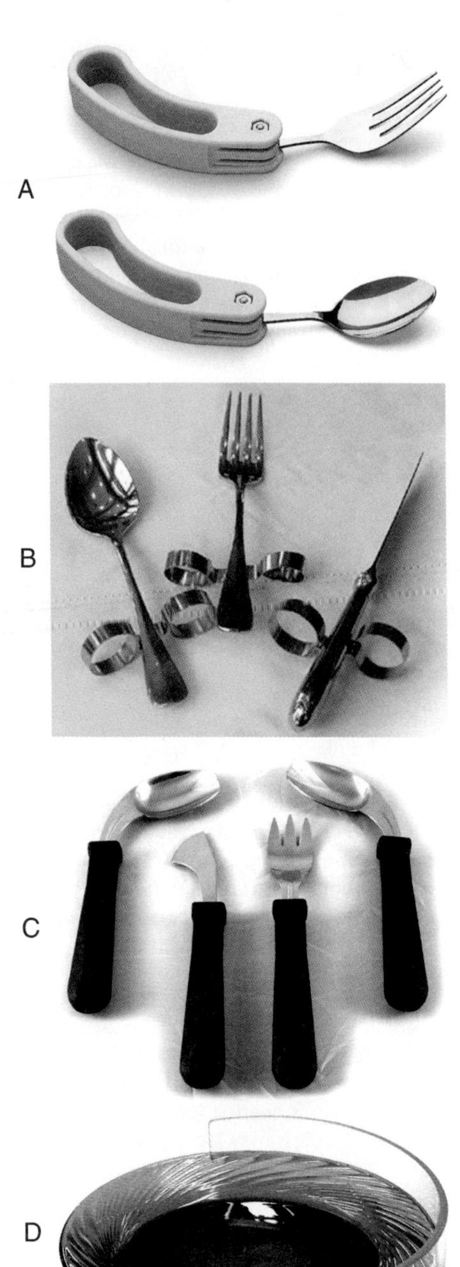

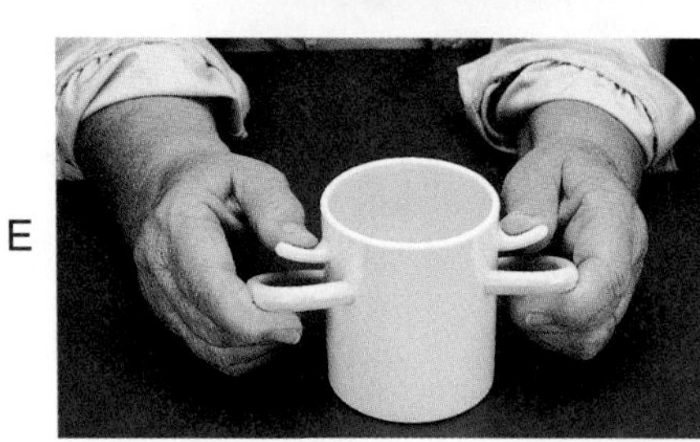

FIGURE 20-2 Assistive devices for eating. **A,** The fork and spoon are angled. Fingers are inserted through the opening or wrapped around the handle. **B,** The utensils can be adjusted for the person's grip strength. **C,** Eating utensils have tapered and angled handles. The knife cuts with slicing and rocking motions. **D,** The plate guard helps keep food on the plate. **E,** The thumb grips on the cup help prevent spilling.

OBRA DIETARY REQUIREMENTS

The Omnibus Budget Reconciliation Act of 1987 (OBRA) has requirements for food served in nursing centers.

- Each person's nutritional and dietary needs are met.
- The person's diet is well-balanced. It is nourishing and tastes good. Food is well-seasoned. It is not too salty or too sweet.
- Food is appetizing. It has an appealing aroma and is attractive.
- Foods vary in color and texture.
- Hot food is served hot. Cold food is served cold.
- Food is served promptly. If not, hot food cools and cold food warms.
- Food is prepared to meet each person's needs. Some people need food cut, ground, or chopped. Others have special diets ordered by the doctor.
- Other foods are offered to residents who refuse the food served. Substituted food must have a similar nutritional value to the first food served.
- Each person receives at least 3 meals a day. A bedtime snack is offered.
- The center provides needed assistive devices and utensils (Fig. 20-2). They promote independence in eating. Make sure the person has needed equipment.

SPECIAL DIETS

Doctors may order special diets for a nutritional deficiency or a disease (Table 20-2). They may also order them for weight control (gain or loss) or to remove or decrease certain substances in the diet. *Regular diet*, *general diet*, and *house diet* mean no dietary limits or restrictions.

The sodium-controlled diet is often ordered. So is a diabetes meal plan (p. 315). Persons with swallowing problems may need a dysphagia diet (p. 315).

The Sodium-Controlled Diet

The average amount of sodium in the daily diet is 3000 to 5000 mg (milligrams). The body needs no more than 2300 mg a day. Healthy people excrete excess sodium in the urine.

Heart, liver, and kidney diseases and certain drugs cause the body to retain extra sodium. Sodium causes the body to retain water. With too much sodium, water is retained. Tissues swell with water. There is excess fluid in the blood vessels. The heart works harder. With heart disease, the extra workload can cause serious problems or death.

Sodium-control decreases the amount of sodium in the body. Less water is retained. Less water in the tissues and blood vessels reduces the heart's workload.

The doctor orders the amount of sodium allowed. Sodium-controlled diets involve:

- Omitting high-sodium foods (Box 20-2, p. 314)
- Not adding salt to food at the table
- Limiting the amount of salt used in cooking
- Diet planning

TABLE 20-2 Special Diets

Diet	Use	Foods Allowed
Clear liquid—foods liquid at body temperature and that leave small amounts of residue; non-irritating and non–gas forming	After surgery, for acute illness, infection, nausea and vomiting, and to prepare for GI exams	Water, tea, and coffee (without milk or cream); carbonated drinks; gelatin; fruit juices without pulp (apple, grape, cranberry); fat-free broth; hard candy, sugar, and Popsicles
Full liquid—foods liquid at room temperature or that melt at body temperature	Advance from clear-liquid diet after surgery; for stomach irritation, fever, nausea, and vomiting; for persons unable to chew, swallow, or digest solid foods	Foods on the clear-liquid diet; custard; eggnog; strained soups; strained fruit and vegetable juices; milk and milk shakes; cooked cereals; plain ice cream and sherbet; pudding; yogurt
Mechanical soft—semi-solid foods that are easily digested	Advance from full-liquid diet, chewing problems, GI disorders, and infections	All liquids; eggs (not fried); broiled, baked, or roasted meat, fish, or poultry that is chopped or shredded; mild cheeses (American, Swiss, cheddar, cream, cottage); strained fruit juices; refined bread (no crust) and crackers; cooked cereal; cooked or pureed vegetables; cooked or canned fruit without skin or seeds; pudding; plain cakes and soft cookies without fruit or nuts
Fiber- and residue-restricted—foods that leave a small amount of residue in the colon	Diseases of the colon and diarrhea	Coffee, tea, milk, carbonated drinks, strained fruit and vegetable juices; refined bread and crackers; creamed and refined cereal; rice; cottage and cream cheese; eggs (not fried); plain puddings and cakes; gelatin; custard; sherbet and ice cream; canned or cooked fruit without skin or seeds; potatoes (not fried); strained cooked vegetables; plain pasta; *no raw fruits or vegetables*
High-fiber—foods that increase residue and fiber in the colon to stimulate peristalsis	Constipation and GI disorders	All fruits and vegetables; whole-wheat bread; whole-grain cereals; fried foods; whole-grain rice; milk, cream, butter, and cheese; meats
Bland—foods that are non-irritating and low in roughage; foods served at moderate temperatures; no strong spices or condiments	Ulcers, gallbladder disorders, and some intestinal disorders; after abdominal surgery	Lean meats; white bread; creamed and refined cereals; cream or cottage cheese; gelatin; plain puddings, cakes, and cookies; eggs (not fried); butter and cream; canned fruits and vegetables without skin and seeds; strained fruit juices; potatoes (not fried); pastas and rice; strained or soft cooked carrots, peas, beets, spinach, squash, and asparagus tips; creamed soups from allowed vegetables; no fried or spicy foods
High-calorie—3000 to 4000 calories daily; includes 3 full meals and between-meal snacks	Weight gain and some thyroid problems	Dietary increases in all foods; large portions of regular diet with 3 between-meal snacks
Calorie-controlled—adequate nutrients while controlling calories to promote weight loss and reduce body fat	Weight loss	Foods low in fats and carbohydrates and lean meats; avoid butter, cream, rice, gravies, salad oils, noodles, cakes, pastries, carbonated and alcoholic drinks, candy, potato chips, and similar foods
High-iron—foods high in iron	Anemia, after blood loss, for women during the reproductive years	Liver and other organ meats; lean meats; egg yolks; shellfish; dried fruits; dried beans; green leafy vegetables; lima beans; peanut butter; enriched breads and cereals
Fat-controlled (low cholesterol)—foods low in fat and prepared without adding fat	Heart disease, gallbladder disease, disorders of fat digestion, liver disease, diseases of the pancreas	Skim milk (fat free) or buttermilk; cottage cheese (no other cheeses allowed); gelatin; sherbet; fruit; lean meats, poultry, and fish (baked, broiled, or roasted); fat-free broth; soups made with skim milk (fat-free); margarine; rice, pasta, breads, and cereals; vegetables; potatoes

Continued

TABLE 20-2 Special Diets—cont'd

Diet	Use	Foods Allowed
High-protein—aids and promotes tissue healing	Burns, high fever, infection, and some liver diseases	Meat, milk, eggs, cheese, fish, poultry; breads and cereals; green leafy vegetables
Sodium-controlled—a certain amount of sodium is allowed	Heart disease, fluid retention, liver diseases, and some kidney diseases	Fruits and vegetables and unsalted butter are allowed; adding salt at the table is not allowed; highly salted foods and foods high in sodium are not allowed; the use of salt during cooking may be restricted
Diabetes meal plan—the same amount of carbohydrates, protein, and fat are eaten at the same time each day	Diabetes	Determined by nutritional and energy requirements

BOX 20-2 High-Sodium Foods

Grains
- Baked goods—biscuits, muffins, cakes, cookies, pies, pastries, sweet rolls, donuts, and so on
- Breads and rolls
- Cereals—cold, instant hot
- Noodle mixes
- Pancakes
- Salted snack foods—pretzels, corn chips, popcorn, crackers, chips, and so on
- Stuffing mixes
- Waffles

Vegetables
- Canned vegetables
- Olives
- Pickles and other pickled vegetables
- Relish
- Sauerkraut
- Tomato sauce or paste
- Vegetable juices—tomato, V8, Bloody Mary mixes
- Vegetables with sauces, creams, or seasonings

Fruits
- None—fruits are not high in sodium

Dairy Group
- Buttermilk
- Cheese
- Commercial dips made with sour cream

Protein Foods
- Bacon and Canadian bacon
- Canned meats and fish—chicken, tuna, salmon, anchovies, sardines
- Caviar
- Chipped, dried, and corned beef and other meats
- Deli meats—turkey, ham, bologna, salami, pastrami, and so on

Protein Foods—cont'd
- Dried fish
- Ham
- Herring
- Hot dogs (frankfurters)
- Liverwurst
- Lox and smoked salmon
- Mackerel
- Pepperoni
- Salt pork
- Sausages
- Scrapple
- Shellfish—shrimp, crab, clams, oysters, scallops, lobster

Other
- Asian foods—Chinese, Japanese, East Indian Thai, Vietnamese
- Baking soda and baking powder
- Catsup (ketchup)
- Cocoa mixes
- Commercially prepared dinners—frozen, canned, boxed, and so on
- Mayonnaise
- Mexican foods
- Mustard
- Pasta dishes—lasagna, manicotti, ravioli
- Peanut butter
- Pizzas
- Pot pies
- Salad dressings
- Salted nuts or seeds
- Sauces—soy, teriyaki, Worcestershire, steak, barbecue, pasta, chili, cocktail
- Seasoning salts—garlic, onion, celery, meat tenderizers, monosodium glutamate (MSG), and so on
- Soups—canned, packaged, instant, dried, bouillon

Diabetes Meal Plan

Diabetes is a chronic illness in which the body cannot produce or use insulin properly (Chapter 28). The pancreas produces and secretes insulin. Insulin lets the body use sugar. Without enough insulin, sugar builds up in the bloodstream. It is not used by cells for energy. Diabetes is usually treated with insulin or other drugs, diet, and exercise.

A meal plan for healthy eating is developed. Consistency is key. It involves:

- Food preferences (likes, eating habits, meal times, culture, and life-style). Food amounts and preparation methods may be restricted.
- Calories needed. The same amount of carbohydrates, protein, and fat are eaten each day.
- Eating meals and snacks at regular times. The person eats at regular times every day to maintain a certain blood sugar level.

Serve meals and snacks on time. Always check what was eaten. Report what the person did and did not eat. A between-meal snack makes up for what was not eaten (p. 322). The nurse tells you what to provide.

The Dysphagia Diet

***Dysphagia** means difficulty* (dys) *swallowing* (phagia). See Box 20-3 for signs and symptoms.

- A *slow swallow* means the person has difficulty getting enough food and fluids for good nutrition and fluid balance.
- An *unsafe swallow* means that food enters the airway (aspiration). ***Aspiration** is breathing fluid, food, vomitus, or an object into the lungs* (p. 324).

Food thickness is changed to meet the person's needs (see Box 20-3). Safety and comfort are important when feeding a person with dysphagia. You must:

- Know the signs and symptoms of dysphagia (see Box 20-3).
- Feed the person according to the care plan.
- Follow aspiration precautions (Box 20-4) and the care plan.
- Report changes in how the person eats.
- Observe for signs and symptoms of aspiration: choking, coughing, or difficulty breathing during or after meals; abnormal breathing or respiratory sounds. Report these observations at once.

BOX 20-3 Dysphagia

Signs and Symptoms

The person:

- Avoids food that needs chewing.
- Avoids food with certain textures and temperatures.
- Tires during a meal.
- Has food spill out of the mouth while eating.
- "Pockets" or "squirrels" food in the cheeks. This means that food remains or is hidden in the mouth.
- Eats slowly, especially solid foods.
- Complains that food will not go down or that the food is stuck.
- Coughs or chokes before, during, or after swallowing.
- Regurgitates food after eating (p. 324).
- Spits out food suddenly and almost violently.
- Has food come up through the nose.
- Has hoarseness—especially after eating.
- Makes gurgling sounds while talking or breathing after swallowing.
- Has a runny nose, sneezes, or has excessive drooling.
- Complains of frequent heartburn.
- Has a decreased appetite.

Dysphagia Diet

- *Thickened liquid*—No lumps. Pureed with milk, gravy, or broth to thickness of baby food. Thickener is added to some foods and fluids as needed. Does not mound on a plate. May be called *creamy* or a *sauce*. Stir before serving if the food settles.
- *Medium thick (nectar-like)*—The thickness of nectar or V8 juice (does not hold its shape). Stir right before serving.
- *Extra thick (honey-like)*—Thick like honey. Mounds a bit on a spoon. Can drink from a cup. Stir before serving.
- *Yogurt-like*—Thick like yogurt or pudding. Holds its shape. Served with a spoon.
- *Puree*—No lumps; mounds on a plate. May be thick like mashed potatoes.

BOX 20-4 Aspiration Precautions

- Help the person with meals and snacks. Follow the care plan.
- Position the person upright as the nurse and care plan direct. The person maintains this position for at least 1 hour after eating.
- Support the upper back, shoulders, and neck with a pillow.
- Observe for signs and symptoms of aspiration during meals and snacks.
- Check the person's mouth after eating for pocketing. Check inside the cheeks, under the tongue, and on the roof of the mouth. Remove any food.
- Provide mouth care after eating.
- Report and record your observations.

FLUID BALANCE

Water is needed to live. Death can result from too much or too little water. Water is ingested through fluids and foods. Water is lost through urine, feces, and vomit. It is also lost through the skin (perspiration) and the lungs (expiration).

Fluid balance is needed for health. *The amount of fluid taken in* ***(intake)*** and *the amount of fluid lost* ***(output)*** must be equal. When fluid intake exceeds fluid output *body tissues swell with water* ***(edema)***. Edema is common in people with heart and kidney diseases. ***Dehydration*** *is a decrease in the amount of water in body tissues.* Fluid output exceeds intake. Common causes are poor fluid intake, vomiting, diarrhea, bleeding, excess sweating, and increased urine production.

Normal Fluid Requirements

An adult needs 1500 mL (milliliters) of water daily to survive. About 2000 to 2500 mL are needed for normal fluid balance. Water requirements increase with hot weather, exercise, fever, illness, and excess fluid losses.

See *Focus on Older Persons: Normal Fluid Requirements.*

Special Fluid Orders

The doctor may order the amount of fluid a person can have during a 24-hour period. This is done to maintain fluid balance. Intake and output records are kept (Chapter 21). Common fluid orders are:

- *Encourage fluids.* The person drinks an increased amount of fluid. The order states the amount to ingest. A variety of fluids are offered and kept within the person's reach. Offer fluids often to persons who cannot feed themselves.
- *Restrict fluids.* Fluids are limited to a certain amount. They are offered in small amounts and in small containers. The water mug is removed from the room or kept out of sight. Frequent oral hygiene keeps the mouth moist.
- *Nothing by mouth.* The person cannot eat or drink anything. *NPO* stands for *non per os.* It means nothing *(non)* by *(per)* mouth *(os)*. NPO is ordered before and after surgery, before some laboratory tests and diagnostic procedures, and to treat certain illnesses. An NPO sign is posted above the bed. The water mug is removed. Frequent oral hygiene is needed, but the person must not swallow any fluid. The person is NPO for 6 to 10 hours before surgery and before some laboratory tests and diagnostic procedures. Follow agency policy.
- *Thickened liquids.* All fluids are thickened, including water. The thickness depends on the person's ability to swallow (see Box 20-3). Thickener is added before fluids are served. Or thickened commercial fluids are used.

FOCUS ON OLDER PERSONS

Normal Fluid Requirements

The amount of body water decreases with age. So does the thirst sensation. Older persons need water, but they may not feel thirsty. You need to offer water often.

Older persons are at risk for diseases that affect fluid balance. Dehydration and edema are risks. Some persons have special fluid orders.

MEETING FOOD AND FLUID NEEDS

Weakness, illness, and confusion can affect appetite and ability to eat. So can unpleasant odors, sights, and sounds. An uncomfortable position, oral hygiene needs, elimination needs, and pain also affect appetite.

See *Focus on Communication: Meeting Food and Fluid Needs.*

Preparing for Meals

Preparing patients and residents for meals promotes comfort. If they are ready to eat, you can serve meals faster. Foods stay at the correct temperature.

See *Delegation Guidelines: Preparing for Meals.*
See *Promoting Safety and Comfort: Preparing for Meals.*
See procedure: *Preparing the Person for a Meal.*

FOCUS ON COMMUNICATION

Meeting Food and Fluid Needs

The person may not eat or drink all the food and fluids served. You need to find out why and tell the nurse. Ask the person to explain. You can say:

- "Please tell me why you didn't eat everything."
- "Was there something wrong with your food?"
- "Did your food taste okay?"
- "Was there something you didn't like?"
- "Was your food too hot or too cold?"
- "Would you like something else?"
- "Weren't you hungry?"

DELEGATION GUIDELINES

Preparing for Meals

To prepare a person for a meal, you need this information from the nurse and the care plan.

- How much help the person needs
- Where the person will eat—room or dining room
- What the person uses for elimination—bathroom, commode, bedpan, or urinal
- What type of oral hygiene the person needs
- If the person wears dentures
- If the person wear eyeglasses or hearing aids
- How to position the person—in bed, a chair, or wheelchair
- How the person gets to the dining room—by self or with help
- If the person uses a wheelchair, walker, or cane
- When to report observations
- What patient or resident concerns to report at once

PROMOTING SAFETY AND COMFORT

Preparing for Meals

Safety

Before meals, the person needs to eliminate and have oral hygiene. Follow Standard Precautions and the Bloodborne Pathogen Standard (Chapter 12). Also follow them when cleaning equipment and the room.

Comfort

The meal setting must be free of unpleasant sights, sounds, and odors. If allowed, remove unpleasant equipment from the room.

Preparing the Person for a Meal

QUALITY OF LIFE

- Knock before entering the person's room.
- Address the person by name.
- Introduce yourself by name and title.
- Explain the procedure before starting and during the procedure.
- Protect the person's rights during the procedure.
- Handle the person gently during the procedure.

PRE-PROCEDURE

1 Follow *Delegation Guidelines: Preparing for Meals.* See *Promoting Safety and Comfort: Preparing for Meals.*
2 Practice hand hygiene.
3 Collect the following.
- Equipment for oral hygiene (Chapter 16)
- Bedpan and cover, urinal, or commode
- Toilet tissue
- Wash basin
- Soap
- Washcloth
- Towel
- Gloves

4 Provide for privacy.

PROCEDURE

5 Make sure eyeglasses and hearing aids are in place.
6 Assist with oral hygiene. Make sure dentures are in place. Wear gloves, and practice hand hygiene after removing and discarding them.
7 Assist with elimination. Make sure the incontinent person is clean and dry. Wear gloves, and practice hand hygiene after removing and discarding them.
8 Assist with hand washing. Wear gloves, and practice hand hygiene after removing and discarding them.
9 Do the following if the person will eat in bed.
  a Raise the head of the bed to a comfortable position.
  b Remove items from the over-bed table. Clean the over-bed table.
  c Adjust the over-bed table in front of the person.
10 Do the following if the person will sit in a chair.
  a Position the person in a chair or wheelchair.
  b Remove items from the over-bed table. Clean the table.
  c Adjust the over-bed table in front of the person.
11 Assist the person to the dining area. (This step is for the person who eats in a dining area.)

POST-PROCEDURE

12 Provide for comfort. (See the inside of the front cover.)
13 Place the call light within reach.
14 Empty, clean, rinse, and disinfect equipment. Return equipment to its proper place. Wear gloves and practice hand hygiene after removing and discarding them.
15 Straighten the room. Eliminate unpleasant noise, odors, or equipment.
16 Unscreen the person.
17 Complete a safety check of the room. (See the inside of the front cover.)
18 Practice hand hygiene.

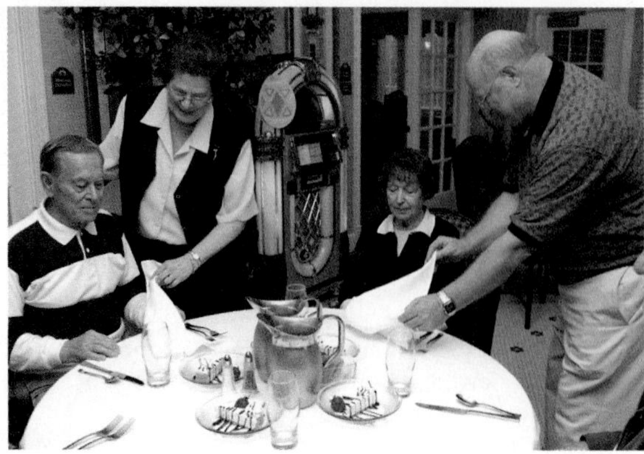

FIGURE 20-3 These residents are eating in the dining room. Volunteers help as needed.

Dining Programs

The needs of nursing center residents vary. The following dining programs are common in nursing centers.

- *Social dining.* A dining room table seats 4 to 6 residents (Fig. 20-3). Food is served as in a restaurant. Residents are oriented and can feed themselves.
- *Family dining.* Food is served in bowls and on platters. Residents serve and feed themselves as at home.
- *Low-stimulation dining.* Meal time distractions are prevented. The health team decides on the best place for each person to sit.
- *Restaurant-style menus.* The person selects food from a menu. This program allows more food choices. The person is served as in a restaurant.
- *Open dining.* A buffet is open for several hours. Residents can eat any time while the buffet is open.

Serving Meals

Food is served in containers that keep foods at the correct temperature. Hot food is kept hot. Cold food is kept cold.

You serve meals after preparing patients and residents for meals. If they are ready to eat, you can serve meals promptly. Doing so keeps food at the correct temperature.

If food is not served within 15 minutes, re-check food temperatures. Follow agency policy. If not at the correct temperature, get fresh food. Temperature guides and food thermometers are in dining rooms and in nursing unit kitchens. Some agencies allow re-heating in microwave ovens.

See *Delegation Guidelines: Serving Meals.*

See *Promoting Safety and Comfort: Serving Meals.*

See procedure: *Serving Meal Trays.*

DELEGATION GUIDELINES

Serving Meals

To serve meal trays, you need this information from the nurse and the care plan.

- The person's food allergies (if any)
- What assistive devices the person uses
- If the person needs help opening cartons, cutting food, buttering bread, and so on
- If the person's intake is measured (Chapter 21)
- If calorie counts are done (p. 322)
- When to report observations
- What patient or resident concerns to report at once

PROMOTING SAFETY AND COMFORT

Serving Meals

Safety

Always check food temperature after re-heating. Food that is too hot can cause burns.

Comfort

Check the person's position when serving a meal. The position may have changed after the person was prepared to eat. Provide other comfort measures as needed. See the inside of the front cover for comfort measures.

Serving Meal Trays

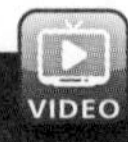

QUALITY OF LIFE

- Knock before entering the person's room.
- Address the person by name.
- Introduce yourself by name and title.
- Explain the procedure before starting and during the procedure.
- Protect the person's rights during the procedure.
- Handle the person gently during the procedure.

PRE-PROCEDURE

1 Follow *Delegation Guidelines: Serving Meals.* See *Promoting Safety and Comfort: Serving Meals.*

2 Practice hand hygiene.

Serving Meal Trays—cont'd

VIDEO

PROCEDURE

3 Make sure the tray is complete. Check items on the tray with the dietary card. Make sure assistive devices are included.
4 Identify the person. Check the ID (identification) bracelet against the dietary card. Also call the person by name.
5 Place the tray within the person's reach. Adjust the over-bed table as needed.
6 Remove food covers. Open cartons, cut food into bite-sized pieces, butter bread, and so on as needed. Season food as the person prefers and is allowed on the care plan.
7 Place the napkin, clothes protector, assistive devices, and eating utensils within reach.
8 Place the call light within reach.
9 Do the following when the person is done eating.
 a Measure and record intake if ordered (Chapter 21).
 b Note the amount and type of foods eaten. (See "Calorie Counts," on p. 322.)
 c Check for and remove any food in the mouth (pocketing). Wear gloves. Practice hand hygiene after removing and discarding them.
 d Remove the tray.
 e Clean spills. Change soiled linen and clothing.
 f Help the person return to bed if needed.
 g Assist with oral hygiene and hand washing. Wear gloves. Practice hand hygiene after removing and discarding the gloves.

POST-PROCEDURE

10 Provide for comfort. (See the inside of the front cover.)
11 Place the call light within reach.
12 Raise or lower bed rails. Follow the care plan.
13 Complete a safety check of the room. (See the inside of the front cover.)
14 Follow agency policy for soiled linen.
15 Practice hand hygiene.
16 Report and record your observations.

Feeding the Person

Weakness, paralysis, casts, confusion, and other limits can make self-feeding impossible. These persons are fed.

Serve food and fluids in the order the person prefers. Offer fluids during the meal. Fluids help the person chew and swallow.

Use teaspoons to feed the person. They are less likely to cause injury than forks. The teaspoon should only be one-third (⅓) full. This portion is chewed and swallowed easily. Some people need smaller portions. Follow the care plan.

Persons who need to be fed are often angry, humiliated, and embarrassed. Some are depressed, resentful, or refuse to eat. Let them do what they can. Some can manage "finger foods" (bread, cookies, crackers). If strong enough, let them hold milk or juice cups (never hot drinks). Follow activity limits ordered by the doctor. Provide support. Encourage them to try, even if food is spilled.

Visually impaired persons are often very aware of food aromas. They may know the food served. Always describe what is on the tray and what you are offering. For persons who feed themselves, describe foods and fluids and their place on the tray. Use the numbers on a clock for the location of foods (Fig. 20-4).

Many people pray before eating. Allow time and privacy for prayer. This shows respect and caring.

Meals provide social contact with others. Engage the person in pleasant conversation. However, allow time for chewing and swallowing. Also, sit facing the person. Sitting is more relaxing. It shows that you have time for the person. By facing the person, you can see how well the person is eating. You can also see swallowing problems.

See *Focus on Older Persons: Feeding the Person*, p. 320.

See *Focus on Surveys: Feeding the Person*, p. 320.

See *Delegation Guidelines: Feeding the Person*, p. 320.

See *Promoting Safety and Comfort: Feeding the Person*, p. 320.

See procedure: *Feeding the Person*, p. 321.

Text continued on p. 322

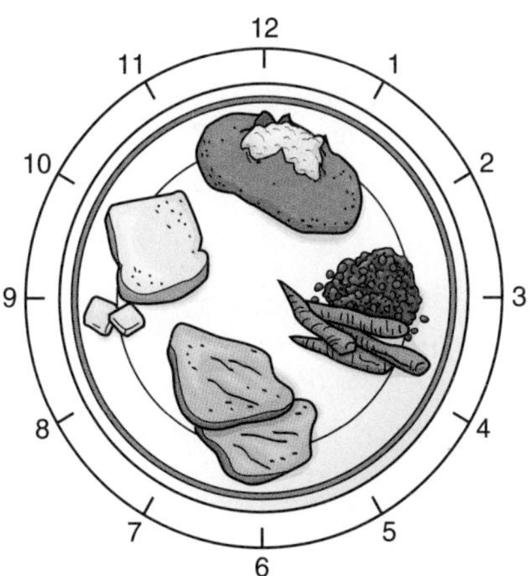

FIGURE 20-4 The numbers on a clock are used to help a visually impaired person locate food.

FOCUS ON OLDER PERSONS

Feeding the Person

Persons with dementia may become distracted during meals. Some cannot sit long enough for a meal. Others forget how to use eating utensils. Some persons resist your efforts to assist them with eating. A confused person may throw or spit food.

The Alzheimer's Disease Education and Referral Center (ADEAR) recommends the following. The measures may be part of the person's care plan.

- Provide a calm, quiet setting. Limit noise and other distractions. This helps the person focus on the meal.
- Limit the number of food choices.
- Offer several small meals throughout the day instead of larger ones.
- Use straws or cups with lids. These make drinking easier.
- Provide finger foods if the person has problems with utensils. A bowl may be easier to use than a plate.
- Provide healthy snacks. Keep snacks where the person can see them.

You must be patient. Talk to the nurse if you feel upset or impatient. Remember, the person has the right to be treated with dignity and respect.

DELEGATION GUIDELINES

Feeding the Person

Before feeding a person, you need this information from the nurse and the care plan.

- The person's food allergies (if any)
- Why the person needs help
- How much help the person needs
- How to position the person
- If the person can manage finger foods
- The person's activity limits
- The person's dietary restrictions
- What size portion to feed the person—⅓ teaspoonful or less
- Needed safety measures if the person has dysphagia
- If the person can use a straw
- What observations to report and record:
  - The amount and kind of food eaten
  - Complaints of nausea or dysphagia
  - Signs and symptoms of dysphagia
  - Signs and symptoms of aspiration
- When to report observations
- What patient or resident concerns to report at once

FOCUS ON SURVEYS

Feeding the Person

Surveyors will focus on nutritional needs. They will assess if staff:

- Provide assistance with eating.
- Encourage the person to eat.
- Help the person use assistive devices.
- Feed the person if necessary.

PROMOTING SAFETY AND COMFORT

Feeding the Person

Safety

Check food temperature. Very hot foods and fluids can burn the person.

Prevent aspiration. Check the person's mouth before offering more food or fluids. The person's mouth must be empty between bites and swallows.

Comfort

The person will eat better if not rushed. Sit to show the person that you have time. Standing communicates that you are in a hurry.

Wipe the person's hands, face, and mouth as needed during the meal. Use the napkin. If necessary, use a wet washcloth. Then dry the person with a towel.

Feeding the Person

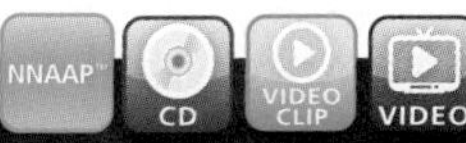

QUALITY OF LIFE

- Knock before entering the person's room.
- Address the person by name.
- Introduce yourself by name and title.
- Explain the procedure before starting and during the procedure.
- Protect the person's rights during the procedure.
- Handle the person gently during the procedure.

PRE-PROCEDURE

1 Follow *Delegation Guidelines: Feeding the Person.* See *Promoting Safety and Comfort: Feeding the Person.*
2 Practice hand hygiene.
3 Position the person in a comfortable position for eating—usually sitting or high-Fowler's. (NOTE: Some state competency tests require that the person sit upright at least 75 to 90 degrees.)
4 Get the tray. Place the tray on the over-bed table or dining table where the person can reach it.

PROCEDURE

5 Identify the person. Check the ID bracelet against the dietary card. Also call the person by name.
6 Drape a napkin across the person's chest and underneath the chin. Clean the person's hands with a hand wipe.
7 Tell the person what foods and fluids are on the tray.
8 Prepare food for eating. Cut food into bite-sized pieces. Season food as the person prefers and is allowed on the care plan.
9 Place the chair where you can sit comfortably. Sit facing the person at eye level.
10 Serve foods in the order the person prefers. Identify foods as you serve them. Alternate between solid and liquid foods. Use a spoon for safety (Fig. 20-5). Allow enough time for chewing and swallowing. Do not rush the person. Also offer water, coffee, tea, or other fluids on the tray.
11 Check the person's mouth before offering more food or fluids. Make sure the person's mouth is empty between bites and swallows. Ask if the person is ready for the next bite or drink.
12 Use straws (if allowed) for liquids if the person cannot drink out of a glass or cup. Have 1 straw for each liquid. Provide short straws for weak persons. Follow the care plan for using straws.
13 Wipe the person's hands, face, and mouth as needed during the meal. Use the napkin or a hand wipe.
14 Follow the care plan if the person has dysphagia. (Some persons with dysphagia do not use straws.) Give thickened liquid with a spoon.
15 Talk with the person in a pleasant manner.
16 Encourage him or her to eat as much as possible.
17 Wipe the person's mouth with a napkin or a hand wipe. Discard the napkin or hand wipe.
18 Note how much and which foods were eaten. See "Calorie Counts" (p. 322).
19 Measure and record intake if ordered (Chapter 21).
20 Remove the tray.
21 Take the person back to his or her room (if in a dining area).
22 Assist with oral hygiene and hand washing. Provide for privacy. Wear gloves. Practice hand hygiene after removing and discarding gloves.

POST-PROCEDURE

23 Provide for comfort. (See the inside of the front cover.)
24 Place the call light within reach.
25 Raise or lower bed rails. Follow the care plan.
26 Complete a safety check of the room. (See the inside of the front cover.)
27 Return the food tray to the food cart.
28 Practice hand hygiene.
29 Report and record your observations.

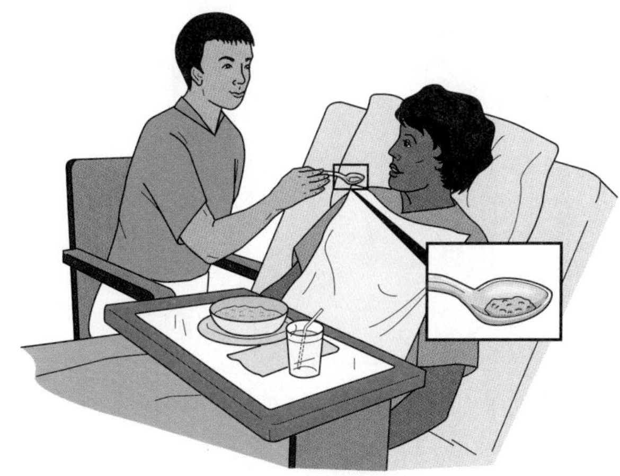

FIGURE 20-5 A spoon is used to feed the person. The spoon is one-third ($^1/_3$) full.

Between-Meal Snacks

Many special diets involve between-meal snacks. Common snacks are crackers, milk, juice, a milkshake, cake, wafers, a sandwich, gelatin, and custard.

Snacks are served upon arrival on the nursing unit. Provide needed utensils, a straw, and a napkin. Follow the same considerations and procedures for serving meals and feeding the person.

Calorie Counts

Calorie records are kept for some people. On a flow sheet, note what the person ate and how much. For example, a chicken breast, rice, beans, a roll, pudding, and 2 pats of butter were served. The person ate all the chicken, half the rice, and the roll. One pat of butter was used. The beans and pudding were not eaten. Note these on the flow sheet. A nurse or dietitian converts these portions into calories.

Providing Drinking Water

Patients and residents need fresh drinking water each shift. They also need water when the water mug is empty (Fig. 20-6).

Some agencies do not use the procedure that follows. Each person's mug is filled as needed. The mug is taken to an ice and water dispenser. If so, fill the mug with ice first. Then add water. Follow the agency's procedure for providing fresh drinking water.

See *Focus on Communication: Providing Drinking Water.*

See *Delegation Guidelines: Providing Drinking Water.*

See *Promoting Safety and Comfort: Providing Drinking Water.*

See procedure: *Providing Drinking Water.*

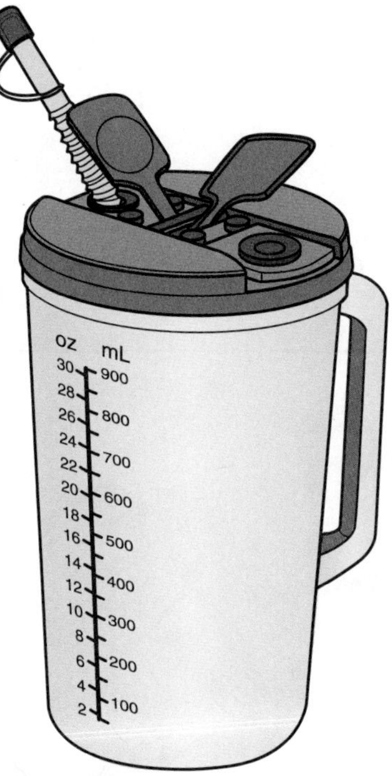

FIGURE 20-6 Water mug with straw. The mug is marked in milliliters (mL) and ounces (oz).

FOCUS ON COMMUNICATION

Providing Drinking Water

Some persons do not like ice in their water. Others like mostly ice with little water. Ask about the person's preferences. You can say:

- "How much ice do you want in your water?"
- "Do you like more ice or more water?"

Also ask the person where to place the mug. Be sure the person can reach it.

DELEGATION GUIDELINES

Providing Drinking Water

To provide water, you need this information from the nurse and the care plan.

- The person's fluid orders
- If the person can have ice
- If the person uses a straw

PROMOTING SAFETY AND COMFORT

Providing Drinking Water

Safety

Water mugs can spread microbes. To prevent the spread of microbes:

- Make sure the mug is labeled with the person's name and room and bed number.
- Do not touch the rim or inside of the mug or lid.
- Do not let the ice scoop touch the mug, lid, or straw.
- Do not place the ice scoop in the ice container or dispenser. Place it in the scoop holder or on a towel for the scoop.
- Keep the ice chest closed when not in use.
- Make sure the mug is clean. Also check for cracks and chips. Provide a new mug as needed.

Providing Drinking Water

QUALITY OF LIFE

- Knock before entering the person's room.
- Address the person by name.
- Introduce yourself by name and title.
- Explain the procedure before starting and during the procedure.
- Protect the person's rights during the procedure.
- Handle the person gently during the procedure.

PRE-PROCEDURE

1 Follow *Delegation Guidelines: Providing Drinking Water.* See *Promoting Safety and Comfort: Providing Drinking Water.*
2 Obtain a list of persons who have special fluid orders from the nurse. Or use your assignment sheet.
3 Practice hand hygiene.
4 Collect the following.
   - Cart
   - Ice chest filled with ice
   - Cover for the ice chest
   - Scoop
   - Paper towels
   - Water mugs for patient and resident use
   - Large water pitcher filled with cold water (optional depending on agency procedure)
   - Towel for the scoop
5 Cover the cart with paper towels. Arrange equipment on top of the paper towels.

PROCEDURE

6 Take the cart to the person's room door. Do not take the cart into the room.
7 Check the person's fluid orders. Use the list from the nurse.
8 Identify the person. Check the ID bracelet against the fluid order sheet or your assignment sheet. Also call the person by name.
9 Take the mug from the person's over-bed table. Empty it into the bathroom sink.
10 Determine if a new mug is needed.
11 Use the scoop to fill the mug with ice (Fig. 20-7). Do not let the scoop touch the mug, lid, or straw.
12 Place the ice scoop on the towel.
13 Fill the mug with water. Get water from the bathroom or the large water pitcher on the cart.
14 Place the mug on the over-bed table.
15 Make sure the mug is within the person's reach.

POST-PROCEDURE

16 Provide for comfort. (See the inside of the front cover.)
17 Place the call light within reach.
18 Complete a safety check of the room. (See the inside of the front cover.)
19 Practice hand hygiene.
20 Repeat steps 6 through 19 for each person.

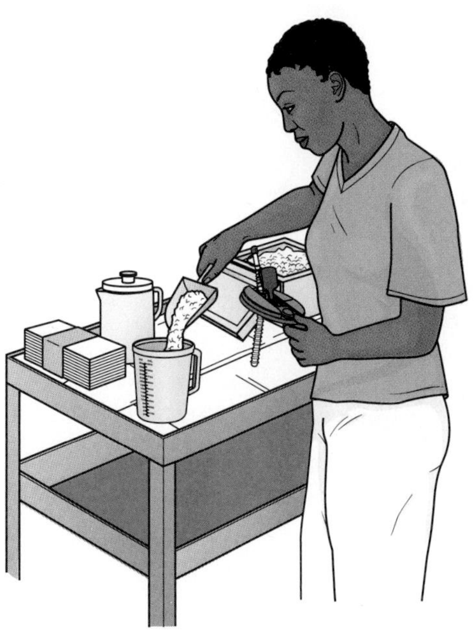

FIGURE 20-7 Providing drinking water.

ASSISTING WITH SPECIAL NEEDS

Many persons cannot eat or drink because of illness, surgery, or injury. The doctor may order nutritional support or IV (intravenous) therapy to meet food and fluid needs.

Enteral Nutrition

Some persons cannot or will not ingest, chew, or swallow food. Or food cannot pass from the mouth into the esophagus and into the stomach or small intestine. They may require enteral nutrition. ***Enteral nutrition*** *is giving nutrients into the gastro-intestinal* (GI) *tract* (enteral) *through a feeding tube.* ***Gavage*** *is the process of giving a tube feeding* (Fig. 20-8).

These feeding tubes are common.

- *Naso-gastric (NG) tube.* A feeding tube is inserted through the nose *(naso)* into the stomach *(gastro)* (Fig. 20-9).
- *Gastrostomy tube.* A feeding tube is inserted through a surgically created opening *(stomy)* in the stomach *(gastro)* (Fig. 20-10).

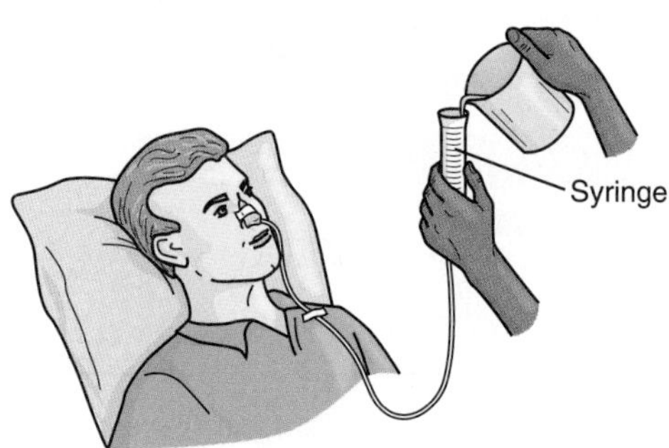

FIGURE 20-8 A tube feeding is given with a syringe.

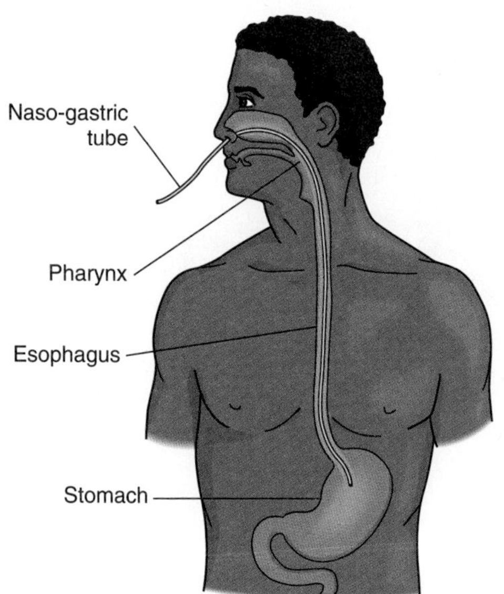

FIGURE 20-9 A naso-gastric (NG) tube is inserted through the nose and esophagus and into the stomach.

Observations. Diarrhea, constipation, delayed stomach emptying, and aspiration (p. 315) are risks. Report the following at once.

- Nausea
- Discomfort during the feeding
- Vomiting
- Distended (enlarged and swollen) abdomen
- Coughing
- Complaints of indigestion or heartburn
- Redness, swelling, drainage, odor, or pain at the ostomy site
- Fever
- Signs and symptoms of respiratory distress (Chapter 26)
- Increased pulse rate
- Complaints of flatulence (Chapter 19)
- Diarrhea (Chapter 19)

Preventing Aspiration. Aspiration is a major risk from tube feedings. It can cause pneumonia and death. Aspiration can occur:

- *During insertion.* An NG tube can slip into the airway. An x-ray is taken after insertion to check tube placement.
- *From tube movement out of place.* Coughing, sneezing, vomiting, suctioning, and poor positioning are common causes. A tube can move from the stomach or intestines into the esophagus and then into the airway. The RN (registered nurse) checks tube placement before a tube feeding. *You never check feeding tube placement.*
- *From regurgitation.* ***Regurgitation*** *is the backward flow of stomach contents into the mouth.* Delayed stomach emptying and over-feeding are common causes.

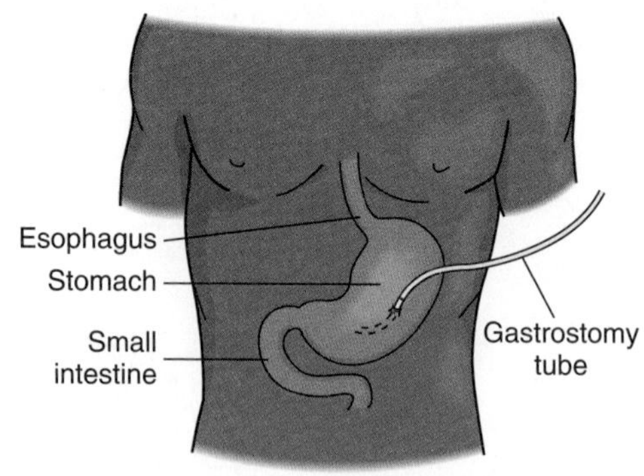

FIGURE 20-10 A gastrostomy tube.

To help prevent regurgitation and aspiration:

- Position the person in Fowler's or semi-Fowler's position before the feeding. Follow the care plan and the nurse's directions.
- Maintain Fowler's or semi-Fowler's position after the feeding. This allows formula to move through the GI tract. The position is required for 1 to 2 hours after the feeding or at all times. Follow the care plan and the nurse's directions.
- Avoid the left side-lying position. It prevents the stomach from emptying into the small intestine.

Comfort Measures. Persons with feeding tubes usually are NPO. Dry mouth, dry lips, and sore throat cause discomfort. Sometimes hard candy or gum is allowed. These measures are common every 2 hours while the person is awake.

- Oral hygiene
- Lubricant for the lips
- Mouth rinses

Feeding tubes can irritate and cause pressure on the nose. These measures are common.

- Clean the nose and nostrils every 4 to 8 hours.
- Secure the tube to the nose (Fig. 20-11). Use tape or a tube holder. Tube holders have foam cushions that prevent pressure on the nose. Re-taping is not needed. Re-taping irritates the nose.
- Secure the tube to the person's garment at the shoulder area (see Fig. 20-8). Do 1 of the following according to agency policy.
  - Loop a rubber band around the tube. Then pin the rubber band to the garment with a safety pin.
  - Tape the tube to the garment.

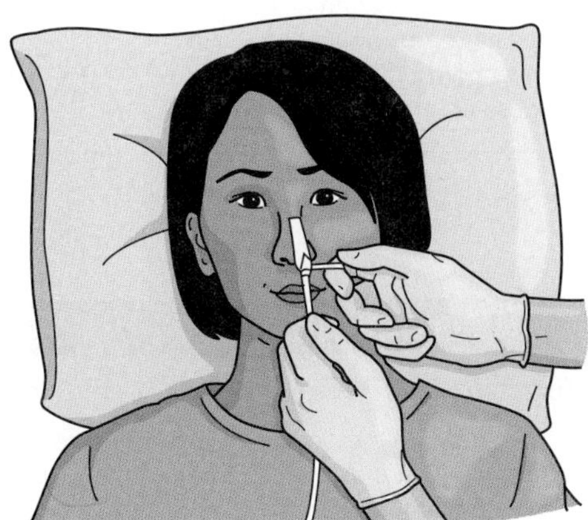

FIGURE 20-11 The feeding tube is secured to the nose.

IV Therapy

***Intravenous (IV) therapy** is giving fluids though a needle or catheter into a vein. IV and IV infusion* also refer to IV therapy. See Figure 20-12 for the basic equipment used.

- The *IV bag* contains the solution.
- A *catheter* or *needle* is inserted into a vein.
- The *IV tube* or *infusion tubing* connects the IV bag to the catheter or needle.
- Fluid drips from the bag into the *drip chamber.*
- The *clamp* is used to regulate the flow rate.
- The IV bag hangs from an IV pole (IV standard) or ceiling hook.

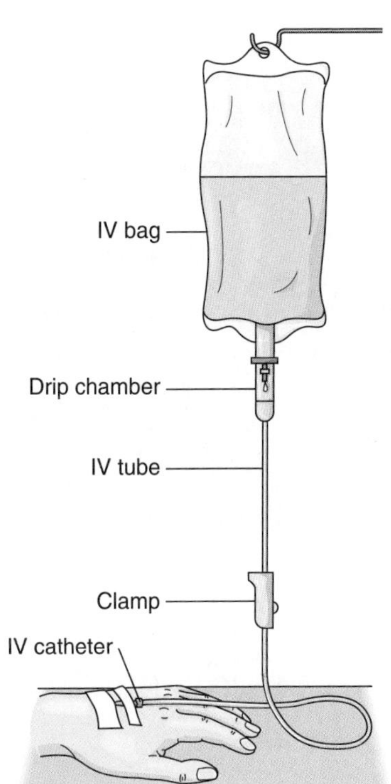

FIGURE 20-12 Equipment for IV therapy.

Flow Rate. The doctor orders the amount of fluid to give (infuse) and the amount of time to give it in. With this information, the RN figures the flow rate. The *flow rate is the number of drops per minute* (gtt/min) *or milliliters per hour* (mL/hr). The abbreviation *gtt* means *drops*. The Latin word *guttae* means *drops*.

The RN sets the clamp for the flow rate. Or an electric pump is used to control the flow rate. The flow rate is displayed in mL/hr. An alarm sounds if something is wrong. Tell the nurse at once if you hear an alarm.

You can check the flow rate if a pump is not used. The RN tells you the number of drops per minute (gtt/min). To check the flow rate, count the number of drops in 1 minute (Fig. 20-13). Tell the RN at once if:

- No fluid is dripping.
- The rate is too fast.
- The rate is too slow.
- The bag is empty or close to being empty.

See *Promoting Safety and Comfort: Flow Rate.*

Assisting With IV Therapy. You help meet the safety, hygiene, and activity needs of persons with IVs. Follow the safety measures in Box 20-5. Report any of the signs and symptoms listed in Box 20-5 at once.

You never start or maintain IV therapy. Nor do you regulate the flow rate or change IV bags. You never give blood or IV drugs.

See *Focus on Communication: Assisting With IV Therapy.*

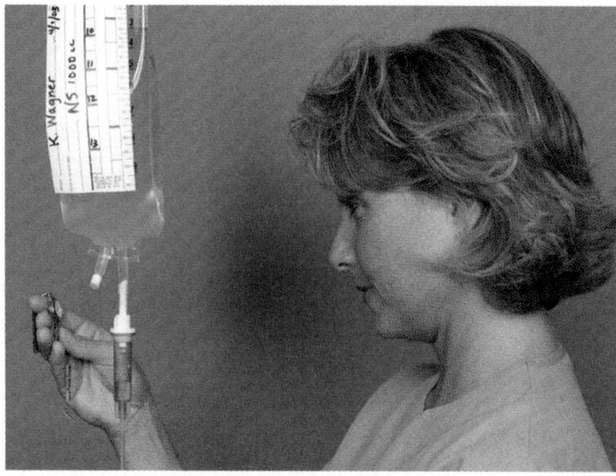

FIGURE 20-13 The flow rate is checked by counting the number of drops per minute.

PROMOTING SAFETY AND COMFORT

Flow Rate

Safety

The person can suffer serious harm if the flow rate is too fast or too slow. The flow rate can change from:

- Position changes
- Kinked tubes
- Lying on the tube

Never change the position of the clamp or adjust any controls on IV pumps. Tell the nurse at once if there is a problem with the flow rate.

BOX 20-5 IV Therapy

- Follow Standard Precautions and the Bloodborne Pathogen Standard.
- Do not move the needle or catheter. Needle or catheter position must be maintained. If the needle or catheter is moved, it may come out of the vein. Then fluid flows into tissues (infiltration). Or the flow stops.
- Follow the safety measures for restraints (Chapter 11). The nurse may splint or restrain the extremity to prevent movement. Or the nurse may apply a protective device. This helps prevent the needle or catheter from moving.
- Protect the IV bag, tubing, and needle or catheter when the person walks. Portable IV stands are rolled along next to the person.
- Assist the person with turning and re-positioning. Move the IV bag to the side of the bed on which the person is lying. Always allow enough slack in the tubing. The needle or catheter can move from pressure on the tube.
- Tell the nurse at once if bleeding occurs from the insertion site. Follow Standard Precautions and the Bloodborne Pathogen Standard.
- Report signs and symptoms of IV therapy complications. Report the following at once.
  - Local—at the IV site
    - Bleeding
    - Blood backing up into the IV tube
    - Puffiness or swelling
    - Pale or reddened skin
    - Complaints of pain at or above the IV site
    - Hot or cold skin near the site
  - Systemic—involving the whole body
    - Fever
    - Itching
    - Drop in blood pressure
    - Pulse rate greater than 100 beats per minute
    - Irregular pulse
    - Cyanosis
    - Confusion or changes in mental function
    - Loss of consciousness
    - Difficulty breathing
    - Shortness of breath
    - Decreasing or no urine output
    - Chest pain
    - Nausea

FOCUS ON COMMUNICATION

Assisting With IV Therapy

The nurse may instruct the person how to position the arm during IV therapy. You may need to remind the person:

- To position the arm a certain way
- About position limits

For example, Mr. Winn has an IV in his arm. If he bends his arm, the tubing is kinked. The flow of fluid stops. You can say: "Mr. Winn, please keep your arm straight. The fluid will not flow through your IV when your arm is bent."

FOCUS ON PRIDE

The Person, Family, and Yourself

Personal and Professional Responsibility

Many agencies serve food in new ways. For example:

- *24-hour catering.* Meals and snacks are served 24 hours a day. This is for persons who cannot or do not want to eat at the usual meal times. Food is ordered directly from the food service department. Food choices must be within the person's ordered diet.
- *Mobile food carts.* Food service staff bring a food cart to the nursing unit. The person selects food and a tray is prepared.

With such systems, you may have new responsibilities. You may have to serve food trays more often. Or you may need to read and fill out menus. Know your role in the agency's food ordering and delivery system. Take pride in helping others meet their nutritional needs.

Rights and Respect

The right to personal choice is important to meet food and fluid needs. Cultural, social, religious, medical, and personal factors affect food choices throughout life. These do not change when in a hospital or nursing center. People often comment about food likes and dislikes. A person may say that the food is cold. Or it is bland. Or the food tastes bad.

People have the right to express what they prefer. Do not become angry or upset. The person should not feel as if he or she is complaining or being picky. Learning the person's likes and dislikes can improve nutrition. It also shows interest and concern for the person. Respect the person's right to express personal food choices.

Independence and Social Interaction

Some persons with IVs can shower or bathe in a tub. This promotes comfort and independence. IV sites must be kept clean and dry. The nurse may have you apply a plastic bag, plastic wrap, or glove to protect the site. Follow agency policy and the nurse's instructions.

Delegation and Teamwork

Some agencies use meal carts for trays. Each tray is in a slot. Trays are served in the order that they appear in the cart. The entire nursing team serves trays. You may serve trays to patients and residents of other staff members. They do the same for you. The team works together to serve food promptly.

Ethics and Laws

Caring for persons with special nutrition needs can be complex. Treatments may require changes in the way you give care. For example, you learned to place a person receiving tube feedings in semi-Fowler's or Fowler's position. If you lower the head of the bed, the person may regurgitate and aspirate. In Chapter 21, you will learn not to take a blood pressure in the arm with an IV infusion.

Each person is different. Consider what special care measures may be needed. If you do not know, ask the nurse. Neglecting safety measures is unethical. The person may be harmed. Legal action can be taken. You can lose your ability to work as a nursing assistant.

REVIEW QUESTIONS

Circle the BEST answer.

1 MyPlate encourages
  a The same diet for everyone
  b Eating less
  c Increasing the amount of high-sodium foods
  d Eating more refined grains

2 On a 2000 calorie diet, what is the amount of grains needed for an adult woman?
  a 1 oz
  b 2 to 2½ oz
  c 3 oz
  d 5 to 6 oz

3 On a 2000 calorie diet, which would meet an adult male's daily dairy needs?
  a 1 slice of bread, 1 cup of cheese, and ½ oz of nuts
  b 2 cups of milk and 1 cup of cooked rice
  c 1 cup of milk, 1 cup of yogurt, and 1½ oz of cheese
  d 2 tablespoons of peanut butter and 1 egg

4 Which food group contains the *most* cholesterol?
  a Grains
  b Vegetables
  c Fruit
  d Protein foods

5 These statements are about oils. Which is *true?*
  a The best oil choices come from fish, nuts, and vegetable oils.
  b Oils are low in calories.
  c Oils from plant sources contain cholesterol.
  d Oils are a food group.

6 Protein is needed for
  a Tissue growth and repair
  b Energy and the fiber for bowel elimination
  c Body heat and to protect organs from injury
  d Improving the taste of food

7 Which foods provide the *most* protein?
  a Butter and cream
  b Tomatoes and potatoes
  c Meats and fish
  d Corn and lettuce

8 The sodium-controlled diet involves
  a Omitting high-sodium foods
  b Adding salt to food at the table
  c Using 2400 mg of salt in cooking
  d A sodium-intake flow sheet

Continued

REVIEW QUESTIONS—cont'd

Circle the BEST answer—cont'd

9 Diabetes meal planning involves
- **a** Changing the thickness of foods
- **b** Varying the amount of carbohydrates each day
- **c** Controlling sodium
- **d** Eating at regular times

10 Which does OBRA require?
- **a** 2 meals a day and a bedtime snack
- **b** Serving food promptly
- **c** Serving food at room temperature to avoid burns
- **d** A sodium-controlled diet

11 For normal fluid balance, an adult requires
- **a** 500 to 1000 mL daily
- **b** 1500 mL daily
- **c** 2000 to 2500 mL daily
- **d** 5000 mL daily

12 A person is NPO. You should
- **a** Provide a variety of fluids
- **b** Offer fluids in small amounts and in small containers
- **c** Remove the water mug from the room
- **d** Remove oral hygiene equipment from the room

13 A person coughs and drools while eating. You should
- **a** Give the person a drink
- **b** Puree the person's food
- **c** Give mouth care and continue feeding
- **d** Tell the nurse

14 When feeding a person
- **a** Ask in what order the person likes foods served
- **b** Use a fork
- **c** Stand facing the person
- **d** Talk with your co-workers

15 Before providing fresh drinking water, you need to know the person's
- **a** Intake
- **b** Fluid orders
- **c** Diet
- **d** Preferred beverages

16 Which position prevents regurgitation after a tube feeding?
- **a** Fowler's or semi-Fowler's position
- **b** The supine position
- **c** The left or right side-lying position
- **d** The prone position

17 A person with a feeding tube is NPO. Which measure should you question?
- **a** Provide oral hygiene.
- **b** Provide mouth rinses.
- **c** Give clear liquids.
- **d** Apply lubricant to the lips.

18 A person has an NG tube. To prevent nasal irritation
- **a** Clean the tube every 4 to 8 hours
- **b** Replace the tape on the nose every 4 hours
- **c** Remove the tube every 4 hours
- **d** Secure the tube to the person's gown

19 A nurse asks you to check an IV flow rate. A pump is not used. What should you do?
- **a** Count the drops in 30 seconds. Multiply the number by 2.
- **b** Count the drops for 1 minute.
- **c** Check if the fluid is dripping too fast or slow.
- **d** Measure the amount of fluid.

20 You see bleeding from an IV site. You should
- **a** Tell the nurse
- **b** Move the needle or catheter
- **c** Remove the IV
- **d** Clamp the IV tubing

Answers to these questions are on p. 505.

FOCUS ON PRACTICE

Problem Solving

Mr. Lund has Parkinson's disease (Chapter 28). This affects his movement, swallowing, and speech. When you try to feed him, he closes his mouth and shakes his head. He refuses all of the foods on his tray. He takes only small sips of thickened liquid. What do you do? What measures might be included in his care plan to meet nutrition and fluid needs?

CHAPTER

21

Assisting With Assessment

OBJECTIVES

- Define the key terms and key abbreviations listed in this chapter.
- Explain why vital signs are measured.
- List the factors affecting vital signs.
- Identify the normal ranges for each temperature site.
- Explain when to use each temperature site.
- Explain how to use thermometers.
- Identify the pulse sites.
- Describe a normal pulse and normal respirations.
- Describe the practices to follow when measuring blood pressure.
- Describe the 4 types of pain.
- Explain why pain is personal.
- List the signs and symptoms of pain.
- Identify the fluids counted as intake and the fluids counted as output.
- Explain how to prepare the person for weight and height measurements.
- Explain how you assist with assessment.
- Perform the procedures described in this chapter.
- Explain how to promote PRIDE in the person, the family, and yourself.

KEY TERMS

blood pressure (BP) The amount of force exerted against the walls of an artery by the blood

body temperature The amount of heat in the body that is a balance between the amount of heat produced and the amount lost by the body

diastolic pressure The pressure in the arteries when the heart is at rest

discomfort See "pain"

fever Elevated body temperature

hypertension When the systolic pressure is 140 mm Hg or higher *(hyper)*, or the diastolic pressure is 90 mm Hg or higher

hypotension When the systolic pressure is below *(hypo)* 90 mm Hg, or the diastolic pressure is below 60 mm Hg

intake The amount of fluid taken in

output The amount of fluid lost

pain To ache, hurt, or be sore; discomfort

pulse The beat of the heart felt at an artery as a wave of blood passes through the artery

pulse rate The number of heartbeats or pulses felt or heard in 1 minute

respiration Breathing air into *(inhalation)* and out of *(exhalation)* the lungs

stethoscope An instrument used to listen to the sounds produced by the heart, lungs, and other body organs

systolic pressure The pressure in the arteries when the heart contracts

thermometer A device used to measure *(meter)* temperature *(thermo)*

vital signs Temperature, pulse, respirations, and blood pressure; and pain in some agencies

KEY ABBREVIATIONS

BP	Blood pressure
C	Centigrade
F	Fahrenheit
Hg	Mercury
ID	Identification
I&O	Intake and output
IV	Intravenous
mL	Milliliter
mm	Millimeter
mm Hg	Millimeters of mercury
oz	Ounce

You assist the nurse with the assessment step of the nursing process. Some observations involve measurements.

VITAL SIGNS

Vital signs reflect the function of 3 body processes—regulation of body temperature, breathing, and heart function. The ***vital signs*** *of body function are:*

- *Temperature*
- *Pulse*
- *Respirations*
- *Blood pressure*
- *Pain* (in some agencies, p. 347)

Vital signs are often called TPR (temperature, pulse, and respirations) and BP (blood pressure). A person's vital signs vary within certain limits. Box 21-1 lists the factors affecting vital signs.

Vital signs are measured to detect changes in normal body function. They show even minor changes in the person's condition. They tell about treatment responses. Vital signs often signal life-threatening events.

Accuracy is essential when you measure, record, and report vital signs. If unsure of your measurements, promptly ask the nurse to take them again. Unless otherwise ordered, take vital signs with the person at rest—lying or sitting. Report the following at once.

- Any vital sign that is changed from a prior measurement
- Vital signs above or below the normal range

See *Focus on Communication: Vital Signs.*

See *Focus on Older Persons: Vital Signs.*

BOX 21-1 Factors Affecting Vital Signs

- Activity
- Anger
- Anxiety
- Drugs
- Eating
- Exercise
- Fear
- Illness
- Noise
- Pain
- Sleep
- Weather

FOCUS ON COMMUNICATION

Vital Signs

Patients and residents like to know their measurements. If agency policy allows, tell the person the measurements. If the person consents, you can tell family members if they ask. This information is private and confidential. Roommates and visitors must not hear what you say.

Sometimes measurements are abnormal. Sometimes you cannot feel a pulse or hear a blood pressure. Do not alarm the person. You can say:

- "I'm not sure if I counted your pulse correctly. I'll ask the nurse to take it."
- "I'm not sure if I heard your blood pressure correctly. I'll ask the nurse to take it again."
- "Your pulse is a little slow (or fast). I'll ask the nurse to check it."
- "Your temperature is higher than normal. I'll use another thermometer and ask the nurse to check you."

FOCUS ON OLDER PERSONS

Vital Signs

Measuring vital signs on persons with dementia may be difficult. The person may move about, hit at you, and grab equipment. This is not safe for the person or you. Two staff may be needed. One uses touch and a soothing voice to calm and distract the person. The other measures the vital signs.

Trying the procedure when the person is calmer may help. Or take the pulse and respirations at one time. Then take the temperature and blood pressure at another time.

Approach the person calmly. Use a soothing voice. Tell the person what you will do. Do not rush the person. Follow the care plan. If you cannot measure vital signs, tell the nurse.

Body Temperature

***Body temperature** is the amount of heat in the body. It is a balance between the amount of heat produced and the amount lost by the body.* Heat is produced as cells use food for energy. It is lost through the skin, breathing, urine, and feces. Body temperature stays fairly stable. It is lower in the morning and higher in the afternoon and evening. See Box 21-1 for the factors affecting body temperature.

You use thermometers to measure temperature. A ***thermometer** is a device used to measure* (meter) *temperature* (thermo). Thermometers have Fahrenheit (F) or centigrade (C) scales.

Temperature Sites. Temperature sites are the mouth, rectum, axilla (underarm), tympanic membrane (ear), and temporal artery (forehead) (Box 21-2). Each site has a normal range (Table 21-1). ***Fever** means an elevated body temperature.* Always report temperatures that are above or below the normal range.

See *Focus on Communication: Temperature Sites.*
See *Focus on Older Persons: Temperature Sites.*
See *Promoting Safety and Comfort: Temperature Sites.*

BOX 21-2 Temperature Sites

Oral Site
Oral temperatures are not taken if the person:
- Is under 4 or 5 years of age.
- Is unconscious.
- Has had surgery or an injury to the face, neck, nose, or mouth.
- Is receiving oxygen.
- Breathes through the mouth.
- Has a naso-gastric tube.
- Is delirious, restless, confused, or disoriented.
- Is paralyzed on 1 side of the body.
- Has a sore mouth.
- Has a convulsive (seizure) disorder.

Rectal Site
The rectal site is used for infants and children under 3 years old. Rectal temperatures are taken when the oral site cannot be used. Rectal temperatures are not taken if the person:
- Has diarrhea.
- Has a rectal disorder or injury.
- Has heart disease.
- Had rectal surgery.
- Is confused or agitated.

Tympanic Membrane Site
The site has fewer microbes than the mouth or rectum. The risk of spreading infection is reduced. This site is not used if the person has:
- An ear disorder
- Ear drainage

Temporal Artery Site
Measures body temperature at the temporal artery in the forehead. The site is non-invasive.

Axillary Site
Less reliable than the other sites. It is used when the other sites cannot be used.

TABLE 21-1 Normal Body Temperatures

Site	Baseline	Normal Range
Oral	98.6°F (37.0°C)	97.6°F to 99.6°F (36.5°C to 37.5°C)
Rectal	99.6°F (37.5°C)	98.6°F to 100.6°F (37.0°C to 38.1°C)
Axillary	97.6°F (36.5°C)	96.6°F to 98.6°F (35.9°C to 37.0°C)
Tympanic membrane	98.6°F (37.0°C)	98.6°F (37.0°C)
Temporal artery	99.6°F (37.5°C)	99.6°F (37.5°C)

FOCUS ON COMMUNICATION

Temperature Sites

Using the rectal site can be embarrassing and uncomfortable. Be professional. Tell the person what you are going to do. Explain why you must use the site. For example:

> Mr. Presney, I need to check your temperature. I must use the rectal site because oxygen changes the temperature in your mouth. This thermometer has to stay in place for 2 minutes. Please tell me if you feel pain.

A glass thermometer remains in the rectum for at least 2 minutes. This can cause discomfort. To promote comfort, talk the person through the procedure. You can say: "I'm almost done. There's about 1 minute left. Are you doing okay?"

FOCUS ON OLDER PERSONS

Temperature Sites

Older persons have lower body temperatures than younger persons. An oral temperature of 98.6°F (37.0°C) may signal fever in an older person.

PROMOTING SAFETY AND COMFORT

Temperature Sites

Safety
The rectal site is dangerous for persons with heart disease. The thermometer can stimulate the vagus nerve. This nerve affects the heart. Stimulation of the vagus nerve slows the heart rate. The heart rate can slow to dangerous levels in some persons.

Thermometers. Follow the manufacturer's instructions and agency procedures to use, clean, and store thermometers.

- *Electronic thermometers* are battery operated. The temperature is shown on the front of the device. See "Electronic Thermometers."
    - *Standard electronic thermometer*—measures body temperature at the oral, rectal, and axillary sites. See Figure 21-1, *A*.
    - *Tympanic membrane thermometer*—measures body temperature at the tympanic membrane in the ear (Fig. 21-1, *B*).
    - *Temporal artery thermometer*—measures body temperature at the temporal artery in the forehead (Fig. 21-1, *C*).
    - *Digital thermometer*—measures body temperature at the oral, rectal, and axillary sites. Depending on the type, the temperature is measured in 6 to 60 seconds. See Figure 21-1, *D*.
- *Glass thermometers* have a hollow glass tube and a bulb tip (Fig. 21-1, *E*). The device is filled with a substance. When heated, the substance expands and rises in the tube. When cooled, the substance contracts and moves down the tube. See "Glass Thermometers" on p. 336.

Taking Temperatures. The nurse and care plan tell you:

- When to take the person's temperature
- What site to use
- What thermometer to use

See *Delegation Guidelines: Taking Temperatures.*
See *Promoting Safety and Comfort: Taking Temperatures.*

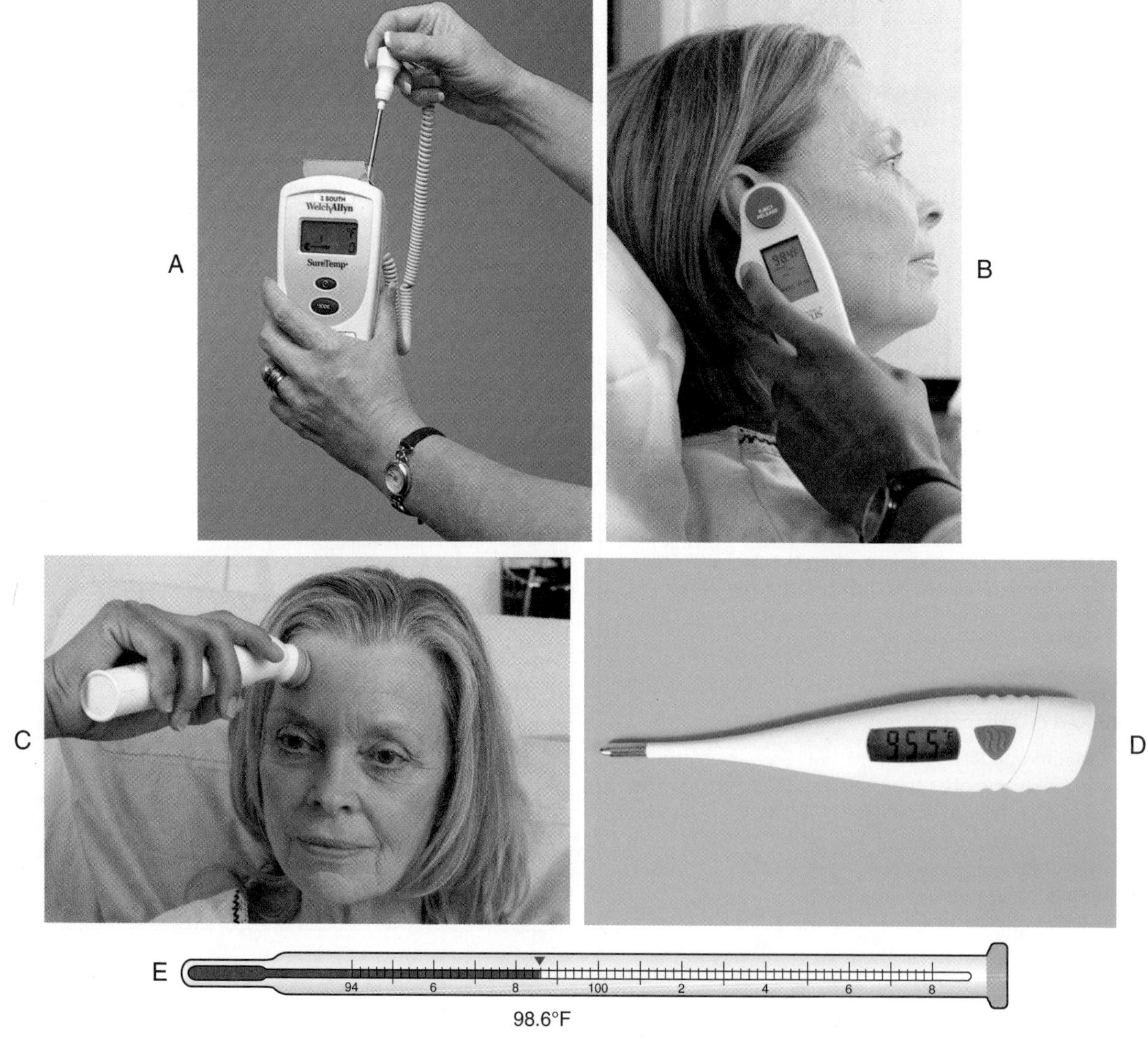

FIGURE 21-1 Types of thermometers. **A,** Standard electronic thermometer. **B,** Tympanic membrane thermometer. **C,** Temporal artery thermometer. **D,** Digital thermometer. **E,** Glass thermometer.

DELEGATION GUIDELINES

Taking Temperatures

Before taking temperatures, you need this information from the nurse and the care plan.

- What site to use for each person—oral, rectal, axillary, tympanic membrane, or temporal artery
- What thermometer to use for each person
- How long to leave a glass thermometer in place (p. 336)
- When to take temperatures
- What persons are at risk for elevated temperatures
- What observations to report and record
- When to report observations
- What patient or resident concerns to report at once
  - A temperature that is changed from a past measurement
  - A temperature above or below the normal range for the site used

PROMOTING SAFETY AND COMFORT

Taking Temperatures

Safety

Thermometers are inserted into the mouth, rectum, axilla, and ear. Each area has many microbes. The area may contain blood. Therefore each person has his or her own glass or digital thermometer. Disposable covers (sheaths) or caps are used for other electronic thermometers. This prevents the spread of microbes and infection. Follow Standard Precautions and the Bloodborne Pathogen Standard (Chapter 12).

With rectal temperatures, your gloved hands may have contact with feces. If so, remove gloves and practice hand hygiene. Then note the temperature on your note pad or assignment sheet. Put on clean gloves to complete the procedure.

Comfort

Remove the thermometer promptly. Do not leave it in place longer than needed. This affects comfort. For example, an oral glass thermometer is left in place for 2 or 3 minutes. Do not leave it in place longer than that.

Electronic Thermometers. Electronic thermometers are commonly used. Probe covers or caps prevent the spread of infection.

Electronic thermometers have batteries. Some are kept in chargers when not in use.

- Standard electronic thermometers (see Fig. 21-1, *A*) measure temperature in a few seconds. They have oral (blue) and rectal (red) probes. The oral (blue) probe is used for axillary temperatures.
- Tympanic membrane thermometers measure temperature in 1 to 3 seconds. They are comfortable and not invasive. There are fewer microbes in the ear than in the mouth or rectum. The risk of spreading infection is reduced. To use one, gently insert the covered probe into the ear (see Fig. 21-1, *B*).
- Temporal artery thermometers measure body temperature in 3 to 4 seconds. Non-invasive, they measure the temperature of the blood in the temporal artery. It is the same temperature of the blood coming from the heart. To use one:
  1. Use the side of the head that is exposed. Do not use the side covered by hair, a dressing, a hat, or other covering. Do not use the side that was on a pillow.
  2. Place a disposable cap or cover on the thermometer.
  3. Place the device in the center of the forehead.
  4. Press the scan button.
  5. Slide the device across the forehead and across the temporal artery (see Fig. 21-1, *C*).
  6. Release the scan button.
  7. Read the temperature display.

See *Focus on Older Persons: Electronic Thermometers.*

See procedure: *Taking a Temperature With an Electronic Thermometer*, p. 334.

Text continued on p. 336

FOCUS ON OLDER PERSONS

Electronic Thermometers

Tympanic membrane and temporal artery thermometers are used for persons who are confused and resist care. They are fast and comfortable. Oral and rectal glass and electronic thermometers are unsafe.

- A glass thermometer can break if the person moves, resists care, or bites down on it. Serious injury can occur.
- An electronic thermometer can injure the mouth and teeth if the person bites down on it. Injuries also can occur if the person moves quickly and without warning.

Taking a Temperature With an Electronic Thermometer

QUALITY OF LIFE

- Knock before entering the person's room.
- Address the person by name.
- Introduce yourself by name and title.
- Explain the procedure before starting and during the procedure.
- Protect the person's rights during the procedure.
- Handle the person gently during the procedure.

PRE-PROCEDURE

1 Follow *Delegation Guidelines: Taking Temperatures,* p. 333. See *Promoting Safety and Comfort: Taking Temperatures,* p. 333.
2 For an oral temperature, ask the person not to eat, drink, smoke, or chew gum for at least 15 to 20 minutes before the measurement or as required by agency policy.
3 Practice hand hygiene.
4 Collect the following.
   - Thermometer—electronic or tympanic membrane
   - Probe (blue for an oral or axillary temperature; red for a rectal temperature)
   - Probe covers
   - Toilet tissue (rectal temperature)
   - Water-soluble lubricant (rectal temperature)
   - Gloves
   - Towel (axillary temperature)

5 Plug the probe into the thermometer if using a standard electronic thermometer.
6 Practice hand hygiene.
7 Identify the person. Check the identification (ID) bracelet against the assignment sheet. Also call the person by name.

PROCEDURE

8 Provide for privacy. Position the person for an oral, rectal, axillary, or tympanic membrane temperature. The Sims' position is used for a rectal temperature.
9 Put on gloves if contact with blood, body fluids, secretions, or excretions is likely.
10 Insert the probe into a probe cover.
11 *For an oral temperature:*
   a Ask the person to open the mouth and raise the tongue.
   b Place the covered probe at the base of the tongue and to 1 side (Fig. 21-2).
   c Ask the person to lower the tongue and close the mouth.
12 *For a rectal temperature:*
   a Put a small amount of lubricant on a tissue.
   b Lubricate the end of the covered probe.
   c Expose the anal area.
   d Raise the upper buttock.
   e Insert the probe ½ inch into the rectum (Fig. 21-3).
   f Hold the probe in place.
13 *For an axillary temperature:*
   a Help the person remove an arm from the gown. Do not expose the person.
   b Dry the axilla with the towel.
   c Place the covered probe in the center of the axilla (Fig. 21-4).
   d Place the person's arm over the chest.
   e Hold the probe in place.
14 *For a tympanic membrane temperature:*
   a Ask the person to turn his or her head so the ear is in front of you.
   b Pull up and back on the adult's ear to straighten the ear canal (Fig. 21-5).
   c Insert the covered probe gently.
15 Start the thermometer.
16 Hold the probe in place until you hear a tone or see a flashing or steady light.
17 Read the temperature on the display.
18 Remove the probe. Press the eject button to discard the cover.
19 Note the person's name, temperature, and temperature site on your note pad or assignment sheet.
20 Return the probe to the holder.
21 Help the person put the gown back on (axillary temperature). For a rectal temperature:
   a Wipe the anal area with toilet tissue to remove lubricant.
   b Cover the person.
   c Dispose of used toilet tissue.
   d Remove and discard the gloves. Practice hand hygiene.

POST-PROCEDURE

22 Provide for comfort. (See the inside of the front cover.)
23 Place the call light within reach.
24 Unscreen the person.
25 Complete a safety check of the room. (See the inside of the front cover.)
26 Return the thermometer to the charging unit.
27 Practice hand hygiene.
28 Report and record the temperature. Note the temperature site when reporting and recording. Report an abnormal temperature at once.

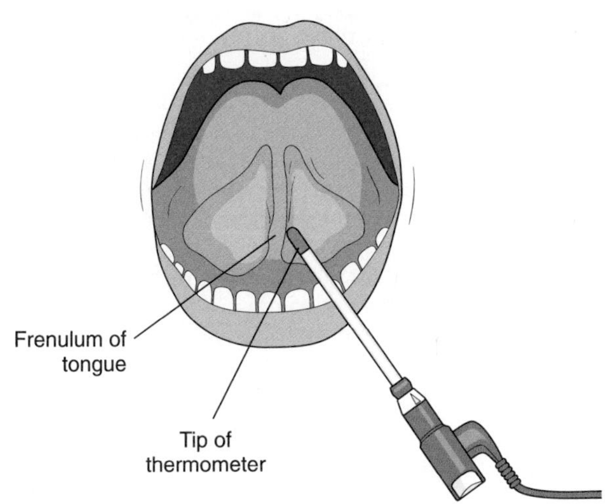

FIGURE 21-2 The thermometer is placed at the base of the tongue and to 1 side.

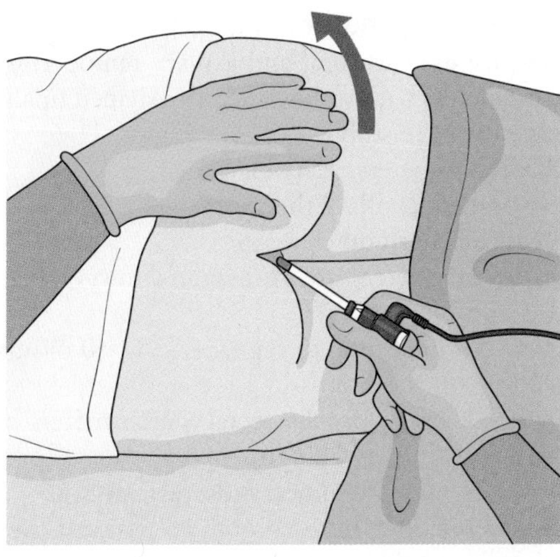

FIGURE 21-3 The rectal temperature is taken with the person in Sims' position. The buttock is raised to expose the anus.

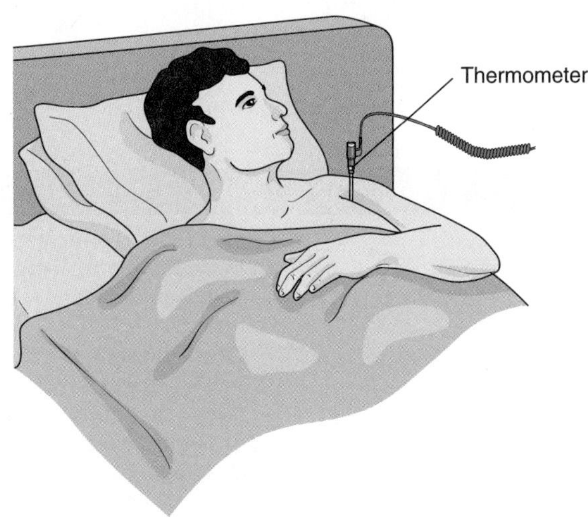

FIGURE 21-4 The thermometer is held in place in the axilla by bringing the person's arm over the chest.

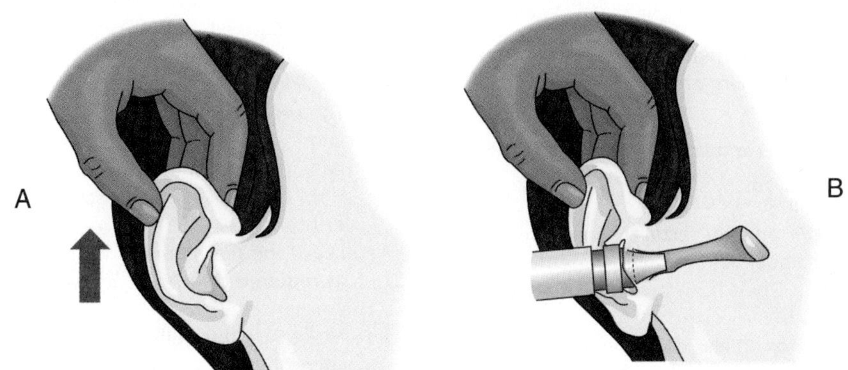

FIGURE 21-5 Using a tympanic membrane thermometer. **A,** The ear is pulled up and back. **B,** The probe is inserted into the ear canal.

Glass Thermometers.

Glass Thermometers. Long- or slender-tip thermometers are used for oral and axillary temperatures. So are thermometers with stubby and pear-shaped tips. Rectal thermometers have stubby tips. See Figure 21-6.

Glass thermometers are color-coded.

- Blue—oral and axillary thermometers
- Red—rectal thermometers

Glass thermometers are re-usable. However, the following are problems.

- They take a long time to register—3 to 10 minutes depending on the site.
- They break easily. Broken rectal thermometers can injure the rectum and colon.
- The person may bite down and break an oral thermometer. Cuts in the mouth are risks. If the thermometer contains mercury, swallowed mercury can cause mercury poisoning.

See Box 21-3 for how to use and read glass thermometers.

See *Promoting Safety and Comfort: Glass Thermometers.*

See procedure: *Taking a Temperature With a Glass Thermometer,* p. 338.

PROMOTING SAFETY AND COMFORT

Glass Thermometers

Safety

Mercury-glass thermometers are rarely used today. However, do not assume that a glass thermometer contains a mercury-free mixture. If a thermometer breaks, tell the nurse at once.

Mercury is a hazardous substance. Do not touch the substance. Do not let the person do so. The agency follows special procedures for handling hazardous materials. See Chapter 9.

BOX 21-3 Glass Thermometers

Reading a Glass Thermometer

- Fahrenheit thermometers (see Fig. 21-6, *A* and *C*):
  - Every other long line is an even degree from 94°F to 108°F.
  - The short lines mean 0.2 (two-tenths) of a degree.
- Centigrade thermometers (see Fig. 21-6, *B*):
  - Each long line means 1 degree. Degrees range from 34°C to 42°C.
  - Each short line means 0.1 (one-tenth) of a degree.
- To read a glass thermometer:
  - Hold it at the stem (Fig. 21-7). Bring it to eye level.
  - Turn it until you can see the numbers and the long and short lines.
  - Turn it back and forth slowly until you can see the silver or red line.
  - Read the nearest degree (long line).
  - Read the nearest tenth of a degree (short line)—an even number on a Fahrenheit thermometer.

Using a Glass Thermometer

- Follow Standard Precautions and the Bloodborne Pathogen Standard.
- Use the person's thermometer.
- Use a rectal thermometer only for rectal temperatures.
- Rinse the thermometer under cold, running water if it was soaking in a disinfectant. Dry it from the stem to the bulb end with tissues.
- Check the thermometer for breaks, cracks, and chips. Discard it following agency policy if it is broken, cracked, or chipped.
- Shake down the thermometer to move the substance down in the tube. Hold it at the stem and stand away from the walls, tables, or other hard surfaces. Flex and snap your wrist until the substance is below 94°F or 34°C. See Figure 21-8.

Using a Glass Thermometer—cont'd

- Insert the thermometer into a plastic cover (Fig. 21-9). Remove the cover to read the device. Discard the cover after use.
- Clean and store the thermometer following agency policy. Wipe it with tissues first to remove mucus, feces, or sweat. Do not use hot water. It causes the substance to expand so much that the thermometer could break. After cleaning, rinse the thermometer under cold, running water. Then store it in a container with a disinfectant solution.

Taking Temperatures

- The oral site:
  - The glass thermometer remains in place 2 to 3 minutes or as required by agency policy.
- The rectal site:
  - Provide for privacy. The buttocks and anus are exposed. The procedure embarrasses many people.
  - Lubricate the bulb end of the rectal thermometer for easy insertion and to prevent injury.
  - Hold the device in place so it is not lost into the rectum or broken.
  - Leave the thermometer in the rectum for 2 minutes or as required by agency policy.
- The axillary site:
  - Make sure the axilla (underarm) is dry. Do not use the site right after bathing.
  - Leave the thermometer in place for 5 to 10 minutes or as required by agency policy.

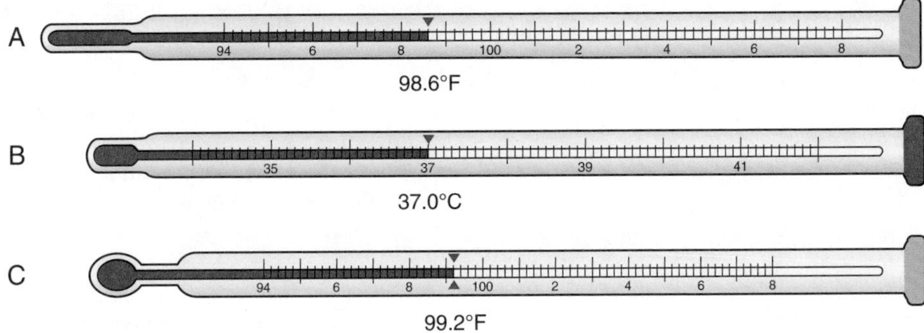

FIGURE 21-6 Glass thermometers. **A,** A Fahrenheit thermometer with a long or slender tip. The temperature measurement is 98.6°F. **B,** Centigrade thermometer with a stubby tip (rectal thermometer). The temperature measurement is 37.0°C. **C,** Fahrenheit thermometer with a pear-shaped tip. The temperature measurement is 99.2°F.

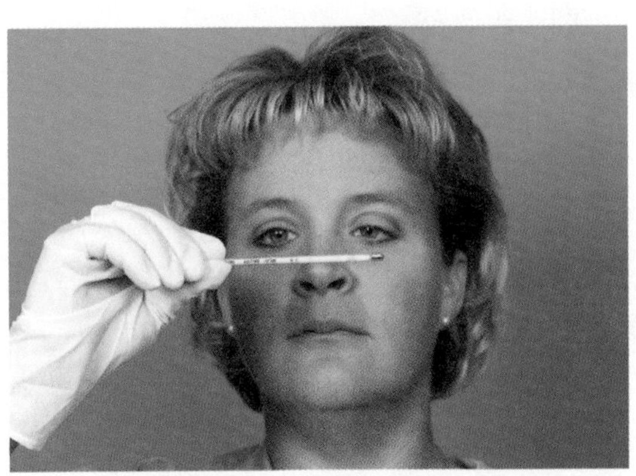

FIGURE 21-7 The thermometer is held at the stem. It is read at eye level.

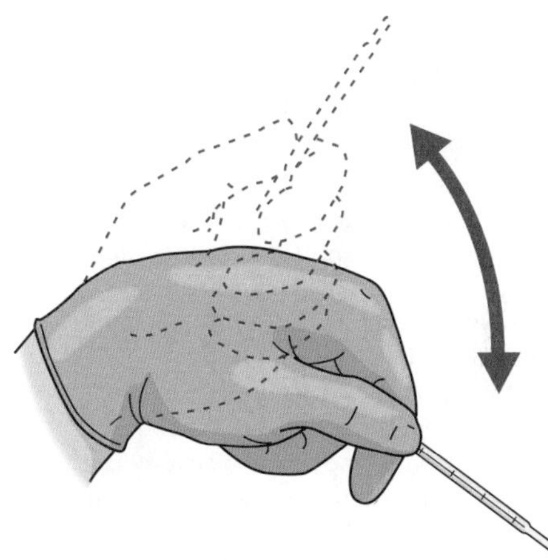

FIGURE 21-8 The wrist is snapped to shake down the thermometer.

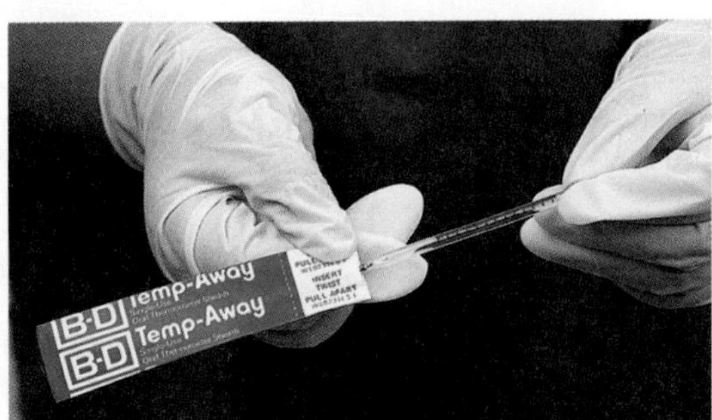

FIGURE 21-9 The thermometer is inserted into a plastic cover.

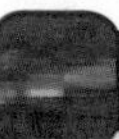

Taking a Temperature With a Glass Thermometer

QUALITY OF LIFE

- Knock before entering the person's room.
- Address the person by name.
- Introduce yourself by name and title.
- Explain the procedure before starting and during the procedure.
- Protect the person's rights during the procedure.
- Handle the person gently during the procedure.

PRE-PROCEDURE

1 Follow *Delegation Guidelines: Taking Temperatures,* p. 333. See *Promoting Safety and Comfort:*
  a *Taking Temperatures,* p. 333
  b *Glass Thermometers,* p. 336
2 For an oral temperature, ask the person not to eat, drink, smoke, or chew gum for at least 15 to 20 minutes before the measurement or as required by agency policy.
3 Practice hand hygiene.
4 Collect the following.
  - Oral or rectal thermometer and holder
  - Tissues
  - Plastic covers if used
  - Gloves
  - Toilet tissue (rectal temperature)
  - Water-soluble lubricant (rectal thermometer)
  - Towel (axillary temperature)
5 Practice hand hygiene.
6 Identify the person. Check the ID bracelet against the assignment sheet. Also call the person by name.
7 Provide for privacy.

PROCEDURE

8 Put on the gloves.
9 Rinse the thermometer under cold running water if it was soaking in a disinfectant. Dry it with tissues.
10 Check for breaks, cracks, or chips.
11 Shake down the thermometer below the lowest number. Hold the device by the stem.
12 Insert it into a plastic cover if used.
13 *For an oral temperature:*
  a Ask the person to moisten his or her lips.
  b Place the bulb end of the thermometer under the tongue and to 1 side (see Fig. 21-2).
  c Ask the person to close the lips around the thermometer to hold it in place.
  d Ask the person not to talk. Remind the person not to bite down on the thermometer.
  e Leave it in place for 2 to 3 minutes or as required by agency policy.
14 *For a rectal temperature:*
  a Position the person in the Sims' position.
  b Put a small amount of lubricant on a tissue.
  c Lubricate the bulb end of the thermometer.
  d Fold back top linens to expose the anal area.
  e Raise the upper buttock to expose the anus (see Fig. 21-3).
  f Insert the thermometer 1 inch into the rectum. Do not force the thermometer.
  g Hold the thermometer in place for 2 minutes or as required by agency policy. Do not let go of it while it is in the rectum.
15 *For an axillary temperature:*
  a Help the person remove an arm from the gown. Do not expose the person.
  b Dry the axilla with the towel.
  c Place the bulb end of the thermometer in the center of the axilla.
  d Ask the person to place the arm over the chest to hold the thermometer in place (see Fig. 21-4). Hold it and the arm in place if he or she cannot help.
  e Leave the thermometer in place for 5 to 10 minutes or as required by agency policy.
16 Remove the thermometer.
17 *For an oral or axillary temperature:*
  a Use a tissue to remove the plastic cover.
  b Wipe the thermometer with a tissue if no cover was used. Wipe from the stem to the bulb end.
  c Discard the tissue and cover (if used).
  d Read the thermometer.
  e Note the person's name and temperature on your note pad or assignment sheet.
  f Help the person put the gown back on (axillary temperature).
18 *For a rectal temperature:*
  a Use toilet tissue to remove the plastic cover.
  b Wipe the thermometer with toilet tissue if no cover was used. Wipe from the stem to the bulb end.
  c Place used toilet tissue on several thicknesses of clean toilet tissue. Discard the cover (if used).
  d Read the thermometer.
  e Place the thermometer on clean toilet tissue.
  f Wipe the anal area with toilet tissue to remove lubricant and any feces. Set the used toilet tissue on several thicknesses of clean toilet tissue.
  g Cover the person.
  h Discard tissue and dispose of toilet tissue in the toilet.
19 Note the person's name and temperature on your note pad or assignment sheet.
20 Shake down the thermometer.
21 Clean the thermometer following agency policy. Return it to the holder.
22 Remove and discard the gloves. Practice hand hygiene.

POST-PROCEDURE

23 Provide for comfort. (See the inside of the front cover.)
24 Place the call light within reach.
25 Unscreen the person.
26 Complete a safety check of the room. (See the inside of the front cover.)
27 Practice hand hygiene.
28 Report and record the temperature. Note the temperature site when reporting and recording. Report an abnormal temperature at once.

Pulse

The ***pulse*** *is the beat of the heart felt at an artery as a wave of blood passes through the artery.* A pulse is felt every time the heart beats.

The temporal, carotid, brachial, radial, femoral, popliteal, posterior tibial, and dorsalis pedis (pedal) pulses are felt on each side of the body (Fig. 21-10). The radial pulse is used most often. It is easy to reach and find. The person is not exposed.

The apical pulse is over the heart. The apex (apical) of the heart is at the tip of the heart, just below the left nipple. This pulse is taken with a stethoscope.

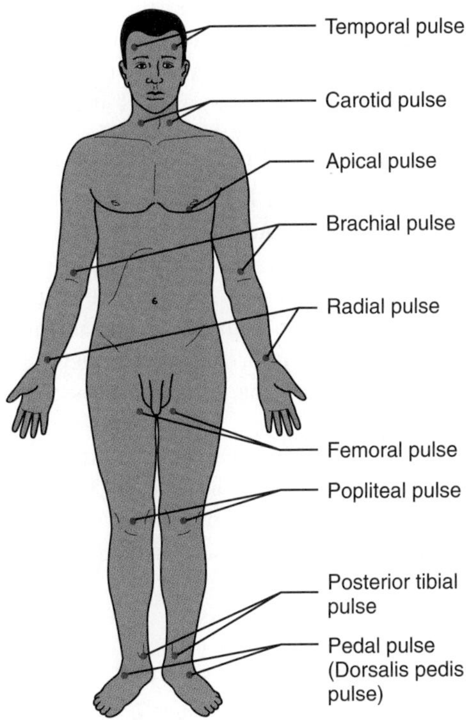

FIGURE 21-10 The pulse sites.

Using a Stethoscope. A ***stethoscope*** *is an instrument used to listen to the sounds produced by the heart, lungs, and other body organs* (Fig. 21-11). You use it for apical pulses and blood pressures.

To use a stethoscope:

- Wipe the ear-pieces and diaphragm with antiseptic wipes before and after use.
- Place the ear-piece tips in your ears. The bend of the tips points forward. Ear-pieces should fit snugly to block out noises. They should not cause pain or discomfort.
- Tap the diaphragm gently. You should hear the tapping. If not, turn the chest piece at the tubing. Gently tap the diaphragm again. Proceed if you hear the tapping sound. Check with the nurse if you do not hear the tapping.
- Place the diaphragm over the pulse site. Hold it in place as in Figure 21-12.
- Prevent noise. Do not let anything touch the tubing. Ask the person to be silent.

See *Focus on Communication: Using a Stethoscope*, p. 340.

See *Promoting Safety and Comfort: Using a Stethoscope*, p. 340.

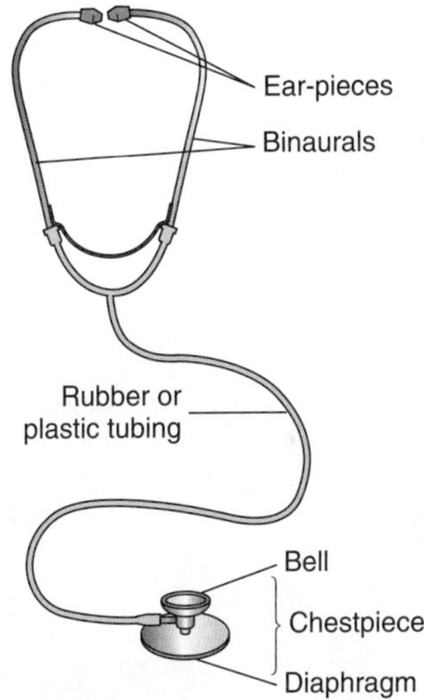

FIGURE 21-11 Parts of a stethoscope.

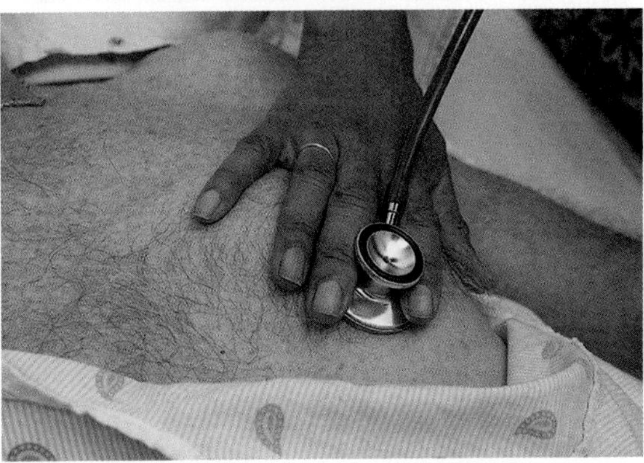

FIGURE 21-12 The stethoscope is held in place with the fingertips of the index and middle fingers.

FOCUS ON COMMUNICATION

Using a Stethoscope

Hearing through the stethoscope is hard if the person is talking. Politely ask the person to be silent. Explain the procedure. Tell the person when and for how long to remain silent. You can say:

> Mr. Bradley, I am going to check your pulse with a stethoscope. It is hard for me to hear your heart beat when you talk. Please do not talk when my stethoscope is on your chest. It will take about 1 minute.

The person may forget and begin talking. You can politely say: "This will only take 1 minute. Please stay quiet until I tell you that I'm done." Thank the person when you are done.

PROMOTING SAFETY AND COMFORT

Using a Stethoscope

Safety

Stethoscopes are in contact with many persons and staff. You must prevent infection. Wipe the ear-pieces and diaphragm with antiseptic wipes before and after use.

Comfort

Stethoscope diaphragms tend to be cold. Warm the diaphragm in your hand before applying it to the person (Fig. 21-13). Cold diaphragms can startle the person.

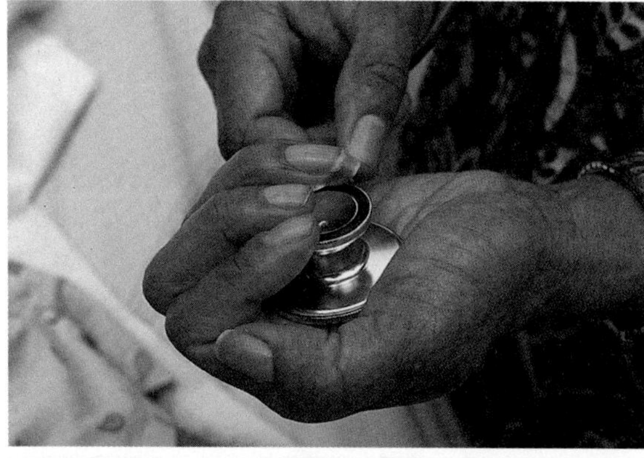

FIGURE 21-13 The diaphragm of the stethoscope is warmed in the palm of the hand.

Pulse Rate. The *pulse rate is the number of heartbeats or pulses felt or heard in 1 minute.* The pulse rate is affected by the factors listed in Box 21-1. Some drugs increase the pulse rate. Other drugs slow down the pulse.

The adult pulse rate is between 60 and 100 beats per minute. A rate of less than 60 or more than 100 is considered abnormal. Report abnormal pulses to the nurse at once.

Rhythm and Force of the Pulse. The pulse *rhythm* should be regular. That is, pulses are felt in a pattern. The same interval occurs between beats. An irregular pulse occurs when the beats are not evenly spaced or beats are skipped (Fig. 21-14).

Force relates to pulse strength. A forceful pulse is easy to feel. It is described as *strong, full,* or *bounding.* Hard-to-feel pulses are described as *weak, thready,* or *feeble.*

Taking Pulses. You will take radial and apical pulses. You must count, report, and record accurately.

The radial pulse is used for routine vital signs. Place the first 2 or 3 fingertips against the radial artery. The radial artery is on the thumb side of the wrist (Fig. 21-15). Count the pulse for 30 seconds. Then multiply the number by 2. This gives the number of beats per minute (pulses in 60 seconds). For example, you count 36 beats in 30 seconds. For the number of beats per minute, multiply 36 by 2 ($36 \times 2 = 72$). The pulse is 72. If the pulse is irregular, count it for 1 minute. In some agencies, all radial pulses are taken for 1 minute. Follow agency policy.

The apical pulse is on the left side of the chest slightly below the nipple (Fig. 21-16). Use a stethoscope and count the pulse for 1 minute. The heartbeat normally sounds like a *lub-dub.* Count each *lub-dub* as 1 beat. Do not count the *lub* as 1 beat and the *dub* as another.

Apical pulses are taken on persons who:

- Have heart disease.
- Have irregular heart rhythms.
- Take drugs that affect the heart.

See *Delegation Guidelines: Taking Pulses.*

See *Promoting Safety and Comfort: Taking Pulses.*

See procedure: *Taking a Radial Pulse.*

See procedure: *Taking an Apical Pulse,* p. 342.

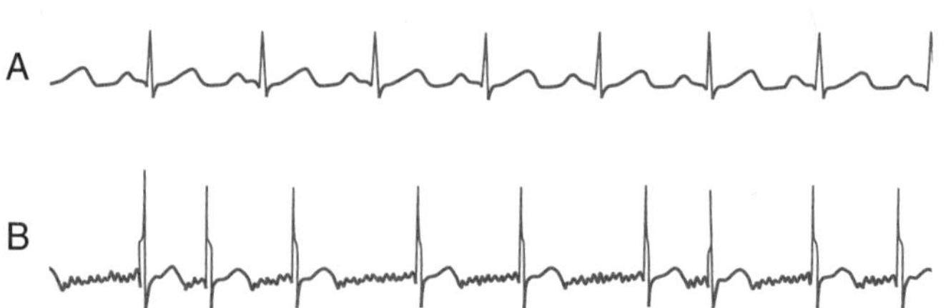

FIGURE 21-14 A, The electrocardiogram shows a regular pulse. The beats occur at regular intervals. **B,** These beats are at irregular intervals.

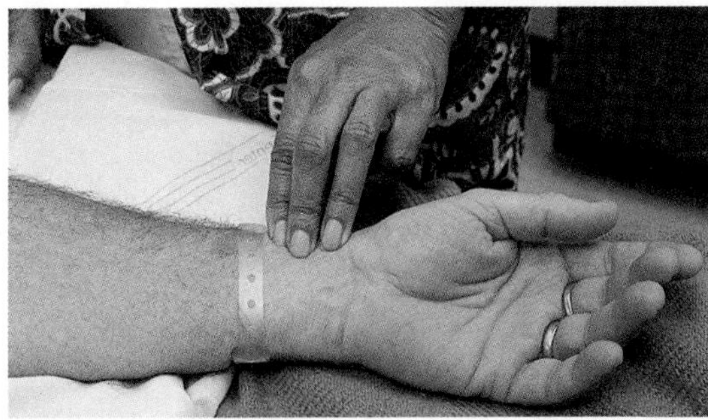

FIGURE 21-15 The 3 middle fingers are used to take the radial pulse.

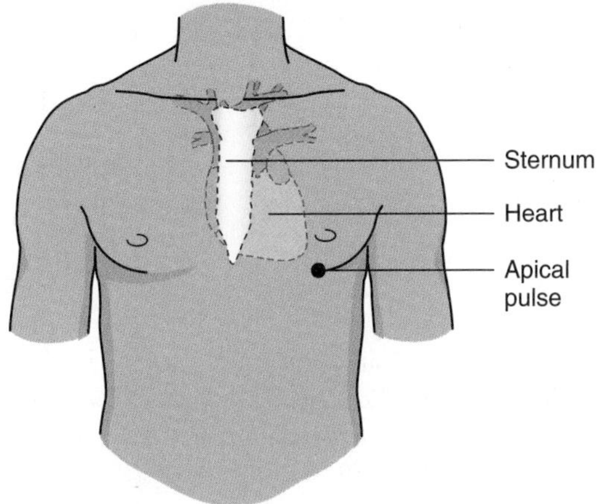

FIGURE 21-16 The apical pulse is located 2 to 3 inches to the left of the sternum (breastbone) and below the left nipple.

DELEGATION GUIDELINES

Taking Pulses

Before taking a pulse, you need this information from the nurse and the care plan.

- What pulse to take for each person—radial or apical
- When to take the pulse
- What other vital signs to measure
- How long to count the pulse—30 seconds or 1 minute
- If the nurse has concerns about certain patients or residents
- What observations to report and record:
  - The pulse site
  - The pulse rate—report a pulse rate less than 60 (bradycardia) or more than 100 (tachycardia) beats per minute at once
  - If the pulse is regular or irregular
  - Pulse force—strong, full, bounding, weak, thready, or feeble
- When to report the pulse rate
- What patient or resident concerns to report at once

PROMOTING SAFETY AND COMFORT

Taking Pulses

Safety

Use your first 2 or 3 fingertips to take a pulse. Do not use your thumb. The thumb has a pulse. You could mistake the pulse in your thumb for the person's pulse. Reporting and recording the wrong pulse rate can harm the person.

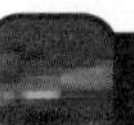

Taking a Radial Pulse

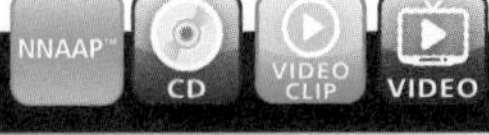

QUALITY OF LIFE

- Knock before entering the person's room.
- Address the person by name.
- Introduce yourself by name and title.
- Explain the procedure before starting and during the procedure.
- Protect the person's rights during the procedure.
- Handle the person gently during the procedure.

PRE-PROCEDURE

1 Follow *Delegation Guidelines: Taking Pulses*. See *Promoting Safety and Comfort: Taking Pulses.*
2 Practice hand hygiene.
3 Identify the person. Check the ID bracelet against the assignment sheet. Also call the person by name.
4 Provide for privacy.

PROCEDURE

5 Have the person sit or lie down.
6 Locate the radial pulse on the thumb side of the person's wrist. Use your first 2 or 3 middle fingertips (see Fig. 21-15).
7 Note if the pulse is strong or weak, and regular or irregular.
8 Count the pulse for 30 seconds. Multiply the number of beats by 2 for the number of pulses in 60 seconds (1 minute). (For example, you count 45 beats in 30 seconds. Multiply 45 by 2. 45 × 2 = 90. The pulse is 90 beats per minute.)
9 Count the pulse for 1 minute if:
   a Directed by the nurse and the care plan.
   b Required by agency policy.
   c The pulse was irregular.
   d Required for your state competency test.
10 Note the following on your note pad or assignment sheet.
   a The person's name
   b Pulse rate
   c Pulse strength
   d If the pulse was regular or irregular

POST-PROCEDURE

11 Provide for comfort. (See the inside of the front cover.)
12 Place the call light within reach.
13 Unscreen the person.
14 Complete a safety check of the room. (See the inside of the front cover.)
15 Practice hand hygiene.
16 Report and record the pulse rate and your observations. Report an abnormal pulse at once.

Taking an Apical Pulse

VIDEO

QUALITY OF LIFE

- Knock before entering the person's room.
- Address the person by name.
- Introduce yourself by name and title.
- Explain the procedure before starting and during the procedure.
- Protect the person's rights during the procedure.
- Handle the person gently during the procedure.

PRE-PROCEDURE

1 Follow *Delegation Guidelines: Taking Pulses,* p. 341. See *Promoting Safety and Comfort: Using a Stethoscope,* p. 340.
2 Practice hand hygiene.
3 Collect a stethoscope and antiseptic wipes.
4 Practice hand hygiene.
5 Identify the person. Check the ID bracelet against the assignment sheet. Also call the person by name.
6 Provide for privacy.

PROCEDURE

7 Clean the ear-pieces and diaphragm with the wipes.
8 Have the person sit or lie down.
9 Expose the nipple area of the left chest. Expose a woman's breasts only to the extent necessary.
10 Warm the diaphragm in your palm.
11 Place the ear-pieces in your ears.
12 Find the apical pulse. Place the diaphragm 2 to 3 inches to the left of the breastbone and below the left nipple (see Fig. 21-16).
13 Count the pulse for 1 minute. Note if it was regular or irregular.
14 Cover the person. Remove the ear-pieces.
15 Note the person's name and pulse on your note pad or assignment sheet. Note if the pulse was regular or irregular.

POST-PROCEDURE

16 Provide for comfort. (See the inside of the front cover.)
17 Place the call light within reach.
18 Unscreen the person.
19 Complete a safety check of the room. (See the inside of the front cover.)
20 Clean the ear-pieces and diaphragm with the wipes.
21 Return the stethoscope to its proper place.
22 Practice hand hygiene.
23 Report and record your observations. Record the pulse rate with *Ap* for apical. Report an abnormal pulse at once.

Respirations

***Respiration** means breathing air into* (inhalation) *and out of* (exhalation) *the lungs.* Each respiration involves 1 inhalation and 1 exhalation. The chest rises during inhalation. It falls during exhalation.

The healthy adult has 12 to 20 respirations per minute. See Box 21-1 for the factors affecting vital signs. Heart and respiratory diseases often increase the respiratory rate.

Respirations are normally quiet, effortless, and regular. Both sides of the chest rise and fall equally. See Chapter 26 for abnormal respiratory patterns.

People tend to change their breathing patterns when they know their respirations are being counted. Therefore do not tell the person that you are counting them. Count respirations right after taking a pulse. Keep your fingers or stethoscope over the pulse site. The person assumes you are taking the pulse.

To count respirations, watch the chest rise and fall. Count them for 30 seconds. Multiply the number by 2 for the number of respirations in 1 minute. For example, you count 8 breaths in 30 seconds. For the number of respirations in 1 minute, multiply 8 by 2 ($8 \times 2 = 16$). The respiratory rate is 16. If you note an abnormal pattern, count respirations for 1 minute.

In some agencies, respirations are counted for 1 minute. Follow agency policy.

See *Delegation Guidelines: Respirations.*

See procedure: *Counting Respirations.*

DELEGATION GUIDELINES

Respirations

Before counting respirations, you need this information from the nurse and the care plan.

- How long to count respirations for each person—30 seconds or 1 minute
- When to count respirations
- If the nurse has concerns about certain patients or residents
- What other vital signs to measure
- What observations to report and record:
  - The respiratory rate
  - Equality and depth of respirations
  - If the respirations were regular or irregular
  - If the person has pain or difficulty breathing
  - Any respiratory noises
  - An abnormal respiratory pattern (Chapter 26)
- When to report observations
- What patient or resident concerns to report at once

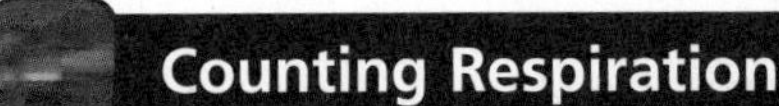

Counting Respirations

NNAAP CD VIDEO CLIP VIDEO

PROCEDURE

1. Follow *Delegation Guidelines: Respirations.*
2. Keep your fingers or stethoscope over the pulse site.
3. Do not tell the person you are counting respirations.
4. Begin counting when the chest rises. Count each rise and fall of the chest as 1 respiration.
5. Note the following.
   a. If respirations are regular
   b. If both sides of the chest rise equally
   c. The depth of respirations
   d. If the person has any pain or difficulty breathing
   e. An abnormal respiratory pattern
6. Count respirations for 30 seconds. Multiply the number by 2 for the number of respirations in 60 seconds (1 minute). (For example, you count 9 breaths in 30 seconds. Multiply 9 × 2. 9 × 2 = 18. The respiratory rate is 18 breaths per minute.)
7. Count respirations for 1 minute if:
   a. Directed by the nurse and the care plan.
   b. Required by agency policy.
   c. They are abnormal or irregular.
   d. Required for your state competency test.
8. Note the person's name, respiratory rate, and other observations on your note pad or assignment sheet.

POST-PROCEDURE

9. Provide for comfort. (See the inside of the front cover.)
10. Place the call light within reach.
11. Unscreen the person.
12. Complete a safety check of the room. (See the inside of the front cover.)
13. Practice hand hygiene.
14. Report and record the respiratory rate and your observations. Report abnormal respirations at once.

Blood Pressure

Blood pressure (BP) *is the amount of force exerted against the walls of an artery by the blood. Systole* is the period of heart muscle contraction. The heart is pumping blood. *Diastole* is the period of heart muscle relaxation. The heart is at rest.

You measure systolic and diastolic pressures. The ***systolic pressure*** *is the pressure in the arteries when the heart contracts.* It is the higher pressure. The ***diastolic pressure*** *is the pressure in the arteries when the heart is at rest.* It is the lower pressure.

Blood pressure is measured in millimeters (mm) of mercury (Hg). The systolic pressure is recorded over the diastolic pressure. A systolic pressure of 120 mm Hg (millimeters of mercury) and a diastolic pressure of 80 mm Hg are written as 120/80 mm Hg.

Normal and Abnormal Blood Pressures. Blood pressure can change from minute to minute. Therefore, blood pressure has normal ranges.

- *Systolic pressure*—90 mm Hg or higher but lower than 120 mm Hg
- *Diastolic pressure*—60 mm Hg or higher but lower than 80 mm Hg

  Treatment is indicated for:
- ***Hypertension****—The systolic pressure is 140 mm Hg or higher* (hyper), *or the diastolic pressure is 90 mm Hg or higher.* Report any systolic measurement at or above 120 mm Hg. Also report a diastolic pressure at or above 80 mm Hg.
- ***Hypotension****—The systolic pressure is below* (hypo) *90 mm Hg, or the diastolic pressure is below 60 mm Hg.* Report a systolic pressure below 90 mm Hg. Also report a diastolic pressure below 60 mm Hg.

See *Focus on Communication: Normal and Abnormal Blood Pressures.*

FOCUS ON COMMUNICATION

Normal and Abnormal Blood Pressures

Many persons want to know their blood pressures. If agency policy allows, you can tell the person. If the blood pressure is high or low, the person may worry. He or she may say: "That is higher (lower) than normal for me." Respond in a calm and professional manner. You can say: "Yes, it was a little high (low). I will tell the nurse." Report abnormal blood pressures to the nurse.

You must report some concerns at once. For example, Mr. Turner's blood pressure is 82/58. Mr. Turner says he is dizzy. You help him lie down. You need to stay with Mr. Turner and report the concern. You press the call light and identify yourself. You say: "Please have Mr. Turner's nurse come to room 216 right away." When the nurse arrives, you say: "Mr. Turner's blood pressure was 82/58. He said he was dizzy. Please check him."

Equipment. You use a stethoscope and a sphygmomanometer to measure blood pressure. The *sphygmomanometer* has a cuff and a measuring device.

- The *aneroid type* has a round dial and a needle that points to the numbers (Fig. 21-17, *A*).
- The *mercury type* has a column of mercury within a calibrated tube (Fig. 21-17, *B*).
- The *electronic type* shows the systolic and diastolic pressures (Fig. 21-17, *C*). It also shows the pulse rate. To use the device, follow the manufacturer's instructions.

You wrap the blood pressure cuff around the upper arm. Tubing connects the cuff to the manometer. Another tube connects the cuff to a small, hand-held bulb (aneroid and mercury types). To inflate the cuff, turn the valve on the bulb clockwise to close the valve and then squeeze the bulb. The inflated cuff causes pressure over the brachial artery. Turn the valve counter-clockwise to open the valve to deflate the cuff. Measure BP as the cuff deflates.

Blood flowing through the arteries produces sounds. Use the stethoscope to listen to the sounds in the brachial artery as you deflate the cuff. You do not need a stethoscope for an electronic manometer.

See *Promoting Safety and Comfort: Equipment.*

PROMOTING SAFETY AND COMFORT

Equipment

Safety

Mercury is a hazardous substance. Some agencies still use mercury manometers. Handle mercury manometers carefully. If one breaks, call for the nurse at once. Do not touch the mercury. Do not let the person touch it. The agency follows special procedures for handling all hazardous substances. See Chapter 9.

Comfort

Inflate the cuff only to the extent necessary (see procedure: *Measuring Blood Pressure).* The inflated cuff causes discomfort. The higher the inflation, the greater the discomfort.

A

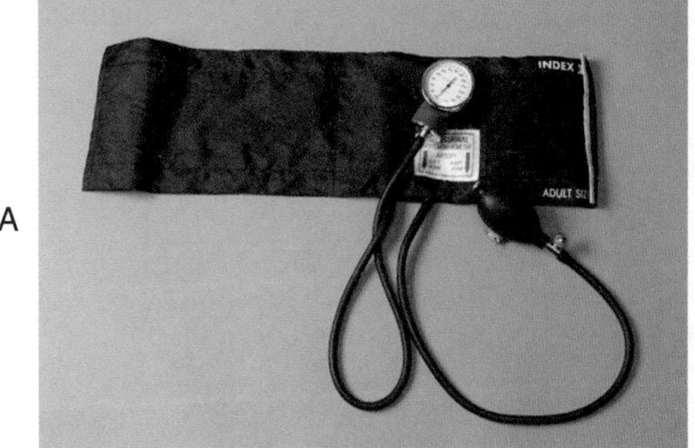

B

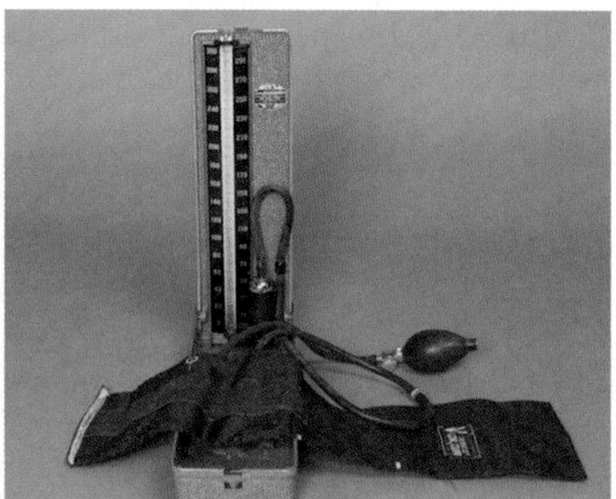

C

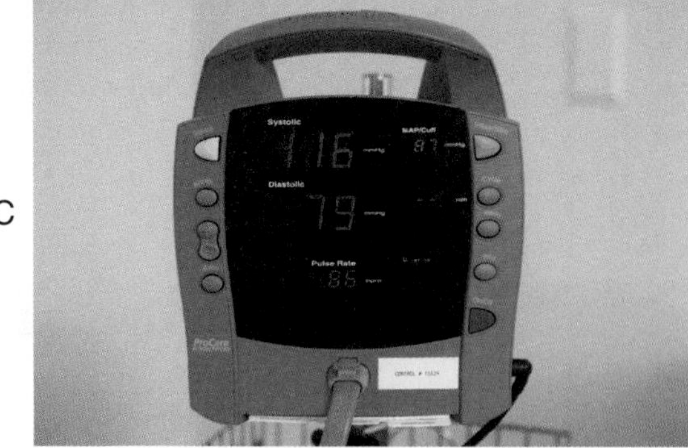

FIGURE 21-17 Blood pressure equipment. **A,** Aneroid manometer and cuff. **B,** Mercury manometer and cuff. **C,** Electronic manometer.

Measuring Blood Pressure. You measure blood pressure in the brachial artery. Follow the guidelines in Box 21-4.

See *Delegation Guidelines: Measuring Blood Pressure.*
See procedure: *Measuring Blood Pressure.*

BOX 21-4 Guidelines for Measuring Blood Pressure

- Do not take BP on an arm:
  - With an IV infusion
  - With an arm cast
  - With a dialysis access site
  - On the side of breast surgery
  - That is injured
- Ask the nurse if you are not sure which arm to use.
- Let the person rest for 10 to 20 minutes before measuring BP.
- Measure BP with the person sitting or lying. Sometimes BP is measured in the standing position.
- Apply the cuff to the bare upper arm. Clothing can affect the measurement.
- Make sure the cuff is snug. The reading will be wrong if the cuff is loose.
- Use a larger cuff if the person is obese or has a large arm. Use a small cuff if the person has a very small arm. Ask the nurse what size to use. Also check the care plan.
- Make sure the room is quiet. Talking, TV, music, and sounds from the hallway can affect an accurate measurement.
- Place the diaphragm of the stethoscope firmly over the brachial artery. The entire diaphragm must have contact with the skin. Do not place it under the cuff.
- Have the manometer where you can clearly see it.
- Measure the systolic and diastolic pressures.
  - Expect to hear the first sound at the point where you last felt the pulse. The first sound is the systolic pressure.
  - The point where the sound disappears is the diastolic pressure.
- Take the BP again if you are not sure of accuracy. Wait 30 to 60 seconds to repeat the measurement. Ask the nurse to take the BP if you are unsure of the measurement.
- Tell the nurse at once if you cannot hear the blood pressure.

DELEGATION GUIDELINES

Measuring Blood Pressure

Before measuring BP, you need this information from the nurse and the care plan.

- When to measure BP
- What arm to use
- The person's normal blood pressure range
- If the nurse has concerns about certain patients or residents
- If the person needs to be lying down, sitting, or standing
- What size cuff to use—regular, child-size, extra large
- What observations to report and record
- When to report the BP measurement
- What patient or resident concerns to report at once

Measuring Blood Pressure

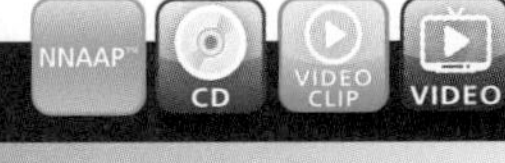

QUALITY OF LIFE

- Knock before entering the person's room.
- Address the person by name.
- Introduce yourself by name and title.
- Explain the procedure before starting and during the procedure.
- Protect the person's rights during the procedure.
- Handle the person gently during the procedure.

PRE-PROCEDURE

1 Follow *Delegation Guidelines: Measuring Blood Pressure.* See *Promoting Safety and Comfort:*
   a *Using a Stethoscope,* p. 340
   b *Equipment*
2 Practice hand hygiene.
3 Collect the following.
   - Sphygmomanometer
   - Stethoscope
   - Antiseptic wipes
4 Practice hand hygiene.
5 Identify the person. Check the ID bracelet against the assignment sheet. Also call the person by name.
6 Provide for privacy.

Continued

Measuring Blood Pressure—cont'd

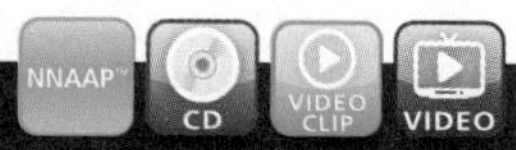

PROCEDURE

7 Wipe the stethoscope ear-pieces and diaphragm with the wipes. Warm the diaphragm in your palm.
8 Have the person sit or lie down.
9 Position the person's arm level with the heart. The palm is up.
10 Stand no more than 3 feet away from the manometer. The mercury type is vertical, on a flat surface, and at eye level. The aneroid type is directly in front of you.
11 Expose the upper arm.
12 Squeeze the cuff to expel any air. Close the valve on the bulb.
13 Find the brachial artery at the inner aspect of the elbow. (The brachial artery is on the little finger side of the arm.) Use your fingertips.
14 Locate the arrow on the cuff (Fig. 21-18, *A*). Align the arrow on the cuff with the brachial artery (Fig. 21-18, *B*). Wrap the cuff around the upper arm at least 1 inch above the elbow. It is even and snug.
15 Place the stethoscope ear-pieces in your ears. Place the diaphragm over the brachial artery (Fig. 21-18, *C*). Do not place it under the cuff.
16 Find the radial pulse. This step is for Methods 1 and 2.
17 *Method 1:*
   a Inflate the cuff until you cannot feel the pulse. Note this point.
   b Inflate the cuff 30 mm Hg beyond where you last felt the pulse.
18 *Method 2:*
   a Inflate the cuff until you cannot feel the pulse. Note this point.
   b Inflate the cuff 30 mm Hg beyond where you last felt the pulse.
   c Deflate the cuff slowly. Note the point when you feel the pulse.
   d Wait 30 seconds.
   e Inflate the cuff again, 30 mm Hg beyond where you felt the pulse return.
19 *Method 3:*
   a Inflate the cuff 160 mm Hg to 180 mm Hg.
   b Deflate the cuff if you hear a blood pressure sound. Re-inflate the cuff to 200 mm Hg.
20 Deflate the cuff at an even rate of 2 to 4 millimeters per second. Turn the valve counter-clockwise to deflate the cuff.
21 Note the point where you hear the first sound (Fig. 21-19). This is the systolic reading. It is near the point where the pulse disappeared (Method 1) or returned (Method 2).
22 Continue to deflate the cuff completely. Note the point where the sound disappears. This is the diastolic reading.
23 Deflate the cuff completely. Remove it from the person's arm. Remove the stethoscope ear-pieces from your ears.
24 Note the person's name and blood pressure on your note pad or assignment sheet.
25 Return the cuff to the case or wall holder.

POST-PROCEDURE

26 Provide for comfort. (See the inside of the front cover.)
27 Place the call light within reach.
28 Unscreen the person.
29 Complete a safety check of the room. (See the inside of the front cover.)
30 Clean the ear-pieces and diaphragm with the wipes.
31 Return the equipment to its proper place.
32 Practice hand hygiene.
33 Report and record the BP. Note which arm was used. Report an abnormal blood pressure at once.

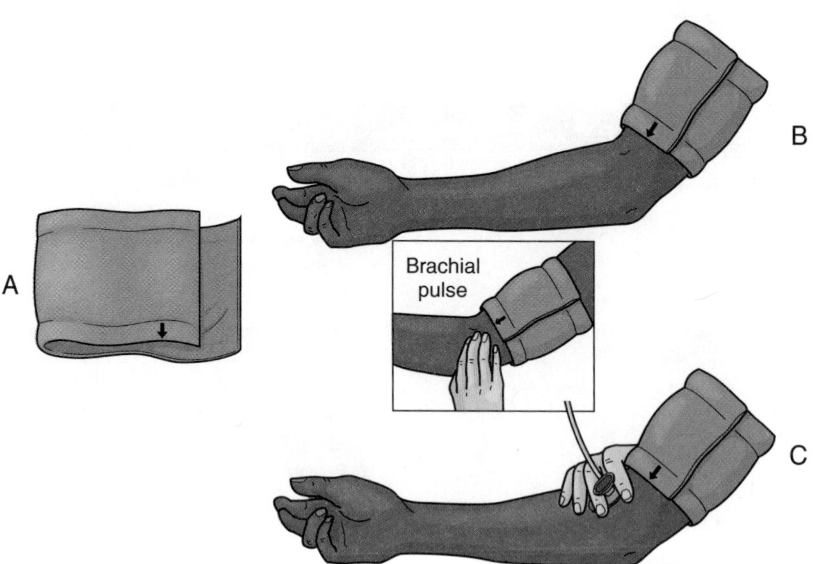

FIGURE 21-18 Measuring blood pressure. **A,** The *arrow* is used for correct cuff alignment. **B,** The cuff is placed so the *arrow* is aligned with the brachial artery. **C,** The diaphragm of the stethoscope is over the brachial artery.

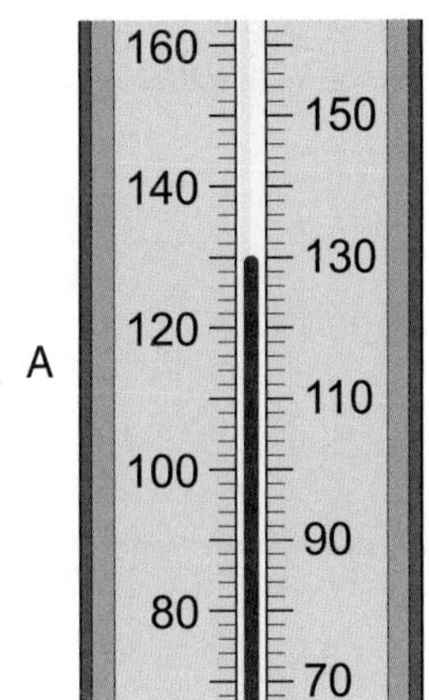

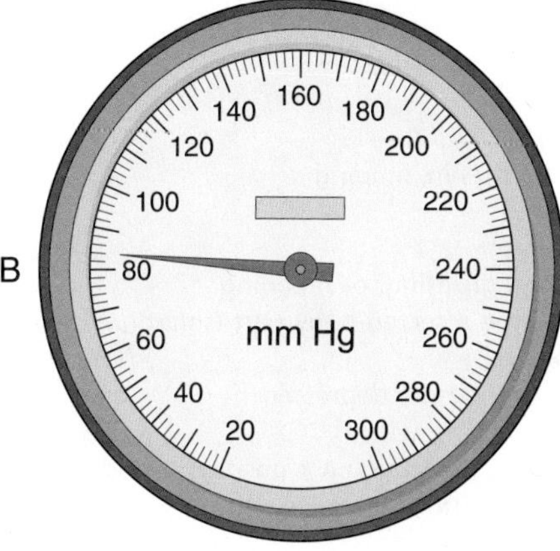

FIGURE 21-19 Reading the manometer. Long lines mark 10 mm Hg values. Short lines mark 2 mm Hg values. **A,** This mercury manometer is at 130 mm Hg. **B,** This aneroid manometer is at 84 mm Hg.

PAIN

Pain *or* ***discomfort*** *means to ache, hurt, or be sore.* Often called the fifth vital sign, pain signals tissue damage. Pain often causes the person to seek health care.

Pain is personal. It differs for each person. What *hurts* to one person may *ache* to another. What one person calls *sore,* another may call *aching.* If a person complains of pain or discomfort, the person *has* pain or discomfort. Believe the person.

See *Focus on Communication: Pain.*

FOCUS ON COMMUNICATION

Pain

Communicating about pain promotes comfort. You can say:

- "I want you to be comfortable. Please tell me if you have any pain."
- "I will tell the nurse about your pain."

If a person complains of pain, the person has pain. Rely on what the person tells you. Promptly report any complaints of pain.

Types of Pain

There are different types of pain.

- *Acute pain* is felt suddenly from injury, disease, trauma, or surgery. There is tissue damage. Acute pain lasts a short time. It lessens with healing.
- *Chronic pain (persistent pain)* continues for a long time (months or years) or occurs off and on. There is no longer tissue damage. Chronic pain remains long after healing. Arthritis is a common cause.
- *Radiating pain* is felt at the site of tissue damage and in nearby areas. Pain from a heart attack is often felt in the left chest, left jaw, left shoulder, and left arm. Gallbladder disease can cause pain in the right upper abdomen, the back, and the right shoulder (Fig. 21-20).
- *Phantom pain* is felt in a body part that is no longer there. A person with an amputated leg may still sense leg pain.

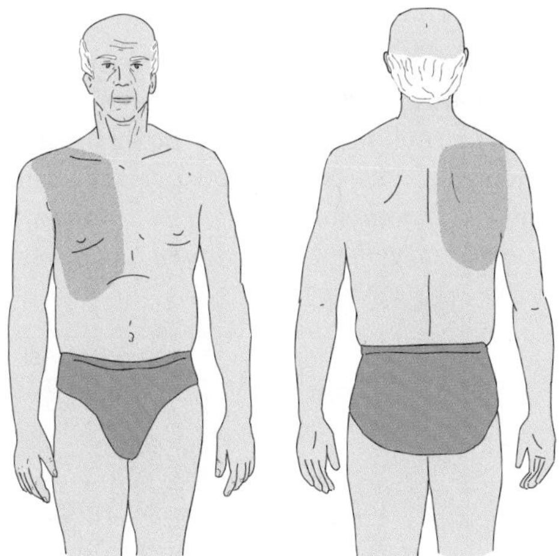

FIGURE 21-20 Gallbladder pain may radiate to the right upper abdomen, the back, and the right shoulder.

Signs and Symptoms of Pain

You cannot see, hear, feel, or smell the person's pain. Rely on what the person tells you. Promptly report any information you collect about pain. Write down what the person says. Use the person's exact words to report and record. The nurse needs the following information.

- *Location.* Where is the pain? Ask the person to point to the area of pain. Pain can radiate. Ask the person if the pain is anywhere else and to point to those areas.
- *Onset and duration.* When did the pain start? How long has it lasted?
- *Intensity.* Does the person complain of mild, moderate, or severe pain? Ask the person to rate the pain on a scale of 0 to 10, with 10 as the most severe (Fig. 21-21). Or use the *Wong-Baker Faces Pain Rating Scale* (Fig. 21-22). Designed for children, the scale is useful for all age-groups. To use the scale, tell the person that each face shows how a person feels. Read the description for each face. Then ask the person to choose the face that best describes how he or she feels.
- *Description.* Ask the person to describe the pain. Ache, dull, and sharp are examples.
- *Factors causing pain.* These are called *precipitating* factors. To *precipitate* means *to cause.* Such factors include moving or turning in bed, coughing or deep breathing, and exercise. Ask what the person was doing before the pain started and when it started.
- *Factors affecting pain.* Ask the person what makes the pain better. Also ask what makes it worse.
- *Vital signs.* Measure the person's pulse, respirations, and blood pressure. Increases in these vital signs often occur with acute pain. Vital signs may be normal with chronic pain.
- *Other signs and symptoms.* Does the person have other symptoms—dizziness, nausea, vomiting, weakness, numbness or tingling, or others? Box 21-5 lists the signs and symptoms that often occur with pain.

See *Focus on Communication: Signs and Symptoms of Pain.*
See *Focus on Older Persons: Signs and Symptoms of Pain.*

BOX 21-5 Signs and Symptoms of Pain

Body Responses
- Appetite: changes in
- Dizziness
- Nausea
- Numbness
- Skin: pale (pallor)
- Sleep: difficulty with
- Sweating (diaphoresis)
- Tingling
- Vital signs (pulse, respirations, and blood pressure): increased
- Vomiting
- Weakness
- Weight loss

Behaviors
- Clenching of the jaw
- Crying
- Frowning
- Gait: changes in; limping
- Gasping
- Grimacing
- Groaning, grunting, or moaning
- Holding the affected body part (splinting; guarding)
- Irritability
- Mood: changes in; depressed
- Pacing
- Positioning: maintaining 1 position; refusing to move; frequent position changes
- Quietness
- Resisting care
- Restlessness
- Rubbing a body part or area
- Screaming
- Speech: slow or rapid; loud or quiet
- Whimpering

PAIN: Ask patient to rate pain on scale of 0-10

No pain — Worst pain imaginable

0	1	2	3	4	5	6	7	8	9	10

FIGURE 21-21 Pain rating scale.

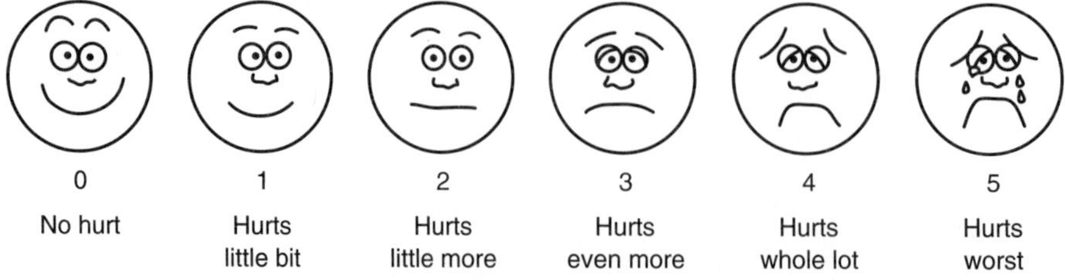

FIGURE 21-22 Wong-Baker Faces Pain Rating Scale.

FOCUS ON COMMUNICATION

Signs and Symptoms of Pain

A person may use words like "hurt" or "discomfort" instead of "pain." Use words that the person uses.

Some persons have trouble rating pain intensity on a 0 to 10 scale. Instead, ask if the pain is mild, moderate, or severe.

FOCUS ON OLDER PERSONS

Signs and Symptoms of Pain

Some older persons have many painful health problems. Chronic pain may mask new pain. Older persons may ignore or deny new pain. They may think it relates to a known health problem. Older persons often deny or ignore pain because of what it may mean.

Thinking and reasoning are affected in some older persons. Some cannot tell you about pain. Changes in behavior may signal pain. Increased confusion, grimacing, restlessness, and loss of appetite are examples. A person who normally moans and groans may become quiet and withdrawn. A person who is friendly and outgoing may become agitated and aggressive. One who is nonverbal and quiet may become restless and cry easily.

You must be alert for the signs of pain. Always report changes in the person's behavior.

All persons have the right to correct pain management. The nurse does a pain assessment when behavior changes.

INTAKE AND OUTPUT

The doctor or nurse may order intake and output (I&O) measurements.

- ***Intake** is the amount of fluid taken in.* All oral fluids are measured and recorded—water, milk, coffee, tea, juices, soups, and soft drinks. So are foods that melt at room temperature—ice cream, sherbet, custard, pudding, gelatin, and Popsicles. The nurse measures and records intravenous (IV) fluids and tube feedings (Chapter 20).
- ***Output** is the amount of fluid lost.* Output includes urine, vomitus, diarrhea, and wound drainage.

I&O records are kept. They are used to evaluate fluid balance and kidney function. They also are kept when the person has special fluid orders.

Measuring Intake and Output. Intake and output are measured in milliliters (mL). You need to know these amounts.

- 1 ounce (oz) equals 30 mL.
- 1 pint is about 500 mL.
- 1 quart is about 1000 mL.

You also need to know the serving sizes of bowls, dishes, cups, pitchers, glasses, and other containers. This information may be on the I&O record (Fig. 21-23, p. 350). Or the serving size is on the container. You may need to convert (change) the amount into milliliters. For example, a juice container holds 4 oz. The person drank all of the juice. Each oz equals 30 mL. To convert to mL, multiply 4 oz by 30 (the number of mL in each oz). The person drank 120 mL of juice (4 × 30 = 120).

A measuring container for fluid is called a *graduate.* It is used to measure left-over fluids, urine, vomitus, and drainage from suction. Like a measuring cup, the graduate is marked in ounces and milliliters (Fig. 21-24, p. 350). Plastic urinals and kidney basins also have amounts marked. Hold the measuring device on a flat surface at eye level to read the amount.

An I&O record is kept at the bedside. When I&O is measured, the amount is recorded in the correct column (see Fig. 21-23). Amounts are totaled at the end of the shift. The totals are recorded in the person's chart.

The urinal, commode, bedpan, or specimen pan (Chapter 22) is used for voiding. Remind the person not to void into the toilet. Also remind the person not to put toilet tissue into the receptacle.

See *Delegation Guidelines: Intake and Output,* p. 351.

See *Promoting Safety and Comfort: Intake and Output,* p. 351.

See procedure: *Measuring Intake and Output,* p. 351.

Text continued on p. 352

OSF℠
ST. JOSEPH MEDICAL CENTER
Bloomington, Illinois

DATE *6/15*

FLUID BALANCE CHART

Water Glass	250mL	Ice Cream	120mL
Styrofoam Cup	180mL	Ice Chips	1/2 amt. of mL's in cup
Cup (coffee)	250mL		
Milk Carton	240mL	Pitcher (Yellow)	1000mL
Pop (1 can)	360mL		
Broth-Soup	175mL		
Juice Carton	120mL		
Juice Glass	120mL		
Jello	120mL		

INTAKE				OUTPUT					
				URINE		OTHER		CONT. IRRIGATION	
TIME	ORAL	Parenteral	Amt. mL Absbd.	Method Collected	Amt. (mL)	Method Collected	Amt. (mL)	In	Out
2400-0100		mL from previous shift		*V*	*150*				
0100-0200						*Vom.*	*150*		
0200-0300									
0300-0400									
0400-0500									
0500-0600	*125*			*V*	*200*				
0600-0700									
0700-0800									
	125	8 - hour Sub total		8-hr T	*350*	8-hr T	*150*		
0800-0900	*100*	mL from previous shift		*V*	*250*				
0900-1000	*100*								
1000-1100									
1100-1200									
1200-1300	*400*			*V*	*250*				
1300-1400									
1400-1500	*200*								
1500-1600									
	1100	8 - hour Sub-total		8-hr T	*500*	8-hr T			
1600-1700		mL from previous shift		*V*	*270*				
1700-1800	*350*								
1800-1900	*50*								
1900-2000	*200*								
2000-2100				*V*	*400*				
2100-2200									
2200-2300									
2300-2400									
	600	8 - hour Sub-total		8-hr T	*670*	8-hr T			
	1825	24 - hour Sub-total		24-hr T	*1520*	24-hr T	*150*		

310' Marie Mills

Source Key:
URINE
V - Voided
C - Catheter
INC - Incontinent
U.C. - Ureteral Catheter

Source Key:
OTHER
G.I.T. - Gastric Intestinal Tube
T.T. - T. Tube
Vom. - Vomitus
Liq S. - Liquid Stool
H.V. - Hemovac

Form No. MF36722 (Rev. 5/97) *MFI*

FIGURE 21-23 A sample intake and output record.

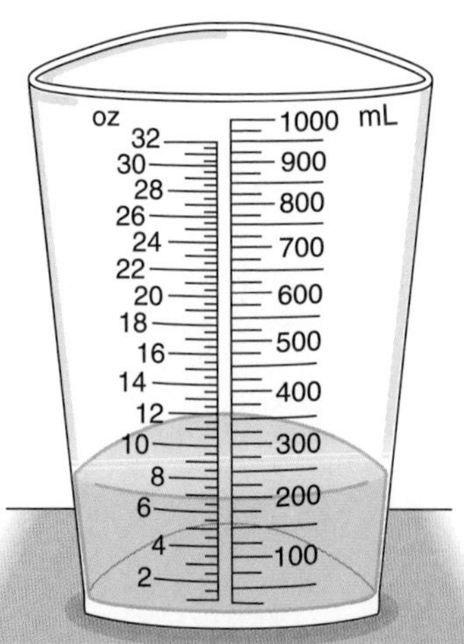

FIGURE 21-24 A graduate marked in ounces (oz) and milliliters (mL).

DELEGATION GUIDELINES

Intake and Output

When measuring I&O, you need this information from the nurse and the care plan.

- If the person has a special fluid order (Chapter 20)
- When to report measurements—hourly or end-of-shift
- What the person uses for voiding—urinal, bedpan, commode, or specimen pan (Chapter 22)
- If the person has a catheter (Chapter 22)
- What patient or resident concerns to report at once

PROMOTING SAFETY AND COMFORT

Intake and Output

Safety

Urine may contain microbes and blood. Microbes can grow in urinals, commodes, bedpans, specimen pans, and drainage systems. Follow Standard Precautions and the Bloodborne Pathogen Standard when handling such equipment. Thoroughly clean the item with a disinfectant after it is used.

Comfort

Promptly measure the contents of urinals, bedpans, commodes, and specimen pans. This helps prevent or reduce odors. Odors can disturb the person.

Measuring Intake and Output

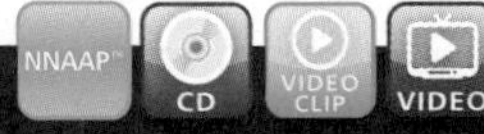

QUALITY OF LIFE

- Knock before entering the person's room.
- Address the person by name.
- Introduce yourself by name and title.
- Explain the procedure before starting and during the procedure.
- Protect the person's rights during the procedure.
- Handle the person gently during the procedure.

PRE-PROCEDURE

1 Follow *Delegation Guidelines: Intake and Output*. See *Promoting Safety and Comfort: Intake and Output*.
2 Practice hand hygiene.
3 Collect the following.
- I&O record
- Graduates
- Gloves

PROCEDURE

4 Put on gloves.
5 Measure intake.
  a Pour liquid remaining in the container into the graduate. Avoid spills and splashes on the outside of the graduate.
  b Measure the amount at eye level on a flat surface. Keep the graduate level.
  c Check the serving amount on the I&O record. Or check the serving size of each container.
  d Subtract the remaining amount from the full serving amount. Note the amount. (For example, a cup holds 250 mL. The amount in the graduate is 50 mL. 250 mL – 50 mL = 200 mL.)
  e Pour fluid in the graduate back into the container.
  f Repeat step 5, a–e for each liquid.
  g Add the amounts from each liquid together.
  h Record the time and amount on the I&O record.
6 Measure output as follows.
  a Pour the fluid into the graduate used to measure output. Avoid spills and splashes on the outside of the graduate.
  b Measure the amount at eye level on a flat surface. Keep the graduate level.
  c Dispose of fluid into the toilet. Avoid splashes.
7 Clean and rinse the graduates. Dispose of rinse into the toilet and flush. Return the graduates to their proper place.
8 Clean, rinse, and disinfect the voiding receptacle or drainage container. Dispose of the rinse into the toilet and flush. Return the item to its proper place.
9 Remove and discard the gloves. Practice hand hygiene.
10 Record the output amount on the person's I&O record.

POST-PROCEDURE

11 Provide for comfort. (See the inside of the front cover.)
12 Make sure the call light is within reach.
13 Complete a safety check of the room. (See the inside of the front cover.)
14 Report and record your observations.

WEIGHT AND HEIGHT

Weight and height are measured on admission to the agency. Then the person is weighed daily, weekly, or monthly. This is done to measure weight gain or loss.

Standing scales are common. Chair, wheelchair, bed, and lift scales are used for persons who cannot stand. Follow the manufacturer's instructions and agency procedures.

When measuring weight and height, follow these guidelines.

- The person wears only a gown or pajamas. Clothes add weight. No footwear is worn. Footwear adds to the weight and height measurements.
- The person voids before being weighed. A full bladder adds weight.
- A dry incontinence product is worn. A wet product adds weight.
- Weigh the person at the same time of day. Before breakfast is the best time. Food and fluids add weight.
- Use the same scale for daily, weekly, and monthly weights. Scales weigh differently.
- Balance the scale at zero (0) before weighing the person. For balance scales, move the weights to zero. A digital scale should read at zero.

See *Focus on Communication: Weight and Height.*
See *Delegation Guidelines: Weight and Height.*
See *Promoting Safety and Comfort: Weight and Height.*
See procedure: *Measuring Weight and Height.*

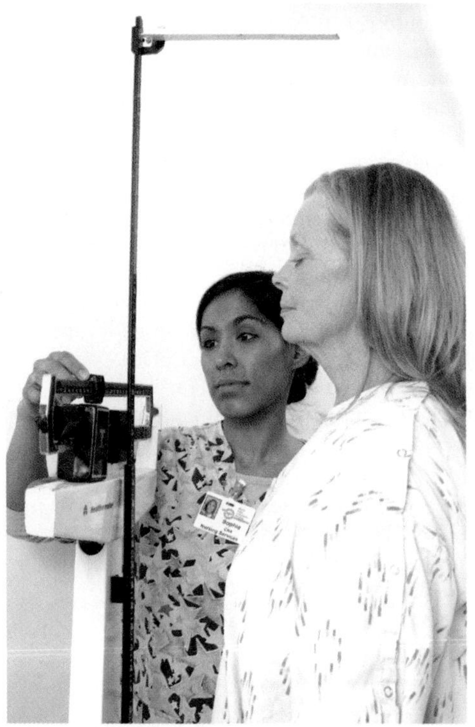

FIGURE 21-25 The person is weighed.

FOCUS ON COMMUNICATION

Weight and Height

Safe care depends on accurate reporting and recording. Some agencies use pounds (lb) for weight. Others use kilograms (kg). For height, some agencies use feet and inches. Others only use inches.

If you do not know what measurements to use, ask the nurse. Follow agency policy to report and record weight and height.

DELEGATION GUIDELINES

Weight and Height

To measure weight and height, you need this information from the nurse and the care plan.

- When to measure weight and height
- What scale to use
- When to report the measurements
- What patient or resident concerns to report at once

PROMOTING SAFETY AND COMFORT

Weight and Height

Safety

Follow the manufacturer's instructions when using chair, wheelchair, bed, or lift scales. Also follow the agency's procedures. Practice safety measures to prevent falls.

Comfort

The person wears only a gown or pajamas for the weight measurement. Prevent chilling and drafts (Chapter 15).

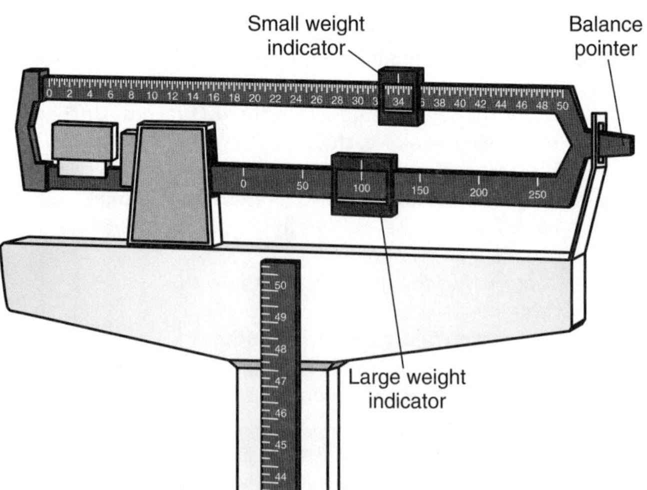

FIGURE 21-26 Balance scale. The lower bar is divided into 50 lb values. The long lines on the upper bar are 1 lb values. The shorter lines are ¼, ½, and ¾ lb values. The lower and upper weights are moved until the balance pointer is in the middle. The values on the lower and upper bars are added for the weight. In this figure, the lower bar is at 100 lb. The upper bar is at 34 lb. The weight is 134 lb (100 lb + 34 lb = 134 lb).

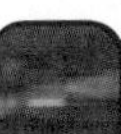

Measuring Weight and Height

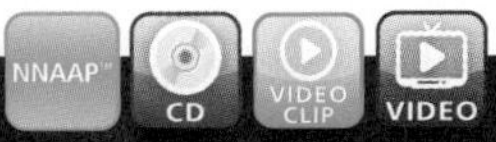

QUALITY OF LIFE

- Knock before entering the person's room.
- Address the person by name.
- Introduce yourself by name and title.
- Explain the procedure before starting and during the procedure.
- Protect the person's rights during the procedure.
- Handle the person gently during the procedure.

PRE-PROCEDURE

1 Follow *Delegation Guidelines: Weight and Height.* See *Promoting Safety and Comfort: Weight and Height.*
2 Ask the person to void.
3 Practice hand hygiene.
4 Bring the scale and paper towels (for a standing scale) to the person's room.
5 Practice hand hygiene.
6 Identify the person. Check the ID bracelet against the assignment sheet. Also call the person by name.
7 Provide for privacy.

PROCEDURE

8 Place the paper towels on the scale platform.
9 Raise the height rod.
10 Move the weights to zero (0). The pointer is in the middle.
11 Have the person remove the robe and footwear. Assist as needed. (NOTE: For some state competency tests, shoes are worn.)
12 Help the person stand on the scale. The person stands in the center of the scale. Arms are at the sides. See Figure 21-25.
13 Move the lower and upper weights until the balance pointer is in the middle (Fig. 21-26).
14 Note the weight on your note pad or assignment sheet.
15 Ask the person to stand very straight.
16 Lower the height rod until it rests on the person's head (Fig. 21-27).
17 Read the height at the movable part of the height rod. Record the height in inches or in feet and inches to the nearest ¼ inch. See Figure 21-28.
18 Note the height on your note pad or assignment sheet.
19 Raise the height rod. Help the person step off of the scale.
20 Help the person put on a robe and non-skid footwear if he or she will be up. Or help the person back to bed.
21 Lower the height rod. Adjust the weights to zero (0) if this is your agency's policy.

POST-PROCEDURE

22 Provide for comfort. (See the inside of the front cover.)
23 Place the call light within reach.
24 Raise or lower bed rails. Follow the care plan.
25 Unscreen the person.
26 Complete a safety check of the room. (See the inside of the front cover.)
27 Discard the paper towels.
28 Return the scale to its proper place.
29 Practice hand hygiene.
30 Report and record the measurements.

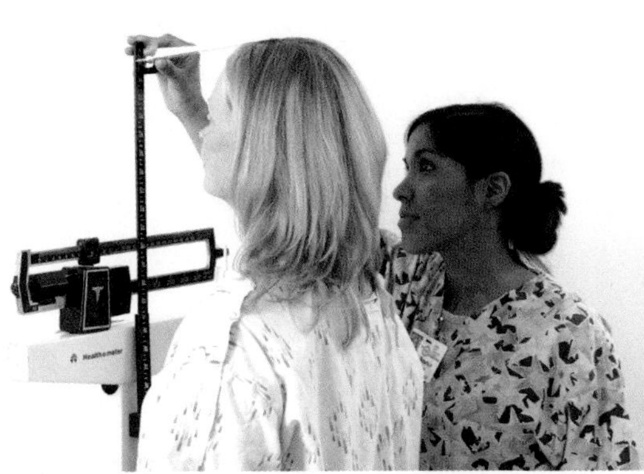

FIGURE 21-27 The height rod rests on the person's head.

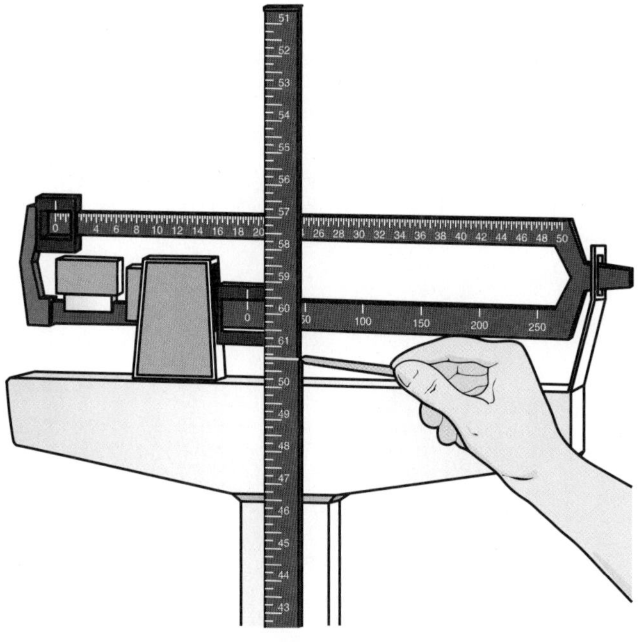

FIGURE 21-28 The height is read at the movable part of the height rod. It is read at the nearest ¼ inch. This height rod measures 61¼ inches (5 feet 1¼ inches).

FOCUS ON PRIDE

The Person, Family, and Yourself

Personal and Professional Responsibility

Measurements are important for the nursing process. They help the nurse plan for and evaluate the person's care. You are responsible for knowing normal vital sign ranges. Report abnormal measurements.

Measurements must be accurate. Tell the nurse if you are unsure of any measurement. For example, you cannot feel a pulse or hear a blood pressure. Never make up a measurement. The person can be harmed. Take pride in safely assisting with the nursing process.

Rights and Respect

When you report abnormal vital signs, the nurse may ask you to repeat the measurements. The nurse may ask you to use different equipment, change the person's position, or check a measurement at a later time. Follow the nurse's directions.

The nurse may re-check the measurements. Do not be offended. Show respect. Avoid negative thoughts or statements about the nurse or yourself. It does not mean the nurse cannot trust you or that you have done something wrong. The nurse needs to check the measurements for safe care.

Independence and Social Interaction

Personal choice promotes independence. The person may prefer that you use the right or left arm for pulses and blood pressures. If safe to do so, use the arm the person prefers. Unless orders direct otherwise, allow the person to choose to sit or lie when vital signs are measured.

Delegation and Teamwork

You may care for persons needing Transmission-Based Precautions (Chapter 12). Know your agency's policy for measuring vital signs on persons with isolation precautions.

Some agencies have isolation carts or kits that contain equipment. A stethoscope, blood pressure cuff, and thermometer are common. The equipment is taken into the person's room and left there. You use that equipment when measuring vital signs. You do not use your own stethoscope or bring other equipment into the room. If equipment must be brought in, it is cleaned after use. Special cleansers may be needed. Follow agency policy to protect others from infection.

Ethics and Laws

You may question what the person tells you about his or her pain. For example, Mrs. Watson rates her headache pain as 9 on the 0 to 10 pain rating scale. She is working a crossword puzzle and listening to music. When you have a headache that severe, you rest in a dark, quiet room. You doubt that her pain is really a 9 on the scale. You decide not to tell the nurse.

Mrs. Watson's pain really was severe. She was trying to distract herself from the pain. She did not receive prompt pain relief because the pain was not reported to the nurse.

Pain is personal. It is handled in different ways. Ignoring a person's pain is wrong. Reporting a different pain rating is wrong. Avoid making judgments about the person's pain. Accurate reporting is needed for proper pain management.

REVIEW QUESTIONS

Circle the BEST answer.

1 Which should you report at once?
   a An oral temperature of 98.4°F
   b A rectal temperature of 101.6°F
   c An axillary temperature of 97.6°F
   d An oral temperature of 99.0°F

2 A rectal temperature is taken when the person
   a Is unconscious
   b Has heart disease
   c Is confused
   d Has diarrhea

3 Which is usually used to take an adult's pulse?
   a The radial pulse
   b The apical pulse
   c The carotid pulse
   d The brachial pulse

4 For an adult, which pulse do you report at once?
   a A regular pulse at 64 beats per minute
   b A strong pulse at 78 beats per minute
   c A regular pulse at 90 beats per minute
   d An irregular pulse at 124 beats per minute

5 In an adult, normal respirations are
   a 10 to 18 per minute
   b 12 to 20 per minute
   c Less than 20 per minute
   d More than 20 per minute

6 Respirations are usually counted
   a After taking the temperature
   b Before taking the pulse
   c After taking the pulse
   d After taking the blood pressure

7 Which blood pressure is normal for an adult?
   a 88/54 mm Hg
   b 140/90 mm Hg
   c 100/58 mm Hg
   d 112/78 mm Hg

8 When measuring BP
   a Use the arm with an IV infusion
   b Apply the cuff to the bare upper arm
   c Make sure the cuff is loose
   d Place the stethoscope under the cuff

9 The systolic blood pressure is the point
   a Where the pulse is no longer felt
   b 30 mm Hg above where the pulse was felt
   c Where the first sound is heard
   d Where the last sound is heard

10 You are not sure you heard an accurate BP measurement. You should
   a Record what you think you heard
   b Measure the BP again after 60 seconds
   c Repeat the BP using the bell part of the stethoscope
   d Ask another nursing assistant to take the BP

11 A person has pain in the left chest, the left jaw, and the left shoulder and arm. This is
   a Acute pain
   b Chronic pain
   c Radiating pain
   d Phantom pain

12 A person is restless and complains of pain. You should
   a Rate the intensity based on the person's behavior
   b Give a pain-relief drug and tell the nurse
   c Report the complaint if you think the person has pain
   d Ask about the pain's location, intensity, onset, and description

13 Which are *not* counted as fluid intake?
   a Butter, sauces, and melted cheese
   b Coffee, tea, juices, and soft drinks
   c Ice cream, sherbet, custard, and pudding
   d Popsicles and gelatin

14 A person drank all of an 8 oz carton of milk. How many mL of fluid would you chart on the I&O record?
   a 8 mL
   b 60 mL
   c 120 mL
   d 240 mL

15 A person was served 250 mL of coffee and 120 mL of juice. You measure 50 mL of coffee and 60 mL of juice left. What do you chart for intake on the I&O record?
   a 110 mL
   b 260 mL
   c 370 mL
   d 480 mL

16 For an accurate weight measurement, the person
   a Wears footwear
   b Wears a robe and gown
   c Voids first
   d Chooses what scale to use

Answers to these questions are on p. 505.

FOCUS ON PRACTICE

Problem Solving

You measure a patient's vital signs. The pulse is 110. The respiratory rate is 24. The oral temperature is 100.8°F. You think you heard the blood pressure at 86/52. You are unsure of the measurement. What will you do? Which, if any, of these vital signs are abnormal? What must you do?

CHAPTER

22 Assisting With Specimens

OBJECTIVES

- Define the key terms and key abbreviations listed in this chapter.
- Explain why specimens are collected.
- Explain the rules for collecting specimens.
- Describe the different types of urine specimens.
- Perform the procedures described in this chapter.
- Explain how to promote PRIDE in the person, the family, and yourself.

KEY TERMS

acetone See "ketone"
glucosuria Sugar *(glucos)* in the urine *(uria)*; glycosuria
glycosuria Sugar *(glycos)* in the urine *(uria)*: glucosuria
hematuria Blood *(hemat)* in the urine *(uria)*
hemoptysis Bloody *(hemo)* sputum (*ptysis* means *to spit*)
ketone A substance that appears in urine from the rapid breakdown of fat for energy; acetone; ketone body
ketone body See "ketone"
sputum Mucus from the respiratory system that is expectorated (expelled) through the mouth

KEY ABBREVIATIONS

BM Bowel movement
ID Identification
I&O Intake and output
mL Milliliter
oz Ounce

Specimens *(samples)* are collected and tested to prevent, detect, and treat disease. Most specimens are tested in the laboratory. All specimens sent to the laboratory require requisition slips. The slip has the person's identifying information and the test ordered. And the specimen container is labeled according to agency policy. Some tests are done at the bedside. When collecting specimens, follow the rules in Box 22-1.

See *Promoting Safety and Comfort: Assisting With Specimens.*

PROMOTING SAFETY AND COMFORT

Assisting With Specimens

Safety

Blood, body fluids, secretions, and excretions may contain blood and microbes. This includes urine, stool, and sputum specimens. Follow Standard Precautions and the Bloodborne Pathogen Standard when collecting, testing, and handling specimens.

BOX 22-1 Rules for Collecting Specimens

- Follow the rules for medical asepsis.
- Follow Standard Precautions and the Bloodborne Pathogen Standard (Chapter 12).
- Use a clean container for each specimen.
- Use the correct container.
- Do not touch the inside of the container or the inside of the lid.
- Identify the person. Check the ID (identification) bracelet against the laboratory requisition slip or assignment sheet. Compare all information.
- Label the container in the person's presence. Provide clear, accurate information.
- Collect the specimen at the correct time.
- Ask a female if she is having a menstrual period. Tell the nurse. Menstruating may cause blood to be in the urine specimen.
- Ask the person not to have a bowel movement (BM) when collecting a urine specimen. The specimen must not contain stools.
- Ask the person to void before collecting a stool specimen. The specimen must not contain urine.
- Ask the person to put toilet tissue in the toilet or wastebasket. Urine and stool specimens must not contain tissue.
- Secure the lid on the specimen container tightly.
- Place the specimen container in a labeled *BIOHAZARD* plastic bag. Do not let the container touch the outside of the bag. Seal the bag.
- Take the specimen and requisition slip to the laboratory or storage area.

URINE SPECIMENS

Urine specimens are collected for urine tests. Follow the rules in Box 22-1.

See *Delegation Guidelines: Urine Specimens.*

See *Promoting Safety and Comfort: Urine Specimens.*

The Random Urine Specimen

The random urine specimen is used for routine urinalysis (UA). No special measures are needed. It is collected any time during a 24-hour period. Many people can collect the specimen themselves. Weak and very ill persons need help.

See procedure: *Collecting a Random Urine Specimen*, p. 358.

DELEGATION GUIDELINES

Urine Specimens

To collect a urine specimen, you need this information from the nurse and the care plan.

- Voiding device used—bedpan, urinal, commode, or toilet with specimen pan
- The type of specimen needed
- What time to collect the specimen
- What special measures are needed
- If you need to test the specimen (p. 360)
- If measuring intake and output (I&O) is ordered (Chapter 21)
- What observations to report and record:
  - Problems obtaining the specimen
  - Color, clarity, and odor of urine
  - Blood in the urine
  - Particles in the urine
  - Complaints of pain, burning, urgency, difficulty voiding, or other problems
  - The time the specimen was collected
- When to report observations
- What patient or resident concerns to report at once

PROMOTING SAFETY AND COMFORT

Urine Specimens

Comfort

Urine specimens may embarrass some people. They do not like clear specimen containers that show urine. It may be helpful to place the specimen container in a paper bag. Or provide a paper towel or washcloth to wrap around the container.

Collecting a Random Urine Specimen

QUALITY OF LIFE

- Knock before entering the person's room.
- Address the person by name.
- Introduce yourself by name and title.
- Explain the procedure before starting and during the procedure.
- Protect the person's rights during the procedure.
- Handle the person gently during the procedure.

PRE-PROCEDURE

1 Follow *Delegation Guidelines: Urine Specimens,* p. 357. See *Promoting Safety and Comfort:*
   a *Assisting With Specimens,* p. 356
   b *Urine Specimens,* p. 357
2 Practice hand hygiene.
3 Collect the following before going to the person's room.
   - Laboratory requisition slip
   - Specimen container and lid
   - Voiding device—bedpan and cover, urinal, commode, or specimen pan (Fig. 22-1)
   - Specimen label
   - Plastic bag
   - *BIOHAZARD* label (if needed)
   - Gloves
4 Arrange collected items in the person's bathroom.
5 Practice hand hygiene.
6 Identify the person. Check the ID bracelet against the requisition slip. Also call the person by name.
7 Label the container in the person's presence.
8 Put on gloves
9 Collect a graduate to measure output.
10 Provide for privacy.

PROCEDURE

11 Ask the person to void into the device. Remind him or her to put toilet tissue into the wastebasket or toilet. Toilet tissue is not put in the bedpan or specimen pan.
12 Take the voiding device to the bathroom.
13 Pour about 120 mL (milliliters) (4 oz [ounces]) into the specimen container.
14 Place the lid on the specimen container. Put the container in the plastic bag. Do not let the container touch the outside of the bag. Apply a *BIOHAZARD* label.
15 Measure urine if I&O are ordered. Include the specimen amount.
16 Empty, rinse, clean, disinfect, and dry equipment. Return equipment to its proper place.
17 Remove and discard the gloves. Practice hand hygiene. Put on clean gloves.
18 Assist with hand washing.
19 Remove and discard the gloves. Practice hand hygiene.

POST-PROCEDURE

20 Provide for comfort. (See the inside of the front cover.)
21 Place the call light within reach.
22 Raise or lower bed rails. Follow the care plan.
23 Unscreen the person.
24 Complete a safety check of the room. (See the inside of the front cover.)
25 Practice hand hygiene.
26 Take the specimen and requisition slip to the laboratory or storage area. Wear gloves.
27 Remove and discard the gloves. Practice hand hygiene.
28 Report and record your observations.

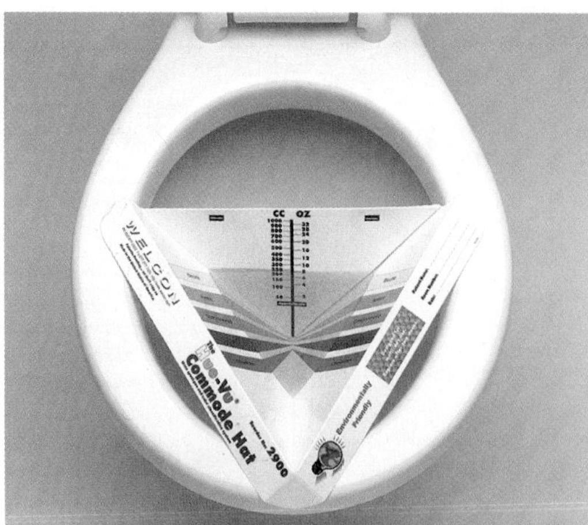

FIGURE 22-1 The specimen pan is placed at the front of the toilet on the toilet rim. This pan has a color chart for urine.

The Midstream Specimen

The midstream specimen is also called a *clean-voided specimen* or *clean-catch specimen.* The perineal area is cleaned before collecting the specimen. This reduces the number of microbes in the urethral area. The person starts to void into a device. Then the person stops the urine stream, and a sterile specimen container is positioned. The person voids into the container until the specimen is obtained.

Stopping the urine stream is hard for many people. You may need to position and hold the specimen container in place after the person starts to void (Fig. 22-2).

See *Focus on Communication: The Midstream Specimen.*

See procedure: *Collecting a Midstream Specimen.*

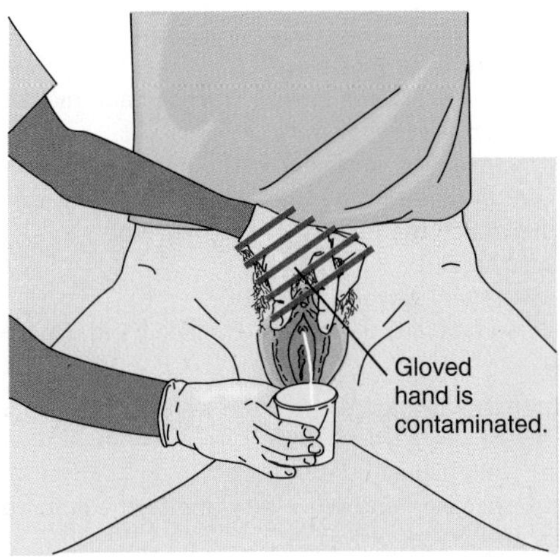

FIGURE 22-2 The labia are separated to collect a midstream specimen.

FOCUS ON COMMUNICATION

The Midstream Specimen

Some persons can collect the midstream specimen without help. You may need to explain the procedure. Use words the person understands. Show what supplies to use. Also, ask if the person has questions. For example:

> *Ms. Jacobs, I need a midstream urine specimen from you. This means I need urine from the middle of your urine stream. First, wipe well with this towelette (show the towelette). Wipe from front to back. The specimen goes in this cup (show the specimen cup). Please do not touch the inside of the cup. Start your urine stream and then stop. Position the cup to catch urine and begin your stream again. If you cannot stop your stream, just position the cup during the middle of the stream. I need at least this much urine in the cup if possible (point to the 30 mL measure on the cup). Remove the cup when it is about that full. Finish urinating. Secure the lid on top of the cup. Please do not touch the inside of the lid. I will take the specimen when you are done. Do you have any questions?*

Collecting a Midstream Specimen

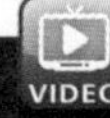

QUALITY OF LIFE

- Knock before entering the person's room.
- Address the person by name.
- Introduce yourself by name and title.
- Explain the procedure before starting and during the procedure.
- Protect the person's rights during the procedure.
- Handle the person gently during the procedure.

PRE-PROCEDURE

1 Follow *Delegation Guidelines: Urine Specimens,* p. 357. See *Promoting Safety and Comfort:*
   a *Assisting With Specimens,* p. 356
   b *Urine Specimens,* p. 357
2 Practice hand hygiene.
3 Collect the following before going to the person's room.
   - Laboratory requisition slip
   - Midstream specimen kit—specimen container, label, towelettes, sterile gloves
   - Plastic bag
   - Sterile gloves if not part of the kit
   - Disposable gloves
   - BIOHAZARD label (if needed)
4 Arrange your work area.
5 Practice hand hygiene.
6 Identify the person. Check the ID bracelet against the requisition slip. Also call the person by name.
7 Put on disposable gloves.
8 Collect the following.
   - Voiding device—bedpan and cover, urinal, commode, or specimen pan if needed
   - Supplies for perineal care (Chapter 16)
   - Graduate to measure output
   - Paper towels
9 Provide for privacy.

Continued

Collecting a Midstream Specimen—cont'd

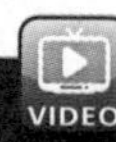

PROCEDURE

10 Provide perineal care (Chapter 16). (Wear gloves for this step. Practice hand hygiene after removing and discarding them.)
11 Open the sterile kit.
12 Put on the sterile gloves.
13 Open the packet of towelettes.
14 Open the sterile specimen container. Do not touch the inside of the container or lid. Set the lid down so the inside is up.
15 *For a female*—clean the perineal area with towelettes.
  a Spread the labia with your thumb and index finger. Use your non-dominant hand. (This hand is now contaminated. It must not touch anything sterile.)
  b Clean down the urethral area from front to back. Use a clean towelette for each stroke.
  c Keep the labia separated to collect the urine specimen (steps 17 through 20).
16 *For a male*—clean the penis with towelettes.
  a Hold the penis with your non-dominant hand. (This hand is now contaminated. It must not touch anything sterile.)
  b Clean the penis starting at the meatus. (Retract the foreskin if the male is uncircumcised.) Clean in a circular motion. Start at the center and work outward.
  c Keep holding the penis (and foreskin retracted in the uncircumcised male) until the specimen is collected (steps 17 through 20).
17 Ask the person to void into a device.
18 Pass the specimen container into the urine stream. Keep the labia separated (see Fig. 22-2).
19 Collect about 30 to 60 mL (1 to 2 oz) of urine.
20 Remove the specimen container before the person stops voiding. Release the foreskin of the uncircumcised male.
21 Release the labia or penis. Let the person finish voiding into the device.
22 Put the lid on the specimen container. Touch only the outside of the container and lid. Wipe the outside of the container. Set the container on a paper towel.
23 Provide toilet tissue when the person is done voiding.
24 Take the voiding device to the bathroom.
25 Measure urine if I&O are ordered. Include the specimen amount.
26 Empty, rinse, clean, disinfect, and dry equipment. Return equipment to its proper place.
27 Remove and discard the gloves. Practice hand hygiene. Put on clean disposable gloves.
28 Label the specimen container in the person's presence. Place the container in the plastic bag. Do not let the container touch the outside of the bag. Apply a *BIOHAZARD* label.
29 Assist with hand washing.
30 Remove and discard the gloves. Practice hand hygiene.

POST-PROCEDURE

31 Provide for comfort. (See the inside of the front cover.)
32 Place the call light within reach.
33 Raise or lower the bed rails. Follow the care plan.
34 Unscreen the person.
35 Complete a safety check of the room. (See the inside of the front cover.)
36 Practice hand hygiene.
37 Take the specimen and requisition slip to the laboratory or storage area. Wear gloves.
38 Remove and discard the gloves. Practice hand hygiene.
39 Report and record your observations.

The 24-Hour Urine Specimen

All urine voided during a 24-hour period is collected for a 24-hour urine specimen. Urine is chilled on ice or refrigerated during this time. This prevents the growth of microbes. For some tests, a preservative is added to the collection container.

The person voids to begin the test with an empty bladder. Discard this voiding. Save *all voidings* for the next 24 hours. The person and nursing staff must clearly understand the procedure and the test period. The test is restarted if:

- A voiding was not saved.
- Toilet tissue was discarded into the specimen.
- The specimen contains stools.

Testing Urine

The doctor orders the type and frequency of urine tests. Random urine specimens are usually needed. The nurse may ask you to do these simple tests.

- *Testing for pH*—Urine pH measures if urine is acidic or alkaline. Changes in normal pH (4.6 to 8.0) occur from illness, food, and drugs.
- *Testing for blood*—Injury and disease can cause hematuria. ***Hematuria*** *means blood* (hemat) *in the urine* (uria). Sometimes blood is seen in the urine. At other times it is unseen *(occult)*.
- *Testing for glucose and ketones*—In diabetes, the pancreas does not secrete enough insulin (Chapter 28). The body needs insulin to use sugar for energy. If not used, sugar builds up in the blood. Some sugar appears in the urine. ***Glucosuria (glycosuria)*** *means sugar* (glucos, glycos) *in the urine* (uria).The diabetic person may also have ketones in the urine. ***Ketones (ketone bodies, acetone)*** *are substances that appear in urine from the rapid breakdown of fat for energy.* The body uses fat for energy if it cannot use sugar. Tests for glucose and ketones are usually done 4 times a day—30 minutes before each meal and at bedtime. The doctor uses the test to make drug and diet decisions.

Using Reagent Strips. Reagent strips (dipsticks) have sections that change color when they react with urine. To use a reagent strip:

- Do not touch the test area on the strip.
- Dip the strip into urine.
- Compare the strip with the color chart on the bottle (Fig. 22-3).

See *Delegation Guidelines: Testing Urine.*
See *Promoting Safety and Comfort: Testing Urine.*

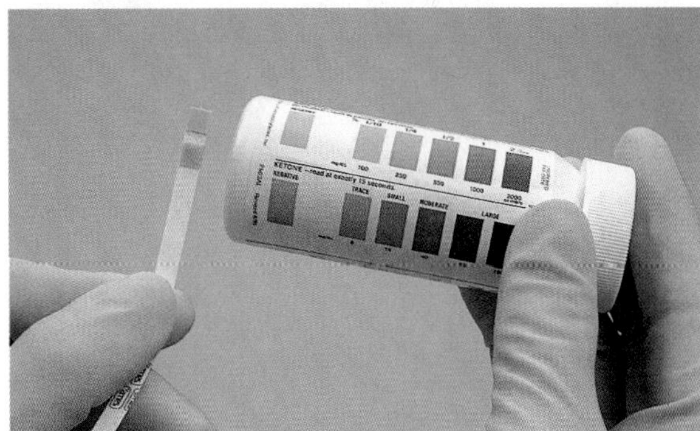

FIGURE 22-3 Reagent strip for sugar and ketones.

DELEGATION GUIDELINES

Testing Urine

When testing urine is delegated to you, you need this information from the nurse and the care plan.

- What test is needed
- What equipment to use
- When to test urine
- Instructions for the test ordered
- If the nurse wants to observe the results of each test
- What observations to report and record
  - The time you collected and tested the specimen
  - Test results
  - Problems obtaining the specimen
  - Color, clarity, and odor of urine
  - Blood in the urine
  - Particles in the urine
  - Complaints of pain, burning, urgency, difficulty voiding, or other problems
- When to report test results and observations
- What patient or resident concerns to report at once

PROMOTING SAFETY AND COMFORT

Testing Urine

Safety

You must be accurate when testing urine. Promptly report the results to the nurse. Ordered drugs may depend on the results.

When using reagent strips:

- Check the color of the reagent strips. Do not use discolored strips.
- Check the expiration date on the bottle. Do not use the strips if the date has passed.
- Follow the manufacturer's instructions. Otherwise you could get the wrong result. The doctor uses the test results in diagnosing and treating the person. A wrong result can cause serious harm.

Testing Urine With Reagent Strips

QUALITY OF LIFE

- Knock before entering the person's room.
- Address the person by name.
- Introduce yourself by name and title.
- Explain the procedure before starting and during the procedure.
- Protect the person's rights during the procedure.
- Handle the person gently during the procedure.

PRE-PROCEDURE

1 Follow *Delegation Guidelines: Testing Urine*. See *Promoting Safety and Comfort:*
   a *Assisting With Specimens,* p. 356
   b *Testing Urine*
2 Practice hand hygiene.
3 Collect gloves and the reagent strips ordered.
4 Practice hand hygiene.
5 Identify the person. Check the ID bracelet against the assignment sheet. Also call the person by name.
6 Put on gloves
7 Collect equipment for the urine specimen. (See procedure: *Collecting a Random Urine Specimen,* p. 358.)
8 Provide for privacy.

Continued

Testing Urine With Reagent Strips—cont'd

PROCEDURE

9 Collect the urine specimen. (See procedure: *Collecting a Random Urine Specimen,* p. 358.)
10 Remove a strip from the bottle. Put the cap on the bottle at once. It must be on tight.
11 Dip the strip test areas into the urine.
12 Remove the strip after the correct amount of time. See the manufacturer's instructions.
13 Tap the strip gently against the urine container. This removes excess urine.
14 Wait the required amount of time. See the manufacturer's instructions.
15 Compare the strip with the color chart on the bottle (see Fig. 22-3). Read the results.
16 Discard disposable items and the specimen.
17 Empty, rinse, clean, disinfect, and dry equipment. Return equipment to its proper place.
18 Remove and discard the gloves. Practice hand hygiene.

POST-PROCEDURE

19 Provide for comfort. (See the inside of the front cover.)
20 Place the call light within reach.
21 Raise or lower bed rails. Follow the care plan.
22 Unscreen the person.
23 Complete a safety check of the room. (See the inside of the front cover.)
24 Practice hand hygiene.
25 Report and record the test results and other observations.

STOOL SPECIMENS

Stools are studied for fat, microbes, worms, blood, and other abnormal contents. Urine must not contaminate the stool specimen. The person uses 1 device for voiding and another for a BM. Some tests require a warm stool. The specimen is taken at once to the laboratory or storage area. Follow the rules in Box 22-1.

See *Focus on Communication: Stool Specimens.*
See *Delegation Guidelines: Stool Specimens.*
See *Promoting Safety and Comfort: Stool Specimens.*
See procedure: *Collecting a Stool Specimen.*

FOCUS ON COMMUNICATION

Stool Specimens

Always explain the procedure before you begin. Explain what the person needs to do and what you will do. Also show the equipment and supplies. For example:

The doctor wants your stools tested. So we need a specimen from a bowel movement. I'm going to place the specimen pan (show specimen pan) at the back of the toilet bowl. You will urinate into the toilet. Your bowel movement will collect in the specimen pan. Please put toilet tissue in the toilet, not in the specimen pan. After your bowel movement, put your call light on right away. I'll put some stool in this specimen container (show the specimen container).

After explaining the procedure, ask if the person has questions. If you do not know the answer, refer the question to the nurse.

Also make sure the person understands what to do. You can say: "Mrs. Clark, please tell me what you're going to do so I know you understand what I said."

DELEGATION GUIDELINES

Stool Specimens

Before collecting a stool specimen, you need this information from the nurse.

- What time to collect the specimen
- What equipment to use
- What special measures are needed
- If the nurse wants to observe the stool
- What observations to report and record:
  - The time you collected the specimen
  - Problems obtaining the specimen
  - Color, amount, consistency, and odor of stools
  - Blood in the stools
  - Complaints of pain or discomfort
- When to report observations
- What patient or resident concerns to report at once

PROMOTING SAFETY AND COMFORT

Stool Specimens

Comfort

Stools normally have an odor. A person may be embarrassed that you need to collect a specimen. Complete the task quickly and carefully. Also act in a professional manner.

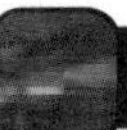

Collecting a Stool Specimen

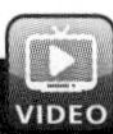

VIDEO

QUALITY OF LIFE

- Knock before entering the person's room.
- Address the person by name.
- Introduce yourself by name and title.
- Explain the procedure before starting and during the procedure.
- Protect the person's rights during the procedure.
- Handle the person gently during the procedure.

PRE-PROCEDURE

1 Follow *Delegation Guidelines: Stool Specimens.* See *Promoting Safety and Comfort:*
   a *Assisting With Specimens,* p. 356
   b *Stool Specimens*
2 Practice hand hygiene.
3 Collect the following before going to the person's room.
   - Laboratory requisition slip
   - Specimen pan for the toilet
   - Specimen container and lid
   - Specimen label
   - Tongue blades
   - Disposable bag
   - Plastic bag
   - *BIOHAZARD* label (if needed)
   - Gloves
4 Arrange collected items in the person's bathroom.
5 Practice hand hygiene.
6 Identify the person. Check the ID bracelet against the requisition slip. Also call the person by name.
7 Label the specimen container in the person's presence.
8 Put on gloves.
9 Collect the following.
   - Device for voiding—bedpan and cover, urinal, commode, or specimen pan
   - Toilet tissue
10 Provide for privacy.

PROCEDURE

11 Ask the person to void. Provide the voiding device if the person does not use the bathroom. Empty, rinse, clean, disinfect, and dry the device. Return it to its proper place.
12 Put the specimen pan on the toilet if the person will use the bathroom. Place it at the back of the toilet (Fig. 22-4, p. 364). Or provide the bedpan or commode.
13 Ask the person not to put toilet tissue into the bedpan, commode, or specimen pan. Provide a bag for toilet tissue if the person uses the bedpan or commode.
14 Place the call light and toilet tissue within reach. Raise or lower bed rails. Follow the care plan.
15 Remove and discard the gloves. Practice hand hygiene. Leave the room if the person can be left alone.
16 Return when the person signals. Or check on the person every 5 minutes. Knock before entering.
17 Practice hand hygiene. Put on clean gloves.
18 Lower the bed rail near you if up. Remove the bedpan (if used). Provide perineal care if needed.
19 Assist the person off of the toilet or commode (if used).
20 Note the color, amount, consistency, and odor of stools.
21 Collect the specimen.
   a Use a tongue blade to take about 2 tablespoons of stool to the specimen container (Fig. 22-5, p. 364). Take the sample from the middle of a formed stool.
   b Include pus, mucus, or blood present in the stool.
   c Take stool from 2 different places in the BM if required by agency policy.
   d Put the lid on the specimen container.
   e Place the container in the plastic bag. Do not let the container touch the outside of the bag. Apply a *BIOHAZARD* label according to agency policy.
   f Wrap the tongue blade in toilet tissue. Discard it in the disposable bag.
22 Remove and discard the gloves. Practice hand hygiene. Put on clean gloves.
23 Empty, rinse, clean, disinfect, and dry equipment. Return equipment to its proper place.
24 Remove and discard the gloves. Practice hand hygiene. Put on clean gloves.
25 Assist with hand washing.
26 Remove and discard the gloves. Practice hand hygiene.

POST-PROCEDURE

27 Provide for comfort. (See the inside of the front cover.)
28 Place the call light within reach.
29 Raise or lower bed rails. Follow the care plan.
30 Unscreen the person.
31 Complete a safety check of the room. (See the inside of the front cover.)
32 Deliver the specimen and requisition slip to the laboratory or storage area. Follow agency policy. Wear gloves.
33 Remove and discard the gloves. Practice hand hygiene.
34 Report and record your observations.

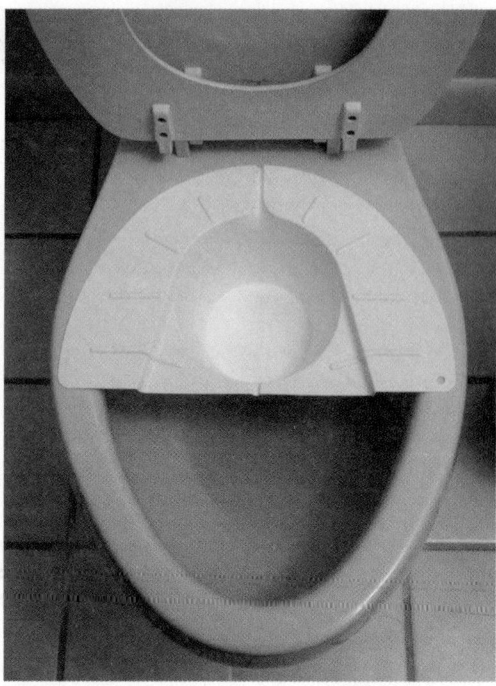

FIGURE 22-4 The specimen pan is placed at the back of the toilet for a stool specimen.

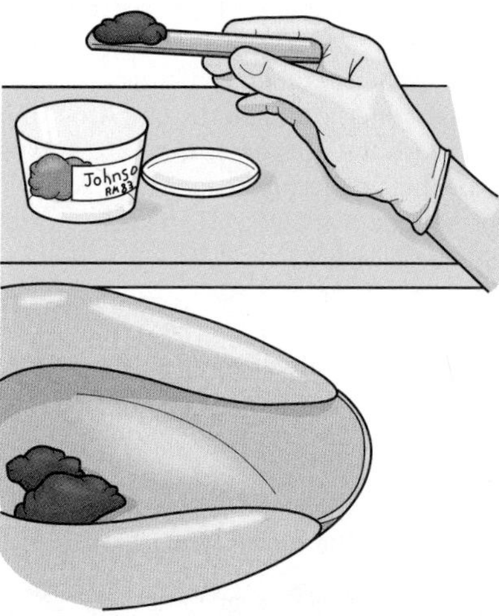

FIGURE 22-5 A tongue blade is used to transfer a small amount of stool from the bedpan to the specimen container.

SPUTUM SPECIMENS

Respiratory disorders cause the lungs, bronchi, and trachea to secrete mucus. *Mucus from the respiratory system is called* ***sputum*** *when expectorated (expelled) through the mouth.* Sputum specimens are studied for blood, microbes, and abnormal cells.

The person coughs up sputum from the bronchi and trachea. This is often painful and hard to do. It is easier to collect a specimen in the morning. Secretions collect in the trachea and bronchi during sleep. They are coughed up on awakening.

To collect a specimen, follow the rules in Box 22-1. Also have the person rinse the mouth with water. Rinsing decreases saliva and removes food particles. Mouthwash is not used. It destroys some of the microbes in the mouth.

See *Delegation Guidelines: Sputum Specimens.*

See *Promoting Safety and Comfort: Sputum Specimens.*

See procedure: *Collecting a Sputum Specimen.*

DELEGATION GUIDELINES

Sputum Specimens

To collect a sputum specimen, you need this information from the nurse.

- When to collect the specimen
- How much sputum is needed—usually 1 to 2 teaspoons
- If the person uses the bathroom
- If the person can hold the sputum container
- What observations to report and record:
    - The time the specimen was collected
    - The amount of sputum collected
    - How easily the person raised the sputum
    - Sputum color—clear, white, yellow, green, brown, or red
    - Sputum odor—none or foul odor
    - Sputum consistency—thick, watery, or frothy (with bubbles or foam)
    - ***Hemoptysis***—*bloody* (hemo) *sputum* (ptysis *means* to spit)
    - If the person was not able to produce sputum
    - Any other observations
- When to report observations
- What patient or resident concerns to report at once

PROMOTING SAFETY AND COMFORT

Sputum Specimens

Safety

The doctor may order isolation precautions if the person has or may have tuberculosis (TB) (Chapter 28). Protect yourself by wearing a TB respirator (Chapter 12).

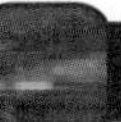

Collecting a Sputum Specimen

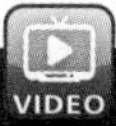

VIDEO

QUALITY OF LIFE

- Knock before entering the person's room.
- Address the person by name.
- Introduce yourself by name and title.
- Explain the procedure before starting and during the procedure.
- Protect the person's rights during the procedure.
- Handle the person gently during the procedure.

PRE-PROCEDURE

1 Follow *Delegation Guidelines: Sputum Specimens.* See *Promoting Safety and Comfort:*
   a *Assisting With Specimens,* p. 356
   b *Sputum Specimens*
2 Practice hand hygiene.
3 Collect the following before going to the person's room.
   - Laboratory requisition slip
   - Sputum specimen container and lid
   - Specimen label
   - Plastic bag
   - *BIOHAZARD* label (if needed)
4 Arrange collected items in the person's bathroom.
5 Practice hand hygiene.
6 Identify the person. Check the ID bracelet against the requisition slip. Also call the person by name.
7 Label the specimen container in the person's presence.
8 Collect gloves and tissues.
9 Provide for privacy. If able, the person uses the bathroom for the procedure.

PROCEDURE

10 Put on gloves.
11 Ask the person to rinse the mouth out with clear water.
12 Have the person hold the container. Only the outside is touched.
13 Ask the person to cover the mouth and nose with tissues when coughing. Follow agency policy for used tissues.
14 Ask him or her to take 2 or 3 breaths and cough up the sputum.
15 Have the person expectorate directly into the container (Fig. 22-6). Sputum should not touch the outside of the container.
16 Collect 1 to 2 teaspoons of sputum unless told to collect more.
17 Put the lid on the container.
18 Place the container in the plastic bag. Do not let the container touch the outside of the bag. Apply a *BIOHAZARD* label according to agency policy.
19 Remove and discard the gloves. Practice hand hygiene. Put on clean gloves.
20 Assist with hand washing.
21 Remove and discard the gloves. Practice hand hygiene.

POST-PROCEDURE

22 Provide for comfort. (See the inside of the front cover.)
23 Place the call light within reach.
24 Raise or lower bed rails. Follow the care plan.
25 Unscreen the person.
26 Complete a safety check of the room. (See the inside of the front cover.)
27 Practice hand hygiene.
28 Deliver the specimen and the requisition slip to laboratory or storage area. Follow agency policy. Wear gloves.
29 Remove and discard the gloves. Practice hand hygiene.
30 Report and record your observations.

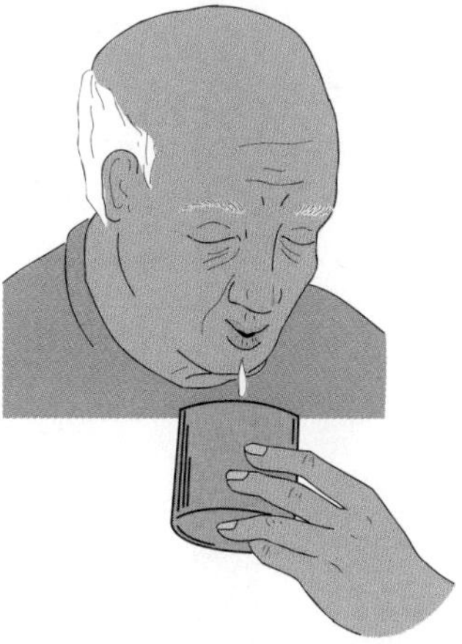

FIGURE 22-6 The person expectorates into the center of the specimen container.

FOCUS ON PRIDE

The Person, Family, and Yourself

Personal and Professional Responsibility
You must collect and test specimens on the right person. Otherwise, 1 or both persons could be harmed. Before collecting or testing a specimen, carefully identify the person. Check the ID bracelet against the laboratory requisition slip or assignment sheet. Compare all information, not just the person's name.

In some agencies, you write collection information on the specimen container. Date, time, and the collector's name or initials are examples. Follow agency policy to label specimens. Take pride in collecting and testing specimens properly.

Rights and Respect
Specimen collection embarrasses many people. Respect the person's right to privacy. To promote comfort and privacy:

- Politely ask visitors to leave the room.
- Close doors, privacy curtains, and window coverings.
- Leave the room if it is safe to do so. If you cannot leave, explain this to the person.
- Place the specimen container in a paper bag or wrap it in a paper towel or washcloth so others do not see the specimen.
- Act professionally. Do not make statements that may embarrass the person.

Independence and Social Interaction
Some persons can collect their own urine and sputum specimens. This promotes independence. It also helps reduce embarrassment.

Explain the procedure to the person. This helps the person know how to correctly collect the specimen. Show the person the specimen container and how it is used. Also, ask the person where you should place the container. When ready to collect the specimen, the person knows where to find the container.

Delegation and Teamwork
You may need to take a specimen to the laboratory. Before you go, tell the nurse and your co-workers that you are leaving the area. Also, ask if other staff need specimens taken to the laboratory. Doing so saves staff time. This also prevents having too many staff members off the unit at the same time. Return from the laboratory promptly.

Ethics and Laws
Ethics is concerned with right and wrong behavior. If you did not collect a specimen correctly, do not send it to the laboratory. Tell the nurse what happened. Then collect the specimen at the next opportunity. Test results must be accurate for correct diagnosis and treatment. Take pride in honestly reporting mistakes.

REVIEW QUESTIONS

Circle the BEST answer.

1 Which specimen was collected correctly?
- a A stool specimen that contains urine
- b A urine specimen that contains toilet tissue
- c A sputum specimen with a label and requisition slip
- d A urine specimen with a loose lid in a biohazard bag

2 A random urine specimen is collected
- a After sleep
- b Before meals
- c After meals
- d Any time

3 Perineal care is given before collecting a
- a Random urine specimen
- b Midstream specimen
- c Sputum specimen
- d Stool specimen

4 To collect a midstream specimen on a female
- a Spread the labia to expose the urethral area
- b Clean the urethral area from back to front
- c Collect urine at the start of the urine stream
- d Collect about 10 mL of urine

5 Urine is tested for glucose
- a To measure the pH
- b To check for blood
- c To check for sugar
- d To check for ketones

6 A stool specimen must be kept warm. After collecting the specimen
- a Wrap it in a warm, moist washcloth
- b Put it in a paper bag
- c Cover it with a towel
- d Take it to the laboratory or storage area

7 The best time to collect a sputum specimen is
- a On awakening
- b After meals
- c At bedtime
- d After oral hygiene

8 A sputum specimen is needed. You should ask the person to
- a Use mouthwash
- b Rinse the mouth with clear water
- c Brush the teeth
- d Remove dentures

Answers to these questions are on p. 505.

FOCUS ON PRACTICE

Problem Solving

You collect and send a specimen to the laboratory. Later, you realize that you placed the wrong label on the container. What do you do? Why is it important to label specimens properly?

Assisting With Exercise and Activity

CHAPTER 23

OBJECTIVES

- Define the key terms and key abbreviations listed in this chapter.
- Describe bedrest.
- Explain how to prevent the complications from bedrest.
- Describe the devices used to support and maintain body alignment.
- Describe range-of-motion exercises.
- Describe 4 walking aids.
- Perform the procedures described in this chapter.
- Explain how to promote PRIDE in the person, the family, and yourself.

KEY TERMS

abduction Moving a body part away from the mid-line of the body
adduction Moving a body part toward the mid-line of the body
ambulation The act of walking
atrophy The decrease in size or the wasting away of tissue
contracture The lack of joint mobility caused by abnormal shortening of a muscle
dorsiflexion Bending the toes and foot up at the ankle
extension Straightening a body part
external rotation Turning the joint outward
flexion Bending a body part
footdrop The foot falls down at the ankle; permanent plantar flexion
hyperextension Excessive straightening of a body part
internal rotation Turning the joint inward
opposition Touching an opposite finger with the thumb
orthostatic hypotension Abnormally low *(hypo)* blood pressure when the person suddenly stands up (*ortho* and *static*); postural hypotension
plantar flexion The foot *(plantar)* is bent *(flexion);* bending the foot down at the ankle
postural hypotension See "orthostatic hypotension"
pronation Turning the joint downward
range of motion (ROM) The movement of a joint to the extent possible without causing pain
rotation Turning the joint
supination Turning the joint upward

KEY ABBREVIATIONS

ADL Activities of daily living
ID Identification
ROM Range of motion

Illness, surgery, injury, pain, and aging can limit activity. Inactivity, whether mild or severe, affects every body system. And it affects mental well-being.

You assist the nurse in promoting exercise and activity in all persons to the extent possible. The care plan and your assignment sheet include the person's activity level and needed exercises.

See *Focus on Older Persons: Assisting With Exercise and Activity.*

FOCUS ON OLDER PERSONS

Assisting With Exercise and Activity

Persons with dementia may resist exercise and activity. They do not understand what is happening and may fear harm. They may become agitated and combative. Some cry out for help. Do not force the person to exercise or take part in activities. Stay calm and ask the nurse for help. Follow the care plan.

BEDREST

The doctor orders bedrest to treat a health problem. Or it is a nursing measure if the person's condition changes. Generally bedrest is ordered to:

- Reduce physical activity.
- Reduce pain.
- Encourage rest.
- Regain strength.
- Promote healing.

The types of bedrest are:

- *Strict bedrest.* Everything is done for the person. The person stays in bed for all activities of daily living (ADL).
- *Bedrest.* The person can perform some ADL. Self-feeding, oral hygiene, bathing, shaving, and hair care are often allowed.
- *Bedrest with commode privileges.* The commode is used for elimination.
- *Bedrest with bathroom privileges (bedrest with BRP).* The bathroom is used for elimination.

The person's care plan and your assignment sheet tell you the activities allowed. Always ask the nurse what bedrest means for each person. Check with the nurse if you have questions about a person's activity limits.

Complications From Bedrest

Bedrest and lack of exercise and activity can cause serious complications. Pressure ulcers, constipation, and fecal impaction can result. Urinary tract infections and renal calculi (kidney stones) can occur. So can blood clots (thrombi) and pneumonia (inflammation and infection of the lung).

The musculo-skeletal system is affected by lack of exercise and activity. You help prevent the following to maintain normal movement.

- A ***contracture*** *is the lack of joint mobility caused by abnormal shortening of a muscle.* The contracted muscle is fixed into position, is deformed, and cannot stretch (Fig. 23-1). Common sites are the fingers, wrists, elbows, toes, ankles, knees, and hips. They can also occur in the neck and spine. The site is deformed and stiff.
- ***Atrophy*** *is the decrease in size or the wasting away of tissue.* Tissues shrink in size. *Muscle atrophy* is a decrease in size or a wasting away of muscle (Fig. 23-2).

Orthostatic hypotension *is abnormally low* (hypo) *blood pressure when the person suddenly stands up* (ortho *and* static). When a person moves from lying or sitting to a standing position, the blood pressure drops. The person is dizzy and weak, has spots before the eyes, and may faint. *Orthostatic hypotension also is called* ***postural hypotension.*** (*Postural* relates to *posture* or *standing.*) Slowly changing positions is key to preventing orthostatic hypotension. Return the person to a sitting or lying position if orthostatic hypotension occurs.

Good nursing care prevents complications from bedrest. Good alignment, range-of-motion exercises (p. 370), and frequent position changes are important measures. These are part of the care plan.

See *Focus on Communication: Complications From Bedrest.*

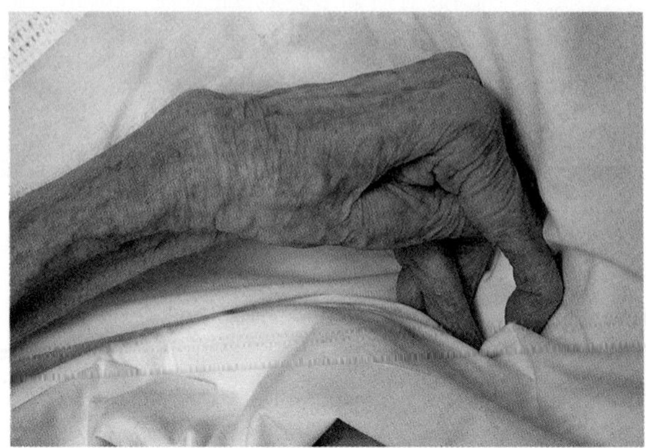

FIGURE 23-1 A contracture.

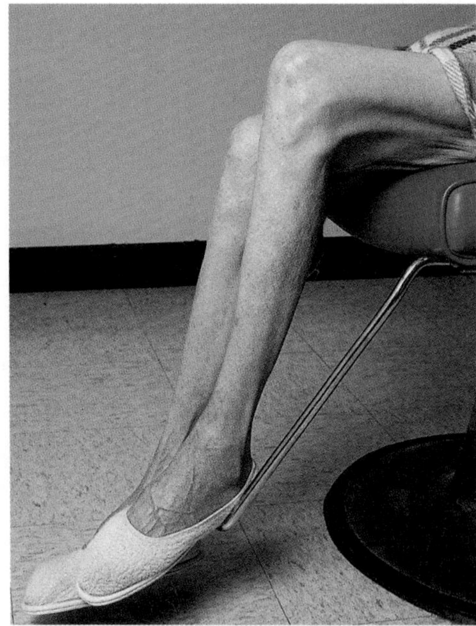

FIGURE 23-2 Muscle atrophy.

FOCUS ON COMMUNICATION

Complications From Bedrest

Orthostatic hypotension can occur when the person moves from lying or sitting to standing. To check for orthostatic hypotension, ask these questions.

- "Do you feel weak?"
- "Do you feel dizzy?"
- "Do you see spots before your eyes?"
- "Do you feel like fainting?"

Positioning

Body alignment and positioning were discussed in Chapter 13. Supportive devices are often used to support and maintain the person in a certain position.

- *Bed-boards*—are placed under the mattress to prevent it from sagging (Fig. 23-3).
- *Foot-boards*—prevent plantar flexion that can lead to footdrop. In ***plantar flexion,*** *the foot* (plantar) *is bent* (flexion). ***Footdrop*** *is when the foot falls down at the ankle (permanent plantar flexion).* The foot-board is placed so the soles of the feet are flush against it (Fig. 23-4). Foot-boards also keep top linens off the feet and toes.
- *Trochanter rolls*—prevent the hips and legs from turning outward (external rotation) (Fig. 23-5). A bath blanket is folded to the desired length and rolled up. The loose end is placed under the person from the hip to the knee. Then the roll is tucked alongside the body.
- *Hip abduction wedges*—keep the hips abducted (apart) (Fig. 23-6). The wedge is placed between the person's legs. These are common after hip replacement surgery.
- *Hand rolls or hand grips*—prevent contractures of the thumb, fingers, and wrist (Fig. 23-7, p. 370). Foam rubber sponges, rubber balls, and finger cushions (Fig. 23-8, p. 370) also are used.
- *Splints*—keep the elbows, wrists, thumbs, fingers, ankles, and knees in normal position. They are usually secured in place with Velcro (Fig. 23-9, p. 370).
- *Bed cradles*—keep the weight of top linens off the feet and toes (Fig. 23-10, p. 370). The weight of top linens can cause footdrop and pressure ulcers.

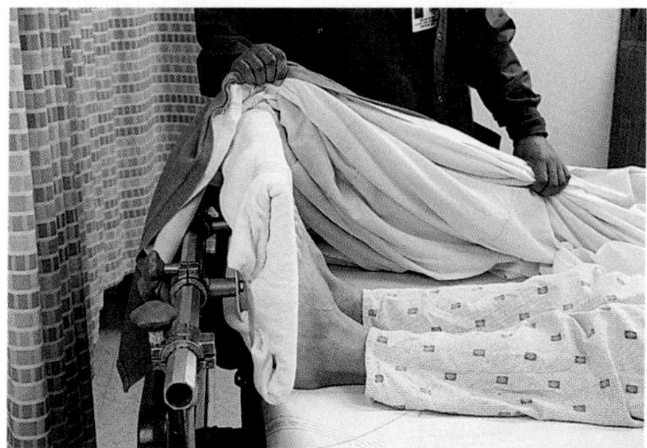

FIGURE 23-4 A foot-board. Feet are flush with the board to keep them in normal alignment.

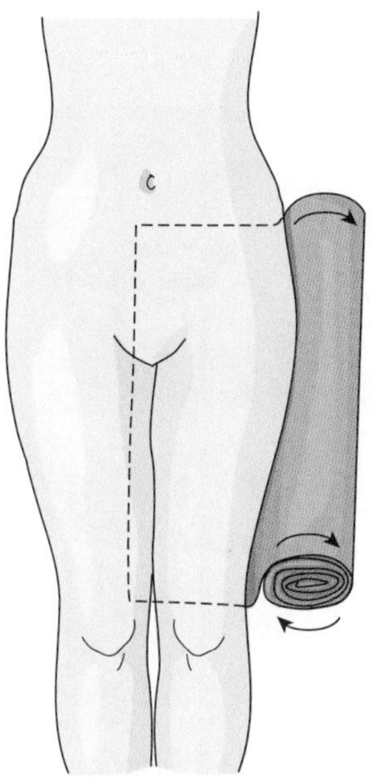

FIGURE 23-5 A trochanter roll is made from a bath blanket. It extends from the hip to the knee.

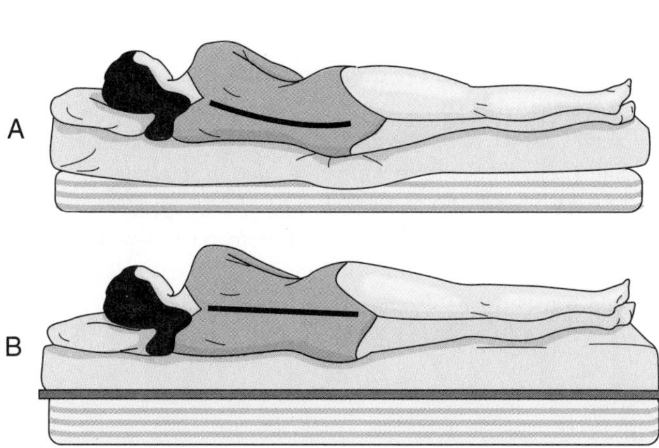

FIGURE 23-3 Bed-boards. **A,** Mattress sagging without bed-boards. **B,** Bed-boards are under the mattress. No sagging occurs.

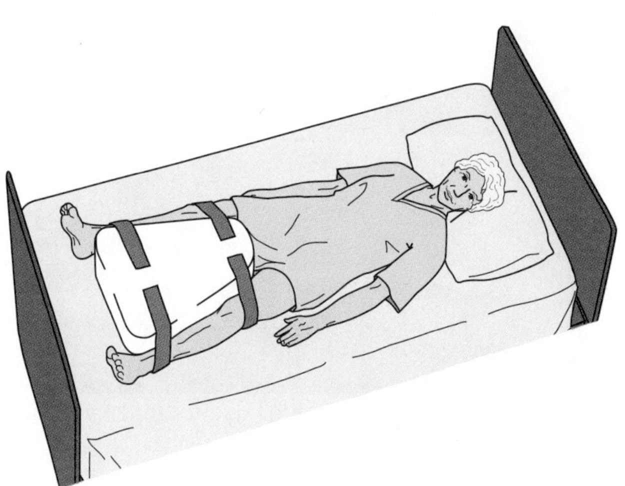

FIGURE 23-6 Hip abduction wedge.

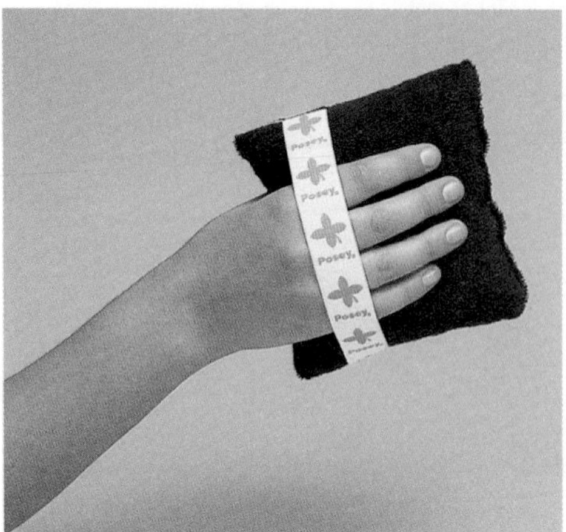

FIGURE 23-7 Hand grip.

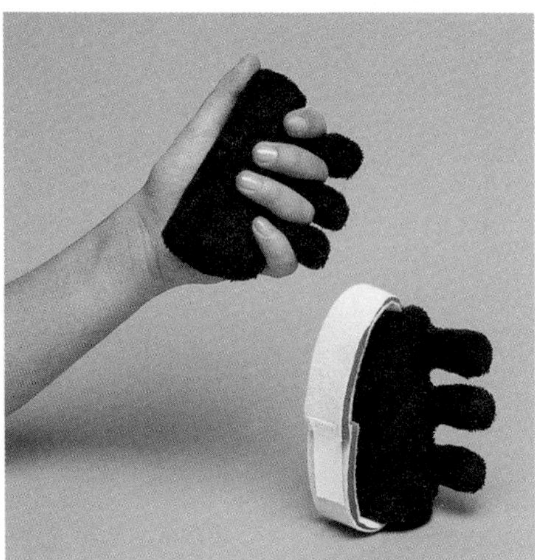

FIGURE 23-8 Finger cushion.

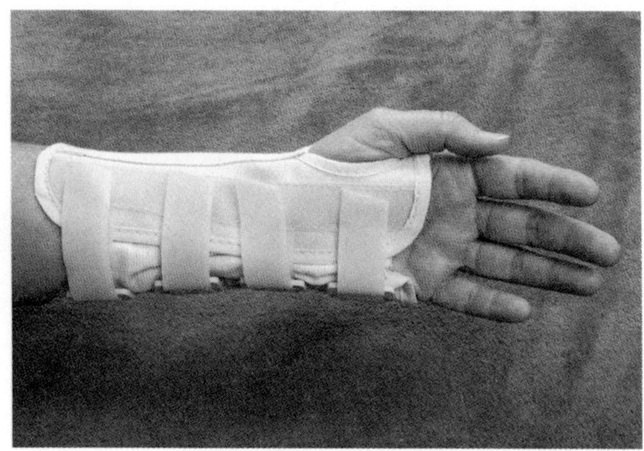

FIGURE 23-9 A splint.

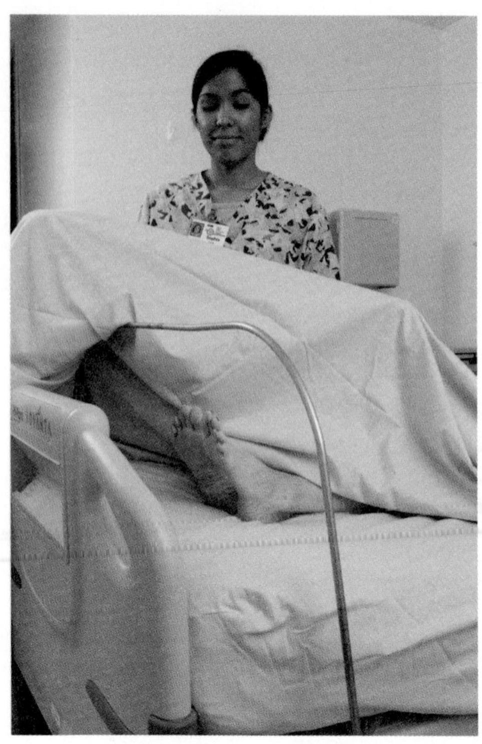

FIGURE 23-10 A bed cradle.

Exercise

Exercise helps prevent contractures, muscle atrophy, and other complications from bedrest. Some exercise occurs with ADL and when turning and moving in bed without help. Other exercises are needed for muscles and joints. (See "Range-of-Motion Exercises.")

RANGE-OF-MOTION EXERCISES

*The movement of a joint to the extent possible without causing pain is the **range of motion (ROM)*** of the joint. Range-of-motion exercises involve moving the joints through their complete range of motion (Box 23-1). They are usually done at least 2 times a day.

- *Active* ROM exercises—are done by the person.
- *Passive* ROM exercises—you move the joints through their range of motion.
- *Active-assistive* ROM exercises—the person does the exercises with some help.

See *Focus on Communication: Range-of-Motion Exercises*.

See *Focus on Surveys: Range-of-Motion Exercises*.

See *Delegation Guidelines: Range-of-Motion Exercises*.

See *Promoting Safety and Comfort: Range-of-Motion Exercises*.

See procedure: *Performing Range-of-Motion Exercises*, p. 372.

Text continued on p. 375

BOX 23-1 Range-of-Motion Exercises

Joint Movements

- ***Abduction***—*moving a body part away from the mid-line of the body*
- ***Adduction***—*moving a body part toward the mid-line of the body*
- ***Opposition***—*Touching an opposite finger with the thumb*
- ***Flexion***—*bending a body part*
- ***Extension***—*straightening a body part*
- ***Hyperextension***—*excessive straightening of a body part*
- ***Dorsiflexion***—*bending the toes and foot up at the ankle*
- ***Plantar flexion***—*bending the foot down at the ankle*
- ***Rotation***—*turning the joint*
- ***Internal rotation***—*turning the joint inward*
- ***External rotation***—*turning the joint outward*
- ***Pronation***—*turning the joint downward*
- ***Supination***—*turning the joint upward*

Safety Measures

- Cover the person with a bath blanket for warmth and privacy.
- Exercise only the joints the nurse tells you to exercise.
- Expose only the body parts being exercised.
- Use good body mechanics.
- Support the part being exercised.
- Move the joint slowly, smoothly, and gently.
- Do not force a joint beyond its present range of motion.
- Do not force a joint to the point of pain.
- Ask the person if he or she has pain or discomfort.

FOCUS ON COMMUNICATION

Range-of-Motion Exercises

Do not force a joint beyond its present range of motion or to the point of pain. Ask the person to tell you if he or she:

- Feels that the joint cannot move any farther.
- Feels pain or discomfort in the joint.
- Needs to stop or rest.

The person may not be able to tell you about discomfort or limited joint movement. Observe for signs of pain (Chapter 21). Restlessness and grimacing are examples. Stop if you suspect pain or meet resistance. Tell the nurse.

FOCUS ON SURVEYS

Range-of-Motion Exercises

The person's care plan must focus on his or her ROM. The goal may be 1 of the following.

- Increase range of motion.
- Prevent loss or further decreases in range of motion.

During a survey, surveyors may observe you performing ROM activities.

DELEGATION GUIDELINES

Range-of-Motion Exercises

When delegated ROM exercises, you need this information from the nurse and the care plan.

- The ROM exercises ordered—active, passive, active-assistive
- Which joints to exercise
- How often the exercises are done
- How many times to repeat each exercise
- What observations to report and record:
  - The time the exercises were performed
  - The joints exercised
  - The number of times the exercises were performed on each joint
  - Complaints of pain or signs of stiffness or spasm
  - The degree to which the person took part in the exercises
- When to report observations
- What patient or resident concerns to report at once

PROMOTING SAFETY AND COMFORT

Range-of-Motion Exercises

Safety

ROM exercises can cause injury if not done properly. Muscle strain, joint injury, and pain are possible. Practice the measures in Box 23-1. Remind the person to tell you if he or she has pain during the procedure.

ROM exercises to the neck can cause serious injury if not done properly. Some agencies provide nursing assistants with special training before doing such exercises. Other agencies do not let nursing assistants do them. Know your agency's policy. *Perform ROM exercises to the neck only if allowed by your agency and if the nurse instructs you to do so.* In some agencies, only physical therapists do neck exercises.

Comfort

To promote physical comfort during ROM exercises, see Box 23-1. Provide privacy to promote mental comfort.

Performing Range-of-Motion Exercises

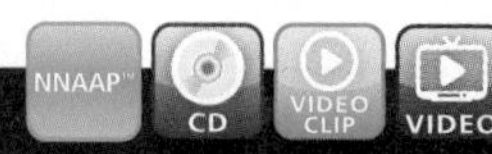

QUALITY OF LIFE

- Knock before entering the person's room.
- Address the person by name.
- Introduce yourself by name and title.
- Explain the procedure before starting and during the procedure.
- Protect the person's rights during the procedure.
- Handle the person gently during the procedure.

PRE-PROCEDURE

1 Follow *Delegation Guidelines: Range-of-Motion Exercises,* p. 371. See *Promoting Safety and Comfort: Range-of-Motion Exercises,* p. 371.
2 Practice hand hygiene.
3 Identify the person. Check the ID (identification) bracelet against the assignment sheet. Also call the person by name.
4 Obtain a bath blanket.
5 Provide for privacy.
6 Raise the bed for body mechanics. Bed rails are up if used.

PROCEDURE

7 Lower the bed rail near you if up.
8 Position the person supine.
9 Cover the person with the bath blanket. Fan-fold top linens to the foot of the bed.
10 Exercise the neck *if allowed by your agency and if the nurse instructs you to do so* (Fig. 23-11).
  a Place your hands over the person's ears to support the head. Support the jaw with your fingers.
  b Flexion—bring the head forward. The chin touches the chest.
  c Extension—straighten the head.
  d Hyperextension—bring the head backward until the chin points up.
  e Rotation—turn the head from side to side.
  f Lateral flexion—move the head to the right and to the left.
  g Repeat flexion, extension, hyperextension, rotation, and lateral flexion 5 times—or the number of times stated on the care plan.
11 Exercise the shoulder (Fig. 23-12).
  a Grasp the wrist with 1 hand. Grasp the elbow with the other hand.
  b Flexion—raise the arm straight in front and over the head.
  c Extension—bring the arm down to the side.
  d Hyperextension—move the arm behind the body. (Do this if the person sits in a straight-backed chair or is standing.)
  e Abduction—move the straight arm away from the side of the body.
  f Adduction—move the straight arm to the side of the body.
  g Internal rotation—bend the elbow. Place it at the same level as the shoulder. Move the forearm down toward the body.
  h External rotation—move the forearm toward the head.
  i Repeat flexion, extension, hyperextension, abduction, adduction, and internal and external rotation 5 times—or the number of times stated on the care plan.
12 Exercise the elbow (Fig. 23-13).
  a Grasp the person's wrist with 1 hand. Grasp the elbow with your other hand.
  b Flexion—bend the arm so the same-side shoulder is touched.
  c Extension—straighten the arm.
  d Repeat flexion and extension 5 times—or the number of times stated on the care plan.
13 Exercise the forearm (Fig. 23-14, p. 374).
  a Continue to support the wrist and elbow.
  b Pronation—turn the hand so the palm is down.
  c Supination—turn the hand so the palm is up.
  d Repeat pronation and supination 5 times—or the number of times stated on the care plan.
14 Exercise the wrist (Fig. 23-15, p. 374).
  a Hold the wrist with both of your hands.
  b Flexion—bend the hand down.
  c Extension—straighten the hand.
  d Hyperextension—bend the hand back.
  e Radial flexion—turn the hand toward the thumb.
  f Ulnar flexion—turn the hand toward the little finger.
  g Repeat flexion, extension, hyperextension, radial flexion, and ulnar flexion 5 times—or the number of times stated on the care plan.
15 Exercise the thumb (Fig. 23-16, p. 374).
  a Hold the person's hand with 1 hand. Hold the thumb with your other hand.
  b Abduction—move the thumb out from the inner part of the index finger.
  c Adduction—move the thumb back next to the index finger.
  d Opposition—touch each fingertip with the thumb.
  e Flexion—bend the thumb into the hand.
  f Extension—move the thumb out to the side of the fingers.
  g Repeat abduction, adduction, opposition, flexion, and extension 5 times—or the number of times stated on the care plan.
16 Exercise the fingers (Fig. 23-17, p. 374).
  a Abduction—spread the fingers and thumb apart.
  b Adduction—bring the fingers and thumb together.
  c Flexion—make a fist.
  d Extension—straighten the fingers so the fingers, hand, and arm are straight.
  e Repeat abduction, adduction, flexion, and extension 5 times—or the number of times stated on the care plan.

Performing Range-of-Motion Exercises—cont'd

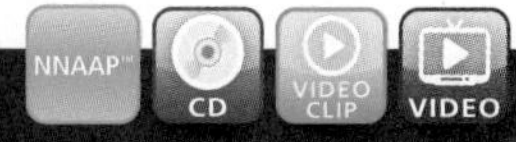

PROCEDURE—cont'd

17 Exercise the hip (Fig. 23-18, p. 374).
  a Support the leg. Place 1 hand under the knee. Place your other hand under the ankle.
  b Flexion—raise the leg.
  c Extension—straighten the leg.
  d Hyperextension—move the leg behind the body. (Do this if the person is standing.)
  e Abduction—move the leg away from the body.
  f Adduction—move the leg toward the other leg.
  g Internal rotation—turn the leg inward.
  h External rotation—turn the leg outward.
  i Repeat flexion, extension, hyperextension, abduction, adduction, and internal and external rotation 5 times—or the number of times stated on the care plan.

18 Exercise the knee (Fig. 23-19, p. 374).
  a Support the knee. Place 1 hand under the knee. Place your other hand under the ankle.
  b Flexion—bend the knee.
  c Extension—straighten the knee.
  d Repeat flexion and extension 5 times—or the number of times stated on the care plan.

19 Exercise the ankle (Fig. 23-20, p. 375).
  a Support the foot and ankle. Place 1 hand under the foot. Place your other hand under the ankle.
  b Dorsiflexion—pull the foot upward. Push down on the heel at the same time.
  c Plantar flexion—turn the foot down. Or point the toes.
  d Repeat dorsiflexion and plantar flexion 5 times—or the number of times stated on the care plan.

20 Exercise the foot (Fig. 23-21, p. 375).
  a Continue to support the foot and ankle.
  b Pronation—turn the outside of the foot up and the inside down.
  c Supination—turn the inside of the foot up and the outside down.
  d Repeat pronation and supination 5 times—or the number of times stated on the care plan.

21 Exercise the toes (Fig. 23-22, p. 375).
  a Flexion—curl the toes.
  b Extension—straighten the toes.
  c Abduction—spread the toes.
  d Adduction—put the toes together.
  e Repeat flexion, extension, abduction, and adduction 5 times—or the number of times stated on the care plan.

22 Cover the leg. Raise the bed rail if used.

23 Go to the other side. Lower the bed rail near you if up.

24 Repeat steps 11 through 21.

POST-PROCEDURE

25 Provide for comfort. (See the inside of the front cover.)

26 Remove the bath blanket.

27 Place the call light within reach.

28 Lower the bed to a comfortable and safe level for the person. Follow the care plan.

29 Raise or lower bed rails. Follow the care plan.

30 Fold and return the bath blanket to its proper place.

31 Unscreen the person.

32 Complete a safety check of the room. (See the inside of the front cover.)

33 Practice hand hygiene.

34 Report and record your observations.

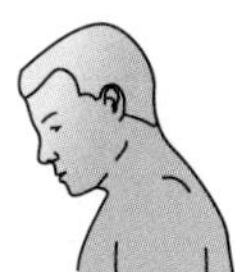

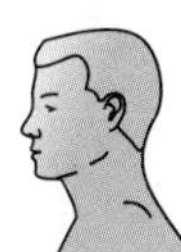

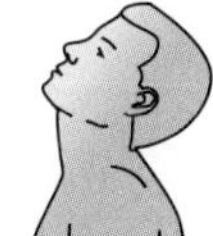

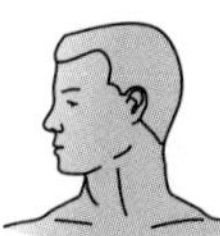

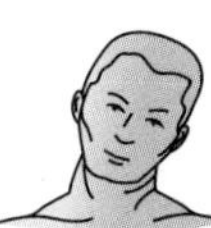

FIGURE 23-11 Range-of-motion exercises for the neck.

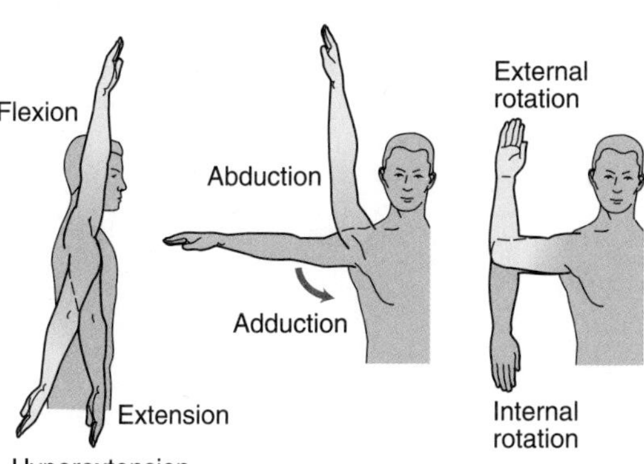

FIGURE 23-12 Range-of-motion exercises for the shoulder.

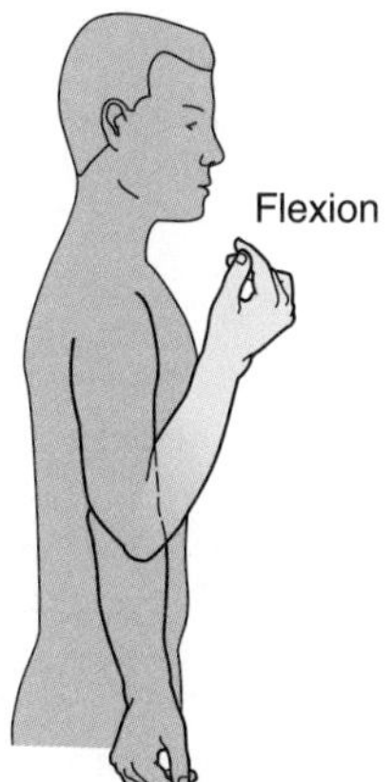

FIGURE 23-13 Range-of-motion exercises for the elbow.

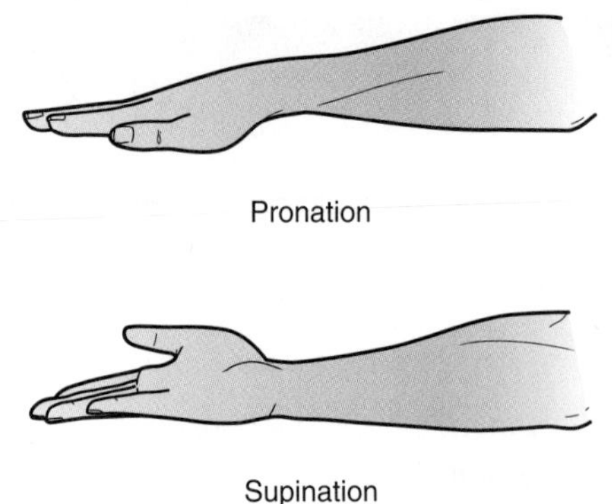

FIGURE 23-14 Range-of-motion exercises for the forearm.

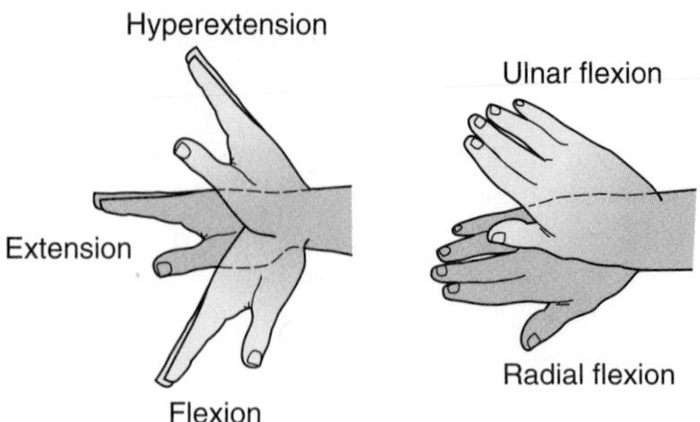

FIGURE 23-15 Range-of-motion exercises for the wrist.

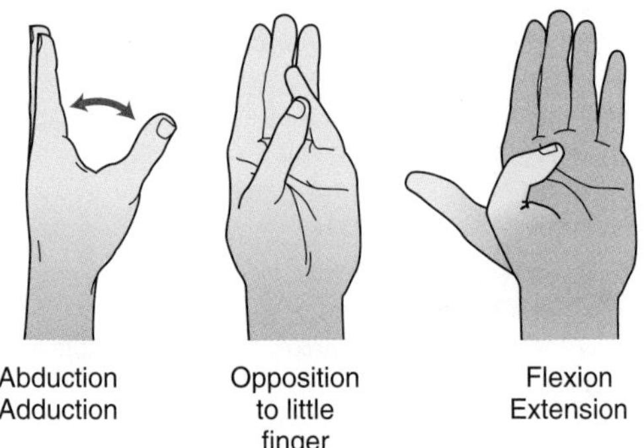

FIGURE 23-16 Range-of-motion exercises for the thumb.

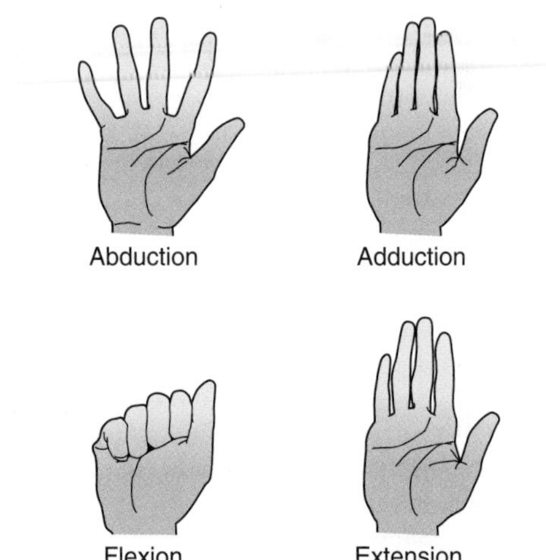

FIGURE 23-17 Range-of-motion exercises for the fingers.

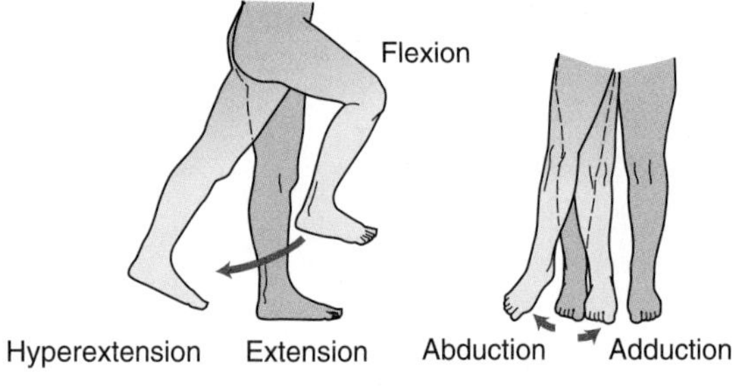

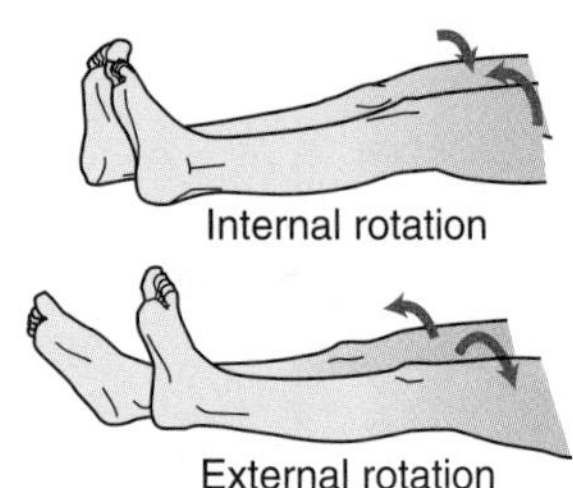

FIGURE 23-18 Range-of-motion exercises for the hip.

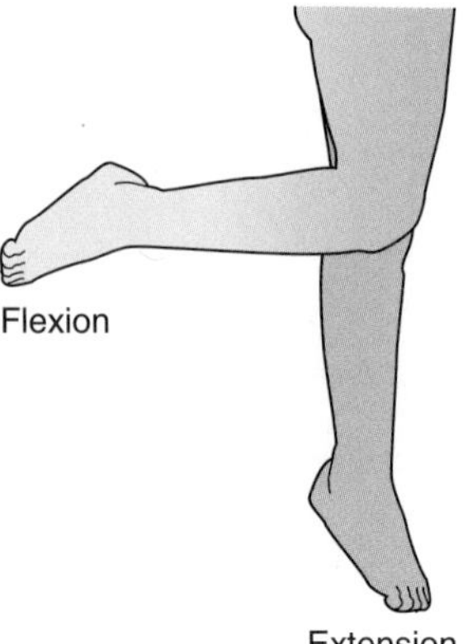

FIGURE 23-19 Range-of-motion exercises for the knee.

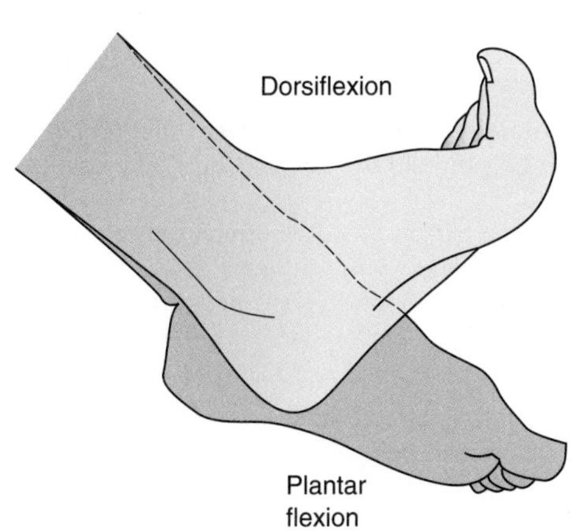

FIGURE 23-20 Range-of-motion exercises for the ankle.

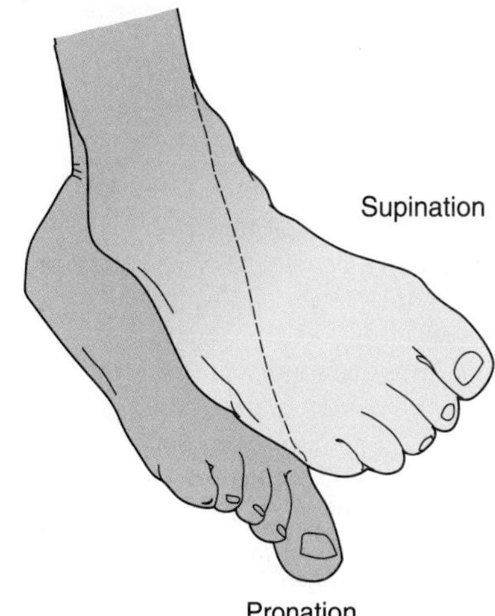

FIGURE 23-21 Range-of-motion exercises for the foot.

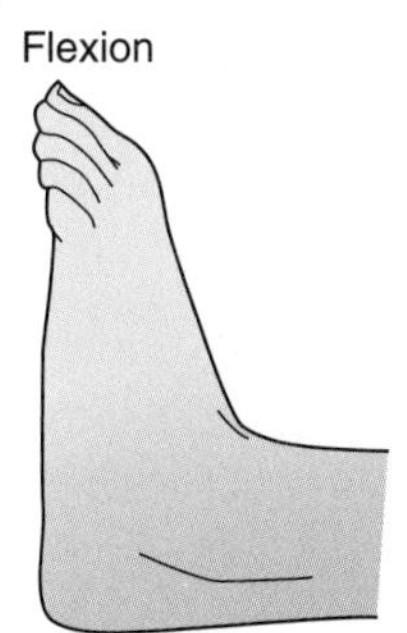

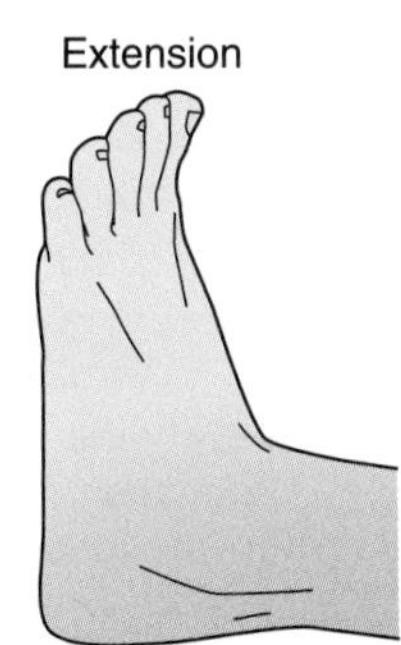

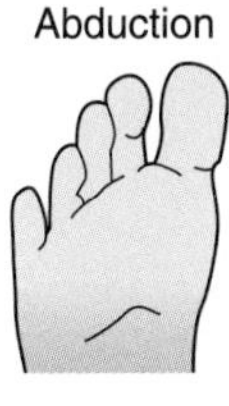

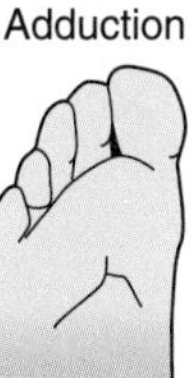

FIGURE 23-22 Range-of-motion exercises for the toes.

AMBULATION

Ambulation is the act of walking. Some people are weak and unsteady from bedrest, illness, surgery, or injury. They need help walking.

After bedrest, activity increases slowly and in steps. First the person sits on the side of the bed (dangles). Sitting in a bedside chair follows. Next the person walks in the room and then in the hallway.

Follow the care plan when helping a person walk. Use a gait (transfer) belt if the person is weak or unsteady. The person also uses hand rails along the wall. Always check for orthostatic hypotension (p. 368).

See *Focus on Communication: Ambulation.*

See *Delegation Guidelines: Ambulation*, p. 376.

See *Promoting Safety and Comfort: Ambulation*, p. 376

See procedure: *Helping the Person Walk*, p. 376.

FOCUS ON COMMUNICATION

Ambulation

Before ambulating, explain the activity. This promotes comfort and reduces fear. Explain:

- How far to walk
- What assistive devices are used
- How you will assist
- What the person should report to you
- How you will help if the person begins to fall

For example, you can say:

Mr. Owens, I am going to help you walk from your bed to the doorway and back. This belt helps support you while you walk. I will always be at your side and hold the belt. Tell me right away if you feel unsteady, dizzy, weak, or faint. Also tell me if you feel pain or discomfort. If you begin to fall, I will use the belt to pull you close to me and gently lower you to the floor. Do you have any questions?

DELEGATION GUIDELINES

Ambulation

Before helping with ambulation, you need this information from the nurse and the care plan.

- How much help the person needs
- If the person uses a cane, walker, crutches, or a brace
- Areas of weakness—right arm or leg, left arm or leg
- How far to walk
- What observations to report and record:
  - How well the person tolerated the activity
  - Shuffling, sliding, limping, or walking on tip-toes
  - Complaints of pain or discomfort
  - Complaints of orthostatic hypotension—weakness, dizziness, spots before the eyes, feeling faint
  - The distance walked
- When to report observations
- What patient or resident concerns to report at once

PROMOTING SAFETY AND COMFORT

Ambulation

Safety

Practice the safety measures to prevent falls (Chapter 10). Use a gait belt to help the person stand. Also use it during ambulation.

Remind the person to walk normally. Encourage the person to stand erect with the head up and the back straight. Discourage shuffling, sliding, and walking on tip-toes.

Comfort

The fear of falling affects mental comfort. Explain the purpose of the gait belt. Also explain how you will help the person if he or she starts to fall (Chapter 10).

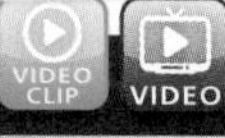

Helping the Person Walk

QUALITY OF LIFE

- Knock before entering the person's room.
- Address the person by name.
- Introduce yourself by name and title.
- Explain the procedure before starting and during the procedure.
- Protect the person's rights during the procedure.
- Handle the person gently during the procedure.

PRE-PROCEDURE

1 Follow *Delegation Guidelines: Ambulation*. See *Promoting Safety and Comfort: Ambulation*.
2 Practice hand hygiene.
3 Collect the following.
- Robe and non-skid footwear
- Paper or towel to protect bottom linens
- Gait (transfer) belt

4 Identify the person. Check the ID bracelet against the assignment sheet. Also call the person by name.
5 Provide for privacy.

PROCEDURE

6 Lower the bed to a safe and comfortable level for the person. Follow the care plan. Lock the bed wheels. Lower the bed rail if up.
7 Fan-fold top linens to the foot of the bed.
8 Place the paper or towel under the person's feet. Put the shoes on the person. Fasten the shoes.
9 Help the person sit on the side of the bed. (See procedure: *Sitting on the Side of the Bed [Dangling]*, Chapter 14.)
10 Make sure the person's feet are flat on the floor.
11 Help the person put on the robe.
12 Apply the gait belt at the waist over clothing. (See procedure: *Applying a Transfer/Gait Belt*, Chapter 10.)
13 Help the person stand. (See procedure: *Transferring the Person to a Chair or Wheelchair*, Chapter 14.) Grasp the gait belt at each side. If no gait belt, place your arms under the person's arms around to the shoulder blades.
14 Stand at the person's weak side while he or she gains balance. Hold the belt at the side and back. If not using a gait belt, have 1 arm around the back and the other at the elbow to support the person.
15 Encourage the person to stand erect with the head up and the back straight.
16 Help the person walk. Walk to the side and slightly behind the person on the person's weak side. Provide support with the gait belt (Fig. 23-23). If not using a gait belt, have 1 arm around the back and the other at the elbow to support the person. Encourage the person to use the hand rail on his or her strong side.
17 Encourage the person to walk normally. The heel strikes the floor first. Discourage shuffling, sliding, or walking on tip-toes.
18 Walk the required distance if the person tolerates the activity. Do not rush the person.
19 Help the person return to bed. Remove the gait belt. (See procedure: *Transferring the Person From a Chair or Wheelchair to Bed*, Chapter 14.)
20 Lower the head of the bed. Help the person to the center of the bed.
21 Remove the shoes. Remove the paper or towel over the bottom sheet.

POST-PROCEDURE

22 Provide for comfort. (See the inside of the front cover.)
23 Place the call light within reach.
24 Raise or lower bed rails. Follow the care plan.
25 Return the robe and shoes to their proper place.
26 Unscreen the person.
27 Complete a safety check of the room. (See the inside of the front cover.)
28 Practice hand hygiene.
29 Report and record your observations.

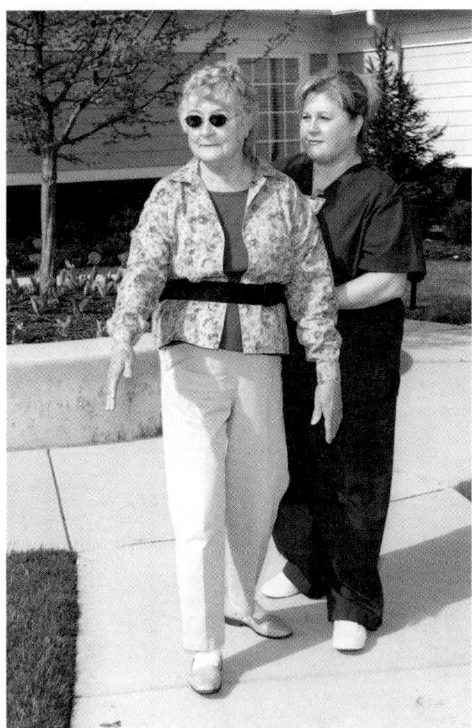

FIGURE 23-23 Assisting with ambulation. The nursing assistant walks at the person's side and slightly behind her. A gait belt is used for safety.

Walking Aids

Walking aids support the body. The type ordered depends on the person's condition, the support needed, and the disability. The physical therapist measures and teaches the person to use the device.

Crutches. Crutches are used when the person cannot use 1 leg or when 1 or both legs need to gain strength. Some persons with permanent leg weakness can use crutches. Falls are a risk. Follow these safety measures.

- Check the crutch tips. They must not be worn down, torn, or wet. Replace worn or torn crutch tips. Dry wet tips with paper towels.
- Check crutches for flaws. Check wooden crutches for cracks and metal crutches for bends.
- Tighten all bolts.
- Have the person wear street shoes. They must be flat and have non-skid soles.
- Make sure clothes fit well. Loose clothes may get caught between the crutches and underarms. Loose clothes and long skirts can hang forward and block the person's view of the feet and crutch tips.
- Practice safety rules to prevent falls (Chapter 10).
- Keep crutches within the person's reach. Put them by the person's chair or against a wall.

Walkers. Walkers give more support than canes (p. 378). Wheeled walkers are common (Fig. 23-24). They have wheels on the front legs and rubber tips on the back legs. The person pushes the walker about 6 to 8 inches in front of his or her feet. Rubber tips on the back legs prevent the walker from moving while the person is standing. Some have a braking action when weight is applied to the walker's back legs.

Baskets, pouches, and trays attach to the walker. They are used for needed items. This allows more independence. They also free the hands to grip the walker.

See *Promoting Safety and Comfort: Walkers.*

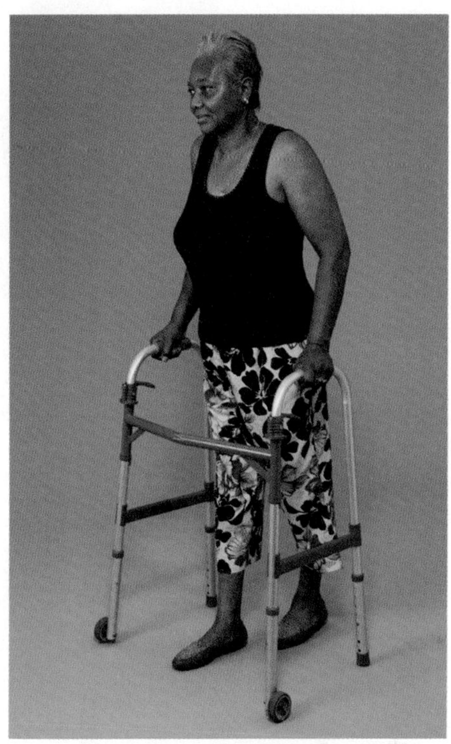

FIGURE 23-24 Wheeled walker.

PROMOTING SAFETY AND COMFORT

Walkers

Safety

Walker wheels are usually on the outside of the walker (see Fig. 23-24). With the wheels on the outside, the walker may be too wide for some doorways. The wheels can be moved to the inside of the walker. This reduces the width of the walker. It is easier for the person to go through some doorways.

Some walkers have seats. The person sits when a rest is needed. Never push the walker when the person is seated. Use a wheelchair instead.

Canes. Canes are used for weakness on 1 side of the body. They help provide balance and support (Fig. 23-25).

A cane is held on the *strong side* of the body. (If the left leg is weak, the cane is held in the right hand.) The cane tip is about 6 to 10 inches to the side of the foot. It is about 6 to 10 inches in front of the foot on the strong side. The grip is level with the hip. The person walks as follows.

- *Step A:* The cane is moved forward 6 to 10 inches (Fig. 23-26, *A*).
- *Step B:* The weak leg (opposite the cane) is moved forward even with the cane (Fig. 23-26, *B*).
- *Step C:* The strong leg is moved forward and ahead of the cane and the weak leg (Fig. 23-26, *C*).

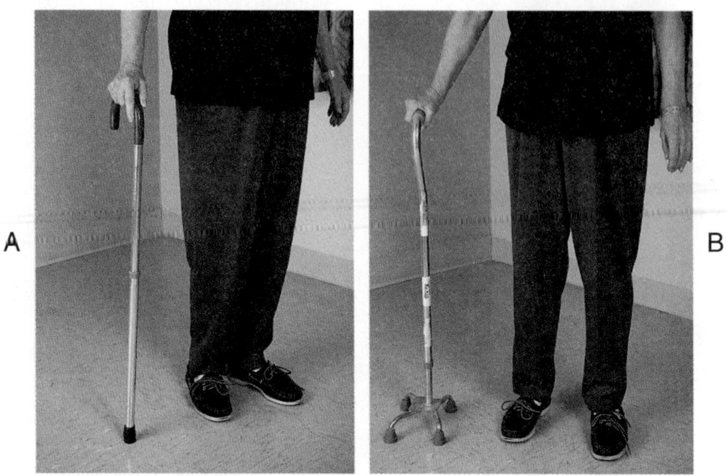

FIGURE 23-25 A, Single-tip cane. **B,** Four-point cane.

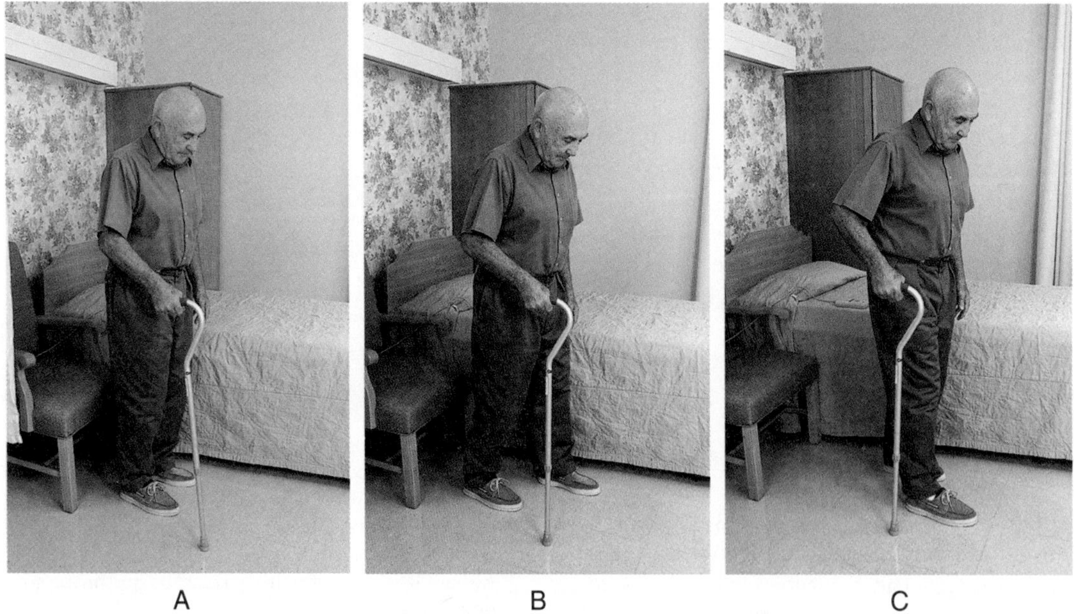

FIGURE 23-26 Walking with a cane. **A,** The cane is moved forward about 6 to 10 inches. **B,** The leg opposite the cane (weak leg) is brought forward even with the cane. **C,** The leg on the cane side (strong side) is moved ahead of the cane and the weak leg.

Braces. Braces support weak body parts. They also prevent or correct deformities or prevent joint movement. Metal, plastic, or leather is used for braces. A brace is applied over the ankle, knee, or back (Fig. 23-27).

Keep skin and bony points under braces clean and dry. This prevents skin breakdown. Report redness or signs of skin breakdown at once. Also report complaints of pain or discomfort. The nurse assesses the skin under braces every shift. The care plan tells you when to apply and remove a brace.

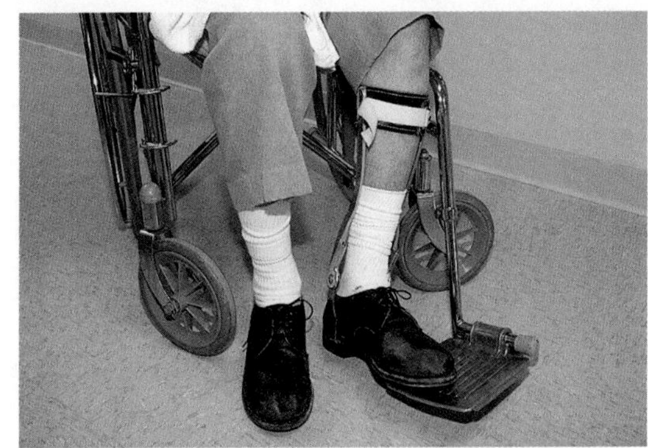

FIGURE 23-27 Leg brace.

FOCUS ON PRIDE

The Person, Family, and Yourself

Personal and Professional Responsibility

Exercise and activity have positive long-term effects. Every person has a responsibility to stay active. Disease, injury, pain, and aging affect activity levels. Even with such limits, you can promote activity, exercise, and well-being. You can:

- Encourage the person to be as active as possible.
- Resist the urge to do things that the person can safely do alone or with some help.
- Focus on the person's abilities.
- Tell the person when he or she is doing well or making progress.
- Tell the person you are proud of what he or she did or tried to do.

Rights and Respect

Make sure garments provide privacy during exercise and activity. When ambulating, the person must not walk in the room or hallway with a gown open in the back. During range-of-motion exercises, cover the person with a bath blanket. Expose only the body part being exercised. Protect the right to privacy. Privacy promotes dignity and mental comfort.

Independence and Social Interaction

Nursing center activity programs promote physical and mental well-being. Joints and muscles are exercised. Circulation is stimulated. Social interaction is mentally stimulating.

Activities must meet the person's interests and physical, mental, and social needs. Bingo, dances, exercise groups, shopping trips, concerts, and guest speakers are common. Some centers have gardening activities. Residents may share ideas with you or talk about favorite pastimes. Share these and your ideas with the health team. They are given to the resident group that plans activities.

Encourage involvement in activities. Listen to the person's interests. Suggest options that the person may like. Allow personal choice. Independence and well-being are promoted when the person chooses activities. Do not force the person to take part in activities that do not interest him or her.

Delegation and Teamwork

You must know the person's activity limits. The person's care plan and your assignment sheet tell you the activities allowed. Ask the nurse what bedrest means for each person. Ask the nurse if you have questions about a person's activity limits. Take pride in providing safe care by knowing and following the person's activity level.

Ethics and Laws

Persons with contractures must be moved slowly and carefully. Pain and injury occur if the person is moved carelessly. You can lose your ability to work as a nursing assistant for handling persons in ways that cause harm. Always work carefully. Move patients and residents in a way that shows you care for their comfort, safety, and well-being.

REVIEW QUESTIONS

Circle T if the statement is TRUE or F if it is FALSE.

1 **T F** You must know the person's activity level.

2 **T F** A hip abduction wedge keeps the legs together.

3 **T F** A person is dizzy when walking. Help the person to sit.

4 **T F** A walker and a cane give the same support.

5 **T F** When using a cane, the feet move first.

6 **T F** When using a wheeled walker, the walker is pushed in front of the person's feet.

7 **T F** A person has a brace. Bony areas need protection from skin breakdown.

Circle the BEST answer.

8 The purpose of bedrest is to
  a Prevent orthostatic hypotension
  b Reduce pain and promote healing
  c Prevent pressure ulcers, constipation, and blood clots
  d Cause contractures and muscle atrophy

9 Which helps prevent plantar flexion?
  a Bed-boards
  b A foot-board
  c A trochanter roll
  d Hand rolls

10 Which prevents the hip from turning outward?
  a A cane
  b A foot-board
  c A trochanter roll
  d A leg brace

11 A contracture is
  a The loss of muscle strength from inactivity
  b A blood clot in the muscle
  c A decrease in the size of a muscle
  d The lack of joint mobility from shortening of a muscle

12 Active ROM exercises are performed by
  a The physical therapist
  b The person
  c You
  d The person with the help of another

13 When performing ROM exercises, which may cause injury?
  a Supporting the part being exercised
  b Moving the joint slowly, smoothly, and gently
  c Forcing the joint through its full range of motion
  d Exercising only the joints indicated by the nurse

14 Flexion involves
  a Bending the body part
  b Straightening the body part
  c Moving the body part toward the body
  d Moving the body part away from the body

15 Turning the joint downward is called
  a Dorsiflexion
  b Rotation
  c Supination
  d Pronation

16 When ambulating a person
  a The person can shuffle or slide when walking after bedrest
  b A gait belt is used if the person is weak or unsteady
  c Encourage the person to walk quickly
  d You walk on the person's strong side

17 A person uses crutches. Which is a safety problem?
  a Crutch tips are wet.
  b The person is wearing non-skid shoes.
  c Crutches are kept within the person's reach.
  d Crutch bolts are tight.

18 A cane is held
  a At waist level
  b On the strong side
  c On the weak side
  d On either side

Answers to these questions are on p. 505.

FOCUS ON PRACTICE

Problem Solving

You are ambulating a resident in the hallway with a walker and gait belt. The resident says: "I feel dizzy." There is not a chair nearby. You see a wheelchair at the nurses' station at the end of the hallway. What will you do? How might you use planning and teamwork to avoid this problem in the future?

Assisting With Wound Care

CHAPTER 24

OBJECTIVES

- Define the key terms and key abbreviations listed in this chapter.
- Describe skin tears, circulatory ulcers, and diabetic foot ulcers.
- Explain how to assist in preventing skin tears, circulatory ulcers, and diabetic foot ulcers.
- Describe what to observe about wounds.
- Explain how to secure dressings.
- Explain the rules for applying dressings.
- Explain the purpose, effects, and complications of heat and cold applications.
- Describe the rules for applying heat and cold.
- Perform the procedures described in this chapter.
- Explain how to promote PRIDE in the person, the family, and yourself.

KEY TERMS

constrict To narrow
dilate To expand or open wider
skin tear A break or rip in the outer layers of the skin; the epidermis (top skin layer) separates from the underlying tissues
ulcer A shallow or deep crater-like sore of the skin or mucous membrane
wound A break in the skin or mucous membrane

KEY ABBREVIATIONS

C	Centigrade
F	Fahrenheit
ID	Identification
PPE	Personal protective equipment

A *wound is a break in the skin or mucous membrane.* Common causes are:

- Surgery
- *Trauma*—an accident or violent act that injures the skin, mucous membranes, bones, and organs
- Unrelieved pressure or friction (Chapter 25)
- Decreased blood flow through arteries or veins
- Nerve damage

The wound is a portal of entry for microbes. Infection is a major threat. Wound care includes preventing infection and further injury to the wound and nearby tissues.

See *Delegation Guidelines: Assisting With Wound Care.*

DELEGATION GUIDELINES

Assisting With Wound Care

Your state and agency may not allow you to perform the procedures in this chapter. Before performing a procedure, make sure that:

- Your state allows you to perform the procedure.
- The procedure is in your job description.
- You have the necessary education and training.
- You review the procedure with a nurse.
- A nurse is available to answer questions and to supervise you.

SKIN TEARS

A ***skin tear*** *is a break or rip in the outer layers of the skin* (Fig. 24-1). *The epidermis (top skin layer) separates from the underlying tissues.* The hands, arms, and lower legs are common sites for skin tears. Causes include:

- Friction, shearing (Chapter 13), pulling, or pressure on the skin.
- Falls or bumping a hard surface. Beds, bed rails, chairs, wheelchair footplates, and tables are dangers.
- Holding an arm or leg too tight.
- Removing tape or adhesives.
- Bathing, dressing, and other tasks.
- Pulling buttons and zippers across fragile skin.
- Jewelry—yours or the person's. Rings, watches, and bracelets are examples.
- Long or jagged fingernails (yours or the person's) and long or jagged toenails.

Skin tears are painful. They are portals of entry for microbes. Infection is a risk. Tell the nurse at once if you cause or find a skin tear. To prevent skin tears, follow the care plan and the measures in Box 24-1.

See *Focus on Older Persons: Skin Tears.*

BOX 24-1 Preventing Skin Tears

- Follow the care plan and safety rules to:
  - Move, turn, position, or transfer the person.
    - Prevent shearing and friction.
    - Use an assist device to move and turn the person in bed.
    - Use pillows to support arms and legs.
  - Pad bed rails and wheelchair arms, footplates, and leg supports.
  - Bathe the person.
  - Keep the skin moisturized and apply lotion.
  - Offer fluids.
- Keep your fingernails short and smoothly filed.
- Keep the person's fingernails short and smoothly filed. Report long, tough, or jagged toenails.
- Do not wear rings with large or raised stones. Do not wear bracelets.
- Be patient and calm when the person is confused, is agitated, or resists care.
- Dress and undress the person carefully.
- Dress the person in soft clothes with long sleeves and long pants.
- Provide good lighting so the person can see. The person needs to avoid bumping into furniture, walls, and equipment.
- Provide a safe area for wandering (Chapter 30).
- Remove tape carefully (p. 388).
- Do not apply adhesive tape (p. 388).

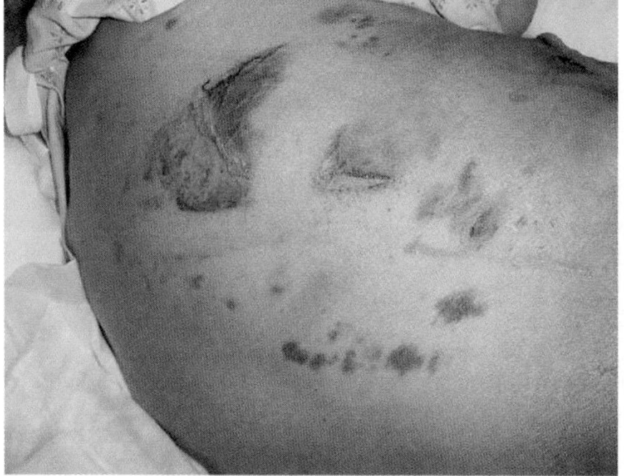

FIGURE 24-1 Skin tear.

FOCUS ON OLDER PERSONS

Skin Tears

Older persons are at risk for skin tears because of thin and fragile skin. Some persons are confused and may resist care. They often move quickly and without warning. Or they pull away during care. Some try to hit or kick. These sudden movements can cause skin tears.

Never force care on a person. Chapter 30 describes how to care for persons who are confused and resist care. Always follow the care plan.

CIRCULATORY ULCERS

An **ulcer** *is a shallow or deep crater-like sore of the skin or mucous membrane. Circulatory ulcers (vascular ulcers)* are open sores on the lower legs or feet. They are caused by decreased blood flow through the arteries or veins. Persons with diseases affecting blood flow to and from the legs and feet are at risk. These wounds are painful and hard to heal. Infection and gangrene can develop. *Gangrene* is a condition in which there is death of tissue.

Circulatory ulcers include:

- *Venous ulcers (stasis ulcers)* are open sores on the lower legs or feet caused by poor venous blood flow (Fig. 24-2). *Stasis* means *stopped or slowed fluid flow.* The heels and inner part of the ankles are common sites. They can occur from skin injury. Scratching and trauma are examples. Venous ulcers are painful. Infection is a risk. Healing is slow.
- *Arterial ulcers* are open wounds on the lower legs or feet caused by poor arterial blood flow. They are found between the toes, on top of the toes, and on the outer side of the ankle (Fig. 24-3).
- *Diabetic foot ulcers* are open wounds on the foot caused by complications from diabetes. Diabetes (Chapter 28) can affect the nerves and blood vessels. When nerves are affected, the person can lose complete or partial sensation in a foot or leg. The person may not feel pain, heat, or cold. When blood vessels are affected, blood flow decreases. Tissues and cells do not get needed oxygen and nutrients. Sores heal poorly. Common foot problems (Fig. 24-4) can cause infection and tissue death (gangrene). Sometimes the affected part must be amputated.

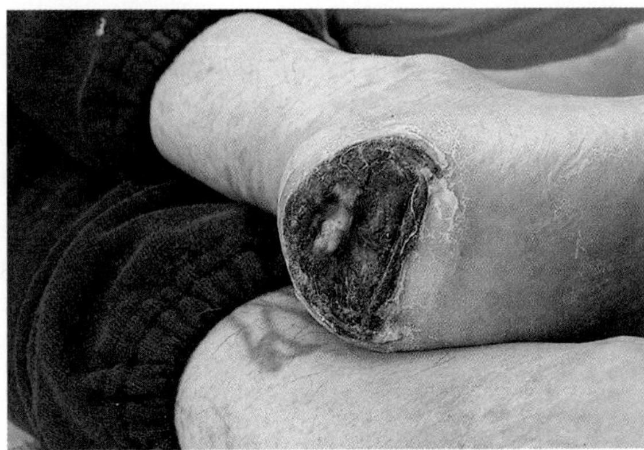

FIGURE 24-2 Venous ulcer.

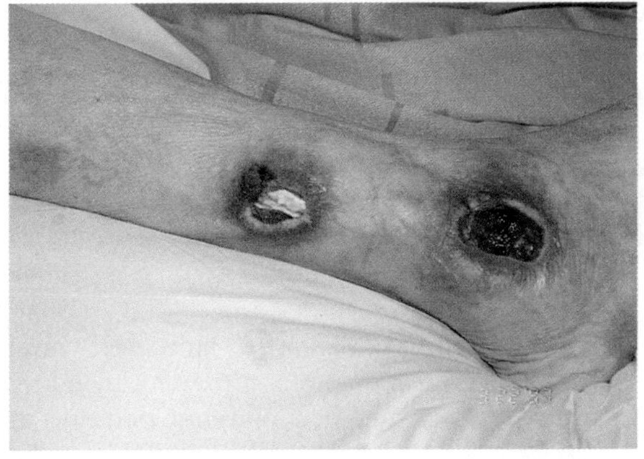

FIGURE 24-3 Arterial ulcer.

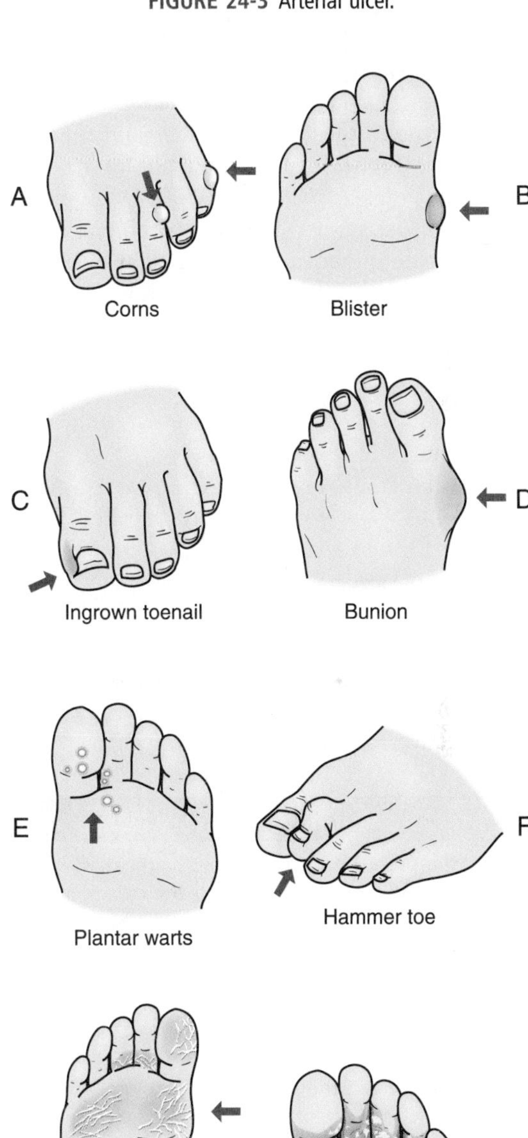

FIGURE 24-4 Foot problems common with diabetes.

Prevention and Treatment

Check the person's feet and legs every day. Report any sign of a foot problem at once. You must help prevent skin breakdown on the legs and feet. Follow the care plan to prevent and treat circulatory ulcers (Box 24-2). The doctor orders drugs and treatments as needed.

Persons at risk need professional foot care. *You do not cut the toenails of persons with diseases affecting circulation.*

Elastic Stockings. Elastic stockings exert pressure on the veins. The pressure promotes venous blood return to the heart. The stockings help prevent blood clots in leg veins *(thrombi)*. A blood clot is called a *thrombus.*

If blood flow is sluggish, blood clots *(thrombi)* may form in the deep veins in the lower leg or thigh (Fig. 24-5, *A*). A blood clot *(thrombus)* can break loose and travel through the bloodstream. It then becomes an *embolus*—a blood clot that travels through the vascular system until it lodges in a blood vessel (Fig. 24-5, *B*). An embolus from a vein lodges in the lungs *(pulmonary embolism)*. A pulmonary embolism can cause severe respiratory problems and death. Report chest pain or shortness of breath at once.

Persons at risk for thrombi include those who:

- Have heart and circulatory disorders.
- Are on bedrest.
- Have had surgery.
- Are older.
- Are pregnant.

Elastic stockings also are called AE stockings (AE means *anti-embolic* or *anti-emboli*). They also are called TED hose (TED means *thrombo-embolic disease*).

The person usually has 2 pairs of stockings. Wash 1 pair while the other pair is worn. Wash them by hand with a mild soap. Hang them to dry.

See *Delegation Guidelines: Elastic Stockings.*

See *Promoting Safety and Comfort: Elastic Stockings.*

See procedure: *Applying Elastic Stockings.*

BOX 24-2 Preventing Circulatory Ulcers

- Remind the person not to sit with the legs crossed.
- Re-position the person according to the care plan—at least every 2 hours.
- Do not use elastic or rubber band–type garters to hold socks or hose in place.
- Do not dress the person in tight clothes.
- Provide good skin care daily. Keep the feet clean and dry. Clean and dry between the toes.
- Do not scrub or rub the skin during bathing and drying.
- Keep linens clean, dry, and wrinkle-free.
- Avoid injury to the legs and feet.
- Make sure shoes fit well.
- Keep pressure off the heels and other bony areas. Use pillows or other devices as directed.
- Check the person's legs and feet. Report skin breaks or changes in skin color.
- Do not massage over pressure points (Chapter 25). *Never rub or massage reddened areas.*
- Use protective devices as directed.
- Follow the care plan for walking and exercises.

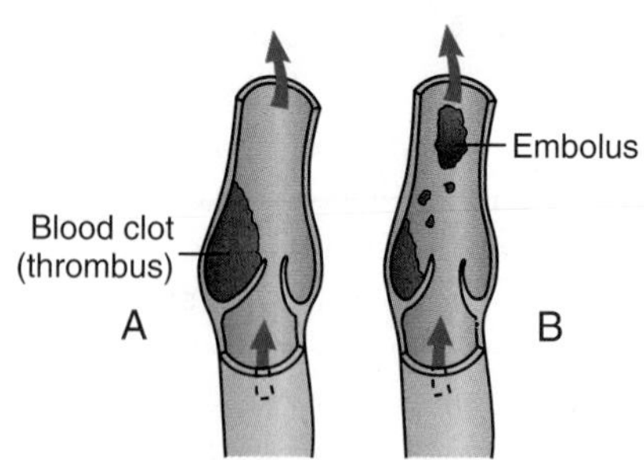

FIGURE 24-5 **A,** A blood clot is attached to the wall of a vein. The *arrow* shows the direction of blood flow. **B,** Part of the thrombus breaks off and becomes an embolus. The embolus travels in the bloodstream until it lodges in a distant vessel.

DELEGATION GUIDELINES
Elastic Stockings

To apply elastic stockings, you need this information from the nurse and the care plan.

- What size to use—small, medium, large, or extra-large
- What length to use—thigh-high or knee-high
- When to remove them and for how long—usually every 8 hours for 30 minutes
- What observations to report and record:
  - The size and length of stockings applied
  - When you applied the stockings
  - Skin color and temperature
  - Leg and foot swelling
  - Skin tears, wounds, or signs of skin breakdown
  - Complaints of pain, tingling, or numbness
  - When you removed the stockings and for how long
  - When you re-applied the stockings
  - When you washed the stockings
- When to report observations
- What patient or resident concerns to report at once

PROMOTING SAFETY AND COMFORT
Elastic Stockings

Safety

Apply the stocking so the toe opening is over the top of the toes or under the toes. Follow the manufacturer's instructions. Use the opening to check circulation, skin color, and skin temperature in the toes.

Stockings should not have twists, creases, or wrinkles after you apply them. Twists can affect circulation. So can stockings that roll or bunch up. Creases and wrinkles can cause skin breakdown.

Loose stockings do not promote venous blood return to the heart. Stockings that are too tight can affect circulation. Tell the nurse if the stockings are too loose or too tight.

Comfort

Apply stockings before the person gets out of bed. Otherwise the person's legs can swell from sitting or standing. Stockings are hard to put on when the legs are swollen. The person lies in bed while they are off. This prevents the legs from swelling.

Gently handle and move the person's foot and leg. Do not force the joints (toes, foot, ankle, knee, and hip) beyond their range of motion or to the point of pain.

Applying Elastic Stockings

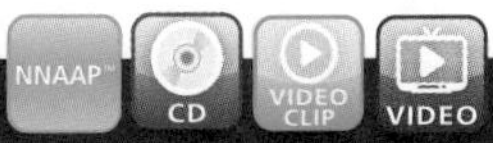

QUALITY OF LIFE

- Knock before entering the person's room.
- Address the person by name.
- Introduce yourself by name and title.
- Explain the procedure before starting and during the procedure.
- Protect the person's rights during the procedure.
- Handle the person gently during the procedure.

PRE-PROCEDURE

1 Follow *Delegation Guidelines:*
  a *Assisting With Wound Care,* p. 381
  b *Elastic Stockings*
  See *Promoting Safety and Comfort: Elastic Stockings.*
2 Practice hand hygiene.
3 Obtain elastic stockings in the correct size and length. Note the location of the toe opening.
4 Identify the person. Check the ID (identification) bracelet against the assignment sheet. Also call the person by name.
5 Provide for privacy.
6 Raise the bed for body mechanics. Bed rails are up if used.

PROCEDURE

7 Lower the bed rail.
8 Position the person supine.
9 Expose the legs. Fan-fold top linens up toward the thighs.
10 Turn the stocking inside out down to the heel.
11 Slip the foot of the stocking over the toes, foot, and heel (Fig. 24-6, *A*). Make sure the heel pocket is properly positioned on the person's heel. The toe opening is over or under the toes.
12 Grasp the stocking top. Pull the stocking up the leg. It turns right side out as it is pulled up. The stocking is even and snug (Fig. 24-6, *B*).
13 Remove twists, creases, or wrinkles.
14 Repeat steps 10 through 13 for the other leg.

POST-PROCEDURE

15 Cover the person.
16 Provide for comfort. (See the inside of the front cover.)
17 Place the call light within reach.
18 Lower the bed to a comfortable and safe level for the person. Follow the care plan.
19 Raise or lower bed rails. Follow the care plan.
20 Unscreen the person.
21 Complete a safety check of the room. (See the inside of the front cover.)
22 Practice hand hygiene.
23 Report and record your observations.

A
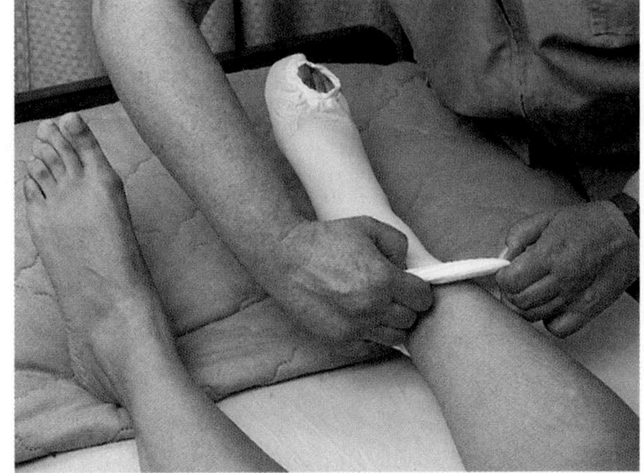

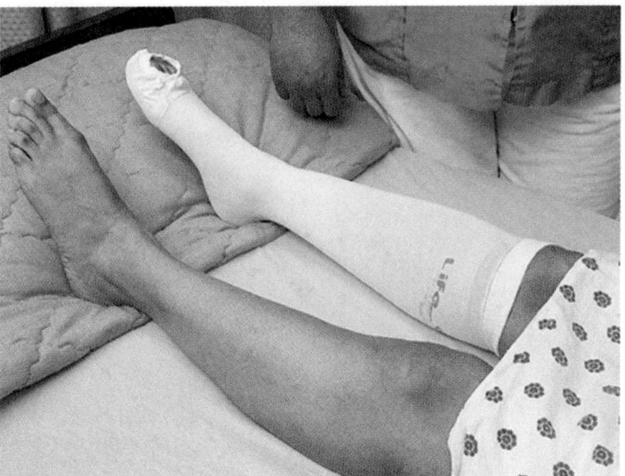
B

FIGURE 24-6 Applying elastic stockings. **A,** The stocking is slipped over the toes, foot, and heel. **B,** The stocking turns right side out as it is pulled up over the leg. The heel is positioned in the heel pocket of the stocking.

Elastic Bandages. Elastic bandages have the same purposes as elastic stockings. They provide support and reduce swelling from injuries. Sometimes they are used to hold dressings in place. They are applied to arms and legs. To apply bandages:

- Use the correct size—length and width.
- Position the person in good alignment.
- Face the person during the procedure.
- Start at the lower *(distal)* part of the extremity. Work upward to the top *(proximal)* part.
- Expose the fingers or toes if possible. This allows circulation checks.
- Apply the bandage with firm, even pressure.
- Check the color and temperature of the extremity every hour.
- Re-apply a loose or wrinkled bandage.
- Replace a moist or soiled bandage.

See *Focus on Communication: Elastic Bandages.*
See *Delegation Guidelines: Elastic Bandages.*
See *Promoting Safety and Comfort: Elastic Bandages.*
See procedure: *Applying an Elastic Bandage.*

DELEGATION GUIDELINES

Elastic Bandages

To apply elastic bandages, you need this information from the nurse and the care plan.

- Where to apply the bandage
- What width and length to use
- When to remove the bandage and for how long—usually every 8 hours for 30 minutes
- What to do if the bandage is wet or soiled
- What observations to report and record:
  - The width and length applied
  - When you applied the bandage
  - Skin color and temperature
  - Swelling of the part
  - Skin tears, wounds, or signs of skin breakdown
  - Complaints of pain, itching, tingling, or numbness
  - When you removed the bandage and for how long
  - When you re-applied the bandage
- When to report observations
- What patient or resident concerns to report at once

FOCUS ON COMMUNICATION

Elastic Bandages

Elastic bandages should promote comfort. To check for comfort, you can ask:

- "Does the bandage feel too tight?"
- "Do you feel pain, itching, or numbness?" If yes: "What do you feel? Where do you feel it?"

PROMOTING SAFETY AND COMFORT

Elastic Bandages

Safety

Elastic bandages must be firm and snug, but not tight. A tight bandage can affect circulation.

Bandages are secured in place with clips, tape, or Velcro. Clips are metal or plastic. Clips can injure the skin if they are loose, fall off, or cause pressure. Use clips only if the nurse tells you to. Check the bandage often to make sure the clips are correctly in place.

Some agencies do not allow you to apply elastic bandages. Know your agency's policy.

Comfort

A tight bandage can cause pain and discomfort. Apply it with firm, even pressure. Remove the bandage if the person complains of pain, tingling, or numbness. Tell the nurse at once.

Applying an Elastic Bandage

QUALITY OF LIFE

- Knock before entering the person's room.
- Address the person by name.
- Introduce yourself by name and title.
- Explain the procedure before starting and during the procedure.
- Protect the person's rights during the procedure.
- Handle the person gently during the procedure.

PRE-PROCEDURE

1 Follow *Delegation Guidelines:*
   a *Assisting With Wound Care,* p. 381
   b *Elastic Bandages*
   See *Promoting Safety and Comfort: Elastic Bandages.*
2 Practice hand hygiene.
3 Collect the following.
   - Elastic bandage as directed by the nurse
   - Tape or clips (unless the bandage has Velcro)
4 Identify the person. Check the ID bracelet against the assignment sheet. Also call the person by name.
5 Provide for privacy.
6 Raise the bed for body mechanics. Bed rails are up if used.

PROCEDURE

7 Lower the bed rail near you if up.
8 Help the person to a comfortable position. Expose the part you will bandage.
9 Make sure the area is clean and dry.
10 Hold the bandage so the roll is up. The loose end is on the bottom (Fig. 24-7, *A*).
11 Apply the bandage to the smallest part of the wrist, foot, ankle, or knee.
12 Make 2 circular turns around the part (Fig. 24-7, *B*).
13 Make over-lapping spiral turns in an upward direction. Each turn over-laps ½ to ¾ of the previous turn (Fig. 24-7, *C*). Each over-lap is equal.
14 Apply the bandage smoothly with firm, even pressure. It is not tight.
15 End the bandage with 2 circular turns.
16 Secure the bandage in place with Velcro, tape, or clips. Clips are not under the body part.
17 Check the fingers or toes for coldness or cyanosis (bluish color). Ask about pain, itching, numbness, or tingling. Remove the bandage if any are noted. Report your observations.

POST-PROCEDURE

18 Provide for comfort. (See the inside of the front cover.)
19 Place the call light within reach.
20 Lower the bed to a comfortable and safe level for the person. Follow the care plan.
21 Raise or lower bed rails. Follow the care plan.
22 Unscreen the person.
23 Complete a safety check of the room. (See the inside of the front cover.)
24 Practice hand hygiene.
25 Report and record your observations.

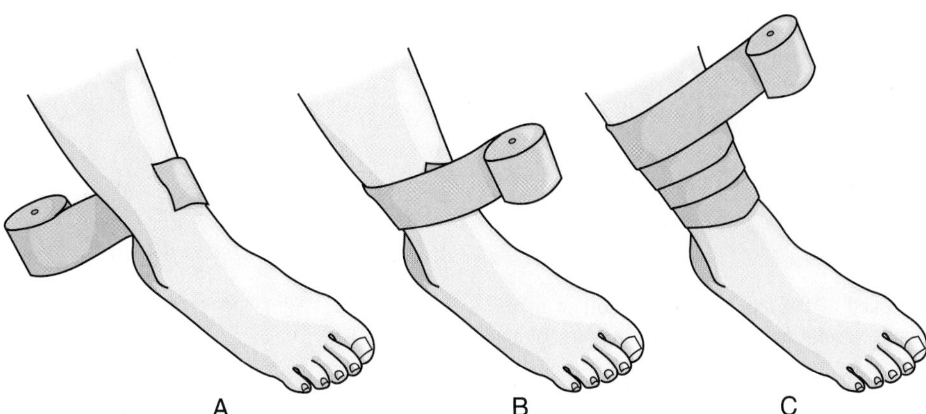

FIGURE 24-7 Applying an elastic bandage. **A,** The bandage roll is up. The loose end is at the bottom. **B,** The bandage is applied to the smallest part with 2 circular turns. **C,** The bandage is applied with spiral turns in an upward direction.

DRESSINGS

Wound dressings have many functions. They:

- Protect wounds from injury and microbes.
- Absorb drainage.
- Remove dead tissue.
- Promote comfort.
- Cover unsightly wounds.
- Provide a moist environment for wound healing.
- Apply pressure (pressure dressings) to control bleeding.

Securing Dressings

Dressings must be secured over wounds. Microbes can enter the wound and drainage can escape if the dressing is dislodged. Tape and Montgomery ties are used to secure dressings. Binders (p. 391) hold dressings in place.

Tape. Adhesive, paper, plastic, cloth, and elastic tapes are common. Adhesive tape sticks well. However, problems with adhesive include:

- It is hard to remove if it remains on the skin.
- It can irritate the skin.
- Skin tears occur if skin is removed with tape.
- Many people are allergic to adhesive tape.

Paper, plastic, and cloth tapes usually do not cause allergic reactions. Elastic tape allows movement of the body part.

Tape is applied to the top, middle, and bottom of the dressing. The tape extends several inches beyond each side of the dressing (Fig. 24-8). *Do not apply tape to circle the entire body part. If swelling occurs, circulation to the part is impaired.*

See *Focus on Communication: Tape.*

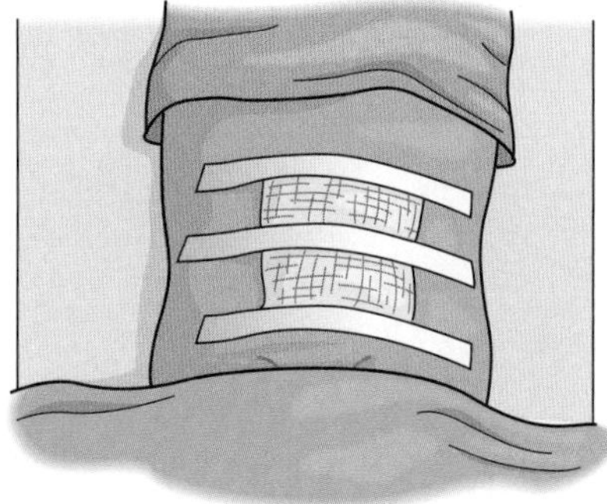

FIGURE 24-8 Tape is applied at the top, middle, and bottom of the dressing. The tape extends several inches beyond both sides of the dressing.

FOCUS ON COMMUNICATION

Tape

Before applying tape, ask if the person has an allergy to tape. You can ask:

- "Do any types of tape irritate your skin?"
- "Do you have an allergy to tape?"

Montgomery Ties. Montgomery ties (Fig. 24-9) are used for large dressings and frequent dressing changes. A Montgomery tie has an adhesive strip and cloth tie. With the dressing in place, the adhesive strips are placed on both sides of the dressing. Then the cloth ties are secured over the dressing.

A wound may need 2 or 3 Montgomery ties on each side. The ties are undone for the dressing change. The adhesive strips stay in place. They are not removed unless soiled. Montgomery ties protect the skin from frequent tape application and removal.

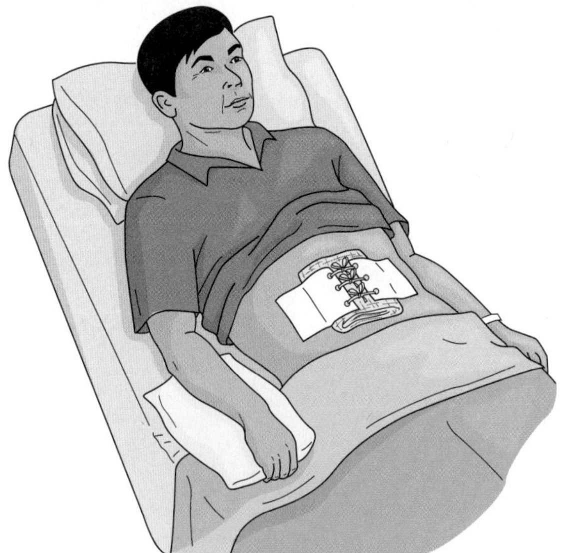

FIGURE 24-9 Montgomery ties.

Applying Dressings

Some agencies let you apply simple, dry, non-sterile dressings to simple wounds. Follow the rules in Box 24-3.

See *Focus on Older Persons: Applying Dressings.*

See *Delegation Guidelines: Applying Dressings.*

See *Promoting Safety and Comfort: Applying Dressings.*

See procedure: *Applying a Dry, Non-Sterile Dressing,* p. 390.

BOX 24-3 Applying Dressings

- Let pain-relief drugs take effect, usually 30 minutes. The dressing change can cause discomfort. The nurse gives the drug and tells you how long to wait.
- Meet fluid and elimination needs before you begin.
- Collect equipment and supplies before you begin.
- Do not bend or reach over your work area.
- Control your nonverbal communication. Wound odors, appearance, and drainage may be unpleasant. Do not communicate your thoughts or reactions to the person.
- Remove soiled dressings so the person cannot see the soiled side. The drainage and its color may upset the person.
- Do not force the person to look at the wound. A wound can affect body image and self-esteem. The nurse helps the person deal with the wound.
- Remove tape by pulling it toward the wound.
- Remove dressings gently. They may stick to the wound, drain, or surrounding skin. If the dressing sticks, the nurse may have you wet the dressing with a saline solution. A wet dressing is easier to remove.
- Touch only the outer edges of old and new dressings.
- Report and record your observations. See *Delegation Guidelines: Applying Dressings.*

FOCUS ON OLDER PERSONS

Applying Dressings

Older persons have thin, fragile skin. Skin tears must be prevented. Extreme care is necessary when removing tape.

DELEGATION GUIDELINES

Applying Dressings

When applying a dressing is delegated to you, you need this information from the nurse.

- When to change the dressing
- When the person received a pain-relief drug; when it will take effect
- What to do if the dressing sticks to the wound
- How to clean the wound
- What dressings to use
- How to secure the dressing—tape or Montgomery ties
- What kind of tape to use—adhesive, paper, plastic, cloth, or elastic
- What size tape to use—½, ¾, 1, 2, or 3 inch width
- What observations to report and record:
  - What you used to dress the wound and secure the dressing
  - A red or swollen wound
  - An area around the wound that is warm to touch
  - If wound edges are closed or separated
  - A wound that has broken open
  - Drainage appearance—clear, bloody, or watery and blood-tinged; thick and green, yellow, or brown
  - The amount of drainage
  - Wound or drainage odor
  - Intactness and color of surrounding tissues
  - Possible dressing contamination—urine; feces; other body fluids, secretions, or excretions; dislodged dressing
  - Pain
  - Fever
- When to report observations
- What patient or resident concerns to report at once

PROMOTING SAFETY AND COMFORT

Applying Dressings

Safety

Contact with blood, body fluids, secretions, or excretions is likely. Follow Standard Precautions and the Bloodborne Pathogen Standard. Wear personal protective equipment (PPE) as needed.

Do not apply tape to irritated, injured, or non-intact skin. Tape can further damage the skin.

Comfort

Wounds and dressing changes can cause discomfort or pain. The nurse may give a pain-relief drug before the dressing change. Allow time for the drug to take effect. Gently apply and remove tape and dressings.

The person may not report discomfort from a dressing. You should ask:

- "Is the dressing comfortable?"
- "Does the tape cause pain or itching?"

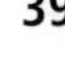

Applying a Dry, Non-Sterile Dressing

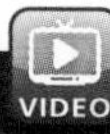
VIDEO

QUALITY OF LIFE

- Knock before entering the person's room.
- Address the person by name.
- Introduce yourself by name and title.
- Explain the procedure before starting and during the procedure.
- Protect the person's rights during the procedure.
- Handle the person gently during the procedure.

PRE-PROCEDURE

1 Follow *Delegation Guidelines:*
   a *Assisting With Wound Care,* p. 381
   b *Applying Dressings,* p. 389
   See *Promoting Safety and Comfort: Applying Dressings,* p. 389.
2 Practice hand hygiene.
3 Collect the following.
   - Gloves
   - PPE as needed
   - Tape or Montgomery ties
   - Dressings as directed by the nurse
   - Saline solution as directed by the nurse
   - Cleaning solution as directed by the nurse
   - Adhesive remover
   - Dressing set with scissors and forceps
   - Plastic bag
   - Bath blanket
4 Practice hand hygiene.
5 Identify the person. Check the ID bracelet against the assignment sheet. Also call the person by name.
6 Provide for privacy.
7 Arrange your work area. You should not have to reach over or turn your back on your work area.
8 Raise the bed for body mechanics. Bed rails are up if used.

PROCEDURE

9 Lower the bed rail near you if up.
10 Help the person to a comfortable position.
11 Cover the person with a bath blanket. Fan-fold top linens to the foot of the bed.
12 Expose the affected body part.
13 Make a cuff on the plastic bag. Place the bag within reach.
14 Practice hand hygiene.
15 Put on needed PPE. Put on gloves.
16 Remove tape or undo Montgomery ties.
   a *Tape:* hold the skin down. Gently pull the tape toward the wound.
   b *Montgomery ties:* fold ties away from the wound.
17 Remove any adhesive from the skin. Wet a 4 × 4 gauze dressing with adhesive remover. Clean away from the wound.
18 Remove gauze dressings. Start with the top dressing and remove each layer. Keep the soiled side away from the person's sight. Put dressings in the plastic bag. They must not touch the outside of the bag.
19 Remove the dressing over the wound very gently. It may stick to the wound or drain site. Moisten the dressing with saline if it sticks to the wound.
20 Observe the wound, drain site, and wound drainage.
21 Remove the gloves and put them in the bag. Practice hand hygiene.
22 Open the new dressings.
23 Cut the length of tape needed.
24 Put on clean gloves.
25 Clean the wound with saline as directed by the nurse. See Figure 24-10.
26 Apply dressings as directed by the nurse.
27 Secure the dressings. Use tape or Montgomery ties.
28 Remove the gloves. Put them in the bag.
29 Remove and discard PPE.
30 Practice hand hygiene.
31 Cover the person. Remove the bath blanket.

POST-PROCEDURE

32 Provide for comfort. (See the inside of the front cover.)
33 Place the call light within reach.
34 Lower the bed to a comfortable and safe level for the person. Follow the care plan.
35 Raise or lower bed rails. Follow the care plan.
36 Return equipment and supplies to their proper place. Leave extra dressings and tape in the room.
37 Discard used supplies in the bag. Tie the bag closed. Discard the bag following agency policy. (Wear gloves for this step.)
38 Clean your work area. Follow the Bloodborne Pathogen Standard.
39 Unscreen the person.
40 Complete a safety check of the room. (See the inside of the front cover.)
41 Remove and discard the gloves. Practice hand hygiene.
42 Report and record your observations.

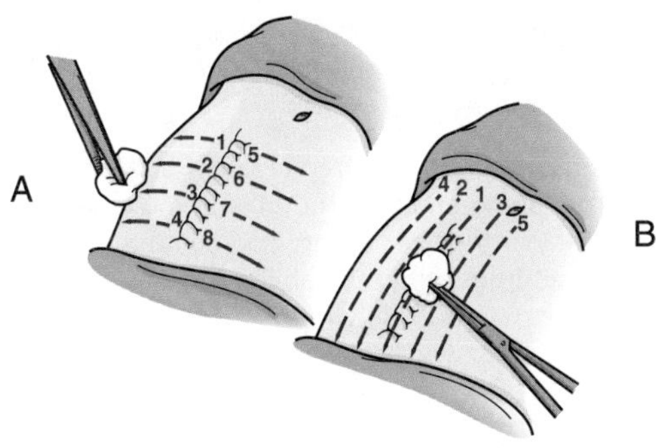

FIGURE 24-10 Cleaning a wound. **A,** Clean starting at the wound and stroking out to the surrounding skin. Use new gauze for each stroke. **B,** Clean the wound from the top to the bottom. Start at the wound. Then clean the surrounding areas. Use new gauze for each stroke.

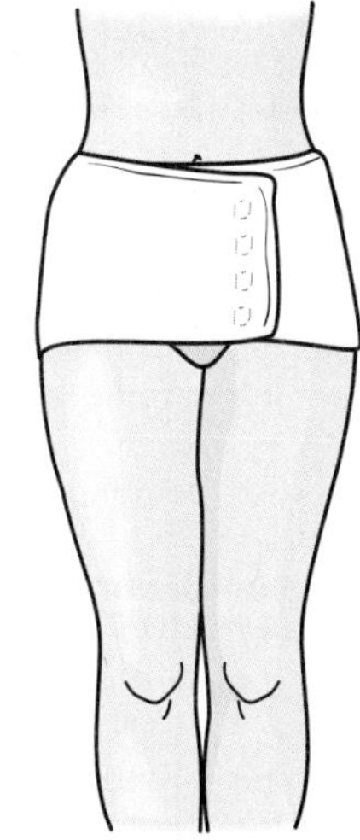

FIGURE 24-11 Abdominal binder.

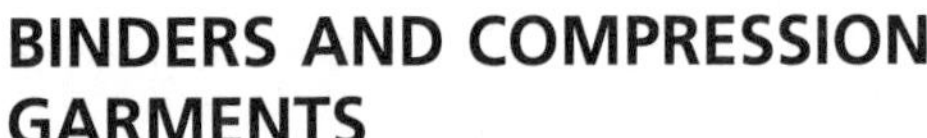

BINDERS AND COMPRESSION GARMENTS

Binders are wide bands of elastic fabric. They are applied to the abdomen, chest, or perineal area. Binders promote healing by supporting wounds and holding dressings in place. They also prevent or reduce swelling, promote comfort, and prevent injury. These binders are common.

- *Abdominal binder*—provides abdominal support and holds dressings in place (Fig. 24-11). The top part is at the waist. The lower part is over the hips. Binders are secured with Velcro or with hook and loop closures.
- *Breast binder*—supports the breasts after surgery (Fig. 24-12). It is secured with Velcro or padded zippers.

Compression garments are made of a tight, stretchy fabric (Fig. 24-13). They help:

- Reduce swelling.
- Prevent fluid buildup at the surgical site.
- Hold the skin against the body.
- Achieve the desired shape.

Box 24-4, p. 392 lists the rules for applying binders and compression garments.

See *Focus on Communication: Binders and Compression Garments*, p. 392.

See *Promoting Safety and Comfort: Binders and Compression Garments*, p. 392.

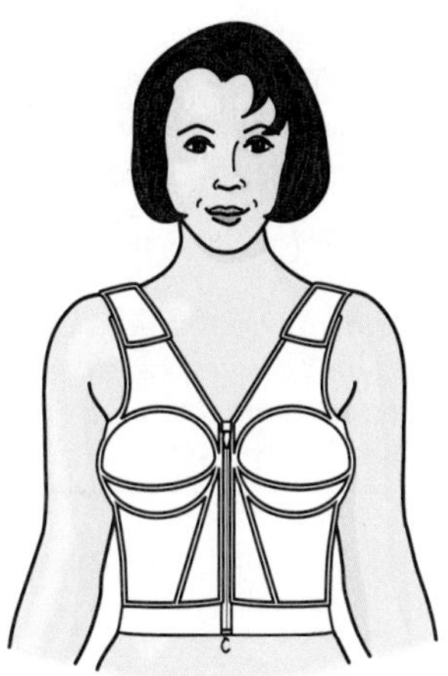

FIGURE 24-12 Breast binder.

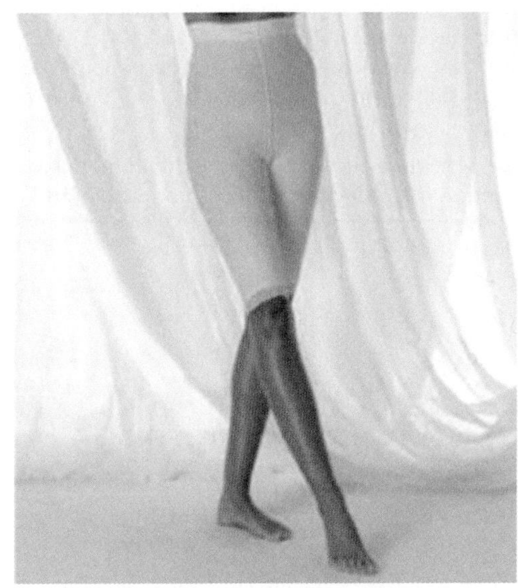

FIGURE 24-13 Compression garment.

BOX 24-4 Applying Binders and Compression Garments

- Follow the manufacturer's instructions.
- Apply the device for firm, even pressure over the area.
- Apply the device so it is snug. It must not interfere with breathing or circulation.
- Position the person in good alignment.
- Re-apply the device if it is out of position or causes discomfort.
- Secure safety pins, if used, pointing away from the wound.
- Change the device if it is moist or soiled. This prevents the growth of microbes.
- Tell the nurse at once if there is a change in the person's breathing.
- Check the skin under and around the device. Tell the nurse at once if there is redness, irritation, or other signs of a skin problem.

FOCUS ON COMMUNICATION

Binders and Compression Garments

The person may not tell you about pain or discomfort. You need to ask:
- "Is the binder (or garment) too tight or too loose?"
- "Does the binder (or garment) cause pain?"
- "Do you feel pressure from the binder (or garment)?" If yes: "Where? Please show me."

PROMOTING SAFETY AND COMFORT

Binders and Compression Garments

Safety

Apply binders and compression garments properly. Otherwise, severe discomfort, skin irritation, and circulatory and respiratory problems can occur. Correct application is needed for safety and for the device to work properly.

Comfort

A binder or compression garment should promote comfort. Tell the nurse if the device causes pain or discomfort.

HEAT AND COLD APPLICATIONS

Heat and cold applications promote healing and comfort. They also reduce tissue swelling. Heat and cold have opposite effects on body functions.

See *Focus on Older Persons: Heat and Cold Applications.*

FOCUS ON OLDER PERSONS

Heat and Cold Applications

Older persons have thin and fragile skin. Burns are a risk. Changes from aging and health problems increase the risk for burns. They include circulatory and nervous system changes. Some drugs affect the ability to sense pain. Confused persons and those with dementia may not recognize pain. Look for behavior changes. Behavior changes can signal pain.

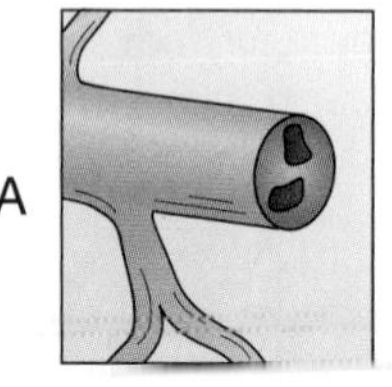

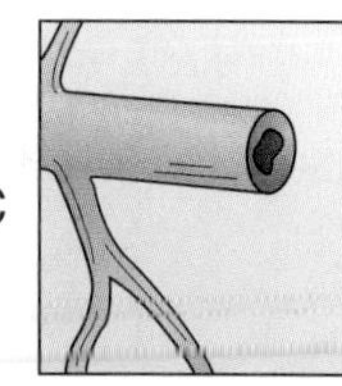

FIGURE 24-14 A, A blood vessel under normal conditions. **B,** Dilated blood vessel. **C,** Constricted blood vessel.

Heat Applications

Heat applications can be applied to almost any body part. They are often used for musculo-skeletal injuries or problems (sprains, arthritis). Heat:
- Relieves pain.
- Relaxes muscles.
- Promotes healing.
- Reduces tissue swelling.
- Decreases joint stiffness.

When heat is applied to the skin, blood vessels in the area dilate. ***Dilate*** *means to expand or open wider* (Fig. 24-14). Blood flow increases. Tissues have more oxygen and nutrients for healing. Excess fluid is removed from the area faster. The skin is red and warm.

Complications. High temperatures can cause burns. Report pain, excessive redness, and blisters at once. Also observe for pale skin. When heat is applied too long, blood vessels ***constrict*** *(narrow)* (see Fig. 24-14). Blood flow decreases. Tissues receive less blood. Tissue damage occurs and the skin is pale.

Metal implants pose risks. Metal conducts heat. Deep tissues can be burned. Pacemakers (cardiac devices) and joint replacements are made of metal. Do not apply heat to an implant area.

Heat is not applied to a pregnant woman's abdomen. The heat can affect fetal growth.

Moist and Dry Heat Applications. With a *moist heat application,* water is in contact with the skin. Water conducts heat. Moist heat has greater and faster effects than dry heat. Heat penetrates deeper with a moist application. To prevent injury, moist heat applications have lower

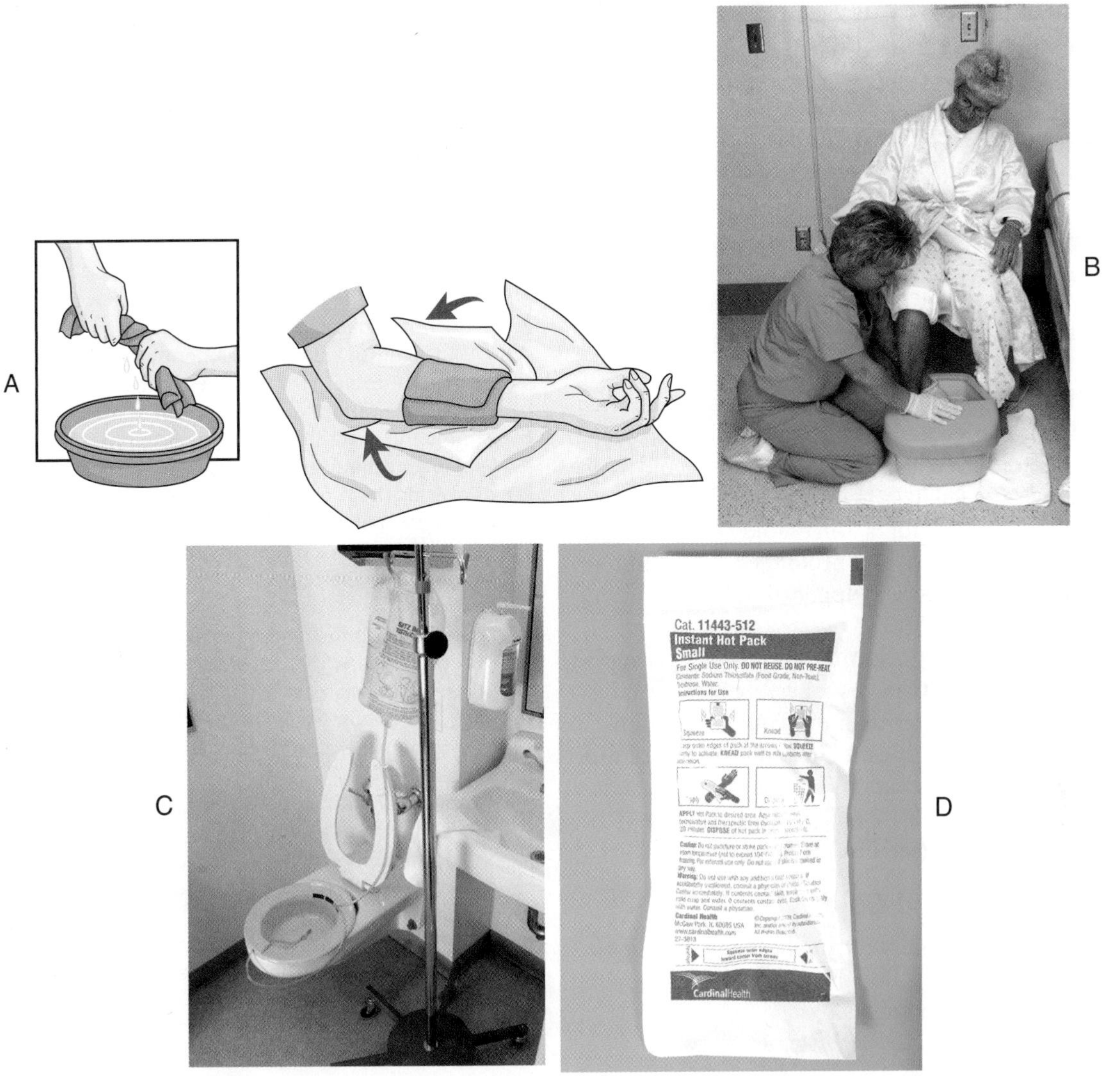

FIGURE 24-15 Moist heat applications. **A,** Compress. **B,** Hot soak. **C,** Disposable sitz bath. **D,** Hot pack. (NOTE: Compresses can be hot or cold. And some hot packs can also be used as cold packs.)

(cooler) temperatures than dry heat applications. Moist heat applications (Fig. 24-15) include:

- *Hot compress.* A *compress* is a soft pad applied over a body area. It is usually made of cloth.
- *Hot soak.* A body part is put into water.
- *Sitz bath.* The perineal and rectal areas are immersed in warm or hot water. (*Sitz* means *seat* in German.)
- *Hot pack.* A *pack* involves wrapping a body part.

With *dry heat applications,* water is not in contact with the skin. A dry heat application stays at the desired temperature longer. Dry heat does not penetrate as deep as moist heat. Because water is not used, dry heat needs higher (hotter) temperatures for the desired effect. Therefore burns are still a risk.

Some *hot packs* and the *aquathermia pad* (Aqua-K, K-Pad) are dry heat applications (Fig. 24-16). The aquathermia pad is an electrical device. Tubes inside the pad are filled with distilled water. Heated water flows to the pad through a hose. Another hose returns water to the heating unit. The water is re-heated and returned back into the pad.

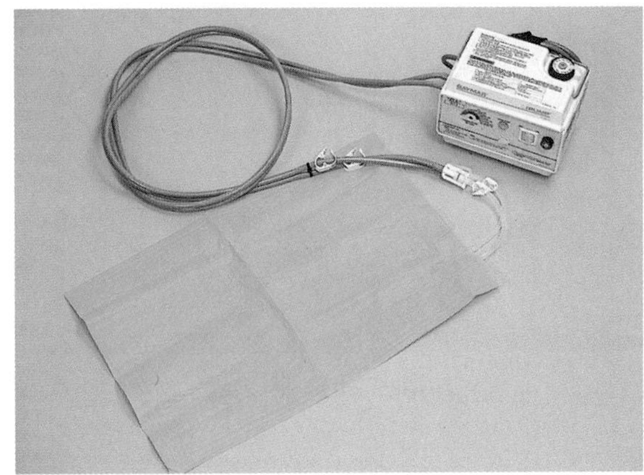

FIGURE 24-16 The aquathermia pad.

Cold Applications

Cold applications are often used to treat sprains and fractures. Cold applications reduce pain, prevent swelling, and decrease circulation and bleeding. Cold has the opposite effect of heat. When cold is applied to the skin, blood vessels constrict (see Fig. 24-14). Blood flow decreases. Less oxygen and nutrients are carried to the tissues.

Cold applications are useful right after an injury. Decreased blood flow reduces the amount of bleeding. Less fluid collects in the tissues. Cold has a numbing effect on the skin. This helps reduce or relieve pain in the part.

Complications. Complications include pain, burns, blisters, and poor circulation. Burns and blisters occur from intense cold. They also occur when dry cold is in direct contact with the skin.

When cold is applied for a long time, blood vessels dilate. Blood flow increases. The prolonged application of cold has the same effect as heat applications.

Moist and Dry Cold Applications. Moist cold applications penetrate deeper than dry ones. Therefore moist cold applications are warmer than dry cold applications.

The cold compress is a moist cold application (see Fig. 24-15, *A*). Dry cold applications include ice bags, ice collars, and ice gloves (Fig. 24-17). Cold packs can be moist or dry applications (see Fig. 24-15, *D*).

Applying Heat and Cold

Protect the person from injury during heat and cold applications. Follow the rules in Box 24-5. See Table 24-1 for heat and cold temperature ranges.

See *Focus on Communication: Applying Heat and Cold.*

See *Delegation Guidelines: Applying Heat and Cold.*

See *Promoting Safety and Comfort: Applying Heat and Cold.*

See procedure: *Applying Heat and Cold Applications,* p. 396.

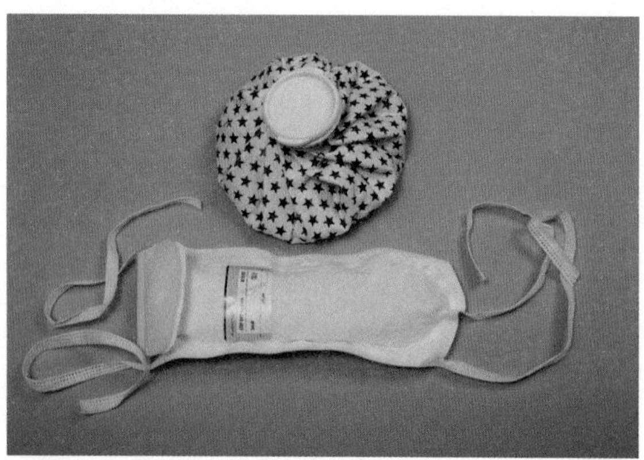

FIGURE 24-17 Ice bags.

BOX 24-5 Applying Heat and Cold

- Know how to use the equipment. Follow the manufacturer's instructions for commercial devices.
- Measure the temperature of moist applications. Use a bath thermometer. Or follow agency policy for measuring temperature.
- Follow agency policies for safe temperature ranges. See Table 24-1.
- Do not apply *very hot* (above 106°F or 41.1°C) applications. Tissue damage can occur. A nurse applies *very hot* applications.
- Ask the nurse what the temperature should be.
  - Heat—cooler temperatures for persons at risk
  - Cold—warmer temperatures for persons at risk
- Know the exact site of the application. Have the nurse show you the site.
- Cover dry heat or cold applications before applying them. Use a flannel cover, towel, or other cover as directed.
- Provide for privacy. Properly screen and drape the person. Expose only the body part involved. Avoid unnecessary exposure.
- Maintain comfort and body alignment during the procedure.
- Observe the skin every 5 minutes during the procedure. See *Delegation Guidelines: Applying Heat and Cold.*
- Do not let the person change the temperature of the application.
- Know how long to leave the application in place. See *Delegation Guidelines: Applying Heat and Cold.* Heat and cold are applied no longer than 15 to 20 minutes.
- Follow the rules for electrical safety when using electrical appliances to apply heat.
- Place the call light within the person's reach.
- Complete a safety check before leaving the room. (See the inside of the front cover.)

TABLE 24-1 Heat and Cold Temperature Ranges

Temperature	Fahrenheit (F) Range	Centigrade (C) Range
Hot	98°F to 106°F	36.6°C to 41.1°C
Warm	93°F to 98°F	33.8°C to 36.6°C
Tepid	80°F to 93°F	26.6°C to 33.8°C
Cool	65°F to 80°F	18.3°C to 26.6°C
Cold	50°F to 65°F	10.0°C to 18.3°C

Modified from Perry AG, Potter PA: Clinical nursing skills and techniques, *ed 7, St Louis, 2010, Mosby.*

FOCUS ON COMMUNICATION

Applying Heat and Cold

The person may not tell you about pain or discomfort. The person may not know what symptoms to report. For heat and cold applications, you need to ask:

- "Does the application feel too hot or too cold?"
- "Do you feel any pain, numbness, or burning?"
- "Do you feel weak, faint, or drowsy?" If yes: "Tell me how you feel."

DELEGATION GUIDELINES

Applying Heat and Cold

To apply heat or cold, you need this information from the nurse and the care plan.

- The type of application—hot compress or pack, commercial compress, hot soak, sitz bath, aquathermia pad; ice bag, ice collar, ice glove, cold pack, or cold compress
- How to cover the application
- What temperature to use (see Table 24-1)
- The application site
- How long to leave the application in place
- What observations to report and record:
  - Complaints of pain or discomfort, numbness, or burning
  - Excessive redness
  - Blisters
  - Pale, white, or gray skin
  - Cyanosis (bluish color)
  - Shivering
  - Rapid pulse, weakness, faintness, and drowsiness (sitz bath)
  - Time, site, and length of application
- When to report observations
- What patient or resident concerns to report at once

PROMOTING SAFETY AND COMFORT

Applying Heat and Cold

Safety

Check the person every 5 minutes. Also follow these safety measures.

- *Sitz bath.* Blood flow increases to the perineum and rectum. Therefore less blood flows to other body parts. The person may become weak or feel faint. Drowsiness can occur from the bath's relaxing effect. Observe for signs of weakness, fainting, or fatigue. Also protect the person from injury. Check the person often. Keep the call light within reach and prevent chills and burns.
- *Commercial hot and cold packs.* Read warning labels and follow the manufacturer's instructions.
- *Aquathermia pad:*
  - Follow electrical safety precautions (Chapter 9).
  - Check the device for damage or flaws.
  - Follow the manufacturer's instructions.
  - Place the heating unit on an even, uncluttered surface. This prevents it from being knocked over or knocked off of the surface.
  - Make sure the hoses do not have kinks or bubbles. Water must flow freely.
  - Use a flannel cover to insulate the pad. It absorbs perspiration at the application site. (Some agencies use towels or pillowcases.)
  - Secure the pad in place with ties, tape, or rolled gauze. Do not use pins. They can puncture the pad and cause leaks.
  - Do not place the pad under the person or under a body part. This prevents the escape of heat. Burns can result if heat cannot escape.
  - Give the key used to set the temperature to the nurse. This prevents anyone from changing the temperature. The temperature is usually set at 105°F (40.5°C) with a key.

Some persons have medicated patches or ointments applied to the skin. Do not apply heat over such areas.

Comfort

Cold applications can cause chills and shivering. Provide for warmth. Use bath blankets or other blankets as needed.

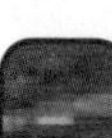

Applying Heat and Cold Applications

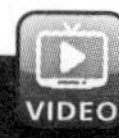

VIDEO

QUALITY OF LIFE

- Knock before entering the person's room.
- Address the person by name.
- Introduce yourself by name and title.
- Explain the procedure before starting and during the procedure.
- Protect the person's rights during the procedure.
- Handle the person gently during the procedure.

PRE-PROCEDURE

1 Follow *Delegation Guidelines:*
  a *Assisting With Wound Care,* p. 381
  b *Applying Heat and Cold,* p. 395
  See *Promoting Safety and Comfort: Applying Heat and Cold,* p. 395.
2 Practice hand hygiene.
3 Collect equipment.
  - *For a hot compress:*
    - Basin
    - Bath thermometer
    - Small towel, washcloth, or gauze squares
    - Plastic wrap or aquathermia pad
    - Ties, tape, or rolled gauze
    - Bath towel
    - Waterproof pad
  - *For a hot soak:*
    - Water basin or arm or foot bath
    - Bath thermometer
    - Waterproof pad
    - Bath blanket
    - Towel
  - *For a sitz bath:*
    - Disposable sitz bath
    - Bath thermometer
    - Two bath blankets, bath towels, and a clean gown
  - *For a hot or cold pack:*
    - Commercial pack
    - Pack cover
    - Ties, tape, or rolled gauze (if needed)
    - Waterproof pad
  - *For an aquathermia pad:*
    - Aquathermia pad and heating unit
    - Distilled water
    - Flannel cover or other cover as directed
    - Ties, tape, or rolled gauze
  - *For an ice bag, ice collar, ice glove, or dry cold pack:*
    - Ice bag, collar, glove, or cold pack
    - Crushed ice (except for a cold pack)
    - Flannel cover or other cover as directed
    - Paper towels
  - *For a cold compress:*
    - Large basin with ice
    - Small basin with cold water
    - Gauze squares, washcloths, or small towels
    - Waterproof pad
4 Identify the person. Check the ID bracelet against the assignment sheet. Also call the person by name.

PROCEDURE

5 Provide for privacy.
6 Position the person for the procedure.
7 Place the waterproof pad (if needed) under the body part.
8 *For a hot compress:*
  a Fill the basin ½ to ⅔ full with hot water as directed. Measure water temperature.
  b Place the compress in the water.
  c Wring out the compress.
  d Apply the compress over the area. Note the time.
  e Cover the compress as directed. Do 1 of the following.
    1 Apply plastic wrap and then a bath towel. Secure the towel in place with ties, tape, or rolled gauze.
    2 Apply an aquathermia pad.
9 *For a hot soak:*
  a Fill the container ½ full with hot water. Measure water temperature.
  b Place the body part into the water. Pad the edge of the container with a towel. Note the time.
  c Cover the person with a bath blanket for warmth.
10 *For a sitz bath:*
  a Place the disposable sitz bath on the toilet seat.
  b Fill the sitz bath ⅔ full with water. Measure water temperature.
  c Secure the gown above the waist.
  d Help the person sit on the sitz bath. Note the time.
  e Provide for warmth. Place 1 bath blanket around the shoulders. Place the other over the legs.
  f Stay with the person if he or she is weak or unsteady.
11 *For a hot or cold pack:*
  a Squeeze, knead, or strike the pack as directed by the manufacturer.
  b Place the pack in the cover.
  c Apply the pack. Note the time.
  d Secure the pack in place with ties, tape, or rolled gauze. Some packs are secured with Velcro straps.
12 *For an aquathermia pad:*
  a Fill the heating unit to the fill line with distilled water.
  b Remove the bubbles. Place the pad and tubing below the heating unit. Tilt the heating unit from side to side.
  c Set the temperature as the nurse directs (usually 105°F [40.5°C]). Remove the key.
  d Place the pad in the cover.
  e Plug in the unit. Let water warm to the desired temperature.
  f Set the heating unit on the bedside stand. Keep the pad and connecting hoses level with the unit. Hoses must not have kinks.
  g Apply the pad to the part. Note the time.
  h Secure the pad in place with ties, tape, or rolled gauze. Do not use pins.

Applying Heat and Cold Applications—cont'd

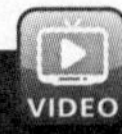

PROCEDURE—cont'd

13 *For an ice bag, collar, or glove:*
  a Fill the device with water. Put in the stopper. Turn the device upside down to check for leaks.
  b Empty the device.
  c Fill the device ½ to ⅔ full with crushed ice or ice chips.
  d Remove excess air. Bend, twist, or squeeze the device. Or press it against a firm surface.
  e Place the cap or stopper on securely.
  f Dry the device with paper towels.
  g Place the device in the cover.
  h Apply the device. Note the time.
  i Secure the device in place with ties, tape, or rolled gauze.

14 *For a cold compress:*
  a Place the small basin with cold water into the large basin with ice.
  b Place the compresses into the cold water.
  c Wring out a compress.
  d Apply the compress to the part. Note the time.

15 Place the call light within reach. Unscreen the person.
16 Raise or lower bed rails. Follow the care plan.
17 Check the person every 5 minutes. Check for signs and symptoms of complications (see *Delegation Guidelines: Applying Heat and Cold,* p. 395). Remove the application if any occur. Tell the nurse at once.
18 Check the application every 5 minutes. Change the application if cooling (hot application) or warming (cold application) occurs.
19 Remove the application at the specified time. Heat and cold applications are left on for 15 to 20 minutes.

POST-PROCEDURE

20 Provide for comfort. (See the inside of the front cover.)
21 Place the call light within reach.
22 Raise or lower bed rails. Follow the care plan.
23 Unscreen the person.
24 Clean, rinse, dry, and return re-usable items to their proper place. Follow agency policy for soiled linen. Wear gloves for this step.
25 Complete a safety check of the room. (See the inside of the front cover.)
26 Remove and discard the gloves. Practice hand hygiene.
27 Report and record your observations.

FOCUS ON PRIDE

The Person, Family, and Yourself

Personal and Professional Responsibility

You are responsible for the tasks you perform. If unsure if you are allowed to do a task, ask the nurse. If you do not know how to use the equipment, tell the nurse. Never perform a task you are not comfortable doing. The person may be harmed. Do not be afraid, embarrassed, or ashamed to tell the nurse about your concerns. Take pride in acting responsibly.

Rights and Respect

A person may ask about the need for a wound care measure. For example: "Why do I need to wear a bandage?" or "What is the reason for the cold pack?" Avoid answers like: "It's to help you get better" or "The doctor (nurse) says you need it." The person has the right to be informed.

Be kind, caring, and patient when the person asks questions. Refer questions to the nurse. Tell the person that you will ask the nurse to explain the reason. Wait until the person's questions are answered before performing the procedure.

Independence and Social Interaction

Remember to explain procedures to patients and residents. They can plan if they know what will happen. For example, a person wants to make a phone call before a hot compress is applied. Or a person wants a dressing changed by a certain time—before visitors arrive or before an activity. You promote independence when you involve the person in planning.

Delegation and Teamwork

Wound care can be painful and tiring. The team coordinates care to promote comfort and rest. To assist:

- Plan care with the nurse. Ask when drugs for pain will be given and when they will take effect. Allow rest periods before and after care that is tiring.
- Be prepared. Gather supplies. Leaving to get supplies causes delays. Care and procedures take longer than planned.
- Work with the nurse as instructed. You may need to position the person or raise a body part while the nurse changes a dressing. Teamwork reduces the amount of energy the person must use.

Ethics and Laws

Agencies have rules for charging for supplies used. The person's name and the type and amount of items used are recorded. Ethical practice involves honestly following agency rules. Not charging supplies correctly costs the nursing unit and agency money. Taking supplies home for your own use is unethical. This is stealing. Take pride in following agency rules and being an honest and reliable member of the nursing team.

REVIEW QUESTIONS

Circle the BEST answer.

1 Which can cause skin tears?
  a Keeping your nails trimmed and smooth
  b Dressing the person in soft clothing
  c Wearing rings
  d Padding wheelchair footplates

2 A person has a circulatory ulcer. Which measure should you question?
  a Hold socks in place with elastic garters.
  b Do not cut or trim toenails.
  c Apply elastic stockings.
  d Re-position the person every hour.

3 Diabetic foot ulcers are caused by
  a Gangrene
  b Amputation
  c Infection
  d Nerve and blood vessel damage

4 A person has diabetes. The person's feet are checked every
  a 2 hours
  b Day
  c Week
  d Month

5 Elastic stockings are applied
  a Before the person gets out of bed
  b When the person is standing
  c After the person's shower or bath
  d For 30 minutes and then removed

6 When applying an elastic bandage
  a Apply it from the large to the small part of the extremity
  b Apply it from the upper to lower part of the extremity
  c Cover the fingers or toes if possible
  d Position the part in good alignment

7 Dressings
  a Protect the wound from injury
  b Prevent drainage
  c Provide a dry environment for wound healing
  d Support the wound and reduce swelling

8 To secure a dressing, apply tape
  a Around the entire part
  b Along the sides of the dressing
  c To the top, middle, and bottom of the dressing
  d As the person prefers

9 To remove tape
  a Pull it toward the wound
  b Pull it away from the wound
  c Use an adhesive remover
  d Use a saline solution

10 An abdominal binder is used to
  a Prevent blood clots
  b Prevent wound infection
  c Provide support and hold dressings in place
  d Decrease swelling and circulation

11 The *greatest* threat from heat applications is
  a Infection
  b Burns
  c Chilling
  d Skin tears

12 The nurse asks you to apply a hot pack. Which should you question?
  a Check that the pack's temperature is at least 110°F (43.3°C).
  b Place the pack in a cover.
  c Secure the pack in place with ties.
  d Check the person for complications every 5 minutes.

13 When using an aquathermia pad
  a Place the pad under the body part
  b Avoid covering the pad
  c Secure the pad in place with pins
  d Follow electrical safety precautions

14 Which signals a complication of a cold application?
  a Cool skin
  b Cyanosis
  c Decreased swelling
  d Fever

15 Before applying an ice bag
  a Place the bag in the freezer
  b Measure the temperature of the bag
  c Place the bag in a cover
  d Provide perineal care

16 Moist cold compresses are left in place no longer than
  a 20 minutes
  b 30 minutes
  c 45 minutes
  d 60 minutes

Answers to these questions are on p. 505.

FOCUS ON PRACTICE

Problem Solving

You are dressing an older resident with thin, fragile skin. You notice a new skin tear on the person's arm. What do you do? How can you prevent skin tears?

CHAPTER 25

Assisting With Pressure Ulcers

OBJECTIVES

- Define the key terms and key abbreviation listed in this chapter.
- Describe the causes and risk factors for pressure ulcers.
- Identify the persons at risk for pressure ulcers.
- Describe the stages of pressure ulcers.
- Identify the sites for pressure ulcers.
- Explain how to prevent pressure ulcers.
- Identify the complications from pressure ulcers.
- Explain how to promote PRIDE in the person, the family, and yourself.

KEY TERMS

bony prominence An area where the bone sticks out or projects from the flat surface of the body

eschar Thick, leathery dead tissue that may be loose or adhered to the skin; it is often black or brown

friction The rubbing of 1 surface against another

pressure ulcer A localized injury to the skin and/or underlying tissue, usually over a bony prominence, resulting from pressure or pressure in combination with shear; any lesion caused by unrelieved pressure that results in damage to underlying tissues

shear When layers of the skin rub against each other; when the skin remains in place and underlying tissues move and stretch and tear underlying capillaries and blood vessels causing tissue damage

slough Dead tissue that is shed from the skin; it is usually light colored, soft, and moist; may be stringy at times

KEY ABBREVIATION

CMS Centers for Medicare & Medicaid Services

Before defining pressure ulcer, you need to understand these terms.

- ***Bony prominence****—an area where the bone sticks out or projects from the flat surface of the body.* The back of the hand, shoulder blades, elbows, hips, spine, sacrum, knees, ankles, heels, and toes are bony prominences (Fig. 25-1, p. 400). These areas also are called *pressure points.*
- ***Shear****—when layers of the skin rub against each other. Or shear is when the skin remains in place and underlying tissues move and stretch and tear underlying capillaries and blood vessels. Tissue damage occurs.* See Chapter 14.
- ***Friction****—the rubbing of 1 surface against another.* The skin is dragged across a surface. Friction is always present with shearing.

The National Pressure Ulcer Advisory Panel (NPUAP) defines ***pressure ulcer*** *as a localized injury to the skin and/or underlying tissue, usually over a bony prominence* (Fig. 25-2, p. 401). *It is the result of pressure or pressure in combination with shear.* Decubitus ulcer, bed sore, and pressure sore are other terms for pressure ulcer.

The Centers for Medicare & Medicaid Services (CMS) defines ***pressure ulcer*** *as any lesion caused by unrelieved pressure that results in damage to underlying tissues.* According to the CMS, friction and shear are not the main causes of pressure ulcers. However, friction and shear are important contributing factors.

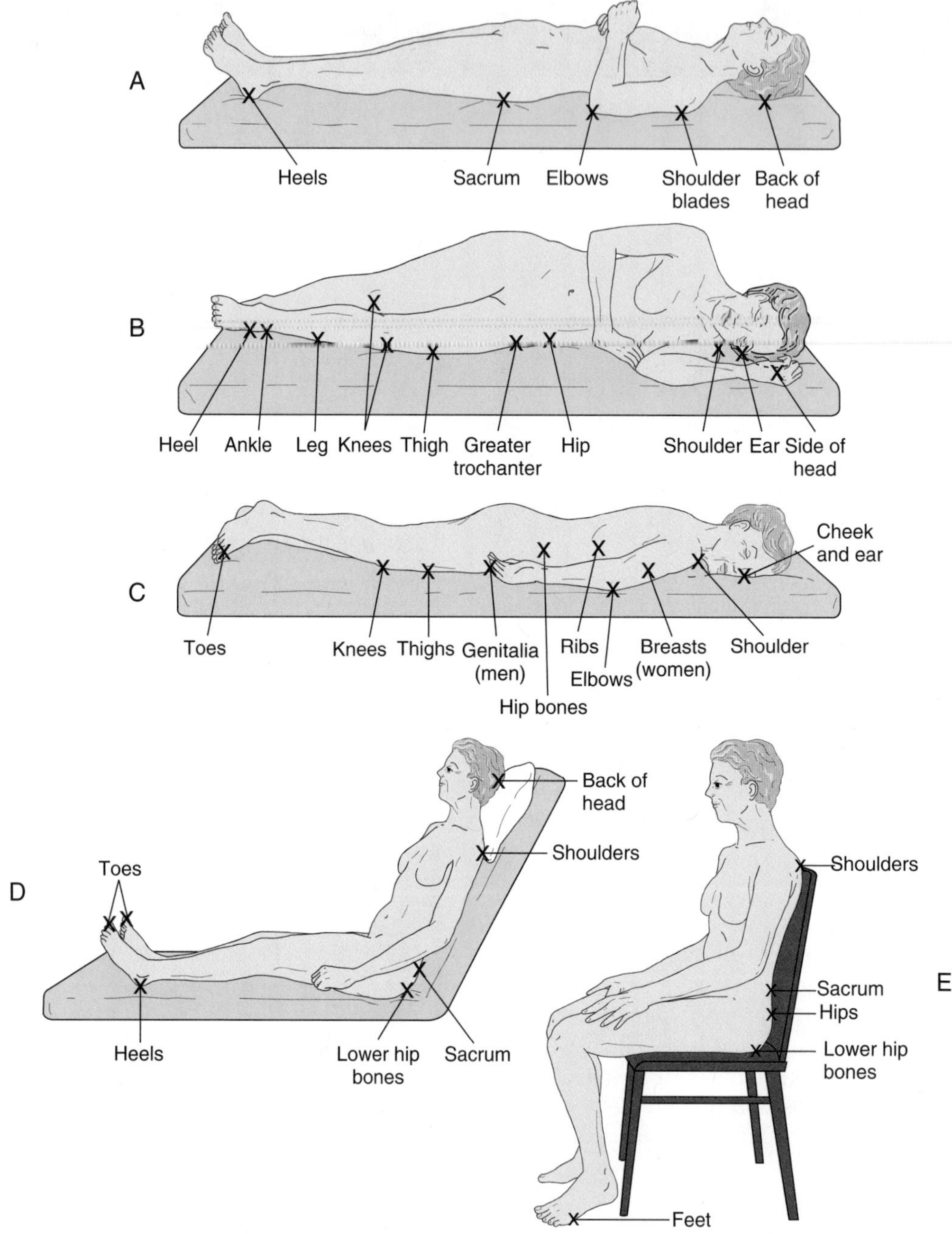

FIGURE 25-1 Bony prominences (pressure points). **A,** The supine position. **B,** The lateral position. **C,** The prone position. **D,** Fowler's position. **E,** Sitting position.

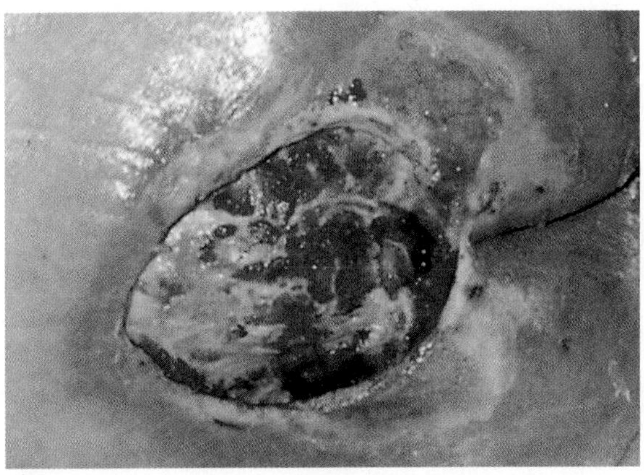

FIGURE 25-2 A pressure ulcer.

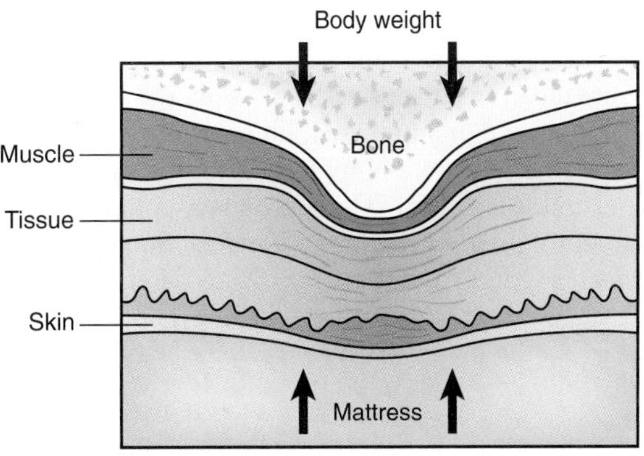

FIGURE 25-3 Tissue under pressure. The skin is squeezed between 2 hard surfaces—the bone and the mattress.

RISK FACTORS

Pressure is the major cause of pressure ulcers. Shearing and friction are important factors. Risk factors include breaks in the skin and skin breakdown, poor circulation to an area, moisture, dry skin, and irritation by urine and feces.

Unrelieved pressure squeezes tiny blood vessels. For example, pressure occurs when the skin over a bony area is squeezed between hard surfaces (Fig. 25-3). The bone is 1 hard surface. The other is usually the mattress or chair seat. Squeezing or pressure prevents blood flow to the skin and underlying tissues. Oxygen and nutrients cannot get to the cells. Skin and tissues die.

Friction scrapes the skin, causing an open area. The open area needs to heal. A good blood supply is needed. A poor blood supply or an infection can lead to a pressure ulcer.

Shear occurs when the person slides down in the bed or chair. Blood vessels and tissues are damaged. Blood flow to the area is reduced.

PERSONS AT RISK

Persons at risk for pressure ulcers are those who:

- Are *bedfast* (confined to bed) or *chairfast* (confined to a chair).
- Need some or total help moving.
- Are agitated or have involuntary muscle movements.
- Have urinary or fecal incontinence.
- Are exposed to moisture—urine, feces, wound drainage, sweat, or saliva.
- Have poor nutrition or poor fluid balance.
- Have lowered mental awareness.
- Have problems sensing pain or pressure.
- Have circulatory problems.
- Are obese or very thin.
- Have a healed pressure ulcer.
- Take drugs that affect wound healing.
- Refuse some care and treatment measures.
- Have health problems such as kidney failure, thyroid disease, or diabetes.
- Smoke.

See *Focus on Older Persons: Persons at Risk.*

FOCUS ON OLDER PERSONS

Persons at Risk

Older persons have fragile skin. Such skin is easily injured. They may have chronic diseases that affect mobility, nutrition, circulation, and mental awareness.

PRESSURE ULCER STAGES

In persons with light skin, a red area is the first sign of a pressure ulcer. In persons with dark skin, the skin may have no color change or appear red, blue, or purple. Color does not fade when pressure is applied. The area may feel warm or cool and soft or firm. The person may complain of pain, burning, tingling, or itching in the area. Some persons do not feel anything unusual. Box 25-1 describes pressure ulcer stages. The stages are shown in Figure 25-4.

See *Focus on Communication: Pressure Ulcer Stages.*

BOX 25-1 Pressure Ulcer Stages

Suspected deep tissue injury: A purple or maroon area of intact skin or a blood-filled blister. Pressure or shear has damaged underlying soft tissue. Involved tissue may be painful, firm, mushy, boggy, warm, or cool. Skin changes may be hard to see in persons with dark skin. See Figure 25-4, *A*.

Stage 1: Intact skin with redness over a bony prominence. The color does not fade with pressure. In persons with dark skin, skin color may differ from surrounding areas. It may appear pale, blue, or purple. See Figure 25-4, *B*.

Stage 2: Partial-thickness skin loss (Fig. 25-4, *C*). The wound may involve a blister or shallow ulcer. An ulcer may appear to be reddish-pink. A blister may be intact or open.

Stage 3: Full-thickness tissue loss (Fig. 25-4, *D*). The skin is gone. Subcutaneous fat may be exposed. Slough may be present. ***Slough*** *is dead tissue that is shed from the skin. It is usually light colored, soft, and moist. It may be stringy at times.*

Stage 4: Full-thickness tissue loss with muscle, tendon, and bone exposure (Fig. 25-4, *E*). Slough and eschar may be present. ***Eschar*** *is thick, leathery dead tissue that may be loose or adhered to the skin. It is often black or brown.*

Unstageable: Full-thickness tissue loss with the ulcer covered by slough and/or eschar (Fig. 25-4, *F*). Slough is yellow, tan, gray, green, or brown. Eschar is tan, brown, or black. The stage (Stage 3 or 4) cannot be determined until enough slough and eschar are removed.

FOCUS ON COMMUNICATION

Pressure Ulcer Stages

Tell the nurse if you see areas of redness, skin color changes, blisters, or skin or tissue loss. Describe what you see as best as you can. Tell the nurse the site. For example, you can say:

- "I saw a reddened area on Mr. Drake's left heel. It was about the size of a quarter. The skin looked intact. Would you please look at it?"
- "I just gave Ms. Richards a bath. I noticed a reddened area with a blister on her left hip. I didn't see any drainage. Would you please look at it? I'll help you turn her."

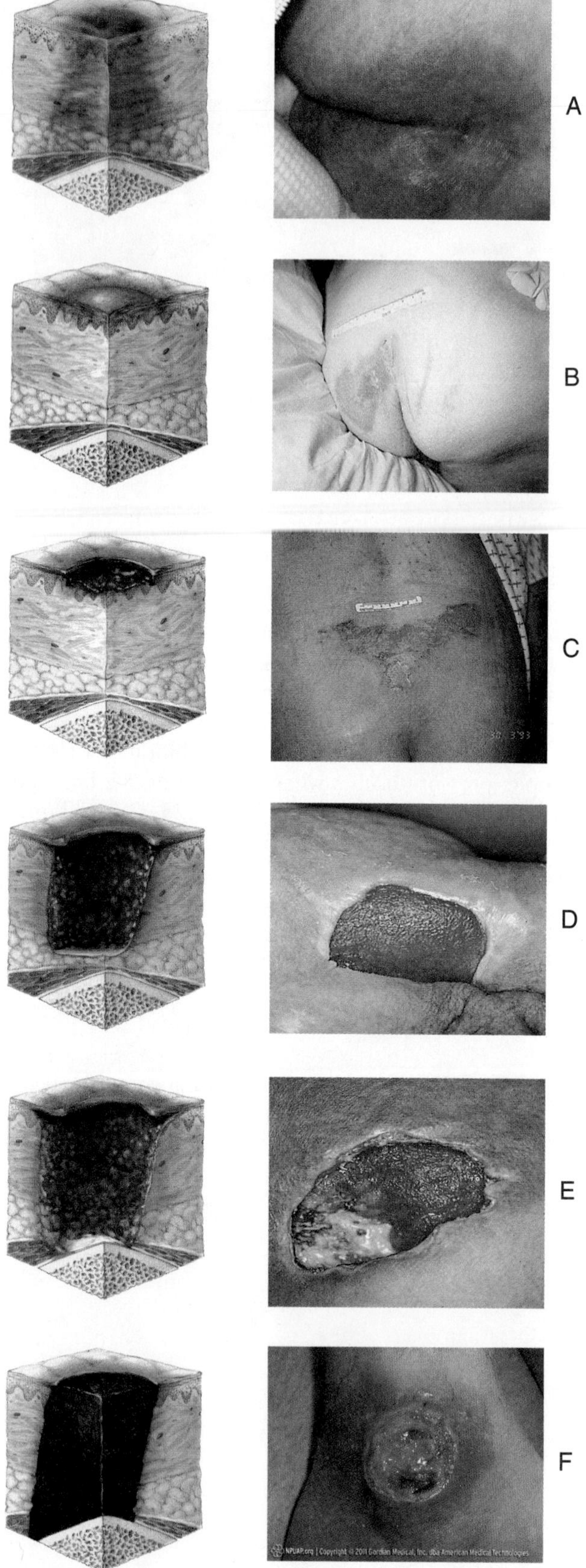

FIGURE 25-4 Pressure ulcer stages. **A,** Suspected deep tissue injury. **B,** Stage 1. **C,** Stage 2. **D,** Stage 3. **E,** Stage 4. **F,** Unstageable.

SITES

Pressure ulcers usually occur over bony prominences (pressure points). These areas bear the weight of the body in certain positions (see Fig. 25-1). Pressure from body weight can reduce the blood supply to the skin. According to the CMS, the sacrum is the most common site for a pressure ulcer. However, pressure ulcers on the heels often occur.

The ears also are sites for pressure ulcers. This is from pressure on the ear from the mattress when in the side-lying position. Eyeglasses and oxygen tubing (Chapter 26) also can cause pressure on the ears. A urinary catheter can cause pressure and friction on the meatus. Tubes, casts, braces, and other devices can cause pressure on arms, hands, legs, and feet. A pressure ulcer can develop where medical equipment is attached to the skin.

For people who are obese, pressure ulcers can occur in areas where skin has contact with skin. Common sites are between abdominal folds, the legs, the buttocks, the thighs, and under the breasts. Friction occurs in these areas.

PREVENTION AND TREATMENT

Preventing pressure ulcers is much easier than trying to heal them. Good nursing care, cleanliness, and skin care are essential. The measures in Box 25-2 help prevent skin breakdown and pressure ulcers. Always follow the person's care plan.

Some agencies use symbols or colored stickers as pressure ulcer alerts. They are placed on the person's door or chart. They remind the staff that the person is at risk for a pressure ulcer.

See *Focus on Surveys: Prevention and Treatment,* p. 404.

BOX 25-2 Preventing Pressure Ulcers

Moving and Positioning

- Follow the person's re-positioning schedule (Fig. 25-5, p. 404). Re-position bedfast persons at least every 1 to 2 hours. Re-position chairfast persons every hour. Some persons are re-positioned every 15 minutes.
- Remind persons sitting in chairs to shift their positions every 15 minutes.
- Position the person according to the care plan. Use pillows for support as directed. The 30-degree lateral position is recommended (Fig. 25-6, p. 404).
- Do not position the person:
    - On a pressure ulcer
    - On a reddened area
    - On tubes or other medical devices
- Do not leave a person on a bedpan longer than needed.
- Do not let the person sit on donut-shaped cushions.
- Prevent shearing and friction during moving and transfer procedures. Do not drag the person during positioning and transfers. Use assist devices as directed. See Chapter 14.
- Prevent friction in bed. Powder sheets lightly to prevent friction if directed to do so by the nurse.
- Prevent shearing. Do not raise the head of the bed more than 30 degrees. Follow the care plan for:
    - When to raise the head of the bed
    - How far to raise the head of the bed
    - How long (in minutes) to raise the head of the bed
- Use pillows, foam wedges, or other devices to prevent bony areas from contact with bony areas. The ankles, knees, hips, and sacrum are examples.
- Keep the heels and ankles off the bed. Use pillows or other devices as directed. Place the pillows or devices under the lower legs from mid-calf to the ankles.
- Use protective devices as directed.

Moving and Positioning—cont'd

- Support the person's feet properly. Use a footrest if the person's feet do not touch the floor when sitting in a chair. The body slides forward when feet do not touch the floor. For the person in a wheelchair, position the feet on the footrests.

Skin Care

- Inspect the skin every time you provide care. This includes during or after transfers, re-positioning, bathing, and elimination procedures. Report any concern at once.
- Follow the person's bathing schedule. Some persons do not need a bath every day.
- Do not use hot water to bathe or clean the skin. Hot water can irritate the skin.
- Use a cleansing agent as directed. Soap can dry and irritate the skin.
- Provide good skin care.
    - The skin is clean and dry after bathing.
    - The skin is free of moisture from a bath, urine, stools, sweat, wound drainage, and other secretions.
    - The areas under the breasts and the groin area are clean and dry.
- Follow measures to prevent incontinence.
- Prevent skin exposure to moisture. Check persons who are incontinent of urine or feces often. Provide good skin care and change linens and garments at the time of soiling. Use incontinence products as directed.
- Apply an ointment or moisture barrier if the person is incontinent of urine or feces.
- Check persons who perspire heavily or have wound drainage often. Change linens and garments as needed. Provide good skin care.
- Apply moisturizer to dry areas—hands, elbows, hips, ankles, heels, and so on. The nurse tells you what to use and what areas need attention.

Continued

BOX 25-2 Preventing Pressure Ulcers—cont'd

Skin Care—cont'd

- Give a back massage when re-positioning the person. Do not massage bony areas.
- Do not massage over pressure points. *Never rub or massage reddened areas.*
- Keep linens clean, dry, and wrinkle-free.
- Make sure the person's bed or chair is free of objects. Crumbs, pins, pencils, pens, and coins are examples.
- Do not irritate the skin. Avoid scrubbing or vigorous rubbing when bathing or drying the person.
- Use pillows and blankets to prevent skin from being in contact with skin. They also reduce moisture and friction.

Skin Care—cont'd

- Make sure clothes do not increase the risk for pressure ulcers.
  - Avoid thick seams, buttons, or zippers that press against the skin.
  - Avoid tight clothes.
  - Keep clothes from bunching up or wrinkling.
- Make sure socks and shoes are in good repair. Socks should not have wrinkles or creases. Make sure there is nothing in the shoes before the person puts them on.
- Do not apply heat or cold (Chapter 24) directly on a pressure ulcer.

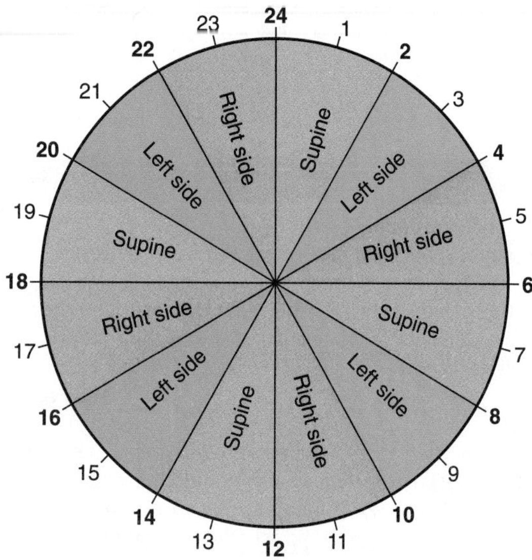

FIGURE 25-5 Turn clock. The clock shows the times to turn the person and to what position.

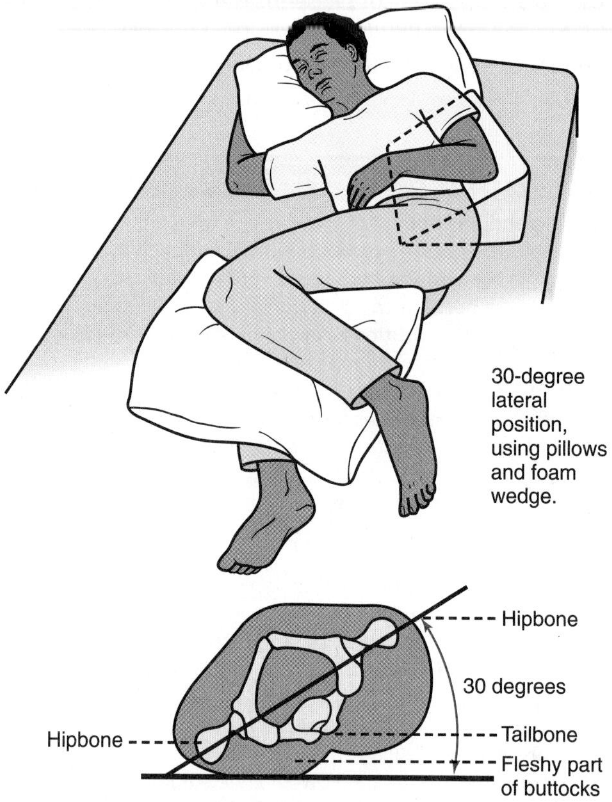

30-degree lateral position, using pillows and foam wedge.

Hipbone
30 degrees
Tailbone
Fleshy part of buttocks
Hipbone

FIGURE 25-6 The 30-degree lateral position. Pillows are placed under the head, shoulder, and leg. This position inclines (lifts up) the hip to avoid pressure on the hip. The person does not lie on the hip as in the side-lying position.

FOCUS ON SURVEYS

Prevention and Treatment

Some pressure ulcers are *avoidable*. That is, they develop because of improper use of the nursing process. Some pressure ulcers are *unavoidable*—they develop despite efforts to prevent them. Because pressure ulcers are very serious, they are a focus of surveys.

You may be interviewed during a site survey. You might be asked about:

- How you are involved in the person's care.
- What measures the agency uses to prevent pressure ulcers.
- What skin changes you should report and when.
- To whom you should report skin changes.
- Your knowledge of pressure ulcer prevention measures in the person's care plan.

Protective Devices

The doctor orders wound care products, drugs, treatments, and special equipment to promote healing. Support surfaces are used to relieve or reduce pressure. Such surfaces include foam, air, alternating air, gel, or water mattresses. The best surface for the person is used.

Protective devices are often used to prevent and treat pressure ulcers and skin breakdown. These devices are common.

- *Bed cradle.* A bed cradle is a metal frame placed on the bed and over the person (Chapter 23). Top linens are brought over the cradle to prevent pressure on the legs, feet, and toes.
- *Heel and elbow protectors.* These devices are made of foam padding, pressure-relieving gel, sheepskin, and other cushion materials. They fit the shape of heels and elbows (Fig. 25-7).
- *Heel and foot elevators.* These raise the heels and feet off of the bed (Fig. 25-8). They prevent pressure. Some also prevent footdrop (Chapter 23).
- *Gel or fluid-filled pads and cushions.* These devices involve a pressure-relieving gel or fluid (Fig. 25-9). They are used for chairs and wheelchairs to prevent pressure. The outer case is vinyl. The pad or cushion is placed in a fabric cover to protect the person's skin.
- *Special beds.* Some beds have air flowing through the mattresses (Fig. 25-10, p. 406). The person *floats* on the mattress. Body weight is distributed evenly. There is little pressure on body parts. Some beds allow re-positioning without moving the person. The person is turned to the prone or supine position or the bed is tilted various degrees. Alignment does not change. Pressure points change as the position changes. There is little friction. Some beds constantly rotate from side to side. They are useful for persons with spinal cord injuries.
- *Other equipment.* Pillows, trochanter rolls, foot-boards, and other positioning devices are used (Chapter 23). They help keep the person in good alignment.
- *Dressings.* Sometimes dressings are used. The wound must be moist enough to promote healing. If too moist, the dressing can interfere with healing. If a pressure ulcer has drainage, a dressing that absorbs drainage is used. The dressing absorbs slough. The slough is removed when the dressing is removed.

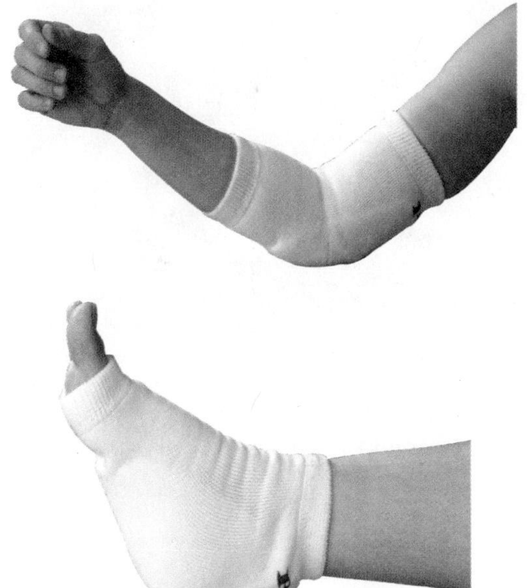

FIGURE 25-7 Heel and elbow protectors.

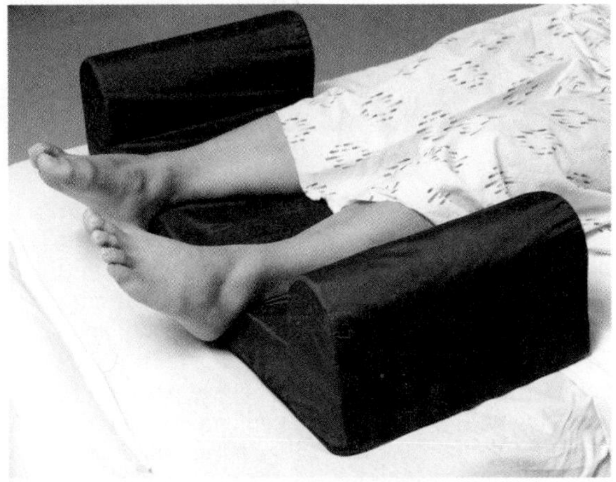

FIGURE 25-8 Heel elevator.

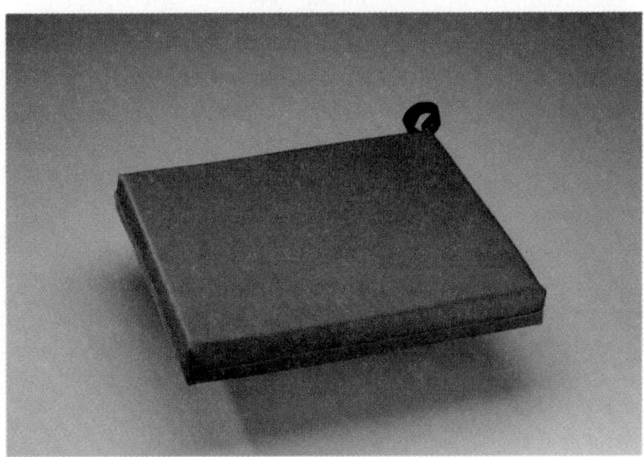

FIGURE 25-9 Gel and foam cushion with a 2-color cover. The colors remind the staff to re-position the person.

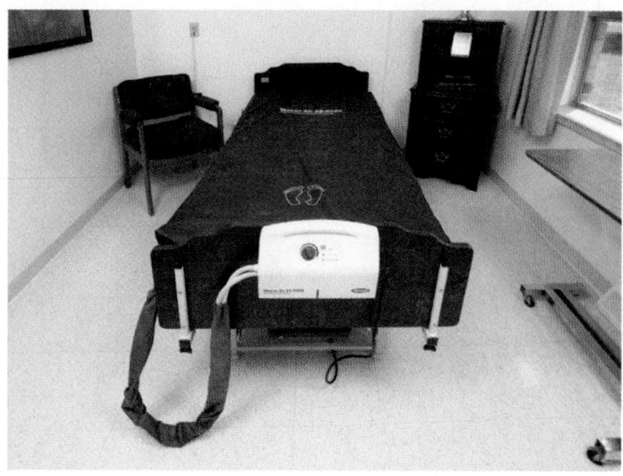

FIGURE 25-10 Air flotation bed.

COMPLICATIONS

Infection is the most common complication. According to the CMS, all Stage 2, 3, and 4 pressure ulcers are colonized with bacteria. *Colonized* refers to the presence of bacteria in a wound surface or in wound tissue. The person does not have signs and symptoms of an infection. A wound is *infected* when bacteria invade the tissue around or in the pressure ulcer. The person has signs and symptoms of infection (Chapter 12). Pain and delayed healing may signal an infection.

Osteomyelitis is a risk if the pressure ulcer is over a bony prominence. *Osteomyelitis* means inflammation *(itis)* of the bone *(osteo)* and bone marrow *(myel)*. Pain is severe. The person is treated with bedrest and antibiotics. Careful and gentle positioning is needed. Surgery may be needed to remove dead bone and tissue.

Pressure ulcers can cause pain. Pain management is important. Pain may affect movement and activity. Immobility is a risk factor for pressure ulcers. And it may delay healing of an existing pressure ulcer.

FOCUS ON PRIDE

The Person, Family, and Yourself

Personal and Professional Responsibility

You have an important role in preventing and treating pressure ulcers. Tasks like positioning, applying protective devices, and skin care may be delegated to you. Your care must improve the person's quality of life, health, and safety. Your attitude and the quality of your work affect the person. If you take your role seriously and believe you have a positive impact, the person will benefit. If you are careless and lack concern for the person's well-being, harm can result.

You are an important member of the nursing team. Take pride in your role. Work to the best of your ability. The person will benefit and you will find joy in your work.

Rights and Respect

You have the right and responsibility to speak for patients and residents. This is called being an advocate. When you see or suspect a problem, tell the nurse. You may be the first to notice a pressure ulcer. Telling the nurse can prevent further harm and result in prompt actions to promote healing. Take pride in being a voice for patients and residents.

Independence and Social Interaction

A pressure ulcer is a serious matter. Infection, pain, and longer hospital or nursing center stays are complications. Healing can be a very long process. As time passes, family and friends may not be able to visit often. Or the person may feel like a burden to others. Loneliness and depression can occur.

The person's physical needs are great. Do not neglect mental and social needs. Be kind. Show compassion. Take time to listen. Provide care in a way that improves the person's quality of life.

Delegation and Teamwork

You must report and record the completion of delegated tasks. Be accurate and honest. Never report or record something you did not do. Also, do not report or record before completing a task.

For example, Mrs. Scott was placed on the bedpan at 2250 (10:50 PM). The nursing assistant did not report this to the nurse. The next shift began at 2300 (11:00 PM). At 0700 (7:00 AM), the day shift found Mrs. Scott still on the bedpan. A pressure ulcer had developed. At risk for pressure ulcers, Mrs. Scott was to be re-positioned every 2 hours. Mrs. Scott's chart showed that she had been re-positioned every 2 hours from 2300 (11:00 PM) to 0700 (7:00 AM).

Poor communication, false recording, and negligence will cause harm. You must be thorough, honest, and careful when completing, reporting, and recording delegated tasks.

Ethics and Laws

Agencies must have a plan to predict, prevent, and treat pressure ulcers early. Many agencies use a form or screening tool to identify persons at risk. Assessments are done on admission and regularly. The agency must take action to address risks.

Know your agency's policies and procedures for identifying those at risk for pressure ulcers. Follow the measures in Box 25-2 and the person's care plan to do your part to prevent pressure ulcers.

REVIEW QUESTIONS

Circle* T *if the statement is TRUE or* F *if it is FALSE.

1 **T F** Unrelieved pressure squeezes tiny blood vessels. Tissues do not receive needed oxygen and nutrients.

2 **T F** Persons who are bedfast or chairfast are at risk for pressure ulcers.

3 **T F** Pressure ulcers can involve muscles, tendons, and bones.

4 **T F** Pressure ulcers can develop on the ears.

5 **T F** All pressure ulcers are avoidable.

6 **T F** To prevent pressure ulcers, the head of the bed is raised higher than 30 degrees.

7 **T F** You should inspect the person's skin every time you provide care.

8 **T F** You are giving a bath. You must dry under the breasts and in the groin area well.

9 **T F** You are giving a back massage. You should massage bony areas.

10 **T F** All Stage 2, 3, and 4 pressure ulcers are infected.

Circle the BEST answer.

11 Pressure ulcers are the result of
- **a** Unrelieved pressure
- **b** Moisture
- **c** Medical devices
- **d** Aging

12 Which can contribute to the development of pressure ulcers?
- **a** Shear
- **b** Slough
- **c** Bony prominences
- **d** Eschar

13 Which is *not* a risk factor for pressure ulcers?
- **a** Incontinence
- **b** Lowered mental awareness
- **c** Moisture
- **d** Balanced diet

14 The following are sources of moisture *except*
- **a** Urine and feces
- **b** Wound drainage
- **c** Sweat
- **d** Barrier ointment

15 In a light-skinned person, the first sign of a pressure ulcer is
- **a** A blister
- **b** A reddened area
- **c** Drainage
- **d** Gangrene

16 Which is the *most* common site for a pressure ulcer?
- **a** Back of the head
- **b** Hip
- **c** Sacrum
- **d** Heel

17 A care plan includes the following. Which should you question?
- **a** Re-position the person every 2 hours.
- **b** Scrub and rub the skin during bathing.
- **c** Apply lotion to dry areas.
- **d** Keep linens clean, dry, and wrinkle-free.

18 You should position the person
- **a** On an existing pressure ulcer
- **b** On a reddened area
- **c** On tubes or other medical devices
- **d** Using assist devices

19 What is the preferred position for preventing pressure ulcers?
- **a** 30-degree lateral position
- **b** Semi-Fowler's position
- **c** Prone position
- **d** Supine position

20 Which skin care measure should you question?
- **a** Use pillows to prevent skin to skin contact.
- **b** Apply a moisture barrier for incontinence.
- **c** Apply a hot compress to a pressure ulcer.
- **d** Change moist garments as often as needed.

21 Persons sitting in chairs should shift their positions every
- **a** 15 minutes
- **b** 30 minutes
- **c** Hour
- **d** 2 hours

22 You see a reddened area on the person's skin. What should you do?
- **a** Rub or massage the area.
- **b** Apply a moisturizer.
- **c** Apply a moisture barrier.
- **d** Tell the nurse.

Answers to these questions are on p. 505.

FOCUS ON **PRACTICE**

Problem Solving

Mr. Russell is at risk for pressure ulcers. He is to be re-positioned every 2 hours. He complains when you awaken him to provide care. You and a co-worker enter his room to re-position him. He is asleep. What will you do? What is the risk of waiting to re-position him? How can you provide safe, quality care that avoids causing him frustration?

CHAPTER

26 Assisting With Oxygen Needs

OBJECTIVES

- Define the key terms and key abbreviations listed in this chapter.
- Describe hypoxia and abnormal respirations.
- Explain the measures that promote oxygenation.
- Describe the devices used to give oxygen.
- Explain how to safely assist with oxygen therapy.
- Perform the procedures described in this chapter.
- Explain how to promote PRIDE in the person, the family, and yourself.

KEY TERMS

apnea The lack or absence *(a)* of breathing *(pnea)*
bradypnea Slow *(brady)* breathing *(pnea);* respirations are fewer than 12 per minute
Cheyne-Stokes respirations Respirations gradually increase in rate and depth and then become shallow and slow; breathing may stop *(apnea)* for 10 to 20 seconds
cyanosis Bluish color to the skin, lips, mucous membranes, and nail beds
dyspnea Difficult, labored, or painful *(dys)* breathing *(pnea)*
hyperventilation Breathing *(ventilation)* is rapid *(hyper)* and deeper than normal
hypoventilation Breathing *(ventilation)* is slow *(hypo),* shallow, and sometimes irregular
hypoxia Cells do not have enough *(hypo)* oxygen *(oxia)*
Kussmaul respirations Very deep and rapid respirations
orthopnea Breathing *(pnea)* deeply and comfortably only when sitting *(ortho)*
orthopneic position Sitting up *(ortho)* and leaning over a table to breathe *(pneic)*
oxygen concentration The amount (percent) of hemoglobin containing oxygen
tachypnea Rapid *(tachy)* breathing *(pnea);* respirations are more than 20 per minute

KEY ABBREVIATIONS

CO_2 Carbon dioxide
ID Identification
L/min Liters per minute
O_2 Oxygen
SpO_2 Saturation of peripheral oxygen (oxygen concentration)

Oxygen (O_2) is a gas. It has no taste, odor, or color. It is a basic need required for life. Death occurs within minutes if breathing stops. Brain damage and serious illness can occur without enough oxygen. Illness, surgery, and injuries affect the amount of oxygen in the body.

ALTERED RESPIRATORY FUNCTION

Hypoxia *means that cells do not have enough* (hypo) *oxygen* (oxia). Without enough O_2, cells cannot function properly. Anything affecting respiratory function can cause hypoxia. The brain is very sensitive to inadequate O_2. Restlessness is an early sign. So are dizziness and disorientation. Report the signs and symptoms in Box 26-1 at once.

Hypoxia threatens life. All organs need O_2 to function. Oxygen is given (p. 412). The cause of hypoxia is treated.

BOX 26-1 Altered Respiratory Function

- Hypoxia: signs and symptoms of
  - Restlessness
  - Dizziness
  - Confusion and disorientation
  - Behavior and personality changes
  - Concentrating and following directions: problems with
  - Anxiety and apprehension
  - Fatigue
  - Agitation
  - Pulse rate: increased
  - Respirations: increased rate and depth
  - Sitting position: often leaning forward
  - *Cyanosis (bluish color to the skin, lips, mucous membranes, and nail beds)*
  - Dyspnea
- Breathing pattern: abnormal
- Shortness of breath or complaints of being "winded" or "short-winded"
- Cough (note frequency and time of day)
  - Dry and hacking
  - Harsh and barking
  - Productive (produces sputum) or non-productive
- Sputum (mucus from the respiratory system)
  - Color: clear, white, yellow, green, brown, or red
  - Odor: none or foul odor
  - Consistency: thick, watery, or frothy (with bubbles or foam)
  - *Hemoptysis:* bloody *(hemo)* sputum (*ptysis* means *to spit*)
- Respirations: noisy—wheezing, wet-sounding, crowing sounds
- Chest pain (note location)
  - Constant or comes and goes
  - Person's description: stabbing, knife-like, aching
  - What makes it worse: movement, coughing, yawning, sneezing, sighing, deep breathing
- Position
  - Sitting upright
  - Leaning forward or hunched over a table

Abnormal Respirations

Adults normally breathe 12 to 20 times per minute. Normal respirations are quiet, effortless, and regular. Both sides of the chest rise and fall equally. These breathing patterns are abnormal (Fig. 26-1):

- ***Tachypnea***—*rapid* (tachy) *breathing* (pnea). *Respirations are more than 20 per minute.*
- ***Bradypnea***—*slow* (brady) *breathing* (pnea). *Respirations are fewer than 12 per minute.*
- ***Apnea***—*lack or absence* (a) *of breathing* (pnea).
- ***Hypoventilation***—*breathing* (ventilation) *is slow* (hypo), *shallow, and sometimes irregular.*
- ***Hyperventilation***—*breathing* (ventilation) *is rapid* (hyper) *and deeper than normal.*
- ***Dyspnea***—*difficult, labored, or painful* (dys) *breathing* (pnea).
- ***Cheyne-Stokes respirations***—*respirations gradually increase in rate and depth and then become shallow and slow. Breathing may stop* (apnea) *for 10 to 20 seconds.*
- ***Orthopnea***—*breathing* (pnea) *deeply and comfortably only when sitting* (ortho).
- ***Kussmaul respirations***—*very deep and rapid respirations.*

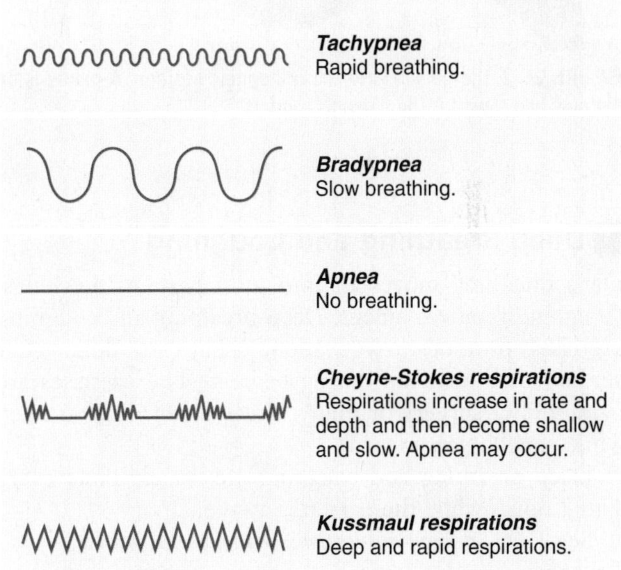

FIGURE 26-1 Some abnormal breathing patterns.

MEETING OXYGEN NEEDS

Air must move deep into the lungs to alveoli where O_2 and CO_2 (carbon dioxide) are exchanged. Disease, injury, and surgery can prevent air from reaching the alveoli. Pain, immobility, and some drugs interfere with deep breathing and coughing.

Positioning

Breathing is usually easier in the semi-Fowler's and Fowler's positions. Persons with difficulty breathing often prefer *sitting up and leaning over a table to breathe. This is called the* ***orthopneic position.*** (*Ortho* means *sitting* or *standing*. *Pneic* means *breathing*.) Place a pillow on the table to increase the person's comfort (Fig. 26-2).

Position changes are needed at least every 2 hours. Follow the care plan.

FOCUS ON COMMUNICATION

Deep Breathing and Coughing

To encourage cough etiquette (Chapter 12), you can say:

Please remember to cover your nose and mouth when coughing. I'll put these tissues where you can reach them. Here is a waste container to dispose of your tissues. Where would you like me to place it? Also, please remember to wash your hands often. Let me know if you need help.

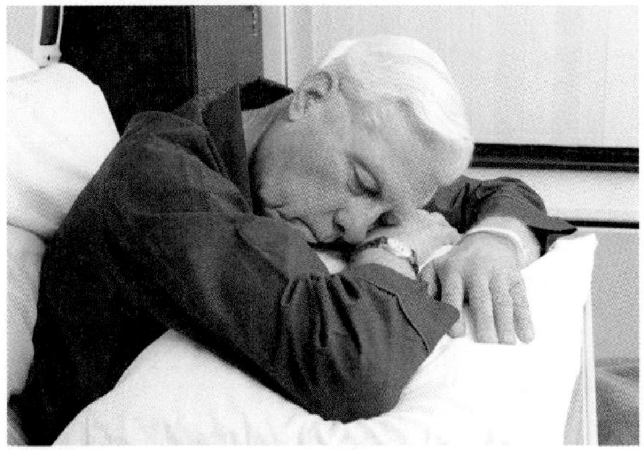

FIGURE 26-2 The person is in the orthopneic position. A pillow is on the over-bed table for the person's comfort.

DELEGATION GUIDELINES

Deep Breathing and Coughing

When delegated deep-breathing and coughing exercises, you need this information from the nurse and the care plan.

- When to do them and how often
- How many deep breaths and coughs the person needs to do
- What observations to report and record:
  - The number of deep breaths and coughs
  - How the person tolerated the procedure
- When to report observations
- What patient or resident concerns to report at once

Deep Breathing and Coughing

Deep breathing moves air into most parts of the lungs. Coughing removes mucus. Deep-breathing and coughing exercises promote oxygenation. They are done after surgery or injury and during bedrest. The exercises are painful after surgery or injury. Breaking an incision open while coughing is a fear.

Deep breathing and coughing are usually done every 1 to 2 hours while the person is awake.

See *Focus on Communication: Deep Breathing and Coughing.*

See *Delegation Guidelines: Deep Breathing and Coughing.*

See *Promoting Safety and Comfort: Deep Breathing and Coughing.*

See procedure: *Assisting With Deep-Breathing and Coughing Exercises.*

PROMOTING SAFETY AND COMFORT

Deep Breathing and Coughing

Safety

Respiratory hygiene and cough etiquette are needed if the person has a productive cough (Chapter 12). The person needs to:

- Cover the nose and mouth when coughing or sneezing.
- Use tissues to contain respiratory secretions.
- Dispose of tissues in the nearest waste container after use.
- Wash his or her hands after coughing or contact with respiratory secretions.

While the person is covering the nose and mouth, you need to splint his or her incision with your hands or a pillow. See step 8a in procedure: *Assisting With Deep-Breathing and Coughing Exercises.* Make sure you wear gloves to splint the incision.

Assisting With Deep-Breathing and Coughing Exercises

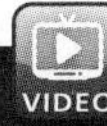

VIDEO

QUALITY OF LIFE

- Knock before entering the person's room.
- Address the person by name.
- Introduce yourself by name and title.
- Explain the procedure before starting and during the procedure.
- Protect the person's rights during the procedure.
- Handle the person gently during the procedure.

PRE-PROCEDURE

1 Follow *Delegation Guidelines: Deep Breathing and Coughing*. See *Promoting Safety and Comfort: Deep Breathing and Coughing*.
2 Practice hand hygiene.
3 Identify the person. Check the identification (ID) bracelet against the assignment sheet. Also call the person by name.
4 Provide for privacy.

PROCEDURE

5 Lower the bed rail if up.
6 Help the person to a comfortable sitting position: sitting on the side of the bed, semi-Fowler's, or Fowler's.
7 Have the person deep breathe.
 a Have the person place the hands over the rib cage (Fig. 26-3).
 b Have the person breathe as deeply as possible. Remind the person to inhale through the nose.
 c Ask the person to hold the breath for 2 to 3 seconds.
 d Ask the person to exhale slowly through pursed lips (Fig. 26-4, p. 412). Ask the person to exhale until the ribs move as far down as possible.
 e Repeat this step 4 more times.
8 Ask the person to cough.
 a Have the person place both hands over the incision. One hand is on top of the other (Fig. 26-5, *A*, p. 412). The person can hold a pillow or folded towel over the incision (Fig. 26-5, *B*, p. 412). If the person is covering the nose and mouth for respiratory hygiene, splint the incision with your hands or a pillow. Wear gloves.
 b Have the person take in a deep breath as in step 7.
 c Ask the person to cough strongly twice with the mouth open.

POST-PROCEDURE

9 Provide for comfort. (See the inside of the front cover.)
10 Place the call light within reach.
11 Raise or lower bed rails. Follow the care plan.
12 Unscreen the person.
13 Complete a safety check of the room. (See the inside of the front cover.)
14 Practice hand hygiene.
15 Report and record your observations.

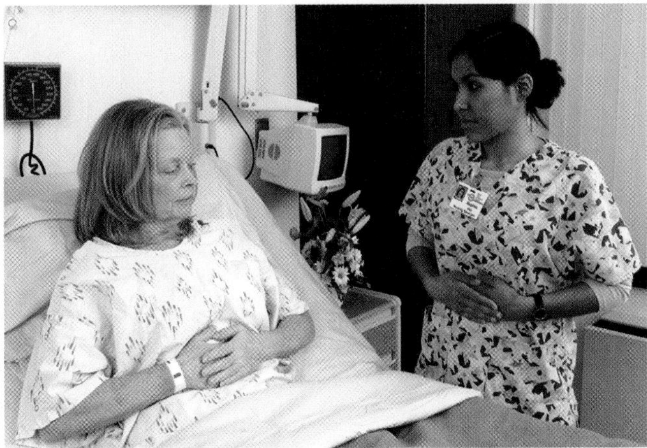

FIGURE 26-3 The hands are over the rib cage for deep breathing.

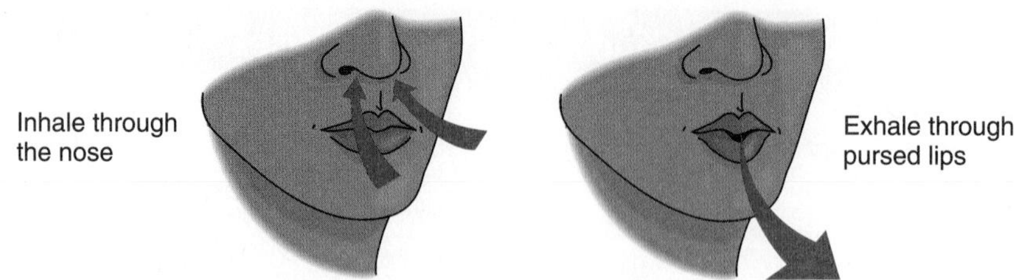

FIGURE 26-4 The person inhales through the nose and exhales through pursed lips during the deep-breathing exercise.

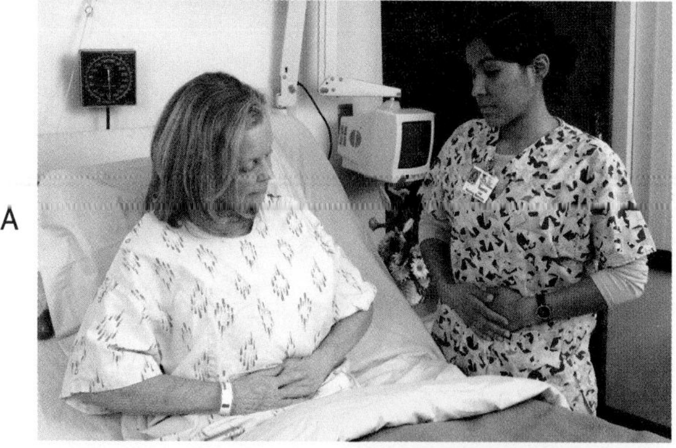

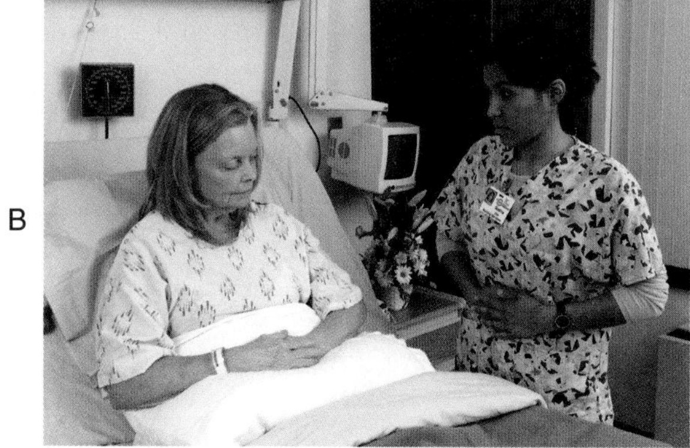

FIGURE 26-5 The incision is supported for the coughing exercise. **A,** The hands are over the incision. **B,** A pillow is held over the incision.

ASSISTING WITH OXYGEN THERAPY

Disease, injury, and surgery often interfere with breathing. The amount of O_2 in the blood may be less than normal *(hypoxemia)*. If so, the doctor orders oxygen therapy.

Oxygen is treated as a drug. The doctor orders when to give O_2, the amount, and the device to use. Some people need oxygen constantly. Others need it for symptom relief—chest pain or shortness of breath. Oxygen helps relieve chest pain. Persons with respiratory diseases may have enough oxygen at rest. With mild exercise or activity, they become short of breath. Oxygen helps to relieve shortness of breath.

You do not give oxygen. The nurse and respiratory therapist start and maintain oxygen therapy. You help provide safe care.

Pulse Oximetry

Pulse oximetry measures *(metry)* the oxygen *(oxi)* concentration in arterial blood. ***Oxygen concentration** is the amount (percent) of hemoglobin containing O_2.* The normal range is 95% to 100%. For example, if 97% of all hemoglobin (100%) carries O_2, tissues get enough oxygen. If only 90% contains O_2, tissues do not get enough oxygen.

A sensor attaches to a finger, toe, earlobe, nose, or forehead (Fig. 26-6). A good sensor site is needed. Avoid swollen sites and sites with skin breaks. Sometimes blood flow to the fingers or toes is poor. Then the earlobe, nose, and forehead sites are used.

Nail polish, fake nails, and movements affect measurements. Remove nail polish or use another site. Do not use a finger site if the person has fake nails. Blood pressure cuffs affect blood flow. If using a finger site, do not measure blood pressure on that side.

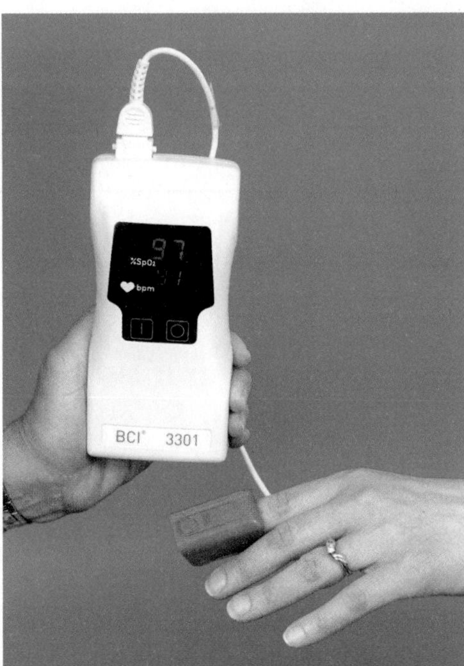

FIGURE 26-6 A pulse oximetry sensor is attached to a finger. The device displays the O_2 concentration and pulse.

Oxygen concentration is often measured with vital signs. Or it is monitored continuously. Alarms are set for continuous monitoring. An alarm sounds if O_2 concentration is low. Report and record oxygen concentration according to agency policy. An agency may use 1 of these terms.

- Pulse oximetry or pulse ox
- O_2 saturation or O_2 sat
- SpO_2 (saturation of peripheral oxygen)

See *Delegation Guidelines: Pulse Oximetry.*
See *Promoting Safety and Comfort: Pulse Oximetry.*
See procedure: *Using a Pulse Oximeter,* p. 414.

DELEGATION GUIDELINES

Pulse Oximetry

To assist with pulse oximetry, you need this information from the nurse and the care plan.

- What site to use
- How to use the equipment
- What sensor to use
- What type of tape to use (if needed)
- The person's normal range of SpO_2
- Alarm limits for SpO_2 and pulse rate (if set)
- When to do the measurement
- What pulse site to use: apical or radial
- How often to check the sensor site (usually every 2 hours)
- What observations to report and record:
  - The date and time
  - The SpO_2 and display pulse rate
  - Apical or radial pulse rate
  - What the person was doing at the time
  - Oxygen flow rate (p. 416) and the device used (p. 416)
  - Reason for the measurement: routine, continuous monitoring, or condition change
- When to report observations
- What patient or resident concerns to report at once:
  - An SpO_2 below the alarm limit (usually 95%)
  - A pulse rate above or below the alarm limit
  - The signs and symptoms listed in Box 26-1

PROMOTING SAFETY AND COMFORT

Pulse Oximetry

Safety

The person's condition can change quickly. Pulse oximetry does not lessen the need for good observations. Observe for signs and symptoms of hypoxia and altered respiratory system function (see Box 26-1).

Comfort

A clip-on sensor feels like a clothespin. It should not hurt or cause discomfort. Ask the person to tell you at once if it causes pain, discomfort, or too much pressure. Change the sensor site as directed by the nurse.

Using a Pulse Oximeter

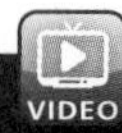

QUALITY OF LIFE

- Knock before entering the person's room.
- Address the person by name.
- Introduce yourself by name and title.
- Explain the procedure before starting and during the procedure.
- Protect the person's rights during the procedure.
- Handle the person gently during the procedure.

PRE-PROCEDURE

1 Follow *Delegation Guidelines: Pulse Oximetry,* p. 413. See *Promoting Safety and Comfort: Pulse Oximetry,* p. 413.
2 Practice hand hygiene.
3 Collect the following before going to the person's room.
- Oximeter
- Tape (if needed)
- Towel

4 Arrange your work area.
5 Practice hand hygiene.
6 Identify the person. Check the ID bracelet against your assignment sheet. Also call the person by name.
7 Provide for privacy.

PROCEDURE

8 Provide for comfort.
9 Dry the site with a towel.
10 Clip or tape the sensor to the site.
11 Turn on the oximeter.
12 Set the high and low alarm limits for SpO_2 and pulse rate. Turn on audio and visual alarms. (This step is for continuous monitoring.)
13 Check the person's pulse (apical or radial) with the pulse on the display. The pulse rates should be about the same. Note both pulses on your assignment sheet.
14 Read the SpO_2 on the display. Note the value on the flow sheet and your assignment sheet.
15 Leave the sensor in place for continuous monitoring. Otherwise, turn off the device and remove the sensor.

POST-PROCEDURE

16 Provide for comfort. (See the inside of the front cover.)
17 Place the call light within reach.
18 Unscreen the person.
19 Complete a safety check of the room. (See the inside of the front cover.)
20 Return the device to its proper place (unless monitoring is continuous).
21 Practice hand hygiene.
22 Report and record the SpO_2, the pulse rates, and your other observations.

Oxygen Sources

Oxygen is supplied as follows.

- *Wall outlet.* O_2 is piped into each person's unit (Fig. 26-7).
- *Oxygen tank.* The oxygen tank is placed at the bedside. Small tanks are used for emergencies and transfers. They also are used by persons who walk or use wheelchairs (Fig. 26-8). A gauge tells how much O_2 is left (Fig. 26-9).
- *Oxygen concentrator.* The machine removes O_2 from the air (Fig. 26-10). A power source is needed. A portable oxygen tank is needed for power failures and mobility.
- *Liquid oxygen system.* A portable unit is filled from a stationary unit. The portable unit has enough O_2 for about 8 hours of use. A dial shows the amount of O_2 in the unit. The portable unit is worn over the shoulder (Fig. 26-11).

See *Promoting Safety and Comfort: Oxygen Sources.*

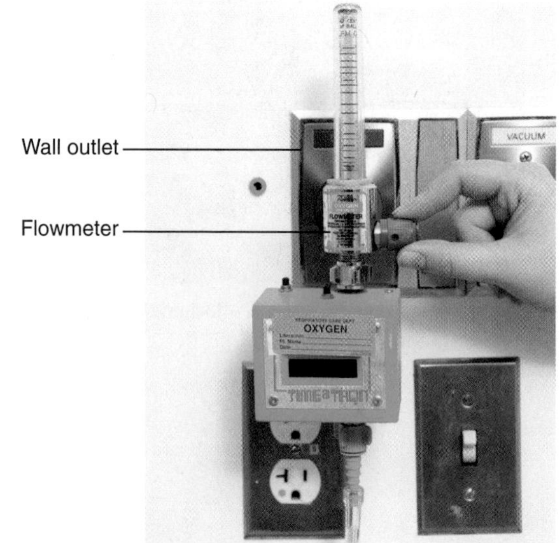

FIGURE 26-7 Wall oxygen outlet. The flowmeter is used to set the oxygen flow rate.

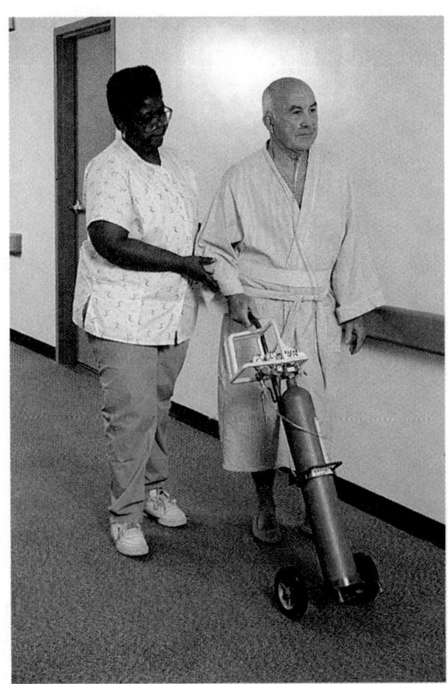

FIGURE 26-8 A portable oxygen tank is used when walking.

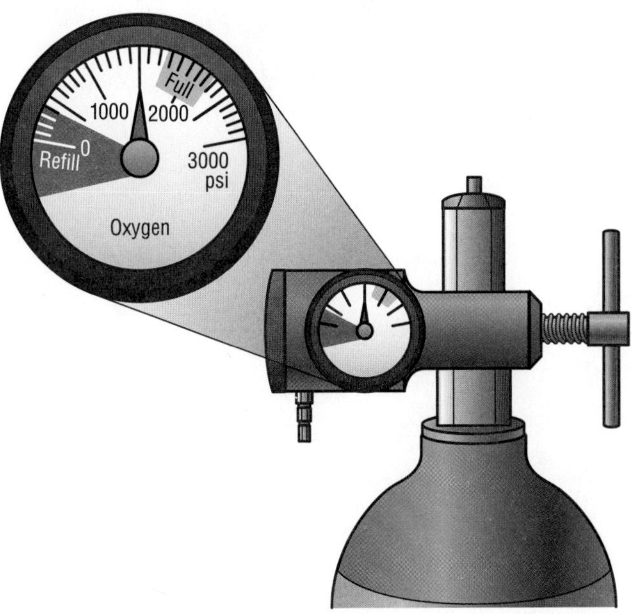

FIGURE 26-9 The gauge shows the amount of oxygen in the tank.

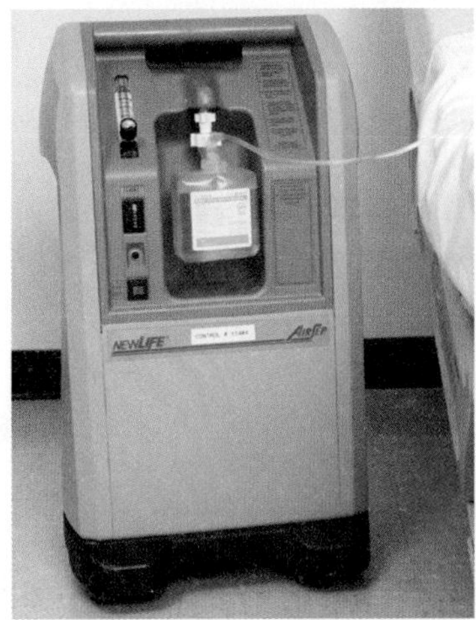

FIGURE 26-10 Oxygen concentrator.

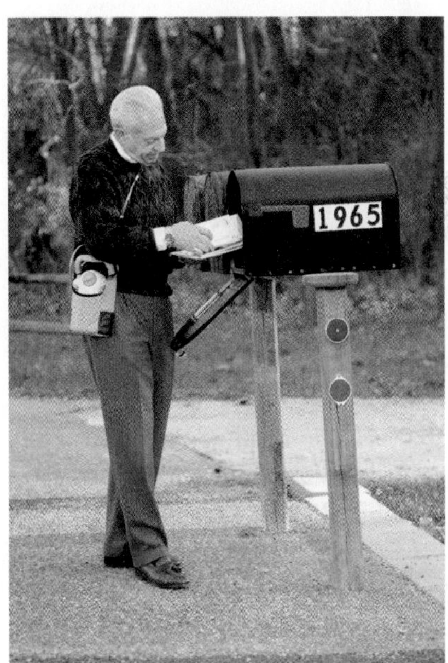

FIGURE 26-11 A portable liquid oxygen unit is worn over the shoulder.

PROMOTING SAFETY AND COMFORT

Oxygen Sources

Safety

Liquid oxygen is very cold. If touched, it can freeze the skin. Never tamper with the equipment. Doing so is unsafe and could damage the equipment. Follow agency procedures and the manufacturer's instructions when working with liquid oxygen.

Oxygen tanks and liquid oxygen systems contain a certain amount of O_2. When the O_2 level is low, a new tank is needed or the liquid oxygen system is refilled. Always check the O_2 level when you are with or near persons using these oxygen sources. Report a low O_2 level at once.

Oxygen Devices

The doctor orders the device for giving O_2. These devices are common:

- *Nasal cannula* (Fig. 26-12). The prongs are inserted into the nostrils (Fig. 26-13). A band goes behind the ears and under the chin to keep the device in place. A cannula allows eating and drinking. Tight prongs can irritate the nose. Pressure on the ears and cheekbones is possible.
- *Simple face mask* (Fig. 26-14). It covers the nose and mouth. The mask has small holes in the sides. CO_2 escapes when exhaling. Talking and eating are hard to do with a mask. Listen carefully. Moisture can build up under the mask. Keep the face clean and dry. This helps prevent irritation from the mask. For eating, the nurse changes the oxygen mask to a cannula.

Oxygen Flow Rates

The *flow rate* is the amount of oxygen given. It is measured in liters per minute (L/min). The doctor orders 1 to 15 liters of O_2 per minute. The nurse or respiratory therapist sets the flow rate with a flowmeter (see Fig. 26-7).

The nurse and care plan tell you the person's flow rate. When giving care and checking the person, always check the flow rate. Tell the nurse at once if it is too high or too low. A nurse or respiratory therapist will adjust the flow rate.

Oxygen Safety

You assist the nurse with oxygen therapy. *You do not give oxygen. You do not adjust the flow rate unless allowed by your state and agency.* However, you must give safe care. Follow the rules in Box 26-2. Also follow the rules for fire and the use of oxygen (Chapter 9).

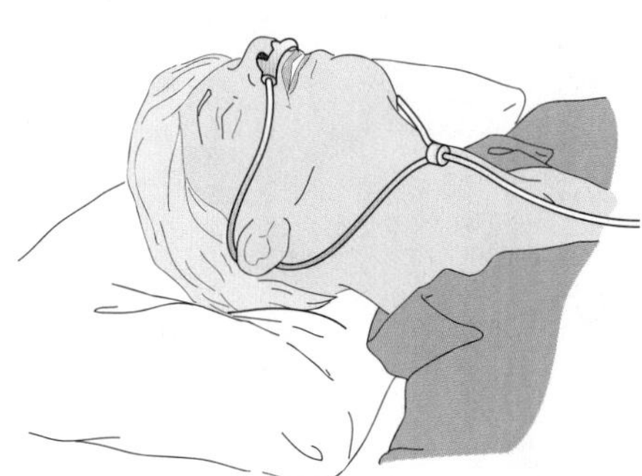

FIGURE 26-12 Nasal cannula.

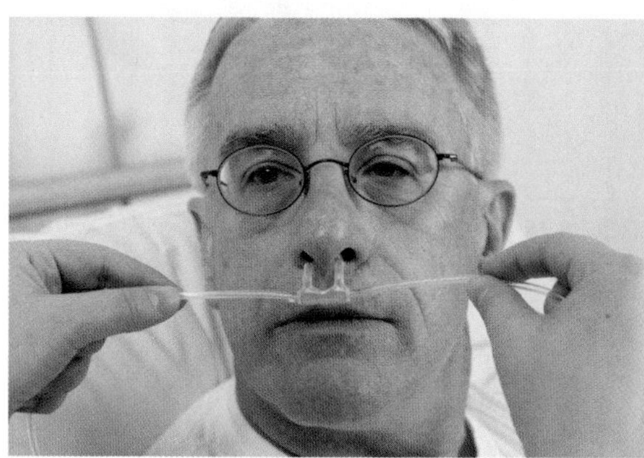

FIGURE 26-13 Cannula prongs are inserted. The prong openings face downward.

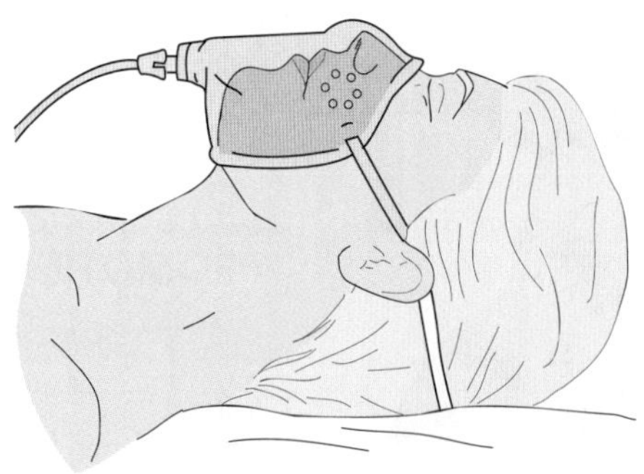

FIGURE 26-14 Simple face mask.

BOX 26-2 Oxygen Safety

- Do not remove the oxygen device.
- Make sure the oxygen device is secure but not tight.
- Check for signs of irritation from the device. Check behind the ears, under the nose (cannula), and around the face (mask). Also check the cheekbones.
- Keep the face clean and dry when a mask is used.
- Do not shut off the oxygen flow. *However, turn off the oxygen flow if there is a fire. Remove the oxygen device.*
- Do not adjust the flow rate unless allowed by your state and agency.
- Tell the nurse at once if the flow rate is too high or too low.
- Tell the nurse at once if a humidifier is not bubbling (Fig. 26-15). Humidified (moist) oxygen prevents drying of the airway's mucous membranes. Bubbling in the humidifier means that moisture is being produced.
- Maintain an adequate water level in the humidifier.
- Secure tubing in place. Tape or pin it to the person's garment following agency policy. Do not puncture the tubing.
- Make sure there are no kinks in the tubing.
- Make sure the person does not lie on any part of the tubing.
- Make sure the oxygen tank is secure in its holder.
- Report signs and symptoms of hypoxia, respiratory distress, or abnormal breathing patterns to the nurse at once (see Box 26-1).
- Give oral hygiene as directed. Follow the care plan.
- Make sure the oxygen device is clean and free of mucus.

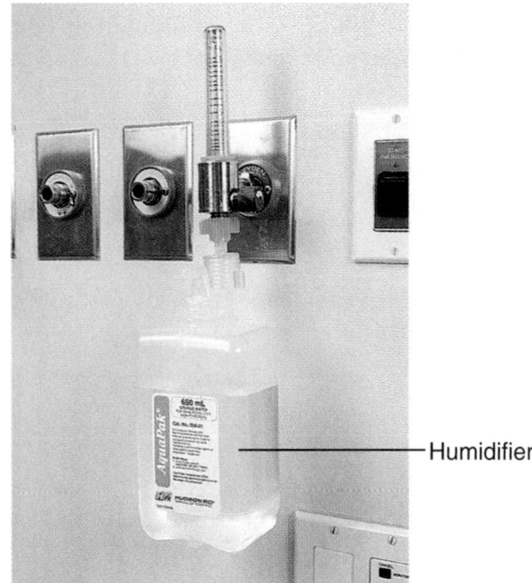

FIGURE 26-15 Oxygen set-up with a humidifier.

FOCUS ON PRIDE

The Person, Family, and Yourself

Personal and Professional Responsibility

You are responsible for reporting the person's complaints. A person may say: "I can't breathe" or "I'm not getting enough air." Yet you see the person breathing. Do not dismiss the complaint. Tell the nurse at once. You cannot feel what the person does. Trust what the person tells you.

Rights and Respect

People have the right to a safe setting. For safety, smoking is not allowed where oxygen is used and stored. NO SMOKING signs are common in rooms and hallways. You may need to remind the person or visitors not to smoke. Be polite and respectful. Show the person where smoking is allowed.

Independence and Social Interaction

The need for long-term oxygen therapy changes a person's life. Work, daily activities, and hobbies may be a challenge. The person may feel alone and depressed. Social support from family and friends is important.

Portable oxygen sources increase independence. Small oxygen tanks and portable liquid oxygen units are examples. Such devices allow freedom and promote quality of life.

Delegation and Teamwork

Activities increase the need for O_2. Moving in bed, transferring, and walking are examples. Persons receiving oxygen therapy need O_2 during activities. Plan ahead. If needed, ask the nurse to change to a portable oxygen tank. Or ask the nurse for longer tubing. Do not remove the person's device.

Before starting a procedure, plan ahead. Know what you need to collect, how you will perform the procedure, and if you need help.

Ethics and Laws

Oxygen is treated as a drug. State nurse practice acts allow nurses to give drugs. You assist the nurse with oxygen therapy. You do not give oxygen. You do not adjust the flow rate unless allowed by your state and agency and instructed to do so by the nurse.

If asked to give oxygen or adjust a flow rate, politely refuse. Remember, refusing to perform a task is your right and duty when the task is beyond the legal limits of your role. Do not ignore the request. Tell the nurse that you can assist. For example, you can gather and set up the supplies. Or ask if you can help with another task instead.

REVIEW QUESTIONS

Circle the BEST answer.

1 Hypoxia is
 a Not enough oxygen in the blood
 b The amount of hemoglobin that contains oxygen
 c Not enough oxygen in the cells
 d The lack of carbon dioxide

2 An early sign of hypoxia is
 a Cyanosis
 b Increased pulse and respiratory rates
 c Restlessness
 d Dyspnea

3 A person can breathe deeply and comfortably only while sitting. This is called
 a Apnea
 b Orthopnea
 c Bradypnea
 d Kussmaul respirations

4 Tachypnea means that respirations are
 a Slow
 b Rapid
 c Absent
 d Difficult or painful

5 Which should you report to the nurse at once?
 a A respiratory rate of 18 per minute
 b An SpO_2 of 97%
 c Bubbling in a humidifier
 d Dyspnea

6 A person has an SpO_2 of 98%. Which is *true?*
 a The pulse oximeter is wrong.
 b The pulse is 98 beats per minute.
 c The measurement is within normal range.
 d The person has hypoxia.

7 Which is *not* a site for a pulse oximetry sensor?
 a Toe
 b Finger
 c Earlobe
 d Upper arm

8 You are assisting with deep breathing and coughing. You need to explain the procedure again if the person
 a Inhales through pursed lips
 b Sits in a comfortable position
 c Inhales deeply through the nose
 d Holds a pillow over an incision

9 When assisting with oxygen therapy, you can
 a Turn the oxygen on and off
 b Start the oxygen
 c Decide what device to use
 d Keep connecting tubing secure and free of kinks

10 A person is receiving oxygen therapy. Which measure should you question?
 a Provide oral hygiene.
 b Check for signs of irritation.
 c Adjust the flow rate if it is too high or too low.
 d Secure tubing in place.

Answers to these questions are on p. 505.

FOCUS ON PRACTICE

Problem Solving

You are a student training in the clinical setting. You are helping a nursing assistant transfer a resident to a wheelchair. The nursing assistant asks you to connect the person's nasal cannula to the portable oxygen tank and turn it on to 2 L/min. Nursing assistants in your state are not allowed to adjust oxygen flow rates. How will you respond? What will you do if the nursing assistant adjusts the flow rate?

Assisting With Rehabilitation and Restorative Nursing Care

CHAPTER 27

OBJECTIVES

- Define the key terms and key abbreviations listed in this chapter.
- Describe how rehabilitation and restorative care involve the whole person.
- Identify the complications to prevent.
- Identify the common reactions to rehabilitation.
- Explain your role in rehabilitation and restorative nursing care.
- List the common rehabilitation programs and services.
- Explain how to promote PRIDE in the person, the family, and yourself.

KEY TERMS

activities of daily living (ADL) The activities usually done during a normal day in a person's life

disability Any lost, absent, or impaired physical or mental function

prosthesis An artificial replacement for a missing body part

rehabilitation The process of restoring the person to his or her highest possible level of physical, psychological, social, and economic function

restorative aide A nursing assistant with special training in restorative nursing and rehabilitation skills

restorative nursing care Care that helps persons regain health, strength, and independence

KEY ABBREVIATIONS

ADL Activities of daily living

ROM Range of motion

Disease, injury, birth defects, and surgery can affect body function. Often more than 1 function is lost. A ***disability*** *is any lost, absent, or impaired physical or mental function.*

Some disabilities are short-term. Others are permanent. Daily activities are hard or seem impossible. The person may depend totally or in part on others for basic needs. The degree of disability affects how much function is possible.

Rehabilitation *is the process of restoring the person to his or her highest possible level of physical, psychological, social, and economic function.* The goal is to improve abilities and function at the highest level of independence. Some persons have the goal of returning to work. For others, self-care is the goal. Sometimes improved function is not possible. Then the goal is to prevent further loss of function for the best possible quality of life.

Some people have suffered strokes, fractures, amputations, or other diseases and injuries. Some have had joint replacement surgery. All need to regain function. Some must adjust to a long-term disability. Some need home care or nursing center care.

RESTORATIVE NURSING

Some persons are weak. Many cannot perform daily functions. ***Restorative nursing care*** *is care that helps persons regain health, strength, and independence.* With progressive illnesses, disabilities increase. Restorative nursing:

- Helps maintain the highest level of function.
- Prevents unnecessary decline in function.

Restorative nursing measures promote:

- Self-care
- Elimination
- Positioning
- Mobility
- Communication
- Cognitive function

Many persons need both restorative nursing and rehabilitation. In many agencies, they mean the same thing. Both focus on the whole person.

Restorative Aides

Some agencies have restorative aides. A *restorative aide is a nursing assistant with special training in restorative nursing and rehabilitation skills.* These aides assist the nursing and health teams as needed. Required training varies among states. If there are no state requirements, the agency provides needed training.

REHABILITATION AND THE WHOLE PERSON

A health problem has physical, psychological, and social effects. So does a disability. The person needs to adjust physically, psychologically, socially, and economically. Abilities—what the person can do—are stressed. Complications are prevented. They can cause further disability.

See *Focus on Older Persons: Rehabilitation and the Whole Person.*

Physical Aspects

Rehabilitation starts when the person first seeks health care. Complications are prevented. They can occur from bedrest, a long illness, or recovery from surgery or injury. Bowel and bladder problems are prevented. So are contractures and pressure ulcers. Good alignment, turning and re-positioning, range-of-motion (ROM) exercises, and supportive devices are needed (Chapters 13, 14, and 23). Good skin care also prevents pressure ulcers (Chapters 16 and 25).

Elimination. Some persons need bladder training (Chapter 18). The method depends on the person's problems, abilities, and needs. Some need bowel training (Chapter 19). Control of bowel movements and regular elimination are goals. Fecal impaction, constipation, and fecal incontinence are prevented.

FOCUS ON OLDER PERSONS

Rehabilitation and the Whole Person

Rehabilitation takes longer in older persons than in other age groups. Changes from aging affect healing, mobility, vision, hearing, and other functions. Chronic health problems can slow recovery. Older persons are at risk for injuries. Fast-paced rehabilitation programs are hard for them. Their programs usually are slower-paced.

Self-Care. Self-care is a major goal. *Activities of daily living (ADL) are the activities usually done during a normal day in a person's life.* ADL include bathing, oral hygiene, dressing, eating, elimination, and moving about. The health team evaluates the person's ability to perform ADL. The need for self-help devices is considered.

Sometimes the hands, wrists, and arms are affected. Self-help devices are often needed. Equipment is changed, made, or bought to meet the person's needs.

- Eating devices include glass holders, plate guards, and silverware with curved handles or cuffs (Chapter 20). Some devices attach to splints (Fig. 27-1).
- Electric toothbrushes have back-and-forth brushing motions for oral hygiene.
- Adaptive devices for hygiene promote independence. Some are shown in Figure 27-2.
- Self-help devices are useful for cooking, dressing, writing, phone calls, and other tasks. Some are shown in Figure 27-3.

See *Focus on Surveys: Self-Care.*

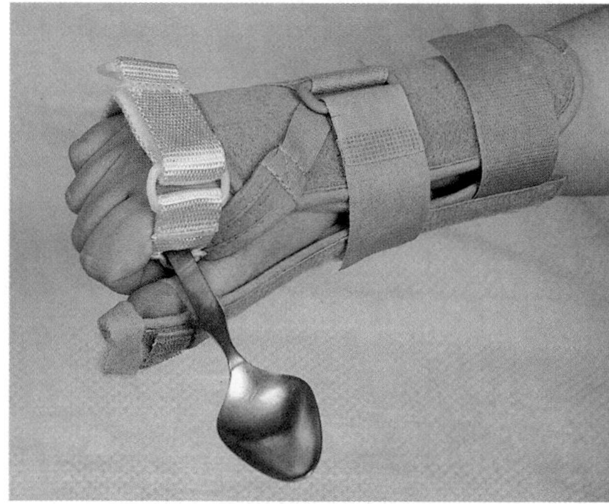

FIGURE 27-1 Eating device attached to a splint.

FOCUS ON SURVEYS

Self-Care

During a survey, attention is given to rehabilitation goals. The ability to perform self-care—bathing, dressing, and grooming—is an example. Surveyors will try to determine if:

- Care measures address the person's needs and rehabilitation goals. For example, a person needs a bath mitt. Is the mitt available? Does the person use the mitt to bathe? Does staff bathe the person instead of the person doing so?
- The care plan is followed by all staff.

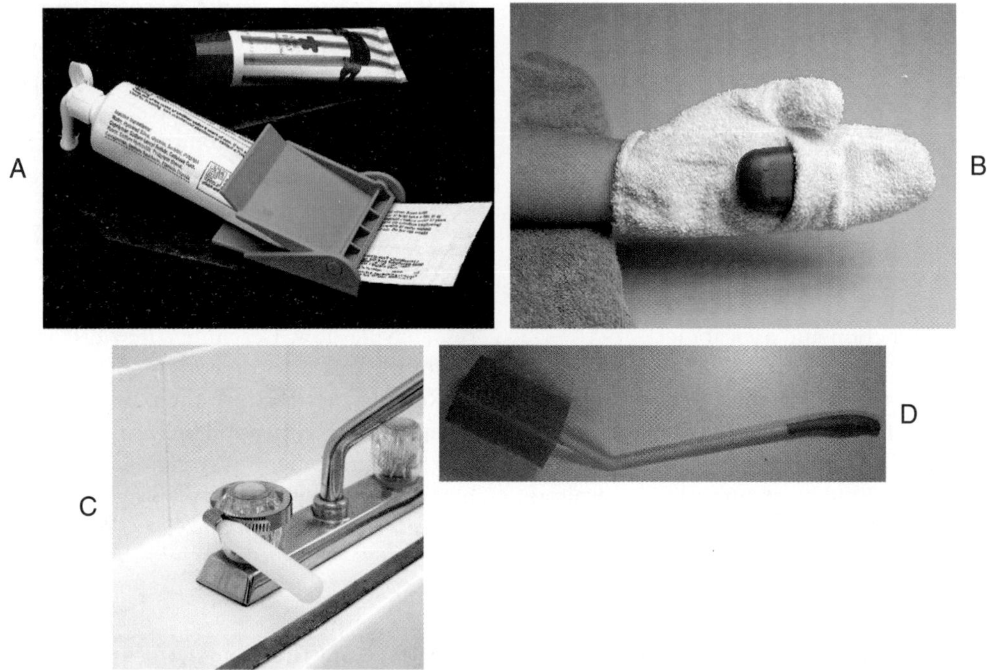

FIGURE 27-2 Adaptive devices for hygiene. **A,** Tube squeezer for toothpaste. **B,** The mitt holds a bar of soap. **C,** A tap turner makes round knobs easy to turn. **D,** A long-handled sponge is used for hard to reach body parts.

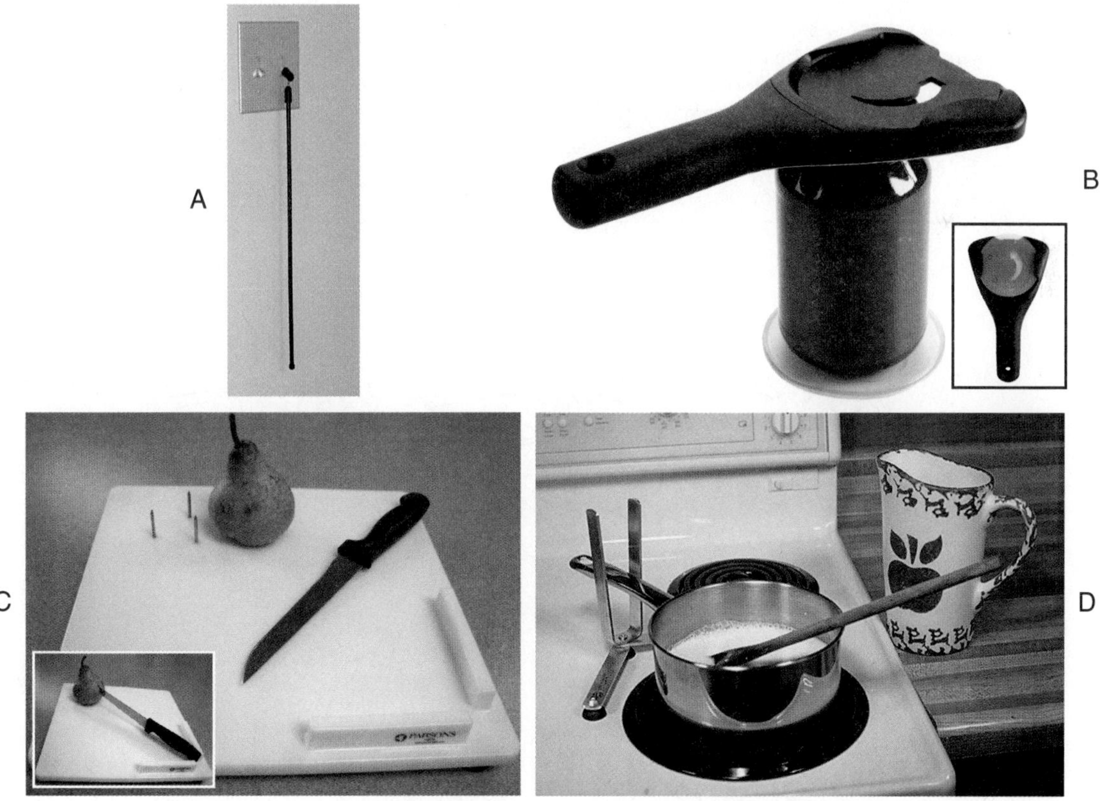

FIGURE 27-3 **A,** Light switch extender. **B,** Jar opener. **C,** Cutting board. **D,** Pot stabilizer.

Mobility. The person may need crutches or a walker, cane, or brace (Chapter 23). Physical and occupational therapies are common for musculo-skeletal and nervous system problems. Some people need wheelchairs. If possible, they learn wheelchair transfers to and from the bed, toilet, bathtub, sofa, and chair and in and out of vehicles (Fig. 27-4).

A ***prosthesis*** *is an artificial replacement for a missing body part.* The person learns how to use the artificial arm or leg (Chapter 28). The goal is for the device to be like the missing body part in function and appearance.

Nutrition. Difficulty swallowing *(dysphagia)* may occur after a stroke. The person may need a dysphagia diet (Chapter 20). When possible, the person learns exercises to improve swallowing. Some persons cannot swallow. They need enteral nutrition (Chapter 20).

Communication. *Aphasia* may occur from a stroke (Chapter 28). Aphasia is the total or partial loss *(a)* of the ability to use or understand language *(phasia).* Speech therapy and communication devices are helpful (Chapter 6).

See *Focus on Communication: Communication.*

FOCUS ON COMMUNICATION

Communication

Speaking is difficult or impossible for some persons. Persons with speech disorders may need other communication methods. Pictures, reading, writing, facial expressions, and gestures are examples. The person and health team decide on the best method. All health team members and the family use the same method with the person. Changing methods can cause confusion and delay progress.

Psychological and Social Aspects

A disability can affect function and appearance. Self-esteem and relationships may suffer. Some persons may feel unwhole, useless, unattractive, unclean, or undesirable. They may deny the disability and expect therapy to correct the problem. Some persons are depressed, angry, and hostile.

A good attitude is important. The person must accept his or her limits and be motivated. The focus is on abilities and strengths. Despair and frustration are common. Progress may be slow. Learning a new task is a reminder of the disability. Old fears and emotions may recur.

Remind persons of their *progress.* They need help accepting disabilities and limits. Give support, reassurance, and encouragement. Psychological and social needs are part of the care plan. Spiritual support helps some persons.

See *Focus on Communication: Psychological and Social Aspects.*

FOCUS ON COMMUNICATION

Psychological and Social Aspects

Denial, anger, depression, fear, and frustration are common during rehabilitation. Good communication and support provide encouragement. To deal with such emotions:

- Listen to the person.
- Show concern not pity.
- Focus on what the person can do. Point out even slight progress.
- Be polite but firm. Do not let the person control you.
- Do not shout at or insult the person. Such behaviors are abuse and mistreatment.
- Do not argue with the person.
- Tell the nurse. The person may need other support measures.

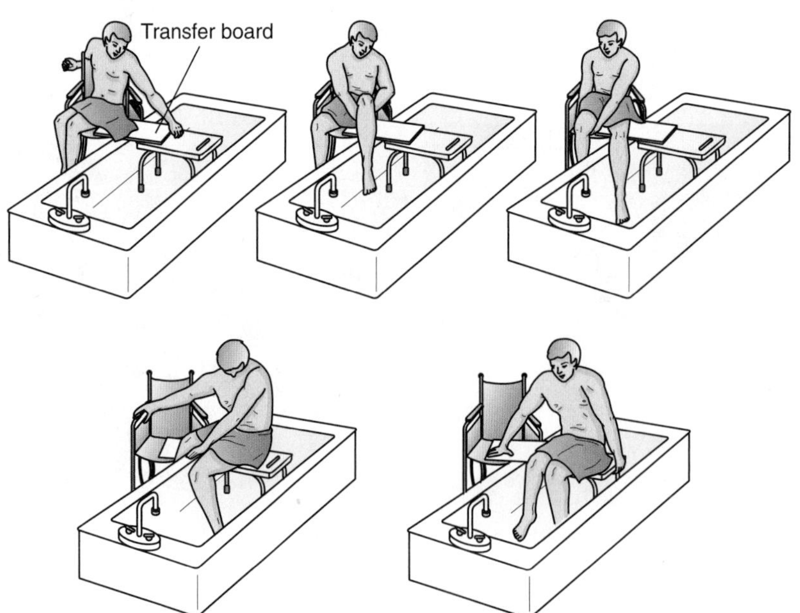

FIGURE 27-4 The person transfers from the wheelchair to the tub. A transfer board (sliding board) is used.

THE REHABILITATION TEAM

Rehabilitation is a team effort. The person is the key team member. The family, doctor, and nursing and health teams help the person set goals and plan care. The focus is on regaining function and independence.

The team meets often to discuss the person's progress. The rehabilitation plan is changed as needed. The person and family attend the meetings when possible. Families provide support and encouragement. Often they help with home care.

Your Role

You focus on promoting the person's independence. Preventing decline in function also is a goal. The many procedures, care measures, and rules in this book apply. Safety, communication, legal, and ethical aspects apply. So do the measures in Box 27-1.

See *Focus on Communication: Your Role.*

BOX 27-1 Assisting With Rehabilitation and Restorative Care

- Follow the care plan and the nurse's instructions.
- Follow the person's daily routine.
- Provide for safety.
- Protect the person's rights. Privacy and personal choice are very important.
- Report early signs and symptoms of complications. They include pressure ulcers, contractures, and bowel and bladder problems.
- Keep the person in good alignment at all times.
- Turn and re-position the person as directed.
- Use safe transfer methods.
- Practice measures to prevent pressure ulcers.
- Perform ROM exercises as instructed.
- Apply assistive devices as ordered.
- Provide needed self-help devices.
- Do not pity the person or give sympathy.
- Encourage the person to perform ADL to the extent possible.
- Give the person time to complete tasks. Do not rush the person.
- Give praise when even a little progress is made.
- Provide emotional support and reassurance.
- Try to understand and appreciate the person's situation, feelings, and concerns.
- Provide for spiritual needs.
- Practice the methods developed by the rehabilitation team. This helps you better assist the person.
- Practice the task that the person must do. This helps you guide and direct the person.
- Know how to apply the person's self-help devices.
- Know how to use the person's equipment.
- Stress what the person can do. Focus on abilities and strengths. Do not focus on disabilities and weaknesses.
- Remember that muscles will atrophy if not used. And contractures can develop.
- Have a hopeful outlook.

FOCUS ON COMMUNICATION

Your Role

You may need to guide and direct the person during care measures. First, listen to how the nurse or therapist guides and directs the person. Use those words. Hearing the same thing helps the person learn and remember what to do.

REHABILITATION PROGRAMS AND SERVICES

Rehabilitation begins when the person first needs health care. Often this is in the hospital. Common rehabilitation programs include:

- *Cardiac rehabilitation*—for heart disorders
- *Brain injury rehabilitation*—for nervous system disorders including traumatic brain injury
- *Spinal cord rehabilitation*—for spinal cord injuries
- *Stroke rehabilitation*—after a stroke
- *Respiratory rehabilitation*—for respiratory system disorders such as chronic obstructive pulmonary disease, after lung surgery, or for respiratory complications from other health problems
- *Musculo-skeletal rehabilitation*—for fractures, joint replacement surgery, and other musculo-skeletal problems
- *Rehabilitation for complex medical and surgical conditions*—for wound care, diabetes, burns, and other complex problems

The process often continues after hospital discharge. The person may need home care or care in a nursing center or rehabilitation agency. There are agencies for persons who are blind or deaf, have intellectual disabilities (formerly called mental retardation), are physically disabled, or have speech problems. Some agencies are for persons who are mentally ill. Substance abuse programs are common.

QUALITY OF LIFE

Successful rehabilitation and restorative care improves quality of life. The goal is independence to the greatest extent possible. A hopeful and winning outlook is needed. The more the person can do alone, the better his or her quality of life. To promote quality of life:

- Protect the right to privacy.
- Encourage personal choice.
- Protect the right to be free from abuse and mistreatment.
- Learn to deal with your anger and frustration.
- Encourage activities.
- Provide a safe setting.
- Show patience, understanding, and sensitivity.

FOCUS ON PRIDE

The Person, Family, and Yourself

Personal and Professional Responsibility

In some agencies, nursing assistants can advance to restorative aides. Some states require special training for certification. Students learn the knowledge and skills needed to assist with rehabilitation.

Professional behaviors are highly valued when considering which nursing assistants to promote. Those with a positive attitude, good work ethic, and excellent job performance are considered first. Restorative aides require patience, kindness, and good communication skills.

Seek out learning opportunities and practice positive work habits. Take pride in continuing to learn and improve as a nursing assistant.

Rights and Respect

Rehabilitation is challenging for the person, the family, and the nursing staff. No matter how difficult the situation, you must protect the person's rights.

- *Right to privacy*—The person re-learns old skills or practices new skills in private. No one needs to watch. They do not need to see mistakes, falls, spills, or clumsiness. Nor do they need to see anger or tears. Privacy protects dignity and promotes self-respect.
- *Right to be free from abuse and mistreatment*—Improvement may not be seen for weeks. Learning to use self-help devices and re-learning how to speak and dress take time. Simple things are often very hard to do. Repeated explanations and demonstrations may have no or little results. You, other staff, or the family may become upset and short-tempered. Protect the person from abuse and mistreatment. No one can shout at, scream at, yell at, or call the person names. They cannot hit or strike the person. Unkind remarks are not allowed. Report signs of abuse or mistreatment to the nurse.
- *Right to a safe setting*—The setting must meet the person's needs. Needed changes are made. The over-bed table, bedside stand, call light, and other needed items are moved to the person's strong side. If unable to use the call light, another form of communication is used.

Independence and Social Interaction

The more the person can do for himself or herself, the better his or her quality of life. To promote independence:

- Focus on what the person can do. Stress abilities and strengths. Do not show pity or sympathy.
- Encourage activities. Let the person do things of interest. The person usually chooses activities that he or she can do.
- Remain patient. Avoid rushing the person.
- Resist the urge to do things for the person that he or she can do. This hinders the person's ability to regain function. Remind the family to resist as well.
- Offer encouragement and support. The person may worry about how others view the disability. Remind the person that others have disabilities. They can give support and understanding. Persons who are sad and depressed may rely on others and not try to improve. Encourage them. Have a caring and positive attitude.
- Have the person use self-help devices as needed.
- Encourage personal choice. Not being able to control body movements or functions is very frustrating. Personal choice gives the person control.

Delegation and Teamwork

Disability affects the whole person. Anger and frustration are common. Many persons are upset and discouraged. Some have trouble controlling such feelings. They may have outbursts.

You may feel short-tempered. You must learn to deal with your anger and frustration. The person does not choose loss of function. If the process upsets you, think how the person must feel. You must show patience, understanding, sensitivity, and respect. You must be calm and professional. Control your words and actions. And give the person support and encouragement.

Managing your feelings can be a challenge. Share your feelings with the nurse. The nurse can suggest ways to help you control or express your feelings. You may need to assist with other persons for a while. Take pride in being a part of a strong, supportive team.

Ethics and Laws

The person may not want to practice rehabilitation procedures or methods. He or she may want you to provide care instead. Personal choice is important. However, the person needs to follow the rehabilitation plan. Otherwise, he or she will not make progress. Letting the person control you is the wrong thing to do. Report any problems to the nurse.

REVIEW QUESTIONS

Circle* T *if the statement is TRUE and* F *if it is FALSE.

1 T F You should give praise for even slight progress.

2 T F Speech therapy should be done in private.

3 T F A person is not allowed dessert until exercises are done. This is mistreatment.

4 T F A person refuses to attend a concert at the nursing center. The person must attend. It is part of the rehabilitation plan.

5 T F Rehabilitation for older persons is usually slower-paced than for younger persons.

6 T F You do not need to know how to apply self-help devices.

7 T F You need to know how to use the person's care equipment.

8 T F You need to convey hopefulness to the person.

Circle the BEST answer.

9 Rehabilitation and restorative nursing care focus on
- a What the person cannot do
- b Self-care
- c The whole person
- d Mobility and communication

10 Rehabilitation begins with preventing
- a Angry feelings
- b Contractures and pressure ulcers
- c Illness and injury
- d Loss of self-esteem

11 A person has weakness on the right side. ADL are
- a Done by the person to the extent possible
- b Done by you
- c Postponed until the right side can be used
- d Supervised by a therapist

12 To provide emotional support during rehabilitation
- a Remind the person of his or her limits
- b Give sympathy and show pity
- c Politely correct mistakes
- d Listen and give praise

13 During therapy, a person wants music played. You should
- a Explain that music is not allowed
- b Choose some music
- c Ask the person to choose some music
- d Ask a therapist to choose some music

14 A person's right side is weak. You moved the call light to the left side. You promoted quality of life by
- a Protecting the person from abuse and mistreatment
- b Allowing personal choice
- c Providing for safety
- d Taking part in activities

Answers to these questions are on p. 505.

FOCUS ON PRACTICE

Problem Solving

Ms. Mills requires rehabilitation after a hip fracture. The care plan includes long-handled devices for dressing and bathing. While helping Ms. Mills bathe, you give her the long-handled sponge. She says: "I don't feel like using that today. Will you wash my feet for me?" What will you say and do? How will your response affect her progress?

CHAPTER

28 Caring for Persons With Common Health Problems

OBJECTIVES

- Define the key terms and key abbreviations listed in this chapter.
- Describe cancer and how it is treated.
- Describe musculo-skeletal and nervous system disorders and the care required.
- Describe hearing loss and eye disorders and the care required.
- Describe cardiovascular and respiratory disorders and the care required.
- Describe digestive, urinary, and reproductive disorders and the care required.
- Describe endocrine, immune system, and skin disorders and the care required.
- Explain how to promote PRIDE in the person, the family, and yourself.

KEY TERMS

aphasia The total or partial loss *(a)* of the ability to use or understand language *(phasia)*
arthritis Joint *(arthr)* inflammation *(itis)*
arthroplasty The surgical replacement *(plasty)* of a joint *(arthro)*
benign tumor A tumor that does not spread to other body parts
cancer See "malignant tumor"
emesis See "vomitus"
fracture A broken bone
hemiplegia Paralysis *(plegia)* on 1 side *(hemi)* of the body
malignant tumor A tumor that invades and destroys nearby tissues and can spread to other body parts; cancer
metastasis The spread of cancer to other body parts
paralysis Loss of muscle function, sensation, or both
paraplegia Paralysis in the legs and lower trunk
quadriplegia Paralysis in the arms, legs, and trunk; tetraplegia
tetraplegia See "quadriplegia"
tumor A new growth of abnormal cells
vomitus The food and fluids expelled from the stomach through the mouth; emesis

KEY ABBREVIATIONS

AIDS	Acquired immunodeficiency syndrome
ALS	Amyotrophic lateral sclerosis
BPH	Benign prostatic hyperplasia
CAD	Coronary artery disease
CO_2	Carbon dioxide
COPD	Chronic obstructive pulmonary disease
CVA	Cerebrovascular accident
HBV	Hepatitis B virus
HIV	Human immunodeficiency virus
IV	Intravenous
MI	Myocardial infarction
mm Hg	Millimeters of mercury
MS	Multiple sclerosis
O_2	Oxygen
RA	Rheumatoid arthritis
ROM	Range of motion
STD	Sexually transmitted disease
TB	Tuberculosis
TIA	Transient ischemic attack
UTI	Urinary tract infection

Understanding common health problems gives meaning to the required care. The nurse gives you more information as needed. Refer to Chapter 7 as you study this chapter.

CANCER

Cells reproduce for tissue growth and repair. Cells divide in an orderly way. Sometimes cell division and growth are out of control. A mass or clump of cells develops. This *new growth of abnormal cells is called a* ***tumor***. Tumors are benign or malignant (Fig. 28-1).

- ***Benign tumors*** *do not spread to other body parts.* They can grow to a large size, but rarely threaten life. They usually do not grow back when removed.
- ***Malignant tumors (cancer)*** *invade and destroy nearby tissues. They can spread to other body parts.* They may be life-threatening. Sometimes they grow back after removal.

Metastasis *is the spread of cancer to other body parts* (Fig. 28-2). Cancer cells break off the tumor and travel to other body parts. New tumors grow at those sites. This occurs if cancer is not treated and controlled.

Cancer can occur almost anywhere. Common sites are the skin, lung and bronchus, colon and rectum, breast, prostate, uterus, ovary, urinary bladder, kidney, mouth and pharynx, pancreas, and thyroid gland.

Cancer Risk Factors

Cancer is the second leading cause of death in the United States. The National Cancer Institute describes these risk factors.

- *Growing older.* Cancer occurs in all age-groups. However, most cancers occur in persons over 65 years of age.
- *Tobacco.* This includes using tobacco (smoking, snuff, and chewing tobacco) and being around tobacco (second-hand smoke).
- *Sunlight.* Sun, sunlamps, and tanning booths cause early aging of the skin and skin damage. These can lead to skin cancer.
- *Ionizing radiation.* This can cause cell damage that leads to cancer. Sources are x-rays and radon gas that forms in the soil and some rocks. Radioactive fallout is another source. It can come from the production, testing, or use of atomic weapons.
- *Certain chemicals and other substances.* Examples include paint, pesticides, and used engine oil.
- *Some viruses and bacteria.* Certain viruses increase the risk of cancers—cervical, liver, lymphoma, leukemia, Kaposi's sarcoma (associated with AIDS, p. 452), stomach.
- *Certain hormones.* Hormone replacement for menopause is an example. It may increase the risk of breast cancer.
- *Family history of cancer.* Certain cancers tend to occur in families. They include melanoma and cancers of the breast, ovary, prostate, and colon.
- *Alcohol.* More than 2 drinks a day increases the risk of certain cancers—mouth, throat, esophagus, larynx, liver, and breast.
- *Poor diet, lack of physical activity, and being over-weight.* A high-fat diet increases the risk of cancers of the colon, uterus, and prostate. Lack of physical activity and being over-weight increase the risk for cancers of the breast, colon, esophagus, kidney, and uterus.

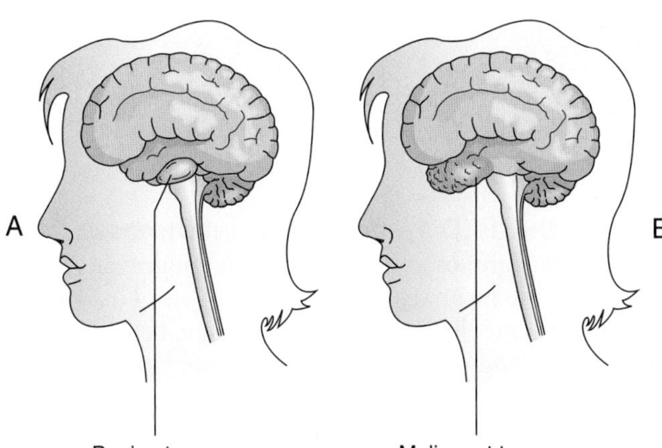

FIGURE 28-1 Tumors. **A,** A benign tumor grows within a local area. **B,** A malignant tumor invades other tissues.

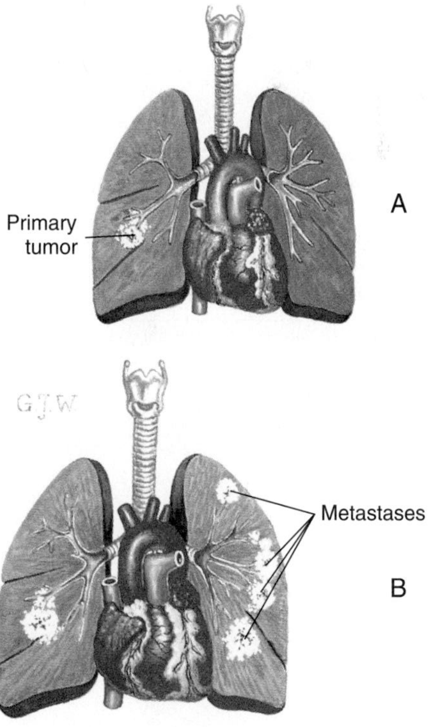

FIGURE 28-2 **A,** Tumor in the lung. **B,** Tumor has metastasized to the other lung.

Cancer Treatment

If detected early, cancer can be treated and controlled (Box 28-1). Treatment depends on the tumor type, its site and size, and if it has spread. The treatment goal may be to:

- Cure the cancer.
- Control the disease.
- Reduce symptoms for as long as possible.

Surgery, radiation therapy, and chemotherapy are the most common treatments.

- Surgery removes tumors.
- Radiation therapy kills cells. X-ray beams are aimed at the tumor. Sometimes radioactive material is implanted in or near the tumor. Cancer cells and normal cells receive radiation. Both are destroyed. Burns, skin breakdown, and hair loss can occur at the treatment site. Special skin care measures are ordered. Extra rest is needed for fatigue. Discomfort, nausea, vomiting, diarrhea, and loss of appetite *(anorexia)* are other side effects.
- *Chemotherapy* involves drugs that kill cells. Cancer cells and normal cells are affected. Side effects include hair loss *(alopecia)*, poor appetite, nausea, vomiting, diarrhea, and *stomatitis*—inflammation *(itis)* of the mouth *(stomat)*. Bleeding and infection are risks from decreased blood cell production.

BOX 28-1 Some Signs and Symptoms of Cancer

General Signs and Symptoms

- Thickening or lump in the breast or any other body part
- New mole or a change in an existing mole
- A sore that does not heal
- Hoarseness or cough that does not go away
- Changes in bowel or bladder habits
- Discomfort after eating
- A hard time swallowing
- Weight gain or loss with no known reason
- Unusual bleeding or discharge
- Feeling weak or very tired *(fatigue)*

Modified from National Cancer Institute: What you need to know about cancer,™ *NIH Publication No. 06-1566, Bethesda, Md, revised February 2005.*

The Person's Needs

Persons with cancer have many needs. They include:

- Pain relief or control
- Rest and exercise
- Fluids and nutrition
- Preventing skin breakdown
- Preventing bowel problems—constipation from pain-relief drugs; diarrhea from some cancer treatments
- Dealing with treatment side effects
- Psychological and social needs
- Spiritual needs
- Sexual needs

Anger, fear, and depression are common. Some surgeries are disfiguring. The person may feel unwhole, unattractive, or unclean. The person and family need support.

Spiritual needs are important. A spiritual leader may provide comfort. To many people, spiritual needs are just as important as physical needs.

Persons dying of cancer often receive hospice care (Chapters 1 and 32). Support is given to the person and family.

See *Focus on Communication: The Person's Needs.*

FOCUS ON COMMUNICATION

The Person's Needs

Knowing what to say to a person with cancer can be hard. Do not avoid the person. Talk as you would with any other person. Avoid comments like "I'm sure you will be fine" or "It will be okay."

Often the person needs to talk and have someone listen. Listen and use touch to show that you care. Being there when needed is important. You may not have to say anything. Just listen.

MUSCULO-SKELETAL DISORDERS

Musculo-skeletal disorders affect movement. Activities of daily living, social activities, and quality of life are affected. Injury and aging are common causes of musculo-skeletal disorders.

Arthritis

***Arthritis** means joint* (arthr) *inflammation* (itis). Pain, swelling, and stiffness occur in the affected joints. The joints are hard to move.

Osteoarthritis (Degenerative Joint Disease). This is the most common type of arthritis. Aging, being overweight, and joint injury are common causes. The fingers, spine (neck and lower back), and weight-bearing joints (hips, knees, and feet) are often affected.

Joint stiffness occurs with rest and lack of motion. Pain occurs with weight-bearing and motion. Or pain is constant or occurs from lack of motion. Pain can affect rest, sleep, and mobility. Cold weather and dampness seem to increase symptoms.

There is no cure. Treatment involves:

- *Pain relief.* Drugs decrease swelling and inflammation and relieve pain.
- *Heat and cold.* Heat relieves pain, increases blood flow, and reduces swelling. Cold applications may be used after joint use.
- *Exercise.* Exercise decreases pain, increases flexibility, and improves blood flow. It helps with weight control and promotes fitness. Mental well-being improves. The person is taught what exercises to do.
- *Rest and joint care.* Good body mechanics, posture, and regular rest protect the joints. Relaxation methods are helpful. Canes and walkers provide support. Splints support weak joints and keep them in alignment.
- *Weight control.* If over-weight, weight loss reduces stress on weight-bearing joints. And it helps prevent further joint injury.
- *Healthy life-style.* The focus is on fitness, exercise, rest, managing stress, and good nutrition.

Falls are prevented. Help is given with activities of daily living (ADL) as needed. Toilet seat risers are helpful when hips and knees are affected. So are chairs with higher seats and armrests. Some people need joint replacement surgery.

Rheumatoid Arthritis. Rheumatoid arthritis (RA) is a chronic inflammatory disease. It causes joint pain, swelling, stiffness, and loss of function. More common in women, it usually develops between the ages of 20 and 50.

RA occurs on both sides of the body. For example, if the right wrist is involved, so is the left wrist. The wrist and finger joints near the hand are often affected (Fig. 28-3). Other joints affected are the neck, shoulders, elbows, hips, knees, ankles, and feet. Joints are tender, warm, and swollen. Other body parts may be affected. Fatigue and fever are common. The person does not feel well. Symptoms may last for many years.

Treatment goals are to:

- Relieve pain.
- Reduce inflammation.
- Slow down or stop joint damage.

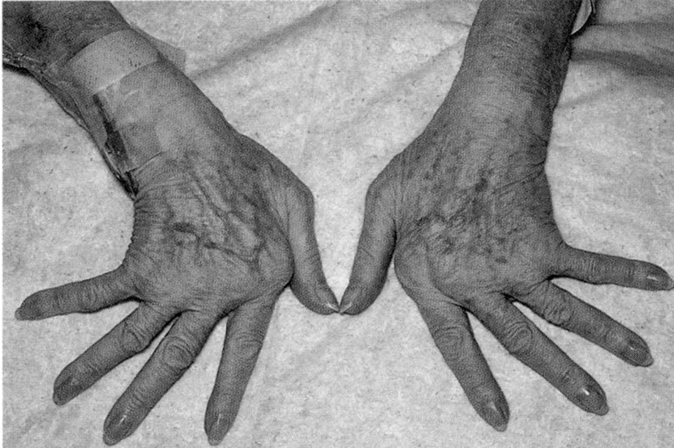

FIGURE 28-3 Deformities caused by rheumatoid arthritis.

The person's care plan may include:

- *Rest balanced with exercise.* Short rest periods during the day are better than long times in bed. An exercise program is prescribed. Range-of-motion (ROM) exercises are included. Exercise helps maintain healthy and strong muscles, joint mobility, and flexibility. It also promotes sleep, reduces pain, and helps weight control.
- *Proper positioning.* Contractures and deformities are prevented. Bed-boards, a bed cradle, trochanter rolls, and pillows are used.
- *Joint care.* Good body mechanics and body alignment, wrist and hand splints, and self-help devices reduce stress on joints. Some need walking aids.
- *Weight control.* Excess weight places stress on the weight-bearing joints. Exercise and a healthy diet help control weight.
- *Measures to reduce stress.* Relaxation, distraction, exercise, and regular rest help reduce stress.
- *Measures to prevent falls.* See Chapter 10.

Drugs are given for pain relief and inflammation. Heat and cold applications may be ordered. Some persons need joint replacement surgery.

Emotional support is needed. A good outlook is important. Persons with RA need to stay as active as possible. The more they can do for themselves, the better off they are. Give encouragement and praise. Listen when the person needs to talk.

Joint Replacement Surgery. *Arthroplasty is the surgical replacement* (plasty) *of a joint* (arthro). The damaged joint is removed and replaced with an artificial joint *(prosthesis)*.

Hip and knee replacements are common. See Box 28-2. Ankle, foot, shoulder, elbow, and finger joints also can be replaced.

BOX 28-2 Care Measures After Joint Replacement Surgery—Hip and Knee

- Deep-breathing and coughing exercises to prevent respiratory complications (Chapter 26).
- Elastic stockings to prevent thrombi (blood clots) in the legs.
- Exercises to strengthen the hip or knee. These are taught by a physical therapist.
- Measures to protect the hip as shown in Figure 28-4, p. 430.
- Food and fluids for tissue healing and to restore strength.
- Safety measures to prevent falls.
- Measures to prevent infection. Wound, urinary tract, and skin infections must be prevented.
- Measures to prevent pressure ulcers (Chapter 25).
- Assist devices for moving, turning, re-positioning, and transfers.
- Assistance with walking and a walking aid. The person may need a cane, walker, or crutches.

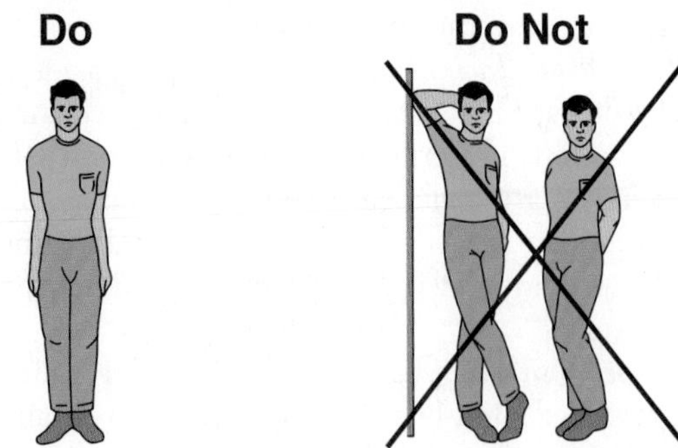

Do not cross your operated leg past the mid-line of the body or turn your kneecap in toward your body.

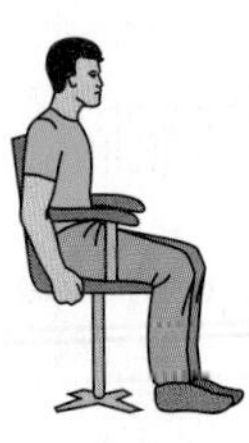

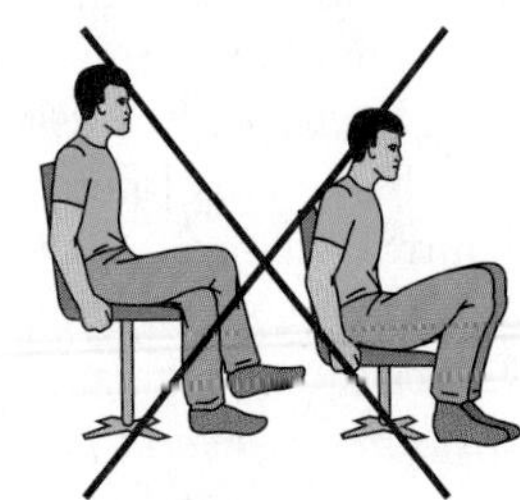

Do not sit in low chairs or cross your legs.

To sit: Use a high chair with arms or add pillows to elevate the seat.

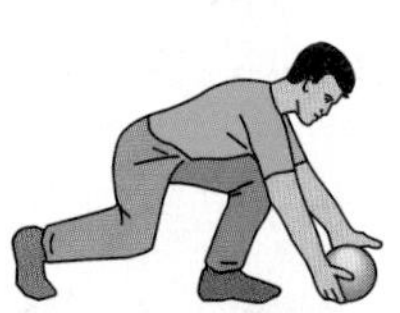

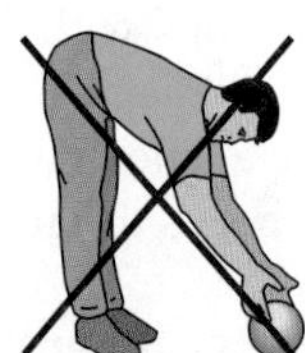

Avoid flexing your hips past 90 degrees.

To bend: Keep the operative leg behind you or as instructed by your therapist.

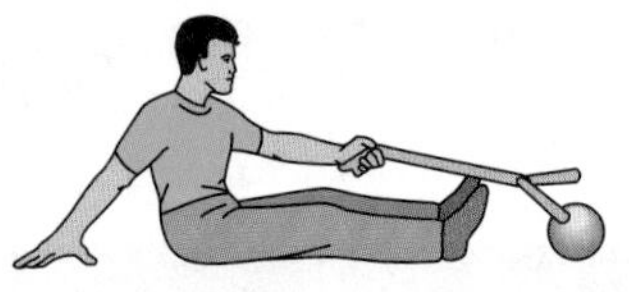

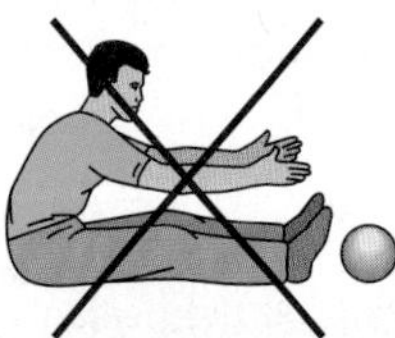

To reach: Use long-handled grabbers or as your therapist advises.

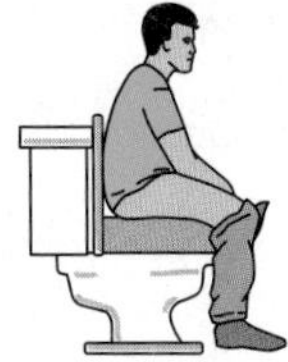

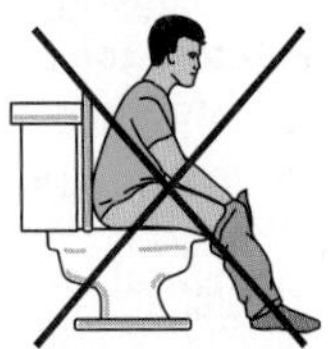

Use an elevated toilet.

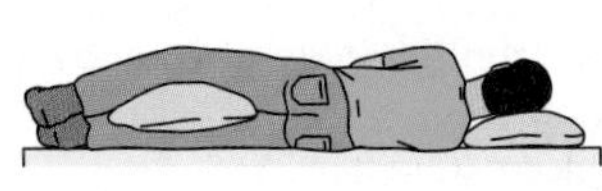

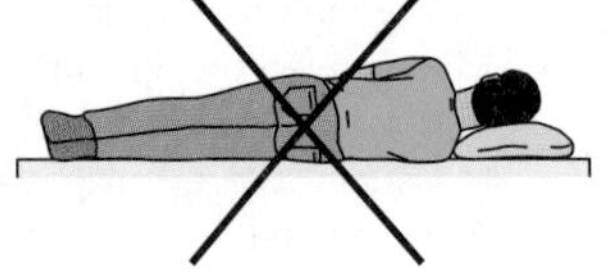

Sleep with a pillow between the legs.

FIGURE 28-4 Measures to protect the hip after hip replacement surgery.

Osteoporosis

With osteoporosis, the bone *(osteo)* becomes porous and brittle *(porosis)*. Bones are fragile and break easily. Spine, hip, wrist, and rib fractures are common.

Older people are at risk. The risk for women increases after menopause because the ovaries do not produce estrogen. The lack of estrogen and low levels of dietary calcium cause bone changes.

All ethnic groups are at risk. Other risk factors include a family history of the disease, being thin or having a small frame, eating disorders (Chapter 29), tobacco use, alcoholism, lack of exercise, bedrest, and immobility. Exercise and activity are needed for bone strength. Bone must bear weight to form properly. If not, calcium is lost from the bone. The bone becomes porous and brittle.

Back pain, gradual loss of height, and stooped posture occur. Fractures are a major threat. Even slight activity can cause fractures. They can occur from turning in bed, getting up from a chair, or coughing. Fractures are great risks from falls and accidents.

Prevention is important. Doctors often order calcium and vitamin supplements. Estrogen is ordered for some women. Other preventive measures include:

- Exercising weight-bearing joints—walking, jogging, stair climbing
- No smoking
- Limiting alcohol and caffeine
- Back supports or corsets for good posture
- Walking aids if needed
- Safety measures to prevent falls and accidents
- Good body mechanics
- Safe moving, transferring, turning, and positioning procedures

Fractures

A *fracture is a broken bone.* Fractures are open or closed (Fig. 28-5).

- *Open fracture (compound fracture).* The broken bone has come through the skin.
- *Closed fracture (simple fracture).* The bone is broken but the skin is intact.

Falls, accidents, bone tumors, and osteoporosis are some causes. Signs and symptoms of a fracture are:

- Pain
- Swelling
- Loss of function or movement
- Movement where motion should not occur
- Deformity (the part is in an abnormal position)
- Bruising and skin color changes at the fracture site
- Bleeding (internal or external)

For healing, bone ends are brought into and held in normal position. This is called *reduction* and *fixation.*

- *Closed reduction and external fixation.* The bone is moved back into place. The bone is not exposed.
- *Open reduction and internal fixation.* This requires surgery. The bone is exposed and moved into alignment. Nails, rods, pins, screws, plates, or wires keep the bone in place.

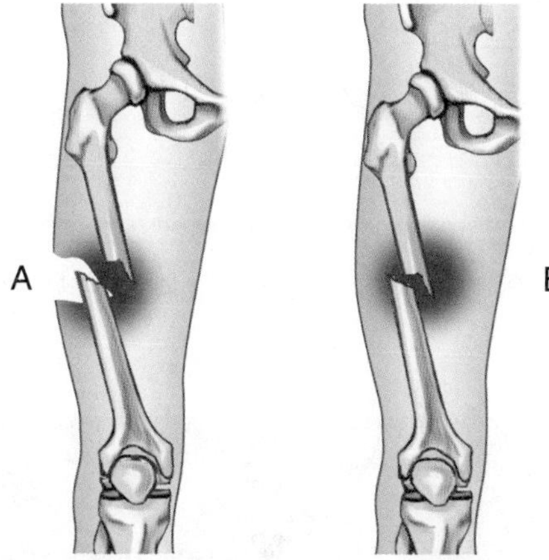

FIGURE 28-5 A, Open fracture. **B,** Closed fracture.

After reduction, the bone ends must not move. The person has a cast or traction. Splints, walking boots, and external fixators also are used.

- *Casts.* Casts are made of plaster of Paris, plastic, or fiberglass. Plastic and fiberglass casts dry quickly. A plaster of Paris cast dries in 24 to 48 hours. It is odorless, white, and shiny when dry. When wet, it is gray and cool and has a musty smell. The nurse may ask you to assist with care (Box 28-3).
- *Traction.* A steady pull from 2 directions keeps the bone in place. Weights, ropes, and pulleys are used (Fig. 28-8). Traction is applied to the neck, arms, legs, or pelvis. To assist with the person's care, see Box 28-4, p. 432.

BOX 28-3 Cast Care

- Do not cover the cast with blankets, plastic, or other material. A cast gives off heat as it dries. Covers prevent the escape of heat. Burns can occur if heat cannot escape.
- Turn the person every 2 hours or as directed. All cast surfaces need exposure to air. Turning promotes even drying.
- Do not place a wet cast on a hard surface. It flattens the cast. The cast must keep its shape. Use pillows to support the entire length of the cast (Fig. 28-6, p. 432).
- Support the wet cast with your palms to turn and position the person (Fig. 28-7, p. 432). Fingertips can dent the cast. The dents can cause pressure areas and skin breakdown.
- Report rough cast edges. The nurse needs to cover the cast edges with tape.
- Keep the cast dry. A wet cast loses its shape. Some casts are near the perineal area. The nurse may apply a waterproof material around the perineal area after the cast dries.
- Do not let the person insert anything into the cast. Itching under the cast causes an intense desire to scratch. Items used for scratching (pencils, coat hangers, knitting needles, back scratchers, and so on) can open the skin. Infection is a risk. Scratching items can wrinkle the stockinette or cotton padding. Or they can be lost into the cast. Both can cause pressure and skin breakdown.
- Elevate a casted arm or leg on pillows. This reduces swelling.
- Have enough help to turn and re-position the person. Plaster casts are heavy and awkward. Balance is lost easily.
- Position the person as directed.
- Follow the care plan for elimination needs. Some persons use a fracture pan.
- Report these signs and symptoms at once.
  - *Pain*—pressure ulcer, poor circulation, nerve damage
  - *Swelling and a tight cast*—reduced blood flow to the part
  - *Pale skin*—reduced blood flow to the part
  - *Cyanosis (bluish skin color)*—reduced blood flow to the part
  - *Odor*—infection
  - *Inability to move the fingers or toes*—pressure on a nerve
  - *Numbness*—pressure on a nerve, reduced blood flow to the part
  - *Temperature changes*—cool skin means poor circulation; hot skin means inflammation
  - *Drainage on or under the cast*—infection or bleeding
  - *Chills, fever, nausea, and vomiting*—infection
- Complete a safety check before leaving the room. (See the inside of the front cover.)

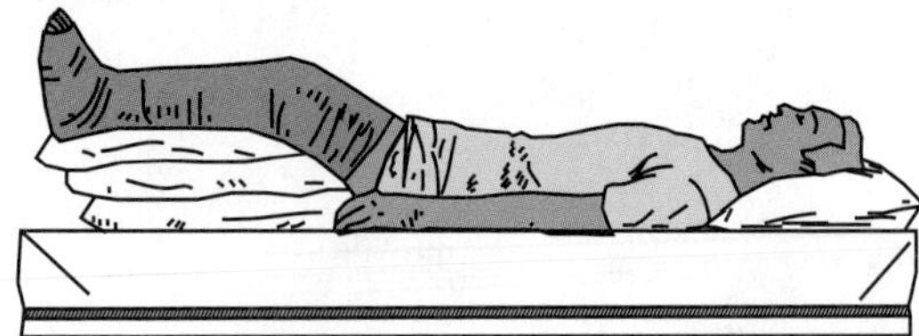

FIGURE 28-6 Pillows support the entire length of the wet cast.

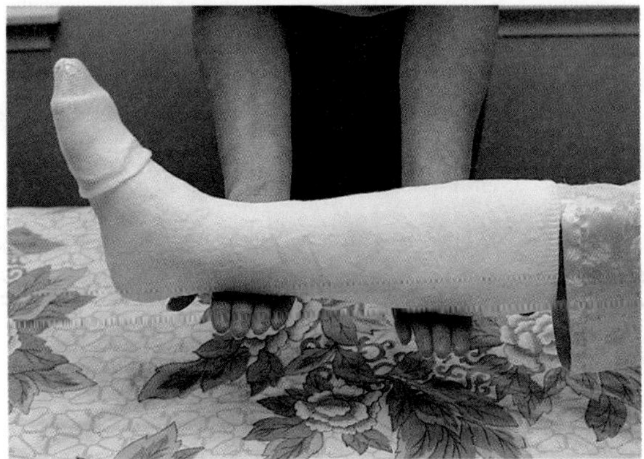

FIGURE 28-7 The cast is supported with the palms.

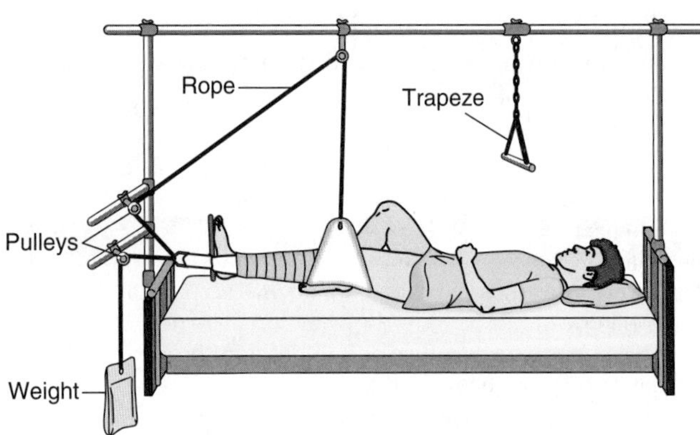

FIGURE 28-8 Traction set-up. Note the weight, pulleys, and rope. A trapeze is used to raise the upper body off the bed.

BOX 28-4 Caring for Persons in Traction

- Keep the person in good alignment.
- Do not remove the traction.
- Keep the weights off the floor. Weights must hang freely from the traction set-up (see Fig. 28-8).
- Do not add or remove weights.
- Check for frayed ropes. Report fraying at once.
- Perform ROM exercises for the uninvolved joints as directed.
- Position the person as directed. Usually only the supine position is allowed. Slight turning may be allowed.
- Provide the fracture pan for elimination.
- Give skin care as directed.
- Put bottom linens on the bed from the top down. The person uses a trapeze to raise the upper body off the bed (see Fig. 28-8).
- Check pin, nail, wire, or tong sites for redness, drainage, and odors. Report observations at once.
- Observe for the signs and symptoms listed under cast care (see Box 28-3). Report them at once.
- Complete a safety check before leaving the room. (See the inside of the front cover.)

Hip Fractures. Fractured hips are common in older persons (Fig. 28-9). The fracture requires internal fixation (p. 431) or partial or total hip replacement. Adduction, internal rotation, external rotation, and severe hip flexion are avoided after surgery. Rehabilitation is usually needed.

Post-operative problems present life-threatening risks. They include respiratory complications, urinary tract infections, and thrombi (blood clots) in the leg veins. Pressure ulcers, constipation, and confusion are other risks. Box 28-5 describes the required care.

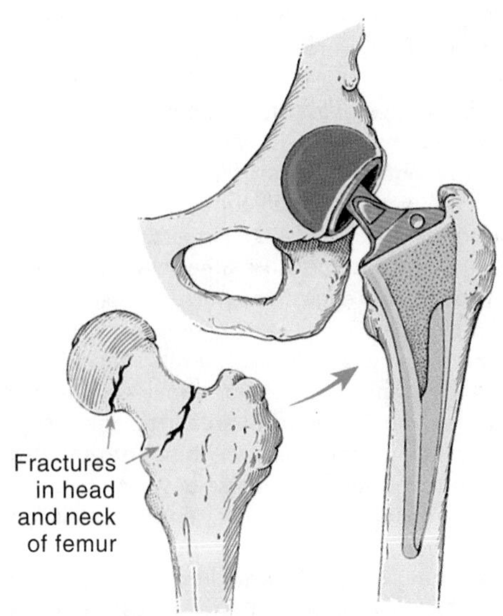

FIGURE 28-9 Hip fracture repaired with a prosthesis.

BOX 28-5 Hip Fracture Care

- Give good skin care. Skin breakdown can be rapid.
- Prevent pressure ulcers.
- Prevent wound, skin, and urinary tract infections.
- Encourage deep-breathing and coughing exercises as directed.
- Turn and position the person as directed. Turning and positioning depend on the type of fracture and the surgery. Usually the person is not positioned on the operative side.
- Prevent external rotation of the hip. Use trochanter rolls, pillows, or sandbags.
- Keep the leg abducted at all times. Use pillows (Fig. 28-10) or a hip abduction wedge (abductor splint). Do not exercise the affected leg.
- Provide a straight-back chair with armrests. The person needs a high, firm seat.
- Place the chair on the unaffected side.
- Use assist devices to move, turn, re-position, and transfer the person.
- Do not let the person stand on the operated leg unless allowed by the doctor.
- Elevate the leg following the care plan. With an internal fixation device, the leg is not elevated when the person sits in a chair. Elevating the leg puts strain on the device.
- Apply elastic stockings to prevent thrombi (blood clots) in the legs.
- Remind the person not to cross his or her legs.
- Assist with walking according to the care plan. The person uses a walker or crutches.
- Follow measures to protect the hip. See Box 28-2 and Figure 28-4.
- Practice safety measures to prevent falls.
- Complete a safety check before leaving the room. (See the inside of the front cover.)

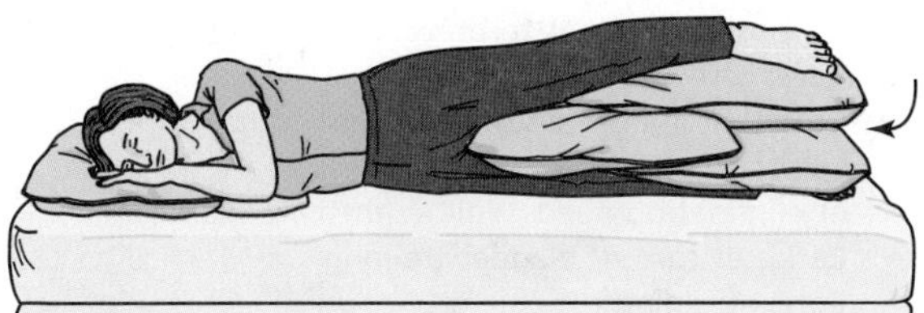

FIGURE 28-10 Pillows are used to keep the hip in abduction.

Loss of Limb

An *amputation* is the removal of all or part of an extremity. Severe injuries, tumors, severe infection, gangrene, and vascular disorders are common causes. Diabetes can cause vascular changes leading to amputation.

Gangrene is a condition in which there is death of tissue. Causes include infection, injuries, and vascular disorders. Blood flow is affected. Tissues do not get enough oxygen and nutrients. Tissues become black, cold, and shriveled (Fig. 28-11). Surgery is needed to remove dead tissue. Gangrene can cause death.

The person is fitted with a prosthesis—an artificial replacement for a missing body part (Fig. 28-12). Occupational and physical therapists help the person use the prosthesis.

The person may feel that the limb is still there. Aching, tingling, and itching are common sensations. Or the person complains of pain in the amputated part *(phantom pain)*. This is a normal reaction. It may occur for a short time or for many years.

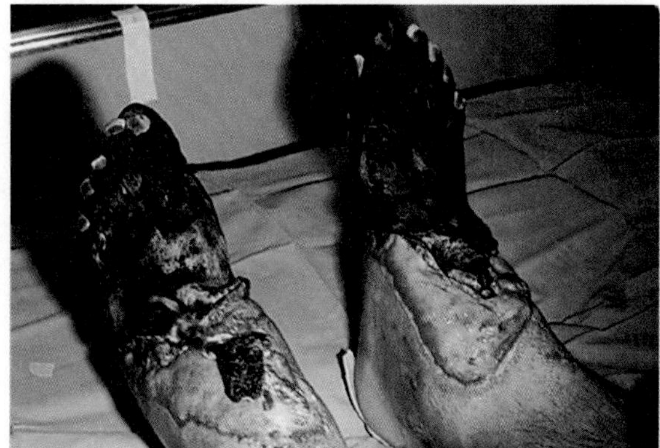

FIGURE 28-11 Gangrene.

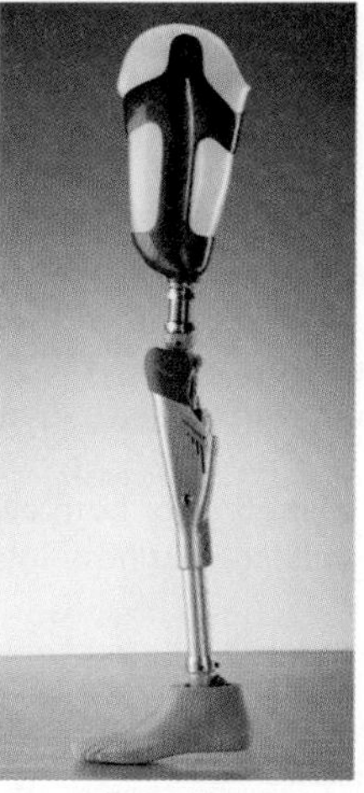

FIGURE 28-12 Leg prosthesis.

NERVOUS SYSTEM DISORDERS

Nervous system disorders can affect mental and physical function. They can affect the ability to speak, understand, feel, see, hear, touch, think, control bowels and bladder, and move.

Stroke

Stroke is a disease that affects the arteries that supply blood to the brain. It also is called a *brain attack* or *cerebrovascular accident (CVA)*. It occurs when 1 of these happens:

- A blood vessel in the brain bursts. Bleeding occurs in the brain (cerebral hemorrhage).
- A blood clot blocks blood flow to the brain.

Brain cells in the affected area do not get enough oxygen and nutrients. Brain damage occurs. Functions controlled by that part of the brain are lost (Fig. 28-13).

Stroke is a leading cause of death and disability among adults in the United States. See Box 28-6 for warning signs. The person needs emergency care. Blood flow to the brain must be restored as soon as possible.

Warning signs may last a few minutes. This is called a *transient ischemic attack (TIA). (Transient* means *temporary* or *short term. Ischemic* means *to hold back* [ischein] *blood* [hemic].) Blood supply to the brain is interrupted for a short time. A TIA may occur before a stroke. The person also may have nausea, vomiting, and memory loss. Unconsciousness, noisy breathing, high blood pressure, slow pulse, redness of the face, and seizures may occur. So can ***hemiplegia***—*paralysis* (plegia) *on 1 side* (hemi) *of the body.* The person may lose bowel and bladder control and the ability to speak. (See "Aphasia.") All stroke-like symptoms signal the need for emergency care.

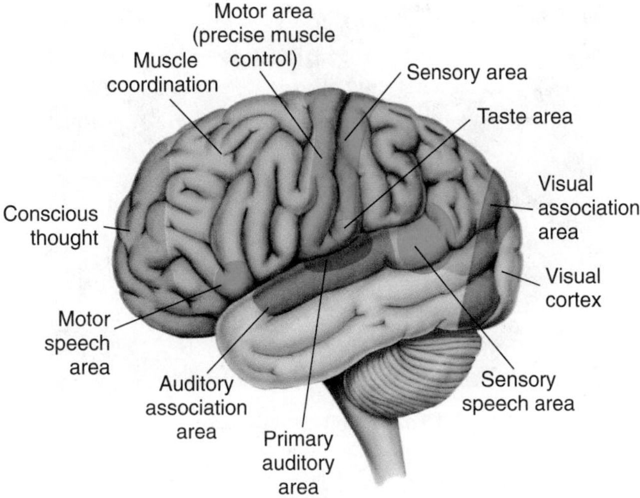

FIGURE 28-13 Functions lost from a stroke depend on the area of brain damage.

BOX 28-6 Warning Signs of Stroke

- Sudden numbness or weakness of the face, arm, or leg (especially on 1 side of the body)
- Sudden confusion, trouble speaking or understanding speech
- Sudden trouble seeing in 1 or both eyes
- Sudden trouble walking, dizziness, loss of balance or coordination
- Sudden severe headache with no known cause

From National Institute of Neurological Disorders and Stroke: Know stroke. Know the signs. Act in time, *National Institutes of Health, NIH Publication Number 13-4872, Bethesda, Md, July 2013.*

BOX 28-7 Stroke Care Measures

- Position the person in the lateral (side-lying) position to prevent aspiration.
- Keep the bed in semi-Fowler's position.
- Approach the person from the strong (unaffected) side. Place objects on the strong (unaffected side). The person may have loss of vision on the affected side.
- Turn and re-position the person at least every 2 hours.
- Use assist devices to move, turn, re-position, and transfer the person.
- Encourage deep breathing and coughing.
- Prevent contractures.
- Prevent pressure ulcers (Chapter 25).
- Meet food and fluid needs. The person may need a dysphagia diet (Chapter 20).
- Apply elastic stockings to prevent thrombi (blood clots) in the legs.
- Assist with ROM exercises to prevent contractures. They also strengthen affected extremities.
- Meet elimination needs. Follow the care plan for:
  - Catheter care or bladder training
  - Bowel training
- Practice safety precautions.
  - Keep the call light within reach on the person's strong (unaffected) side.
  - Check the person often if he or she cannot use the call light. Follow the care plan.
  - Use bed rails according to the care plan.
  - Prevent falls and other injuries.
- Have the person do as much self-care as possible. This includes turning, positioning, and transferring. The person uses assistive, self-help, and ambulating aids as needed.
- Do not rush the person. Movements are slower after a stroke.
- Follow established communication methods.
- Give support, encouragement, and praise.
- Complete a safety check before leaving the room. (See the inside of the front cover.)

The effects of stroke include:

- Loss of face, hand, arm, leg, or body control
- Hemiplegia
- Changing emotions (crying easily or mood swings, sometimes for no reason)
- Difficulty swallowing (dysphagia)
- Aphasia or slowed or slurred speech
- Changes in sight, touch, movement, and thought
- Impaired memory
- Urinary frequency, urgency, or incontinence
- Loss of bowel control or constipation
- Depression and frustration

Rehabilitation starts at once. The person may depend in part or totally on others for care. The health team helps the person regain the highest possible level of function (Box 28-7).

Aphasia

***Aphasia** is the total or partial loss* (a) *of the ability to use or understand language* (phasia). Aphasia is a language disorder. Parts of the brain responsible for language are damaged. Stroke, head injury, brain infections, and cancer are common causes. Two types of aphasia are:

- *Expressive aphasia (motor aphasia, Broca's aphasia)* is difficulty expressing or sending out thoughts. Thinking is clear. The person knows what to say but has difficulty speaking or cannot speak the words. There are problems speaking, spelling, counting, gesturing, or writing. The person may:
  - Omit small words such as "is," "and," "of," and "the."
  - Speak in single words or short sentences. "Walk dog" can mean "I will take the dog for walk" or "You take the dog for a walk."
  - Put words in the wrong order. Instead of "bathroom," the person may say "room bath."
  - Think 1 thing but say another. The person may want food but asks for a book.
  - Call people by the wrong names.
  - Make up words.
  - Produce sounds and no words.
  - Cry or swear for no reason.
- *Receptive aphasia (Wernicke's aphasia)* is difficulty understanding language. The person has trouble understanding what is said or read. People and common objects are not recognized. The person may not know how to use a fork, toilet, cup, TV, phone, or other items.

Some people have both types. This is called *expressive-receptive aphasia (global aphasia, mixed aphasia)*. The person has problems speaking and understanding language.

Parkinson's Disease

Parkinson's disease is a slow, progressive disorder with no cure. Movement is affected. Persons over the age of 50 are at risk. Signs and symptoms become worse over time (Fig. 28-14). They include:

- *Tremors*—often start in the hand. Pill-rolling movements—rubbing the thumb and index finger—may occur. The person may have trembling in the hands, arms, legs, jaw, and face.
- *Rigid, stiff muscles*—in the arms, legs, neck, and trunk.
- *Slow movements*—the person has a slow, shuffling gait.
- *Stooped posture and impaired balance*—it is hard to walk. Falls are a risk.
- *Mask-like expression*—the person cannot blink and smile. A fixed stare is common.

Other signs and symptoms develop over time. They include swallowing and chewing problems, constipation, and bladder problems. Sleep problems, depression, and emotional changes (fear, insecurity) can occur. So can memory loss and slow thinking. The person may have slurred, monotone, and soft speech. Some people talk too fast or repeat what they say.

Drugs are ordered to treat and control the disease. Exercise and physical therapy help improve strength, posture, balance, and mobility. Therapy is needed for speech and swallowing problems. The person may need help with eating and self-care. Normal elimination is a goal. Safety measures are needed to prevent falls and injuries.

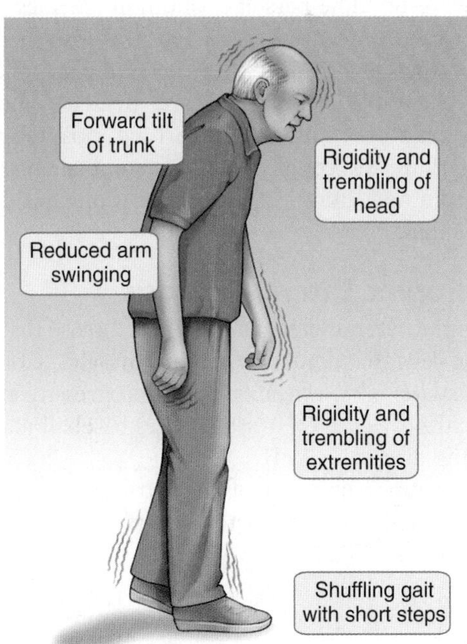

FIGURE 28-14 Signs of Parkinson's disease.

Multiple Sclerosis

Multiple sclerosis (MS) is a chronic disease. *Multiple* means *many*. *Sclerosis* means *hardening* or *scarring*. The myelin (which covers nerve fibers) in the brain and spinal cord is destroyed. Nerve impulses are not sent to and from the brain in a normal way. Functions are impaired or lost. There is no cure.

Symptoms usually start between the ages of 20 and 40. The risk increases if a family member has MS.

Signs and symptoms may include:

- Blurred or double vision; blindness in 1 eye
- Muscle weakness in the arms and legs
- Balance and coordination problems
- Tingling, prickling, or numb sensations
- Partial or complete paralysis
- Pain
- Speech problems
- Tremors
- Dizziness
- Concentration, attention, memory, and judgment problems
- Depression
- Bowel and bladder problems
- Problems with sexual function
- Hearing loss
- Fatigue

MS can present in many ways. For example:

- The symptoms last for a few weeks or a few months. The symptoms gradually disappear with partial or complete recovery. The person is in *remission*. At some point, symptoms flare up again *(relapse)*.
- The person's condition gradually declines with more and more symptoms. There are no remissions.
- Symptoms become worse. More symptoms occur with each flare-up. The person's condition declines.

Persons with MS are kept as active as long as possible and as independent as possible. The care plan reflects the person's changing needs. Skin care, hygiene, and ROM exercises are important. So are turning, positioning, and deep breathing and coughing. Bowel and bladder elimination is promoted. Injuries and complications from bedrest are prevented.

Amyotrophic Lateral Sclerosis

Amyotrophic lateral sclerosis (ALS) is a disease that attacks the nerve cells that control voluntary muscles. Commonly called *Lou Gehrig's disease*, it is rapidly progressive and fatal. (Lou Gehrig was a New York Yankees baseball player. He died of the disease in 1941.)

More common in men, it usually strikes between 40 and 60 years of age. Most die 3 to 5 years after onset. Some live for 10 years or more.

Motor nerve cells in the brain, brainstem, and spinal cord are affected. These cells stop sending messages to the muscles. The muscles weaken, waste away (atrophy), and twitch. Over time, the brain cannot start voluntary movements or control them. The person cannot move the arms, legs, and body. Muscles for speaking, chewing and swallowing, and breathing also are affected. Eventually respiratory muscles fail.

The disease usually does not affect the mind, intelligence, or memory. Sight, smell, taste, hearing, and touch are not affected. Usually bowel and bladder functions remain intact.

ALS has no cure. Some drugs can slow the disease and improve symptoms. However, damage cannot be reversed. The person is kept active and independent to the extent possible. The care plan reflects the person's changing needs.

Head Injury

Head injuries result from trauma to the scalp, skull, or brain. Some minor injuries do not need health care. Or the person needs some emergency treatment.

Traumatic brain injury (TBI) occurs when a sudden trauma damages the brain. Brain tissue is bruised or torn. Bleeding can be in the brain or in nearby tissues. Spinal cord injuries are likely. Motor vehicle crashes, falls, assaults, and firearms are common causes. So are sports and recreation injuries.

If the person survives, some permanent damage is likely. Disabilities depend on the severity and site of injury. They include:

- *Cognitive problems*—thinking, memory, and reasoning.
- *Sensory problems*—sight, hearing, touch, taste, and smell.
- *Communication problems*—expressing or understanding language.
- *Behavior or mental health problems*—depression, anxiety, personality changes, aggressive behavior, socially inappropriate behavior.
- *Stupor*—an unresponsive state; the person can be briefly aroused.
- *Coma*—the person is unconscious, does not respond, is unaware, and cannot be aroused.
- *Vegetative state*—the person is unconscious and unaware of surroundings. He or she has sleep-wake cycles and periods of being alert.
- *Persistent vegetative state (PVS)*—the person is in a vegetative state for more than 1 month.

Rehabilitation is required. Nursing care depends on the person's needs and abilities.

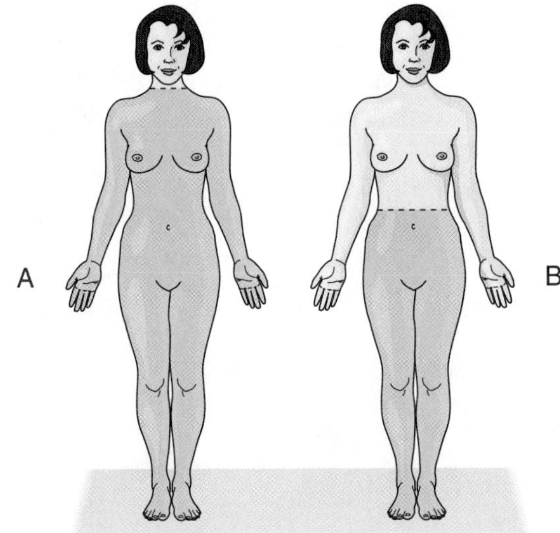

FIGURE 28-15 The *shaded areas* show the area of paralysis. **A,** Quadriplegia (tetraplegia). **B,** Paraplegia.

BOX 28-8 Care of Persons With Paralysis

- Practice safety measures to prevent falls. Use bed rails as directed.
- Keep the bed in a low position. Follow the care plan.
- Keep the call light within reach. If unable to use the call light, check the person often.
- Prevent burns. Check bath water, heat applications, and food for proper temperature.
- Turn (logroll) and re-position the person at least every 2 hours.
- Prevent pressure ulcers. Follow the care plan.
- Use supportive devices to maintain good alignment.
- Follow bowel and bladder training programs.
- Keep intake and output records.
- Maintain muscle function and prevent contractures. Assist with ROM exercises.
- Assist with food and fluid needs as needed. Provide self-help devices as ordered.
- Give emotional and psychological support.
- Follow the person's rehabilitation plan.
- Complete a safety check of the room. (See the inside of the front cover.)

Spinal Cord Injury

Spinal cord injuries can seriously damage the nervous system. ***Paralysis*** *(loss of muscle function, sensation, or both)* can result. Common causes are stab or gunshot wounds, motor vehicle crashes, falls, and sports injuries.

Problems depend on the amount of damage to the spinal cord and the level of injury. The higher the level of injury, the more functions lost (Fig. 28-15).

- *Lumbar injuries*—sensory and muscle function in the legs is lost. The person has paraplegia. ***Paraplegia*** *is paralysis in the legs and lower trunk. (Para* means *beyond; plegia* means *paralysis).*
- *Thoracic injuries*—sensory and muscle function below the chest is lost. The person has paraplegia.
- *Cervical injuries*—sensory and muscle function of the arms, legs, and trunk is lost. *Paralysis in the arms, legs, and trunk is called* ***quadriplegia*** *or* ***tetraplegia****. (Quad* and *tetra* mean *four. Plegia* means *paralysis.)*

Cervical traction with a special bed may be needed. The spine is kept straight at all times. See Box 28-8 for care measures. Emotional needs are great. Reactions to paralysis and loss of function are often severe. If the person lives, rehabilitation is needed.

HEARING LOSS

Hearing loss is not being able to hear the normal range of sounds associated with normal hearing. Deafness is the most severe form. *Deafness* is hearing loss in which it is impossible for the person to understand speech through hearing alone. Clear speech, responding to others, safety, and awareness of surroundings require hearing.

A person may not notice gradual hearing loss. Others may see changes in the person's behavior or attitude. Obvious signs and symptoms of hearing loss include:

- Speaking too loudly
- Leaning forward to hear
- Turning and cupping the better ear toward the speaker
- Answering questions or responding inappropriately
- Asking for words to be repeated
- Asking others to speak louder or to speak more slowly and clearly
- Having trouble hearing over the phone
- Having problems following conversations when 2 or more people are talking
- Turning up the TV, radio, or music volume so loud that others complain

Persons with hearing loss may wear hearing aids or lip-read (speech-read). They watch facial expressions, gestures, and body language. Some people learn American Sign Language (ASL) (Fig. 28-16, p. 438).

Some people have *hearing assistance dogs* (hearing dogs). The dog alerts the person to sounds. Phones, doorbells, smoke detectors, alarm clocks, sirens, and on-coming cars are examples.

See *Focus on Communication: Hearing Loss,* p. 438.

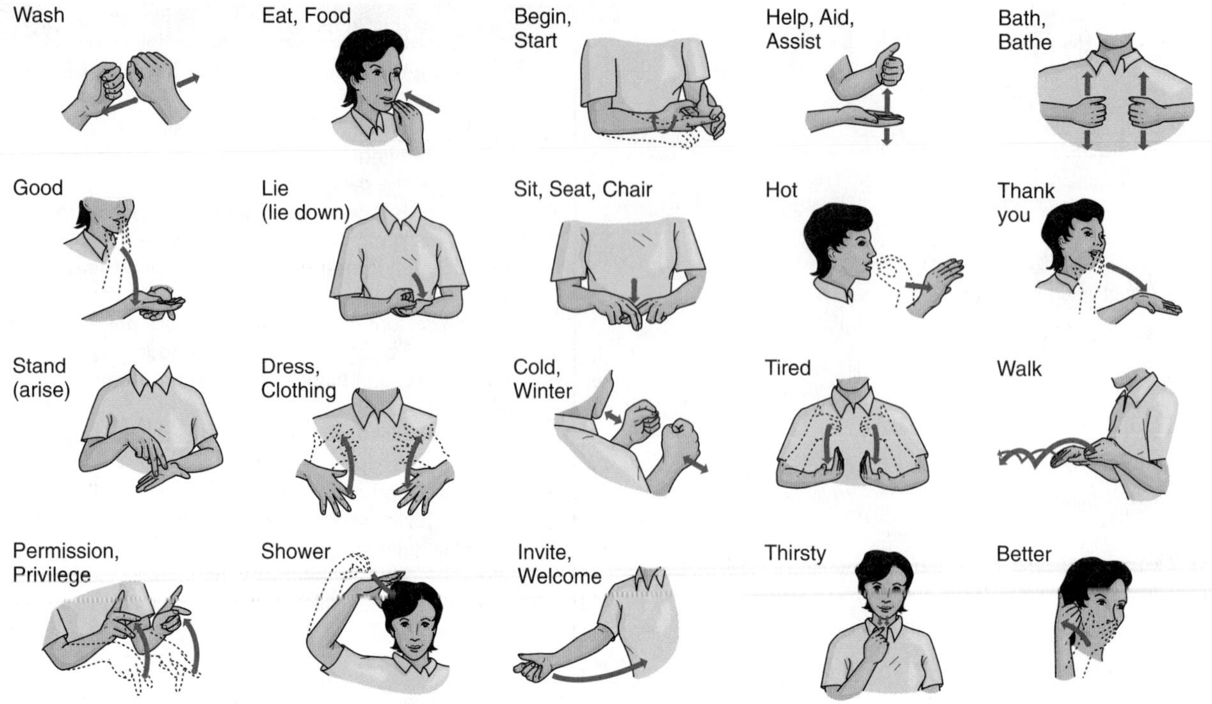

FIGURE 28-16 American Sign Language examples.

> **FOCUS ON COMMUNICATION**
>
> ***Hearing Loss***
>
> The National Association of the Deaf (NAD) uses the terms *deaf* and *hard-of-hearing* to describe persons with hearing loss. Do not use the terms *deaf and dumb, deaf-mute,* or *hearing-impaired.* Such terms offend persons who are hard-of-hearing.
>
> There are many ways to communicate with persons who have hearing loss. Some use American Sign Language (ASL). The nurse can contact a sign language interpreter. Some persons write notes, use a computer, or use pictures. Others lip-read (speech-read). Another method may be used with lip-reading so that messages are understood.
>
> Follow the care plan or ask the nurse which method to use. See Box 28-9 for measures to promote communication.

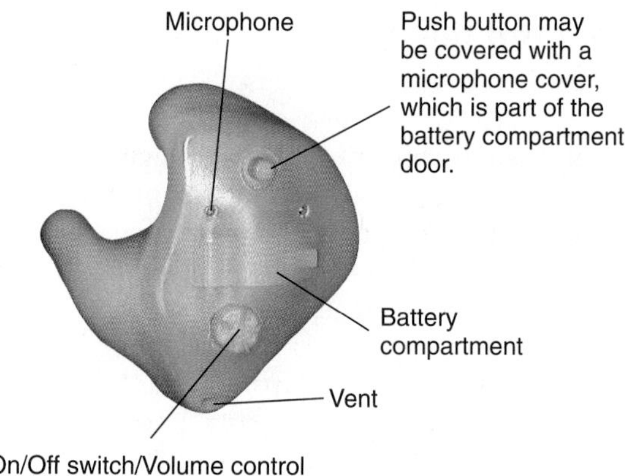

FIGURE 28-17 A hearing aid.

Hearing Aids

Hearing aids fit inside or behind the ear (Fig. 28-17). They make sounds louder. They do not correct, restore, or cure hearing problems. Background noise and speech are louder. The measures in Box 28-9 apply.

Hearing aids are battery-operated. If the device does not seem to work properly:

- Check if the hearing aid is *on.* It has an *on* and *off* switch.
- Check the battery position.
- Insert a new battery if needed.
- Clean the hearing aid. *Follow the nurse's directions and the manufacturer's instructions.*

Hearing aids are turned off when not in use. And the battery is removed.

Hearing aids are costly. Handle and care for them properly. When not in the ear, store a hearing aid in its case. Place the case in the top drawer of the bedside stand.

BOX 28-9 Measures to Promote Hearing

The Environment
- Reduce or eliminate background noises. Turn off radios, stereos, music players, TVs, air conditioners, fans, and so on.
- Provide a quiet place to talk.
- Have the person sit in small groups or where he or she hears best.

The Person
- Have the person wear his or her hearing aid. It must be turned on and working.
- Have the person wear needed eyeglasses or contact lenses. The person needs to see your face to lip-read (speech-read).

You
- Gain attention. Alert the person to your presence. Raise an arm or hand, or lightly touch the person's arm. Do not startle or approach the person from behind.
- Position yourself at the person's level. Sit if the person is sitting. Stand if the person is standing.
- Face the person when speaking. Do not turn or walk away while you are talking. Do not talk to the person from the doorway or another room.
- Stand or sit in good light. Shadows and glares affect the person's ability to see your face clearly.
- Speak clearly, distinctly, and slowly.
- Speak in a normal tone of voice. Do not shout.

You—cont'd
- Adjust the pitch of your voice as needed. Ask if the person can hear you better.
  - If the person does not wear a hearing aid, lower the pitch if you are a female. Women's voices are higher-pitched and harder to hear than lower-pitched male voices.
  - If the person wears a hearing aid, raise the pitch slightly.
- Do not cover your mouth, smoke, eat, or chew gum while talking. Mouth movements are affected.
- Keep your hands away from your face. The person needs to see your face clearly.
- Stand or sit on the side of the better ear.
- State the topic of conversation first.
- Tell the person when you are changing the subject. State the new topic.
- Use short sentences and simple words.
- Use gestures and facial expressions to give useful clues.
- Write out important names and words.
- Say things in another way if the person does not seem to understand.
- Keep conversations and discussions short. This avoids tiring the person.
- Repeat and re-phrase statements as needed.
- Be alert to messages sent by your facial expressions, gestures, and body language.

EYE DISORDERS

Vision loss occurs at all ages. Problems range from mild loss to complete blindness. *Blindness* is the absence of sight. Vision loss is sudden or gradual. One or both eyes are affected. The following are common.

- *Cataract* is a clouding of the lens (Fig. 28-18). The normal lens is clear. *Cataract* comes from the Greek word for *waterfall.* Trying to see is like looking through a waterfall. A cataract can occur in 1 or both eyes. Surgery is the only treatment (Box 28-10). Signs and symptoms include:
  - Cloudy, blurry, or dimmed vision (Fig. 28-19, *A* and *B*, p. 440).
  - Colors seem faded. Blues and purples are hard to see.
  - Sensitivity to light and glares.
  - Poor vision at night.
  - Halos around lights.
  - Double vision in the affected eye.
- *Age-related macular degeneration (AMD)* blurs central vision. *Central vision* is what you see "straight-ahead." AMD causes a blind spot in the center of vision. See Figure 28-19, *A* and *C*, p. 440. Laser surgery may help.
- *Diabetic retinopathy* is a complication of diabetes. Tiny blood vessels in the retina are damaged. It is a leading cause of blindness. Usually both eyes are affected. Vision blurs. See Figure 28-19, *A* and *D*, p. 440. The person may see spots "floating." Often there are no early warning signs. The person needs to control diabetes, blood pressure, and cholesterol. Laser surgery may help.
- *Glaucoma* results when fluid builds up in the eye and causes pressure on the optic nerve. The optic nerve is damaged. Vision loss with eventual blindness occurs. Glaucoma can develop in 1 or both eyes. Peripheral vision (side vision) is lost. The person sees through a tunnel (Fig. 28-20, p. 440), has blurred vision, and sees halos around lights. Drugs and surgery can control glaucoma and prevent further damage. Prior damage cannot be reversed.

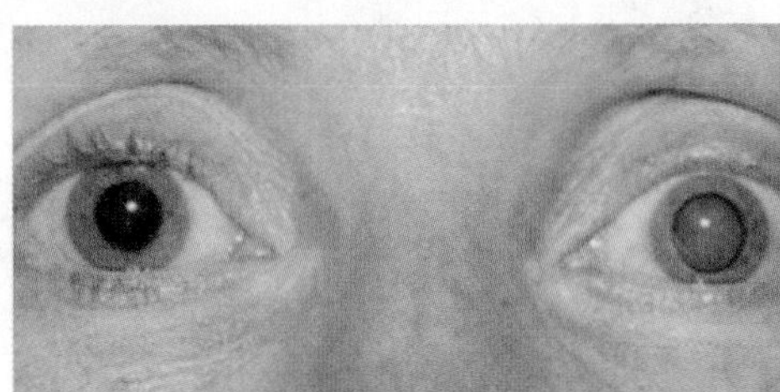

FIGURE 28-18 The right eye is normal. The left eye has a cataract.

BOX 28-10 Nursing Measures After Cataract Surgery

- Keep the eye shield in place as directed. The shield is worn for sleep, including naps.
- Follow measures for persons who are visually impaired or blind when an eye shield is worn (p. 441). The person may have vision loss in the other eye.
- Remind the person not to rub or press the affected eye.
- Do not bump the eye.
- Place the over-bed table and the bedside stand on the un-operative side.
- Place the call light within reach.
- Report eye drainage or complaints of pain at once.

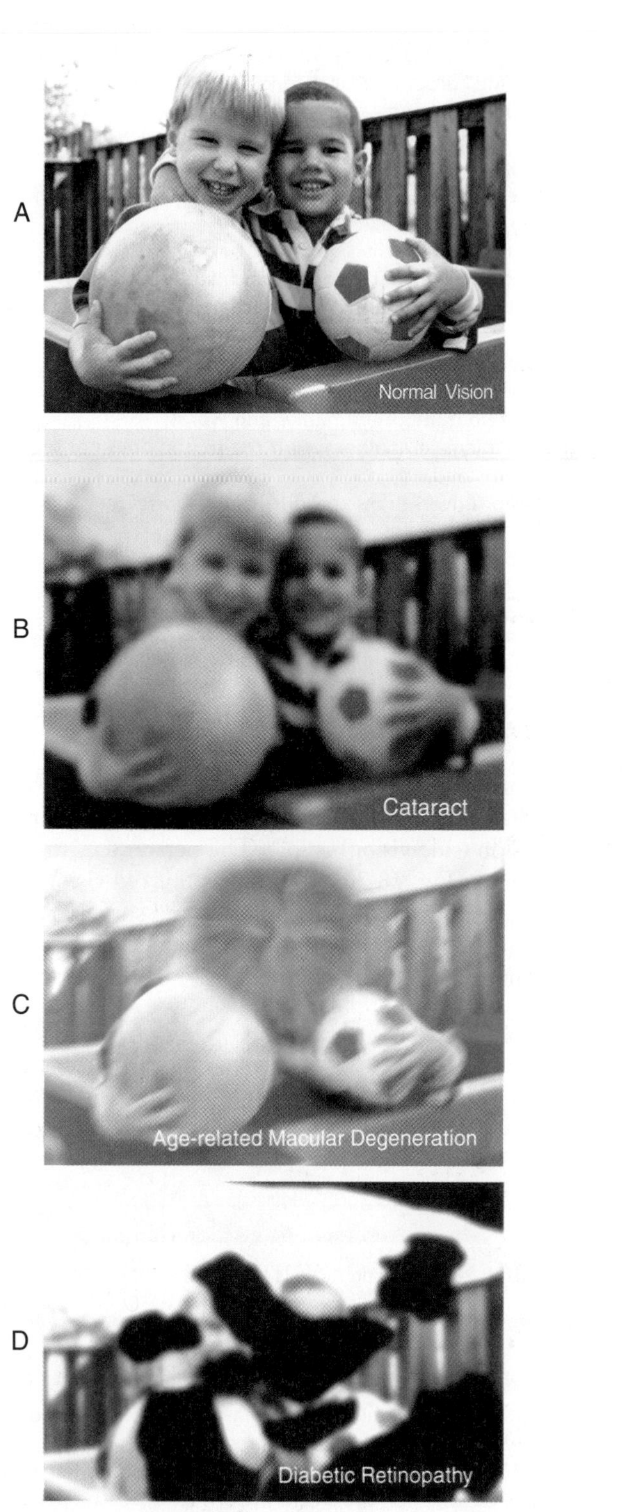

FIGURE 28-19 Vision loss with eye disorders. **A,** Normal vision. **B,** Vision loss from a cataract. **C,** Vision loss from macular degeneration. **D,** Vision loss from diabetic retinopathy.

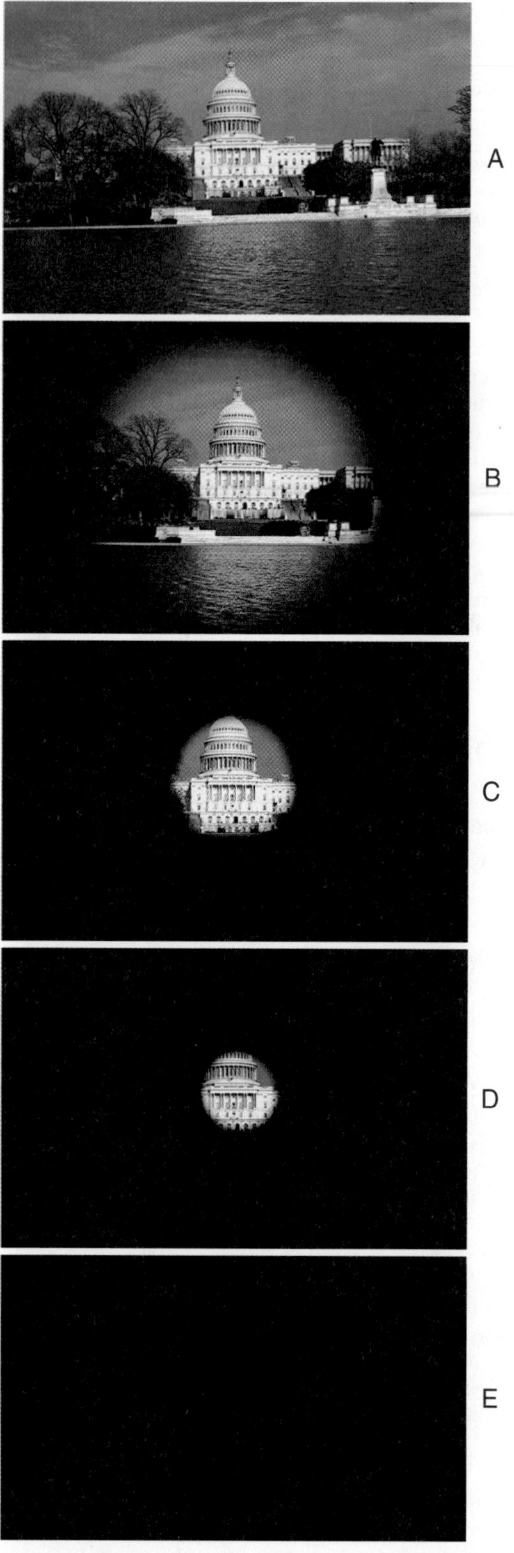

FIGURE 28-20 Vision loss from glaucoma. **A,** Normal vision. **B,** Loss of peripheral vision begins. **C, D, and E,** Vision loss continues, with eventual blindness.

Impaired Vision and Blindness

Birth defects, injuries, and eye diseases are among the causes of impaired vision and blindness. They also are complications of some diseases. Some people are totally blind. Others sense some light but have no usable vision. Others have some usable vision but cannot read newsprint. The legally blind person sees at 20 feet what a person with normal vision sees at 200 feet.

Loss of sight is serious. Adjustments can be hard and long. The person may need to learn to move about, perform daily tasks, read and write, communicate with others, and use a guide dog.

Rehabilitation programs help the person adjust to the vision loss and learn to be independent. The goal is for the person to be as active as possible and to have quality of life. The person learns to use visual and adaptive devices, braille, long canes, and guide dogs.

Braille is a touch reading and writing system using raised dots for each letter of the alphabet (Fig. 28-21). The first 10 letters also represent the numbers 0 through 9. Braille is read by moving the hands from left to right along each line of braille.

Special devices allow computer access. A "braille display" lets the person read information. Braille printers allow printing computer information in braille.

Blind and visually impaired persons learn to move about using a long cane with a red tip or a guide dog. Both are used world-wide.

When caring for blind or visually impaired persons, follow the practices in Box 28-11.

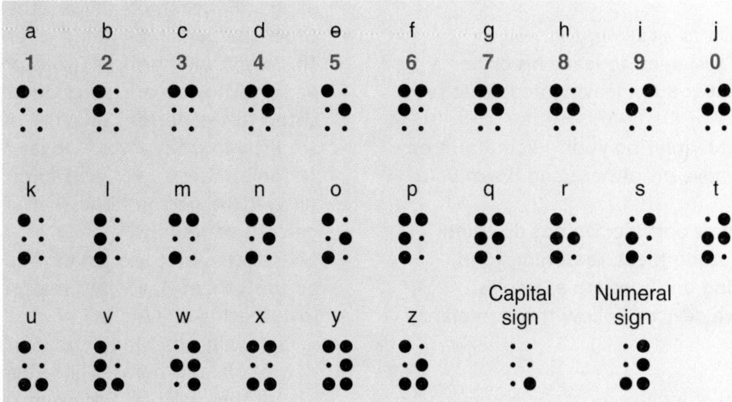

FIGURE 28-21 Braille.

BOX 28-11 Caring for Blind and Visually Impaired Persons

The Environment

- Report worn carpeting and other flooring.
- Keep furniture, equipment, and electrical cords out of areas where the person will walk.
- Keep chairs pushed in under the table or desk.
- Keep doors fully open or fully closed. This includes room, closet, and cabinet doors.
- Keep drawers fully closed.
- Report burnt-out light bulbs.
- Provide lighting as the person prefers. Tell the person when the lights are on or off.
- Adjust window coverings to prevent glares. Sunny days and bright, snowy days cause glares.
- Keep the call light and TV, light, and other controls within reach.
- Turn on night-lights in the person's room and bathroom and in hallways.
- Practice safety measures to prevent falls (Chapter 10).
- Orient the person to the room. Describe the layout. Include the location and purpose of furniture and equipment.
- Let the person move about. Let him or her touch and find furniture and equipment.
- Do not re-arrange furniture and equipment.

The Environment—cont'd

- Provide a consistent meal-time setting.
    - Avoid plates, napkins, placemats, and tablecloths with patterns and designs. Use solid colors and provide contrast. For example, place a white plate on a dark placemat or tablecloth.
    - Have the person sit in good light.
    - Keep place settings the same.
        - The knife and spoon are to the right of the plate.
        - The fork and napkin are to the left of the plate.
        - The glass or cup is to the right of the plate if the person is right-handed. It is to the left of the plate if the person is left-handed.
    - Arrange main dishes, side dishes, seasonings, and condiments in a straight line or in a semi-circle just beyond the person's place setting. Arrange things in the same way for each meal.
    - Explain the location of food and beverages. Use the face of a clock (Chapter 20). Or guide the person's hand to each item on the tray or place setting.
    - Cut meat, open containers, butter bread, and perform other tasks as needed.
- Complete a safety check before leaving the room. (See the inside of the front cover.)

Modified from American Foundation for the Blind.

Continued

BOX 28-11 Caring for Blind and Visually Impaired Persons—cont'd

The Person

- Have the person use railings when climbing stairs.
- Have the person wear comfortable shoes that fit correctly.
- Assist with walking as needed. Offer to guide the person. Ask if he or she would like help. Respect the person's answer. If your help is accepted:
  - Offer your arm. Tell the person which arm is offered. Tap the back of your hand against the person's hand.
  - Have the person hold on to your arm just above the elbow (Fig. 28-22). Do not grab the person's arm.
  - Walk at a normal pace. Walk 1 step ahead of the person. Stand next to the person at the top and bottom of stairs and when crossing streets.
  - Never push, pull, or guide the person in front of you.
  - Pause when changing direction, stepping up, and stepping down.
  - Tell the person about stairs, elevators, escalators, doors, turns, furniture, and other obstructions. State if steps are up or down.
  - Have the person hold on to a railing, the wall, or other strong surface if you need to leave his or her side. Tell the person that you are leaving and what to hold on to.
- Guide the person to a seat by placing your guiding arm on the seat. The person will move his or her hand down your arm to the seat.
- Let the person do as much as possible. Do not do things that the person can do. Cutting meat, seasoning food, getting dressed, and putting on shoes are examples.
- Provide visual and adaptive devices. Follow the care plan.

You

- Identify yourself when you enter the room. Give your name, title, and reason for being there. Do not touch the person until you have indicated your presence.
- Ask the person how much he or she can see. Do not assume that the person is totally blind or that the person has some vision.
- Identify others. Explain where each person is located and what the person is doing.
- Offer to help. Simply say: "May I help you?" Respect the person's answer.
- Leave the person's belongings in the same place that you found them. Do not move or re-arrange things. If you have to move things, tell the person what you moved and where.

Communication

- Face the person when speaking. Speak slowly and clearly.
- Use a normal tone of voice. Do not shout or speak loudly. Vision loss does not mean the person has hearing loss.
- Address the person by name. This tells the person that you are directing a comment or question to him or her.
- Speak directly to the person. Do not talk to just family and friends who are present.
- Feel free to use words such as "see," "look," "read," or "watch TV." You also can use "blind" and "visually impaired."
- Feel free to refer to colors, sizes, shapes, patterns, designs, and so on.
- Describe people, places, and things thoroughly. Do not leave out a detail because you do not think it is important.
- Warn the person of dangers. Give a calm and clear warning. You can say "wait" first. Then describe the danger. For example: "Wait, there is ice on the walk."
- Greet the person by name when he or she enters a room. This alerts the person to your presence in the room. Tell the person who you are. Also identify others in the room.
- Listen to the person. Give the person verbal cues that you are listening. Say: "yes," "okay," "I see," "tell me more," "I don't understand," and so on.
- Answer the person's questions. Provide specific and descriptive responses.
- Give step-by-step explanations of procedures as you perform them. Say when the procedure is over.
- Give specific directions.
  - Say: "right behind you," "on your left," or "in front of you." Avoid phrases like "over here" or "over there."
  - Tell the distance. For example: "Three steps in front of you" or "At the end of the hallway by the nurses' station."
  - Give landmarks if possible. Sounds and scents can serve as "landmarks." "By the kitchen" is an example.
- Tell the person when you are leaving the room or the area. If appropriate, tell the person where you are going. For example: "I'm going to go into your bathroom now."
- Tell the person when you are ending a conversation. For example: "I enjoyed hearing about your children. Thank you for sharing stories with me."

Corrective Lenses

Eyeglasses and contact lenses can correct many vision problems. Some people wear eyeglasses for reading or seeing at a distance. Others wear them for all activities. Contact lenses are usually worn while awake. Some contacts can be worn day and night for up to 30 days.

Eyeglass lenses are hardened glass or plastic. Clean them daily and as needed. Wash glass lenses with warm water. Dry them with a lens cloth or cotton cloth. Plastic lenses scratch easily. Use special cleaning solutions and cloths.

Contact lenses fit on the eye. They are cleaned, removed, and stored according to the manufacturer's instructions.

See *Delegation Guidelines: Corrective Lenses.*

See *Promoting Safety and Comfort: Corrective Lenses.*

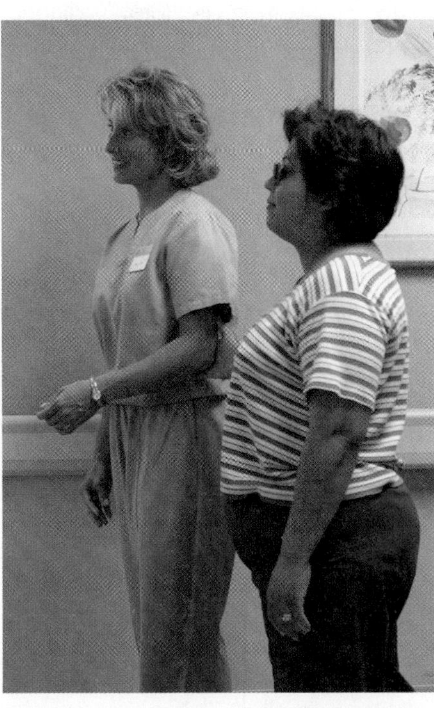

FIGURE 28-22 The blind person walks slightly behind the nursing assistant. She touches the nursing assistant's arm lightly.

DELEGATION GUIDELINES

Corrective Lenses

Cleaning eyeglasses is a routine care measure. Do not wait until the nurse tells you to clean them. Clean them daily and as needed.

To clean eyeglasses, find out if you need a special cleaning solution. Then follow the manufacturer's instructions.

PROMOTING SAFETY AND COMFORT

Corrective Lenses

Safety

Eyeglasses are costly. Protect them from loss or damage (Fig. 28-23). When not worn, put them in their case. Place the case in the top drawer of the bedside stand.

Some agencies let nursing assistants remove and insert contact lenses. Others do not. Know your agency's policy. If allowed to insert and remove contacts, follow agency procedures.

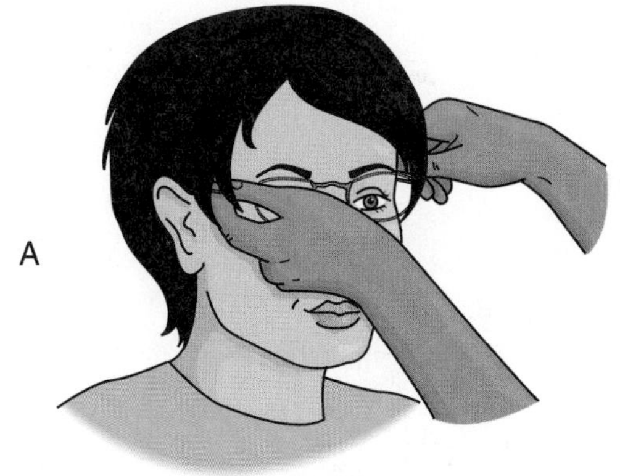

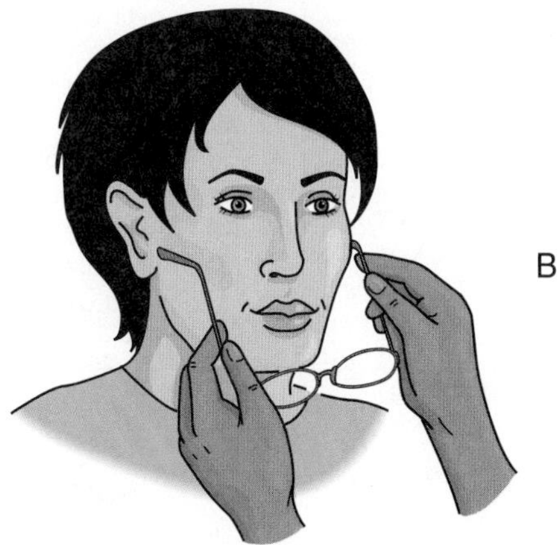

FIGURE 28-23 Removing eyeglasses. **A,** Hold the frames in front of the ears. **B,** Lift the frames from the ears. Bring the glasses down and away from the face.

CARDIOVASCULAR DISORDERS

Cardiovascular disorders are leading causes of death in the United States. Problems occur in the heart or blood vessels.

Hypertension

With *hypertension* (high blood pressure), the resting blood pressure is too high. The systolic pressure is 140 mm Hg (millimeters of mercury) or higher *(hyper)*. Or the diastolic pressure is 90 mm Hg or higher. Such measurements must occur several times. *Pre-hypertension* is when the systolic pressure is between 120 and 139 mm Hg, or the diastolic pressure is between 80 and 89 mm Hg. Pre-hypertension will likely develop into hypertension in the future. See Box 28-12 for risk factors.

Narrowed blood vessels are a common cause. The heart pumps with more force to move blood through narrowed vessels. Kidney disorders, head injuries, some pregnancy problems, and adrenal gland tumors are causes.

Signs and symptoms develop over time. Headache, blurred vision, dizziness, and nose bleeds occur. Hypertension can lead to stroke, hardening of the arteries, heart attack, heart failure, kidney failure, and blindness.

Life-style changes can lower blood pressure. A diet low in fat and salt, a healthy weight, and regular exercise are needed. No smoking is allowed. Alcohol and caffeine are limited. Managing stress and sleeping well also lower blood pressure. Certain drugs lower blood pressure.

Coronary Artery Disease

The coronary arteries supply the heart muscle with blood. In coronary artery disease (CAD), the coronary arteries become hardened and narrow. One or all are affected. The heart muscle gets less blood and oxygen (O_2). CAD also is called *coronary heart disease* and *heart disease.*

The most common cause is atherosclerosis (Fig. 28-24). Plaque—made up of cholesterol, fat, and other substances—collects on artery walls. The narrowed arteries block blood flow. Blockage may be total or partial. Blood clots can form along the plaque and block blood flow.

The major complications of CAD are angina, myocardial infarction (heart attack) (p. 446), irregular heartbeats, and sudden death. The more risk factors (see Box 28-12), the greater the chance of CAD and its complications.

CAD can be treated. Treatment goals are to:

- Relieve symptoms (see "Angina").
- Slow or stop atherosclerosis.
- Lower the risk of blood clots.
- Widen or bypass clogged arteries.
- Reduce cardiac events (see "Angina" and "Myocardial Infarction," p. 446).

CAD requires life-style changes. Drugs may be used to decrease the heart's workload, relieve symptoms, prevent a heart attack or sudden death, or to delay the need for procedures that open or bypass diseased arteries (Fig. 28-25).

BOX 28-12 Risk Factors for Cardiovascular Disorders

Factors You *Cannot* Change

- Age—45 years or older for men; 55 years or older for women
- Gender—men are at greater risk than women; risk increases for women after menopause
- Race—African-Americans are at greater risk
- Family history—tends to run in families

Factors You *Can* Change

- Being over-weight
- Stress
- Smoking and tobacco use
- High-salt diet
- Excessive alcohol
- Lack of exercise
- Atherosclerosis
- Blood pressure
- High blood cholesterol
- Diabetes

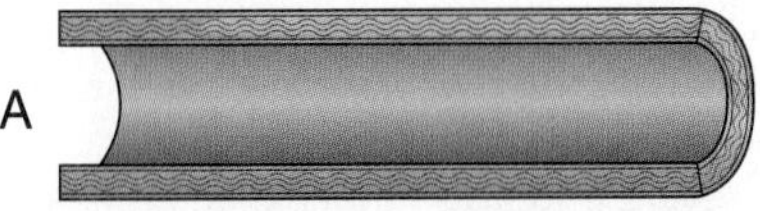

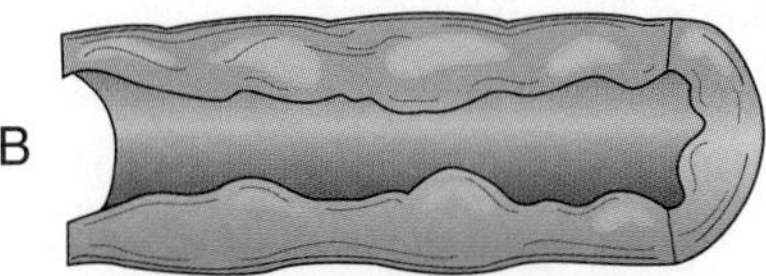

FIGURE 28-24 **A,** Normal artery. **B,** Plaque on the artery wall in atherosclerosis.

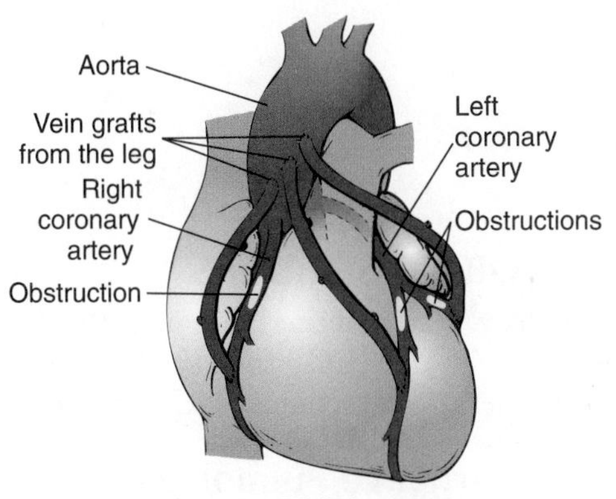

FIGURE 28-25 Coronary artery bypass surgery.

Angina

Angina (pain) is chest pain from reduced blood flow to part of the heart muscle (myocardium). It occurs when the heart needs more O_2. Normally blood flow to the heart increases when O_2 needs increase. Exertion, a heavy meal, stress, and excitement increase the heart's need for O_2. So do smoking and very hot or very cold temperatures. In CAD, narrowed vessels prevent increased blood flow.

Chest pain is described as a tightness, pressure, squeezing, or burning in the chest (Fig. 28-26). Pain can occur in the shoulders, arms, neck, jaw, or back. Pain in the jaw, neck, and down 1 or both arms is common. The person may be pale, feel faint, and perspire. Dyspnea is common. Nausea, fatigue, and weakness may occur. Some persons complain of "gas" or indigestion. Rest often relieves symptoms in 3 to 15 minutes.

Besides rest, a *nitroglycerin* tablet is taken when angina occurs. It is placed under the tongue. There it dissolves and is rapidly absorbed into the bloodstream. Tablets are kept within the person's reach at all times. The person takes a tablet and then tells the nurse. Some persons have nitroglycerin patches. The nurse applies and removes them.

Things that cause angina are avoided. These include over-exertion, heavy meals and over-eating, and emotional stress. The person stays indoors during cold weather or during hot, humid weather. A doctor-supervised exercise program (cardiac rehabilitation) is helpful.

See "Coronary Artery Disease" for the treatment of angina. The goal is to increase blood flow to the heart. Doing so may prevent or lower the risk of heart attack and death. Chest pain lasting longer than a few minutes and not relieved by rest and nitroglycerin may signal heart attack. The person needs emergency care.

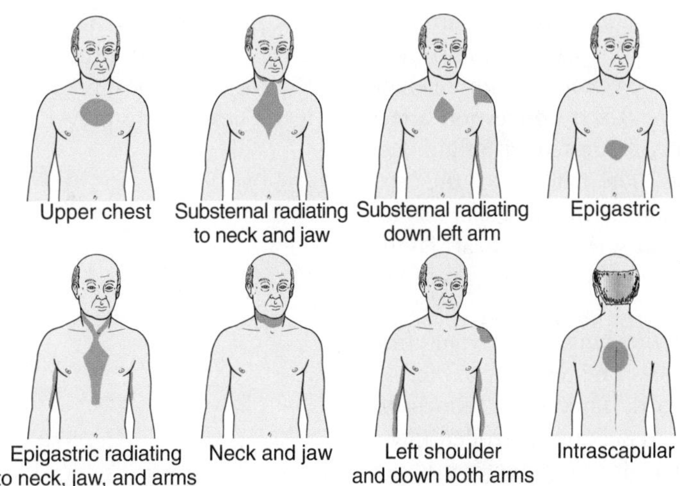

FIGURE 28-26 *Shaded areas* show where the pain of angina is located.

Myocardial Infarction

Myocardial refers to the *heart muscle. Infarction* means *tissue death*. With myocardial infarction (MI), blood flow to the heart muscle is suddenly blocked. Part of the heart muscle dies. Sudden cardiac death *(sudden cardiac arrest)* can occur (Chapter 31).

MI also is called:

- Heart attack
- Acute myocardial infarction (AMI)
- Acute coronary syndrome (ACS)

See Box 28-13 for signs and symptoms. MI is an emergency. Efforts are made to:

- Relieve pain.
- Restore blood flow to the heart.
- Stabilize vital signs.
- Give O_2.
- Calm the person.
- Prevent death and life-threatening problems.

The person may need medical or surgical procedures to open or bypass the diseased artery. Cardiac rehabilitation is needed. The goals are to:

- Recover and resume normal activities.
- Prevent another MI.
- Prevent complications such as heart failure or sudden cardiac arrest.

BOX 28-13 Signs and Symptoms of Myocardial Infarction

- Chest pain
  - Sudden, severe; usually on the left side
  - Described as crushing, stabbing, squeezing, or as someone sitting on the chest
  - More severe and lasts longer than angina
  - Not relieved by rest or nitroglycerin
- Pain or numbness in 1 or both arms, the back, neck, jaw, or stomach
- Indigestion or "heartburn"
- Dyspnea
- Nausea
- Dizziness
- Perspiration and cold, clammy skin
- Pallor or cyanosis
- Blood pressure: low
- Pulse: weak and irregular
- Fear, apprehension, and a feeling of doom

Heart Failure

Heart failure or congestive heart failure (CHF) occurs when the weakened heart cannot pump normally. Blood backs up. Tissue congestion occurs.

When the left side of the heart cannot pump blood normally, blood backs up into the lungs. Respiratory congestion occurs. The person has dyspnea, increased sputum, cough, and gurgling sounds in the lungs. The body does not get enough blood. Signs and symptoms occur from the effects on other organs. Poor blood flow to the brain causes confusion, dizziness, and fainting. The kidneys produce less urine. The skin is pale. Blood pressure falls.

When the right side of the heart cannot pump blood normally, blood backs up into the venous system. Feet and ankles swell. Neck veins bulge. Liver congestion affects liver function. The abdomen is congested with fluid. Less blood is pumped to the lungs. The left side of the heart receives less blood from the lungs. The left side has less blood to pump to the body. As with left-sided heart failure, organs receive less blood. The signs and symptoms of left-sided failure occur.

Pulmonary edema (fluid in the lungs) can result from heart failure. It is an emergency. The person can die.

Drugs strengthen the heart. They also reduce the amount of fluid in the body. A sodium-controlled diet is ordered. Oxygen is given. Semi-Fowler's position is preferred for breathing. Intake and output (I&O), daily weight, elastic stockings, and ROM exercises are part of the care plan.

RESPIRATORY DISORDERS

The respiratory system brings O_2 into the lungs and removes carbon dioxide (CO_2) from the body. Respiratory disorders interfere with this function and threaten life.

Chronic Obstructive Pulmonary Disease

Chronic obstructive pulmonary disease (COPD) involves 2 disorders—chronic bronchitis and emphysema. These disorders interfere with O_2 and CO_2 exchange in the lungs. They obstruct air flow. Less air gets into the lungs; less air leaves the lungs. Lung function is gradually lost.

Cigarette smoking is the most important risk factor. Pipe, cigar, and other smoking tobaccos are also risk factors. So is exposure to second-hand smoke. Not smoking is the best way to prevent COPD. COPD has no cure.

Chronic Bronchitis. Chronic bronchitis occurs after repeated episodes of bronchitis. *Bronchitis* means *inflammation (itis)* of the *bronchi (bronch)*. Smoking is the major cause.

Smoker's cough in the morning is often the first symptom. At first the cough is dry. Over time, the person coughs up mucus. Mucus may contain pus. The cough becomes more frequent. The person has difficulty breathing and tires easily. Mucus and inflamed breathing passages obstruct airflow into the lungs. The body cannot get normal amounts of O_2.

The person must stop smoking. Oxygen therapy and breathing exercises are often ordered. Respiratory tract infections are prevented. If one occurs, the person needs prompt treatment.

Emphysema. In emphysema, the alveoli enlarge. They become less elastic. They do not expand and shrink normally with breathing in and out. As a result, some air is trapped in the alveoli when exhaling. Trapped air is not exhaled. Over time, more alveoli are involved. O_2 and CO_2 exchange cannot occur in the affected alveoli. As more air is trapped in the lungs, the person develops a *barrel chest* (Fig. 28-27).

Smoking is the most common cause. The person has shortness of breath and a cough. At first, shortness of breath occurs with exertion. Over time, it occurs at rest. Sputum may contain pus. Fatigue is common. The person works hard to breathe in and out. And the body does not get enough O_2. Breathing is easier when the person sits upright and slightly forward (Chapter 26).

The person must stop smoking. Respiratory therapy, breathing exercises, oxygen, and drug therapy are ordered.

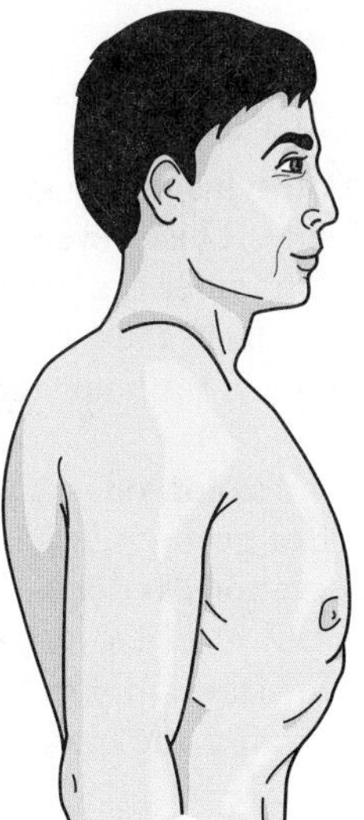

FIGURE 28-27 Barrel chest from emphysema.

Asthma

With asthma, the airway becomes inflamed and narrow. Extra mucus is produced. Dyspnea results. Wheezing and coughing are common. So are pain and tightness in the chest. Symptoms are mild to severe.

Asthma usually is triggered by allergies. Other triggers include air pollutants and irritants, smoking and secondhand smoke, respiratory infections, exertion, and cold air.

Sudden attacks *(asthma attacks)* can occur. There is shortness of breath, wheezing, coughing, rapid pulse, sweating, and cyanosis. The person gasps for air and is very frightened.

Asthma is treated with drugs. Severe attacks may require emergency care.

Influenza

Influenza *(flu)* is a respiratory infection caused by viruses. Older persons are at great risk. Pneumonia is a common complication.

Signs and symptoms of flu include:

- High fever (100°F to 102°F) for 3 to 4 days
- Headache
- General aches and pains
- Fatigue and weakness that can last 2 to 3 weeks
- Chest discomfort
- Cough
- Stuffy nose, sneezing, and sore throat may occur

Treatment involves fluids and rest. The doctor orders drugs for symptom relief and to shorten the flu episode.

Coughing and sneezing spread flu viruses. Follow Standard Precautions. The flu vaccine is the best prevention.

See *Focus on Older Persons: Influenza.*

FOCUS ON OLDER PERSONS

Influenza

Older persons may not have the usual signs and symptoms. The following may signal flu in older persons.

- Changes in mental status or behavior
- Worsening or other health problems
- A body temperature below the normal range
- Fatigue
- Decreased appetite and fluid intake

Pneumonia

Pneumonia is an inflammation and infection of lung tissue. (*Pneumo* means *lungs*.) Affected tissues fill with fluid. O_2 and CO_2 exchange is affected.

Bacteria, viruses, and other microbes are causes. The person is very ill. Signs and symptoms of pneumonia include:

- High fever
- Chills
- Painful cough
- Chest pain on breathing
- Rapid pulse and breathing
- Shortness of breath
- Cyanosis
- Thick and white, green, yellow, or rust-colored sputum
- Nausea and vomiting
- Headache
- Tiredness
- Muscle aches

Drugs are ordered for infection and pain. Fluid intake is increased because of fever and to thin secretions. Thin secretions are easier to cough up. Intravenous (IV) therapy and oxygen may be needed. Semi-Fowler's position eases breathing. Rest is important. Standard Precautions are followed. Transmission-Based Precautions are used depending on the cause.

See *Focus on Older Persons: Pneumonia.*

> **FOCUS ON OLDER PERSONS**
>
> ***Pneumonia***
>
> Changes from aging, diseases, and decreased mobility increase the risk of pneumonia in older persons. Older adults are at great risk of dying from pneumonia.
>
> Older persons may not have the usual signs and symptoms. Drugs and other diseases can mask signs and symptoms. Older persons may show signs of confusion, dehydration, and rapid respirations.

Tuberculosis

Tuberculosis (TB) is a bacterial infection in the lungs. TB is spread by airborne droplets with coughing, sneezing, speaking, singing, or laughing (Chapter 12). Nearby persons can inhale the bacteria. Those who have close, frequent contact with an infected person are at risk. TB is more likely to occur in close, crowded areas. Age, poor nutrition, and HIV (human immunodeficiency virus) infection are other risk factors.

TB can be present in the body but not cause signs and symptoms. An active infection may not occur for many years. Only persons with an active infection can spread the disease to others.

Chest x-rays and TB testing can detect the disease. Signs and symptoms are tiredness, loss of appetite, weight loss, fever, and night sweats. Cough and sputum increase over time. Sputum may contain blood. Chest pain occurs.

Drugs for TB are given. Standard Precautions and Transmission-Based Precautions are needed (Chapter 12). The person must cover the mouth and nose with tissues when sneezing, coughing, or producing sputum. Tissues are flushed down the toilet, placed in a *BIOHAZARD* bag, or placed in a paper bag and burned. Hand washing after contact with sputum is essential.

DIGESTIVE DISORDERS

The digestive system breaks down food for the body to absorb. Solid wastes are eliminated. Diarrhea, constipation, flatulence, and fecal incontinence are discussed in Chapter 19. So is ostomy care.

Vomiting

Vomitus (emesis) *is the food and fluids expelled from the stomach through the mouth.* Vomiting signals illness or injury. Aspirated vomitus can obstruct the airway. Vomiting large amounts of blood can lead to shock (Chapter 31). These measures are needed.

- Follow Standard Precautions and the Bloodborne Pathogen Standard.
- Turn the person onto his or her side with the head turned well to 1 side. This prevents aspiration.
- Place a kidney basin under the person's chin.
- Move vomitus away from the person.
- Provide oral hygiene. This helps remove the bitter taste of vomitus.
- Observe vomitus for color, odor, and undigested food. If it looks like coffee grounds, it contains blood. Report your observations at once.
- Measure, report, and record the amount of vomitus.
- Save a specimen for laboratory study.
- Dispose of vomitus after the nurse observes it.
- Eliminate odors.
- Provide for comfort. (See the inside of the front cover.)

Diverticular Disease

Small pouches can develop in the colon. The pouches bulge outward through weak spots in the colon (Fig. 28-28). Each pouch is called a *diverticulum*. (*Diverticulare* means to turn *inside out*). *Diverticulosis* is the condition of having these pouches. (*Osis* means *condition of.*) The pouches can become infected or inflamed—*diverticulitis*. (*Itis* means *inflammation.*)

Many people over 60 years of age have diverticulosis. Age, a low-fiber diet, and constipation are risk factors.

When feces enter the pouches, they can become inflamed and infected. The person has abdominal pain and tenderness in the lower left abdomen. Fever, nausea and vomiting, chills, cramping, and constipation are likely. Bloating, rectal bleeding, frequent urination, and pain while voiding can occur.

Diet changes are ordered. Sometimes antibiotics are ordered. Surgery is done for severe disease, obstruction, and ruptured pouches. The diseased part of the bowel is removed. A colostomy may be needed (Chapter 19).

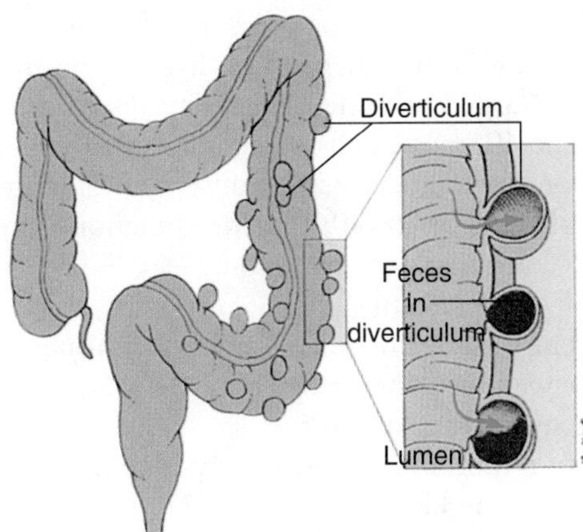

FIGURE 28-28 Diverticulosis.

Hepatitis

Hepatitis is an inflammation *(itis)* of the liver *(hepat)*. It can be mild or cause death. See Box 28-14 for signs and symptoms. Some people have no symptoms. Treatment involves rest, a healthy diet, fluids, and no alcohol. Recovery takes 1 to 2 months.

Protect yourself and others. Follow Standard Precautions and the Bloodborne Pathogen Standard. Transmission-Based Precautions are ordered as necessary (Chapter 12). Assist the person with hygiene and hand washing as needed.

There are 5 major types of hepatitis.

- *Hepatitis A* is spread by the fecal-oral route. The hepatitis A virus is ingested when eating or drinking food or water contaminated with feces. It is also ingested when eating or drinking from a contaminated vessel. Causes include poor sanitation, crowded living condition, poor nutrition, and poor hygiene. Anal sex and IV drug use also are causes. Handle bedpans, feces, and rectal thermometers carefully. Good hand washing is needed by everyone, including the person.
- *Hepatitis B* is caused by the hepatitis B virus (HBV). It is spread through contact with infected blood and body fluids (saliva, semen, vaginal secretions). HBV is not spread through food or water, breast-feeding, hugging or kissing, coughing, sneezing, holding hands, or sharing eating utensils. It can be spread by:
  - IV drug use and sharing needles and syringes
  - Accidental needle sticks
  - Sex without a condom, especially anal sex
  - Contaminated tools used for tattoos or body piercings
  - Sharing a toothbrush, razor, or nail clippers with an infected person
- *Hepatitis C* is spread by blood contaminated with the hepatitis C virus. A person may have no symptoms but can transmit the disease. Serious liver disease and damage may show up years later. The virus can be spread by blood contaminated with the virus through:
  - IV drug use and sharing needles and syringes
  - Inhaling cocaine through contaminated straws
  - Contaminated tools used for tattoos or body piercings
  - High-risk sexual activity—sex with an infected person, multiple sex partners
  - Sharing a toothbrush, razor, or nail clippers with an infected person
- *Hepatitis D* occurs only in people infected with hepatitis B. It is spread the same way as HBV.
- *Hepatitis E* is spread through food or water contaminated by feces from an infected person. It is spread by the fecal-oral route. This disease is not common in the United States.

BOX 28-14 Signs and Symptoms of Hepatitis

- Jaundice (yellowish color of the skin or whites of the eyes)
- Fatigue, weakness
- Pain and discomfort: abdominal, joint, muscles
- Appetite: loss of
- Nausea and vomiting
- Diarrhea
- Bowel movements: light, clay-colored
- Urine: dark
- Fever and chills
- Headache
- Itching
- Weight loss
- Skin rash

URINARY SYSTEM DISORDERS

The kidneys, ureters, bladder, and urethra are the major urinary system structures. Disorders can occur in these structures.

- *Urinary tract infection (UTI).* UTIs are common. Microbes can enter the system through the urethra. Catheterization, urological exams, intercourse, poor perineal hygiene, immobility, and poor fluid intake are common causes. UTI is a common healthcare-associated infection (Chapter 12).
    - *Cystitis* is a bladder *(cyst)* infection *(itis)* caused by bacteria. Urinary frequency, urgency, difficult or painful urination, foul-smelling urine, blood or pus in the urine, and fever may occur. Antibiotics are ordered. Fluids are encouraged. If untreated, cystitis can lead to pyelonephritis.
    - *Pyelonephritis* is inflammation *(itis)* of the kidney *(nephr)* pelvis *(pyelo)*. Cloudy urine may contain pus, mucus, and blood. Chills, fever, back pain, and nausea and vomiting occur. So do the signs and symptoms of cystitis. Treatment involves antibiotics and fluids.
- *Kidney stones (calculi).* These are hard deposits in the kidney. Stones vary in size from grains of sand to golf-ball size (Fig. 28-29). Bedrest, immobility, and poor fluid intake are risk factors. Signs and symptoms are listed in Box 28-15. Drugs are given for pain relief. The person needs to drink 2000 to 3000 mL (milliliters) a day. The fluids help stones pass from the body through the urine. All urine is strained. Medical or surgical removal of the stone may be necessary. Some diet changes can prevent stones.
- *Kidney failure.* The kidneys do not function or are severely impaired. Waste products are not removed from the blood. Fluid is retained. Heart failure and hypertension easily result. Kidney failure may be acute or chronic. The person is very ill.

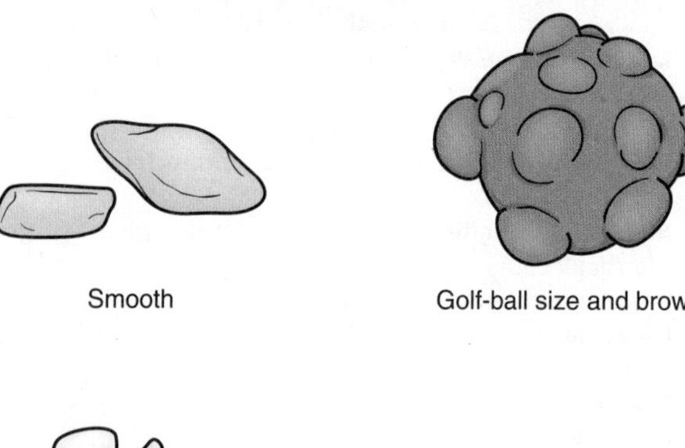

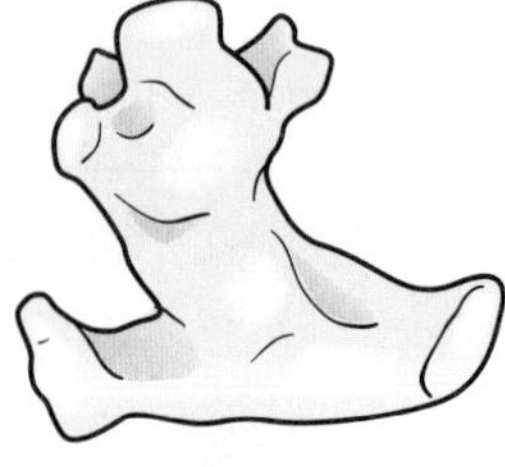

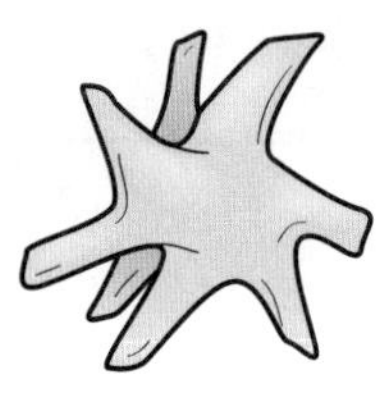

FIGURE 28-29 Kidney stones.

BOX 28-15 Signs and Symptoms of Kidney Stones

- Severe, cramping pain in the back and side just below the ribs
- Pain in the lower abdomen, thigh, and urethra
- Nausea and vomiting
- Fever and chills
- Dysuria—difficult or painful *(dys)* urination *(uria)*
- Urinary urgency
- Burning on urination
- Hematuria—blood *(hemat)* in the urine *(uria)*
- Cloudy urine
- Foul-smelling urine

Prostate Enlargement

The prostate is a gland in men. It lies in front of the rectum and just below the bladder (Chapter 7). The prostate surrounds the urethra. About the size of a walnut, the prostate grows larger (enlarges) as the man grows older. This is called benign prostatic hyperplasia (BPH). *Benign* means *non-malignant. Hyper* means *excessive. Plasia* means *formation* or *development.* Benign prostatic hypertrophy is another name for enlarged prostate. (*Trophy* means *growth.*)

After age 60, most men have some symptoms of BPH. The enlarged prostate presses against the urethra obstructing urine flow (Fig. 28-30). Bladder function is gradually lost. These problems are common:

- A weak urine stream
- Frequent voidings of small amounts of urine
- Urgency and leaking or dribbling of urine
- Frequent voiding at night
- Urinary retention (The man cannot void. Urine remains in the bladder.)

The doctor may order drugs to shrink the prostate or stop its growth. Some microwave and laser treatments destroy the excess prostate tissue. Or surgery is done to remove tissue.

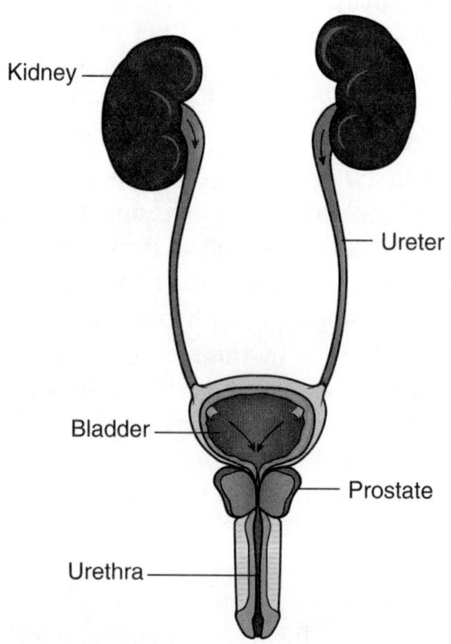

FIGURE 28-30 Enlarged prostate. The prostate presses against the urethra. Urine flow is obstructed.

REPRODUCTIVE DISORDERS

Aging affects the reproductive system (Chapter 8). Injuries, diseases, and surgeries can affect reproductive structures and functions.

Sexually Transmitted Diseases

A sexually transmitted disease (STD) is spread by oral, vaginal, or anal sex. Some people do not have signs and symptoms or are not aware of an infection. Others know but do not seek treatment because of embarrassment.

STDs often occur in the genital and rectal areas. They also occur in the ears, mouth, nipples, throat, tongue, eyes, and nose. Condom use helps prevent the spread of STDs, especially the human immunodeficiency virus (HIV) and acquired immunodeficiency syndrome (AIDS). Some STDs are also spread through skin breaks, by contact with infected body fluids (blood, semen, saliva), or by contaminated blood or needles.

Standard Precautions and the Bloodborne Pathogen Standard are followed.

See *Focus on Older Persons: Sexually Transmitted Diseases.*

> **FOCUS ON OLDER PERSONS**
>
> ***Sexually Transmitted Diseases***
>
> Many older people are sexually active. They get and can spread STDs in the same ways that younger persons do. However, many do not think they are at risk. Always practice Standard Precautions and follow the Bloodborne Pathogen Standard. Do not assume that older people are too old to have sex.

ENDOCRINE DISORDERS

The endocrine system is made up of glands. The endocrine glands secrete hormones that affect other organs and glands. Diabetes is the most common endocrine disorder.

Diabetes

In diabetes, the body cannot produce or use insulin properly. Insulin is needed for glucose to move from the blood into the cells. The pancreas secretes insulin. Without enough insulin, sugar builds up in the blood. Blood glucose (sugar) is high. Cells do not have enough sugar for energy and cannot function.

The 3 types of diabetes are:

- *Type 1 diabetes.* Occurs most often in children. The pancreas produces little or no insulin. Onset is rapid.
- *Type 2 diabetes.* This type is more common in older persons. However, it is becoming more common in children, teens, and young adults. Being over-weight, lack of exercise, and hypertension are risk factors. The pancreas secretes insulin. However, the body cannot use it well. Onset is slow. Infections are frequent. Wounds heal slowly.
- *Gestational diabetes.* Develops during pregnancy. (*Gestation* comes from *gestare*. It means *to bear*.) It usually goes away after the baby is born. However, the mother is at risk for type 2 diabetes later in life.

Risk factors include a family history of the disease. For type 1, whites are at greater risk than non-whites. Type 2 is more common in older and over-weight persons. African-American, Native American, and Hispanics are at risk for type 2.

Signs and Symptoms of Diabetes. Signs and symptoms of diabetes are:

- Being very thirsty
- Urinating often
- Feeling very hungry or tired
- Losing weight without trying
- Having sores that heal slowly
- Having dry, itchy skin
- Tingling or loss of feeling in the feet
- Blurred vision

Complications of Diabetes. Diabetes must be controlled to prevent complications. They include blindness, renal failure, nerve damage, and damage to the gums and teeth. Heart and blood vessel diseases are very serious problems. They can lead to stroke, heart attack, and slow healing. Foot and leg wounds and ulcers are very serious (Chapter 24). Infection and gangrene can occur. Amputation may be necessary.

Diabetes Treatment. Type 1 diabetes is treated with daily insulin therapy, healthy eating (Chapter 20), and exercise. Type 2 diabetes is treated with healthy eating and exercise. Many persons with type 2 take oral drugs. Some need insulin. Over-weight persons need to lose weight. Types 1 and 2 involve controlling blood pressure, cholesterol, and the risk factors for CAD.

Good foot care is needed. Corns, blisters, calluses, and other foot problems can lead to an infection and amputation. See Chapters 17 and 24.

The person's blood sugar level can fall too low or go too high. Blood glucose is monitored daily or 3 or 4 times a day for:

- *Hypoglycemia*—low *(hypo)* sugar *(glyc)* in the blood *(emia)*
- *Hyperglycemia*—high *(hyper)* sugar *(glyc)* in the blood *(emia)*

See Table 28-1, p. 452 for the causes, signs, and symptoms of hypoglycemia and hyperglycemia. Both can lead to death if not corrected. You must call for the nurse at once.

TABLE 28-1 Hypoglycemia and Hyperglycemia

Hypoglycemia (Low Blood Sugar)		Hyperglycemia (High Blood Sugar)	
Causes	**Signs and Symptoms**	**Causes**	**Signs and Symptoms**
Too much insulin or diabetic drugs	Fatigue; weakness	Not enough insulin or diabetic drugs	Weakness
Increased exercise	Dizziness; faintness	Too little exercise	Drowsiness
Omitting or missing a meal	Vision changes	Eating too much food	Vision: blurred
Delayed meal	Hunger	Emotional stress	Hunger; thirst
Eating too little food	Tingling around the mouth	Infection or sickness	Dry mouth (very)
Vomiting	Headache	Undiagnosed diabetes	Headache
Drinking alcohol	Skin: cold and clammy		Skin: dry
	Sweating		Face: flushed
	Respirations: rapid and shallow		Respirations: rapid, deep, and labored
	Pulse: rapid		Pulse: rapid, weak
	Blood pressure: low		Blood pressure: low
	Motions: clumsy and jerky		Breath odor: sweet
	Trembling; shakiness		Leg cramps
	Confusion		Urination: frequent
	Convulsions		Nausea; vomiting
	Unconsciousness		Convulsions
			Coma

IMMUNE SYSTEM DISORDERS

The immune system protects the body from microbes, cancer cells, and other harmful substances. It defends against threats inside and outside the body. Immune system disorders occur from problems with the immune response. The response may be inappropriate, too strong, or lacking.

Autoimmune Disorders

Autoimmune disorders can occur. The immune system attacks the body's own *(auto)* normal cells, tissues, or organs. Most autoimmune disorders are chronic. Signs and symptoms depend on the disease. Common autoimmune disorders include:

- *Graves' disease.* The immune system attacks the thyroid gland. The thyroid gland produces excess amounts of the hormone thyroxine.
- *Lupus.* This is an inflammatory disease affecting the blood cells, joints, skin, kidneys, lungs, heart, or brain.
- *Multiple sclerosis.* See p. 436.
- *Rheumatoid arthritis.* See p. 429.
- *Type 1 diabetes.* See p. 451.

Acquired Immunodeficiency Syndrome

Acquired immunodeficiency syndrome (AIDS) is caused by the *human immunodeficiency virus (HIV).* The virus attacks the immune system. Therefore it destroys the body's ability to fight infections and certain cancers. Some infections are life-threatening.

The virus is spread through body fluids—blood, semen, vaginal secretions, and breast milk. HIV is not spread by saliva, tears, sweat, sneezing, coughing, insects, or casual contact. HIV is spread mainly by:

- Unprotected anal, vaginal, or oral sex with an infected person. "Unprotected" is without a new latex or polyurethane condom.
- Needle and syringe sharing among IV drug users.
- HIV-infected mothers. Babies can become infected during pregnancy, shortly after birth, and through breast-feeding.

Box 28-16 lists the signs and symptoms of AIDS. Some HIV-infected persons have symptoms within a few months. Others are symptom-free for more than 10 years. However, they carry the virus. They can spread it to others.

Persons with AIDS are at risk for pneumonia, TB, Kaposi's sarcoma (a cancer), and nervous system damage. Memory loss, loss of coordination, paralysis, mental health disorders, and dementia signal nervous system damage.

Many new drugs help slow the spread of HIV in the body. They also reduce complications and prolong life. AIDS has no vaccine and no cure at present. It is a life-threatening disease.

You may care for persons with AIDS or for persons who are HIV carriers (Box 28-17). You may have contact with the person's blood or body fluids. Protect yourself and others. Follow Standard Precautions and the Bloodborne Pathogen Standard. A person may have the HIV virus but no symptoms. In some persons, HIV or AIDS is not yet diagnosed.

See *Focus on Older Persons: Acquired Immunodeficiency Syndrome.*

BOX 28-16 Signs and Symptoms of AIDS

- Appetite: loss of
- Cough
- Depression
- Diarrhea
- Energy: lack of
- Fatigue
- Fever
- Headache
- Memory loss, confusion, and forgetfulness
- Mouth or tongue:
  - Brown, red, pink, or purple spots or blotches
  - Sores or white patches
- Night sweats
- Pneumonia
- Shortness of breath
- Skin:
  - Rashes or flaky skin
  - Brown, red, pink, or purple spots or blotches on the skin, eyelids, or nose
- Swallowing: painful or difficult
- Swollen glands: neck, underarms, and groin
- Vision loss
- Weight loss

BOX 28-17 The Person With AIDS

- Follow Standard Precautions and the Bloodborne Pathogen Standard.
- Provide daily hygiene. Avoid irritating soaps.
- Follow the care plan for oral hygiene. A toothbrush with soft bristles is best.
- Provide oral fluids as ordered.
- Measure and record intake and output.
- Measure weight daily.
- Encourage deep-breathing and coughing exercises as ordered.
- Prevent pressure ulcers.
- Assist with ROM exercises and ambulation as ordered.
- Encourage self-care. The person may use assistive devices (walker, commode, eating devices).
- Encourage the person to be as active as possible.
- Change linens and garments when damp or wet.
- Listen and provide emotional support.

FOCUS ON OLDER PERSONS

Acquired Immunodeficiency Syndrome

Older persons get and spread HIV through sexual contact and IV drug use. Aging and some diseases mask the signs and symptoms of AIDS. Older persons are less likely to be tested for HIV/AIDS. Often the person dies without the disease being diagnosed.

SKIN DISORDERS

There are many types of skin disorders. Alopecia, hirsutism, dandruff, lice, and scabies are discussed in Chapter 17. Skin tears and pressure ulcers are discussed in Chapters 24 and 25. Burns are discussed in Chapter 31.

Shingles

Shingles (herpes zoster) is caused by the same virus that causes chicken pox. The virus lies dormant in nerve tissue. (*Dormant* means *to be inactive.*) The virus can become active years later.

The person has a rash with fluid-filled blisters on 1 side of the body (Fig. 28-31). Burning or tingling pain, numbness, and itching can occur.

Persons who have had chicken pox are at risk. So are persons with weakened immune systems from HIV infections, cancer treatments, transplant surgeries, and stress.

The doctor orders anti-viral drugs and drugs for pain relief. For many healthy people, blisters heal and pain is gone in 3 to 5 weeks. A vaccine is available to prevent shingles.

According to the Centers for Disease Control and Prevention, shingles lesions are infectious until they crust over. Follow Standard Precautions and any Transmission-Based Precautions as ordered.

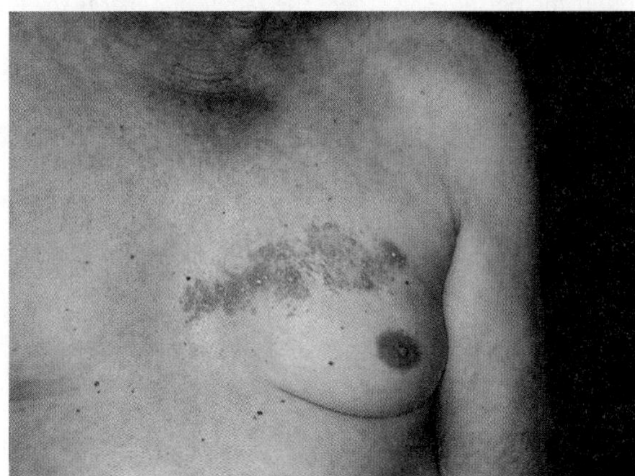

FIGURE 28-31 Shingles rash.

FOCUS ON PRIDE

The Person, Family, and Yourself

Personal and Professional Responsibility

You are responsible for having a basic understanding of common health problems. This knowledge allows you to safely assist with care. Only common health problems were presented in this chapter. And only basic information was given.

You may want to know more about a health problem. Or a person may have a disorder not discussed in this chapter. Ask the nurse to explain the problem and the care required. Also look up the problem in a medical dictionary. Take pride in learning more.

Rights and Respect

Persons have the right to make choices for themselves. Some choices are unhealthy. For example, a person with COPD continues to smoke. Or a person with CAD refuses to exercise or make diet changes. The health team teaches the person the risks and encourages healthy changes. They cannot force changes. However, they must be sure the person understands the risks.

Some persons believe that unhealthy choices improve their quality of life. They know the risks but choose not to change. You may not respect the person's decision, but you must respect the person. Treat the person with dignity and respect.

Independence and Social Interaction

The person and family have many reactions to health problems. Fear, anger, worry, and guilt are common. Families respond in different ways. A helpful and encouraging family provides motivation and support. Family bonds are stronger when everyone shares responsibility and relies on each other. The person's health and quality of life also benefit. Some families refuse to help. Or only 1 or 2 members help and support the person. This strains the family and places stress on the person. Report concerns to the nurse.

Promote pride in the family. Compliment their efforts. Encourage the family's help and support.

Delegation and Teamwork

A person's condition can change quickly. A person with angina may have an MI. A person with asthma may have an asthma attack. A person may begin vomiting.

Sudden changes in a person's condition require the nurse's attention. Assist the nurse as directed. You may need to help other patients or residents while the nurse provides care. Help willingly. The entire nursing team must give that "extra effort" during an emergency.

Ethics and Laws

With chronic health problems, staff often care for persons many times. Staff get to know the person. They learn about likes, dislikes, and preferences. Staff learn about the person's family, school or work, hobbies, and so on. Interest in the person adds to quality of care.

However, staff must avoid crossing professional boundaries (Chapter 3). Maintaining boundaries can be hard when caring for persons you see often and get to know well. However, you must protect the person's privacy and rights. Watch your behavior closely to avoid crossing boundaries. Tell the nurse if you suspect a person is crossing boundaries.

REVIEW QUESTIONS

Circle the BEST answer.

1 Which is a warning sign of cancer?
- **a** Painful, swollen joints
- **b** Feeling weak or very tired
- **c** A rash with blisters
- **d** Chest pain relieved by rest

2 Chemotherapy will likely cause
- **a** Nausea and vomiting
- **b** Burns
- **c** Skin breakdown
- **d** Weight gain

3 A person has arthritis. Care includes
- **a** Keeping joints abducted
- **b** Applying traction to affected joints
- **c** Wearing a cast to prevent joint movement
- **d** Rest balanced with exercise

4 A person had hip replacement surgery. Which should you question?
- **a** Provide a chair with a low seat.
- **b** Do not cross the legs.
- **c** Keep a hip abduction wedge between the legs.
- **d** Provide a long-handled brush for bathing.

5 A person with osteoporosis is at risk for
- **a** An amputation
- **b** Phantom pain
- **c** Fractures
- **d** Paralysis

6 A cast needs to dry. Which should you question?
- **a** Turn the person so the cast dries evenly.
- **b** Cover the cast with blankets and plastic.
- **c** Elevate the cast on pillows.
- **d** Support the cast by the palms when lifting.

7 A person is in traction. Care includes
- **a** Avoiding ROM exercises
- **b** Keeping the weights on the floor
- **c** Removing the weights if the person is uncomfortable
- **d** Giving skin care at frequent intervals

8 After a hip fracture repair, the operated leg is
- **a** Abducted at all times
- **b** Adducted at all times
- **c** Externally rotated at all times
- **d** Flexed at all times

9 A person had a stroke. Which should you question?
- **a** Leave the bed in semi-Fowler's position.
- **b** Perform ROM exercises every 2 hours.
- **c** Turn and re-position the person every 2 hours.
- **d** Place needed items on the weak (affected) side.

10 A person has aphasia. You know that
- **a** The person cannot speak
- **b** The person cannot hear
- **c** The person has a language disorder
- **d** Mouth and face muscles are affected

11 In Parkinson's disease
- **a** Symptoms progress rapidly
- **b** Mental function is affected first
- **c** Tremors, slow movements, and a shuffling gait occur
- **d** Paralysis occurs but mental function is intact

12 A person has multiple sclerosis. Which is *true?*
- **a** There is a cure.
- **b** Only voluntary muscles are affected.
- **c** Persons over the age of 50 are at risk.
- **d** Over time, the person depends on others for care.

13 A person has tetraplegia from a spinal cord injury. Which should you question?
- **a** Keep the bed in a low position.
- **b** Assist with active ROM exercises.
- **c** Follow the bowel training program.
- **d** Turn and re-position every hour.

14 When talking to a person with hearing loss
- **a** Shout
- **b** Change the subject if the person does not seem to understand
- **c** Avoid using gestures and facial expressions
- **d** Use short sentences and simple words

15 A hearing aid does not seem to be working. Your *first* action is to
- **a** See if it is turned on
- **b** Wash it with soap and water
- **c** Have it repaired
- **d** Remove the batteries

16 A person has a cataract. Which is *true?*
- **a** Central vision is lost.
- **b** Peripheral vision is lost.
- **c** Vision is cloudy, blurry, or dimmed.
- **d** Blindness occurs.

17 When eyeglasses are not worn, they should be
- **a** Soaked in a cleansing solution
- **b** Put in the eyeglass case
- **c** Taken to the nurses' station
- **d** Placed on the over-bed table

18 Which are dangers to persons who are blind or visually impaired?
- **a** Drawers that are fully closed
- **b** Doors that are fully open
- **c** Burnt-out bulbs
- **d** Night-lights

19 A person is blind. You should
- **a** Avoid using colors to describe things
- **b** Move furniture to provide variety
- **c** Have the person walk in front of you
- **d** Explain procedures step-by-step

20 In hypertension, the systolic blood pressure is
- **a** 140 mm Hg or higher
- **b** 120 mm Hg or higher
- **c** 90 mm Hg or higher
- **d** 80 mm Hg or higher

21 A person is being treated for hypertension. Which would you question?
- **a** No smoking
- **b** A high-sodium diet
- **c** Regular exercise
- **d** A low-fat diet

Continued

REVIEW QUESTIONS—cont'd

Circle the BEST answer.—cont'd

22 A person has angina. Which is *true?*
- **a** There is heart muscle damage.
- **b** Pain is described as crushing or stabbing.
- **c** Pain is relieved with rest and nitroglycerin.
- **d** Pain is always on the left side of the chest.

23 A person complains of sudden squeezing chest pain. You should
- **a** Report the pain if it is not relieved in 15 minutes
- **b** Report the pain at once
- **c** Give the person a nitroglycerin tablet
- **d** Give the person oxygen

24 A person has heart failure. Which measure should you question?
- **a** Encourage fluids.
- **b** Measure intake and output.
- **c** Measure weight daily.
- **d** Perform range-of-motion exercises.

25 The most common cause of COPD is
- **a** Smoking
- **b** Allergies
- **c** Being over-weight
- **d** A high-sodium diet

26 A person has emphysema. Which is *true?*
- **a** The person has an infection.
- **b** Breathing is usually easier lying down.
- **c** The person has dyspnea.
- **d** Wheezing and chest-tightness occur.

27 Which position eases breathing in the person with pneumonia?
- **a** Supine
- **b** Prone
- **c** Trendelenburg's
- **d** Semi-Fowler's

28 Tuberculosis is spread by
- **a** Contaminated drinking water
- **b** Coughing and sneezing
- **c** Contact with wound drainage
- **d** The fecal-oral route

29 A person has TB. You had contact with the person's sputum. You should
- **a** Put on gloves
- **b** Wash your hands
- **c** Use an alcohol-based hand rub
- **d** Tell the nurse

30 A person is vomiting. Which position is *best?*
- **a** Supine
- **b** Prone
- **c** Semi-Fowler's
- **d** Lying with the head turned to the side

31 Hepatitis is an inflammation of the
- **a** Liver
- **b** Gallbladder
- **c** Pancreas
- **d** Stomach

32 Hepatitis A is spread by
- **a** Needle sharing
- **b** Coughing and sneezing
- **c** Contaminated blood
- **d** The fecal-oral route

33 Hepatitis requires
- **a** Sterile gloving
- **b** Double-bagging
- **c** Standard Precautions
- **d** Masks, gowns, and goggles

34 A person has cystitis. This is a
- **a** Kidney infection
- **b** Kidney stone
- **c** Sexually transmitted disease
- **d** Bladder infection

35 Urinary problems with BPH are caused by
- **a** A weak urine stream
- **b** An enlarged prostate pressing against the urethra
- **c** Frequent voiding at night
- **d** Voiding in small amounts

36 These statements are about STDs. Which is *true?*
- **a** Some people do not have signs and symptoms.
- **b** STDs affect only the genital area.
- **c** Condoms do not prevent the spread of STDs.
- **d** STDs cannot cause death.

37 A person with diabetes is vomiting after a meal. The person is at risk for
- **a** Hypoglycemia
- **b** Hyperglycemia
- **c** Jaundice
- **d** Bleeding

38 HIV is spread through
- **a** Coughing and sneezing
- **b** Using public phones and restrooms
- **c** Body fluids
- **d** Hugging an infected person

39 HIV and AIDS are prevented by
- **a** Transmission-Based Precautions
- **b** Radiation therapy
- **c** Chemotherapy
- **d** Standard Precautions

40 A person has shingles. Which is *true?*
- **a** Healing takes 3 to 5 days.
- **b** Persons who have had chicken pox are at risk.
- **c** Lesions are not infectious.
- **d** A rash with blisters covers the body.

Answers to these questions are on p. 505.

FOCUS ON PRACTICE

Problem Solving

A resident with diabetes is confused, weak, and shaky. What do you do? What might these signs and symptoms indicate? How does understanding the person's health problems help you give better care?

Caring for Persons With Mental Health Disorders

CHAPTER 29

OBJECTIVES

- Define the key terms and key abbreviations listed in this chapter.
- Explain the difference between mental health and mental illness.
- List the causes of mental health disorders.
- Describe 5 anxiety disorders.
- Explain the defense mechanisms used to relieve anxiety.
- Explain schizophrenia.
- Describe bipolar disorder and depression.
- Describe personality disorders.
- Describe substance abuse and addiction.
- Describe suicide and the persons at risk.
- Describe the care required by persons with mental health disorders.
- Explain how to promote PRIDE in the person, the family, and yourself.

KEY TERMS

anxiety A vague, uneasy feeling in response to stress
compulsion Repeating an act over and over again (a ritual)
defense mechanism An unconscious reaction that blocks unpleasant or threatening feelings
delusion A false belief
delusion of grandeur An exaggerated belief about one's importance, wealth, power, or talents
delusion of persecution A false belief that one is being mistreated, abused, or harassed
flashback Reliving a trauma in thoughts during the day and in nightmares during sleep
hallucination Seeing, hearing, smelling, or feeling something that is not real
mental Relating to the mind; something that exists in the mind or is done by the mind
mental health The person copes with and adjusts to everyday stresses in ways accepted by society
mental health disorder A disturbance in the ability to cope with or adjust to stress; behavior and function are impaired; mental illness, psychiatric disorder
mental illness See "mental health disorder"
obsession A recurrent, unwanted thought, idea, or image
panic An intense and sudden feeling of fear, anxiety, terror, or dread
paranoia A disorder *(para)* of the mind *(noia);* false beliefs (delusions) and suspicion about a person or a situation
phobia An intense fear
psychiatric disorder See "mental health disorder"
stress The response or change in the body caused by any emotional, physical, social, or economic factor
suicide To kill oneself
suicide contagion Exposure to suicide or suicidal behaviors within one's family, one's peer group, or media reports of suicide
withdrawal syndrome The person's physical and mental response after stopping or severely reducing the use of a substance that was used regularly

KEY ABBREVIATIONS

BPD	Borderline personality disorder
GI	Gastro-intestinal
OCD	Obsessive-compulsive disorder
PTSD	Post-traumatic stress disorder

The whole person has physical, social, psychological, and spiritual parts. Each part affects the other.

- A physical problem can have social, mental, and spiritual effects.
- A mental health problem can have physical, social, and spiritual effects.
- A social problem can have physical, mental, and spiritual effects.

BASIC CONCEPTS

***Mental** relates to the mind. It is something that exists in the mind or is done by the mind.* Therefore mental health involves the mind. Mental health and mental health disorders involve stress.

- ***Stress**—is the response or change in the body caused by any emotional, physical, social, or economic factor.*
- ***Mental health**—means that the person copes with and adjusts to everyday stresses in ways accepted by society.*
- ***Mental health disorder**—is a disturbance in the ability to cope with or adjust to stress. Behavior and function are impaired. **Mental illness** and **psychiatric disorder*** are other names.

Causes of mental health disorders include:

- Not being able to cope with or adjust to stress
- Chemical imbalances
- Genetics
- Physical, biological, or psychological factors
- Drug or substance abuse
- Social and cultural factors

BOX 29-1 Signs and Symptoms of Anxiety

- Appetite: loss of
- Apprehension
- Attention span: poor
- Blood pressure: increased
- "Butterflies" in the stomach
- Diarrhea
- Directions: difficulty following
- "Lump" in the throat
- Mouth: dry
- Nausea
- Pulse: rapid
- Respirations: rapid
- Sleep: difficulty
- Speech: rapid, voice changes
- Sweating
- Tiredness
- Trembling
- Urinary frequency and urgency
- Weakness

ANXIETY DISORDERS

***Anxiety** is a vague, uneasy feeling in response to stress.* The person senses danger or harm—real or imagined. The person acts to relieve the unpleasant feeling. Often anxiety occurs when needs are not met.

Some anxiety is normal. Persons with mental health disorders have higher levels of anxiety. Signs and symptoms depend on the degree of anxiety (Box 29-1).

Coping and defense mechanisms may help to relieve anxiety. Some are healthy, others are not—eating, drinking, smoking, and fighting are examples. Healthy coping includes discussing the problem, exercising, playing music, taking a hot bath, and wanting to be alone.

***Defense mechanisms** are unconscious reactions that block unpleasant or threatening feelings* (Box 29-2). Some use of defense mechanisms is normal. In mental health disorders, they are used poorly.

Some common anxiety disorders are:

- *Generalized anxiety disorder.* The person has at least 6 months of extreme anxiety. He or she worries about health, money, or family problems, often for no reason. Getting through the day can be difficult. Worry can prevent the person from normal function.
- *Panic disorder. **Panic** is an intense and sudden feeling of fear, anxiety, terror, or dread.* Signs and symptoms of anxiety are severe and usually last a few minutes (see Box 29-1). The person may also have chest pain, shortness of breath, numbness and tingling in the hands, and dizziness. The person may feel that he or she is having a heart attack, losing his or her mind, or on the verge of death. Attacks can occur at any time, even during sleep. A *panic attack* is when symptoms last longer than a few minutes.
- *Phobias. **Phobia** means an intense fear.* The person has an intense fear of an object, situation, or activity that has little or no actual danger. The person avoids what is feared. When faced with the fear, the person has high anxiety and cannot function. Common phobias are fear of:
  - Being in an open, crowded, or public place (*agoraphobia—agora* means *marketplace*)
  - Water (*aquaphobia—aqua* means *water*)
  - Being in or trapped in an enclosed or narrow space (*claustrophobia—claustro* means *closing*)
  - The slightest uncleanliness (*mysophobia—myso* means *anything that is disgusting*)
- *Obsessive-compulsive disorder (OCD).* The person may have both obsessive and compulsive behaviors. An ***obsession** is a recurrent, unwanted thought, idea, or image. **Compulsion** is repeating an act over and over again (a ritual).* The act may not make sense. Anxiety is great if the act is not done. Common rituals are hand washing, cleaning, counting things to a certain number, or touching things in a certain order. Such rituals can take over an hour every day. They are very distressing and affect daily life.
- *Post-traumatic stress disorder (PTSD).* PTSD occurs after a terrifying event. PTSD can develop at any age. See Box 29-3 for signs and symptoms. PTSD can develop:
  - After being harmed or after a loved one was harmed—mugging, rape, torture, kidnapping, abuse
  - After seeing a harmful event happen—war, terrorist attack, crash (vehicle, train, plane), bombing, flood, tornado, hurricane, earthquake

BOX 29-2 Defense Mechanisms

Compensation. *Compensate* means *to make up for, replace, or substitute.* The person makes up for or substitutes a strength for a weakness.
EXAMPLE: Not good in sports, a child develops another talent.

Conversion. *Convert* means *to change.* An emotion is shown as a physical symptom or changed into a physical symptom.
EXAMPLE: Not wanting to read out loud in school, a child complains of a headache.

Denial. *Deny* means *refusing to accept or believe something that is true.* The person refuses to face or accept unpleasant or threatening things.
EXAMPLE: After a heart attack, a person continues to smoke.

Displacement. *Displace* means *to move or take the place of.* An individual moves behaviors or emotions from one person, place, or thing to a safe person, place, or thing.
EXAMPLE: Angry at your boss, you yell at a friend.

Identification. *Identify* means *to relate* or *recognize.* A person assumes the ideas, behaviors, and traits of another person.
EXAMPLE: A neighbor is a high school cheerleader. A little girl practices cheerleading in her backyard.

Projection. *Project* means *to blame another.* An individual blames another person or object for unacceptable behaviors, emotions, ideas, or wishes.
EXAMPLE: Sleeping too long, a worker blames the traffic when late for work.

Rationalization. *Rational* means *sensible, reasonable,* or *logical.* An acceptable reason or excuse is given for behaviors or actions. The real reason is not given.
EXAMPLE: Often late for work, an employee does not get a raise. The employee thinks: "My boss doesn't like me."

Reaction formation. A person acts in a way opposite to what he or she truly feels.
EXAMPLE: A worker does not like his boss. He buys the boss a gift.

Regression. *Regress* means *to move back* or *to retreat.* The person retreats or moves back to an earlier time or condition.
EXAMPLE: A 3-year-old wants a baby bottle when a new baby comes into the family.

Repression. *Repress* means *to hold down* or *keep back.* The person keeps unpleasant or painful thoughts or experiences from the conscious mind. They cannot be recalled or remembered.
EXAMPLE: A child was sexually abused. Now 33 years old, there is no memory of the event.

BOX 29-3 Signs and Symptoms of Post-Traumatic Stress Disorder

- Affection: problems with
- Aggressive and violent behaviors
- Anger: gets mad easily; outbursts
- Avoidance of situations that remind of the harmful event
- Closeness: problems with
- Difficulty around the anniversary of the harmful event
- Emotionally numb: especially to those with whom the person used to be close
- ***Flashbacks:*** *reliving the trauma in thoughts during the day and in nightmares during sleep;* may involve images, sounds, smells, or feelings; the person may believe that the trauma is happening all over again
- Guilt: intense
- Irritability
- Loss of interest in things he or she used to enjoy
- Physical symptoms:
  - Headache
  - Gastro-intestinal (GI) distress
  - Immune system problems
  - Dizziness
  - Chest pain
  - Discomfort in other body parts
- Sleeping: problems with
- Startles easily
- Trusting people: problems with

SCHIZOPHRENIA

Schizophrenia means split *(schizo)* mind *(phrenia)*. It is a severe, chronic, disabling brain disorder. It involves:

- ***Hallucinations***—*seeing, hearing, smelling, or feeling something that is not real.* A person may see animals, insects, or people that are not real. "Voices" are a common type of hallucination. "Voices" may comment on behavior or order the person to do things, warn of danger, or talk to other voices.
- ***Delusions***—*false beliefs.* For example, the person believes that a radio station is airing the person's thoughts. Some people have ***delusions of grandeur***—*exaggerated beliefs about one's importance, wealth, power, or talents.* For example, a man believes he is Superman. Or a woman believes she is the Queen of England. ***Delusions of persecution*** *are false beliefs that one is being mistreated, abused, or harassed.* For example, a person believes that someone is "out to get" him or her.
- ***Paranoia***—*a disorder* (para) *of the mind* (noia). *The person has false beliefs (delusions) and suspicion about a person or situation.* For example, a person believes that others are cheating, harassing, poisoning, spying on, or plotting against him or her.
- *Thought disorders.* The person has trouble organizing thoughts or connecting thoughts logically. Speech may be garbled and hard to understand. The person may suddenly stop speaking in the middle of a thought. Some persons make up words that have no meaning.
- *Movement disorders.* These include:
  - Being clumsy and uncoordinated
  - Involuntary movements
  - Grimacing
  - Unusual mannerisms
  - Sitting for hours without moving, speaking, or responding
- *Emotional and behavioral problems.* Normal functions are impaired or absent. The person may:
  - Lose motivation or interest in daily activities.
  - Be unable to plan or do activities.
  - Seem to lack emotional responses.
  - Neglect personal hygiene.
  - Withdraw socially.
- *Cognitive problems. Cognitive* relates to *understanding, remembering,* and *reasoning.* The person may have trouble paying attention or understanding or remembering information. Symptoms make it hard for the person to perform daily tasks.

Some persons regress. To *regress* means *to retreat* or *move back to an earlier time or condition.* For example, a 5-year-old wets the bed when there is a new baby. This is normal. Healthy adults do not act like infants or children.

FOCUS ON COMMUNICATION

Schizophrenia

Delusions, hallucinations, and paranoia can frighten a person. Good communication is important. Remember to:

- Speak slowly and calmly.
- Do not pretend you experience what the person does. Help the person focus on reality.
- Do not try to convince the person that the experience is not real. To the person, it is real.

For example, a person hears voices. You can say: "I don't hear the voices, but I believe you do. Try to listen to my voice and not the other voices."

Symptoms usually begin between the ages of 16 and 30. The onset tends to be earlier in men than in women. People with schizophrenia do not tend to be violent. However, if a person becomes violent, it is often directed at family members in the home setting. Some persons with schizophrenia attempt suicide (p. 463).

See *Focus on Communication: Schizophrenia.*

BIPOLAR DISORDER

Bipolar means 2 *(bi)* poles or ends *(polar)*. The person with bipolar disorder has severe extremes in mood, energy, and ability to function. There are emotional lows (depression) and emotional highs (mania). Therefore the disorder is also called manic-depressive illness.

The disorder tends to run in families. It usually develops during the late teens or early adulthood. Life-long management is required.

Signs and symptoms range from mild to severe (Box 29-4). Mood changes are called "episodes." Some people are suicidal.

DEPRESSION

Depression involves the body, mood, and thoughts. Symptoms (see Box 29-4) affect work, study, sleep, eating, and other activities. The person is very sad. Interest in daily activities is lost.

Some types of depression tend to run in families. Some physical disorders can cause depression. Stroke, heart attack, cancer, and Parkinson's disease are examples. Hormonal factors may cause depression. Thyroid problems, the menstrual cycle, pregnancy, miscarriage, childbirth (post-partum depression), and menopause involve hormonal changes. A stressful event such as the death of a partner, parent, or child may cause depression. So can divorce or job loss.

BOX 29-4 Signs and Symptoms of Bipolar Disorder

Mania (Manic Episode)
- Increased energy, activity, and restlessness
- Excessively "high," overly happy mood
- Extreme irritability
- Feeling "jumpy" or "wired"
- Racing thoughts and rapid speech
- Jumping from 1 idea to another
- Easily distracted, problems concentrating
- Little sleep needed
- Unrealistic beliefs in one's abilities and powers
- Poor judgment
- Spending sprees
- A lasting period of behavior that is different from usual
- Increased sex drive
- Drug or alcohol abuse
- Aggressive behavior
- Denial that anything is wrong
- Frequent absences or poor performance at work or school

Depression (Depressive Episode)
- Sadness
- Hopelessness
- Empty mood
- Worry and anxiety
- Guilt
- Loss of interest in activities once enjoyed
- Loss of interest in sex
- Feeling tired or "slowed down"
- Problems concentrating, remembering, or making decisions
- Restlessness or irritability
- Sleep problems
- Change in appetite: low or increased
- Chronic pain or other symptoms without a cause
- Frequent absences or poor performance at work or school
- Thoughts of death or suicide
- Suicide attempts

Depression in Older Persons

Depression is common in older persons. They have many losses—death of family and friends, loss of body functions, loss of independence. See Box 29-5 for the signs and symptoms of depression in older persons.

Some medical conditions and drug side effects can cause symptoms of depression. Depression in older persons is often overlooked or a wrong diagnosis is made. Often the person is thought to have a cognitive disorder (Chapter 30). Therefore depression is often not treated.

PERSONALITY DISORDERS

Personality disorders involve rigid and maladaptive behaviors. To *adapt* means *to change* or *adjust. Mal* means *bad, wrong, or ill. Maladaptive* means *to change or adjust in the wrong way.* Because of behavior, persons with personality disorders cannot function well in society.

BOX 29-5 Signs and Symptoms of Depression in Older Persons

- Fatigue
- Inability to experience pleasure
- Feelings of uselessness, hopelessness, or helplessness
- Decreased sexual interest
- Increased dependency
- Anxiety
- Slow or unreliable memory
- Paranoia
- Agitation
- Focus on the past
- Thoughts of death or suicide
- Difficulty completing activities of daily living
- Changes in sleep patterns
- Poor grooming
- Withdrawal from people or interests
- Muscle aches, abdominal pain, and headaches
- Nausea and vomiting
- Dry mouth
- Loss of appetite
- Weight loss

Antisocial Personality Disorder

The person has a long-term pattern of thinking and behaviors that violates the rights of others. He or she has no regard for right and wrong and the safety of others. The person has poor judgment, lacks responsibility, has no guilt, and is hostile. The person is not loyal to any person or group. Morals and ethics are lacking. The person lies, charms, or cons others for personal gain or pleasure. Stealing, fighting, and drug abuse are common criminal acts.

Borderline Personality Disorder

Borderline personality disorder (BPD) involves unstable moods, behaviors, and relationships. The person has a long-term pattern of at least 5 of the following.

- Extreme reactions. These involve panic, depression, and rage.
- Intense and stormy relationships with loved ones, family, and friends. The person has extremes from love and closeness to dislike and anger.
- Unstable self-image. The person has sudden changes in feelings, opinions, values, and goals.
- Impulsive and dangerous behaviors. Spending sprees, unsafe sex, substance abuse, reckless driving, and binge eating are examples.
- Suicidal behaviors or threats of self-harm. Self-harm behaviors include cutting, burning, and hitting oneself; head banging; and hair pulling.
- Intense and changing moods.
- Feelings of emptiness or boredom.
- Intense anger or anger control problems.
- Paranoid thoughts or severe dissociative symptoms. *Dissociate* means *to disconnect* or *separate.* The person feels cut-off from oneself, observes oneself from outside the body, or loses touch with reality.

SUBSTANCE ABUSE AND ADDICTION

Substance abuse or addiction occurs when a person overuses or depends on alcohol or drugs. Physical and mental health are affected. So is the welfare of others.

The substances involved affect the nervous system. Some depress the nervous system. Others stimulate it. All affect the mind and thinking.

Alcoholism and Alcohol Abuse

Alcohol slows down brain activity. It affects alertness, judgment, coordination, and reaction time. Over time, heavy drinking damages the brain, central nervous system, liver, kidneys, heart, blood vessels, and stomach. It also can cause forgetfulness and confusion.

Alcoholism is when a person has signs of physical addiction to alcohol and continues to drink. The person continues to drink despite problems with physical and mental health and social, family, and job responsibilities. *Alcohol abuse* is when drinking leads to problems, but not physical addiction.

Alcoholism (alcohol dependence) includes these symptoms.

- *Craving*—a strong need or urge to drink
- *Loss of control*—cannot control the amount of time spent drinking, the amount of alcohol, or what happens while drinking
- *Physical dependence*—withdrawal symptoms (nausea, sweating, shakiness, anxiety) when drinking is stopped
- *Tolerance*—greater amounts of alcohol are needed to get "high"

Alcoholism is a chronic disease. It lasts throughout life. Alcoholism can be treated but not cured. Counseling and drugs are used to help the person stop drinking. The person must avoid all alcohol to prevent a relapse.

See *Focus on Older Persons: Alcoholism and Alcohol Abuse.*

FOCUS ON OLDER PERSONS

Alcoholism and Alcohol Abuse

Alcohol effects vary with age. Even small amounts can make older persons feel "high." Older persons are at risk for falls, vehicle crashes, and other injuries from drinking. They have:

- Slower reaction times
- Hearing and vision problems
- A lower tolerance for alcohol

Older persons tend to take more prescribed drugs than younger persons. Mixing alcohol with some drugs can be harmful, even fatal. Alcohol also makes some health problems worse. High blood pressure is an example.

Drug Abuse and Addiction

Drugs affect normal brain function. While they create intense feelings of pleasure, they have long-term effects on the brain. Changes in the brain can turn drug abuse into addiction.

- *Drug abuse*—is using a drug for non-medical or non-therapy effects.
- *Drug addiction*—is a chronic, relapsing brain disease. The person has an overwhelming desire to take the drug because it affects mental awareness. The person has to have the drug. Often higher doses are needed. The person cannot stop taking the drug without treatment. A diagnosis is based on 3 or more of the following during a 12-month period.
  - The drug is often taken in larger amounts. Or it is taken longer than intended.
  - The person tries to cut down or stop using the drug.
  - Much time is spent using the drug or recovering from its effects. Or a great deal of time is spent trying to obtain the drug. The person gave up or reduced social, job, or recreational events because of drug use.
  - The person continues to use the drug. The person does so despite knowing that problems are caused by or made worse by using the drug.
  - The person has tolerance to the drug.
    - The drug has less and less effect on the person.
    - The person needs more of the drug to get high.
  - The person has withdrawal symptoms (withdraw means to stop, remove, or take away).
    - ***Withdrawal syndrome*** *is the person's physical and mental response after stopping or severely reducing the use of a substance that was used regularly.* The body responds with anxiety, restlessness, insomnia, irritability, impaired attention, and physical illness.
    - The same (or similar) drug is taken to relieve or avoid withdrawal symptoms.

Drug abuse and addiction affect social and mental function. They are linked to crimes, violence, car crashes, and suicide. Family, work, school, legal, and financial issues can result. Physical effects can occur from 1 use, high doses, or prolonged use—HIV and AIDS, cardiovascular disease, stroke, sudden death, hepatitis, lung disease, cancer.

Legal and illegal drugs are abused. Legal drugs are approved for use in the United States. Doctors prescribe them. Illegal drugs are not approved for use. They are obtained through illegal means. And some persons obtain legal drugs through illegal means.

A drug treatment program combines various therapies and services to meet the person's needs. Drug abuse and addiction are chronic problems. Relapses can occur. A short-term, one-time treatment is often not enough. Treatment is a long-term process.

EATING DISORDERS

An eating disorder involves extremes in eating patterns. The person has a severe disturbance in eating behavior. Eating disorders are more common in women and girls.

- *Anorexia nervosa. Anorexia* means no *(an)* appetite *(orexia). Nervosa* relates to *nerves* or *emotions*. The person has an intense fear of weight gain or obesity. A fat body image is felt despite being dangerously thin. The person avoids food and meals or eats food in small amounts. Intense exercise and vomiting are common. So is enema and laxative use to rid the body of food. Laxatives are drugs that promote defecation. Diuretic abuse also may occur. These drugs cause the kidneys to produce large amounts of urine. Extra fluid in the body is lost. Weight loss results. Serious health problems can result. Death is a risk from cardiac arrest or suicide.
- *Bulimia nervosa*. Binge eating occurs. That is, the person eats large amounts of food. Then the body is purged (rid) of the food to prevent weight gain. Vomiting, laxatives, enemas, diuretics, fasting, and intense exercise are some methods used.
- *Binge eating disorder*. The person often eats large amounts of food. Eating is out of control. Binge eating is not followed by purging, fasting, or exercise. Often the person is over-weight or obese. High blood pressure, heart disease, diabetes, and joint pain can occur.

SUICIDE

Suicide *means to kill oneself.* Risk factors are listed in Box 29-6. *If a person mentions or talks about suicide, take the person seriously. Call for the nurse at once. Do not leave the person alone.*

Agencies treating persons with mental health disorders must identify persons at risk for suicide. They must:

- Identify specific factors or features that increase or decrease the risk for suicide.
- Meet the person's immediate safety needs.
- Provide the most appropriate setting to treat the person.
- Provide crisis information to the person and family. A crisis "hotline" phone number is an example.

See *Focus on Communication: Suicide.*

See *Focus on Older Persons: Suicide.*

Suicide Contagion

Suicide contagion *is exposure to suicide or suicidal behaviors within one's family, one's peer group, or media reports of suicide.* The exposure has led to more suicides and suicidal behaviors in persons at risk. Adolescents and young adults are at risk for suicide contagion.

Following suicide exposure, those close to the victim need evaluation by a mental health professional. They include family, friends, peers, and co-workers. Persons at risk for suicide need mental health services.

BOX 29-6 Suicide Risk Factors

- Depression and other mental health disorders
- Substance abuse disorder
- Prior suicide attempt
- Family history of a mental health disorder or substance abuse
- Family history of suicide
- Family violence (including physical or sexual abuse)
- Firearms in the home
- Incarceration (prison or jail)
- Exposure to the suicidal behavior of others (family, friends, media figures)

Modified from National Institute of Mental Health: Suicide in the U.S.: statistics and prevention, *National Institutes of Health, NIH publication No. 06-4594.*

FOCUS ON COMMUNICATION

Suicide

Persons thinking of suicide may talk about their thoughts. A person may say:

- "I just don't want to live anymore."
- "I wish I was dead."
- "I wish I had never been born."
- "Everyone would be better off without me."

Call for the nurse at once if a person mentions thoughts of suicide.

A person may ask you not to tell anyone about the suicidal thoughts. Protecting personal information is important. But the person's safety is the priority. Never promise that you will not tell anyone. Report the statement to the nurse at once.

FOCUS ON OLDER PERSONS

Suicide

According to the National Institute of Mental Health, suicide rates are higher in older persons than in other age groups. White men age 85 and older are at risk. Depression in older persons is a common risk factor.

Many older persons suffer from depression (p. 461). Depression often occurs with other serious illnesses. Heart disease, stroke, diabetes, cancer, and Parkinson's disease are examples. The person also may have social and financial problems.

Most older victims did not report depression to their doctors. Or depression was not diagnosed.

CARE AND TREATMENT

Treatment of mental health disorders involves having the person explore thoughts and feelings. Psychotherapy and behavior, group, occupational, art, and family therapies are used. Often drugs are ordered.

The care plan reflects the person's needs. The needs of the total person must be met. This includes physical, safety and security, and emotional needs.

Communication is important. Be alert to nonverbal communication. This includes the person's nonverbal communication and your own.

Persons with mental health disorders may respond to stress with anxiety, panic, or anger. Some become violent. You must protect yourself. Once you are safe, the health team can protect the person and others. To protect yourself:

- Call for help. Do not try to handle the situation on your own.
- Keep a safe distance between you and the person.
- Be aware of your setting. Do not let the person between you and the exit.

See *Focus on Communication: Care and Treatment.*

FOCUS ON COMMUNICATION

Care and Treatment

Nonverbal communication involves eye contact, tone of voice, facial expressions, body movements, and posture. Persons with depression often have little eye contact, poor posture, and speak softly. Some do not speak much at all. Facial expressions may not change. Some persons cry.

Persons with anxiety feel uneasy. They may be restless, unable to sit still, and talk fast. Eye contact may be prolonged and intense. Others have poor eye contact. The eyes may dart from one place to another. Be alert to nonverbal cues. Report what you observe.

Your nonverbal communication is also important. When interacting with persons with mental health disorders:

- Face the person.
- Maintain eye contact.
- Position yourself near the person but not too close. Do not invade the person's space.
- Crouch, sit, or stand at the person's level if safe to do so.
- Show interest and concern through your posture and facial expressions.
- Speak calmly.

FOCUS ON PRIDE

The Person, Family, and Yourself

Personal and Professional Responsibility

People do not choose to have physical or mental health disorders. Just as a person does not choose to have diabetes, a person does not choose anxiety or depression. How you view the illness affects how you treat the person. Treat the person with kindness, respect, and compassion. Provide quality care. Tell the nurse about any concerns.

Rights and Respect

Agencies have strict rules to protect the person's rights to privacy and confidentiality. Do not talk about the person with your family or friends. This violates the person's rights. Never give information to someone not involved in the person's care. This includes the person's family. Direct questions to the nurse. Follow agency policies and procedures. Take pride in protecting the person's rights.

Independence and Social Interaction

Social support is important in the treatment of mental health disorders. Interacting with others offers a healthy way to deal with stress. Family and friends provide a sense of worth and belonging. The care plan includes how they are involved in the person's care.

Providing support for a person with a mental health disorder can be demanding. The family needs support. Many communities offer support groups. You can also offer encouragement. Tell the family that you value the support they give.

Delegation and Teamwork

Caring for persons with mental health disorders requires great teamwork. A person may become hostile or violent. Or the person may threaten or attempt suicide. The team must react quickly to protect the person and others. If someone calls for help, respond at once. Assist as the nurse directs. Take pride in working as a team to ensure safety.

Ethics and Laws

Persons with mental health disorders may say or do things that seem strange or odd to you. Do not laugh at or insult the person. Do not joke with others about the person.

Ethics deals with right and wrong conduct. Be professional. Treat the person with dignity and respect. Take pride in the way you treat others.

REVIEW QUESTIONS

Circle the BEST answer.

1 Stress is
  a A way to cope with or adjust to everyday living
  b A response or change in the body caused by some factor
  c A mental health disorder
  d An unwanted thought or idea

2 Defense mechanisms are used to
  a Blame others
  b Make excuses for behavior
  c Return to an earlier time
  d Block unpleasant feelings

3 These statements are about defense mechanisms. Which is *true?*
  a Using them signals a mental health disorder.
  b They relieve anxiety.
  c They prevent mental health disorders.
  d Persons with mental health disorders use them well.

4 A phobia is
  a The event that causes stress
  b A false belief
  c An intense fear of something
  d A feeling or emotion

5 A person cleans and cleans. This behavior is
  a A delusion
  b A hallucination
  c A compulsion
  d An obsession

6 A person has nightmares about a trauma. The person is having
  a Flashbacks
  b Phobias
  c Panic attacks
  d Anxiety

7 Schizophrenia
  a Involves obsessions and compulsions
  b Can be cured with drugs and therapy
  c Usually begins in late adulthood
  d Is a disabling brain disorder

8 Bipolar disorder means that the person
  a Is very suspicious
  b Has anxiety
  c Is very unhappy and feels unwanted
  d Has severe extremes in mood

9 In bipolar disorder, an "emotional high" is called
  a Depression
  b A hallucination
  c Mania
  d An obsession

10 In antisocial personality disorder, the person
  a Is hostile and lacks morals
  b Has a sad, anxious, or empty mood
  c Withdraws from people and interests
  d Has regard for right and wrong

11 These statements are about alcoholism. Which is *true?*
  a The person has a strong craving for alcohol.
  b The disease can be cured.
  c After treatment, the person can have a social drink.
  d The person can control the amount and time spent drinking.

12 With drug addiction
  a Physical and social function are not affected
  b The person has to have the drug
  c Lower doses are needed for the effect
  d The person can stop taking the drug without treatment

13 Binge eating followed by purging occurs in
  a Anorexia nervosa
  b Binge-eating disorder
  c Bulimia nervosa
  d Borderline personality disorder

14 A person talks about suicide. What should you do?
  a Identify factors that increase the risk of suicide.
  b Ask what method the person intends to use.
  c Restrain the person.
  d Call for the nurse.

15 Which is a sign of depression in older persons?
  a Hallucinations
  b Withdrawal from people and interests
  c Increased energy and activity
  d Weight gain

Answers to these questions are on p. 505.

FOCUS ON PRACTICE

Problem Solving

Ms. Ellis is being treated for bipolar disorder. At 0300, you see her pacing in her room. She appears restless. You ask if she needs anything. She begins to talk very fast about work that needs to be done at home. She says: "I don't need to be here. I'm leaving, and you can't stop me!" What will you do? Is Ms. Ellis showing signs and symptoms of mania or depression? How will you protect yourself if she becomes violent?

CHAPTER

30 Caring for Persons With Confusion and Dementia

OBJECTIVES

- Define the key terms and key abbreviations listed in this chapter.
- Describe confusion and its causes.
- List the measures that help confused persons.
- Explain the differences between delirium, depression, and dementia.
- Describe the signs, symptoms, and behaviors of Alzheimer's disease (AD).
- Explain the care required by persons with AD and other dementias.
- Describe the effects of AD on the family.
- Explain validation therapy.
- Explain how to promote PRIDE in the person, the family, and yourself.

KEY TERMS

cognitive function Involves memory, thinking, reasoning, ability to understand, judgment, and behavior

confusion A mental state of being disoriented to person, time, place, situation, or identity

delirium A state of sudden, severe confusion and rapid changes in brain function

delusion A false belief

dementia The loss of cognitive function that interferes with routine personal, social, and occupational activities

elopement When a person leaves the agency without staff knowledge

hallucination Seeing, hearing, smelling, or feeling something that is not real

paranoia A disorder *(para)* of the mind *(noia);* false beliefs (delusions) and suspicion about a person or situation

pseudodementia False *(pseudo)* dementia

sundowning Signs, symptoms, and behaviors of AD increase during hours of darkness

KEY ABBREVIATIONS

AD	Alzheimer's disease
ADL	Activities of daily living
NIA	National Institute on Aging
OBRA	Omnibus Budget Reconciliation Act of 1987

Changes in the brain and nervous system occur with aging and certain diseases (Box 30-1). Cognitive function may be affected. (*Cognitive* relates to *knowledge.*) Quality of life is affected. *Cognitive function involves memory, thinking, reasoning, ability to understand, judgment, and behavior.*

CONFUSION

Confusion is a mental state of being disoriented to person, time, place, situation, or identity. Disease, brain injury, infections, hearing and vision loss, and drug side effects are some causes. With aging, blood supply to the brain is reduced. Personality and mental changes can result. Memory and ability to make good judgments are lost. A person may not know people, the time, or the place. Daily activities may be affected. Behavior changes are common. The person may be angry, restless, depressed, and irritable.

Acute confusion (*delirium*—p. 468) occurs suddenly. It is usually temporary. Causes include infection, illness, injury, drugs, and surgery. Treatment is aimed at the cause.

Confusion from physical changes cannot be cured. Some measures help improve function (Box 30-2). You must meet the person's basic needs.

BOX 30-1 Nervous System Changes From Aging

- Nerve cells are lost.
- Nerve conduction slows.
- Responses and reaction times are slower.
- Reflexes are slower.
- Vision and hearing decrease.
- Taste and smell decrease.
- Touch and sensitivity to pain decrease.
- Blood flow to the brain is reduced.
- Sleep patterns change.
- Memory is shorter.
- Forgetfulness occurs.
- Dizziness can occur.

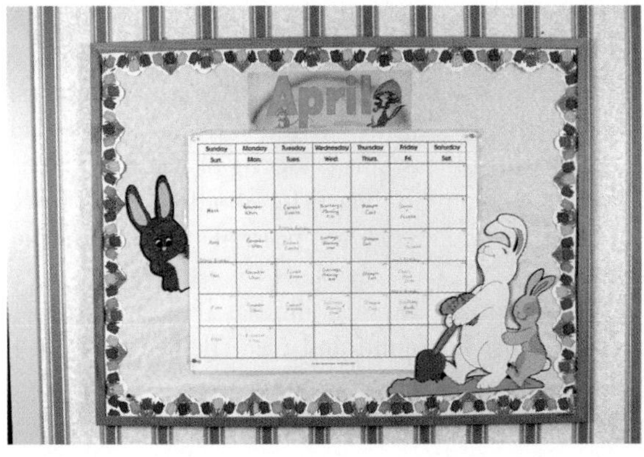

FIGURE 30-1 A large calendar can help persons who are confused.

BOX 30-2 Caring for Persons With Confusion

- Follow the person's care plan.
- Provide for safety.
- Face the person. Speak clearly.
- Call the person by name every time you have contact with him or her.
- State your name. Show your name tag.
- Give the date and time each morning. Repeat as needed during the day or evening.
- Explain what you are going to do and why.
- Give clear, simple directions and answers to questions.
- Ask clear and simple questions. Give the person time to respond.
- Keep calendars and clocks with large numbers in the person's room and in nursing areas (Fig. 30-1). Remind the person of holidays, birthdays, and other events.
- Have the person wear eyeglasses and hearing aids as needed.
- Use touch to communicate (Chapter 6).
- Place familiar objects and pictures within view.
- Provide newspapers, magazines, TV, and radio. Read to the person if appropriate.
- Discuss current events with the person.
- Maintain the day-night cycle.
  - Open window coverings during the day. Close them at night.
  - Use night-lights at night. Use them in rooms, bathrooms, hallways, and other areas.
  - Have the person wear regular clothes during the day—not sleepwear.
- Provide a calm, relaxed, and peaceful setting. Prevent loud noises, rushing, and crowded hallways and dining rooms.
- Follow the person's routine. Meals, bathing, exercise, TV, bedtime, and other activities have a schedule. This promotes a sense of order and what to expect.
- Break tasks into small steps when helping the person.
- Do not re-arrange furniture or the person's belongings.
- Encourage the person to take part in self-care.
- Be consistent.

DEMENTIA

***Dementia** is the loss of cognitive function that interferes with routine personal, social, and occupational activities.* (*De* means *from. Mentia* means *mind.*) Changes in personality, mood, behavior, and communication are common. Dementia occurs when the brain is damaged by disease or injury.

Dementia is not a normal part of aging. Most older people do not have dementia. Early warning signs include:

- Memory loss (losing things, forgetting names)
- Problems with common tasks (for example, dressing, cooking, driving)
- Problems with language and communication; forgetting simple words
- Getting lost in familiar places
- Misplacing things and putting things in odd places (for example, putting a watch in the oven)
- Personality, mood, and behavior changes
- Poor or decreased judgment (for example, going outdoors in the snow without shoes)

If brain changes have not occurred, some dementias can be reversed. When the cause is removed, so are the signs and symptoms. Treatable causes include:

- Drugs and alcohol
- Delirium and depression (p. 468)
- Tumors
- Heart, lung, and blood vessel problems
- Head injuries
- Infection
- Vision and hearing problems

Permanent dementias result from changes in the brain. The causes in Box 30-3, p. 468 have no cure. Function declines over time. Alzheimer's disease is the most common type of permanent dementia.

***Pseudodementia** means false* (pseudo) *dementia.* The person has signs and symptoms of dementia. However, there are no changes in the brain. This can occur with delirium and depression. Both can be mistaken for dementia.

Delirium

Delirium *is a state of sudden, severe confusion and rapid changes in brain function.* Usually temporary and reversible, it occurs with physical or mental illness. Causes include acute or chronic illness, surgery, drug or alcohol abuse, and infections. Delirium often lasts for about 1 week. However, it may take several weeks for normal mental function to return.

Delirium signals physical illness. It is an emergency. The cause must be found and treated. See Box 30-4 for signs and symptoms.

BOX 30-3 Causes of Permanent Dementia

- AIDS-related dementia
- Alcohol-related dementia and Korsakoff's syndrome
- Alzheimer's disease
- Brain tumors
- Cerebrovascular disease
- Huntington's disease (a nervous system disease)
- Multi-infarct dementia (MID)—many *(multi)* strokes leave areas of damage *(infarct)*
- Multiple sclerosis
- Parkinson's disease
- Stroke
- Syphilis
- Trauma and head injury

BOX 30-4 Signs and Symptoms of Delirium

- Alertness: changes in. The person is usually more alert in the morning and less alert at night.
- Sensation: changes in.
- Awareness: changes in.
- Movement: very active or slow moving.
- Drowsiness.
- Confusion about time or place.
- Memory:
  - Decreased short-term memory and recall. Cannot remember events since the delirium began.
  - Cannot remember past events.
- Thinking and behavior are without purpose.
- Problems concentrating.
- Speech does not make sense.
- Emotional changes:
  - Agitation
  - Anger
  - Anxiety
  - Apathy
  - Depression
  - Euphoria
  - Irritability
- Incontinence.
- Restlessness.

Modified from MedlinePlus: Delirium, *Bethesda, Md, updated March 22, 2013, U.S. National Library of Medicine, National Institutes of Health.*

Depression

Depression is the most common mental health disorder in older persons. It is often overlooked. Depression, aging, and some drug side effects have similar signs and symptoms. See Chapter 29 for signs and symptoms of depression in older persons.

ALZHEIMER'S DISEASE

Alzheimer's disease (AD) is a brain disease. Many brain cells are destroyed and die (Fig. 30-2). These functions are affected:

- Memory
- Thinking
- Reasoning
- Judgment
- Language
- Behavior
- Mood
- Personality

The person has problems with work and everyday functions. Problems with family and social relationships occur. There is a slow, steady decline in memory and mental function.

The onset is gradual. Usually symptoms first appear after age 60. The person can live 3 to 4 years or as long as 10 or more years. Nearly half of persons age 85 and older have AD. More women than men have AD. Women live longer than men.

AD is not a normal part of aging. The cause is unknown. A family history of AD increases a person's risk of developing the disease.

Signs of AD

According to the Alzheimer's Association, the most common early symptom of AD is difficulty remembering newly learned information. The classic sign of AD is a gradual loss of short-term memory. At first, the only symptom may be forgetfulness. Box 30-5 lists the warning and other signs of AD. See Box 30-6 for the differences between AD and normal age-related changes.

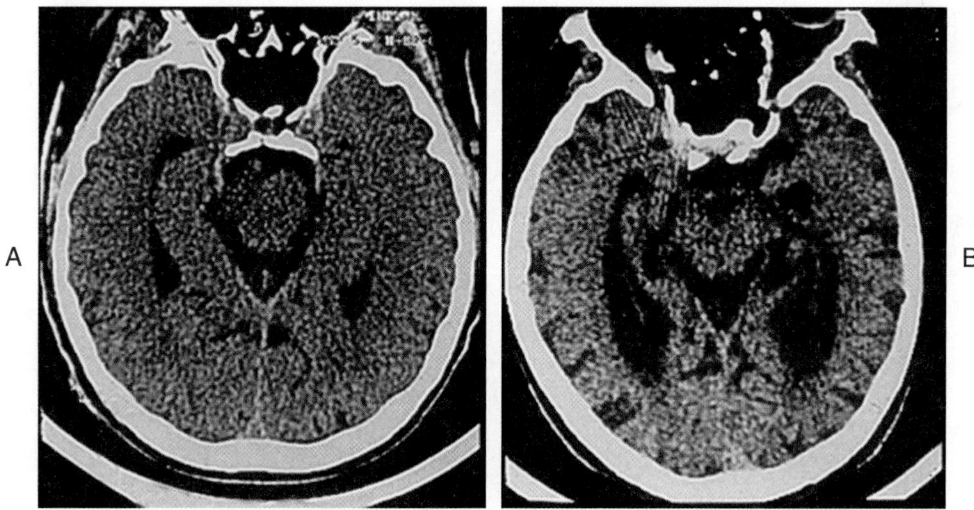

FIGURE 30-2 **A,** Normal brain. **B,** Dark patches show damage to brain tissue.

BOX 30-5 Signs of Alzheimer's Disease

Warning Signs

- Asks the same question over and over again.
- Repeats the same story—word for word, again and again.
- Forgets activities that were once done regularly and with ease—cooking, repairs, playing cards, and so on.
- Loses the ability to pay bills or balance a checkbook.
- Gets lost in familiar places.
- Misplaces household items.
- Neglects to bathe. Or wears the same clothes over and over again.
- Relies on someone else to make decisions or answer questions that he or she would have handled.

Other Signs

- Forgets recent events, conversations, and appointments.
- Forgets simple directions.
- Forgets names of family members and the names of everyday things (clock, TV, and so on).
- Forgets words, cannot find the right word, or loses train of thought.
- Substitutes unusual words and names for what is forgotten.
- Speaks in a native language.
- Curses or swears.
- Forgets important dates and events.

Other Signs—cont'd

- Takes longer to do things.
- Misplaces things. Puts things in odd places.
- Has problems keeping track of bills and writing checks.
- Gives away large amounts of money.
- Does not recognize or understand numbers.
- Has problems following conversations.
- Has problems reading and writing.
- Has problems driving to familiar places.
- Forgets where he or she is.
- Forgets how he or she got to a certain place.
- Does not know how to get back home.
- Wanders from home.
- Cannot tell or understand time or dates.
- Cannot solve everyday problems (iron left on, stove burners left on, food burning on the stove, and so on).
- Cannot perform everyday tasks (dressing, bathing, brushing teeth, and so on).
- Distrusts others.
- Is stubborn.
- Does not want to do things and withdraws socially.
- Is restless.
- Becomes suspicious and fearful.
- Sleeps more than usual.

Warning signs modified from Eric Pfeiffer, MD: The seven warning signs of Alzheimer's disease, *University of South Florida Suncoast Alzheimer's and Gerontology Center. Reprinted with permission.*

BOX 30-6 Alzheimer's Disease and Normal Aging

Signs of AD	Normal Age-Related Changes
• Poor judgment and decision making.	• Makes a bad decision once in a while.
• Cannot manage a budget.	• Misses a monthly payment.
• Loses track of the date or season.	• Forgets which day it is but remembers later.
• Problems having a conversation.	• Sometimes forgets which word to use.
• Misplaces things. Cannot retrace steps to find them.	• Loses things from time to time.

Modified from Alzheimer's Association: 10 early signs and symptoms of Alzheimer's, *2013*

BOX 30-7 Three Stages of Alzheimer's Disease—National Institute on Aging

Mild AD
- Memory problems
- Getting lost
- Problems handling money and paying bills
- Repeating questions
- Taking longer to complete daily tasks
- Poor judgment
- Losing things or misplacing them in odd places
- Mood and personality changes

Moderate AD
- Increased memory loss and confusion
- Problems recognizing family and friends
- Cannot learn new things
- Problems with tasks having multiple steps—getting dressed is an example
- Problems coping with new situations
- Hallucinations, delusions, and paranoia (p. 472)
- Impulsive behavior

Severe AD
- Depends on others for care
- Cannot communicate
- Weight loss
- Seizures
- Skin infections
- Difficulty swallowing
- Groaning, moaning, or grunting
- Increased sleeping
- In bed most or all of the time
- Lack of bowel and bladder control

Modified from National Institute on Aging: About Alzheimer's disease: symptoms, *National Institutes of Health.*

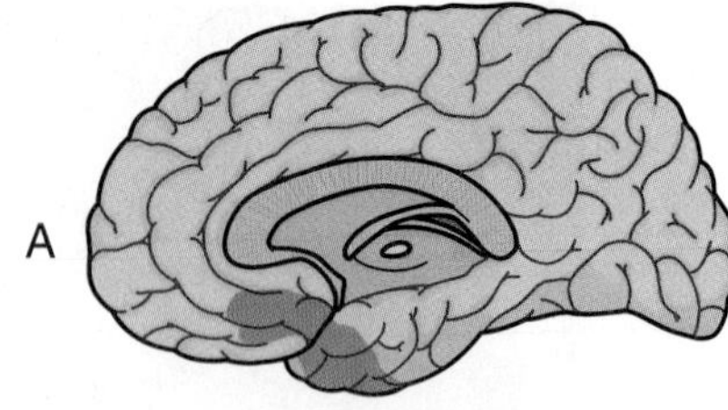

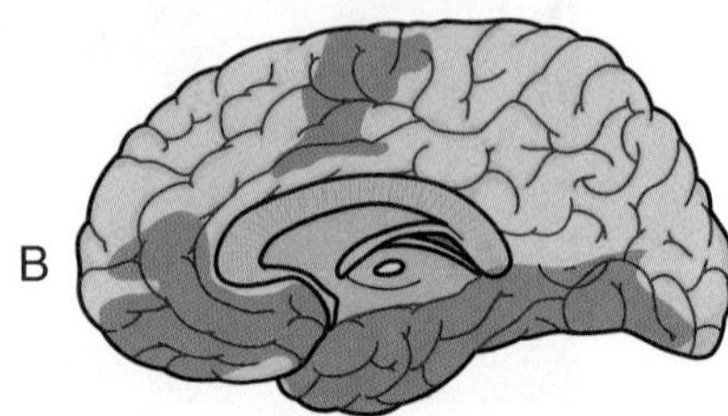

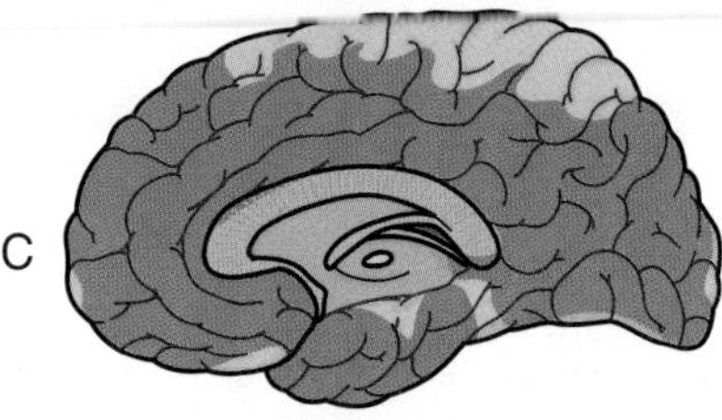

FIGURE 30-3 A, Very early AD. **B,** Mild to moderate AD. **C,** Severe AD. (Note: Blue shading shows the area of brain damage.)

Stages of AD

Signs and symptoms become more severe as the disease progresses. The disease ends in death. AD is often described in 3 stages (Box 30-7; Fig. 30-3). The Alzheimer's Association describes AD in 7 stages (Box 30-8).

Behaviors and Problems

AD changes how a person behaves and acts. Besides the signs and symptoms in Boxes 30-5, 30-7, and 30-8, these changes are common.
- Wandering and getting lost
- Sundowning (p. 472)
- Hallucinations (p. 472)
- Delusions (p. 472)
- Paranoia (p. 472)
- Catastrophic reactions (p. 472)
- Agitation and aggression (p. 472)
- Communication problems (p. 473)
- Screaming (p. 473)
- Repetitive behaviors (p. 474)
- Changes in intimacy and sexuality (p. 474)
- Rummaging and hiding things (p. 474)

Health problems can make the problems worse. Examples include illness, infection, drugs, lack of sleep, constipation, hunger, thirst, poor vision or hearing, alcohol, and caffeine. So can problems in the person's setting. They include:
- A strange setting. The person does not know the setting well.
- Too much noise (TV, radio, music, people talking at once) can cause confusion and frustration.
- Not understanding signs. The person may think that a WET FLOOR sign means to urinate on the floor.
- Mirrors. The person may think that a mirror image is another person in the room.

See *Promoting Safety and Comfort: Behaviors and Problems.*

PROMOTING SAFETY AND COMFORT

Behaviors and Problems

Safety

Some behaviors and problems are not caused by AD. They may be caused by illness, injury, or drugs. If the cause is not treated, it may threaten the person's life. Always report changes in behavior to the nurse.

BOX 30-8 Seven Stages of Alzheimer's Disease—Alzheimer's Association

Stage 1—No Impairment
- No signs of memory problems.

Stage 2—Very Mild Cognitive Decline
- Memory lapses.
- Forgets familiar words.
- Forgets location of everyday things.
- Symptoms are not noticed by others.

Stage 3—Mild Cognitive Decline
- Symptoms are noticed by others.
- Memory or concentration problems.
- Problems with the right words or names.
- Problems remembering names of new people.
- Increased problems with tasks in social or work settings.
- Forgets what was just read.
- Loses or misplaces a valuable object.
- Increased problems planning and organizing.

Stage 4—Moderate Cognitive Decline
- Forgets recent events.
- Problems with arithmetic. Counting backward from 100 by subtracting 7 (100, 93, 86, 79, 72, and so on) is an example.
- Increased difficulty with complex tasks. Paying bills and managing money are examples.
- Forgets things about one's past.
- Becomes moody or withdrawn in social situations.

Stage 5—Moderately Severe Cognitive Decline
- Noticeable gaps in memory and thinking.
- May need help with activities of daily living (ADL).
- Cannot recall his or her address or phone number.
- Confusion about day, time, and place.

Stage 5—Moderately Severe Cognitive Decline—cont'd
- Problems with simple arithmetic. Counting backward from 40 by subtracting 4 (40, 36, 32, 28, 24, and so on) is an example.
- Needs help choosing clothing.
- Can remember things about family and self.
- Can eat and meet elimination needs.

Stage 6—Severe Cognitive Decline
- Memory problems worsen.
- Personality and behavior changes. See "Behaviors and Problems."
- Needs much help with ADL.
- Loses awareness of recent things and the setting.
- Remembers his or her own name but has problems with personal past.
- Can distinguish between familiar and unfamiliar faces.
- Problems remembering the name of a spouse, partner, or caregiver.
- Sleep patterns change. May sleep during the day and be restless at night.
- Bladder and bowel control problems increase.
- Tends to wander and may become lost.

Stage 7—Very Severe Cognitive Decline
- Cannot respond to his or her setting.
- Unable to have a conversation. May say words or phrases.
- Cannot control movement.
- Needs great assistance with ADL.
- Cannot smile.
- Cannot hold the head up or sit without support.
- Muscles become rigid.
- Impaired swallowing.

Modified from Alzheimer's Association: Seven stages of Alzheimer's, *2013.*

Wandering and Getting Lost. Persons with AD are not oriented to person, time, and place. They may wander away and not find their way back. Wandering may be by foot, car, bike, or other means. They may be with you one moment and gone the next.

Judgment is poor. They cannot tell what is safe or dangerous. Life-threatening accidents are great risks. They can walk into traffic or into a nearby river, lake, ocean, or forest. If not properly dressed, heat or cold exposure is a risk.

Wandering may have no cause. Or the person may be looking for something or someone—the bathroom, the bedroom, a child, or a partner. Pain, drug side effects, stress, restlessness, and anxiety are possible causes. Sometimes finding the cause prevents wandering.

See *Promoting Safety and Comfort: Wandering and Getting Lost.*

PROMOTING SAFETY AND COMFORT

Wandering and Getting Lost

Safety

Patients and residents may try to wander to another nursing unit or out of the agency. *Leaving the agency without staff knowledge is called* ***elopement.*** Serious injury and death have resulted from elopement. State and federal guidelines to prevent elopement are followed.

All staff must be alert to persons who wander. They are allowed to wander in safe areas (Fig. 30-4, p. 472). Unsafe areas include kitchens, shower rooms, and utility rooms.

Tell your team members when you are caring for a person who wanders. You cannot be with the person all the time. The team can assist and monitor the person. Help your team members in the same way. If you see a person wandering into an unsafe area, gently guide the person to a safe place (Fig. 30-5, p. 472). Report the problem to the nurse.

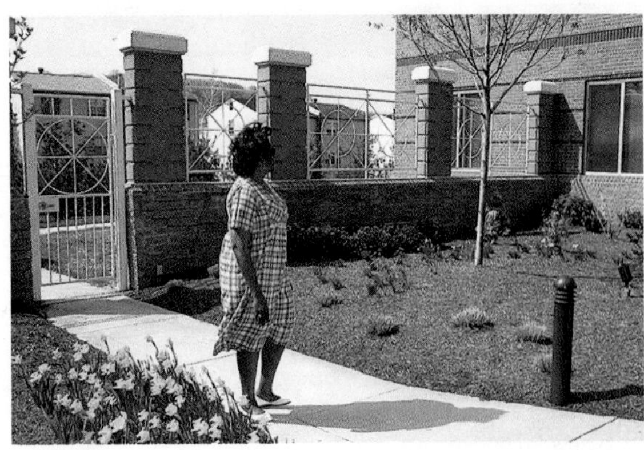

FIGURE 30-4 An enclosed garden allows persons with AD to wander in a safe setting.

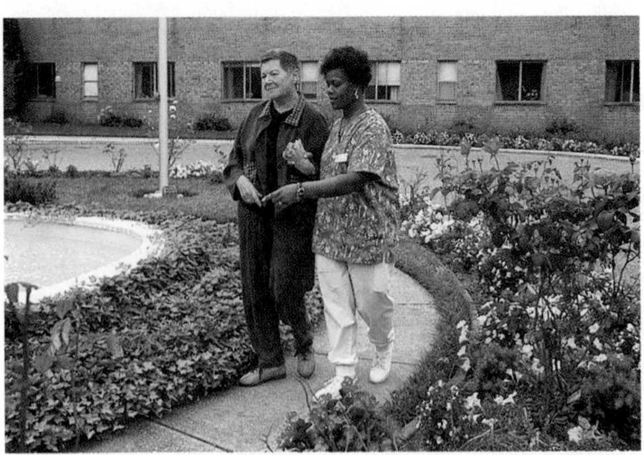

FIGURE 30-5 Guide the person who wanders to a safe area.

MedicAlert® + Alzheimer's Association Safe Return.® *MedicAlert® + Alzheimer's Association Safe Return®* is a 24-hour emergency service for persons who wander or have a medical emergency. The program is nationwide.

The purpose is to find and safely return persons who wander and become lost. A small fee is charged. A family member completes a form and provides a photo. These are entered into a national database. The person receives an ID (wallet card and bracelet or necklace).

When reported missing, the person's information is sent to the police. When the person is found, someone calls the toll-free number on the ID. *MedicAlert® + Alzheimer's Association Safe Return®* then calls the family member or caregiver. The person is returned home safely.

Sundowning. With ***sundowning****, signs, symptoms, and behaviors of AD increase during hours of darkness.* As daylight ends and darkness starts, confusion and restlessness increase. So do anxiety, agitation, and other symptoms. Behavior is worse after the sun goes down. It may continue throughout the night.

Sundowning may relate to being tired or hungry. Poor light and shadows may cause the person to see things that are not there. The person may be afraid of the dark.

Hallucinations and Delusions. A ***hallucination*** *is seeing, hearing, smelling, or feeling something that is not real.* Senses are dulled. Affected persons see animals, insects, or people that are not present. Some hear voices. They may feel bugs crawling or feel that they are being touched.

The problem may be caused by poor vision or hearing. The person needs to wear eyeglasses and hearing aids as prescribed. Other causes include infection, pain, and drugs.

Delusions *are false beliefs.* To the person, the beliefs are real. People with AD may think they are some other person. Some believe that they are in jail, are being killed, or are being attacked. A person may believe that the caregiver is someone else. Many other false beliefs can occur.

Paranoia. ***Paranoia*** *is a disorder* (para) *of the mind* (noia). *The person has false beliefs (delusions) and suspicion about a person or situation.* Paranoia is a type of delusion. The person believes that others are mean, lying, not fair, or "out to get" him or her. The person may be suspicious, fearful, or jealous.

Paranoia may worsen as memory loss gets worse. The National Institute on Aging (NIA) uses these examples:

- The person forgets where he or she put something. The person may believe that someone is taking his or her things.
- The person forgets that you are a caregiver. The person may think that you are a stranger and not trust you.
- The person forgets people whom he or she has met. The person may believe that strangers are harmful.
- The person forgets directions that you give. The person may think that you are trying to trick him or her.

The person may express loss through paranoia. Reasons for the loss do not make sense. Therefore the person blames or accuses others.

See *Promoting Safety and Comfort: Paranoia.*

Catastrophic Reactions. These are extreme responses to normal events or things. The person reacts as if there is a disaster or tragedy. The person may scream, cry, or be agitated or combative. These reactions are common from too many stimuli. Eating, music or TV playing, and being asked questions all at once can overwhelm the person.

Agitation and Aggression. When agitated, the person is restless or worried and cannot settle down. The person may pace, move about, or be unable to sleep. Agitation may lead to aggressive behaviors. The person may yell, scream, swear, hit, pinch, grab, or try to hurt someone. Common causes are:

- Pain or discomfort.
- Anxiety.
- Fatigue.

PROMOTING SAFETY AND COMFORT
Paranoia

Safety

The person's behaviors may not mean paranoia. Fears of harm, strangers, stealing, mistreatment, and so on may be real. Some people take advantage of vulnerable adults (Chapter 3). This includes sexual abuse and financial abuse.

The abuse may be by phone, mail, e-mail, or in person. The abuser may be a friend or family member. According to the NIA, financial abuse occurs when money or belongings are stolen. Financial abuse can include:

- Forging checks or cashing checks without permission
- Taking retirement and Social Security benefits
- Using the person's credit cards or bank accounts
- Changing names on wills, insurance policies, or titles to homes or cars
- "Scams" such as identity theft, phone prizes, and threats
- Borrowing money and not paying it back
- Giving away or selling the person's property without permission
- Forcing the person to sign over property

You must protect the person from harm, abuse, and mistreatment. Report the following at once.

- What the person is saying
- The person seems afraid or worried about money
- Some of the person's items are missing
- The person's behaviors
- Signs and symptoms of problems
- Visitors or family members acting strangely

- Too many or too few stimuli.
- Hunger or thirst.
- Elimination needs, constipation, and incontinence.
- Feeling lost or abandoned.
- Care measures (bathing, dressing) that upset or frighten the person.
- Caregivers. A caregiver may rush the person or be impatient. Or mixed verbal and nonverbal messages are sent. For example, a caregiver talks too fast or too loud. Always consider how your behaviors affect the person.

Communication Problems. People with AD have trouble remembering things. Communication problems include:

- Struggling to find the right word
- Forgetting what he or she wants to say
- Problems understanding the meaning of words
- Attention problems during conversations
- Losing one's train of thought when talking
- Problems blocking background noises—radio, TV, music, phones, and so on
- Frustrations with problems communicating
- Being sensitive to touch, tone, and voice volume

See *Caring About Culture: Communication Problems.* See *Focus on Communication: Communication Problems.*

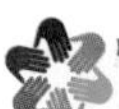

CARING ABOUT CULTURE
Communication Problems

For some people, English is a second language. For example, the first language learned may be Spanish, Italian, French, Russian, Chinese, Japanese, and so on. With AD, the person may forget or no longer understand English. He or she may only use and understand the first language learned.

FOCUS ON COMMUNICATION
Communication Problems

With AD and other dementias, communication abilities decline over time. Some persons can have brief conversations. To promote communication, see Box 30-9. Avoid the following.

- Giving orders. For example: "Sit down and eat." The statement is bossy. It does not show respect for the person. Instead you can say: "Let me help you sit down."
- Wanting the truth. For example, do not say: "Don't you remember?" "What day is it?" Instead you can say: "Today is Friday."
- Correcting the person's errors. For example, do not say: "I just told you that it's time to get dressed. You already had breakfast." Instead you can say: "Let me help you get dressed."
- Pointing out errors. Instead of saying: "You missed a button," say: "Let's try it this way."
- Giving many choices. For example, "What would you like for dinner?" involves many choices. Instead, limit choices. You can say: "Do you want potatoes or rice?"
- Asking open-ended questions. For example, do not say: "How did you sleep last night?" Instead, ask "yes" or "no" questions. You can say: "Did you sleep okay last night?"

Screaming. At first, persons with AD have a hard time finding the right words. As AD progresses, they speak in short sentences or in just words. Often speech is not understandable.

Screaming to communicate is common in persons who are very confused and have poor communication skills. They may scream a word or a name. Or they just make screaming sounds.

Possible causes include hearing and vision problems, pain or discomfort, fear, and fatigue. Too much or not enough stimulation is another cause. A person may react to a caregiver or family member by screaming. See Box 30-9, p. 474.

BOX 30-9 Communicating with Persons Who Have AD or Other Dementias

- Treat the person with dignity and respect.
- Approach the person in a calm, quiet manner.
- Approach the person from the front—not from the side or the back. This avoids startling the person.
- Make eye contact to get the person's attention. Then maintain eye contact.
- Have the person's attention before you start speaking.
- Identify yourself and other people by name.
- Call the person by name.
- Avoid pronouns (he, she, them, it, and so on). For example, instead of saying: "She is here" say: "Mary is here."
- Follow the rules of communication (Chapters 5 and 6).
- Practice measures to promote communication (Chapters 5 and 6).
- Control distractions and noise. TV, radio, and music are examples.
- Speak in a calm, gentle voice.
- Be aware of your body language. Smile and avoid frowning, grimacing, or other negative actions.
- Use gestures or cues. Point to objects.
- Comfort the person with touch. Hold the person's hand while you talk.
- Speak slowly. Use simple words and short sentences.
- Ask or say 1 thing at a time. Present 1 idea, statement, or question at a time.
- Give simple, step-by-step instructions.
- Provide explanations of all procedures and activities.
- Repeat instructions as needed. Give the person time to respond or react.
- Ask simple questions with simple answers. Do not ask complex questions.
- Do not "baby talk" or use a "baby voice."
- Let the person speak. Do not interrupt or rush the person.
- Give the person time to respond.
- Try other words if the person does not seem to understand.
- Provide the word the person is looking for if he or she is struggling to communicate a thought.
- Do not criticize, correct, interrupt, argue, or try to reason with the person.
- Give consistent responses.
- Practice the measures in Chapter 28:
  - To promote hearing
  - To communicate with speech-impaired persons
  - For blind and visually impaired persons
- Try these measures for the screaming person.
  - Provide a calm, quiet setting.
  - Play soft music.
  - Have the person wear hearing aids and eyeglasses.
  - Have a family member or favorite caregiver comfort and calm the person.
  - Use touch to calm the person.

Repetitive Behaviors. *Repetitive* means *to do over and over.* Persons with AD repeat the same motions, words, or questions over and over. For example, the person folds the same napkin over and over. Or the person says the same words or asks the same question over and over. Such behaviors do not harm the person. However, they can annoy caregivers and the family.

Changes in Intimacy and Sexuality. *Intimacy* is a special bond between people who love and respect each other. It involves the way people talk and act toward each other. *Sexuality* is the way partners physically express their feelings for each other. The person with AD may:

- Depend on and cling to his or her partner.
- Not remember life with his or her partner.
- Not remember feelings for his or her partner.
- Fall in love with another person.
- Have side effects from drugs that affect sexual interest.
- Have memory loss, brain changes, or depression that affect sexual interest.
- Have abnormal sexual behaviors.

Sexual behaviors are labeled abnormal because of how and when they occur. Sexual behaviors may involve the wrong person, the wrong place, and the wrong time. Also, persons with AD cannot control behavior.

Healthy persons do not undress or expose themselves in front of others. They do not masturbate or engage in sexual acts in public. They know their sexual partners. Persons with AD often mistake someone else for a sexual partner. The person kisses and hugs the other person.

Being overly *(hyper)* interested in sex is called *hypersexuality.* The person may try to seduce others. Or the person may masturbate often. These behaviors are symptoms of AD. They may not mean that the person wants to have sex. When a person masturbates in public, lead the person to his or her room. Provide for privacy and safety.

The nurse encourages the person's partner to show affection. Their normal practices are encouraged. Examples include hand holding, hugging, kissing, touching, and dancing.

Some behaviors are not sexual. Touching, scratching, and rubbing the genitals can signal infection, pain, or discomfort in the urinary or reproductive systems. Poor hygiene is another cause. So is being wet or soiled from urine or feces. Good hygiene prevents itching. Clean the person quickly and thoroughly after elimination. Do not let the person stay wet or soiled. The nurse assesses the person for urinary or reproductive system problems. The doctor is contacted as necessary.

Rummaging and Hiding Things. *To rummage* means *to search for things by moving things around, turning things over, or looking through something such as a drawer or closet.* The behavior may not have meaning. Or the person may be looking for a certain item but cannot tell you what or why.

The person may hide things, throw things away, or lose things. Eyeglasses, hearing aids, and dentures must stay with the person. Always make sure these items are safe. Money, jewelry, and other important items usually are sent home with the family.

CARE OF PERSONS WITH AD AND OTHER DEMENTIAS

Usually the person is cared for at home until symptoms become severe. Adult day care may help. Often assisted living or nursing center care is required. Other illnesses may require hospital care. You may care for persons with AD or other dementias in such settings. The person and family need your support and understanding.

People with AD do not choose to have the behaviors, signs, and symptoms of the disease. They cannot control what is happening to them. *The disease is responsible, not the person.*

Currently AD has no cure. Symptoms worsen over many years. Over time, the person depends on others for care. Safety, hygiene, food and fluids, elimination, and activity needs must be met. So must comfort and sleep needs. Good skin care and alignment prevent skin breakdown and contractures. The person's care plan will include many of the measures listed in Box 30-10, pp. 476-478.

The person can have other health problems and injuries. However, the person may not be aware of pain, fever, constipation, incontinence, or other signs and symptoms. Carefully observe the person. Report any change in the person's usual behavior.

Infection is a risk. The person cannot fully tend to self-care. Infection can occur from poor hygiene. This includes poor skin care, oral hygiene, and perineal care after bowel and bladder elimination. Inactivity and immobility can cause pneumonia and pressure ulcers.

The person needs to feel useful, worthwhile, and active. This promotes self-esteem. Therapies and activities focus on the person's strengths and past successes. For example:

- A woman used to cook. She helps clean fruit.
- A man was a good dancer. Activities are planned so he can dance.
- A man likes to clean. He helps with dusting.

Supervised activities meet the person's needs and cognitive abilities. Activities are based on what the person enjoys and can do. Some people like crafts, exercise, gardening, and listening and moving to music. Others like sing-alongs, reminiscing, and board games. Some like to string beads, fold towels, or roll dough.

You must treat these persons with dignity and respect. They have the same rights as persons who are alert and active. Talk to them in a calm voice. Always explain what you are going to do. Massage, soothing touch, music, and aromatherapy are comforting and relaxing. The person may need hospice care as death nears (Chapter 32).

See *Focus on Older Persons: Care of Persons With AD and Other Dementias.*

See *Focus on Surveys: Care of Persons With AD and Other Dementias.*

Text continued on p. 479

FOCUS ON OLDER PERSONS

Care of Persons With AD and Other Dementias

Many nursing centers have secured units for persons with AD and other dementias. This means that entrances and exits are locked. Persons in these units cannot wander away. They have a safe setting to move about. Some persons have aggressive behaviors that disrupt or threaten others. They need a secured unit.

According to the Omnibus Budget Reconciliation Act of 1987 (OBRA), secured units are physical restraints. A dementia diagnosis and a doctor's order are needed for placement on a secured unit. At least every 90 days, the health team reviews the person's need for a secured unit. The person's rights are always protected.

At some point, the secured unit is no longer needed for safe care. For example, a person's condition progresses to severe AD (see Box 30-7). The person cannot sit or walk. Wandering is not a concern. The person is transferred to another unit.

FOCUS ON SURVEYS

Care of Persons with AD and Other Dementias

Confusion and dementia affect cognitive function. To ensure quality of life, surveyors will look at all aspects of the person's care. For example:

- Are the person's bathing, dressing, and grooming needs met?
- Is independence promoted? For example, does the staff give the person cues so the person can dress himself or herself?
- Is the person reminded to use the toilet at regular times?
- Is the person in a calm, quiet setting for meals?
- Is the person offered enough fluids to prevent dehydration?
- Does the staff respond to the person in a dignified manner?
- Is a safe setting provided?
- Does the staff provide supervision for safe behaviors?

Federal laws require that nursing assistant education and training include dementia management and preventing abuse. Annual in-service training also is required. Surveyors will review employee records to make sure these requirements are met.

BOX 30-10 Care of Persons with AD and Other Dementias

Environment
- Follow set routines.
- Avoid changing rooms or roommates.
- Place picture signs by room doors, bathrooms, dining rooms, and other areas (Fig. 30-6, p. 478).
- Keep personal items where the person can see and reach them.
- Stay within the person's sight to the extent possible.
- Place memory aids (large clocks and calendars) where the person can see them.
- Keep noise levels low.
- Play music and show movies from the person's past.
- Select tasks and activities that fit the person's abilities and interests.

Safety
- Reassure the person that you are there to help.
- Remove harmful, sharp, and breakable items from the area. This includes knives, scissors, glass, dishes, razors, and tools.
- Provide plastic eating and drinking utensils. They help prevent breakage and cuts.
- Place safety plugs in electrical outlets. Or cover outlets with safety plates.
- Keep cords and electrical items out of reach.
- Remove electric appliances from the bathroom. Hair dryers, curling irons, make-up mirrors, and electric shavers are examples.
- Provide safe storage for:
  - Personal care items (shampoo, deodorant, lotion, and so on)
  - Household cleaners and drugs
  - Dangerous equipment and tools
  - Cigarettes, cigars, pipes, matches, and other smoking materials
  - Car keys
- Keep childproof caps on drug containers and household cleaners.
- Remove knobs from stoves or place safety covers on the knobs (Fig. 30-7, p. 478).
- Remove dangerous appliances, power tools, and firearms from the home.
- Supervise the person who smokes.
- Practice safety measures to prevent:
  - Falls (Chapter 10)
  - Fires (Chapter 9)
  - Burns (Chapter 9)
  - Poisoning (Chapter 9)
- Lock doors to kitchens, utility rooms, and housekeeping closets. Keep them locked.

Wandering
- Follow agency policy for locking doors and windows. Locks are often at the top and bottom of doors (Fig. 30-8, p. 478). The person is not likely to look for a lock in such places.
- Keep door alarms and electronic doors turned on. Respond to alarms at once.
- Follow agency policy for fire exits. Everyone must be able to leave the building if there is a fire.
- Make sure the person wears an ID bracelet or *MedicAlert® + Alzheimer's Association Safe Return®* ID at all times.

Wandering—cont'd
- Know the times of day the person is more likely to wander.
- Follow the person's care plan for daily routine, activities, and exercise. Make sure food, fluid, and elimination needs are met.
- Involve the person in activities—folding napkins, dusting a table, sorting socks, rolling yarn, sweeping, sanding blocks of wood, or watering plants.
- Do not use restraints. Restraints require a doctor's order. They also tend to increase confusion and disorientation.
- Do not argue with the person who wants to leave. The person does not understand what you are saying.
- Go with the person who insists on going outside. Make sure he or she is properly dressed. Guide the person inside after a few minutes.
- Let the person wander in enclosed areas. The agency may have enclosed areas for walking about. They provide a safe place for the person to wander.

Sundowning
- Complete treatments and activities early in the day.
- Encourage exercise and activity early in the day.
- Keep the person on a schedule. Waking up, meal times, and bedtime should involve a set routine.
- Avoid caffeine (coffee, tea, colas, chocolate), sweets, and alcohol late in the day. Provide a calm, quiet setting late in the day.
- Do not restrain the person.
- Meet nutrition and elimination needs. Unmet needs can increase restlessness.
- Use night-lights at night.
- Do not try to reason with the person. He or she cannot understand what you are saying.
- Do not ask the person to tell you what is bothering him or her. Communication is impaired. The person does not understand what you are asking. He or she cannot think or speak clearly.

Hallucinations and Delusions
- Have the person wear eyeglasses and hearing aids as needed.
- Do not argue with the person. He or she does not understand what you are saying.
- Reassure the person. Tell him or her that you will provide protection from harm.
- Distract the person with some item or activity. Go to another room. Taking the person for a walk may be helpful.
- Turn off TV or movies when violent and disturbing programs are on. The person may believe the story is real.
- Comfort the person if he or she seems afraid. Use touch to calm and reassure the person (Fig. 30-9, p. 478).
- Eliminate noises that the person could misinterpret. TV, radio, music, furnaces, air conditioners, and other things could affect the person.
- Check lighting. Make sure there are no glares, shadows, or reflections.
- Cover or remove mirrors. The person could misinterpret his or her reflection.
- Make sure the person cannot reach anything that could be used to hurt the self or others.
- Report behavior changes. They may signal a physical illness.

BOX 30-10 Care of Persons with AD and Other Dementias—cont'd

Paranoia
- Do not react if the person blames you for something.
- Do not argue with the person.
- Let the person know that he or she is safe.
- Use touch or gently hug the person. This shows that you care.
- Search for missing things. This helps distract the person. Talk about what you found. For example, you find a photo. Talk about the photo.

Catastrophic Reactions
- Approach the person from the front. Do not startle the person from behind or the side.
- Be calm. Do not appear rushed. Allow the person time to calm down.
- Use touch appropriately. Know how the person responds to touch. Touch can comfort some people. Others do not like being touched.
- Explain in simple terms what you would like the person to do. For example: "It's time for bed. I'll help you into bed."
- Do not argue with the person.
- Follow the person's care plan for naps and bedtime.
- Follow the person's daily routine.
- Distract the person with an activity.

Agitation and Aggression
- Look at how your behaviors affect the person.
- Provide a calm, quiet setting.
- Follow the person's care plan and a set routine for ADL. Meet the person's basic needs.
- Observe for early signs of agitation and restlessness. Try to remove the cause before the behaviors worsen.
- Do not ignore the problem. Try to find the cause.
- Allow personal choice. Let the person decide things to the extent possible.
- Try to distract the person. A snack, safe object, or activity may help.
- Reassure the person.
  - Speak calmly.
  - Listen to the person's concerns.
  - Try to show that you understand the person's anger or fears.
- Keep personal items within the person's sight. Photos and treasures are examples.
- Reduce glares, noise, and clutter.
- Limit the number of people in the room.
- Use gentle touch.
- Provide soothing music.
- Read to the person using a gentle voice.
- Provide quiet times.
- Limit the amount of caffeine (coffee, tea, colas, chocolate) and sweets that the person eats or drinks.
- See Chapter 6 for dealing with the angry person.
- See Chapter 9 for workplace violence.

Repetitive Behaviors
- Allow harmless acts. Holding a purse, folding napkins, and petting a stuffed animal are examples.
- Distract the person. Music, picture books, exercise, and movies may provide distraction.
- Take the person for a walk.

Repetitive Behaviors—cont'd
- Know when repetitive behaviors are likely to occur. For example, a person constantly calls for a nurse at bedtime.
- Use a calm voice and gentle touch.
- Do not argue with the person.
- Answer the person's question. You may have to answer the same question several times.
- Use memory aids according to the care plan. Clocks, calendars, and photos are examples.

Rummaging and Hiding Things
- Keep harmful items and products out of the person's sight and reach.
- Remove spoiled items from refrigerators and cabinets. The person may look for food and snacks. He or she may not know or be able to taste spoiled food.
- Do not let the person go into the room of another patient or resident.
- Keep wastebaskets covered or out of sight. The person may rummage through a wastebasket or throw things away.
- Check wastebaskets before you empty them. Look for items thrown away or hidden. Do the same before discarding linens or returning food trays.
- Keep bathroom doors closed and toilet seats down. This helps prevent the person from flushing things down the toilet.
- Allow the person to rummage in a safe place. The agency may have a drawer, closet, bag, box, basket, or chest with safe items.

Sleep
- Develop a regular bedtime. Bedtime should be the same each evening.
- Provide a quiet, peaceful mood in the evening—dim lights, low noise level, and music.
- Follow bedtime rituals.
- Use night-lights so the person can see. Use them in rooms, hallways, bathrooms, and other areas. They help prevent accidents and disorientation.
- Limit caffeine during the day.
- Limit naps during the day.
- Follow the person's exercise plan. Play music to the exercise.
- Reduce noises.

Personal Hygiene and Grooming
- Provide good skin care (Chapters 16, 24, and 25). Keep the person's skin free of urine and feces.
- Promote personal hygiene (Chapter 16).
  - Do not force the person into a shower or tub. People with AD are often afraid of bathing. Try bathing the person when he or she is calm.
  - Use the person's preferred bathing method (tub bath, shower).
  - Provide privacy and keep the person warm.
  - Do not rush the person.
- Provide oral hygiene (Chapter 16).
- Choose clothing that is comfortable and simple to put on. Front-opening garments are easy to put on. Pullover tops are harder to put on. And the person may become frightened when his or her head is inside a garment.

Continued

BOX 30-10 Care of Persons with AD and Other Dementias—cont'd

Personal Hygiene and Grooming—cont'd

- Select clothing that closes with Velcro. Such items are easy to put on and take off. Buttons, zippers, snaps, and other closures can frustrate the person.
- Offer simple clothing choices (Fig. 30-10). Let the person choose between 2 shirts or 2 blouses, 2 pants or 2 slacks, and so on.
- Lay clothing out in the order it will be put on. Hand the person 1 item at a time. Tell or show the person what to do. Do not rush him or her.

Other Basic Needs

- Follow a daily routine. This helps the person know when certain things will happen.
- Meet food and fluid needs (Chapter 20). Provide finger foods. Cut food and pour liquids as needed.
- Promote urinary and bowel elimination and prevent incontinence (Chapters 18 and 19).

Other Basic Needs—cont'd

- Provide incontinence care as needed (Chapters 18 and 19).
- Promote exercise and activity during the day (Chapter 23). This helps reduce wandering and sundowning behaviors. The person may also sleep better.
- Reduce intake of coffee, tea, and cola drinks. These contain caffeine. Caffeine is a stimulant. It can increase restlessness, confusion, and agitation.
- Provide a quiet, restful setting. Soft music is better than loud TV programs.
- Play music during care activities such as bathing and during meals.
- Have equipment ready for any procedure. This reduces the amount of time the person is involved in care measures.
- Observe for signs and symptoms of health problems (Chapters 5 and 28).
- Prevent infection (Chapter 12).

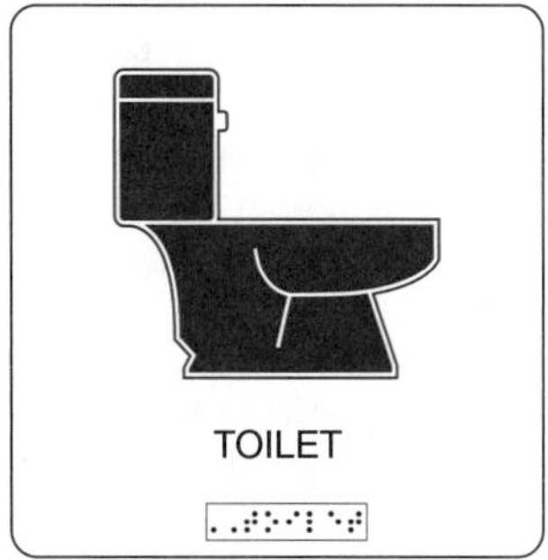

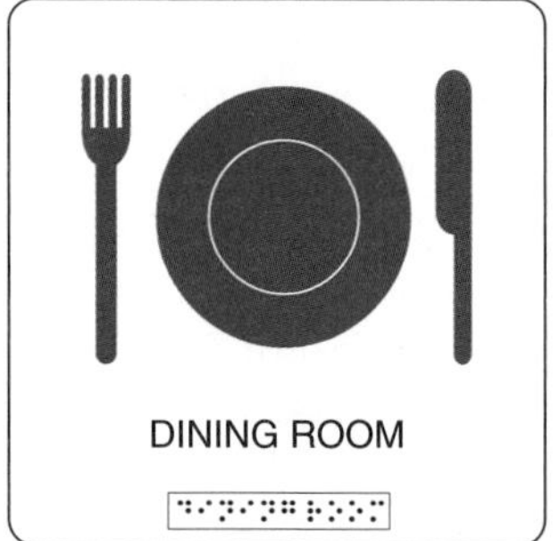

FIGURE 30-6 Signs give cues to persons with dementia.

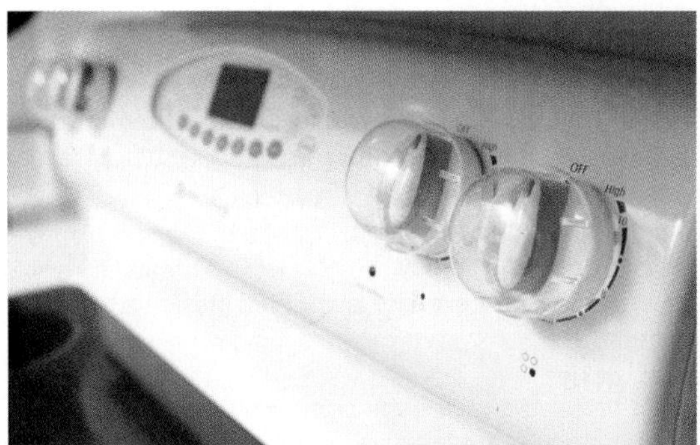

FIGURE 30-7 Safety covers are on stove knobs.

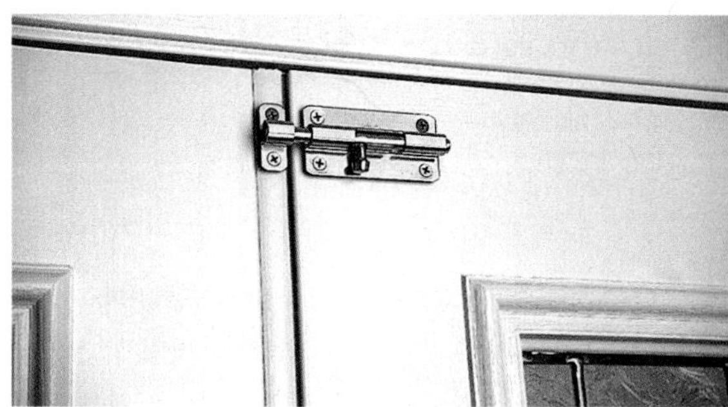

FIGURE 30-8 A slide lock is at the top of the door.

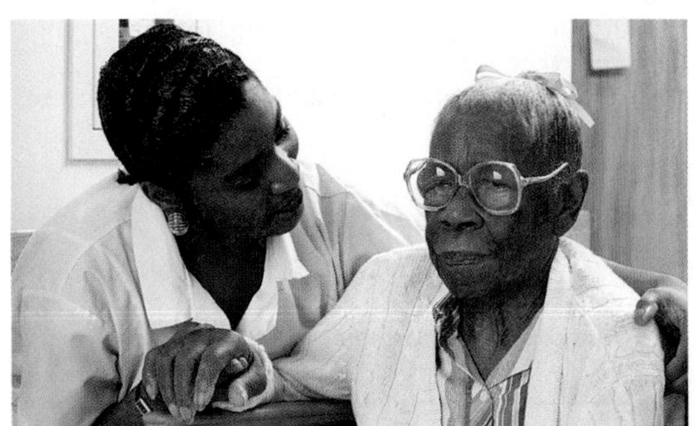

FIGURE 30-9 Use touch to calm the person.

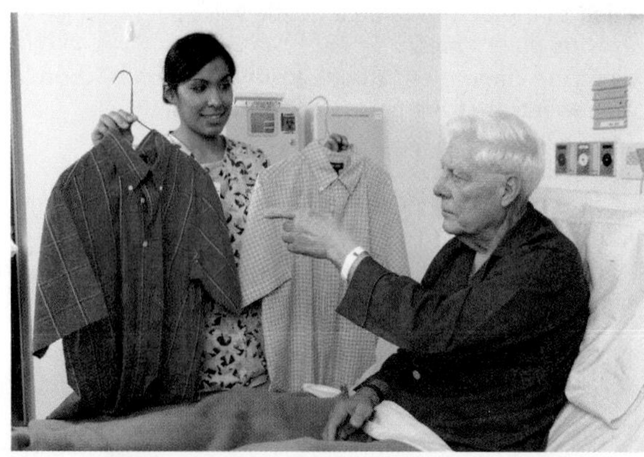

FIGURE 30-10 The person with AD is offered simple clothing choices.

The Family

The person may live at home or with a partner, children, or other family members. Or someone stays with the person. Home health care may help for a while. Adult day care is an option. So is assisted living (Chapter 1). Nursing center care is needed when:

- Family members cannot meet the person's needs.
- The person no longer knows the caregiver.
- Family members have health problems.
- Money problems occur.
- The person's behavior presents dangers to self and others.

Diagnostic tests, doctor's visits, drugs, home care, and assisted living are costly. So is nursing center care. The person's medical care can drain family finances.

Home care and nursing center care are stressful. The family has physical, emotional, social, and financial stresses. Adult children are in the *sandwich generation*. Their own children need attention while an ill parent needs care. Caring for 2 families is stressful. Often adult children have jobs too.

Caregivers can suffer from anger, anxiety, guilt, depression, and sleeplessness. Some cannot concentrate or are irritable. Health problems can develop. They need to focus on their own health. They need a healthy diet, exercise, and plenty of rest. Asking family members and friends for help is important. However, asking for help is hard for some people.

Caregivers need much support and encouragement. AD support groups are sponsored by hospitals, nursing centers, and the Alzheimer's Association. The Alzheimer's Association has chapters across the country. Support groups offer encouragement and advice. Members share their feelings, anger, frustration, guilt, and other emotions. They also share coping and caregiving ideas.

The family often feels hopeless. No matter what is done, the person gets worse. Much time, money, energy, and emotion are needed to care for the person. Anger and resentment may result. Guilt feelings are common. The family knows that the person did not choose the disease and its signs, symptoms, and behaviors. Sometimes behaviors are embarrassing. The family may be upset and angry that the loved one cannot show love or affection.

The family is an important part of the health team. They help plan care when possible. The nurse and support group help the family learn how to give needed care. For home care, they learn how to bathe, feed, dress, and give oral hygiene to the person. They also learn how to provide a safe setting.

In nursing centers, some family members take part in unit activities. For many persons, family members provide comfort. They also need support and understanding from the health team.

The NIA suggests ways that family members can take care of themselves. See Box 30-11.

BOX 30-11 Family Caregivers—Taking Care of Yourself

- Ask for help when you need it. Asking for something specific may be useful. For example:
  - "Can you make Mom's dinner Sunday night?"
  - "Can you stay with Dad from 2 to 4 Monday afternoon?"
  - "Can Mom stay at your house Saturday afternoon?"
- Join a support group.
- Take breaks every day.
- Spend time with friends.
- Maintain hobbies and interests.
- Eat healthy foods.
- Exercise often.
- See a doctor regularly.
- Keep health, legal, and financial information current.
- Remember that these feelings are normal—being sad, lonely, frustrated, confused, angry. Say the following to yourself:
  - "I'm doing the best I can."
  - "What I'm doing would be hard for anyone."
  - "I'm not perfect and that's okay."
  - "I can't control some things."
  - "I need to do what works for right now."
  - "Even when I do everything I can, there will still be problem behaviors. They are caused by the illness, not what I do."
  - "I will enjoy the times when we can be together in peace."
  - "I will get counseling if caregiving becomes too much for me."
- Meet spiritual needs—attending religious services, believing that larger forces or a higher power is at work.
  - Understand that you may feel powerless and hopeless about what is happening.
  - Understand that you are caring for a person with AD. Was the choice made out of love, loyalty, duty, religious obligation, money concerns, fear, habit, or self-punishment?
  - Let yourself feel "uplifts." Examples include good feelings about the person, support from caring people, time for your own interests.
  - Keep connected to something "higher than yourself." This may be believing good comes from every experience.

Modified from National Institute on Aging: Caring for a person with Alzheimer's disease, *Bethesda, Md, July 2012, page last updated July 1, 2013, National Institutes of Health.*

Validation Therapy

The person's care plan may include validation therapy. The therapy is based on these principles.

- All behavior has meaning.
- Development occurs in a sequence, order, and pattern (Chapter 8). Certain tasks must be completed during a stage of development. A stage cannot be skipped. Each stage is the basis of the next stage.
- If a person does not successfully complete a stage of development, unresolved issues and emotions may surface later in life.
- A person may return to the past to resolve such issues and emotions.
- Caregivers need to listen and provide empathy.
- Attempts are not made to correct thoughts or bring the person back to reality. For example:
    - While going from room to room, Mrs. Bell calls for her daughter. In reality, her daughter died 20 years ago. The caregiver does not tell Mrs. Bell that her daughter died. Instead, the caregiver says: "Tell me about your daughter."
    - Mrs. Brown sits all day by the window. She says that she is at the train station waiting to meet her husband. In reality, her husband was killed in a war and never returned home. The caregiver does not remind Mrs. Brown of what happened. Instead, the caregiver asks Mrs. Brown about her husband.
    - Mr. Garcia was 3 years old when his father died. He holds a ball constantly. He is very upset when anyone tries to take the ball from him. He calls for his father and repeats "play ball, play ball." The caregiver does not remind Mr. Garcia that he is 80 years old and that his father died many years ago. Instead, the caregiver says: "Tell me about playing ball."

The health team decides if validation therapy will be part of the person's care plan. If the therapy is used in your agency, you will receive the training needed to use it correctly.

FOCUS ON PRIDE

The Person, Family, and Yourself

Personal and Professional Responsibility

Confusion has many causes. You are responsible for reporting changes in the person's condition. If you notice confusion, do not assume the person has AD. Report the changes at once.

Rights and Respect

The person has the right to privacy and confidentiality. Protect the person from exposure. Only those involved in the person's care are present for care and procedures. The person is allowed to visit in private. Protect confidentiality. Do not share information about the person with others.

The person has the right to keep and use personal items. A pillow, blanket, afghan, or sweater may have meaning to the person. The person may not know why or even recognize the item. Still, it is important and provides comfort. Keep personal items safe. Protect the person's property from loss or damage.

Independence and Social Interaction

Persons with dementia have problems with ADL. Eating, bathing, dressing, and elimination are examples. Maintaining the person's routines can help the person remain independent as long as possible. For example, Mrs. Lund uses the bathroom, washes hands, brushes teeth, puts on make-up, brushes hair, and dresses in the morning. She is more independent when ADL are done in this order. Changing the order causes confusion.

You may need to break down tasks into simple steps. Kindly tell the person each step. Repeat directions as needed. Allow extra time for each task. Resist the urge to take over. Let the person do what is safely possible.

Delegation and Teamwork

Persons with dementia may respond better to certain staff or caregivers. This can vary by day or time of day. Do not be offended if someone else provides care. The team works together to meet the person's needs.

Sometimes the person resists care from everyone. Encouraging the person to allow care is often useless. Use a calm and caring approach. Try giving care at a different time. Never use force.

Ethics and Laws

Persons with AD often have changes in mood, behavior, and personality. The person may become easily agitated or angry. The person does not have control over words and actions. Some behaviors are hard to deal with. You may become short-tempered.

You must control your reactions to stress. Be professional. Tell the nurse if you feel frustrated, angry, or impatient. You may need an assignment change. Never take out your anger on the person or neglect the person's needs. The person must be protected from physical and verbal abuse, mistreatment, and neglect.

REVIEW QUESTIONS

Circle the BEST answer.

1 Cognitive function does *not* involve
 a Memory loss and personality
 b Thinking and reasoning
 c Ability to understand
 d Judgment and behavior

2 A person is confused. Which measure should you question?
 a Restrain in bed at night.
 b Give clear, simple directions.
 c Use touch to communicate.
 d Open drapes during the day.

3 A person has AD. Which is *true?*
 a AD is a normal part of aging.
 b Diet and drugs can cure the disease.
 c AD and delirium are the same.
 d AD ends in death.

4 A person is in the final stage of AD. The person is likely to
 a Wander and become lost
 b Follow simple commands
 c Need total assistance with ADL
 d Repeat questions over and over

5 Which is common in persons with AD?
 a Paralysis
 b Dyspnea
 c Pain
 d Rummaging

6 A person has AD. To communicate, you should
 a Give orders
 b Limit the person's choices
 c Correct the person's mistakes
 d Ask open-ended questions

7 A person with AD is screaming. You know that this is
 a An agitated reaction
 b A way to communicate
 c Caused by a delusion
 d A repetitive behavior

8 The following statements are about sundowning. Which is *true?*
 a Being tired or hungry can increase restlessness.
 b AD behaviors improve at night.
 c Encouraging activity late in the day can help.
 d Dim lighting or darkness is calming.

9 A person has delusions. Which measure should you question?
 a Distract the person with an activity.
 b Tell the person you will provide protection.
 c Tell the person the beliefs are not real.
 d Use touch to calm the person.

10 A person with AD keeps telling you that someone is stealing things. What should you do?
 a Nothing. The person suffers from paranoia.
 b Tell the nurse. Someone could be abusing the person.
 c Replace missing items.
 d Send other items home with the family.

11 A person with AD is at risk for elopement. Which measure should you question?
 a Make sure door alarms are turned on.
 b Make sure an ID bracelet is worn.
 c Assist with exercise as ordered.
 d Tell the person where to wander safely.

12 Safety is important for persons with AD. Which measure is unsafe?
 a Safety plugs are placed in electrical outlets.
 b Cleaners and drugs are kept locked up.
 c The person keeps smoking materials.
 d Sharp and breakable objects are removed from the person's setting.

13 A person with AD is upset. Which is a *correct* response?
 a Try to reason with the person.
 b Ask what is bothering the person.
 c Ignore the problem.
 d Provide reassurance and try to find the cause.

14 You are caring for a person with AD. You should avoid
 a Trying to bring the person back to reality
 b Offering support to the person's family
 c Following a set routine
 d Providing a calm, quiet setting

Answers to these questions are on p. 505.

FOCUS ON PRACTICE

Problem Solving

Mr. Rosin has moderate AD. While preparing him for a bath, he becomes restless and upset. He repeats: "Go away" over and over. How will you respond? How might you meet his hygiene needs?

CHAPTER

31 Assisting With Emergency Care

OBJECTIVES

- Define the key terms and key abbreviations listed in this chapter.
- Describe the rules of emergency care.
- Identify the signs of cardiac arrest and the emergency care required.
- Describe the signs, symptoms, and emergency care for hemorrhage.
- Identify the common causes and emergency care for fainting.
- Identify the signs, symptoms, and emergency care for shock.
- Describe the signs, symptoms, and emergency care for stroke.
- Explain the causes and types of seizures and how to care for a person during a seizure.
- Identify the common causes and emergency care for burns.
- Perform the procedures described in this chapter.
- Explain how to promote PRIDE in the person, the family, and yourself.

KEY TERMS

anaphylaxis A life-threatening sensitivity to an antigen
cardiac arrest See "sudden cardiac arrest"
convulsion See "seizure"
fainting The sudden loss of consciousness from an inadequate blood supply to the brain
first aid Emergency care given to an ill or injured person before medical help arrives
hemorrhage The excessive loss of blood in a short time
respiratory arrest Breathing stops but heart action continues for several minutes
seizure Violent and sudden contractions or tremors of muscle groups; convulsion
shock Results when organs and tissues do not get enough blood
sudden cardiac arrest (SCA) The heart stops suddenly and without warning; cardiac arrest

KEY ABBREVIATIONS

AED Automated external defibrillator
AHA American Heart Association
BLS Basic Life Support
CPR Cardiopulmonary resuscitation
EMS Emergency Medical Services
RRT Rapid Response Team
SCA Sudden cardiac arrest
VF Ventricular fibrillation
V-fib Ventricular fibrillation

Emergencies can occur anywhere. Sometimes you can save a life if you know what to do. You are encouraged to take a first aid course and a Basic Life Support (BLS) course. These courses prepare you to give emergency care.

The BLS procedures in this chapter are given as basic information. They do not replace certification training. You need a BLS course for health care providers.

BOX 31-1 Rules of Emergency Care

- Know your limits. Do not do more than you are able. Do not perform an unfamiliar procedure. Do what you can under the circumstances.
- Stay calm. This helps the person feel more secure.
- Know where to find emergency supplies.
- Follow Standard Precautions and the Bloodborne Pathogen Standard to the extent possible.
- Check for life-threatening problems. Check for breathing, a pulse, and bleeding.
- Keep the person lying down or as you found him or her. Moving the person could make an injury worse.
- Move the person only if the setting is unsafe. Examples include:
  - A burning car or building
  - A building that might collapse
  - Stormy conditions with lightning
  - In water
  - Near electrical wires
- Wait for help to arrive if the scene is not safe enough for you to approach.
- Perform necessary emergency measures.
- Call for help. Or have someone activate the EMS system. *Do not hang up until the operator has hung up.* Give the following information.
  - Your location: street address and city, cross streets or roads, and landmarks
  - Phone number you are calling from
  - What seems to have happened (for example, heart attack, crash, fire)—police, fire equipment, and ambulances may be needed
  - How many people need help
  - Conditions of victims, obvious injuries, and life-threatening situations
  - What aid is being given
- Do not remove clothes unless you have to. If you must remove clothing, tear or cut garments along the seams.
- Keep the person warm. Cover the person with a blanket, coats, or sweaters.
- Reassure the person. Explain what is happening and that help was called.
- Do not give the person fluids.
- Keep on-lookers away. They invade privacy and tend to stare, give advice, and comment about the person's condition. The person may think the situation is worse than it is.

EMERGENCY CARE

First aid *is the emergency care given to an ill or injured person before medical help arrives.* The goals of first aid are to:

- Prevent death.
- Prevent injuries from becoming worse.

In an emergency, the Emergency Medical Services (EMS) system is activated. Emergency personnel (paramedics, emergency medical technicians) rush to the scene. They treat, stabilize, and transport persons with life-threatening problems. Their ambulances have emergency drugs, equipment, and supplies. They have guidelines for care and communicate with doctors in hospital emergency departments. The doctors can tell them what to do. To activate the EMS system, do 1 of the following.

- Dial 911.
- Call the local fire or police department.
- Call the phone operator.

Each emergency is different. The rules in Box 31-1 apply to any emergency. Hospitals and other agencies have procedures for emergencies. Rapid Response Teams (RRTs) are called when a person shows warning signs of a life-threatening condition. An RRT may include a doctor, a nurse, and a respiratory therapist. The RRT's goal is to prevent death.

See *Focus on Communication: Emergency Care.*

See *Promoting Safety and Comfort: Emergency Care.*

FOCUS ON COMMUNICATION

Emergency Care

Some illnesses and injuries are life-threatening. To find out what happened and the person's condition, you can say:

- "Are you okay?"
- "Tell me what's wrong."
- "Where does it hurt?"
- "If you can, please point to where it hurts."
- "Can you move your arms and legs?"

PROMOTING SAFETY AND COMFORT

Emergency Care

Safety

During emergencies, contact with blood, body fluids, secretions, and excretions is likely. Follow Standard Precautions and the Bloodborne Pathogen Standard to the extent possible.

When an emergency occurs in an agency, call for the nurse at once. You may need to activate the EMS system or the RRT. Or you take the person's vital signs (Chapter 21). Assist as instructed by the nurse.

Comfort

Mental comfort is important during emergencies. Help the person feel safe and secure. Give reassurance. Explain the care you provide. Use a calm approach.

BLS FOR ADULTS

When the heart and breathing stop, the person is clinically dead. Blood is not circulated through the body. Heart, brain, and other organ damage occurs within minutes. The American Heart Association's (AHA) BLS procedures support circulation and breathing.

Chain of Survival for Adults

The AHA's BLS courses teach the adult *Chain of Survival.* These actions are taken for heart attack (Chapter 28), sudden cardiac arrest, respiratory arrest, stroke (Chapter 28 and p. 493), and choking (p. 491). They also apply to other life-threatening problems. They are done as soon as possible. Any delay reduces the person's chance of surviving.

Chain of Survival actions for adults are:

- Recognizing cardiac arrest and activating the EMS system at once.
- Early cardiopulmonary resuscitation (CPR).
- Early defibrillation. See p. 487.
- Early advanced care. This is given by EMS staff, doctors, and nurses. They give drugs and perform life-saving measures.
- Organized post–cardiac arrest care. This is care given to improve survival following cardiac arrest.

See *Focus on Communication: Chain of Survival for Adults.*

> **FOCUS ON COMMUNICATION**
>
> ***Chain of Survival for Adults***
>
> Calling for help is a critical step in the Chain of Survival. If others are around, tell a certain person to activate the EMS system. You may not know the person's name. Point to the person. Make eye contact. You can say: "Call 911 and get an AED." (AED stands for automated external defibrillator. See p. 487.) Begin care. Follow up soon. Make sure the person was able to call for help.

Sudden Cardiac Arrest

Sudden cardiac arrest (SCA) or ***cardiac arrest*** *is when the heart stops suddenly and without warning.* Within moments, breathing stops as well. Permanent brain and other organ damage occurs unless circulation and breathing are restored. There are 3 major signs of SCA.

- No response.
- No breathing or no normal breathing. The person may have *agonal gasps* or *agonal respirations* early during SCA. (*Agonal* comes from the Greek word that means *to struggle.* Agonal is used in relation to death and dying.) Agonal gasps do not bring enough oxygen into the lungs. Gasps are not normal breathing.
- No pulse.

The person's skin is cool, pale, and gray. The person is not coughing or moving.

SCA is a sudden, unexpected, and dramatic event. It can occur anywhere and at any time—while driving, shoveling snow, playing golf or tennis, watching TV, eating, or sleeping. Common causes include heart disease, drowning, electric shock, severe injury, choking (Chapter 9), and drug over-dose. These causes lead to an abnormal heart rhythm called ventricular fibrillation (p. 487). The heart cannot pump blood. A normal rhythm must be restored. Otherwise the person will die.

Respiratory Arrest

Respiratory arrest *is when breathing stops but heart action continues for several minutes.* If breathing is not restored, cardiac arrest occurs. Causes of respiratory arrest include:

- Drowning
- Stroke
- Choking
- Drug over-dose
- Electric shock (including lightning strikes)
- Smoke inhalation
- Suffocation
- Heart attack
- Coma
- Other injuries

Rescue Breathing. Rescue breaths are given when there is a pulse but no breathing or only gasping. To give rescue breaths:

- Open the airway (p. 486).
- Give 1 breath every 5 to 6 seconds for adults.
- Give each breath over 1 second. The chest should rise when breaths are given.
- Check the pulse every 2 minutes. If there is no pulse, begin CPR.

CPR for Adults

When the heart and breathing stop, blood and oxygen are not supplied to the body. Brain and other organ damage occurs within minutes.

CPR must be started at once when a person has SCA. CPR supports circulation and breathing. It provides blood and oxygen to the heart, brain, and other organs until advanced emergency care is given. CPR involves:

- Chest compressions
- Airway
- Breathing
- Defibrillation

CPR procedures require speed, skill, and efficiency. Chest compressions and airway and breathing procedures are done until a defibrillator arrives. The defibrillator is used as soon as possible.

See *Promoting Safety and Comfort: CPR for Adults.*

Chest Compressions. The heart, brain, and other organs must receive blood. Otherwise, permanent damage results. In cardiac arrest, the heart has stopped beating. Blood must be pumped through the body in some other way. Chest compressions force blood through the circulatory system.

Before starting chest compressions, check for a pulse. Use the carotid artery on the side near you. To find the carotid pulse, place 2 or 3 fingertips on the trachea (windpipe). Then slide your fingers down off the trachea to the groove of the neck (Fig. 31-1). Check for a pulse for at least 5 seconds but no more than 10 seconds. While checking for a pulse, look for signs of circulation. See if the person has started breathing or is coughing or moving.

The heart lies between the sternum (breastbone) and the spinal column. When pressure is applied to the sternum, the sternum is depressed. This compresses the heart between the sternum and spinal column (Fig. 31-2). For effective chest compressions, the person must be supine on a hard, flat surface—floor or back-board. You are positioned at the person's side.

Hand position is important for effective chest compressions (Fig. 31-3, p. 486). You use the heels of your hands—1 on top of the other—for chest compressions. For proper placement:

- Expose the person's chest. Remove clothing or move it out of the way. You need to see the person's bare skin for proper hand position.
- Place the heel of 1 hand (usually your dominant hand) in the center of the bare chest. The heel of this hand is placed on the sternum between the nipples.
- Place the heel of your other hand on top of the heel of the first hand.

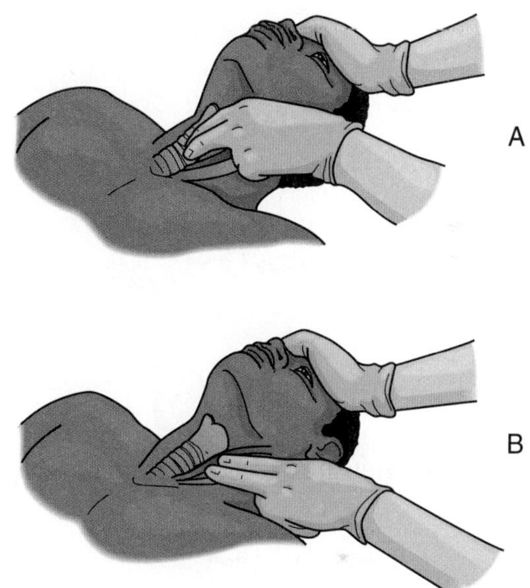

FIGURE 31-1 Locating the carotid pulse. **A,** Two fingers are placed on the trachea. **B,** The fingertips are moved down into the groove of the neck to the carotid artery.

PROMOTING SAFETY AND COMFORT

CPR for Adults

Safety

The discussion and procedures that follow assume that the person does not have injuries from trauma (Chapter 24). If injuries are present, special measures are needed to position the person and open the airway. Such measures are learned during a BLS certification course.

BLS guidelines for infants and children differ from adult guidelines. The procedures also differ. The discussion and procedures in this chapter apply to adults. BLS for infants and children is learned during a BLS certification course.

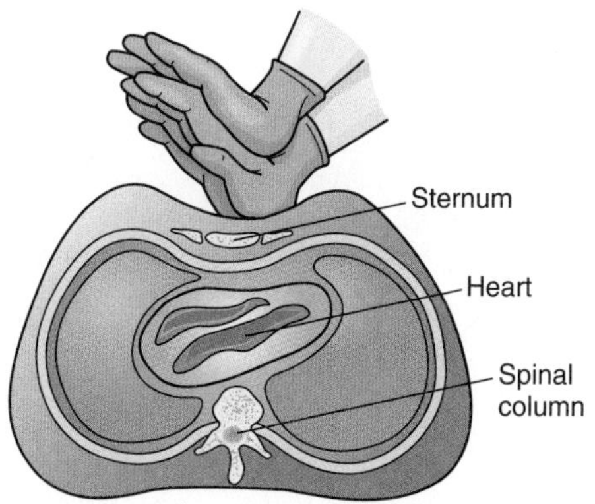

FIGURE 31-2 The heart lies between the sternum and the spinal column. The heart is compressed when pressure is applied to the sternum.

To give chest compressions, your arms are straight. Your shoulders are directly over your hands. And your fingers are interlocked (Fig. 31-4). Exert firm downward pressure to depress the adult sternum at least 2 inches. Then release pressure without removing your hands from the chest. Releasing pressure allows the chest to recoil—to return to its normal position. Recoil lets the heart fill with blood.

The AHA recommends that you:

- Give compressions at a rate of at least 100 per minute.
- Push hard and push fast.
- Push deeply into the chest.
- Interrupt chest compressions only when necessary. Interruptions should be less than 10 seconds. When there are no chest compressions, blood does not flow to the heart, brain, and other organs.

Airway. The respiratory passages (airway) must be open to restore breathing. The airway is often obstructed (blocked) during SCA. The person's tongue falls toward the back of the throat and blocks the airway. The head tilt–chin lift method opens the airway (Fig. 31-5).

- Place the palm of 1 hand on the forehead.
- Tilt the head back by pushing down on the forehead with your palm.
- Place the fingers of your other hand under the lower jaw. Use your index and middle fingers. Do not use your thumb.
- Lift the jaw. This brings the chin forward.
- Do not close the person's mouth. The mouth should be slightly open.

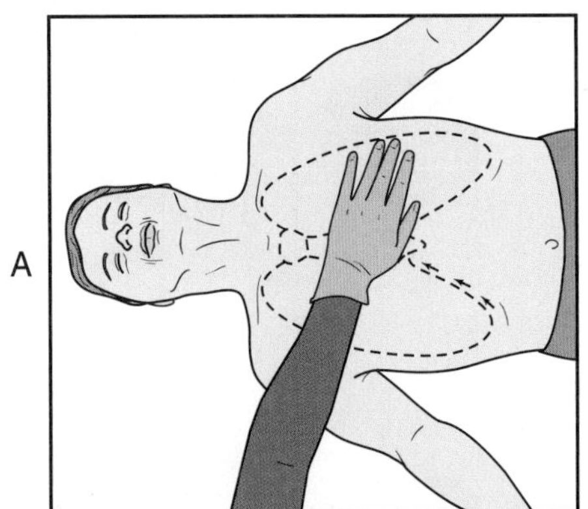

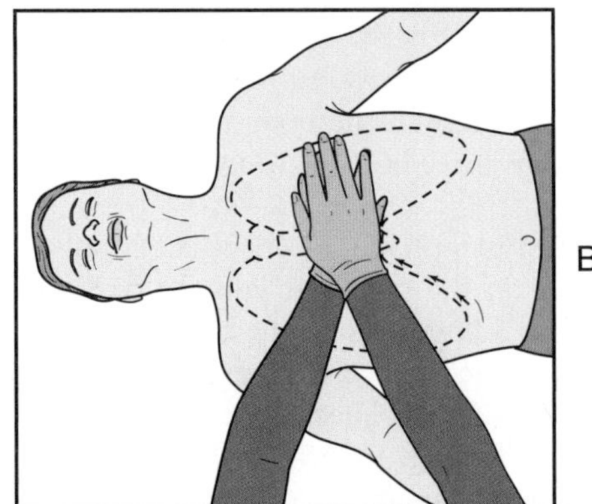

FIGURE 31-3 Proper hand position for CPR. **A,** The heel of the dominant hand is placed in the center of the chest between the nipples. **B,** The heel of the non-dominant hand is placed on top of the dominant hand.

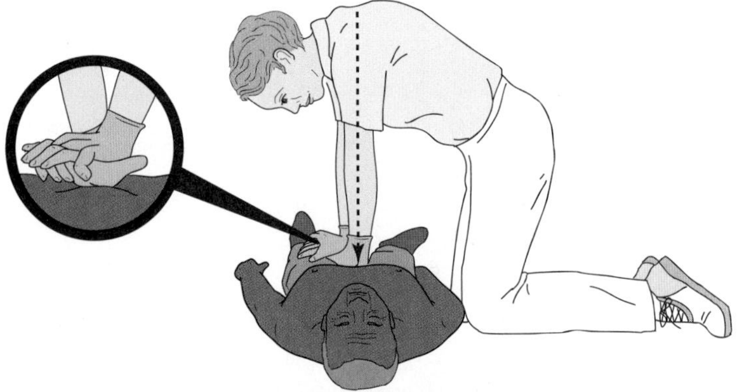

FIGURE 31-4 Giving chest compressions. The arms are straight. The shoulders are over the hands. The fingers are interlocked.

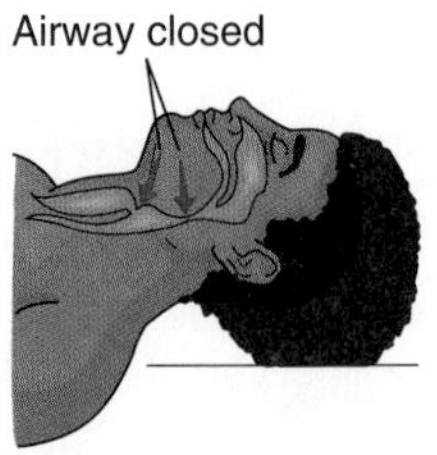

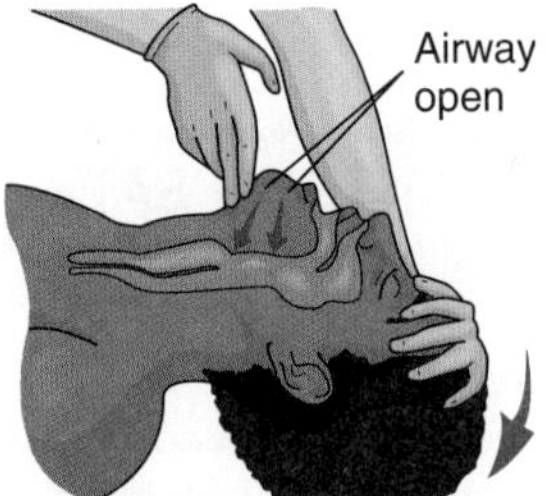

FIGURE 31-5 The head tilt–chin lift method opens the airway. One hand is on the person's forehead. Pressure is applied to tilt the head back. The chin is lifted with the fingers of the other hand.

Breathing. Air is not inhaled when breathing stops. The person must get oxygen. If not, permanent heart, brain, and other organ damage occurs. The person is given *breaths*. That is, a rescuer inflates the person's lungs.

Each breath should take 1 second. *You should see the chest rise with each breath.* Two breaths are given after every 30 chest compressions.

Mouth-to-Mouth Breathing. Mouth-to-mouth breathing (Fig. 31-6) is one way to give breaths. You place your mouth over the person's mouth. Contact with the person's blood, body fluids, secretions, or excretions is likely. To give mouth-to-mouth breathing:

1. Keep the airway open with the head tilt–chin lift method.
2. Pinch the nostrils shut. Use your thumb and index finger. Use the hand on the forehead. Shutting the nostrils prevents air from escaping through the nose.
3. Take a breath. A regular breath is needed, not a deep breath.
4. Place your mouth tightly over the person's mouth. Seal the mouth with your lips.
5. Blow air into the person's mouth. You should see the chest rise as the lungs fill with air. You should also hear the air escape when the person exhales.
6. Repeat the head tilt–chin lift method if the chest did not rise.
7. Remove your mouth from the person's mouth. Then take in a quick breath.
8. Give another breath. You should see the chest rise.

Barrier Device Breathing. A barrier device is used for giving breaths whenever possible. The device prevents contact with the person's mouth and blood, body fluids, secretions, or excretions. A face mask is an example of a barrier device (Fig. 31-7, *A*). When using a barrier device, seal the device against the person's face (Fig. 31-7, *B*). The seal must be tight. Then open the airway with the head tilt–chin lift method.

Defibrillation. *Ventricular fibrillation (VF, V-fib)* is an abnormal heart rhythm (Fig. 31-8, p. 488). It causes sudden cardiac arrest. Rather than beating in a regular rhythm, the heart shakes and quivers like a bowl of Jell-O. The heart does not pump blood. The heart, brain, and other organs do not receive blood and oxygen.

A *defibrillator* is used to deliver a shock to the heart. The shock stops the VF (V-fib). This allows the return of a regular heart rhythm. Defibrillation as soon as possible after the onset of VF (V-fib) increases the person's chance of survival.

For adults, the AHA recommends that rescuers:

- Use an automated external defibrillator (AED) as soon as possible.
- Minimize interruptions in chest compressions before and after a shock is given.
- Give 1 shock. Then resume CPR at once. Begin with chest compressions. Do 5 cycles of 30 compressions and 2 breaths.
- Check for a heart rhythm.

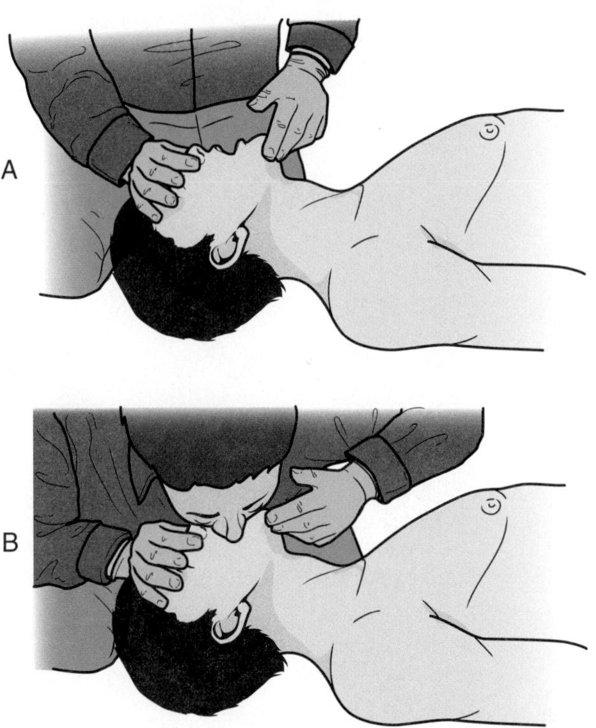

FIGURE 31-6 Mouth-to-mouth breathing. **A,** The person's airway is opened. The nostrils are pinched shut. **B,** The person's mouth is sealed by the rescuer's mouth.

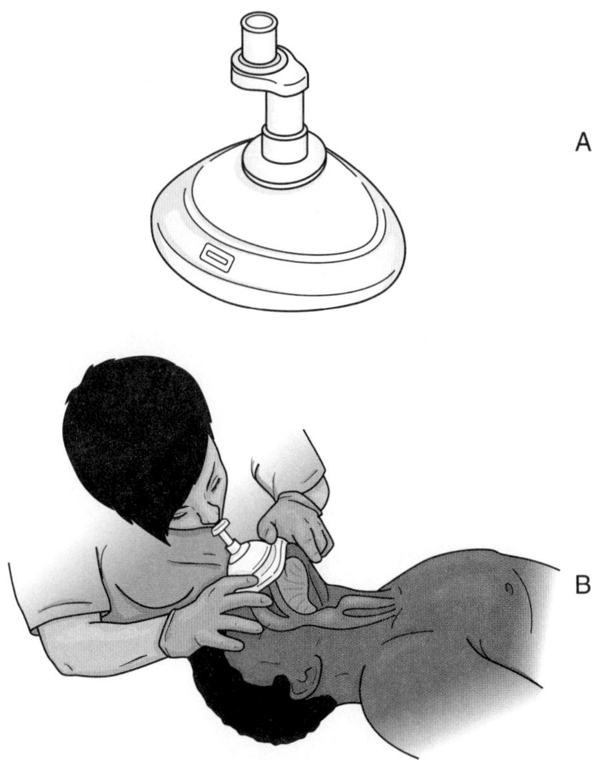

FIGURE 31-7 **A,** Mask for giving breaths. **B,** The mask is in place.

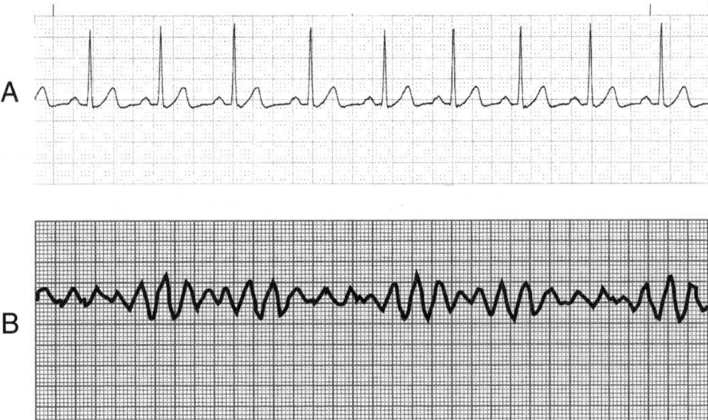

FIGURE 31-8 **A,** Normal rhythm. **B,** Ventricular fibrillation.

AEDs are found in hospitals, nursing centers, dental offices, and other health agencies (Fig. 31-9). They are on airplanes and in airports, health clubs, malls, and many other public places. Some people have them in their homes.

You will learn more about using an AED in the AHA's *BLS for Healthcare Providers* course.

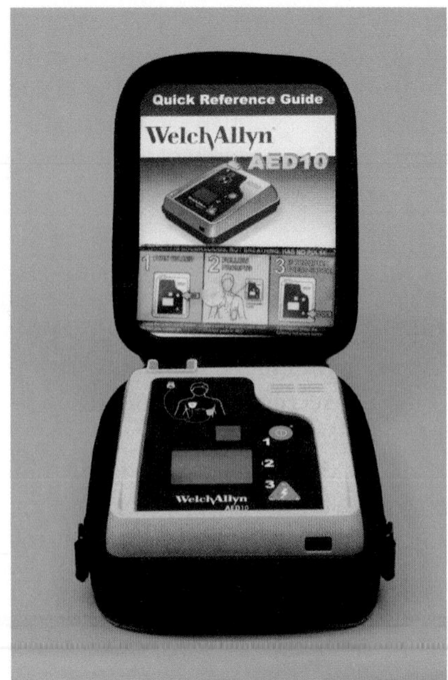

FIGURE 31-9 An automated external defibrillator (AED).

Performing Adult CPR. CPR is done only for cardiac arrest. You must determine if cardiac arrest or fainting (p. 492) has occurred. *CPR is done if the person does not respond, is not breathing (or has no normal breathing), and has no pulse.*

CPR is done alone or with another person. When done alone, chest compressions and rescue breathing are done by 1 rescuer. With 2 rescuers, 1 person gives chest compressions and the other does rescue breathing (Fig. 31-10). Rescuers switch tasks about every 2 minutes to avoid fatigue and inadequate compressions. The second rescuer uses the AED if one is available.

See *Focus on Communication: Performing Adult CPR.*
See *Promoting Safety and Comfort: Performing Adult CPR.*
See procedure: *Adult CPR—One Rescuer.*
See procedure: *Adult CPR With AED—Two Rescuers.*

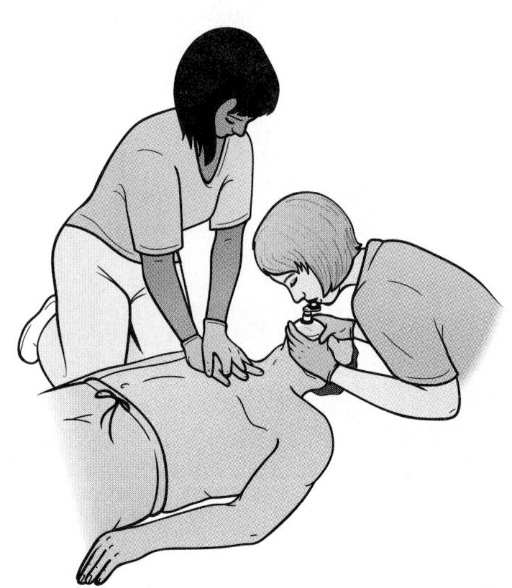

FIGURE 31-10 Two people perform CPR.

FOCUS ON COMMUNICATION

Performing Adult CPR

Good communication is needed when 2 rescuers perform CPR. The rescuer giving compressions must count out loud so the other rescuer is ready to give breaths. Clear communication prevents delays and minimizes interruptions in chest compressions.

PROMOTING SAFETY AND COMFORT

Performing Adult CPR

Safety

Never practice CPR on another person. Serious damage can be done. Mannequins are used to learn and practice CPR.

Make sure you have a safe setting for CPR. Move the person only if the setting is unsafe (see Box 31-1). Do not approach the person if the scene is unsafe for you.

The person must be on a hard, flat surface for CPR. If the person is in bed, place a board under the person. Or move the person to the floor.

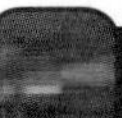

Adult CPR—One Rescuer

PROCEDURE

1 Make sure the scene is safe.
2 Take 5 to 10 seconds to check for a response and breathing.
  a Check if the person is responding. Tap or gently shake the person. Call the person by name, if known. Shout: "Are you okay?"
  b Check for no breathing or no normal breathing (gasping).
3 Call for help. Activate the EMS system or the agency's RRT if the person is not responding and not breathing or not breathing normally (gasping).
4 Get or ask someone to bring an AED if available.
5 Position the person supine on a hard, flat surface. Logroll the person so there is no twisting of the spine. Place the arms alongside the body.
6 Check for a carotid pulse. This should take 5 to 10 seconds. Start chest compressions if you do not feel a pulse.
7 Expose the person's chest.
8 Give chest compressions at a rate of at least 100 per minute. Push hard and fast. Establish a regular rhythm. Count out loud. Press down at least 2 inches. Allow the chest to recoil between compressions. Give 30 chest compressions.
9 Open the airway. Use the head tilt–chin lift method.
10 Give 2 breaths. Each breath should take only 1 second. The chest should rise. (If the first breath does not make the chest rise, try opening the airway again. Use the head tilt–chin lift method.)
11 Continue the cycle of 30 chest compressions followed by 2 breaths. Limit interruptions in compressions to less than 10 seconds. Continue CPR cycles until the AED arrives. See procedure: *Adult CPR With AED—Two Rescuers.* Or continue until help arrives or the person begins to move. If movement occurs, place the person in the recovery position, p. 491.

Adult CPR With AED—Two Rescuers

PROCEDURE

1 Make sure the scene is safe.
2 *Rescuer 1*—Take 5 to 10 seconds to check for a response and breathing.
  a Check if the person is responding. Tap or gently shake the person. Call the person by name, if known. Shout: "Are you okay?"
  b Check for no breathing or no normal breathing (gasping).
3 *Rescuer 2:*
  a Activate the EMS system or the agency's RRT if the person is not responding and not breathing or not breathing normally (gasping).
  b Get a defibrillator (AED) if one is available.
4 *Rescuer 1:*
  a Position the person supine on a hard, flat surface. Logroll the person so there is no twisting of the spine. Place the arms alongside the body.
  b Check for a carotid pulse. This should take 5 to 10 seconds. Start chest compressions if you do not feel a pulse.
  c Expose the person's chest.
  d Give chest compressions at a rate of at least 100 per minute. Push hard and fast. Establish a regular rhythm. Count out loud. Press down at least 2 inches. Allow the chest to recoil between compressions. Give 30 chest compressions.
  e Open the airway. Use the head tilt–chin lift method.
  f Give 2 breaths. Each breath should take only 1 second. The chest should rise. (If the first breath does not make the chest rise, try opening the airway again. Use the head tilt–chin lift method.)
  g Continue the cycle of 30 chest compressions followed by 2 breaths. Limit interruptions in compressions to less than 10 seconds.

Continued

Adult CPR With AED—Two Rescuers—cont'd

PROCEDURE—cont'd

5 *Rescuer 2:*
- a Open the case with the AED.
- b Turn on the AED (Fig. 31-11, *A*).
- c Apply adult electrode pads to the person's chest (Fig. 31-11, *B*). Follow the instructions and diagram provided with the AED.
- d Attach the connecting cables to the AED (Fig. 31-11, *C*).
- e Clear away from the person. Make sure no one is touching the person (Fig. 31-11, *D*).
- f Let the AED check the person's heart rhythm.
- g Make sure everyone is clear of the person if the AED advises a "shock" (see Fig. 31-11, *D*). Loudly instruct others not to touch the person. Say: "I am clear, you are clear, everyone is clear!" Look to make sure no one is touching the person.
- h Press the SHOCK button if the AED advises a "shock" (Fig. 31-11, *E*).

6 *Rescuers 1 and 2:*
- a Perform 2-person CPR.
  1. Begin with compressions. One rescuer gives chest compressions at a rate of at least 100 per minute. Push hard and fast. Establish a regular rhythm. Count out loud. Allow the chest to recoil between compressions. Give 30 chest compressions. Pause to allow the other rescuer to give 2 breaths.
  2. The other rescuer gives 2 breaths after every 30 chest compressions.

7 Repeat steps 5, e–h after 2 minutes of CPR (5 cycles of 30 compressions and 2 breaths). Change positions and continue CPR beginning with compressions.

8 Continue until help takes over or the person begins to move. If movement occurs, place the person in the recovery position.

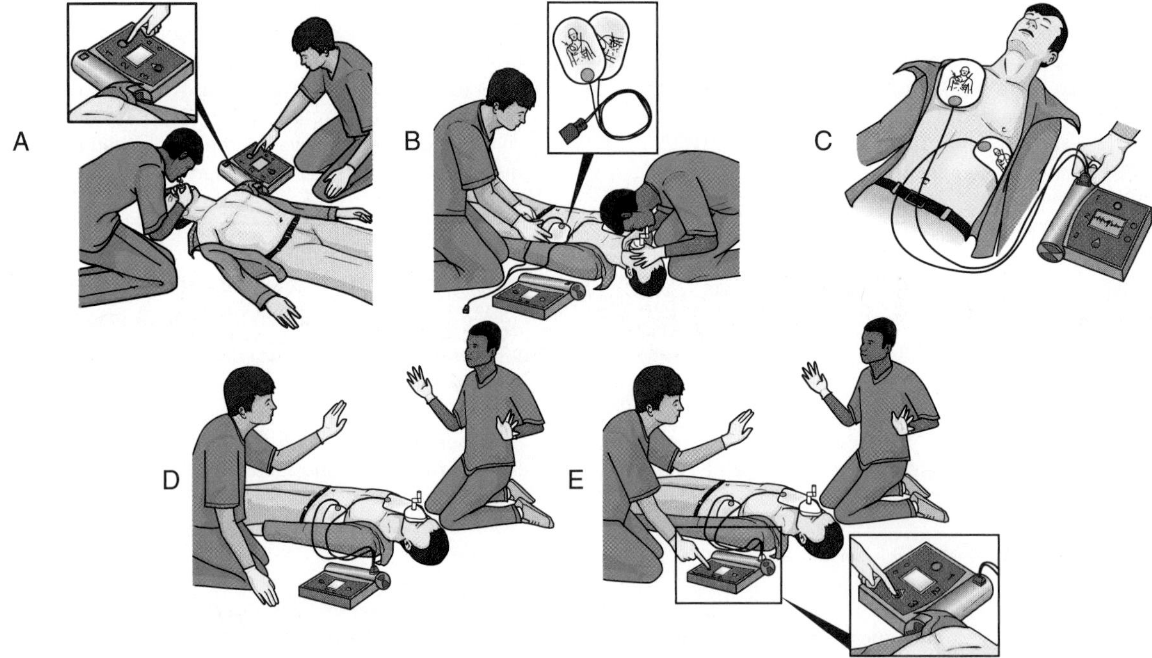

FIGURE 31-11 A, The rescuer turns on the AED. **B,** Electrode pads are placed on the person's chest. **C,** The cables are connected to the AED. **D,** The rescuer says to "clear" the person. The rescuer makes sure no one is touching the person. **E,** The SHOCK button is pressed to deliver a shock.

Hands-Only CPR. When an adult has sudden cardiac arrest, the person's survival depends on others nearby. Outside of the health care setting, persons trained in BLS are often not available. Bystanders may worry that they will not do CPR correctly or that they may injure the person.

The AHA developed "Hands-Only CPR" to improve the response of bystanders who witness an adult collapse suddenly in the out-of-hospital stetting. In "Hands-Only CPR," CPR involves 2 steps.

1 Call 911.
2 Push hard and fast in the center of the chest.

"Hands-Only CPR" is used to educate persons *not* trained in BLS. As a health care provider, use the CPR method presented in this chapter and in a BLS course.

Recovery Position

The recovery position is used when the person is breathing and has a pulse but is not responding (Fig. 31-12). The position helps keep the airway open and prevents aspiration.

Logroll the person into the recovery position. Keep the head, neck, and spine straight. A hand supports the head. *Do not use this position if the person might have neck injuries or other trauma.*

CHOKING

Foreign bodies can obstruct the airway. This is called *choking* or *foreign-body airway obstruction (FBAO).* Air cannot pass through the airways into the lungs. The body does not get enough oxygen. It can lead to cardiac arrest.

Airway obstruction can be mild or severe. With severe airway obstruction, air does not move in and out of the lungs. If the obstruction is not removed, the person will die. Abdominal thrusts are used to relieve severe airway obstruction. See Chapter 9 for emergency care of the choking person.

HEMORRHAGE

Life and body functions require an adequate blood supply. If a blood vessel is cut or torn, bleeding occurs. The larger the blood vessel, the greater the bleeding and blood loss. *Hemorrhage is the excessive loss of blood in a short time.* If bleeding is not stopped, the person will die.

Hemorrhage is internal or external. You cannot see internal hemorrhage. The bleeding is inside body tissues and body cavities. Pain, shock, vomiting blood, coughing up blood, and loss of consciousness signal internal hemorrhage. There is little you can do for internal bleeding.

- Follow the rules in Box 31-1. This includes activating the EMS system.
- Keep the person warm, flat, and quiet until help arrives.
- Do not give fluids.

If not hidden by clothing, external bleeding is usually seen. Bleeding from an artery occurs in spurts. There is a steady flow of blood from a vein. To control bleeding:

- Follow the rules in Box 31-1. This includes activating the EMS system.
- Do not remove any objects that have pierced or stabbed the person.
- Place a sterile dressing directly over the wound. Or use any clean material (handkerchief, towel, cloth, or sanitary napkin).
- Apply firm pressure directly over the bleeding site (Fig. 31-13). Do not release pressure until the bleeding stops. If needed, wrap an elastic bandage firmly over the dressing or material.
- Do not remove the dressing or material. If bleeding continues, apply more dressings or material on top and apply more pressure.
- Bind the wound when bleeding stops. Tape or tie the dressing in place. You can tie the dressing with such things as clothing, a scarf, or a necktie.

See *Promoting Safety and Comfort: Hemorrhage*, p. 492.

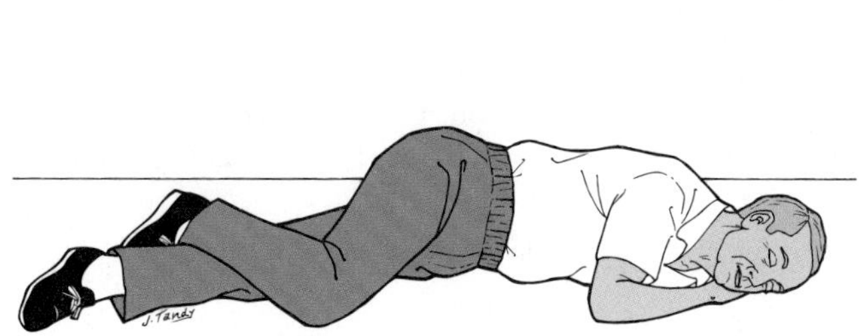

FIGURE 31-12 Recovery position.

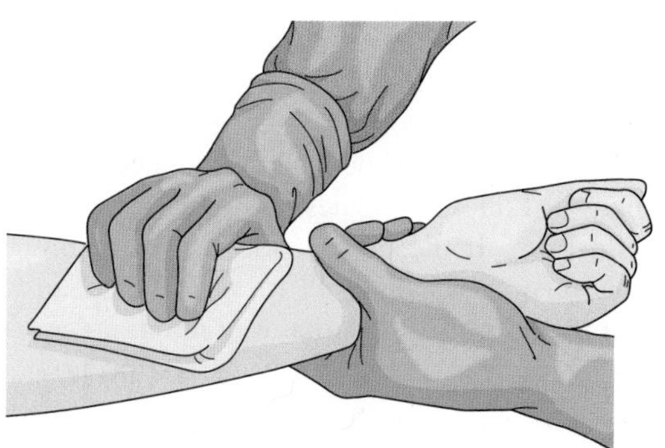

FIGURE 31-13 Direct pressure is applied to the wound to stop bleeding.

PROMOTING SAFETY AND COMFORT

Hemorrhage

Safety

Contact with blood is likely with hemorrhage. Follow Standard Precautions and the Bloodborne Pathogen Standard to the extent possible. Wear gloves if possible. Practice hand hygiene as soon as you can.

FAINTING

***Fainting** is the sudden loss of consciousness from an inadequate blood supply to the brain.* Hunger, fatigue, fear, and pain are common causes. Some people faint at the sight of blood or injury. Standing in 1 position for a long time and being in a warm, crowded room are other causes. Dizziness, perspiration (sweating), and blackness before the eyes are warning signals. The person looks pale. The pulse is weak. Respirations are shallow if consciousness is lost. Emergency care includes the following.

- Have the person sit or lie down before fainting occurs.
- If sitting, the person bends forward and places the head between the knees (Fig. 31-14).
- If the person is lying down, raise the legs.
- Loosen tight clothing (belt, tie, scarf, collar, and so on).
- Keep the person lying down if fainting has occurred. Raise the legs.
- Do not let the person get up until symptoms have subsided for about 5 minutes.
- Help the person to a sitting position after recovery from fainting. Observe for fainting.

SHOCK

***Shock** results when organs and tissues do not get enough blood.* Blood loss, heart attack (myocardial infarction), burns, and severe infection are causes. Signs and symptoms include:

- Low or falling blood pressure
- Rapid and weak pulse
- Rapid respirations
- Cold, moist, and pale skin
- Thirst
- Restlessness
- Confusion and loss of consciousness as shock worsens

Shock is possible in any person who is acutely ill or severely injured. Follow the rules in Box 31-1. Keep the person lying down. If the person does not have injuries from trauma, raise the feet 6 to 12 inches. Lower the feet if the position causes pain. Maintain an open airway and control bleeding. Begin CPR if cardiac arrest occurs.

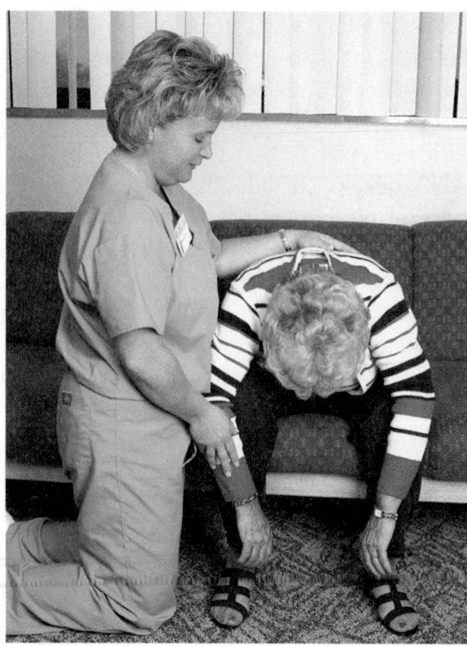

FIGURE 31-14 The person bends forward and lowers her head between her knees to prevent fainting.

Anaphylactic Shock

Some people are allergic or sensitive to foods, insects, chemicals, and drugs. For example, many people are allergic to the drug *penicillin.* An *antigen* is a substance that the body reacts to. The body releases chemicals to fight or attack the antigen. The person may react with an area of redness, swelling, or itching. Or the reaction may involve the entire body.

***Anaphylaxis** is a life-threatening sensitivity to an antigen.* (*Ana* means *without. Phylaxis* means *protection.*) The reaction can occur within seconds. Signs and symptoms include:

- An itchy rash
- Flushed or pale skin
- Feeling warm
- Dyspnea or wheezing from airway narrowing or a swollen tongue or throat
- Feeling that there is a "lump" in the throat
- A fast and weak pulse
- Nausea, vomiting, or diarrhea
- A feeling of dread or doom
- Dizziness or fainting
- Signs and symptoms of shock

Anaphylactic shock is an emergency. The EMS system must be activated. The person needs special drugs to reverse the allergic reaction. Keep the person lying down and the airway open. Start CPR if cardiac arrest occurs.

STROKE

Stroke (cerebrovascular accident) occurs when the brain is suddenly deprived of its blood supply (Chapter 28). Usually only part of the brain is affected. A stroke may be caused by a thrombus, an embolus, or hemorrhage if a blood vessel in the brain ruptures.

Signs of stroke vary (Chapter 28). They depend on the size and location of brain injury. Loss of consciousness or semi-consciousness, rapid pulse, labored respirations, high blood pressure, facial drooping, and hemiplegia (paralysis on 1 side of the body) are signs of a stroke. The person may have sudden confusion, numbness on 1 side of the body or in a body part, slurred speech, and aphasia (the inability to have normal speech). Loss of vision in 1 or both eyes, sudden and severe headache, dizziness, unsteadiness, and falling also are signs and symptoms. Seizures may occur.

Emergency care includes the following.

- Follow the rules in Box 31-1. This includes activating the EMS system.
- Find out when the signs and symptoms began. Tell the EMS staff the time.
- Position the person in the recovery position (see Fig. 31-12).
- Raise the head without flexing the neck.
- Loosen tight clothing (belt, tie, scarf, collar, and so on).
- Keep the person quiet and warm.
- Reassure the person.
- Provide CPR if necessary.
- Provide emergency care for seizures if necessary.

SEIZURES

***Seizures (convulsions)** are violent and sudden contractions or tremors of muscle groups.* Movements are uncontrolled. The person may lose consciousness. Seizures are caused by an abnormality in the brain. Causes include head injury during birth or from trauma, high fever, brain tumors, poisoning, and nervous system disorders or infections. Lack of blood flow to the brain can also cause seizures.

The major types of seizures are:

- *Partial seizure.* Only 1 part of the brain is involved. A body part may jerk. Or the person has a hearing or vision problem or stomach discomfort. The person does not lose consciousness.
- *Generalized tonic-clonic seizure (grand mal seizure).* This type has 2 phases. In the *tonic phase,* the person loses consciousness. If standing or sitting, the person falls to the floor. The body is rigid because all muscles contract at once. The *clonic phase* follows. Muscle groups contract and relax. This causes jerking and twitching movements. Urinary and fecal incontinence may occur. A deep sleep is common after the seizure. Confusion and headache may occur on awakening.
- *Generalized absence (petit mal) seizure.* This type usually lasts a few seconds. There is loss of consciousness, twitching of the eyelids, and staring. No first aid is necessary. However, you should guide the person away from dangers—stairs, streets, a hot stove, fireplaces, and so on.

Emergency Care for Seizures

You cannot stop a seizure. However, you can protect the person from injury.

- Follow the rules in Box 31-1. This includes activating the EMS system.
- Do not leave the person alone.
- Lower the person to the floor. This protects the person from falling.
- Note the time the seizure started.
- Place something soft under the person's head (Fig. 31-15). It prevents the person's head from striking the floor. You can use a pillow, a cushion, or a folded blanket, towel, or jacket. Or cradle the person's head in your lap.
- Loosen tight jewelry and clothing around the person's neck. Ties, scarves, collars, and necklaces are examples.
- Turn the person onto his or her side. Make sure the head is turned to the side.
- Do not put any object or your fingers between the person's teeth. The person can aspirate the object or bite down on your fingers during the seizure.
- Do not try to stop the seizure or control the person's movements.
- Move furniture, equipment, and sharp objects away from the person. He or she may strike these objects during the seizure.
- Note the time the seizure ends.
- Make sure the mouth is clear of food, fluids, and saliva after the seizure.
- Provide BLS if there is no breathing or no normal breathing after the seizure.

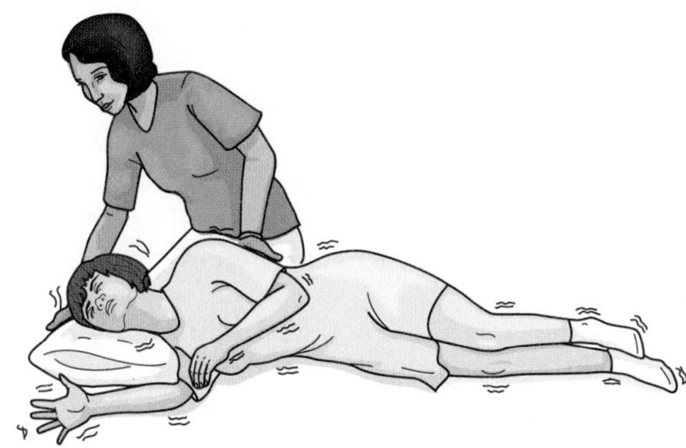

FIGURE 31-15 A pillow protects the person's head during a seizure.

BURNS

Burns can severely disable a person (Fig. 31-16). They can also cause death. Most burns occur in the home. Infants, children, and older persons are at risk. Common causes of burns and fires are:

- Scalds from hot liquids
- Playing with matches and lighters
- Electrical injuries
- Cooking accidents (barbecues, microwave ovens, stoves, ovens)
- Falling asleep while smoking
- Fireplaces
- Space heaters
- No smoke detectors or non-functioning smoke detectors
- Chemicals

Some burns are minor; others are severe. Severity depends on burn size and depth, the body part involved, and the person's age. Burns to the face, eyes, ears, hands, and feet are more serious than burns to an arm or leg. Infants, young children, and older persons are at high risk for death.

Emergency care for severe burns includes the following.

- Follow the rules in Box 31-1. This includes activating the EMS system.
- Do not touch the person if he or she is in contact with an electrical source. Have the power source turned off. Do not approach the person or try to remove the electrical source with any object until the power source is turned off.
- Remove the person from the fire or burn source.
- Stop the burning process. Put out flames with water or roll the person in a blanket. Or smother flames with a coat, sheet, or towel.
- Apply cold or cool water (59°F to 77°F [15°C to 25°C]) until pain is relieved. Do not apply ice directly to the burn.
- Do not remove burned clothing.
- Remove hot clothing that is not sticking to the skin. If you cannot remove hot clothing, cool the clothing with water.
- Remove jewelry and any tight clothing that is not sticking to the skin.
- Provide rescue breathing and CPR as needed.
- Cover burns with sterile, cool, moist coverings. Or use towels, sheets, or any other clean cloth. Keep the covering wet.
- Do not put oil, butter, salve, or ointments on the burns.
- Keep blisters intact. Do not break blisters.
- Cover the person with a blanket or coat to prevent heat loss.

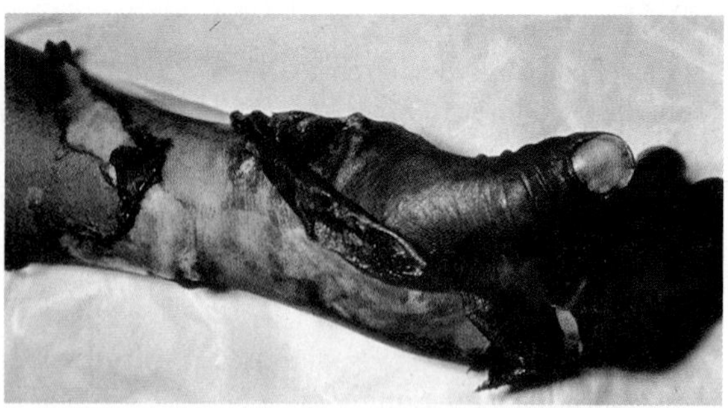

FIGURE 31-16 A burn.

FOCUS ON PRIDE

The Person, Family, and Yourself

Personal and Professional Responsibility

Having an understanding of emergency care is a professional responsibility. This knowledge allows you to safely assist in an emergency situation. This chapter includes basic information on emergency care. BLS courses for health care providers offer further training. The courses allow you to practice emergency procedures. CPR and the use of an AED are examples.

Most agencies require nursing assistants to be certified in BLS. Certification courses often involve a written and skills test. During the skills test, you demonstrate your ability to provide BLS. Take the course seriously. And take pride in receiving this training. What you learn can save a life.

Rights and Respect

During emergencies, protect the right to privacy. Do not expose the person unnecessarily. You may be in a place where you cannot close doors or window coverings. The person may be in a lounge, dining area, or public place. Do what you can to provide privacy. As always, treat the person with dignity and respect.

Independence and Social Interaction

Promoting quality of life and independence in an emergency is important. Choices may be few. However, they are given when possible. Hospital care may be required. The person has the right to choose a hospital.

Sometimes the person may want to refuse care. The EMS staff has guidelines for persons refusing care. For example, the person must be competent and legally able to make his or her own medical decisions. The person must also be informed of the risks, benefits, and alternatives to the care recommended.

Delegation and Teamwork

On-lookers can threaten privacy and confidentiality. During an emergency, your main concern is the person's illness or injuries. You cannot give care and manage on-lookers at the same time. Ask a team member to deal with on-lookers. If someone else is giving care, keep on-lookers away from the person. Take pride in working as a team to protect the person's privacy in an emergency situation.

Ethics and Laws

People are curious. They want to know what happened, the extent of injuries or illness, and if the person will be okay. Do not discuss the situation. Do not offer ideas of what is wrong with the person. Information about the person's care, treatment, and condition is confidential. Keep the person's information private. It is the right thing to do.

REVIEW QUESTIONS

Circle the BEST answer.

1 When giving first aid, you should
  a Know your own limits
  b Move the person
  c Give the person fluids
  d Keep the person cool

2 The signs of sudden cardiac arrest are
  a Restlessness, rapid breathing, and a weak pulse
  b Confusion, hemiplegia, and slurred speech
  c No response, no normal breathing, and no pulse
  d Dizziness, pale skin, and rapid breathing

3 Rescue breathing for an adult involves
  a Giving each breath over 2 seconds
  b Watching the abdomen rise with each breath
  c Giving a breath every 3 to 5 seconds
  d Giving a breath every 5 to 6 seconds

4 In adult CPR, the chest is compressed
  a 1½ inches with the index and middle fingers
  b 2 inches with the heel of 1 hand
  c At least 2 inches with 2 hands
  d At least 1 inch with 2 hands

5 When checking for breathing
  a Use the head tilt–chin lift method to open the airway
  b Look for no breathing or gasping
  c Look, listen, and feel for air moving in and out of the lungs
  d Take 10 to 15 seconds to listen for breathing

6 Which pulse is used during adult CPR?
  a The carotid pulse
  b The apical pulse
  c The brachial pulse
  d The femoral pulse

7 Which compression rate is used for adult CPR?
  a At least 150 compressions per minute
  b At least 100 compressions per minute
  c At least 30 compressions per minute
  d At least 15 compressions per minute

8 When doing adult CPR
  a Give 2 breaths after every 15 compressions
  b Give 2 breaths after every 30 compressions
  c Give 1 breath after every 5 compressions
  d Give 2 breaths when you are tired from giving compressions

9 Two rescuers are giving adult CPR. When should the AED be used?
  a After 5 cycles of CPR
  b After 2 minutes of CPR
  c As soon as the AED arrives
  d When EMS staff arrives

10 A person is hemorrhaging from the left forearm. Your *first* action is to
  a Lower the arm
  b Apply pressure to the brachial artery
  c Tape a dressing in place
  d Apply direct pressure to the wound

11 A person is about to faint. What should you do?
  a Have the person sit or lie down.
  b Take the person outside for fresh air.
  c Have the person stand very still.
  d Raise the head if the person is lying down.

12 Which is a sign of shock?
  a High blood pressure
  b Slow pulse
  c Slow and deep respirations
  d Cold, moist, and pale skin

13 A person in shock needs
  a Rescue breathing
  b Clothes removed
  c To be kept lying down
  d The recovery position

14 A person is having a stroke. Emergency care involves
  a Asking when the person's symptoms began
  b Giving the person sips of water
  c Controlling bleeding
  d Positioning the person bent forward with the head lowered

15 A person is having a tonic-clonic (grand mal) seizure. You should
  a Place an object between the person's teeth
  b Loosen tight jewelry and clothing around the neck
  c Try to stop the person's movements
  d Place the person's head on a firm surface

16 Burns are covered with
  a A clean, moist cloth or dressing
  b Butter or oil
  c Salve or an ointment
  d Nothing

Answers to these questions are on p. 505.

FOCUS ON **PRACTICE**

Problem Solving

A resident has a seizure during an activity. What emergency care will you provide? After the seizure, the person is only gasping. Explain what you would do step-by-step. How will you and the nursing team provide for the person's privacy?

CHAPTER

32 Assisting With End-of-Life Care

OBJECTIVES

- Define the key terms and key abbreviations listed in this chapter.
- Describe palliative care and hospice care.
- Describe the factors affecting attitudes about death.
- Describe the 5 stages of dying.
- Explain how to meet the needs of the dying person and family.
- Describe 3 advance directives.
- Identify the signs of approaching death and the signs of death.
- Explain how to assist with post-mortem care.
- Perform the procedure described in this chapter.
- Explain how to promote PRIDE in the person, the family, and yourself.

KEY TERMS

advance directive A document stating a person's wishes about health care when that person cannot make his or her own decisions

autopsy The examination of the body after death

end-of-life care The support and care given during the time surrounding death

palliative care Care that involves relieving or reducing the intensity of uncomfortable symptoms without producing a cure

post-mortem care Care of the body after *(post)* death *(mortem)*

reincarnation The belief that the spirit or soul is reborn in another human body or in another form of life

rigor mortis The stiffness or rigidity *(rigor)* of skeletal muscles that occurs after death *(mortis)*

terminal illness An illness or injury from which the person will not likely recover

KEY ABBREVIATIONS

DNR Do Not Resuscitate
ID Identification
OBRA Omnibus Budget Reconciliation Act of 1987

End-of-life care describes the support and care given during the time surrounding death. Sometimes death is sudden. Often it is expected. Some people gradually fail. End-of-life care may involve days, weeks, or months.

Your feelings about death affect the care you give. You will help meet the dying person's physical, psychological, social, and spiritual needs. Therefore you must understand the dying process. Then you can approach the dying person with care, kindness, and respect.

TERMINAL ILLNESS

Many illnesses and diseases have no cure. The body cannot function after some injuries. Recovery is not expected. The disease or injury ends in death. *An illness or injury from which the person will not likely recover is a* ***terminal illness.***

Types of Care

Terminally ill persons can choose palliative care or hospice care. The person may opt for palliative care and then change to hospice care.

- *Palliative care. Palliate* means *to soothe or relieve.* ***Palliative care*** *involves relieving or reducing the intensity of uncomfortable symptoms without producing a cure.* The focus is on relief of symptoms. The illness is also treated. The intent is to improve the person's quality of life and provide family support.
- *Hospice care.* The focus is on the physical, emotional, social, and spiritual needs of dying persons and their families (Chapter 1). Often the person has less than 6 months to live. Hospice care does not involve cure or life-saving measures. Pain relief and comfort are stressed. The goal is to improve quality of life. Follow-up care and support groups for survivors are hospice services. Hospice also provides support for the health team to help deal with a person's death.

ATTITUDES ABOUT DEATH

Many people fear death. Others do not believe they will die. Some look forward to and accept death. Attitudes about death often change as a person grows older and with changing circumstances.

Cultural and Spiritual Needs

Practices and attitudes about death differ among cultures. See *Caring About Culture: Death Rites.* In some cultures, dying people are cared for at home by the family. Some families prepare the body for burial.

Spiritual needs relate to the human spirit and to religion and religious beliefs. Many people strengthen their religious beliefs when dying. Religion provides comfort for the dying person and the family.

Attitudes about death are closely related to religion. Some believe that life after death is free of suffering and hardship. They also believe in reunion with loved ones. Many believe sins and misdeeds are punished in the afterlife. Others do not believe in the afterlife. To them, death is the end of life.

There are also religious beliefs about the body's form after death. Some believe the body keeps its physical form. Others believe that only the spirit or soul is present in the afterlife. ***Reincarnation*** *is the belief that the spirit or soul is reborn in another human body or in another form of life.*

Many religions practice rites and rituals during the dying process and at the time of death. Prayers, blessings, scripture readings, and religious music are common sources of comfort. So are visits from a minister, priest, rabbi, or other cleric.

See *Focus on Communication: Cultural and Spiritual Needs.*

Age

Infants and toddlers do not understand the nature or meaning of death. They know or sense that something is different. They sense a caregiver's absence or a different caregiver. They also sense changes in when and how their needs are met. They may feel a sense of loss.

Between 2 and 6 years old, children think death is temporary. It can be reversed. The dead person continues to live and function in some ways and can come back to life. These ideas come from fairy tales, cartoons, movies, video games, and TV. Children this age often blame themselves when someone or something dies. To them, death is punishment for being bad. They know when family members

CARING ABOUT CULTURE

Death Rites

In *Vietnam,* dying persons are helped to recall past good deeds and to achieve a fitting mental state. Death at home is preferred. In some areas, a coin, jewels (a wealthy family), or rice (a poor family) is put in the dead person's mouth. The belief is that they will help the soul go through encounters with gods and devils and the soul will be born rich in the next life.

The *Chinese* have an aversion to death and anything concerning death. Autopsy and disposal of the body are not prescribed by religion. Donating body parts is encouraged. The eldest son makes all arrangements. The body is buried in a coffin. After 7 years, the body is exhumed and cremated. The urn, with the ashes, is buried in the family tomb. White, yellow, or black clothing is worn for mourning.

In *India,* Hindu persons are often accepting of God's will. The person's desire to be clear-headed as death nears must be assessed in planning treatment. A time and place for prayer are essential for the family and the person. Prayer helps them deal with anxiety and conflict. The Hindu priest reads from Holy Sanskrit books. Some priests tie strings (meaning a blessing) around the neck or waist. After death, the son pours water on the mouth of the deceased. Blood transfusions, organ transplants, and autopsies are allowed. Cremation is preferred.

From D'Avanzo CE: Pocket guide to cultural health assessment, *ed 4, St Louis, 2008, Mosby.*

FOCUS ON COMMUNICATION

Cultural and Spiritual Needs

You may have different cultural or religious practices and beliefs about death. You must not judge the person by your standards. Do not make negative comments or insult the person's beliefs. Respect the person as a whole. This includes his or her beliefs and customs.

or pets die. They notice dead birds or bugs. Answers to questions about death often cause fear and confusion. Children who are told "He is sleeping" may be afraid to go to sleep.

Between 6 and 11 years old, children learn that death is final. They do not think they will die. Death happens to others, especially adults. It can be avoided. Children relate death to punishment and body mutilation. It also involves witches, ghosts, goblins, and monsters. Understanding increases as children grow older and have more experiences with death.

Adults fear pain and suffering, dying alone, and the invasion of privacy. They also fear loneliness and separation from loved ones. They worry about the care and support of those left behind. Adults often resent death because it affects plans, hopes, dreams, and ambitions.

Older persons know death will occur. They have had more experiences with dying and death. Many have lost family and friends. Some welcome death as freedom from pain, suffering, and disability. Death also means reunion with those who have died. Like younger adults, many fear dying alone.

THE STAGES OF DYING

Dr. Elisabeth Kübler-Ross described 5 stages of dying. They also are called the "stages of grief." *Grief* is the person's response to loss.

- *Stage 1: Denial.* The person refuses to believe that he or she is dying. "No, not me" is a common response. The person believes a mistake was made.
- *Stage 2: Anger.* The person thinks: "Why me?" There is anger and rage. Dying persons envy and resent those with life and health. Family, friends, and the health team are often targets of anger.
- *Stage 3: Bargaining.* Anger has passed. The person now says: "Yes, me, but...." Often the person bargains with God or a higher power for more time. Promises are made in exchange for more time. Bargaining is usually private and spiritual.
- *Stage 4: Depression.* The person thinks: "Yes, me" and is very sad. The person mourns things that were lost and the future loss of life. The person may cry or say little. Sometimes the person talks about people and things that will be left behind.
- *Stage 5: Acceptance.* The person is calm, at peace, and accepts death. The person has said what needs to be said. Unfinished business is completed. This stage may last for many months or years. Reaching the acceptance stage does not mean death is near.

Dying persons do not always pass through all 5 stages. A person may never get beyond a certain stage. Some move back and forth between stages. For example, Mr. Jones reached acceptance but moves back to bargaining. Then he moves forward to acceptance. Some people stay in one stage.

COMFORT NEEDS

Comfort is a basic part of end-of-life care. It involves physical, mental and emotional, and spiritual needs. For spiritual needs, see "Cultural and Spiritual Needs" on p. 497. Comfort goals are to:

- Prevent or relieve suffering to the extent possible.
- Respect and follow end-of-life wishes.

Dying persons may want family and friends present. They may want to talk about their fears, worries, and anxieties. Some want to be alone. Often they need to talk during the night. Things are quiet, distractions are few, and there is more time to think. You need to listen and use touch.

- *Listening.* The person needs to talk and share worries and concerns. Let the person express feelings and emotions in his or her own way. Do not worry about saying the wrong thing or finding comforting words. You do not need to say anything. Being there for the person is what counts.
- *Touch.* Touch shows care and concern when words cannot. Sometimes the person does not want to talk but needs you nearby. Do not feel that you need to talk. Silence, along with touch, is a powerful and meaningful way to communicate.

Some people may want to see a spiritual leader. Or they want to take part in religious practices. Provide privacy during prayer and spiritual moments. Be courteous to the spiritual leader. The person has the right to have religious objects nearby—medals, pictures, statues, writings, and so on. Handle these valuables with care and respect.

See *Focus on Communication: Comfort Needs.*

See *Focus on Older Persons: Comfort Needs.*

FOCUS ON COMMUNICATION

Comfort Needs

You may not know what to say to the dying person. That is hard for many experienced health team members. Unless you have been near death yourself, do not say: "I understand what you are going through." The statement is a communication barrier. Instead you can say:

- "Would you like to talk? I have time to listen."
- "You seem sad. How can I help?"
- "Is it okay if I quietly sit with you for a while?"

FOCUS ON OLDER PERSONS

Comfort Needs

Persons with Alzheimer's disease (AD) become more and more disabled. Those with advanced AD cannot share their concerns, discomforts, or problems. And it is hard to provide emotional and spiritual comfort.

Focusing on the person's senses—hearing, touch, sight—can promote comfort. Comforting touch or massage can be soothing. So can soft music or sounds from nature—birds chirping, gentle breezes, ocean waves, and so on.

Physical Needs

Dying may take a few minutes, hours, days, or weeks. Body processes slow. The person is weak. Changes occur in levels of consciousness. As the person weakens, basic needs are met. Every effort is made to promote physical and psychological comfort. The person is allowed to die in peace and with dignity.

Pain. Some dying persons do not have pain. Others have severe pain. Always report signs and symptoms of pain at once (Chapter 21). The nurse can give pain-relief drugs to prevent or control pain.

Skin care, personal and oral hygiene, back massages, and good alignment promote comfort. So do frequent position changes and supportive devices. Turn the person slowly and gently. Follow the care plan to prevent and control pain.

Breathing Problems. Shortness of breath and difficulty breathing *(dyspnea)* are common end-of-life problems. Semi-Fowler's position and oxygen (Chapter 26) are helpful. An open window for fresh air may help some people. For others, a fan to circulate air is helpful.

Noisy breathing—called the *death rattle*—is common as death nears. This is caused by mucus collecting in the airway. These measures may help.

- The side-lying position
- Suctioning by the nurse
- Drugs to reduce the amount of mucus

Vision, Hearing, and Speech. Vision blurs and gradually fails. The person turns toward light. A darkened room may frighten the person. The eyes may be half-open. Secretions may collect in the eye corners.

Because of failing vision, explain who you are and what you are doing to the person or in the room. The room should be well lit. However, avoid bright lights and glares.

Good eye care is needed (Chapter 16). If the eyes stay open, a nurse may apply a protective ointment. Then the eyes are covered with moist pads to prevent injury.

Hearing is one of the last functions lost. Many people hear until the moment of death. Even unconscious persons may hear. Always assume that the person can hear. Speak in a normal voice. Provide reassurance and explanations about care. Offer words of comfort. Avoid topics that could upset the person. Do not talk about the person.

Speech becomes harder. It may be hard to understand the person. Sometimes the person cannot speak. Anticipate the person's needs. Do not ask questions that need long answers. Ask a few "yes" or "no" questions. Despite speech problems, you must talk to the person.

Mouth, Nose, and Skin. Oral hygiene promotes comfort. Give routine mouth care if the person can eat and drink. Give frequent oral hygiene as death nears and when taking oral fluids is difficult. Oral hygiene is needed if mucus collects in the mouth and the person cannot swallow. A lip balm may help dry lips.

Crusting and irritation of the nostrils can occur. Nasal secretions, an oxygen cannula, and a naso-gastric tube are common causes. Carefully clean the nose. Apply lubricant as directed by the nurse and the care plan.

Circulation fails and body temperature rises as death nears. The skin is cool, pale, and mottled (blotchy). Sweating increases. Skin care, bathing, and preventing pressure ulcers are necessary. Linens and gowns are changed as needed. Although the skin feels cool, only light bed coverings are needed. Blankets may make the person feel warm and cause restlessness. However, observe for signs of cold. Shivering, hunching shoulders, and pulling covers up may signal that the person is cold. Prevent drafts and provide more blankets.

Nutrition. Nausea, vomiting, and loss of appetite are common at the end of life. The doctor can order drugs for nausea and vomiting.

You may need to feed the person. Favorite foods may help loss of appetite. So may small, frequent meals.

As death nears, loss of appetite is common. The person may choose not to eat or drink. Do not force the person to eat or drink. Report refusal to eat or drink to the nurse.

Elimination. Urinary and fecal incontinence may occur. Use incontinence products or bed protectors as directed. Give perineal care as needed. Constipation and urinary retention are common. Enemas and catheters may be needed. Follow the care plan for catheter care.

The Person's Room. Provide a comfortable and pleasant room. It should be well lit and well ventilated. Remove unnecessary equipment. Some equipment is upsetting to look at (suction machines, drainage containers). If possible, keep these items out of the person's sight.

Mementos, pictures, cards, flowers, and religious items provide comfort. The person and family arrange the room as they wish. This helps meet love, belonging, and esteem needs. The room should reflect the person's choices.

Mental and Emotional Needs

Mental and emotional needs are very personal. Some persons are anxious or depressed. Others have specific fears and concerns. Examples include:

- Severe pain
- When and how death will occur
- What will happen to loved ones
- Dying alone

Simple measures may soothe the person—touch, holding hands, back massage, soft lighting, music at a low volume.

THE FAMILY

This is a hard time for the family. You may find it hard to find comforting words. To show you care, be available, courteous, and considerate. Use touch to show your concern.

Sometimes the family keeps a vigil. That is, someone is with the person at all times including at night. They watch over or pray for the person. Help make them as comfortable as possible.

Respect the right to privacy. The person and family need time together. However, do not neglect care because the family is present. Most agencies let family members help give care. Or you can suggest that they take a break for a beverage or meal.

The family may be very tired, sad, and tearful. Watching a loved one die is very painful. So is dealing with the eventual loss of that person. The family goes through stages like the dying person. They need support, understanding, courtesy, and respect. A spiritual leader may provide comfort. Communicate this request to the nurse at once.

LEGAL ISSUES

Much attention is given to the right to die. Some people make end-of-life wishes known.

Advance Directives

The Patient Self-Determination Act and the Omnibus Budget Reconciliation Act of 1987 (OBRA) give persons the right to accept or refuse treatment. They also give the right to make advance directives. An ***advance directive*** *is a document stating a person's wishes about health care when that person cannot make his or her own decisions.* Advance directives usually forbid certain care if there is no hope of recovery. Quality of care cannot be less because of the person's advance directives.

See *Focus on Surveys: Advance Directives.*

Living Wills. A living will is about measures that support or maintain life when death is likely. Tube feedings, ventilators, and resuscitation are examples. A living will may instruct doctors:

- Not to start measures that prolong dying
- To remove measures that prolong dying

> **FOCUS ON SURVEYS**
>
> ***Advance Directives***
>
> Agencies must comply with federal and state laws about advance directives. One requirement is that agencies educate staff about policies and procedures for advance directives. A surveyor may ask you about advance directives. For example:
>
> - Did you receive information from the agency about advance directives?
> - When did you receive such information?
> - What do advance directives mean to you?
> - What care do you give when a person has an advance directive?

Durable Power of Attorney for Health Care. This advance directive gives the power to make health care decisions to another person. That person is often called a *health care proxy.* Usually this is a family member, friend, or lawyer. When a person cannot make health care decisions, the health care proxy can do so. This advance directive does not cover property or financial matters.

"Do Not Resuscitate" Orders

"Do Not Resuscitate" (DNR) or "No Code" orders mean that the person will not be resuscitated (Chapter 31). The person is allowed to die with peace and dignity. The doctor writes the DNR order after consulting with the person and family. The family and doctor make the decision if the person is not mentally able to do so.

SIGNS OF DEATH

As death nears, these signs may occur fast or slowly.

- Movement, muscle tone, and sensation are lost. This usually starts in the feet and legs. Mouth muscles relax and the jaw drops. The mouth may stay open. The facial expression is often peaceful.
- Peristalsis and other gastro-intestinal functions slow down. Abdominal distention, fecal incontinence, nausea, and vomiting are common.
- Body temperature rises. The person feels cool or cold, looks pale, and perspires heavily.
- Circulation fails. The pulse is fast or slow, weak, and irregular. Blood pressure starts to fall.
- The respiratory system fails. Slow or rapid and shallow respirations are observed. Mucus collects in the airway. Breathing sounds are noisy and gurgling—commonly called the *death rattle.*
- Pain decreases as the person loses consciousness. However, some people are conscious until the moment of death.

The signs of death include no pulse, no respirations, and no blood pressure. The pupils are fixed and dilated. A doctor determines that death has occurred. He or she pronounces the person dead.

CARE OF THE BODY AFTER DEATH

Care of the body after (post) *death* (mortem) *is called* ***post-mortem care.*** You may be asked to assist the nurse. Post-mortem care begins when the person is pronounced dead.

Post-mortem care is done to maintain a good appearance of the body. Discoloration and skin damage are prevented. Valuables and personal items are gathered for the family. The right to privacy and the right to be treated with dignity and respect apply after death.

Within 2 to 4 hours after death, rigor mortis develops. ***Rigor mortis*** *is the stiffness or rigidity* (rigor) *of skeletal muscles that occurs after death* (mortis). The body is positioned in normal alignment before rigor mortis sets in. The family may want to see the body. The body should appear in a comfortable and natural position.

In some agencies, the body is prepared only for viewing by the family. The funeral director completes post-mortem care.

Sometimes an autopsy is done. An ***autopsy*** *is the examination of the body after death.* (*Autos* means *self. Opsis* means *view.*) It is done to determine the cause of death. The coroner or medical examiner can order an autopsy. Or the family can request one. Post-mortem care is not done. Doing so could remove or destroy evidence.

Post-mortem care involves moving the body. For example, soiled areas are bathed and the body is placed in good alignment. Moving the body can cause air in the lungs, stomach, and intestines to be expelled. When air is expelled, sounds are produced. Do not let those sounds alarm or frighten you. They are normal and expected.

See *Delegation Guidelines: Care of the Body After Death.*

See *Promoting Safety and Comfort: Care of the Body After Death.*

See procedure: *Assisting With Post-Mortem Care.*

DELEGATION GUIDELINES

Care of the Body After Death

To assist with post-mortem care, you need this information from the nurse.

- If dentures are inserted or placed in a denture cup
- If tubes and dressings are removed or left in place
- If rings are removed or left in place
- If the family wants to view the body
- Special agency policies and procedures

PROMOTING SAFETY AND COMFORT

Care of the Body After Death

Safety

Standard Precautions and the Bloodborne Pathogen Standard are followed. You may have contact with blood, body fluids, secretions, and excretions.

Assisting With Post-Mortem Care

PRE-PROCEDURE

1 Follow *Delegation Guidelines: Care of the Body After Death.* See *Promoting Safety and Comfort: Care of the Body After Death.*
2 Practice hand hygiene.
3 Collect the following.
- Post-mortem kit (shroud or body bag, gown, ID [identification] tags, gauze squares, safety pins)
- Bed protectors
- Wash basin
- Bath towel and washcloths
- Denture cup
- Tape
- Dressings
- Gloves
- Cotton balls
- Valuables envelope

4 Provide for privacy.
5 Raise the bed for body mechanics.
6 Make sure the bed is flat.

PROCEDURE

7 Put on the gloves.
8 Position the person supine. Arms and legs are straight. A pillow is under the head and shoulders. Or raise the head of the bed 15 to 20 degrees if this is agency policy.
9 Close the eyes. Gently pull the eyelids over the eyes. Apply moist cotton balls gently over the eyelids if the eyes will not stay closed.
10 Insert dentures if it is agency policy to do so. If not, put them in a labeled denture cup.
11 Close the mouth. If necessary, place a rolled towel under the chin to keep the mouth closed.
12 Follow agency policy for jewelry. Remove all jewelry, except for wedding rings if this is agency policy. List the jewelry that you removed. Place the jewelry and the list in a valuables envelope.
13 Place a cotton ball over the rings. Tape them in place.
14 Remove drainage containers.
15 Remove tubes and catheters. Use the gauze squares as needed.
16 Bathe soiled areas with plain water. Dry thoroughly.
17 Place a bed protector under the buttocks.
18 Remove soiled dressings. Replace them with clean ones.
19 Put a clean gown on the body.
20 Brush and comb the hair if necessary.
21 Cover the body to the shoulders with a sheet if the family will view the body.
22 Gather the person's belongings. Put them in a bag labeled with the person's name. Make sure you include eyeglasses, hearing aids, and other valuables.
23 Remove supplies, equipment, and linens. Straighten the room. Provide soft lighting.
24 Remove and discard the gloves. Practice hand hygiene.
25 Let the family view the body. Provide for privacy. Return to the room after they leave.
26 Practice hand hygiene. Put on gloves.
27 Fill out the ID tags. Tie 1 to the ankle or to the right big toe.
28 Place the body in the body bag or cover it with a sheet. Or apply a shroud (Fig. 32-1, p. 502).
  a Position the shroud under the body.
  b Bring the top down over the head.
  c Fold the bottom up over the feet.
  d Fold the sides over the body.
  e Pin or tape the shroud in place.
29 Attach the second ID tag to the body bag, sheet, or shroud.
30 Leave the denture cup with the body.
31 Pull the privacy curtain around the bed. Or close the door.

Continued

Assisting With Post-Mortem Care—cont'd

POST-PROCEDURE

32 Remove and discard the gloves. Practice hand hygiene.
33 Remove all linens and equipment after the body has been removed. Wear gloves for this step.
34 Remove and discard the gloves. Practice hand hygiene.
35 Report the following.
- The time the body was taken by the funeral director
- What was done with jewelry, other valuables, and personal items
- What was done with dentures

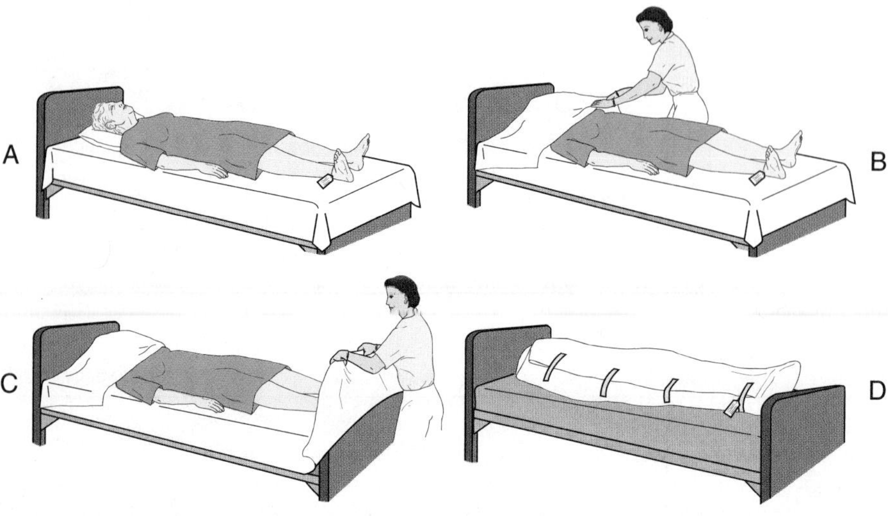

FIGURE 32-1 Applying a shroud. **A,** Position the shroud under the body. **B,** Bring the top of the shroud down over the head. **C,** Fold the bottom up over the feet. **D,** Fold the sides over the body. Tape or pin the sides together. Attach the ID tag.

FOCUS ON PRIDE

The Person, Family, and Yourself

Personal and Professional Responsibility
You may assist with the dying person's care. To give quality care:
- Promote comfort. Report the person's complaints or signs of pain at once. Follow the comfort measures in the care plan.
- Protect the person's privacy.
- Provide support to the person and family. Be kind. Show compassion and respect.
- Offer the family time alone with the person.

Take pride in supporting the person and family during a difficult time.

Rights and Respect
You may not agree with advance directives or resuscitation decisions. However, you must respect the person's or family's wishes. The doctor's orders must be followed. These may be against your personal, religious, or cultural values. If so, discuss the matter with the nurse. You may need an assignment change.

Independence and Social Interaction
The person is encouraged to take part in his or her care to the extent possible. Some days the person can do more than on other days. Follow the nurse's directions and the care plan. Do not force the person to do more than he or she can physically or mentally do.

Delegation and Teamwork
Nurses may spend a lot of time with persons who are dying. Often it is a busy time before and after someone dies. Offer to take equipment and supplies to and from the room. Also help with other patients or residents.

Ethics and Laws
The dying person has rights under OBRA.
- *The right to privacy before and after death.* The person has the right not to have his or her body seen by others. Proper draping and screening are important.
- *The right to visit others in private.* If the person is too weak to leave the room, the roommate may have to do so. A private room provides privacy. The family can stay as long as they like.
- *The right to confidentiality before and after death.* The final moments and cause of death are kept confidential. So are statements, conversations, and family reactions.
- *The right to be free from abuse, mistreatment, and neglect.* The person has the right to receive kind and respectful care before and after death. Report signs of abuse, mistreatment, or neglect at once.
- *Freedom from restraint.* Restraints are used only if ordered by the doctor. Dying persons are often too weak to be dangerous to themselves or others.
- *The right to have personal possessions.* The person may want photos and religious items nearby. Protect the person's property from loss or damage before and after death.
- *The right to a safe and a home-like setting.* Dying persons depend on others for safety. The setting must be safe. A home-like setting provides comfort. Try to keep equipment and supplies out of view. The room should be free from unpleasant odors and noises. Keep the room neat and clean.
- *The right to personal choice.* The person has the right to be involved in treatment and care. The dying person may refuse treatment. The health team must respect choices to refuse treatment or not prolong life.

REVIEW QUESTIONS

Circle the BEST answer.

1 Which is *true?*
  a Death from terminal illness is sudden.
  b Doctors know when death will occur.
  c An illness is terminal when recovery is not likely.
  d All severe injuries end in death.

2 Reincarnation is the belief that
  a There is no afterlife
  b The spirit or soul is reborn into another body or form of life
  c The body keeps its physical form in the afterlife
  d Only the spirit or soul is present in the afterlife

3 Adults and older persons usually fear
  a Dying alone
  b Reincarnation
  c The 5 stages of dying
  d Advance directives

4 Persons in the stage of denial
  a Are angry
  b Are calm and at peace
  c Are sad and quiet
  d Refuse to believe they are dying

5 A person tries to gain more time during the stage of
  a Anger
  b Bargaining
  c Depression
  d Acceptance

6 When caring for the dying person, you should
  a Use touch and listen
  b Do most of the talking
  c Keep the room darkened
  d Speak in a loud voice

7 As death nears, the last sense lost is
  a Sight
  b Taste
  c Smell
  d Hearing

8 The dying person's care includes the following. Which should you question?
  a Eye care
  b Mouth care
  c Active range-of-motion exercises
  d Position changes

9 The dying person is positioned in
  a The supine position
  b Fowler's position
  c Good body alignment
  d The dorsal recumbent position

10 A "DNR" order means that
  a CPR will not be done
  b The person has a living will
  c Life-prolonging measures will be carried out
  d The person is kept alive as long as possible

11 The signs of death are
  a Convulsions and incontinence
  b No pulse, respirations, or blood pressure
  c Loss of consciousness and convulsions
  d The eyes stay open, no muscle movements, and the body is rigid

12 Post-mortem care is done
  a After rigor mortis sets in
  b After the doctor pronounces the person dead
  c When the funeral director arrives for the body
  d After the family has viewed the body

Answers to these questions are on p. 505.

FOCUS ON **PRACTICE**

Problem Solving

Mr. Perez is near the end of his life. You collect supplies to provide mouth care and pillows to position him. When you are ready to give care, his family enters his room. What will you do? Is this a good time to provide care? What will you say to his family?

Review Question Answers

CHAPTER 1
1 a
2 b
3 b
4 a
5 d
6 a
7 b
8 a
9 a
10 d

CHAPTER 2
1 T
2 T
3 F
4 F
5 T
6 F
7 F
8 a
9 b
10 b
11 c
12 d
13 b
14 a
15 a
16 a
17 a
18 d
19 a
20 b
21 d

CHAPTER 3
1 c
2 c
3 d
4 c
5 b
6 c
7 c
8 b
9 a
10 a
11 b
12 d
13 b
14 b
15 c
16 a
17 b
18 c
19 a
20 d
21 b
22 a
23 b
24 d
25 c
26 c

CHAPTER 4
1 T
2 T
3 F
4 T
5 T
6 F
7 T
8 F
9 d
10 c
11 d
12 b
13 b
14 c
15 c
16 d
17 c
18 b
19 a
20 a
21 b
22 d
23 a
24 a
25 c
26 d

CHAPTER 5
1 F
2 F
3 T
4 F
5 F
6 F
7 d
8 b
9 c
10 b
11 b
12 c
13 d
14 d
15 b
16 c
17 a
18 b
19 a
20 d
21 a

CHAPTER 6
1 c
2 d
3 b
4 b
5 c
6 b
7 d
8 c
9 a
10 d
11 a
12 d
13 c
14 b

CHAPTER 7
1 a
2 b
3 a
4 c
5 c
6 a
7 b
8 c
9 d
10 d
11 b
12 a
13 b
14 b
15 b
16 c
17 d
18 a
19 d
20 a
21 b

CHAPTER 8
1 b
2 a
3 a
4 b
5 c
6 d
7 a
8 d
9 b
10 a
11 a
12 c
13 b
14 d

CHAPTER 9
1 d
2 c
3 c
4 d
5 d
6 b
7 a
8 b
9 b
10 c
11 b
12 b
13 a
14 b
15 b
16 c
17 a
18 c
19 b
20 d

CHAPTER 10
1 a
2 c
3 c
4 a
5 b
6 c
7 d
8 c
9 a
10 b
11 a
12 c
13 c
14 a

CHAPTER 11
1 F
2 T
3 T
4 F
5 F
6 T
7 T
8 T
9 F
10 F
11 T
12 F
13 F
14 T
15 F
16 a
17 c
18 b
19 c
20 a
21 b
22 c
23 c
24 d

CHAPTER 12
1 T
2 T
3 F
4 F
5 F
6 F
7 T
8 b
9 b
10 a
11 a
12 b
13 d
14 c
15 a
16 c
17 d
18 c
19 d
20 a

CHAPTER 13
1 a
2 b
3 c
4 a
5 a
6 c
7 d
8 c
9 b
10 b
11 c
12 a

CHAPTER 14
1 b
2 a
3 d
4 a
5 c
6 b
7 a
8 d
9 a
10 c
11 a
12 b
13 b
14 d
15 c

CHAPTER 15
1 F
2 T
3 F
4 T
5 T
6 T
7 b
8 d
9 c
10 b
11 a
12 c
13 c
14 d
15 a
16 b
17 a
18 c
19 b
20 a
21 b
22 d

CHAPTER 16
1 T
2 T
3 F
4 T
5 F
6 F
7 F
8 T
9 T
10 T
11 a
12 c
13 b
14 a
15 c
16 d
17 b
18 a
19 c
20 d
21 b
22 b

CHAPTER 17
1 F
2 T
3 T
4 F
5 F
6 d
7 b
8 c
9 a
10 d
11 c
12 b
13 d
14 b

CHAPTER 18
1 c
2 d
3 a
4 a
5 b
6 a
7 b
8 c
9 c
10 d
11 a
12 a
13 b
14 d
15 c
16 d

CHAPTER 19
1 b
2 a
3 b
4 c
5 a
6 c
7 b
8 d
9 a
10 d
11 c
12 d

CHAPTER 20
1 b
2 d
3 c
4 d
5 a
6 a
7 c
8 a
9 d
10 b
11 c
12 c
13 d
14 a
15 b
16 a
17 c
18 d
19 b
20 a

CHAPTER 21
1 b
2 a
3 a
4 d
5 b
6 c
7 d
8 b
9 c
10 b
11 c
12 d
13 a
14 d
15 b
16 c

CHAPTER 22
1 c
2 d
3 b
4 a
5 c
6 d
7 a
8 b

CHAPTER 23
1 T
2 F
3 T
4 F
5 F
6 T
7 T
8 b
9 b
10 c
11 d
12 b
13 c
14 a
15 d
16 b
17 a
18 b

CHAPTER 24
1 c
2 a
3 d
4 b
5 a
6 d
7 a
8 c
9 a
10 c
11 b
12 a
13 d
14 b
15 c
16 a

CHAPTER 25
1 T
2 T
3 T
4 T
5 F
6 F
7 T
8 T
9 F
10 F
11 a
12 a
13 d
14 d
15 b
16 c
17 b
18 d
19 a
20 c
21 a
22 d

CHAPTER 26
1 c
2 c
3 b
4 b
5 d
6 c
7 d
8 a
9 d
10 c

CHAPTER 27
1 T
2 T
3 T
4 F
5 T
6 F
7 T
8 T
9 c
10 b
11 a
12 d
13 c
14 c

CHAPTER 28
1 b
2 a
3 d
4 a
5 c
6 b
7 d
8 a
9 d
10 c
11 c
12 d
13 b
14 d
15 a
16 c
17 b
18 c
19 d
20 a
21 b
22 c
23 b
24 a
25 a
26 c
27 d
28 b
29 b
30 d
31 a
32 d
33 c
34 d
35 b
36 a
37 a
38 c
39 d
40 b

CHAPTER 29
1 b
2 d
3 b
4 c
5 c
6 a
7 d
8 d
9 c
10 a
11 a
12 b
13 c
14 d
15 b

CHAPTER 30
1 a
2 a
3 d
4 c
5 d
6 b
7 b
8 a
9 c
10 b
11 d
12 c
13 d
14 a

CHAPTER 31
1 a
2 c
3 d
4 c
5 b
6 a
7 b
8 b
9 c
10 d
11 a
12 d
13 c
14 a
15 b
16 a

CHAPTER 32
1 c
2 b
3 a
4 d
5 b
6 a
7 d
8 c
9 c
10 a
11 b
12 b

Appendix A

The Patient Care Partnership: Understanding Expectations, Rights, and Responsibilities

When you need hospital care, your doctor and the nurses and other professionals at our hospital are committed to working with you and your family to meet your health care needs. Our dedicated doctors and staff serve the community in all its ethnic, religious, and economic diversity. Our goal is for you and your family to have the same care and attention we would want for our families and ourselves.

The sections below explain some of the basics about how you can expect to be treated during your hospital stay. They also cover what we will need from you to care for you better. If you have questions at any time, please ask them. Unasked or unanswered questions can add to the stress of being in the hospital. Your comfort and confidence in your care are very important to us.

What to Expect During Your Hospital Stay

- **High quality hospital care.** Our first priority is to provide you the care you need, when you need it, with skill, compassion, and respect. Tell your caregivers if you have concerns about your care or if you have pain. You have the right to know the identity of your doctors, nurses, and others involved in your care, and you have the right to know when they are students, residents, or other trainees.
- **A clean and safe environment.** Our hospital works hard to keep you safe. We use special policies and procedures to avoid mistakes in your care and keep you free from abuse or neglect. If anything unexpected and significant happens during your hospital stay, you will be told what happened, and any resulting changes in your care will be discussed with you.
- **Involvement in your care.** You and your doctor often make decisions about your care before you go to the hospital. Other times, especially in emergencies, those decisions are made during your hospital stay. When decision-making takes place, it should include:
  - *Discussing your medical condition and information about medically appropriate treatment choices.* To make informed decisions with your doctor, you need to understand:
    - The benefits and risks of each treatment.
    - Whether your treatment is experimental or part of a research study.
    - What you can reasonably expect from your treatment and any long-term effects it might have on your quality of life.
    - What you and your family will need to do after you leave the hospital.
    - The financial consequences of using uncovered services or out-of-network providers.

    Please tell your caregivers if you need more information about your treatment choices.
  - *Discussing your treatment plan.* When you enter the hospital, you sign a general consent to treatment. In some cases, such as surgery or experimental treatment, you may be asked to confirm in writing that you understand what is planned and agree to it. This process protects your right to consent to or refuse a treatment. Your doctor will explain the medical consequences of refusing recommended treatment. It also protects your right to decide if you want to participate in a research study.
  - *Getting information from you.* Your caregivers need complete and correct information about your health and coverage so that they can make good decisions about your care. That includes:
    - Past illnesses, surgeries, or hospital stays.
    - Past allergic reactions.
    - Any medicines or dietary supplements (such as vitamins and herbs) that you are taking.
    - Any network or admission requirements under your health plan.
  - *Understanding your health care goals and values.* You may have health care goals and values or spiritual beliefs that are important to your well-being. They will be taken into account as much as possible throughout your hospital stay. Make sure your doctor, your family, and your care team know your wishes.
  - *Understanding who should make decisions when you cannot.* If you have signed a health care power of attorney stating who should speak for you if you become unable to make health care decisions for yourself, or a "living will" or "advance directive" that states your wishes about end-of-life care, give copies to your doctor, your family, and your care team. If you or your family need help making difficult decisions, counselors, chaplains, and others are available to help.
- **Protection of your privacy.** We respect the confidentiality of your relationship with your doctor and other caregivers and the sensitive information about your health and health care that are part of that relationship. State and federal laws and hospital operating policies protect the privacy of your medical information. You will receive a Notice of Privacy Practices that describes the ways that we use, disclose, and safeguard patient information and that explains how you can obtain a copy of information from our records about your care.
- **Preparing you and your family for when you leave the hospital.** Your doctor works with the hospital staff and professionals in your community. You and your family also play an important role in your care. The success of your treatment often depends on your efforts to follow medication, diet, and therapy plans. Your family may need to help care for you at home. You can expect us to help you identify sources of follow-up care and let you know if our hospital has a financial interest in any referrals. As long as you agree we can share information about your care with them, we will coordinate our activities with your caregivers outside the hospital. You can also expect to receive information and, where possible, training about the self-care you will need when you go home.
- **Help with your bill and filing insurance claims.** Our staff will file claims for you with health care insurers or other programs such as Medicare and Medicaid. They also will help your doctor with needed documentation. Hospital bills and insurance coverage are often confusing. If you have questions about your bill, contact our business office. If you need help understanding your insurance coverage or health plan, start with your insurance company or health benefits manager. If you do not have health coverage, we will try to help you and your family find financial help or make other arrangements. We need your help with collecting needed information and other requirements to obtain coverage or assistance.

While you are here, you will receive more detailed notices about some of the rights you have as a hospital patient and how to exercise them. We are always interested in improving. If you have questions, comments, or concerns, please contact ________________________.

Reprinted with permission American Hospital Association, copyright 2003.

Appendix B

National Nurse Aide Assessment Program (NNAAP®) Written Examination Content Outline

The NNAAP® Written Examination is comprised of seventy (70) multiple choice questions. Ten (10) of these questions are pre-test (non-scored) questions on which statistical information will be collected.

I Physical Care Skills

- **A** Activities of Daily Living — 14% of exam
  - **1** Hygiene
  - **2** Dressing and Grooming
  - **3** Nutrition and Hydration
  - **4** Elimination
  - **5** Rest/Sleep/Comfort
- **B** Basic Nursing Skills — 39% of exam
  - **1** Infection Control
  - **2** Safety/Emergency
  - **3** Therapeutic/Technical Procedures
  - **4** Data Collection and Reporting
- **C** Restorative Skills — 7% of exam
  - **1** Prevention
  - **2** Self Care/Independence

II Psychosocial Care Skills

- **A** Emotional and Mental Health Needs — 11% of exam
- **B** Spiritual and Cultural Needs — 2% of exam

III Role of the Nurse Aide

- **A** Communication — 8% of exam
- **B** Client Rights — 7% of exam
- **C** Legal and Ethical Behavior — 3% of exam
- **D** Member of the Health Care Team — 9% of exam

National Nurse Aide Assessment Program (NNAAP®) Skills Evaluation

List of Skills

1. Hand hygiene (Hand washing)
2. Applies one knee-high elastic stocking
3. Assists to ambulate using transfer belt
4. Assists with use of bedpan
5. Cleans upper or lower denture
6. Counts and records radial pulse
7. Counts and records respirations
8. Donning and removing PPE (gown and gloves)
9. Dresses client with affected (weak) right arm
10. Feeds client who cannot feed self
11. Gives modified bed bath (face and one arm, hand and underarm)
12. Measures and records blood pressure
13. Measures and records urinary output
14. Measures and records weight of ambulatory client
15. Performs modified passive range of motion (PROM) for one knee and one ankle
16. Performs modified passive range of motion (PROM) for one shoulder
17. Positions on side
18. Provides catheter care for female
19. Provides foot care on one foot
20. Provides mouth care
21. Provides perineal care (peri-care) for female
22. Transfers from bed to wheelchair using transfer belt

Reproduced and used with permission from the National Council of State Boards of Nursing (NCSBN), Chicago, Ill, ©2012.

*All states do not participate in the program. Such states have other arrangements for nurse aide competency and evaluation programs. The NNAAP® skills identified in this textbook may be evaluated in part, or in full, on the NNAAP® Skills Evaluation.

Appendix C

Job Application

EMPLOYMENT APPLICATION

APPLICANT INSTRUCTIONS

If you need help filling out this application form or for any phase of the employment process, please notify the person that gave you this form and every effort will be made to accommodate your needs in a reasonable amount of time.

1. Please read "APPLICANT NOTE" below.
2. Complete both sides of this page.
3. If more space is needed to complete any question, use comments section at the bottom of this page.
4. Print clearly: incomplete or illegible applications will not be processed. PLEASE NOTE "NOT APPLICABLE" IF NOT ANSWERING A QUESTION.
5. Provide only requested information. Failure to do so may result in disqualification of your application.
6. Some packets may include an AFFIRMATIVE ACTION QUESTIONNAIRE. This information is being gathered for affirmative action under Section 503 of the Rehabilitation Act of 1973. The information requested is voluntary and will be kept confidential. An applicant will not be subject to any adverse treatment for refusing to complete the questionnaire.
7. DO NOT FILL OUT ANY OTHER ATTACHED FORMS OR PAGES UNTIL INSTRUCTED.

TODAY'S DATE: ____________

NAME: ____________ LAST ____________ FIRST ____________ MI

SOCIAL SECURITY NUMBER: ____________

HOME PHONE: ____________ WORK PHONE: ____________

CURRENT ADDRESS: ____________ STREET

____________ CITY ____________ STATE ____________ ZIP

PRIOR ADDRESS: ____________ STREET

____________ CITY ____________ STATE ____________ ZIP

APPLICANT NOTE This application form is intended for use in evaluating your qualifications for employment. This is not an employment contract. Please answer all appropriate questions completely and accurately. False or misleading statements during the interview and on this form are grounds for terminating the application process or, if discovered after employment, terminating employment. All qualified applicants will receive consideration without discrimination based on sex, marital status, race, color, age, creed, national origin, sexual orientation, military reserve membership, ancestry, religion, height, weight, use of a guide or support animal because of blindness, deafness or physical handicap, or the presence of disabilities. A conviction will not necessarily bar an applicant from employment. Additional testing of job-related skills and for the presence of drugs in your body may be required prior to employment. After an offer of employment, and prior to reporting to work, you may be required to submit to a medical review. Depending on company policy and the needs of the job, you will be required to complete a medical history form and may be required to be examined by a medical professional designated by the company.

AVAILABILITY For which position are you applying? ____________

What date can you start? ____________ What category would you prefer? ❑ Full time ❑ Part time ❑ Temporary ❑ Labor pool

For which schedules are you available?* ❑ Weekdays ❑ Weekends ❑ Evenings ❑ Nights ❑ Overtime ❑ Shift ❑ Other________

*reasonable efforts will be made to accommodate sincerely held moral and ethical beliefs, (WI) religious beliefs and practices (All other States)

JOB-RELATED SKILLS NOTE: Do not fill out any part of this section you believe to be non-job related.

❑ Yes ❑ No If the job requires, do you have the appropriate valid drivers license?
Name on license ____________ DL# ____________ Type ____________ State of Issue ____________

❑ Yes ❑ No Have you had any moving violations within the last seven years? Please describe. ____________
Please list any other skills, licenses or certificates that may be job-related or that you feel would be of value to this job or company. ____________

❑ Yes ❑ No Have you been given a job description or had the essential functions of the job explained to you?

❑ Yes ❑ No Do you understand these essential functions?

❑ Yes ❑ No Can you perform the essential functions of this job with or without reasonable accommodation?

SECURITY List states and counties of residence for the past seven years: ____________

❑ Yes ❑ No Have you used any names or Social Security Numbers other than given above? If so, please list in comments, below.

❑ Yes ❑ No Have you been convicted of a crime in the past seven years? If so, please describe in the boxes below. (Conviction will not necessarily be a bar to employment. In accordance with company policy and applicable state and federal laws, factors such as age at time of the offense, remoteness of the offense, time since last conviction, nature of the job sought and rehabilitation effort will be reviewed.)

INCIDENT	CITY/STATE	CHARGE
1.		
2.		

COMMENTS (ASK FOR AN ADDITIONAL PAGE IF NECESSARY)

____

© ADP SCREENING & SELECTION SERVICES 2002

Courtesy ADP Screening and Selection Services, Ft. Collins, Colo.

PREVIOUS EMPLOYERS

PLEASE NOTE: Your application will not be considered unless every question in this section is answered. Since we will make every effort to contact previous employers, the ***correct telephone numbers of past employers are critical.*** Ask for a phone book or call information if necessary. FOR EMPLOYERS OUTSIDE THE U.S., A CURRENT FAX NUMBER IS MANDATORY.

MOST RECENT EMPLOYER ❑ Yes ❑ No Are you currently working for this employer?
❑ Yes ❑ No If yes, may we contact?

PHONE ( )
FAX ( )

COMPANY NAME CITY STATE

FROM TO
DATES EMPLOYED JOB TITLE SUPERVISOR NAME

DUTIES

PER
SALARY (HOUR, WEEK, MONTH) REASON FOR LEAVING

SECOND MOST RECENT EMPLOYER

PHONE ( )
FAX ( )

COMPANY NAME CITY STATE

FROM TO
DATES EMPLOYED JOB TITLE SUPERVISOR NAME

DUTIES

PER
SALARY (HOUR, WEEK, MONTH) REASON FOR LEAVING

THIRD MOST RECENT EMPLOYER

PHONE ( )
FAX ( )

COMPANY NAME CITY STATE

FROM TO
DATES EMPLOYED JOB TITLE SUPERVISOR NAME

DUTIES

PER
SALARY (HOUR, WEEK, MONTH) REASON FOR LEAVING

REFERENCES

Include only individuals familiar with your work ability. Do not include relatives.

NAME	ADDRESS/PHONE	YEARS KNOWN/RELATIONSHIP
1.		
2.		

EDUCATION

NOTE: Do not fill out any part of this section you believe to be non-job related.
Please circle highest grade completed. 7 8 9 10 11 12 13 14 15 16 16+

If your school records are under a different name than listed on page 1, please enter that name__________

NAME	CITY/STATE	GRADUATED	DEGREE?
HIGH SCHOOL			
COLLEGE			
OTHER			

CERTIFICATION AND RELEASE

I certify that I have read and understand the applicant note on page one of this form and that the answers given by me to the foregoing questions and the statements made by me are complete and true to the best of my knowledge and belief. I understand that any false information, omissions or misrepresentations of facts called for in this application, whether on this document or not, may result in rejection of my application or discharge at any time during my employment. I authorize the company and/or its agents, including consumer reporting bureaus, to verify any of this information. I authorize all former employers, persons, schools, companies and law enforcement authorities from any liability for any damage whatsoever for issuing this information. I also understand that the use of illegal drugs is prohibited during employment. If company policy requires, I am willing to submit to drug testing to detect the use of illegal drugs prior to and during employment.

SIGNATURE	DATE

© ADP SCREENING & SELECTION SERVICES 2002

Appendix D

Minimum Data Set: Selected Pages

Sample Pages from Functional Status Form

Resident ______________________ Identifier ______________________ Date ______________

Section G	Functional Status

G0110. Activities of Daily Living (ADL) Assistance
Refer to the ADL flow chart in the RAI manual to facilitate accurate coding

Instructions for Rule of 3

- When an activity occurs three times at any one given level, code that level.
- When an activity occurs three times at multiple levels, code the most dependent, exceptions are total dependence (4), activity must require full assist every time, and activity did not occur (8), activity must not have occurred at all. Example, three times extensive assistance (3) and three times limited assistance (2), code extensive assistance (3).
- When an activity occurs at various levels, but not three times at any given level, apply the following:
  - When there is a combination of full staff performance, and extensive assistance, code extensive assistance.
  - When there is a combination of full staff performance, weight bearing assistance and/or non-weight bearing assistance code limited assistance (2).

If none of the above are met, code supervision.

1. ADL Self-Performance
Code for **resident's performance** over all shifts - not including setup. If the ADL activity occurred 3 or more times at various levels of assistance, code the most dependent - except for total dependence, which requires full staff performance every time

Coding:

Activity Occurred 3 or More Times

0. **Independent** - no help or staff oversight at any time
1. **Supervision** - oversight, encouragement or cueing
2. **Limited assistance** - resident highly involved in activity; staff provide guided maneuvering of limbs or other non-weight-bearing assistance
3. **Extensive assistance** - resident involved in activity, staff provide weight-bearing support
4. **Total dependence** - full staff performance every time during entire 7-day period

Activity Occurred 2 or Fewer Times

7. **Activity occurred only once or twice** - activity did occur but only once or twice
8. **Activity did not occur** - activity did not occur or family and/or non-facility staff provided care 100% of the time for that activity over the entire 7-day period

2. ADL Support Provided
Code for **most support provided** over all shifts; code regardless of resident's self-performance classification

Coding:

0. **No** setup or physical help from staff
1. **Setup** help only
2. **One** person physical assist
3. **Two+** persons physical assist
8. ADL activity itself **did not occur** or family and/or non-facility staff provided care 100% of the time for that activity over the entire 7-day period

	1. Self-Performance	2. Support
	↓ Enter Codes in Boxes ↓	
A. Bed mobility - how resident moves to and from lying position, turns side to side, and positions body while in bed or alternate sleep furniture	☐	☐
B. Transfer - how resident moves between surfaces including to or from: bed, chair, wheelchair, standing position (**excludes** to/from bath/toilet)	☐	☐
C. Walk in room - how resident walks between locations in his/her room	☐	☐
D. Walk in corridor - how resident walks in corridor on unit	☐	☐
E. Locomotion on unit - how resident moves between locations in his/her room and adjacent corridor on same floor. If in wheelchair, self-sufficiency once in chair	☐	☐
F. Locomotion off unit - how resident moves to and returns from off-unit locations (e.g., areas set aside for dining, activities or treatments). **If facility has only one floor,** how resident moves to and from distant areas on the floor. If in wheelchair, self-sufficiency once in chair	☐	☐
G. Dressing - how resident puts on, fastens and takes off all items of clothing, including donning/removing a prosthesis or TED hose. Dressing includes putting on and changing pajamas and housedresses	☐	☐
H. Eating - how resident eats and drinks, regardless of skill. Do not include eating/drinking during medication pass. Includes intake of nourishment by other means (e.g., tube feeding, total parenteral nutrition, IV fluids administered for nutrition or hydration)	☐	☐
I. Toilet use - how resident uses the toilet room, commode, bedpan, or urinal; transfers on/off toilet; cleanses self after elimination; changes pad; manages ostomy or catheter; and adjusts clothes. Do not include emptying of bedpan, urinal, bedside commode, catheter bag or ostomy bag	☐	☐
J. Personal hygiene - how resident maintains personal hygiene, including combing hair, brushing teeth, shaving, applying makeup, washing/drying face and hands (**excludes** baths and showers)	☐	☐

From Centers for Medicare & Medicaid Services: MDS 3.0, http://www.cms.gov/Medicare/Quality-Initiatives-Patient-Assessment-Instruments/NursingHomeQualityInits/MDS30RAIManual.html

Resident ______________________ Identifier ______________ Date ____________

Section G Functional Status

G0120. Bathing

How resident takes full-body bath/shower, sponge bath, and transfers in/out of tub/shower (**excludes** washing of back and hair). Code for **most dependent** in self-performance and support

Enter Code [ ]
A. Self-performance
0. **Independent** - no help provided
1. **Supervision** - oversight help only
2. **Physical help limited to transfer only**
3. **Physical help in part of bathing activity**
4. **Total dependence**
8. **Activity itself did not occur** or family and/or non-facility staff provided care 100% of the time for that activity over the entire 7-day period

Enter Code [ ]
B. Support provided
(Bathing support codes are as defined in item **G0110 column 2, ADL Support Provided**, above)

G0300. Balance During Transitions and Walking

After observing the resident, **code the following walking and transition items for most dependent**

Coding:
0. **Steady at all times**
1. **Not steady, but able to stabilize without staff assistance**
2. **Not steady, only able to stabilize with staff assistance**
8. **Activity did not occur**

↓ **Enter Codes in Boxes**

[ ]	**A. Moving from seated to standing position**
[ ]	**B. Walking** (with assistive device if used)
[ ]	**C. Turning around** and facing the opposite direction while walking
[ ]	**D. Moving on and off toilet**
[ ]	**E. Surface-to-surface transfer** (transfer between bed and chair or wheelchair)

G0400. Functional Limitation in Range of Motion

Code for limitation that interfered with daily functions or placed resident at risk of injury

Coding:
0. **No impairment**
1. **Impairment on one side**
2. **Impairment on both sides**

↓ **Enter Codes in Boxes**

[ ]	**A. Upper extremity** (shoulder, elbow, wrist, hand)
[ ]	**B. Lower extremity** (hip, knee, ankle, foot)

G0600. Mobility Devices

↓ **Check all that were normally used**

[ ]	**A. Cane/crutch**
[ ]	**B. Walker**
[ ]	**C. Wheelchair** (manual or electric)
[ ]	**D. Limb prosthesis**
[ ]	**Z.** None of the above were used

G0900. Functional Rehabilitation Potential

Complete only if A0310A = 01

Enter Code [ ]
A. Resident believes he or she is capable of increased independence in at least some ADLs
0. **No**
1. **Yes**
9. **Unable to determine**

Enter Code [ ]
B. Direct care staff believe resident is capable of increased independence in at least some ADLs
0. **No**
1. **Yes**

Sample Page from Care Assessment (CAA) Summary

Resident ______________________ Identifier ______________ Date ____________

Section V	Care Area Assessment (CAA) Summary

V0200. CAAs and Care Planning

1. Check column A if Care Area is triggered.
2. For each triggered Care Area, indicate whether a new care plan, care plan revision, or continuation of current care plan is necessary to address the problem(s) identified in your assessment of the care area. The Care Planning Decision column must be completed within 7 days of completing the RAI (MDS and CAA(s)). Check column B if the triggered care area is addressed in the care plan.
3. Indicate in the Location and Date of CAA Documentation column where information related to the CAA can be found. CAA documentation should include information on the complicating factors, risks, and any referrals for this resident for this care area.

A. CAA Results

Care Area	A. Care Area Triggered	B. Care Planning Decision	Location and Date of CAA documentation
	↓ Check all that apply ↓		
01. Delirium	☐	☐	
02. Cognitive Loss/Dementia	☐	☐	
03. Visual Function	☐	☐	
04. Communication	☐	☐	
05. ADL Functional/Rehabilitation Potential	☐	☐	
06. Urinary Incontinence and Indwelling Catheter	☐	☐	
07. Psychosocial Well-Being	☐	☐	
08. Mood State	☐	☐	
09. Behavioral Symptoms	☐	☐	
10. Activities	☐	☐	
11. Falls	☐	☐	
12. Nutritional Status	☐	☐	
13. Feeding Tube	☐	☐	
14. Dehydration/Fluid Maintenance	☐	☐	
15. Dental Care	☐	☐	
16. Pressure Ulcer	☐	☐	
17. Psychotropic Drug Use	☐	☐	
18. Physical Restraints	☐	☐	
19. Pain	☐	☐	
20. Return to Community Referral	☐	☐	

B. Signature of RN Coordinator for CAA Process and Date Signed

1. Signature

2. Date ☐☐ – ☐☐ – ☐☐☐☐
Month Day Year

C. Signature of Person Completing Care Plan Decision and Date Signed

1. Signature

2. Date ☐☐ – ☐☐ – ☐☐☐☐
Month Day Year

Illustration Credits

CHAPTER 3 3-1: Courtesy MCN Healthcare, Denver. www.MCNHealthcare.com. All rights reserved. **3-2:** Modified from National Council of State Boards of Nursing, Inc.: *Professional boundaries: a nurse's guide to the importance of appropriate professional boundaries*, Chicago, 1996, Author.

CHAPTER 5 5-2: Courtesy Briggs Corporation, Des Moines.

CHAPTER 6 6-2: From Maslow AH, Frager RD, Fadiman J: *Motivation and personality*, ed 3, Upper Saddle River, NJ, 1987, Pearson Education. Reprinted with permission of Pearson Education, Inc., Upper Saddle River, NJ.

CHAPTER 7 7-9: Redrawn from Thibodeau GA, Patton KT: *The human body in health and disease*, ed 5, St Louis, 2010, Mosby. **7-18:** From Thibodeau GA, Patton KT: *The human body in health and disease*, ed 5, St Louis, 2010, Mosby. **7-28:** From Thibodeau GA, Patton KT: *Structure and function of the body*, ed 11, St Louis, 2000, Mosby.

CHAPTER 10 10-2, 10-3: Images provided courtesy Poesy Company, Arcadia, Calif.

CHAPTER 11 11-1, 11-2, 11-3, 11-5, 11-6, 11-7, 11-8, 11-10, 11-12, 11-13, 11-14, 11-16: Images provided courtesy Poesy Company, Arcadia, Calif.

CHAPTER 12 12-1: Redrawn from Potter PA, Perry AG: *Fundamentals of nursing: concepts, process, and practice*, ed 7, St Louis, 2009, Mosby. **12-13:** From Siegel JD, Rhinehart E, Jackson M, Chiarello L, and the Healthcare Infection Control Practices Advisory Committee: *Guideline for isolation precautions: preventing transmission of infectious agents in healthcare settings 2007*, http://www.cdc.gov/ncidod/dhqp/pdf/isolation2007.pdf.

CHAPTER 13 13-11, 13-12: Images provided courtesy J.T. Poesy Co., Arcadia, Calif.

CHAPTER 14 14-1, 14-2: Courtesy ARJO, Inc., Roselle, Ill. (800-323-1245).

CHAPTER 15 15-9, 15-10: Redrawn from Food and Drug Administration: *Hospital bed system dimensional and assessment guidance to reduce entrapment*, March 10, 2006.

CHAPTER 16 16-18, 16-21: Courtesy ARJO, Inc., Roselle, Ill. (800-323-1245).

CHAPTER 17 17-1: Redrawn from Medline Plus: *Head lice*, Bethesda, Md, updated July 10, 2013, National Institutes of Health. **17-2:** From Marks JG, Miller JJ: *Lookingbill & Marks' principles of dermatology*, ed 4, St Louis, 2006, Saunders.

CHAPTER 18 18-1: Redrawn from Weldon, Inc., Fort Worth, Tex. **18-9, B:** Courtesy Hartmann USA, Inc., Rock Hill, SC. **18-9, C:** Courtesy Hartmann Inc., Heidenheim, Germany. **18-9, D:** Courtesy Principle Business Enterprises, Dunbridge, Ohio. **18-14:** From Potter PA, Perry AG: *Fundamentals of nursing*, ed 7, St Louis, 2009, Mosby.

CHAPTER 19 19-1: Modified from deWit SC: *Fundamental concepts and skills for nursing*, ed 3, Philadelphia, 2009, Saunders.

CHAPTER 20 20-1: Courtesy U.S. Department of Agriculture, Center for Nutrition and Policy Promotion, 2011. **20-2:** Images courtesy Elderstore, Alpharetta, Ga.

CHAPTER 21 21-21: From deWit SC: *Fundamental concepts and skills for nursing*, ed 3, St Louis, 2009, Saunders. **21-22:** From Hockenberry MJ and others: *Wong's nursing care of infants and children*, ed 8, St Louis, 2007, Mosby. **21-23:** Modified from OSF St. Joseph Medical Center, Bloomington, Ill.

CHAPTER 22 22-1: *Courtesy Weldon, Inc., Fort Worth, Tex.*

CHAPTER 23 23-7, 23-8: Images provided courtesy J.T. Posey Co., Arcadia, Calif.

CHAPTER 24 24-1: Used with permission from Rosemary Kohr, RN, PhD, ACNP (cert), www.lhsc.on.ca/wound, Rosemary.Korh@Lhasa.on.ca. **24-3:** From Black JM, Hawks JH: Medical-surgical nursing: clinical management for positive outcomes, ed 7, St Louis, 2005, WB Saunders. **24-4:** Redrawn from National Diabetes Information Clearinghouse (NDICH): *Prevent diabetes problems: keep your feet and skin healthy*, NIH Publication No. 08-4282, Bethesda, Md, May 2008, NDICH. **24-13:** Courtesy Rainey Compression Essentials, Atlanta, Ga.

CHAPTER 25 25-2: From Ostomy wound management, *Proceedings from the November National V.A.C.®* 51(2A, supp):7S, Feb 2005, HMP Communications. Used with permission. **25-3:** Redrawn from U.S. Department of Health and Human Services, Agency for Healthcare Research and Quality: *Understanding your body: what are pressure ulcers?* November 2007. **25-4, A and F [parts 1 & 2] and B, C, D, E [part 1]:** From National Pressure Advisory Panel, 2011. **25-4, B, C, D, and E [part 2]:** Courtesy Laurel Wieresma-Bryant, RN, MSN, Clinical Nurse Specialist, Barnes-Jewish Hospital, St Louis, Mo. **25-7, 25-8, 25-9:** Images provided courtesy Posey Company, Arcadia, Calif.

CHAPTER 26 26-1: Modified from Talbot L, Meyers-Marquardt M: *Pocket guide to critical care assessment*, ed 3, St Louis, 1997, Mosby. **26-11:** Image used by permission from CAIRE Inc., Ball Ground, Georgia.

CHAPTER 27 27-2: Images courtesy ElderStore, Alpharetta, Ga. **27-3, A, C, and D:** Courtesy Parsons ADL, Inc. Tottenham, Ontario. **27-3, B:** Courtesy OXO International, Inc., New York.

CHAPTER 28 **28-2:** Modified from Belcher AE: *Cancer nursing*, St Louis, 1992, Mosby. **28-3, 28-19:** From Swartz MH: *Textbook of physical diagnosis*, ed 6, Philadelphia, 2010, Saunders. **28-4, 28-8, 28-10:** Modified from Monahan FD and others: *Phipps' medical-surgical nursing: health and illness perspectives*, ed 8, St Louis, 2007, Mosby. **28-5, 28-13, 28-14, 28-25:** From Thibodeau GA, Patton KT: *The human body in health & disease*, ed 5, St Louis, 2010, Mosby. **28-6:** Modified from Harkness GA, Dincher JR: *Medical-surgical nursing: total patient care*, ed 10, St Louis, 1999, Mosby.
28-9, 28-28: Modified from Christensen BL, Kockrow EO: *Adult health nursing*, ed 6, St Louis, 2011, Mosby.
28-11: Courtesy Cameron Bangs, MD. From Auerbach PS: *Wilderness medicine, management of wilderness and environmental emergencies*, ed 3, St Louis, 1995, Mosby.
28-12: Courtesy Otto Bock Health Care, Minneapolis.
28-17: Courtesy Siemens Hearing Instruments, Inc., Piscataway, NJ. **28-20, A and B:** From National Eye Institute: *Cataract: what you should know*, Bethesda, Md, September 2013, National Institutes of Health.
28-20, C: Modified from National Eye Institute: *Age-related macular degeneration: what you should know*, Bethesda, Md, August 2013, National Institutes of Health.
28-20, D: Modified from National Eye Institute: *Diabetic retinopathy: what you should know*, Bethesda, Md, September 2013, National Institutes of Health. **28-26:** From Lewis SL, Dirksen SR, Heitkemper MM, Bucher, L, Camera IM: *Medical-surgical nursing: assessment and management of clinical problems*, ed 8, St Louis, 2011, Mosby. **28-30:** From National Kidney and Urologic Diseases Information Clearinghouse: *Prostate enlargement: benign prostatic hyperplasia*, NIH Publication No. 07-3012, Bethesda, Md, June 2006, National Institutes of Health. **28-31:** Courtesy Department of Dermatology, School of Medicine, University of Utah.

CHAPTER 30 **30-2:** From Thibodeau GA, Patton KT: *The human body in health & disease*, ed 5, St Louis, 2010, Mosby.
30-3: From Alzheimer's Disease Education & Referral Center: *Alzheimer's disease fact sheet*, Bethesda, Md, September 2012, updated November 26, 2012, National Institutes of Health.

CHAPTER 31 **31-8:** From Ignatavicius DD, Workman ML: *Medical-surgical nursing: critical thinking for collaborative care*, ed 6, St Louis, 2010, Saunders. **31-16:** From Ignatavicius DD, Workman ML: *Medical-surgical nursing: critical thinking for collaborative care*, ed 6, St Louis, 2010, Saunders.

Glossary

A

abduction Moving a body part away from the mid-line of the body
abuse The willful infliction of injury, unreasonable confinement, intimidation, or punishment that results in physical harm, pain, or mental anguish; depriving the person (or the person's caregiver) of the goods or services needed to attain or maintain well-being
acetone See "ketone"
activities of daily living (ADL) The activities usually done during a normal day in a person's life
acute illness A sudden illness from which a person is expected to recover
adduction Moving a body part toward the mid-line of the body
advance directive A document stating a person's wishes about health care when that person cannot make his or her own decisions
alopecia Hair loss
ambulation The act of walking
anaphylaxis A life-threatening sensitivity to an antigen
anorexia The loss of appetite
antibiotic A drug that kills certain pathogens
anxiety A vague, uneasy feeling in response to stress
aphasia The total or partial loss *(a)* of the ability to use or understand language *(phasia)*
apnea The lack or absence *(a)* of breathing *(pnea)*
artery A blood vessel that carries blood away from the heart
arthritis Joint *(arthr)* inflammation *(itis)*
arthroplasty The surgical replacement *(plasty)* of a joint *(arthr)*
asepsis Being free of disease-producing microbes
aspiration Breathing fluid, food, vomitus, or an object into the lungs
assault Intentionally attempting or threatening to touch a person's body without the person's consent
assisted living residence (ALR) Provides housing, personal care, support services, health care, and social activities in a home-like setting for persons needing help with daily activities
atrophy The decrease in size or the wasting away of tissue
autopsy The examination of the body after death

B

base of support The area on which an object rests
battery Touching a person's body without his or her consent
bed rail A device that serves as a guard or barrier along the side of the bed; side rail
benign tumor A tumor that does not spread to other body parts
biohazardous waste Items contaminated with blood, body fluids, secretions, or excretions; *bio* means *life*, and *hazardous* means *dangerous* or *harmful*
blood pressure (BP) The amount of force exerted against the walls of an artery by the blood
body alignment The way the head, trunk, arms, and legs are aligned with one another; posture
body language Messages sent through facial expressions, gestures, posture, hand and body movements, gait, eye contact, and appearance
body mechanics Using the body in an efficient and careful way
body temperature The amount of heat in the body that is a balance between the amount of heat produced and the amount lost by the body
bony prominence An area where the bone sticks out or projects from the flat surface of the body
boundary crossing A brief act or behavior outside of the helpful zone
boundary sign An act, behavior, or thought that warns of a boundary crossing or boundary violation
boundary violation An act or behavior that meets your needs, not the person's
bradypnea Slow *(brady)* breathing *(pnea)*; respirations are fewer than 12 per minute

C

calorie The fuel or energy value of food
cancer See "malignant tumor"
capillary A tiny blood vessel; food, oxygen, and other substances pass from the capillaries into the cells
cardiac arrest See "sudden cardiac arrest"
carrier A human or animal that is a reservoir for microbes but does not develop the infection
catheter A tube used to drain or inject fluid through a body opening
cell The basic unit of body structure
chart See "medical record"
chemical restraint Any drug used for discipline or convenience and not required to treat medical symptoms
Cheyne-Stokes respirations Respirations gradually increase in rate and depth and then become shallow and slow; breathing may stop *(apnea)* for 10 to 20 seconds
chronic illness An ongoing illness, slow or gradual in onset; it has no known cure; it can be controlled and complications prevented with proper treatment

circumcised The fold of skin (foreskin) covering the glans of the penis was surgically removed
civil law Laws concerned with relationships between people
clean technique See "medical asepsis"
cognitive function Involves memory, thinking, reasoning, ability to understand, judgment, and behavior
colostomy A surgically created opening *(stomy)* between the colon *(colo)* and abdominal wall
coma A state of being unaware of one's setting and being unable to react or respond to people, places, or things
comatose Being unable to respond to stimuli
communicable disease A disease caused by pathogens that spread easily; a contagious disease
communication The exchange of information—a message sent is received and correctly interpreted by the intended person
compulsion Repeating an act over and over again (a ritual)
confidentiality Trusting others with personal and private information
confusion A mental state of being disoriented to person, time, place, situation, or identity
constipation The passage of a hard, dry stool
constrict To narrow
contagious disease See "communicable disease"
contamination The process of becoming unclean
contracture The lack of joint mobility caused by abnormal shortening of a muscle
convulsion See "seizure"
crime An act that violates a criminal law
criminal law Laws concerned with offenses against the public and society in general
culture The characteristics of a group of people—language, values, beliefs, habits, likes, dislikes, customs—passed from one generation to the next
cyanosis Bluish color to the skin, lips, mucous membranes, and nail beds

D

dandruff Excessive amounts of dry, white flakes from the scalp
defamation Injuring a person's name or reputation by making false statements to a third person
defecation The process of excreting feces from the rectum through the anus; a bowel movement
defense mechanism An unconscious reaction that blocks unpleasant or threatening feelings
dehydration A decrease in the amount of water in body tissues
delegate To authorize another person to perform a nursing task in a certain situation
delirium A state of sudden, severe confusion and rapid changes in brain function
delusion A false belief
delusion of grandeur An exaggerated belief about one's importance, wealth, power, or talents
delusion of persecution A false belief that one is being mistreated, abused, or harassed
dementia The loss of cognitive and social function caused by changes in the brain; the loss of cognitive function that interferes with routine personal, social, and occupational activities
denture An artificial tooth or a set of artificial teeth
development Changes in mental, emotional, and social function
developmental task A skill that must be completed during a stage of development
diarrhea The frequent passage of liquid stools
diastolic pressure The pressure in the arteries when the heart is at rest
digestion The process that breaks down food physically and chemically so it can be absorbed for use by the cells
dilate To expand or open wider
disability Any lost, absent, or impaired physical or mental function
disaster A sudden catastrophic event in which people are injured and killed and property is destroyed
discomfort See "pain"
disinfection The process of destroying pathogens
dorsal recumbent position The back-lying or supine position
dorsiflexion Bending the toes and foot up at the ankle
dysphagia Difficulty *(dys)* swallowing *(phagia)*
dyspnea Difficult, labored, or painful *(dys)* breathing *(pnea)*
dysuria Painful or difficult *(dys)* urination *(uria)*

E

edema The swelling of body tissues with water
elder abuse Any knowing, intentional, or negligent act by a caregiver or any other person to an older adult; the act causes harm or serious risk of harm
elopement When a person leaves the agency without staff knowledge
emesis See "vomitus"
enabler A device that limits freedom of movement but is used to promote independence, comfort, or safety
end-of-life care The support and care given during the time surrounding death
end-of-shift report A report that the nurse gives at the end of the shift to the on-coming shift; change-of-shift report
enema The introduction of fluid into the rectum and lower colon
enteral nutrition Giving nutrients into the gastro-intestinal (GI) tract *(enteral)* through a feeding tube
ergonomics The science of designing a job to fit the worker
eschar Thick, leathery dead tissue that may be loose or adhered to the skin; it is often black or brown

ethics Knowledge of what is right conduct and wrong conduct
extension Straightening a body part
external rotation Turning the joint outward

F

fainting The sudden loss of consciousness from an inadequate blood supply to the brain
false imprisonment Unlawful restraint or restriction of a person's freedom of movement
fecal impaction The prolonged retention and buildup of feces in the rectum
fecal incontinence The inability to control the passage of feces and gas through the anus
feces The semi-solid mass of waste products in the colon that is expelled through the anus; also called a *stool*
fever Elevated body temperature
first aid Emergency care given to an ill or injured person before medical help arrives
flashback Reliving a trauma in thoughts during the day and in nightmares during sleep
flatulence The excessive formation of gas or air in the stomach and intestines
flatus Gas or air passed through the anus
flexion Bending a body part
flow rate The number of drops per minute *(gtt/min)* or milliliters per hour *(mL/hr)*
footdrop The foot falls down at the ankle; permanent plantar flexion
Fowler's position A semi-sitting position; the head of the bed is raised between 45 and 60 degrees
fracture A broken bone
fraud Saying or doing something to trick, fool, or deceive a person
freedom of movement Any change in place or position of the body or any part of the body that the person is able to control
friction The rubbing of 1 surface against another
full visual privacy Having the means to be completely free from public view while in bed
functional incontinence The person has bladder control but cannot use the toilet in time

G

gait belt See "transfer belt"
gavage The process of giving a tube feeding
geriatrics The care of aging people
gerontology The study of the aging process
glucosuria Sugar *(glucos)* in the urine *(uria);* glycosuria
glycosuria Sugar *(glycos)* in the urine *(uria);* glucosuria
gossip To spread rumors or talk about the private matters of others
growth The physical changes that are measured and that occur in a steady, orderly manner

H

hallucination Seeing, hearing, smelling, or feeling something that is not real
harassment To trouble, torment, offend, or worry a person by one's behavior or comments
hazardous substance Any chemical in the workplace that can cause harm
healthcare-associated infection (HAI) An infection that develops in a person cared for in any setting where health care is given; the infection is related to receiving health care
health team The many health care workers whose skills and knowledge focus on the person's total care; interdisciplinary health care team
hematuria Blood *(hemat)* in the urine *(uria)*
hemiplegia Paralysis *(plegia)* on 1 side *(hemi)* of the body
hemoglobin The substance in red blood cells that carries oxygen and gives blood its red color
hemoptysis Bloody *(hemo)* sputum *(ptysis* means *to spit)*
hemorrhage The excessive loss of blood in a short time
high-Fowler's position A semi-sitting position; the head of the bed is raised 60 to 90 degrees
hirsutism Excessive body hair
holism A concept that considers the whole person; the whole person has physical, social, psychological, and spiritual parts that are woven together and cannot be separated
hormone A chemical substance secreted by the endocrine glands into the bloodstream
hospice A health care agency or program for persons who are dying
hyperextension Excessive straightening of a body part
hypertension When the systolic pressure is 140 mm Hg or higher *(hyper)*, or the diastolic pressure is 90 mm Hg or higher
hyperventilation Breathing *(ventilation)* is rapid *(hyper)* and deeper than normal
hypotension When the systolic pressure is below *(hypo)* 90 mm Hg, or the diastolic pressure is below 60 mm Hg
hypoventilation Breathing *(ventilation)* is slow *(hypo)*, shallow, and sometimes irregular
hypoxia Cells do not have enough *(hypo)* oxygen *(oxia)*

I

ileostomy A surgically created opening *(stomy)* between the ileum (small intestine *[ileo]*) and the abdominal wall
immunity Protection against a disease or condition; the person will not get or be affected by the disease
infection A disease state resulting from the invasion and growth of microbes in the body
infection control Practices and procedures that prevent the spread of infection
insomnia A chronic condition in which the person cannot sleep or stay asleep all night
intake The amount of fluid taken in
internal rotation Turning the joint inward

intravenous (IV) therapy Giving fluids through a needle or catheter into a vein; IV and IV infusion
invasion of privacy Violating a person's right not to have his or her name, photo, or private affairs exposed or made public without giving consent
involuntary seclusion Separating a person from others against his or her will, keeping the person to a certain area, or keeping the person away from his or her room without consent

J

job description A document that describes what the agency expects you to do
joint The point at which 2 or more bones meet to allow movement

K

ketone A substance that appears in urine from the rapid breakdown of fat for energy; acetone; ketone body
ketone body See "ketone"
Kussmaul respirations Very deep and rapid respirations

L

lateral position The person lies on 1 side or the other; side-lying position
law A rule of conduct made by a government body
libel Making false statements in print, in writing, or through pictures or drawings
lice See "pediculosis"
licensed practical nurse (LPN) A nurse who has completed a 1-year nursing program and has passed a licensing test; called *licensed vocational nurse (LVN)* in some states
licensed vocational nurse (LVN) See "licensed practical nurse (LPN)"
logrolling Turning the person as a unit, in alignment, with 1 motion

M

malignant tumor A tumor that invades and destroys nearby tissues and can spread to other body parts; cancer
malpractice Negligence by a professional person
medical asepsis Practices used to remove or destroy pathogens and to prevent their spread from 1 person or place to another person or place; clean technique
medical record The legal account of a person's condition and response to treatment and care; chart
medical symptom An indication or characteristic of a physical or psychological condition
menopause The time when menstruation stops and menstrual cycles end; there has been at least 1 year without a menstrual period
menstruation The process in which the lining of the uterus *(endometrium)* breaks up and is discharged from the body through the vagina
mental Relating to the mind; something that exists in the mind or is done by the mind
mental health The person copes with and adjusts to everyday stresses in ways accepted by society
mental health disorder A disturbance in the ability to cope with or adjust to stress; behavior and function are impaired; mental illness; psychiatric disorder
mental illness See "mental health disorder"
metabolism The burning of food for heat and energy by the cells
metastasis The spread of cancer to other body parts
microbe See "microorganism"
microorganism A small *(micro)* living thing *(organism)* seen only with a microscope; microbe
mixed incontinence The combination of stress incontinence and urge incontinence

N

need Something necessary or desired for maintaining life and mental well-being
neglect Failure to provide the person with the goods or services needed to avoid physical harm, mental anguish, or mental illness
negligence An unintentional wrong in which a person did not act in a reasonable and careful manner and a person or the person's property was harmed
nocturia Frequent urination *(uria)* at night *(noc)*
non-pathogen A microbe that does not usually cause an infection
nonverbal communication Communication that does not use words
nursing assistant A person who has passed a nursing assistant training and competency evaluation program; performs delegated nursing tasks under the supervision of a licensed nurse
nursing care plan A written guide about the person's nursing care; care plan
nursing diagnosis A health problem that can be treated with nursing measures
nursing process The method nurses use to plan and deliver nursing care; its 5 steps are assessment, nursing diagnosis, planning, implementation, and evaluation
nursing task Nursing care or a nursing function, procedure, activity, or work that can be delegated to nursing assistants when it does not require an RN's professional knowledge or judgment
nursing team Those who provide nursing care—RNs, LPNs/LVNs, and nursing assistants
nutrient A substance that is ingested, digested, absorbed, and used by the body
nutrition The processes involved in the ingestion, digestion, absorption, and use of food and fluids by the body

O

objective data Information that is seen, heard, felt, or smelled by an observer; signs
observation Using the senses of sight, hearing, touch, and smell to collect information
obsession A recurrent, unwanted thought, idea, or image
oliguria Scant amount *(olig)* of urine *(uria);* less than 500 mL in 24 hours
ombudsman Someone who supports or promotes the needs and interests of another person
opposition Touching an opposite finger with the thumb
oral hygiene Mouth care
organ Groups of tissue with the same function
orthopnea Breathing *(pnea)* deeply and comfortably only when sitting *(ortho)*
orthopneic position Sitting up *(ortho)* and leaning over a table to breathe *(pneic)*
orthostatic hypotension Abnormally low *(hypo)* blood pressure when the person suddenly stands up *(ortho* and *static);* postural hypotension
ostomy A surgically created opening; see "colostomy" and "ileostomy"
output The amount of fluid lost
overflow incontinence Small amounts of urine leak from a full bladder
oxygen concentration The amount (percent) of hemoglobin containing oxygen

P

pain To ache, hurt, or be sore; discomfort
palliative care Care that involves relieving or reducing the intensity of uncomfortable symptoms without producing a cure
panic An intense and sudden feeling of fear, anxiety, terror, or dread
paralysis Loss of muscle function, sensation, or both
paranoia A disorder *(para)* of the mind *(noia);* false beliefs (delusions) and suspicion about a person or a situation
paraplegia Paralysis in the legs and lower trunk
pathogen A microbe that is harmful and can cause an infection
pediculosis Infestation with wingless insects; lice
perineal care Cleaning the genital and anal areas; pericare
peristalsis Involuntary muscle contractions in the digestive system that move food down the esophagus through the alimentary canal
phobia An intense fear
physical restraint Any manual method or physical or mechanical device, material, or equipment attached to or near the person's body that he or she cannot remove easily and that restricts freedom of movement or normal access to one's body
planning Setting priorities and goals
plantar flexion The foot *(plantar)* is bent *(flexion);* bending the foot down at the ankle
poison Any substance harmful to the body when ingested, inhaled, injected, or absorbed through the skin
polyuria Abnormally large amounts *(poly)* of urine *(uria)*
post-mortem care Care of the body after *(post)* death *(mortem)*
postural hypotension See "orthostatic hypotension"
posture See "body alignment"
preceptor A staff member who guides another staff member; mentor
pressure ulcer A localized injury to the skin and/or underlying tissue usually over a bony prominence resulting from pressure or pressure in combination with shear; any lesion caused by unrelieved pressure that results in damage to underlying tissues
priority The most important thing at the time
professional boundary That which separates helpful behaviors from behaviors that are not helpful
professionalism Following laws, being ethical, having good work ethics, and having the skills to do your work
professional sexual misconduct An act, behavior, or comment that is sexual in nature
pronation Turning the joint downward
prone position Lying on the abdomen with the head turned to 1 side
prosthesis An artificial replacement for a missing body part
protected health information Identifying information and information about the person's health care that is maintained or sent in any form (paper, electronic, oral)
pseudodementia False *(pseudo)* dementia
psychiatric disorder See "mental health disorder"
pulse The beat of the heart felt at an artery as a wave of blood passes through the artery
pulse rate The number of heartbeats or pulses felt or heard in 1 minute

Q

quadriplegia Paralysis in the arms, legs, and trunk; tetraplegia

R

range of motion (ROM) The movement of a joint to the extent possible without causing pain
recording The written account of care and observations; charting
reflex incontinence Urine is lost at predictable intervals when the bladder is full
registered nurse (RN) A nurse who has completed a 2-, 3-, or 4-year nursing program and has passed a licensing test
regurgitation The backward flow of stomach contents into the mouth

rehabilitation The process of restoring the person to his or her highest possible level of physical, psychological, social, and economic function
reincarnation The belief that the spirit or soul is reborn in another human body or in another form of life
religion Spiritual beliefs, needs, and practices
remove easily The manual method, device, material, or equipment used to restrain the person that can be removed intentionally by the person in the same manner it was applied by the staff
reporting The oral account of care and observations
representative A person who has the legal right to act on the patient's or resident's behalf when he or she cannot do so for himself or herself
respiration The process of supplying the cells with oxygen and removing carbon dioxide from them; breathing air into *(inhalation)* and out of *(exhalation)* the lungs
respiratory arrest Breathing stops but heart action continues for several minutes
restorative aide A nursing assistant with special training in restorative nursing and rehabilitation skills
restorative nursing care Care that helps persons regain health, strength, and independence
reverse Trendelenburg's position The head of the bed is raised and the foot of the bed is lowered
rigor mortis The stiffness or rigidity *(rigor)* of skeletal muscles that occurs after death *(mortis)*
rotation Turning the joint

S

scabies A skin disorder caused by the female mite—a very small spider-like organism
seizure Violent and sudden contractions or tremors of muscle groups; convulsion
self-neglect A person's behaviors and way of living that threaten his or her health, safety, and well-being
semi-Fowler's position The head of the bed is raised 30 degrees; or the head of the bed is raised 30 degrees and the knee portion is raised 15 degrees
semi-prone side position See "Sims'position"
sexuality The physical, emotional, social, cultural, and spiritual factors that affect a person's feelings and attitudes about his or her sex
shear When layers of the skin rub against each other; when the skin remains in place and underlying tissues move and stretch and tear underlying capillaries and blood vessels causing tissue damage
shearing When skin sticks to a surface while muscles slide in the direction the body is moving
shock Results when tissues and organs do not get enough blood
side-lying position See "lateral position"
signs See "objective data"
Sims' position A left side-lying position in which the upper leg (right leg) is sharply flexed so it is not on the lower leg (left leg) and the lower arm (left arm) is behind the person; semi-prone side position
skin tear A break or rip in the outer layers of the skin; the epidermis (top skin layer) separates from the underlying tissues
slander Making false statements orally
sleep deprivation The amount and quality of sleep are decreased
sleepwalking The sleeping person leaves the bed and walks about
slough Dead tissue that is shed from the skin; it is usually light colored, soft, and moist; may be stringy at times
sputum Mucus from the respiratory system that is expectorated (expelled) through the mouth
sterile The absence of *all* microbes—pathogens and non-pathogens
sterilization The process of destroying *all* microbes
stethoscope An instrument used to listen to the sounds produced by the heart, lungs, and other body organs
stoma A surgically created opening seen through the abdominal wall; see "colostomy" and "ileostomy"
stool Excreted feces
stress The response or change in the body caused by any emotional, physical, social, or economic factor
stress incontinence When urine leaks during exercise and certain movements that cause pressure on the bladder
subjective data Things a person tells you about that you cannot observe through your senses; symptoms
sudden cardiac arrest (SCA) The heart stops suddenly and without warning; cardiac arrest
suffocation When breathing stops from the lack of oxygen
suicide To kill oneself
suicide contagion Exposure to suicide or suicidal behaviors within one's family, one's peer group, or media reports of suicide
sundowning Signs, symptoms, and behaviors of Alzheimer's disease increase during hours of darkness
supination Turning the joint upward
supine position The back-lying or dorsal recumbent position
suppository A cone-shaped, solid drug that is inserted into a body opening; it melts at body temperature
symptoms See "subjective data"
system Organs that work together to perform special functions
systolic pressure The pressure in the arteries when the heart contracts

T

tachypnea Rapid *(tachy)* breathing *(pnea);* respirations are more than 20 per minute
teamwork Staff members work together as a group; each person does his or her part to provide safe and effective care
terminal illness An illness or injury from which the person will not likely recover
tetraplegia See "quadriplegia"
thermometer A device used to measure *(meter)* temperature *(thermo)*
tissue A group of cells with similar functions
transfer How a person moves to and from surfaces—bed, chair, wheelchair, toilet, or standing position
transfer belt A device used to support a person who is unsteady or disabled; gait belt
transient incontinence Temporary or occasional incontinence that is reversed when the cause is treated
treatment The care provided to maintain or restore health, improve function, or relieve symptoms
Trendelenburg's position The head of the bed is lowered and the foot of the bed is raised
tumor A new growth of abnormal cells

U

ulcer A shallow or deep crater-like sore of the skin or mucous membrane
uncircumcised The person has foreskin covering the head of the penis
urge incontinence The loss of urine in response to a sudden, urgent need to void; the person cannot get to a toilet in time
urinary frequency Voiding at frequent intervals
urinary incontinence The involuntary loss or leakage of urine
urinary retention The inability to void
urinary urgency The need to void at once
urination The process of emptying urine from the bladder; voiding

V

vein A blood vessel that returns blood to the heart
verbal communication Communication that uses written or spoken words
vital signs Temperature, pulse, respirations, and blood pressure; and pain in some agencies
voiding See "urination"
vomitus The food and fluids expelled from the stomach through the mouth; emesis
vulnerable adult A person 18 years old or older who has a disability or condition that makes him or her at risk to be wounded, attacked, or damaged

W

withdrawal syndrome The person's physical and mental response after stopping or severely reducing the use of a substance that was used regularly
work ethics Behavior in the workplace
workplace violence Violent acts (including assault and threat of assault) directed toward persons at work or while on duty
wound A break in the skin or mucous membrane

Key Abbreviations

AD	Alzheimer's disease
ADL	Activities of daily living
AED	Automated external defibrillator
AHA	American Heart Association
AIDS	Acquired immunodeficiency syndrome
AIIR	Airborne infection isolation room
ALR	Assisted living residence
ALS	Amyotrophic lateral sclerosis
BLS	Basic Life Support
BM	Bowel movement
BP	Blood pressure
BPD	Borderline personality disorder
BPH	Benign prostatic hyperplasia
C	Centigrade
CAD	Coronary artery disease
CDC	Centers for Disease Control and Prevention
CMS	Centers for Medicare & Medicaid Services
CNS	Central nervous system
CO_2	Carbon dioxide
COPD	Chronic obstructive pulmonary disease
CPR	Cardiopulmonary resuscitation
CVA	Cerebrovascular accident
DNR	Do Not Resuscitate
DON	Director of nursing
EMS	Emergency Medical Services
EPHI; ePHI	Electronic protected health information
F	Fahrenheit
FDA	Food and Drug Administration
GI	Gastro-intestinal
gtt	Drops
gtt/min	Drops per minute
HAI	Healthcare-associated infection
HBV	Hepatitis B virus
Hg	Mercury
HIPAA	Health Insurance Portability and Accountability Act of 1996
HIV	Human immunodeficiency virus
HMO	Health maintenance organization
ID	Identification
I&O	Intake and output
IV	Intravenous
L/min	Liters per minute
LPN	Licensed practical nurse
LVN	Licensed vocational nurse
MDRO	Multidrug-resistant organism
mg	Milligram
MI	Myocardial infarction
mL	Milliliter
mL/hr	Milliliters per hour
mm	Millimeter
mm Hg	Millimeters of mercury
MRSA	Methicillin-resistant *Staphylococcus aureus*
MS	Multiple sclerosis
MSD	Musculo-skeletal disorder
MSDS	Material safety data sheet
NATCEP	Nursing assistant training and competency evaluation program
NCSBN	National Council of State Boards of Nursing
NG	Naso-gastric
NIA	National Institute on Aging
NPO	*Non per os;* nothing by mouth
O_2	Oxygen
OBRA	Omnibus Budget Reconciliation Act of 1987
OCD	Obsessive-compulsive disorder
OPIM	Other potentially infectious materials
OSHA	Occupational Safety and Health Administration
oz	Ounce
PASS	*Pull* the safety pin, *aim* low, *squeeze* the lever, *sweep* back and forth
PHI	Protected health information
PPE	Personal protective equipment
PPO	Preferred provider organization
PTSD	Post-traumatic stress disorder
RA	Rheumatoid arthritis
RACE	Rescue, alarm, confine, extinguish
RBC	Red blood cell
RN	Registered nurse
ROM	Range of motion
RRT	Rapid Response Team
SARS	Severe acute respiratory syndrome
SCA	Sudden cardiac arrest
SNF	Skilled nursing facility
SpO_2	Saturation of peripheral oxygen (oxygen concentration)
SSE	Soapsuds enema
STD	Sexually transmitted disease
TB	Tuberculosis
TIA	Transient ischemic attack
TJC	The Joint Commission
USDA	United States Department of Agriculture
UTI	Urinary tract infection
VF	Ventricular fibrillation
V-fib	Ventricular fibrillation
VRE	Vancomycin-resistant *Enterococci*
WBC	White blood cell

Index

Page numbers followed by *"f"* indicate figures, *"t"* indicate tables, and *"b"* indicate boxes.